Get Healthy Now!
with Gary Null

GET HEALTHY NOW!

WITH GARY NULL

Senior Project Editor Amy McDonald

A Complete Guide to
Prevention, Treatment
and Healthy Living

SEVEN STORIES PRESS
New York / Toronto / London

Copyright © 1999 by Gary Null

A Seven Stories Press First Edition.

This book is not intended to replace the services of a physician. Any application of the recommendations set forth in the following pages is at the reader's discretion. The reader should consult with his or her own physician concerning the recommendations in this book.

Portions of *Get Healthy Now!* have been adapted from the following books by Gary Null: *The Woman's Encyclopedia of Natural Healing, The Complete Guide to Sensible Eating (3rd ed.), Healing Your Body Naturally (3rd ed.), Nutrition and the Mind, How to Keep Your Feet and Legs Healthy for a Lifetime* (with Dr. Howard Robins).

All rights reserved. No part of this book may be reproduced, stored in a retrieval system, or transmitted in any form, by any means, including mechanical, electric, photocopying, recording or otherwise, without the prior written permission of the publisher.

In Canada:
Hushion House, 36 Northline Road, Toronto, Ontario M4B 3E2, Canada

In the U.K.:
Turnaround Publisher Services Ltd., Unit 3, Olympia Trading Estate, Coburg Road, Wood Green, London N22 6TZ U.K.

Library of Congress Cataloging-in-Publication Data

Null, Gary.
    Get healthy now! with Gary Null: A complete guide to prevention, treatment, and healthy living. —Seven Stories Press 1st ed.
    p.   cm.
    ISBN: 1-888363-97-5
    1. Alternative medicine—Popular works. I. Title.
R733.N852 1999
615.5—dc21   98-55547
                                                        CIP

9 8 7 6 5 4 3

Book design by Cindy LaBreacht

Seven Stories Press
140 Watts Street
New York, NY 10013
http://www.sevenstories.com

Printed in the U.S.A.

CONTENTS

Part One: Back to the Basics: What is Nutrition?

Part Two: Taking Charge of Your Health

Part Three: Mental Health and Psychological Well-Being

Part Four: Musculoskeletal Fitness

Part Five: Foot and Leg Care

Part Six: Heart, Blood, and Circulation

Part Seven: Allergy and Environmnetal Illness

Part Eight: Cancer Treatment and Prevention
Overview and Historical Perspective

Part Nine: Chronic Conditions

Part Eleven: Of Special Concern to Men

Part Twelve: Health, Beauty, and Longevity

Part Thirteen: Selecting An Alternative Practitioner

PART ONE

Back to the Basics: What Is Nutrition?

1

"You Are What You Eat"

orty years ago, roughly a third of the grocery store was devoted to natural, fresh produce. Today, it is a small fraction of that, and even what appears to be natural has been altered. Fruits and vegetables are routinely grown with artificial fertilizers, sprayed with pesticides, treated with hormones and chemicals to control the time of ripening to facilitate mechanical harvesting, dyed, sprayed with chemicals to prevent them from ripening during shipping or to induce ripening after shipping, and coated with waxes to give a glossy appearance.

Modern bread fares no better. The Western world is built on wheat, which, for thousands of years, has been prepared as bread and known as the staff of life. Wheat (and other whole grains) provides a rich source of nutrients: complex carbohydrates, protein, oils, roughage, and an excellent balance of dozens of vitamins and minerals. Grinding wheat with stone rollers blends these ingredients together, yielding a product so nutritionally rich that it is prone to spoilage and attacks by vermin and fungi if not immediately used. In order to make a product that could be transported over long distances and stored indefinitely, bread less prone to spoiling was necessary. White flour was born.

White flour begins with steel rather than stone rollers, thereby flattening and separating the bran and germ, which carry most of wheat's nutrients and are sold as animal feeds, from a chalklike dust. Chlorine gases are used to bleach out any remaining substance. The product is then "enriched" with synthetic versions of some of the vitamins removed earlier in the processing. The vitamins considered necessary for this "enrichment" are, not coincidentally, those which are most easily synthesized. These are the ingredients commonly listed on loaves of bread made from enriched flour: barley malt, ferrous sulfate, niacin, thiamine mononitrate, riboflavin, corn syrup, partially hydrogenated vegetable shortening, yeast, salt, dicalcium phosphate, calcium propionate, and potassium bromate.

Some of the flour additives and processing chemicals that need not, according to the Code of Federal Regulations, be listed on the package include: oxides of nitrogen, chlorine, nitrosyl chloride, chlorine dioxide, benzoyl peroxide, acetone peroxide, azodicarbonamide, and plaster of Paris.

Sugar

One of the most common additives in processed foods is sugar. The average American eats 160 pounds of sugar a year. After processing, many foods are so lacking in taste that there would be no flavor at all without adding large quantities of sugar or salt.

Sugar is ideal for the processed-food industry because many people like its taste and it is cheap, but primarily because it is addictive. Sugar in large quantities is concealed in many foods; not only in candy, cake, and soft drinks, but in bread, breakfast cereals, cheeses, condiments, and canned or packaged foods. Most processed foods have large amounts of sugar, and those that do not have large amounts of salt. It is not easy to eliminate sugar from your diet.

Water

Americans have grown accustomed to the excellence of their water supplies. Since the turn of the century, treatment of municipal water with chlorine disinfectants has provided protection against disease-causing microorganisms, and private wells are usually tested periodically to assure quality standards. Massive programs to build sewage treatment plants are in effect throughout the country, and standard operation procedures maintain the strict control of disease-causing microorganisms, since much of the water we drink is someone else's sewage.

However, even as the problem of human wastes is being controlled, a larger problem is looming: the industrial pollution of drinking-water supplies. Hundreds of thousands of industrial plants discharge grit, asbestos, phosphates, nitrates, mercury, lead, caustic soda, sulfur, sulfuric acid, oils, and petrochemicals into many of the waterways from which we eventually drink. Treatment plants designed to handle human wastes are unable to remove many of these more toxic, chemically complex, and sometimes unstable substances. Ironically, one of the carcinogens identified as occurring in water results when chlorine mixes with organic matter.

Nationwide, over 700 chemical pollutants have been identified in public water supplies. Most of these are carcinogenic, cause birth defects, or are otherwise toxic. Over 20 scientific studies have documented a consistent link between consumption of trace organic chemical contaminants in drinking water and elevated cancer mortality rates. In spite of mounting evidence, existing United

States public health standards reflect virtually no acknowledgment of toxic and carcinogenic substances in drinking water. As a result, no concerted effort has been made to remove them from public water supplies. Parallel failures to protect drinking water quality and to regulate massive discharges of nonbiodegradable industrial wastes forecast a grim future for the American public. Toxic contamination has already forced many communities to find alternative sources of water. Still, the overwhelming majority of the nation's drinking water systems have never been tested for the presence of toxic pollutants. The response to this dual environmental and health dilemma has been woefully inadequate.

Meat and Poultry

Most of us picture farms as being like those we remember from childhood, or like those we have seen in pictures or on television. We imagine farm animals in their pens, or even roaming around a farmyard. Such farms may exist, but they are not the source of the meat we buy and eat today. Chickens are raised by the tens of thousands in giant buildings where they never see the light of day. They are kept in cages where they cannot move, with conveyor belts bringing them food and water and carrying away their waste. When they do move about, they often slide around on their breasts, as some modern breeds grow too fast for their legs to support them. They are constantly sprayed and their food doused with chemicals, hormones, and medicines. Attempts also are being made to breed featherless chickens.

Many pigs are also raised in cages, without ever seeing daylight. Such conditions are particularly cruel for pigs, which are close to dogs in intelligence and sensitivity. Steers similarly spend most of their lives out of doors, but are no less exposed to chemicals in their upbringing.

Today, a steer is born, taken from its mother and put on a diet of powdered milk, synthetic vitamins, minerals, and antibiotics. Drugs in its food reduce its activities to save on feed. Next, it is permitted to eat some pasture grass, but this is supplemented with processed feed premixed with antibiotics and growth-promoting drugs. At six months, it weighs 500 pounds and is ready for the feed lot. Here it is doused with pesticides and then placed in a pen that is lit around the clock to change natural sleep rhythms and encourage continuous feeding. Food consists of grains, urea, carbohydrates, ground-up newspaper, molasses, plastic pellets, and, most recently, reprocessed manure, a high protein source. After four months in the feed lot, a steer weighs 1,200 pounds. A few more doses of pesticides, antibiotics, and hormones are administered to pretenderize it while it is still alive, and it is ready for slaughter.

Nearly all poultry, pigs, and veal calves, and 60 percent of cattle, get antibiotics added to their feed. Seventy-five percent of pigs eat feed laced with sulfa drugs. Cattle feeders use a variety of hormones and other additives to promote rapid weight gain in their animals.

While farmers rely more and more on chemicals to shore up animal health under factory conditions, dangerous residues are showing up in meat and poultry products. Fourteen percent of meat and poultry sampled by the Agriculture Department in the mid and late 1970s contained illegally high levels of drugs and pesticides. According to a recent General Accounting Office report, "of the 143 drugs and pesticides G.A.O. identified as likely to leave residues in raw meat and poultry, 42 are known to cause or are suspected of causing cancer, 20 of causing birth defects, and six of causing mutations."

Chemical Additives

The average American ate 2 pounds of chemical additives in food in 1960 and 10 pounds in 1978, a fivefold increase in less than 20 years. At the end of 1998, the Food and Drug Administration's (FDA) Everything Added to Food in the United States (EAFUS) Database contained information on more than 3,000 substances that were being added directly to what we eat. The actual number of additives was even higher: Despite its lofty title, the FDA acknowledged that the database did not include "indirect" additives, and may actually have been only a partial compilation of substances that were "lawfully" added to our food supplies. Most of these additives were not put in foods to preserve shelf life or retard spoilage, as is usually claimed; instead, more than 90 percent of the additives (both by weight and by value) were there to deceive—that is, to make the agribusiness product look, taste, feel, and nourish more like the real thing.

No one questions the fact that there are a lot of chemicals in our food. Manufacturers contend, however, that these chemicals are safe, that they have been tested and approved by the Food and Drug Administration. Are all these chemicals really safe? The answer is no.

If food additives can be dangerous, why are we told otherwise? The answer lies in the complex interrelations of the food industry, media, government, and medical research. The food industry is very big business, with annual sales well over $200 billion. Each year, well over $500 million worth of chemicals are added to foods. The food industry is a major advertiser in consumer magazines and on television, so magazines and television too often are careful of being critical. Food industries are major sources of grants for university research departments. Government agencies have close relationships with the industries they are supposed to regulate. Many research scientists and government management personnel eventually enter the industry they previously regulated— and at much higher paying jobs.

There are literally thousands of chemicals added to food. Few of these have been adequately tested, and none have been tested in combination with others. Many that have been tested, have been known to be dangerous for 30 years or more. DES, a synthetic hormone used to fatten cattle, has been known for decades to cause cancer. Industry fights attempts to ban such chemicals every step of the way. When, as in the case of DES, a ban is finally achieved, some producers continue to use it anyway. And by the time the ban is obtained, there are a dozen similar chemicals to replace the one banned, some of which may be worse.

Agribusiness encourages a way of eating that disrupts our physical health and erodes the sense of fulfillment that comes from preparing and eating real food. A fast-food rationale enters the community and the home, with deleterious effects. Agribusiness also undermines all local farmers, who lend economic and ecological stability to the country. And industrialized foods simply do not taste as good as food should. They are dependent upon salt, sugar, chemicals, and billions of dollars in advertising. The fact is, most of us simply have forgotten what real food tastes like.

Basic Nutrition

Basic nutrition begins with six major nutrients: carbohydrates, proteins, fats, vitamins, minerals, and water. Along with an understanding of these basic nutrients, for good health you also need to be aware of the air you breathe, the balance of enzymes in your body, and the function of antioxidants in helping your body to combat disease and degenerative processes. Your body needs all of these nutrients every day. How much you need of each depends on your health as well as your energy needs.

Energy may be why we need food, but it isn't necessarily why we eat sometimes a great deal, sometimes too little, or, all too often, the wrong things in the wrong amounts. When it comes to nourishing our bodies, many of us follow the dictates of myths, fads, or bizarre and exotic diets. We all know the proper kind of gas for a car and the best kind of food for our cat or dog. We may know our carburetors and our Siamese, but we don't know ourselves.

Information about good nutrition abounds. Yet many people don't bother to find out more about it. Some simply don't know where to look or what to trust. The following chapters should help point the way and begin that journey. After reading this section of the book, you will know all about real food and how to make the most of it in living a more healthful life.

2

Carbohydrates

Until recently, carbohydrates have gotten bad press. Highly sugared and refined carbohydrates such as candy, soft drinks, pastries, sugared cereals, as well as refined breads and pastas, have been lumped together with complex carbohydrates such as fruit, nutritious starchy vegetables, whole grains, and tubers. When think of carbohydrates, we tend also to think "calories and fattening."

Most people don't understand that there is a distinction between the two forms of carbohydrates: the *refined starches and sugars* that have given carbohydrates their reputation as food for fat, and the *complex carbohydrates* whose health benefits are finally beginning to be appreciated. Carbohydrates are vital in a proper diet.

Carbohydrates are everywhere. In fact, they are one of the most abundant compounds in living things. The nutrient group includes nondigestible cellulose (the fibrous material that helps give plants their shape), as well as starches and sugars, two of the storable fuels that supply living things with immediate energy. Each gram of carbohydrates supplies the body with four calories of energy when it is burnt up in our cells. In the U.S., half of the calories we get—half of our energy—come from these carbohydrate foods. Many carbohydrate-rich foods also contain substantial amounts of amino acids, the building blocks of protein.

We need carbohydrates. They are the most important source of energy for all our activities. The foods in which they are found are also important sources of the vitamins, minerals, and other nutrients we need to live.

Types of Carbohydrates

Carbohydrate foods come in two forms: complex and refined. Complex carbohydrates are starches and fibers in foods like cereals, legumes, seeds, nuts, vegetables, and tubers. They exist in these foods just as they are found in nature, having undergone minimal or no processing.

Refined carbohydrates, on the other hand, have been substantially tampered with. "Refined" may in fact be an overly refined way of putting it. Having been processed by machinery and industry, they are merely skeletons of the complex carbohydrates found in nature.

While the starches and sugars of all carbohydrates supply energy, complex carbohydrates also offer the fiber necessary for good digestive functioning, supply B and C complex and other vitamins, and manufacture protein, the building blocks of our bodies. In addition, our bodies tolerate and absorb complex carbohydrates best and most effectively.

Refinement, on the other hand, is a recent innovation in our long history of evolution, food consumption, and food delivery. When carbohydrates are refined, they are stripped of both their outer shell (the bran layer that contains most of the fiber) and their oil and a B vitamin-rich germ (found at their cores). Refined carbohydrates may also be bleached, milled, baked (bread), puffed (some cereals), or otherwise processed (sugar).

Unfortunately, these refined carbohydrates predominate in our diet. Breakfast cereals generally are made from wheat, corn, oats, or rice. But, with the exception of real oatmeal and a few hot whole wheat cereals, they are rarely served in their natural forms. Instead they are dried, refined, bleached, steamed, puffed, flaked, or sugared; occasionally a small percentage of the recommended daily allowance of certain minerals and (usually synthetic) vitamins are added. The cereals can then be labeled "enriched."

Most of the nutrients available from such breakfasts come from the milk that people add rather than from the cereal itself. Our breads (even "rye" and "whole wheat") are usually produced from refined flour and are often loaded with chemical additives. The white rice that graces our plates may look pretty, but it lacks the fiber, vitamins, and minerals found in whole-grain brown rice. Even the potato chips we crunch are a far cry from the vitamin- and fiber-rich whole potatoes from which they are made.

Refined carbohydrates may not be good for you. What's worse, they may harm you. They contain little or no fiber, so over-reliance on them as a source of energy can lead to poor intestinal health and myriad digestive disorders. Also, overconsumption of refined sugar is linked to obesity, hypoglycemia, diabetes, and other blood-sugar disorders.

Complex carbohydrates are closer to their natural state. Refined carbohydrates are highly processed foods, depleted of nutrients and fiber, and contain little more than pure starch or sugar, which are energy sources of no practical use.

Danger: Sweets Can Quickly Sour

You need carbohydrates for energy, especially to fuel your brain. But you don't really need refined sugar. Too much glucose in your bloodstream, an aftereffect of a typical high-sugar coffee and doughnut break, for example, may actually worsen fatigue and overburden your vital organs rather picking you up. If you have a well-balanced diet, you should be relying on your liver to send forth new energy from its reserves to your working muscles, not on candy bars or doughnuts. Sugar also has been implicated in cardiovascular problems and diabetes.

We know that anyone with hypertension (high blood pressure) should avoid salt. They should also avoid refined sugar. Animal studies suggest that high blood pressure may even lead to blood-sugar disorders.

Another bonus you receive when you avoid refined sugars is improved resistance to infections. The protective functions of your cells are depressed by all forms of sugar, but especially by sucrose. Also, sugar seems to provoke and worsen skin conditions such as acne. Cutting it out of your diet often results in visible improvement. Omitting refined sugar from your meals will also keep the various acids and other digestive juices in your stomach at normal levels.

Your brain must have a constant supply of glucose in order for its "circuits" to communicate and function properly. Hypoglycemia, or low blood sugar, often caused by overconsumption of refined sugars and flour, can distort perception and alter behavior.

If you suspect you are one of America's hypoglycemia victims, don't take this blood sugar disorder lightly. Consult your doctor for the necessary lab tests. Hypoglycemia not only may lead you to snack too often or to nap too much because of the fatigue and hunger it causes, it could also lead to diabetes or obesity. Remember, if you follow a poor diet high in refined carbohydrates, especially sugars, you are increasing the possibility of damage to your brain and nervous system. Because hypoglycemia interferes with the supply of glucose in your bloodstream, a proper diet can help to regulate it.

Too much refined sugar could be a contributing factor in causing children to become hyperkinetic or learning-disabled. It may also cause young adults to be learning-disabled or delinquent. Some studies even suggest that too much sugar is a causative factor in adults who behave criminally or antisocially.

Even naturally occurring sugars can pose problems. Gastrointestinal complaints, for example, can be caused by a sensitivity to the milk-sugar lactose in dairy products. Cultured dairy products, including yogurt, which are more easily digested, can provide a substitute for less-digestible dairy, while providing the vitamins and minerals you would miss if you avoided milk.

Fructose (the form of sugar predominant in fruits and honey) has been much praised recently as being superior to sucrose (cane sugar) or glucose (corn sugar). Beware: It may be sweeter, so you may use less of it—but a simple sugar is sugar to your body. Watch out for any simple or concentrated sugar!

How Many Carbohydrates Do You Need?

Half the calories Americans consume come from carbohydrates. Unfortunately, most of these are refined carbohydrates. The breads most people eat are 55 percent carbohydrate, since the refined flour from which they are made is 75 percent refined carbohydrate. Most flour cereals are 80 percent refined carbohydrate; our spaghettis and pastas are 75 percent refined carbohydrate. Jams, candies, and some pastries may be 90 percent refined carbohydrate.

In contrast fresh fruit is only 15 percent carbohydrate; dry legumes, even before being doubled in size by the addition of water in cooking, are just 60 percent carbohydrate; and uncooked whole grains, before the absorption of water, are 70 percent carbohydrate. Green leafy vegetables average 8 percent carbohydrate or less. The point is, by eating vegetables, grains, legumes, seeds and some fruits, with moderate to low carbohydrate content, we are actually reducing calories and sugars in our diet.

The ideal diet gets most (85 to 90 percent) of its calories and protein from complex carbohydrates, and 10 to 15 percent from fats found in nuts, seeds, and oils. This ratio allows complex carbohydrates to be the mainstay of the diet, with fewer calories from fats, and fewer from animal protein foods. But, in most cases, that is not what happens.

Our bodies are factories—processing foods, making chemicals, storing materials, and producing energy. Just as plants do, your body factory stores much of its energy in the form of simple sugars and starches. Your backup energy reserve is stored as fat. The form of stored energy immediately available and most easily converted into action comes from carbohydrates. The sugars you absorb from your food may be converted by the body into energy, starch, or fat. At any given time, you usually have available about a 13-hour supply of glycogen (starch) and glucose (a simple sugar). Blood levels of glucose are supposed to remain stable, with about 15 grams circulating at all times. Each gram of glycogen or glucose, when oxidized by the cells, provides four calories of energy for all the body's needs.

Despite what our backgrounds, palates, or emotions may tell us, supplying energy remains the number one purpose of food. Carbohydrates yield immediately available energy; if they are oversupplied, the body builds up its muscle and liver glycogen reserves or converts the extra amount into fat. High-protein diets, on the other hand, can be dangerous. Protein is mainly a building material, not a primary energy source. It can be burnt up as fuel, but this is an inefficient way to provide energy to our systems; it requires extra energy, and it results in a waste product called urea, which must be disposed of through the kidneys. Over the long term, eating too much protein and burning protein as fuel can overstress and even weaken the kidneys.

Complex Carbohydrates

SOURCES Complex carbohydrates are not hard to find. You just have to know where to look. Basic whole grains, for example, include whole wheat (to which, unfortunately, too many people have became allergic because they have consumed so much refined wheat flour in breads, cakes, pastas, and packaged, processed foods), rye, triticale (a cross between rye and wheat you may be able to tolerate if you are allergic to real whole wheat), corn, barley, brown rice, oats, millet, and buckwheat. All these can be served whole, as cereals or side dishes, mixed in soups and casseroles, ground into whole grain flour and baked into bread, or rolled into whole grain pastas.

Legumes, an excellent source of complex carbohydrates, are also more varied than most people realize. Among the common varieties are soybeans and soy products such as tofu, tempeh, and miso, mung beans, lentils, azduki beans, split peas, black-eyed peas, kidney beans, navy beans, red beans, pink beans, pinto beans, black beans, turtle beans, fava beans, chick-peas (garbanzos), and peanuts.

Seeds such as sunflower, pumpkin, chia, and sesame are high in both protein and carbohydrates; alfalfa, chia, and flax seeds (those grown organically for food, not for fabrics, to avoid pesticide contamination) are highly nutritious when sprouted. Most nuts are mainly fat, but almonds, cashews, pistachios, and pine nuts are high in carbohydrates as well.

The entire vegetable family is a rich source of carbohydrates. Those lowest in calories, such as celery, broccoli, and mushrooms, contain mostly water and fiber; the starchier, root vegetables like carrots, beets, potatoes, and yams, tend to be higher in unrefined starches and sugars as well as in fiber.

Fruits are excellent sources of complex carbohydrates, natural sugars, minerals, vitamins, and fiber. Choose from apples, pears, peaches, nectarines, plums, grapes, or citrus fruits. Although the sugar content of these fruits is fairly high, it is diluted with water and released relatively slowly into your system as you chew and digest the cellulose-encased cells of the pulp. Your body doesn't get the kind of sudden jolt it receives from refined, pure sugar. Bananas and other tropical fruits should be eaten in moderation by those sensitive to sugar, since their sugar content is higher. Similarly, dried fruits, including figs, prunes, raisins, dates, apricots, pears, and apples contain three times the sugar dose of fresh fruit; like refined sugar, they are highly concentrated carbohydrates, which should only be eaten occasionally. Hypoglycemics and diabetics should take special note of this precaution.

Eating too much fruit can add extra calories, but as long as you don't eat fatty foods as well, fruit will not make you fat. An apple indeed may contain the equivalent of three teaspoons of sugar and the calories that go with that. But it is much harder to down three whole apples than nine teaspoons of sugar. Some people consume as much sugar in one cup of coffee, one mug of cocoa, or one doughnut—without getting all the beneficial vitamins, minerals, fiber, and enzymes of the apple.

PREPARING COMPLEX CARBOHYDRATE FOODS Grains should be rinsed before use, and the larger legumes—such as beans—should be soaked overnight before cooking. Cooking time can be shortened by using pressure cookers.

People who eat meat and wish to switch to a more complex-carbohydrate-oriented, vegetarian diet often worry that eating will become a boring, asensual experience, limited in variety and taste. Pilgrims, seek no more. There are vegetarian recipes and menus to satisfy every palate and taste. The vegetarian recipes included in later chapters will provide a sampling of their variety and set you on the right nutritional track.

For those who must restrict their sodium intake, a variety of other herbs and spices are available that are even livelier that salt. They include leeks, dill, oregano, cumin, curry, and chili peppers. Vegetables may be mixed with legumes for stews and casseroles as well as soups; seasoned grains, such as millet (perhaps combined with soy granules or lentils for protein enhancement), are delicious stuffed into peppers, tomatoes, or hollowed-out zucchinis.

Digestion of Carbohydrates

Cooked starches are easier to digest than uncooked ones, since heat ruptures the cell walls of plants and allows certain chemicals, called enzymes, to convert the starches to sugars more easily in the mouth and the intestines. These sugars are then used by the body for energy.

Normally, carbohydrates are digested quickly. The carbohydrates in fruit juice may be digested in as little as 40 minutes; starchy foods, such as beans or grains, may take up to 1½ hours. Cooked and eaten properly, the digestion time of a carbohydrate meal may be only 80 to 90 minutes. The more fiber you consume with your meals, the faster the digestion process, since fiber absorbs water and stimulates the actions of the digestive tract.

Animal proteins and fats take much longer to digest, and if sweet or starchy foods are eaten at the same time as meat and fish, they can remain in the stomach for much of the time the protein foods take to digest (up to six hours). This can cause gas and indigestion, since the sugar from the carbohydrates may begin to ferment in the warm acid environment of the stomach. For this reason, it's a good idea if you eat meat, fish, or fowl to serve your meal with only a salad and vegetables, saving primary carbohydrate foods for other meals. Also, as we age we may lose some of our digestive capacities, which increases digestion time. This may vary widely, depending on the size of the animal protein portion, how long it was cooked, how thoroughly the food was chewed, and the age as well as the mental and physical condition of the individual.

If you begin your meal with a beverage, you can briefly dilute the acid in your stomach and slow digestion. Cold beverages can suspend initial digestion for a short time, since the acids and enzymes of your digestive system usually operate at body temperature.

Some people complain that they have trouble digesting beans, and that flatulence is a problem. Partly, this is because these products may ferment in the large intestines, producing gas. Beans should be soaked for at least 15 hours before cooking. Cook them slowly to avoid altering the protein and thoroughly so that their fiber is completely softened. Digestion will then be easier.

Bean sprouts also may be easier to digest than cooked dried beans. Sprouting increases the nutrient content as well as the digestibility of beans, grains, and seeds. Alfalfa and mung beans are two of the most popular types. Alfalfa sprouts are a nutrition powerhouse, containing five times the amount of vitamin C of alfalfa seeds. Two ounces of sprouts a day will supply you with vitamins and live raw enzymes you might not otherwise obtain from your diet, as well as chlorophyll, which is considered an intestine and blood cleanser. Always steam soy bean sprouts briefly before serving them, since the raw beans contain digestion inhibitors, trypsin, and other natural toxins that can only be neutralized by heating.

The typical American dinner, consisting of meat, potatoes, vegetables, and perhaps a salad, with dessert afterwards, mixes up all four digestive processes at once, weakening them all. The acid from the meat's protein neutralizes the enzyme in your mouth that breaks down starches into sugars, so starch digestion is limited and extended. When a sugary dessert is added, its simple refined sugars start fermenting, resulting in too much acid in the stomach. If you then take an antacid, this plays additional havoc with the digestive process. Eventually such habits can lead to chronic indigestion and too much stress for the gastrointestinal tract.

It would be best to eat complex carbohydrates at one meal, protein at another, and fruits as snacks between meals. Protein meals take a long time to digest, and can leave you with less energy for several hours after eating them, since, ironically, much of your energy is used just to digest the protein, with blood channeled from other parts of the body to the digestive organs to help with the work.

If you eat some fruit 10 to 15 minutes before a protein-heavy meal, you can also prevent your blood-glucose levels from declining during the time you are digesting your meal. Someone who eats largely protein at every meal may spend the whole day with part of his or her energy involved in digestion—a strange way to spend a day!

If, on the other hand, you eat three or four small meals that include complex carbohydrates, your energy levels are likely to be higher and more constant throughout the day. What's more, your intestines will be spared the somewhat exhausting, though necessary, process of prolonged digestion.

There are some people who are allergic to one or more grains, legumes, seeds, or nuts; however, most people who in the past have been diagnosed as "carbohydrate intolerant," can actually benefit from complex instead of refined carbohydrates.

What About Fiber?

Fiber, quite simply, is made up of carbohydrates that the human body cannot digest. But just because they are nondigestible does not mean they serve no useful purpose. Fiber substances such as cellulose are in the cell walls, giving plants the power to grow structurally strong. Fiber does a great deal for us, too.

In the last decade fiber has been rediscovered both by the physician and the nutritionist. More and more researchers—at the National Cancer Institute, the American Cancer Society, and elsewhere—are jumping on the fiber bandwagon of digestive health. They have pinpointed the value of fiber in our food to act as a kind of super janitorial service for our intestines, keeping them free of hazardous substances, including some powerful cancer-causing chemicals, that may enter our bodies.

Fiber is not found in meats, cheeses, and minimally in refined carbohydrates, or highly processed foods—that is, in the typical American diet, already too high in fatty meats, bleached breads, and sugary desserts.

Fibrous foods stimulate and exercise your mouth and gums, oral membranes, and facial muscles. Fiber also scrubs the walls of your colon and bowels, cleaning and hastening transit time though the digestive system for the foods you eat, reducing the possibility that your body will harbor toxins longer than it should. Fiber also fills you up, so you don't have to snack so often.

When adequate amounts are missing from your diet, you may develop constipation, and are at risk of colorectal cancer, or one of the other common diseases that attack the gastrointestinal system. This risk becomes greater when your diet is low in fresh, nutritious whole foods and instead is high in fats and sugars.

By contrast, a diet emphasizing moderate amounts of protein, high intake of natural fiber foods, and low fat intake results in better health of the bowels and the whole body, and provides protection against certain types of cancer. Fiber, for the most part, does not even contribute calories.

Fiber should be eaten in its natural form. Our bodies have evolved according to the foods our ancestors ate and are adapted to derive the total nutritional value from the food we eat: protein, fats, carbohydrates, water, vitamins, minerals, trace minerals, and enzymes, along with the bulk necessary for good bowel movements. The processing of most supermarket cereals originally was based on several not necessarily healthful factors. One of these was profit, which continues to play a major role. Another was the erroneous belief that fiber serves no useful purpose. Now that we know better, processing and food industry methods and beliefs are changing. For example, whole-fiber breakfast cereals have begun to be distributed through supermarkets. Read the labels of "natural" cereals carefully to avoid sugar. Some are genuine whole foods, others contain large quantities of sugar in various forms, or are packaged with preservatives.

If you are in fairly good health, 40 to 60 grams, or from one to two ounces a day of fiber from natural sources should be adequate. If occasional periods of irregularity are a problem, a few extra tablespoons of untreated, unheated oat germ, wheat bran, or even a tasty variation such as rice or corn bran can be sprinkled over your morning cereal or evening salad and will provide extra benefits.

If you prefer to use fruits and salad foods to meet your roughage requirements, a raw salad for lunch and a partially cooked grain salad such as tabouli for dinner, plus a big puree of fresh fruit in season, would help fill the bill nicely. Some researchers believe these absorb the most water in your intestines. Oat fiber will absorb up to six times its weight in water, and vegetables generally hold roughly half as much.

All vegetables weren't created equal in terms of fiber. Root vegetables such as carrots are at the top of the list: their crunchy quality and hardness indicate a high fiber yield. They also require beneficial exercise of your jaws and teeth. Buy produce in season, buy it fresh, and eat it raw when possible. Vegetables can be grated for uncooked salads. But do not neglect the less common tubers: yams, kohlrabi, parsnips, and eggplant. Never peel away any vegetable skin if it isn't essential to your recipe to do so, since in and near the skin is stored much of the plant's roughage and nutrients.

The whole legume family deserves special attention. A good way to eat these and profit by the skins is to sprout your peas, chick-peas, mung beans, and lentils rather than cook them. In doing so you are rewarded with the full value of the live food, including minerals, amino acids, and carbohydrate energy. Remember to steam bean sprouts briefly before serving.

A little bran every day will improve your health and regularity, but there's no substitute for a well-balanced diet. And no two fibers are the same. Fiber in fruits and vegetables is different from that in grains. Include them all.

Take, for instance, the fiber in citrus fruits. If you've had a grapefruit or orange for breakfast, you've already had a beneficial two-carbohydrate food factor—protopectin. The pulp of all citrus fruits contains this combination of cellulose plus pectin.

The cellulose in the citrus fruit absorbs fluid from your intestines. So as it enlarges, it quickly pushes along any contents in the intestinal tract. Meanwhile, the pectin becomes gelatinous, and counters to the absorbing effects of cellulose, it provides lubrication and ensures smooth passage for the food.

In addition, protopectin helps you get maximum value out of the other nutritious foods you eat and enhances your system's use of dietary fats. This, in turn, helps provide some protection against the cardiovascular dangers that high cholesterol levels pose.

3

Fats

Americans receive nearly half (45 percent) of their total calories from fats. Our overindulgence in fatty foods has taken its toll by contributing to a high proportion of overweight Americans as well as to the degeneration of our heart and blood vessels, with fats reducing blood flow through our arteries and increasing blood pressure. The American Heart Association recommends that we should reduce the amount of saturated fat and cholesterol in our diet to help prevent heart disease. In 1984, the government's National Heart, Blood and Lung Institute concluded a 10-year study and issued a report conclusively implicating cholesterol in individuals with an increased risk of heart attack. Over the past 15 years, other studies have confirmed this finding. The American Heart Association now states that a high level of cholesterol in the blood is a "major risk factor" for coronary heart disease. And in 1996, the Department of Agriculture issued new rules to set limits on the fat (and cholesterol and sodium) content of school lunches. But we should not avoid fat completely. Reducing the fat in your diet doesn't mean eliminating it. People need not overreact, just act.

Fat provides one of the body's primary nutrients. We need it in small amounts because it allows us to use the fat-soluble vitamins A, D, E, and K, which are essential for the health of our immune system. These vitamins only work when in the presence of fatty molecules or tissue. Fat helps prevent viral infections, protects our heart, blood vessels, and internal organs, slows down the aging process, and helps keep skin healthy. Most importantly, fats, like carbohydrates, are a usable and essential source of energy. They serve as a reserve supply of energy deposited in various parts of the body called adipose tissue.

Fat is a concentrated source of energy. It yields nine calories per gram when it is burned up or oxidized. Proteins and carbohydrates each yield only four calories per gram. Therefore, a little bit of fat goes a long way in carrying out normal body functions.

Body fat acts as an insulator and prevents excessive heat loss. It also acts as a shock absorber. You need some fat around your internal organs to prevent bruising, hemorrhage, or rupture. It also is essential for the utilization of nutrients and the production of hormones. In fact, much of your body's chemistry revolves around the proper utilization of fat. Fat is fine—in limited amounts. But you don't want too much fat, because it may not only surround the organs but can also penetrate them. In excess it can lace itself through the organs, and through the muscle tissue, so your risk of disease (such as heart disease and diabetes) increases.

Not All Fats are Equal

While fats may be equal in calories, as the fat in margarine is no different in terms of its caloric count than the fat in olive oil or butter, they do have unique properties. The omega-3 fatty acids, which are found in fish, for example, have been shown to be healthful to the heart. They also allow the body to use energy more efficiently. The essential fatty acids found in the oil from flaxseed, primrose, sesame seeds, sunflower seeds, safflower seeds, and soy beans are vital for the maintenance of health, growth, maturation, hormone production, and other functions. It is important, therefore, to have a variety of fats in the diet in small amounts. It is not necessary to add tablespoons of fat in the form of oil when grains, legumes, fish, seeds, and nuts are plentiful sources, with a combination of long- and short-chain fatty acids found in each food.

There are two kinds of fats—saturated and unsaturated.

SATURATED FATS Saturated fats are found in animal food sources such as meat and dairy products, constituting half of the USDA's dietary recommendations for the "basic food groups." Technically speaking, fat is saturated if the carbon atom chain that makes it up is also saturated with hydrogen atoms. You can tell if fat is saturated if it turns solid at room temperature. Examples of saturated fats include butter, the fatty part of chicken, fish, veal, lamb, pork, and beef (the actual marbled fat that you can see), lard, and coconut oil.

UNSATURATED FATS Unsaturated fats are primarily found in grains, legumes, seeds, nuts, and the oils derived from them, including corn oil, safflower oil, sunflower oil, and soy oil—all of which are liquid at room temperature. These unsaturated oils should represent the majority of your fat intake. Unsaturated fats should be used because they provide us with certain essential fatty acids. These have several functions: controlling high blood pressure; helping form prostaglandins (important chemicals for a host of bodily functions); and regulating the ability of substances to enter and leave cells. The body cannot easily manufacture those fatty acids not considered "essential" if your diet doesn't provide them.

There are a variety of types of unsaturated fats. The most common are polyunsaturates, such as those found in corn or safflower oil. There are also monounsaturates, such as those in olive oil. There is new evidence suggesting that the latter type actually helps protect your heart by raising levels of certain types of cholesterols (high-density lipoproteins), a blood fat in your body. The omega-3 fish fat mentioned above, for example, is also a monounsaturate.

All fats, however, are combinations of saturated and unsaturated, and we need both each day. But, primarily, the fats in our diet should be of an unsaturated quality. No more than 25 percent should be saturated.

POLYUNSATURATES It is extremely important to know that the *essential* fatty acids—those we need for certain vital functions—are all polyunsaturates. Our systems can manufacture saturated and even some monounsaturated fats from carbohydrates, but not the polyunsaturates. So we must supply these substances from our diet.

What are the vital functions that we need polyunsaturated fatty acids for? First, they are an important part of the membranes that interconnect every cell in our body. Almost all of our cells have both inner and outer membranes. Most of the enzymes in the body are strung along the inner cell membranes, which form a physical locus for the performance of our metabolic functions. And how these membranes influence our enzymes depends largely on the fatty acids in them. A membrane with a high proportion of saturated fat will be very stiff. On the other hand, a higher proportion of mono- and polyunsaturates will allow it to function in a more balanced, responsive way.

A second function performed by fatty acids is to make a special class of hormones, the prostaglandins. A classic hormone is made in one gland—the thyroid, for example—and travels throughout the body giving various signals to cells. Prostaglandins, on the other hand, are made throughout the body. Every single cell, with the exception of the red blood cells, makes prostaglandin. These hormones don't travel far, though, and tend to be destroyed after one passage through the circulatory system. They regulate the local responses of the body to other stimuli, including other hormones, brain chemicals, and drugs.

There are about 50 different biologically active prostaglandins, and the balance between these hormones can have a profound effect on our bodies' functions. Since prostaglandins are manufactured from various fatty acids, an imbalance in the intake of fatty acids can disturb the balance between prostaglandins and trigger a wide range of disorders. These include almost all of the degenerative diseases which have largely emerged in the 20th century. Heart disease, cancer, autoimmune diseases like AIDS, allergies, asthma, and pre-menstrual syndrome are consistently accompanied by prostaglandin imbalances.

How Much Fat Do You Need?

There is considerable disagreement regarding how much fat is necessary and appropriate in the diet. Estimates range from 10 to 30 percent of total caloric intake. To be safe, your consumption of calories from fat probably should be limited to 15 to 20 percent of your total calories. A quarter of these could be saturated. The rest should come from the unsaturated fats found in cooking and salad oils or, more beneficially, from those naturally occurring oils in vegetables, grains, legumes, nuts, and seeds. In their natural state, if they are unbleached, unadulterated, and have not been clarified or chemically altered to destroy their nutritional benefits, oils not only provide you with fat that the body can use, but also supply vitamin E, a substance that has powerful antioxidant properties, preventing the destruction of fatty acids and helping your body heal itself. Vitamin E promotes nerve growth and keeps cells functioning normally.

FATS AND DIETING One of the reasons doctors may prescribe high-fat, high-protein, low-carbohydrate diets is because of the ability of fat and protein to keep you feeling full after a meal, allaying between-meal hunger pangs. If, on the other hand, you eat a complex carbohydrate in the form of a grain or vegetable, it is digested and goes through your system in a matter of 30 to 80 minutes. You benefit from the energy and you're not taxing your digestive system. But it also means there will be a tendency to get hungry sooner.

After all, we tend to gain weight in large part because we get hungry and have snacks between meals. A fatty or high-protein food eaten at mealtime will require one to four hours of digestion just to empty out the stomach. As long as you have that much food in your stomach, your appetite is suppressed so you do not feel hungry. Snacks usually come in the form of high-sugar, refined carbohydrate foods like jelly rolls, candy bars and soft drinks. Bypassing the midmorning, midafternoon, and late evening snack, can mean eliminating 400 to 900 calories. In a period of a week you would be able to knock off a pound just by modifying your diet to reduce snacks and increase the protein and fat content.

The Hazards of Fat

Many people like deep-fried foods such as french fries, onion rings, fried fish, potato chips, and doughnuts. These are prepared with fatty oils heated to high temperatures that alter the chemical structure of the fat, creating free fatty acids that can have an irritating effect upon the stomach and on the sensitive mucous linings of the intestines. Eating fried foods frequently can set into motion the ultimate dysfunction of your intestine. Colitis, spastic colon, or some other form of irritable intestine condition may be the result. Heated fats also slow down digestive time. The longer fat is cooked, the more difficult it is for the enzymes in the stomach and the intestine to break it down. Liquid fats are easier to digest. Oils (or unsaturated fats) go through the system much more rapidly than saturated fats.

As I've said before, when you have a lot of fat in your stomach after a meal, you will have less energy. Your energy is being diverted to facilitating the proper digestion, utilization, absorption, and elimination of food—a lengthy process. Blood and oxygen, also, are diverted, to a degree, even from your brain, just for digestion.

Nearly 95 percent of the fat you consume is digested and used by the body. It is fine to have some amount of fat as reserve, but in the absence of regular, daily exercise the muscles begin to atrophy and fat infiltration into the muscle occurs. Fat then takes the place of unused, atrophied muscles. We lose our strength, endurance, and stamina, and we become more susceptible to body injury, accident, and disease.

Fats are necessary nutrients. We need unsaturated fats from seeds, grains, legumes, and nuts. We don't need all of the oils from salad oil to cooking fats that are typically part of our diet now. Try to keep the fats in your diet to 15 to 20 percent. And be selective, choosing certain types of fish, like salmon, for their healthful fat content.

A Nation at Risk

Almost anyone in the modern United States has a fatty acid problem. We are all at risk, and the reason can be found in the dietary changes we have seen in this country over the past century. We consume no more fat today than our grandparents did 100 years ago. We consume much more sugar and less fiber, however, and we also consume a lot less of the foods that provide fish oils and their plant oil analogues.

As mentioned, one group of essential fatty acids is found in corn oil, as well as safflower, sunflower, liver, and kidney oils. These fatty acids are present to some extent in almost all whole foods, but they are by far most concentrated in these oils. Americans do generally consume a substantial amount of these oils, largely because of publicity from the medical community about the need for fatty acids and the desirability of avoiding saturated fats.

Another group of essential fatty acids, however, is found in foods and oils which Americans seldom use, most typically fish oils, particularly those from oily, cold water fish like salmon, tuna, mackerel, and herring. These fatty acids are also found in some plants; flax seed—which is used to make linseed oil—is the richest plant source. Other northern-climate plants also have seeds which are rich in these fatty acids—the germ of winter wheat, walnuts, and soybean oil, for instance.

One reason for our deficiency in "fish oil" type essential fatty acids is that we now mostly use oils that contain less of these fatty acid groups. Another reason is that we process the oils we do use for convenience. Almost all the oils we buy have been at least partially hydrogenated. This is done to prolong shelf life—but it is a nutritional disaster.

(When reading product labels, it is important to be wary of products made from polyunsaturates, including certain salad oils and margarines, as well as egg and cream substitutes. What labels may fail to mention, however, is that you are eating a saturated fat. The verdict on hydrogenated or partially hydrogenated oils, like margarines, is not yet conclusive concerning their harmful or beneficial effects.)

A century ago, people living near water ate a lot of fish. In England, for example, herring, a good source of this group of fatty acids, was a staple food. But over the years the great schools of herring in the North Sea were wiped out, although efforts have begun to revitalize these food sources. Salmon was another staple—reportedly, workers in one plant in England petitioned not to be served salmon at lunch more than five times in a week! Until World War II, food-grade linseed oil was used widely and frequently in the mountains of northern Europe. Today, salmon is a rare luxury, and linseed oil is something to treat furniture with.

Cod-liver oil is another casualty of changing customs. Not all that long ago cod-liver oil was a common supplement in the winter; we need more of its unsaturated fatty acids when it's cold, and the vitamin A and D it supplied was an additional benefit. The dying away of the popularity of cod-liver oil has also deprived us of a valuable arthritis treatment. The fatty acids found in this oil decrease production of some of the prostaglandin hormones that cause arthritic inflammation.

How can you tell if you are at risk? One sign of essential fatty acid deficiency is dry skin, which tends to get worse in the winter. Another is the rough skin that can appear on the backs of our arms or on our thighs, sometimes called "chicken skin." Brittle or weak fingernails, especially those that tend to split, and dry, unmanageable hair are also warning signs, as is excessive thirst, which usually is not accompanied by a corresponding increase in urination. These are not surefire guides, though; vitamin A, B_6, or zinc deficiencies can produce similar symptoms.

Intense menstrual cramps are signs of an excess production of certain prostaglandins, as well as asthma, eczema, and arthritis. Families with a shared tendency to have allergies often have an inherited dysfunction in the way their bodies process essential fatty acids. This is due to a weak enzymatic link, and these people need more essential fatty acids than the average person.

CORRECTING A DEFICIENCY Americans consume the greatest number of nutritional supplements in the world; to Europeans we're something of a joke in this regard. Taking in fatty acids as supplements is no magic formula; they have to be utilized in the body, and that requires a balance of vitamins and minerals. In fact, without using oil supplements, it's possible to increase the efficiency with which your body uses essential fatty acids by taking extra zinc and B vitamins. Many people have a problem absorbing and metabolizing fatty acids, as noted above. But if the basic levels of these substances aren't provided it is impossible to tell if the problem is metabolic. Many experts state that essential fatty acid deficiencies are rare due to their wide distribution in our diet, but only the corn oil type is actually widely consumed. The first step, then, is to boost your intake of the fish oil type of fatty acids. Sometimes this will bring out the other weak links; once they've been exposed, other supplements can be added more judiciously.

Certain kinds of fish, which themselves are good sources of these fatty acids, have had much of their value in this regard removed by the time they are purchased. For example, sardines are usually canned not in their own oil, but in olive or soybean oil; in fact, due to potential spoilage problems, it's illegal to can sardines in their own oil. Fresh sardines, however, and almost any fresh cold water fish, are a good source.

Nut butters are also rich in these fatty acids, particularly those made from walnuts and chestnuts. So are cold-pressed nut oils—though "cold pressed" is a misnomer; the process does heat the oil to a degree, and some of the valuable fatty acids are lost. This also happens with the processing of nut butters, when some oils are lost or altered through the exposure to air during chopping and grinding. These losses, however, are far outweighed by the food value that does remain.

As mentioned, one of the richest sources of fatty acids is food-grade linseed oil. Whole-grain winter wheat is a palatable and practical source. Vegetable leaves have fish oil type fatty acids in high proportion to other types of fat, but have so little total fat that they are not a very efficient way of supplying these oils. Although olive oil is a good oil to use and may play a role in lowering cholesterol, it does not contain fish oil type fatty acids.

One way to ensure that we get enough essential fatty acids for ideal functioning is to remove foods from our diet which can interfere with their processing. Saturated fats and partially or fully hydrogenated vegetable oils should be avoided. Sugar and alcohol also hamper the efficient metabolizing of fatty acids.

Evening primrose oil is more similar to corn oil than to fish oil in its fatty acids. It has an advantage over corn or safflower oil, though; it bypasses a step in the body's metabolic process that is required to utilize the other oils. Some people who have a weak enzyme which makes it difficult to metabolize essential fatty acids can use evening primrose oil, which doesn't require this enzyme.

Oils lose much of their value when they are used for cooking; heat destroys much of their fatty acid content. So if you're going to rely on oils as supplements, they should be taken in an uncooked form. This can be done by using oils as salad dressing, or mixing them into margarine. In addition, the essential fatty acids in oils oxidize easily, and therefore have a short shelf life. The byproducts of oxidation are dangerous; so as you increase your intake of essential fatty acids it is wise to also take in antioxidants—particularly vitamin A and selenium—to safeguard yourself against oxidation.

All of the substances which supply concentrated essential fatty acids should be used carefully as supplements, as it is possible to "overdose" on essential fatty acid intake. It is also important to be aware of a competitive relationship between some different types of fatty acids in the body's metabolic processes. For example, the fish oil type competes with the corn oil/primrose fatty acids for the enzymes used to metabolize them. Taking too much of either can produce a relative deficiency of the other.

4

Protein

A thick, rare steak, a hamburger, or a platter of fried chicken—the joys of protein? For many of us, protein equals meat, which equals strength, endurance, growth, and health. We have been misled! Meat is only one of several possible dietary sources of protein. Yet it has become the predominant and most expensive source in the average American diet. Our image of protein as the one most important nutrient ("protein" is derived from the Greek "protos," meaning first) has led us to eat so much meat that we often consume more than twice the protein we need each day.

On average, Americans eat nearly 100 grams or 6½ ounces of protein every day when all most of us actually need is three-quarters of that. And despite the legends, even athletes are better off increasing their carbohydrate rather than their protein consumption if they want to increase their endurance and stamina. Eggs, dairy products, grains, legumes, nuts, and seeds are all excellent sources of protein that can supplement meat or replace it in the diet.

Proteins are the building blocks of life. They are the basic material from which all your cells, tissues, and organs are constructed. Only water represents a larger percentage of your total body weight than protein. Proteins are constantly being replaced, 24 hours a day, throughout your entire life, as your body uses and loses cellular materials. The optimal intake of high-quality proteins allows the body to grow and maintain healthy bones, skin, teeth, muscles, and nerves; it keeps the blood count correct; and it allows the metabolism—the body's ability to use food sources—to function at the highest level. Hemoglobin, the part of the red blood cells that provides oxygen to the cells, is made primarily of protein.

When we think of protein, we usually think of it as a body-building substance found in muscles. However, only one-third of our body's protein is concentrated in muscle tissue. Protein is part of every living cell in our body, from the hair on our heads to the nails on our toes. Skin, nails, hair, muscles, cartilage, and tendons all have fibrous protein as their main constituent.

And, with four calories per gram, it is also available as a source of heat and energy. When carbohydrates and fats are in short supply, protein can be converted to glucose, providing necessary energy to the brain and central nervous system.

Protein molecules called enzymes start the metabolic process; they must be present for hundreds of necessary chemical reactions and interactions in our body to occur. Enzymes allow energy to be stored and released in each cell; and they allow protein, fats, carbohydrates, and cholesterol to be synthesized by the liver. Protein is responsible for keeping your blood slightly alkaline, and it is the raw material out of which the antibodies that shield you from infection are created. Hormones, which regulate your metabolism, also contain some protein.

The Essential Amino Acids

The hundreds of proteins your body synthesizes are all made up of chains of only 23 smaller, basic protein substances, called amino acids—composed of nitrogen, carbon, oxygen, hydrogen, and in some cases, sulfur. Of these, the body can synthesize 15 on its own, leaving 8 that must be present in your food to be used. These 8 are called the essential amino acids. A ninth amino acid, histamine, is essential for children.

Amino acids, of which proteins are made, are necessary for certain vitamins and minerals to be utilized. The amino acid tryptophan, for example, initiates the production of the B vitamin, niacin. Proteins help transport fats through the bloodstream by combining with them to form lipoproteins. In fact, the only fluids in your body that do not normally contain protein are perspiration, urine, and bile. It is possible to live without eating protein, but not for very long.

In order for your cells to make the proteins they need for growth, all the necessary amino acids must be present simultaneously in sufficient amounts. This means that if any one amino acid is not present, the protein cannot be constructed. Since protein cannot be stored (except, perhaps, by lactating mothers), it is necessary to eat complete proteins at each meal, or, if you are eating nonanimal products, to mix your protein sources to form complete proteins. To provide your body with only some of the amino acids it needs is like being a baker who buys 100 pounds of flour, 100 pounds of shortening, but only 1 ounce of yeast. Because of the yeast he can bake only one or two cakes. What does he do with all that flour and shortening? In your body, unused amino acids might be excreted or broken down and oxidized for energy and other metabolic needs.

Protein deficiencies occur when we don't consume enough protein for our body's needs, or when the proteins we do consume lack one or more of the eight essential amino acids. These eight are threonine, valine, tryptophan, lysine, methionine, histidine, phenylalanine, and isoleucine. Foods that contain all eight of these essential amino acids are called complete protein foods. Eggs, meat, fowl, fish, grains, legumes, nuts, seeds, vegetables, fruits and dairy products contain complete proteins.

For protein to be absorbed and used by the body, all eight essential amino acids must be present in a certain proportion, actually in about the same proportion in which they occur in eggs, nature's complete food package for chicken embryos. Partially complete proteins may contain all eight, but not in the correct proportions. Thus foods high in partially-complete proteins, such as brewer's yeast (also called nutritional yeast), wheat germ, the soy food tofu, peanuts, and certain micro-sea algae, should be eaten in combination with other protein foods. We have been led to believe that animal products—such as meats, poultry, fish, dairy products, and eggs—are the only adequate sources of protein. This is based on misconceptions that originated over 40 years ago. If we can't thoroughly digest something, we can't utilize its protein, no matter how complete it is. In addition to digestibility, our ability to utilize protein may be influenced by the functioning of our digestive tract, the presence of any disease or infection, and age. Plant sources, once disparaged, are now starting to get higher ratings.

How Much Protein Do You Need?

Generally speaking, adults require .9 grams of protein per kilogram of body weight. (A kilogram is 2.2 pounds.) Thus, a 60-kilogram (132-pound) woman probably needs about 54 grams of protein a day. During spurts of growth, as in infancy, early childhood, and puberty, more protein is needed. Others with higher protein needs include pregnant women and lactating mothers; hypoglycemics; convalescents from surgery and certain types of infection, shock, or fever; and those under any kind of stress. Under certain conditions, such as kidney disease, lower protein intake for a period of time also may be in order.

TOO LITTLE PROTEIN Eating an inadequate amount of high-quality protein forces our bodies to break down more tissue than it can build up, resulting in overall deterioration. Some symptoms of protein deficiency are muscle weakness, loss of endurance, fatigue, growth retardation, loss of weight, irritability, lowered immune response, poor healing, and anemia. Pregnant women must be extra careful to avoid this deficiency, since it will not only affect their health but that of their unborn baby. A protein deficiency can promote a miscarriage, premature delivery, or toxemia. Its effects on the baby's development may set the stage for chronic diseases later in life.

The amino acids in grains are high quality and will maintain life and growth, but when supplemented with foods containing other amino acids, they may yield even higher quality protein in greater quantities. For example, wheat is a fairly good protein. It can maintain life, and millions of poor people have subsisted on bread or cereal alone for long periods of time. However, wheat alone cannot promote optimal growth, and even adults who restrict their protein to one or two food groups or types of foods (a mono-diet) run the very real risk of lowering their body's immune response. Remember, proteins also are needed for the body's natural disease fighters—the antibodies that combat infections. The poor quality of the hair and skin of those on mono-diets reflects their nutritional deficiencies. Their bodies function much as cars do that run on four cylinders when they were built for six or eight.

On the other hand, Americans have been led to think of meat, eggs, fish, and milk as the only real suppliers of protein. We have been led to believe that any meat is a good protein source. Wrong! Cured ham has only 16 percent protein; hot dogs, only 7 percent, less than dried skim milk, which has over 34 percent, or sunflower seeds with 27 percent; lentils have more than 23 percent protein. And while all we need to satisfy our protein needs is a 8 ounces of complete high-quality protein a day, we are getting far more than that.

It is true that incomplete proteins alone do not provide an adequate diet. But one can create complete, or high-quality, proteins by combining foods so that those that are low in some amino acids are eaten together with ones that are high in those same acids. These complementary proteins—all from plant sources—are in this way completed and so can supply protein needs quite nicely. You just have to know how.

Soybeans, for example, are low in the amino acid tryptophan, but high in lysine. To enhance their biological values to you, combine them with complementary proteins like nuts, grains, and seeds, which are low in lysine but high in tryptophan. In countless combinations, they can make satisfying, delicious dishes.

Tofu, for example, made by curdling soybean milk and packing the solids in layers of cloth, has a protein value—in terms of completeness, digestibility and other factors—only slightly less than animal flesh. It can be made even higher in quality by combining it with grains such as brown rice. Soybean sprouts and soy flour can also be used in cooking to enhance the complementary values of other foods.

Other legumes, like chick-peas, lentils, and various kinds of beans, are low in certain amino acids, but high in others. They also can be combined with grains, nuts, and seeds to form complementary proteins of high nutritional value. Consider, after all, how the rest of the world, which has not had the luxury of high meat diets, subsists. Central American and Caribbean nations use beans and rice as staples. Middle Eastern countries combine sesame paste with chick-peas, while Italians mix lentils, chick-peas, and other beans with pasta.

Grains and cereals make ideal complements to legumes because they are generally high in tryptophan and low in isoleucine and lysine. Grains and cereals supply half the world's protein and are great sources of fiber, too. They do not need to be complemented with meat products to raise the protein values. The myth has been that cereals, grains, and seeds are incomplete, poor sources of protein even when combined. This is false. When you combine grains, seeds, and legumes, you can easily exceed animal protein quality. Consider breakfast cereals with soy milk, macaroni and cheese, or tofu eggs—or real eggs if you prefer—served with whole grain breads. These sorts of combinations work well because they complement each other.

Why bother switching from what is easy, the protein found in animal products, to what may take some slight effort or change of habit, creating complementary proteins? Simply because health disadvantages of meats and other animal products should outweigh any slight discomfort in seeking new or improved sources of protein. And because our typical diet is based on an unhealthy protein excess.

TOO MUCH PROTEIN Researchers now agree that American meat eaters and vegetarians alike are generally getting more protein than they need. A study done by the United States Department of Agriculture (USDA) found that the average consumer of animal products gets over 165 percent of their Recommended Daily Allowance for protein. Children fed by their overcautious—and sometimes protein-fanatical—parents, get a whopping 209 percent. Surprisingly, vegetarians get only 15 percent less protein than their nonvegetarian counterparts, still 50 percent more than the Recommended Daily Allowance. Children had identical results in both categories. And in the two groups, women over age 65 consumed the least amount, yet still more than the recommended allotments.

Studies have concluded that vegans (who eat no animal products) and lacto-ovo vegetarians (who include dairy foods and eggs in their diet) both received protein in excess of the established requirements. The plant-eating vegan men ate an average of 128 percent of their protein requirements and the women 111 percent; the egg- and dairy-eating, lacto-ovo vegetarians all ate 150 percent; and the nonvegetarian men ate 192 percent. The nonvegetarian women consumed slightly less than 171 percent of their daily protein requirements. It is not difficult to obtain your protein. One researcher at Harvard, whose studies showed that only 1 ounce, or 30 grams, of protein met daily amino acid requirements, has stated that "it is most unlikely that protein deficiencies will develop in unhealthy adults on a diet in which cereals and vegetables supply adequate calories."

When it comes to certain nutrients, the more the merrier. For example, research indicates that water-soluble vitamin C helps fortify our immune system, and in high doses it may even prevent or reverse certain forms of cancer. In the case of protein, however, more does not mean better. Depending on your age, sex, and the number of calories you require, the total amount of protein needed will average between 30 and 40 grams a day.

In the short run, your body can cope with an excess of protein by burning it for energy. This may be inefficient, since protein takes more energy than carbohydrates or fat to metabolize, but it is not harmful. However, over the long run, too much protein can hurt. Ammonium is released when protein is burned in the cells. The ammonium is turned into urea and excreted through the kidneys. Along with the excess of sodium that generally characterizes the animal-protein diet, this stepped-up excretion process taxes the kidneys. Too much animal protein can also lead to localized edema and generalized dehydration, as people on high-protein diets require more water than others. To process a high-protein diet the body may require up to four times as much water as for a high-carbohydrate diet.

There are numerous other side effects of eating too much protein. Too much protein causes you to lose calcium through the urine, sometimes resulting in a deficiency in that important mineral. High-protein intake has even been linked to osteoporosis, a degenerative disease that causes the demineralization and loss of calcium from our bones by increasing urinary excretion of calcium. Older women suffer most from this condition.

High-protein diets can be dangerous. For example, eight ounces of beef supplies more than 500 calories, while it is only 22 percent protein. But it also contains lots of fat and water. High-protein diets provide too much saturated fats, cholesterol, and sodium, all of which are implicated in heart diseases.

If you eat more protein than you need, your body will have to dispose of extra urea, the nitrogen-containing waste product of protein metabolism. Urea is formed in the liver and excreted through the kidneys. This extra work for your liver and kidneys can be stressful, can make you tired, or cause other problems if you don't drink lots of extra water to flush out the kidneys.

Older people and infants are especially vulnerable if they have to use too much water to flush out this excess urea. They can become dangerously dehydrated. Infants are particularly at risk for such conditions. Protein deficiency is very uncommon in the United States. If anything, as we've said before, we eat too much protein compared to our other food nutrients.

Statistics show that on average, individuals in the United States annually eat approximately 200 pounds of red meat, 50 pounds of chicken and turkey, 10 pounds of assorted fish, 300 eggs, and 250 pounds of various dairy products.

In this country animal sources of protein often contain large amounts of synthetic hormones, saturated fats, antibiotics, pesticide residues, nitrates, and a host of other potentially harmful ingredients. Although we've heard warnings about the nasty ingredients in those plump "butterball" turkeys, about the carcinogenic (or cancer-causing) effects of charcoal broiling or frying fatty beef, the residues in milk, and the mercury and toxic wastes in fish, we're still buying them.

Animal foods are much higher in saturated fats and cholesterol than vegetable protein foods. Especially when combined with the refined carbohydrates of the typical American diet, animal foods have been implicated in increasing our risk of heart disease and arteriosclerosis.

Studies indicate that animal sources contribute to arteriosclerosis much more than vegetable sources. The incidence of arteriosclerosis is substantially higher in those getting their protein from animals than with vegetarians whose protein comes primarily from plant sources.

Preparing Protein Foods

Protein digestion is improved by correct cooking practices. Moderate heating of most protein foods increases their digestibility, particularly in the case of beans, grains, and meat. Beans and other legumes contain several toxins (such as trypsin inhibitors) that can inhibit digestion, but that become harmless when they are cooked or sprouted.

Legumes should never be eaten raw: many contain strong toxins that must be neutralized by heat. All grains and some legumes contain phytic acid in their outer husks. In the intestines, these can form phytates that bind with zinc, calcium, and other minerals and can cause deficiencies in these minerals. Thus, grains should be sprouted, baked with yeast (unleavened breads contain more phytates than leavened), or cooked thoroughly, and vegetarians should supplement their diets with zinc and calcium, or foods containing them. Zinc is present in seafood, peas, corn, egg yolk, carrots, and yeast.

It is also very important to cook meat slowly and thoroughly, because of the microorganisms it contains. Pork harbors a parasite that can cause trichinosis if it is not thoroughly cooked. Other meats should be broiled or roasted. Excessive heating of any protein, whether of animal or plant origin, may cause what are known as cross-linkages (the same mechanisms that cause your hair to stay curled after a permanent wave). Cross-linkages make it difficult for protein-digesting enzymes to break protein down into simple amino acids so they can be absorbed. Therefore, it is best to stay away from deep-fried or overdone protein foods. Milk and milk products are especially sensitive to heat, and should not be heated above the boiling point.

If you have trouble digesting milk, you might try yogurt, buttermilk, or other cultured milk products. These contain live, healthy microorganisms that "predigest" lactose, the sugar in milk that many people cannot tolerate, changing it to more easily absorbed lactic acid.

On the average, about 90 to 93 percent of the amino acids in the foods you eat are absorbed after digestion commences.

Sprinkle brewer's yeast (if you are not allergic to it) on your cereal or blend it with milk, combine tofu with algae in salads, add wheat germ to lentil burgers, and spread peanut butter on whole wheat bread to increase the usability of the protein in these excellent sources.

Protein and Dieting

It is estimated that nearly 80 million Americans in any given year are following some dietary program to lose weight. Regrettably, many will be going on one version or another of a high-protein, low-carbohydrate diet, with the misconception that protein is low in calories. In fact, the protein foods, such as beef or pork, recommended on most of these diets, are very high in calories.

One gram of protein yields 4 calories. Filet mignon, for example, is nearly 40 to 50 percent fat; a single 10 ounce portion can contain up to 1,400 calories. But a certain nutritional sleight of hand makes these diets work for some people. Since meats require six to eight hours to digest, you will probably not be very hungry during digestion. To really control overeating, exercise remains more important than limiting calorie intake, as exercise increases your metabolic efficiency.

Many diet doctors claim high-protein diets melt away fat. When we want to lose weight, they say, we should limit our diets to beef, hard-boiled eggs, chicken, and cottage cheese. But these foods contain substantial amounts of saturated fats and lack carbohydrates. Such low-carbohydrate, high-protein diets create an abnormal biochemical state within the body, resulting in weight loss.

But it is not a healthy weight loss. In effect, these diets prevent proteins from being stored as fat, leading to a buildup of high-calorie compounds called ketones in the bloodstream; this is known as ketosis. Many dieters experience anorexia due to the toxic effects of ketones, eliminating large amounts of water and salt, which contributes to weight reduction. Under normal conditions, our bodies would not excrete this unburned high energy compound. Ketosis, therefore, can lead to dehydration, burning or wasting essential body proteins, kidney infection, kidney stones, renal damage, and in several cases, it has lead to coma and death. These more dangerous conditions usually occur only during starvation or as a metabolic side effect of diabetes.

So, before embarking on the new monthly best-seller's advice, consider the potential long-term health hazards. It is not uncommon for participants in fad diets to experience bleeding gums, depression, lowered resistance to infection, fatigue, weakness, irritability, and dizziness. A high-protein diet has been shown to encourage the onset of degenerative diseases such as arteriosclerosis (hardening of the arteries). Excesses of the amino acid methionine can break down into the nonessential amino acid homocysteine, which can irritate the walls of the arteries, generating fat deposits in these vessels. And if we omit foods with carbohydrates or with fiber, like fruits, grains, and vegetables, we may be inducing vitamin and mineral deficiencies and hurting our digestive system.

Protein and Athletics

One of the most enduring myths about protein is its connection with athletic prowess. Despite scientific evidence to the contrary, many athletes and trainers alike still equate protein with strength. This false notion is based upon the premise that protein, especially animal protein, is turned into muscle when ingested. But what is really needed during a strenuous workout or competition is a quality source of energy. For this, protein is actually a less efficient source than complex carbohydrates, since carbohydrates have more deliverable calories.

Depending on the athletic training schedule a person follows, some extra protein may be advisable. This can amount to about 10 to 30 more grams of high-quality protein daily, which will be used to replace the nitrogen lost by perspiration and to provide the extra protein needed during periods of accelerated muscle growth. However, after the training period, the athlete only needs more calories than the average person, not more protein. Such misconceptions get many a hungry athlete into trouble each year.

Many trainers are well aware of the scientific void behind the "steak and egg" fortification diets, yet they continue high-protein diets because their athletes believe in them, a tradition that has a strong psychological hold and may, in fact, have an effect on their performance.

Yet these athletes are hurting themselves in many ways. As we work, play, or sleep, our systems are maintaining a biochemical balance of amino acids. If we make a habit of consuming more than we need, our bodies may start abnormally increasing the rate of amino acid replacement in our cells. This rapid turnover of cells is believed to accelerate the aging process. A high-protein diet, therefore, may be counterproductive to longevity. Athletes on high-protein diets also run the risk of dehydration. Protein does not give us that extra edge. Complex carbohydrates, if anything, may.

5

Vitamins

Vitamins are organic compounds necessary for life. They have no caloric value, but are important parts of enzymes, which help our bodies use food to supply energy. They also help regulate metabolism, assist in forming bones and tissue, and build major body structures.

There are two categories of vitamins, the oil-soluble and the water soluble. Oil-soluble vitamins (A, D, E, and K) require oil to be absorbed and are stored in the body. When too much of an oil-soluble vitamin builds up in your tissues, it can be dangerous. The water-soluble vitamins (B complex, C, and the bioflavonoids) are not stored by the body and need to be replenished daily.

Vitamin A

Vitamin A, an oil-soluble vitamin, is necessary for growth and repair of your body's tissue. It is essential in the maintenance of your body's immune response, which helps the body fight infections. It helps maintain healthy skin and protects the mucous membranes of the lungs, throat, mouth, and nose. It also helps the body secrete the gastric juices necessary for protein digestion, and it protects the linings of the digestive tract, kidneys, and bladder. Vitamin A is essential in the formation of blood, strong bones, and teeth and in the maintenance of good eyesight.

While abundant in carrots, especially in the form of fresh carrot juice, vitamin A is present in even higher concentrations in such green leafy vegetables as beet greens, spinach, and broccoli. Yellow or orange vegetables are also good sources. Eggs contain vitamin A, as do whole milk and milk products. And while animal livers are concentrated sources of vitamin A, livers also are waste-filtering organs, so one most take care when obtaining nutrients from them. Any hormone or chemical to which the animal was exposed will be concentrated in the liver. It is therefore a problematical food to eat.

One of the first symptoms of vitamin A deficiency is night blindness, and the inability of the eyes to adjust to darkness. Other signs include fatigue, unhealthy skin, loss of appetite, loss of sense of smell, and diarrhea. The recommended daily intake of vitamin A, as established by the National Research Council, is 5,000 IU for adults. It is not difficult to obtain this amount from the foods mentioned above in moderate quantities. During times of disease, trauma, pregnancy, or lactation, supplements may be advisable, but should be administered under a physician's or nutritionist's direction, since megadoses of vitamin A can be harmful.

The B Vitamin Complex

This family of water-soluble vitamins works together to unlock the nutrients in fats, carbohydrates, and protein, making them available as energy. When each component of the B vitamin group is present in the proper ratio, the entire complex will work harmoniously in every cell of the body. B vitamins are found in nutritional yeast, seed germs, eggs, liver, meats, and vegetables. Whenever muscular work increases, when you run or participate in other endurance sports, the need for B vitamin complex increases.

VITAMIN B$_1$ (THIAMINE) Vitamin B$_1$ is essential to normal metabolism and normal nerve function. It converts carbohydrates into glucose, which is the sole source of energy for the brain and nervous system. B$_1$ helps your heart by keeping it firm and resilient. It is found in a variety of foods, including whole grains, legumes, poultry, and fish.

A deficiency of vitamin B$_1$ may result in the degeneration of the insulating protective sheath (myelin) that covers certain nerve fibers. Your nerves can become hypersensitive, causing irritability, sluggishness, forgetfulness, and apathy. If such nerve destruction continues, nerves in the legs may become weakened, and pain may develop in the legs and feet. Paralysis may result. A deficiency may also result in constipation, indigestion, anorexia, swelling, and heart trouble caused by increased blood circulation.

Adult males need a daily minimum of 1.4 mg of vitamin B$_1$, and adult females need at least 1.0 mg. If you drink tea or coffee, perspire a great deal, or if you are under heavy stress, are taking antibiotics, or have a fever, your intake of vitamin B$_1$ should increase. Some nutritionists suggest that athletes should increase their intake to between 10 and 20 mg daily. Such quantities are not easily obtained from food alone. Therefore, a low potency, all-natural vitamin may be good insurance.

VITAMIN B$_2$ (RIBOFLAVIN) Vitamin B$_2$ helps promote proper growth and repair of tissues, and enhances a cell's ability to exchange gases such as oxygen and carbon dioxide in the blood. It helps release energy from the foods you eat, and it also is essential for good digestion, steady nerves, assimilation of iron, and normal vision. It is vital to the health of your entire glandular system, most particularly those involved in stress control, the adrenal glands.

Dairy products, meat, poultry, fish, nutritional yeast, whole grains, leafy green vegetables, and the nutrient-rich soybean can provide ample supplies of vitamin B$_2$.

Lack of vitamin B$_2$ is one deficiency that can be seen readily. If your tongue is purplish red, inflamed, or shiny, you may need more B$_2$. Other symptoms are cracking at the corners of the lips; greasy skin; vision problems such as hypersensitivity to light, itchiness, bloodshot eyes, or blurred sight; headaches; depression; insomnia; or loss of mental alertness. A minimum of 1.6 mg of vitamin B$_2$ daily for adult males and 1.2 mg daily for females is recommended. Two servings of most grains will satisfy this requirement without difficulty.

VITAMIN B$_3$ (NIACIN) Vitamin B$_3$ is essential to every cell in the body. It is the fundamental material of two enzyme systems and helps transform sugar and fat into energy.

Many vital functions in our body's food processing plant would stop without an adequate supply of vitamin B$_3$. Low levels of this vitamin have been linked to mental illness and pellagra, a disease that produces disorders of the skin and intestinal tract.

You can get a reasonable amount of vitamin B$_3$ from green leafy vegetables, wheat germ, brewer's yeast, beans, peas, dried figs, prunes, and dates. Organ meats, salmon, and tuna are also plentiful sources. Adult males need a minimum of 18 mg of vitamin B$_3$ daily, and adult females need 13 mg daily. Studies have shown that excessive amounts of B$_3$ can cause glycogen (a starch that helps the body utilize the energy of sugars like glucose) to be consumed hyperactively by the muscles, resulting in the early onset of fatigue. Again, a low-potency vitamin is a worthwhile investment to be sure you are getting sufficient amounts of niacin.

VITAMIN B$_5$ (PANTOTHENIC ACID) Vitamin B$_5$ also works in all our cells. It converts carbohydrates, fats, and protein to energy, acts as an antistress agent, and manufactures antibodies that fight germs in the blood. B$_5$ is found in many foods including eggs, peanuts, whole grains, beans, and organ meats.

The signs of deficiency include high susceptibility to illness and infection; digestive malfunctions such as abdominal pains and vomiting; muscular and nerve disturbances like leg cramps; insomnia; and mental depression. Although the requirement for pantothenic acid is not yet known, 5 to 10 mg daily for adults is suggested. A low-potency vitamin supplement is suggested.

VITAMIN B$_6$ (PYRIDOXINE) Vitamin B$_6$ nourishes the central nervous system, controls sodium/potassium levels in the blood, and assists in the production of red blood cells and hemoglobin. It helps protect against infection, and assists in manufacturing DNA and RNA, the acids that contain the genetic code for cell growth, repair, and multiplication. It is particularly valuable for those involved in endurance sports.

The best sources of B$_6$ are brewer's yeast, brown rice, bananas, and pears. It is also found in beef, pork liver, and fish such as salmon and herring. Deficiency signs are similar to those of vitamin B$_2$: irritability, nervousness, weakness, dermatitis and other skin changes, and insomnia. The official recommended daily amount for adults is 2 mg of vitamin B$_6$ per 100 grams of protein consumed. This amount is easily obtained from the food sources listed above. I would recommend 50 mg daily.

VITAMIN B$_{12}$ (CYANOCOBALAMIN) Vitamin B$_{12}$ is the most complex of the B vitamins. Every cell in the body depends upon it to function properly. It is especially vital to the cells in your bone marrow, gastrointestinal tract, and nervous system. It helps prevent fatty deposits from accumulating in your liver, and helps maintain normal weight. All B$_{12}$ in its natural state is manufactured by microorganisms, so it is not normally found in fruits and vegetables. Fermented soybean products such as tempeh, nonfat dry milk, poultry, and meat all contain B$_{12}$.

Common symptoms of B$_{12}$ deficiency are motor and mental abnormalities, rapid heartbeat or cardiac pain, facial swelling, jaundice, weakness and fatigue, loss of hair or weight, depression, and impaired memory. Adults need a daily minimum of 30 mcg of vitamin B$_{12}$. If you are a vegetarian, you should include a low-potency vitamin supplement with your diet. I would recommend 500 mcg daily.

FOLIC ACID Folic acid works mostly in the brain and nervous system. It is a vital component of spinal and extracellular fluid, is necessary for the manufacture of DNA and RNA, and helps convert amino acids.

Brewer's yeast, dark green leafy vegetables, wheat germ, oysters, salmon, and chicken all contain folic acid.

Your body needs comparatively minuscule amounts of folic acid; 400 mcg daily are recommended. This is easily obtained from the food sources listed above. If you are pregnant, elderly, or suffer from any nervous disorder, you may benefit from additional amounts.

PARA-AMINOBENZOIC ACID (PABA) Para-aminobenzoic acid is a component of folic acid, and acts as a coenzyme in the body's metabolism of proteins. It helps manufacture healthy blood cells and can help heal skin disorders. In addition, it protects your skin against sunburn by absorbing the portions of those ultraviolet rays of the sun known to cause burns and even skin cancer.

Eggs, brewer's yeast, molasses, wheat germ, and whole grains are good sources of PABA. Signs of deficiency include digestive trouble, nervous tension, emotional instability, and blotchy skin. No official daily requirements have been established for PABA. My recommended daily intake would be 400–600 IU.

CHOLINE Choline is present in all your cellular membranes and works to remove fat. It also helps regulate your cholesterol levels and is vital to the liver's functions. It aids in building and maintaining a healthy nervous system.

If choline is not present in your system, your liver is unable to process any sort of fat. Fatty deposits in the liver interfere with its normal filtering function. A deficiency can also lead to muscle weakness and excessive muscle scarring. Choline is found in a variety of foods, including wheat germ and bran, beans, egg yolks, brewer's yeast, whole grains, nuts, lecithin, meat, and fish.

Your body also produces its own supply of choline, using protein and other B vitamins. Daily requirements are not yet known, but the average daily intake has been estimated to be between 500 and 900 mg. In addition to the foods listed above, two tablespoons of lecithin granules may be taken as a supplement to help meet these requirements. My recommended daily intake would be 500 mg.

INOSITOL Inositol carries the responsibility for breaking down fats, and thus plays an important role in preventing cholesterol buildup and normalizing fat metabolism. Studies indicate that inositol has an anxiety-reducing effect similar to some tranquilizers.

A good supply of inositol can be found in wheat germ, brewer's yeast, whole grains, oranges, nuts, and molasses. Keeping your intestinal tract healthy may be the best way to make sure you are getting enough inositol. The bacteria or intestinal flora found there are indispensable for making inositol in the body. If you suffer from insomnia, hair loss, high cholesterol levels, or cirrhosis of the liver, you may have a deficiency of inositol. A minimum daily requirement for inositol has not yet been established. I recommend 500 mg daily

BIOTIN Biotin helps keep your hair, skin, bone marrow, and glands healthy and growing. It helps produce, and then change into energy, fatty acids, carbohydrates, and amino acids. It is vital to the production of glycogen. Your body manufactures biotin in the intestinal tract. You can also get it from eggs, cheese, nuts, and many other common foods.

Deficiencies are rare. However, when they occur, symptoms include fatigue, depression, skin disorders, slow healing of wounds, muscular pain, anorexia, sensitivity to cold temperatures, and elevated blood-cholesterol levels. Between 150 and 300 mcg of biotin will meet your body's daily needs. This is best obtained from your low-potency vitamin supplement.

Vitamin C

Vitamin C strengthens the immune system, keeps cholesterol levels down, combats stress, promotes fertility, protects against cardiovascular disease and various forms of cancer, maintains mental health, and ultimately may prolong life. Its presence is necessary to build collagen, the "cement" that holds together the connective tissue throughout the body. Athletes, for example, need more vitamin C for collagen synthesis and tissue repair. Vitamin C combats toxic substances in our food, air, and water, and is a natural laxative.

Whole oranges and other citrus fruits, sprouts, berries, tomatoes, sweet potatoes, and green leafy vegetables are important sources of vitamin C. Symptoms of vitamin C deficiency include bleeding gums, a tendency to bruise easily, shortness of breath, impaired digestion, nosebleeds, swollen or painful joints, anemia, lowered resistance to infection, and slow healing of fractures and wounds.

The daily recommended allowance of vitamin C is 45 mg, according to the Food and Nutrition Board. This amount is easily obtained from the fresh fruits and vegetables in your diet, including oranges, sweet peppers, and potatoes. Some nutritionists believe that much higher doses (up to 10 grams daily) can help heal serious illnesses and reduce the risk of cancer (see "The Megadose Controversy" below). Hence, supplements may be beneficial. Those with elevated needs for vitamin C are the elderly, dieters, smokers, heavy drinkers, users of certain medications including oral contraceptives, pregnant and nursing women, and those under any type of stress.

Vitamin D

Vitamin D helps your body utilize calcium and phosphorus to help form strong bones, teeth and healthy skin. Its action also is vital to your nervous system and kidneys.

A prime source of vitamin D is sunshine, but it may be necessary to get this vitamin from food sources and supplements if sunlight is inaccessible, or if sunshine is to be avoided for other health reasons. Food sources include fortified milk and butter, egg yolks, fish liver oils, and seafood such as sardines, salmon, tuna, and herring.

The symptoms of deficiency include brittle and fragile bones, pale skin, some forms of arthritis, insomnia, sensitivity to pain, irregular heartbeat, soft bones and teeth, and injuries that take an abnormally long time to heal. At least 400 IU of vitamin D are needed daily. Greater amounts may be necessary to build strong resistance against bone disease. However, megadoses of this oil-soluble vitamin are not recommended. One-half hour of good sunlight per day is the best supplement.

Vitamin E

Vitamin E is basically an antioxidant; that is, it protects your fatty acids from destruction and maintains the health and integrity of every cell. It is especially important for promoting the health of your muscles, cells, blood, and skin. It is a primary defense against respiratory infection and disease. Vitamin E also is an excellent first aid tonic for burns. It is believed that vitamin E's antioxidant effects make available larger amounts of fats for metabolism, providing the body with extra energy for muscle contractions, and so is useful in exercise as well.

Ideal sources of vitamin E are wheat germ and wheat germ oil. Leafy plant foods eaten with cold-pressed oils, whole grains, seeds, nuts, and fertile eggs are also good sources. Some common symptoms of low vitamin E levels are swelling of the face, ankles, or legs, poor skin condition, muscle cramps, abnormal heartbeat, and respiratory difficulties.

Nutritionists and doctors recommend a daily dosage for adults of between 30 and 400 IU, unless a condition requiring higher amounts is present. It's best to take supplements.

Vitamin K

Vitamin K is an oil-soluble substance that helps your blood clot properly, and aids in proper bone development and function.

The microorganisms and bacteria that naturally live in your large intestine produce vitamin K. You can help them work by eating yogurt and other fermented dairy and soy products. Other good sources include green leaves of plants like kale and spinach, cauliflower, broccoli, and cabbage. A tendency to bruise easily is a symptom of vitamin K deficiency. It can be the symptom of other nutritional deficiencies as well. Little is known about the precise daily minimum need for vitamin K, and supplements are not available over the counter.

Bioflavonoids

Bioflavonoids are a group of water-soluble substances that ensure the strength and proper function of your capillaries. Along with vitamin C, with which they are almost always found in food, the bioflavonoids help manufacture collagen. They also protect your cells against attack and invasion by viruses and bacteria.

Excellent sources of bioflavonoids are grapes, rose hips, prunes, oranges, lemon juice, cherries, black currants, plums, parsley, cabbage, apricots, peppers, papaya, cantaloupe, tomatoes, broccoli, and blackberries. The white pulp of the inside of a grapefruit is also a rich source.

Symptoms of bioflavonoid deficiency include bleeding gums and easily bruised skin. There is no established minimum daily requirement for bioflavonoids, but most nutritionists agree that 900 mg may be an optimum amount. This amount is obtainable from the foods listed above.

Vitamin Supplements

Vitamin supplements may be necessary. The world has changed since our ancestors lived on diets without one-a-day vitamins with iron, special mixtures of stress vitamins, or supplemental vitamins for infants or children. For a variety of reasons, individuals often overlook foods that contain essential vitamins or nutrients. They may just be eating less regularly because of the hectic pace of their lives, they may be unable to eat certain foods for health reasons, or they may be dieting. For many of these people, supplements in controlled, recommended doses, may help to balance one's diet.

Others who may benefit from vitamin supplements include:

❤ Infants—particularly those who are not breast-fed and therefore may be getting uncertain amounts of various vitamins and minerals.

❤ Pregnant or lactating women—pregnant women often have reduced levels of a number of vitamins, even though their caloric intake is usually greater than normal, and therefore, they are getting more foods with more vitamins in them. Vitamin supplements are often prescribed. Iron, as a mineral supplement, is almost always prescribed as well.

❤ Women on oral contraceptives—studies indicate that birth control pills cause shortages of a number of water-soluble vitamins, including thiamin, riboflavin, B_6, B_{12}, folic acid, and vitamin C. Diet changes may not be sufficient and supplements are often suggested.

❤ The elderly—older people tend to absorb less vitamin C and less of the B vitamins than the rest of the population. Also, many older people eat a limited choice of foods. Multivitamin supplements may be in order.

❤ Those with other special problems—people who have had surgery need more vitamin C. Those with certain chronic infections or cancers require more folic acid. Alcoholics require a full range of vitamin supplements because drinking results in poor absorption of all vitamins from foods. Heavy smokers need more vitamin C to repair cells damaged by the toxins in cigarette smoke and tars.

The Megadose Controversy

Dr. Linus Pauling, the Nobel Prize winner, engaged in an ongoing controversy in the media and the scientific press, and with other medical and biochemical researchers, about the possible values of megadoses of vitamin C to help fight the common cold and for use in a number of other health situations. While conflicting research studies support both positions, it would seem logical that Dr. Pauling hit on something substantial. Vitamin C is known to increase the body's ability to ward off infection, to repair tissue damage, and in general to help the body's natural immune system to function properly.

Whether vitamin C is most effective in fighting the common cold or other more serious disorders is debatable. What is clear is that vitamin C plays a role in helping the body fend off diseases—common colds and others.

Vitamin C in large doses seems to have some efficacy in helping treat cancer of the colon, and while not curing the disease, it might slow its development. Research is still minimal in this area.

However, vitamins alone do not work miracles. Megadoses of vitamins should not be used in place of a balanced diet, or to replace days, weeks, or more of neglect of important natural vitamin sources in natural foods. It is important to remember that megadoses as well as vitamin supplements also cannot and should not replace a healthful regular regimen of exercise. Some research does indicate that megadoses of specific vitamins or nutrients can aid in certain specific conditions.

It is possible, for example, that depression can be relieved by taking tryptophan (one of the eight essential amino acids) in elevated doses. However, more than one gram daily, should not be exceeded. Vitamin B_6 may also be useful in larger doses to help women taking the Pill fight depression, a possible side effect, and to help women relieve pre-menstrual syndrome (PMS) effects.

Megadoses of vitamin A for both acne and for deafness has received some experimental attention in recent years. However, large doses of vitamin A can be toxic to the system. Also women who are trying to conceive, or those already pregnant, should avoid taking any excessive doses of vitamin A.

All in all, the case for megadoses of vitamins is valid, however there are a few exceptions. Megadoses of vitamins A or D, for example, can be toxic to the body under certain circumstances. As for vitamin C, researchers are still studying the effects of megadoses and the verdict is not yet in. However, there are indications that substantial healthful effects can sometimes be realized.

6

Minerals

Minerals serve as building materials for bones, teeth, tissue, muscle, blood, and nerve cells. They help spur many biological reactions in the body and maintain the body's fragile balance of fluids.

You need minute amounts of minerals. They constitute only 4 or 5 percent of your total body weight. Although we will examine them individually here, understand that the actions of minerals within your body are interrelated. No one mineral can function in isolation.

Calcium

Calcium is the body's chief mineral. It is the principal component of your bones and teeth, and a vital component of the liquid that bathes your cells. Calcium is one of the raw materials used in the bloodstream. Emotionally, you need it to help cope with stress. An active ingredient of some enzymes, calcium is also an enzyme stimulator, that is, it must be supplied before you can store sugar (glucose) as glycogen in your muscles. Along with several other minerals, calcium also helps maintain the delicate acid/alkaline balance in your blood, protecting it against overacidity.

Without a steady supply of calcium, your bones and teeth would not remain hard and durable. Your brain would not function properly, nor would your muscles be able to store energy. Without enough calcium in your diet, your digestive, circulatory, and immune systems would suffer. Adequate amounts are necessary to avoid the many complications that can come from calcium deposits, which are caused by calcium that has been removed from the body's reserves and lodges in soft tissue. Warnings of calcium deficiency include nervousness, depression, headaches, and insomnia.

Even though milk is one of the best sources of calcium, as are other, more easily absorbed dairy products such as buttermilk, yogurt, acidophilus milk (a healthful bacteria-rich fermented milk product), and kefir (also a milk product), I would suggest not trying to obtain your calcium from dairy. Most cheeses are good sources. Oatmeal, collard greens, and tempeh are also rich in calcium. Sesame seeds, torula yeast, carob flour, and sea vegetables all contain calcium in smaller quantities.

However, the body will not always properly absorb or utilize calcium. For example, if there aren't enough complete proteins in your diet, the necessary substances that allow calcium to be absorbed by your bones won't be available. Also, protein is needed for your body to make collagen. If you eat high-protein foods, you will absorb 15 to 20 percent of the calcium in your food, as opposed to 5 percent if you don't. However, an excessively high protein diet will cause you to lose calcium through the urine. Sugar in the diet (except for lactose or milk sugar) will also antagonize the absorption of calcium.

For a healthy adult, 800 to 1,200 mg of calcium daily is sufficient. This is usually obtainable from foods in the diet such as those listed above. For women who are pregnant or breast-feeding, 1,200 mg is required. As women age, calcium supplements, ideally in forms like amino acid chelate, might be necessary to fight the onset or severity of osteoporosis.

Chromium

Chromium is important to your heart, liver, brain, and glucose metabolism system. It is vital to the production of protein and to white blood cells, where it helps fight bacteria, viruses, toxins, arthritis, cancer, and premature aging. To counteract stress, your adrenal glands must have an adequate supply of chromium.

The best food sources of chromium are whole wheat flour, brewer's yeast, nuts, black pepper, all whole grain cereals except rye and corn, fresh fruit juices, dairy products, root vegetables, legumes, leafy vegetables, and mushrooms.

Without chromium, insulin cannot transport glucose from your bloodstream to your cells, nor can your liver properly remove excess fats from your blood. A deficiency can result in rapid premature aging, since protein production will be seriously impaired. Symptoms of chromium deficiency include fatigue, dizziness, anxiety, insomnia, a craving for alcohol, blurred vision, depression, and panic.

No definitive guidelines have been established by the government on the amount of chromium necessary on a daily basis, but trace-mineral experts suggest that 200 mcg will provide an adequate daily supply. This is usually obtainable from the diet.

Iodine

Iodine is essential to the manufacture of thyroxin, the hormone that controls the speed at which your blood takes the food from your intestines to the cells, where it is used for energy. It is particularly important to your heart, your immune system, and your system of protein synthesis.

Fresh seafood is a good source of iodine, as is garlic. You can enhance the iodine content of your diet by using sea vegetables, such as hijiki, wakame, kelp, or dulse. Dried mushrooms, leafy greens, celery, tomatoes, radishes, carrots, and onions also supply iodine.

Without adequate amounts of iodine, the way your cells use energy would be seriously impaired. Proper growth in childhood could not take place, and maintenance of healthy adult tissue could not occur. An iodine deficiency can lower your resistance to infection and impair metabolism of fat in the bloodstream. Thyroid malfunctions are a direct result of iodine deficiency. Symptoms of inadequate iodine consumption include sluggishness, bad complexion, and unhealthy-looking hair, teeth, and nails. You need 150 mcg of iodine. Some nutritionists believe that 3 mg a day of this trace mineral is necessary to prevent serious thyroid disorders. Sufficient amounts of iodine are generally available in the foods we eat without supplements.

Iron

Without the oxygen-carrier iron, you could not live. The hemoglobin in your red blood cells, the myoglobin in your muscles, and the enzymes tied in with energy release, all depend on iron.

The most concentrated sources of iron are animal livers, but as we have mentioned, the liver is a waste-filtering organ, and any hormone or chemical—like pesticides or antibiotics fed to animals—to which the animal was exposed will be concentrated there. Egg yolks contain more iron than muscle meats. Other good sources include leafy green vegetables, dried beans, peaches, apricots, dates, prunes, cherries, figs, raisins, and blackstrap molasses.

A deficiency of iron can cause certain types of anemia. Deficiency symptoms include chronic fatigue, shortness of breath, headache, pale skin, and opaque or brittle nails. The daily requirements for iron are 10 mg for adult males and 18 mg for women. For pregnant women, 30–60 mg are required. Starting the day with a hot cereal on which you've sprinkled two tablespoons of rice bran, torula yeast, or pumpkin-seed meal will go a long way toward satisfying your iron needs. Daily iron supplements are also recommended.

Magnesium

Magnesium is a versatile, tireless worker in your body's protein production process. In addition, it is one of your body's most important coenzymes. It works with calcium to turn it into something the body can use. It is necessary for the production of hormones, and it works in your muscles, cells, nervous system, digestive system, reproductive system, blood, and immune system.

Leafy green vegetables are one of the best sources for magnesium. Nuts, seeds, avocados, and turnips also contain significant amounts. Whole grains, legumes, organic eggs, and raw milk are excellent sources. Many fruits and natural sweets such as carob, honey, and blackstrap molasses also contain magnesium.

Magnesium deficiency can result in lowered immunity, improper muscle function, and impaired digestion. Without adequate magnesium, your nerves can become ragged and supersensitive to pain. Your bones would be too soft to support you, and production of new protein would be impaired. Without it you would be unable to store energy, synthesize sex hormones, or prevent your blood from clotting. Signs of magnesium deficiency are an irregular heart beat, hair loss, and easily broken nails.

The recommended daily intake of magnesium is 350 mg, but 800–1,200 mg may be a more realistic figure for maintaining optimal health. Sufficient amounts of magnesium can be obtained in the diet from some of the foods listed above.

Manganese

Manganese is a trace mineral that is active in protein production and essential to the correct structure of your bones, teeth, cartilage, and tendons. Vital in the formation of new blood cells in your bone marrow, it is also necessary for transmitting nerve impulses in your brain. Manganese plays an important role in the metabolism of blood sugar and fats, and is necessary for the production of sex hormones.

Nuts, seeds, and whole grains are excellent sources of manganese. Leafy green vegetables, if grown organically in mineral-rich soil, can supply you with manganese. So can rhubarb, broccoli, carrots, potatoes, peas, and beans. Pineapples, blueberries, raisins, cloves, and ginger are also good sources.

Without manganese, a slow deterioration of muscle health—myasthenia gravis—can develop. Protein production and carbohydrate/fat metabolism would be inhibited. Manganese deficiencies can be related to blood-sugar disorders and sexual dysfunction. There is no official recommended daily requirement for manganese, but trace mineral experts suggest up to 7 mg daily. In the case of manganese, it is worthwhile to supplement your diet.

Phosphorous

Phosphorous works in your bones, teeth, collagen, nerves, muscles, metabolic and cellular systems, brain, liver, digestive and circulatory systems, and eyes. It is an important part of your genetic materials, RNA and DNA, and helps maintain your body fluids in the right balance. It is indispensable to the runner since it plays a vital role in supplying energy to muscles by burning carbohydrates.

Phosphorus is available in nearly every food you eat. Eat a lot of refined foods, though, and you are in danger of getting too much. Protein foods like meat, poultry, fish, eggs, dairy products, whole grains, nuts, and seeds supply phosphorus in abundance. Vegetables that contain phosphorus include legumes, whole grains, celery, cabbage, carrots, cauliflower, string beans, cucumber, chard, and pumpkin. Fruits also contain a healthy supply. Too little phosphorus, although rarely seen, is responsible for certain anemias. It might also affect your white blood cells, and immunity to bacteria and viruses would be hampered. The recommended daily intake of phosphorus is 800 mg for adults. Pregnant or lactating women need 1,200 mg. A well-balanced meal plan should provide you with all of this requirement.

Potassium

Potassium, in conjunction with sodium, helps form an electrical pump that speeds nutrients into every cell of your body, while speeding wastes out. It is vital to the function of all cells, helping maintain the proper acid/alkaline balance of your body fluids. Potassium is particularly vital to the workings of your digestive and endocrine systems, your muscles, brain, and nerves.

In general, vegetables, fruits, and other plant foods are far richer sources of potassium than animal foods. Leafy green vegetables are an excellent source. High potassium fruits include bananas, cantaloupes, avocados, dates, prunes, dried apricots, and raisins. Whole grains, beans, legumes, nuts, and seeds are also good sources.

If you find that injuries take a long time to heal, or your skin and other tissues seem "worn out," you may be suffering from a potassium deficiency. Lethargy and insomnia are other early signs of deficiency, along with intestinal spasms, severe constipation, swelling of tissues, thinning of hair, and malfunctioning muscles.

If you eat correctly, you needn't worry about your potassium intake, although studies show that runners can lose extraordinary amounts of potassium through sweating. You can easily consume the 500–1,000 mg needed each day to replace the amount normally lost in your urine. A variety of grains and legumes will meet this requirement easily. Runners can eat extra amounts of potassium-rich foods during times of heavy training. I suggest four medium soy pancakes or two potato fritters as a potassium-rich treat.

Those on certain medications, like diuretics to combat hypertension, also require extra amounts of potassium to replace the mineral that is lost by the diuretic's actions. However, potassium supplements should not be taken without a doctor's advice.

Selenium

Selenium's primary function in your body is as an antioxidant, protecting your cells from being destroyed. It plays a vital role in your enzyme system, and is necessary for the manufacture of prostaglandins, which control blood pressure and clotting. Selenium is needed to protect your eyes against cataracts, contributes to protein production, and protects the artery walls from plaque.

Animal foods tend to have more selenium than plants. Whole grains, mushrooms, asparagus, broccoli, onions, and tomatoes are the best vegetable sources. Eggs are excellent sources of selenium; they also contain sulphur, which helps your body absorb and utilize selenium.

Signs of selenium deficiency include lack of energy, accelerated angina, and the development of degenerative diseases. Deficiencies have been implicated in blood sugar disorders, liver necrosis, arthritis, anemia, heavy metal poisoning, muscular dystrophy, and cancer. There are no official recommended daily amounts for selenium, but the Food and Nutrition Board suggests an intake of 150 mcg daily. It is best to supplement with a 50 mcg vitamin and mineral tablet.

Sodium (Salt)

Sodium, along with potassium, pumps nutrients into cells and waste products out. It also regulates fluid pressure in the cells, thus affecting your blood pressure. With other nutrients, it helps control the acid/alkaline blood levels in the body. Sodium is vital to the ability of nerves to transmit impulses to muscles and to the muscles' ability to contract. It also helps pump glucose into the bloodstream, produces hydrochloric acid for digestion, and keeps calcium suspended in the bloodstream ready for use. Sodium is available in almost every food we eat, including water. Refined foods contain enormous quantities of sodium.

Sodium deficiency is uncommon. But, when it occurs, it is usually caused by stressful situations such as exposure to toxic chemicals, infections, digestive difficulties, allergies, and injuries. Symptoms of deficiency include wrinkles, sunken eyes, flatulence, diarrhea, nausea, vomiting, confusion, fatigue, low blood pressure, irritability, difficulty in breathing, and heightened allergies.

Your body needs between 55 and 440 mg of sodium daily to perform its functions. Under normal conditions, obtaining sufficient quantities is not a problem. Many of us consume between 7,000 and 20,000 mg daily. Too much sodium, however, can result in serious health problems, including hypertension, stress, liver damage, muscle weakness, and pancreatic disease.

Zinc

Zinc plays an important role in the body's production of growth and sex hormones, and in its utilization of insulin. As a coenzyme, zinc helps start many important activities and sparks energy sources. It is an important element in the body's ability to remain in a state of balance, keeping your blood at a proper acidity, producing necessary histamines, removing excess toxic metals, and helping your kidneys maintain a healthy equilibrium of minerals. Zinc works in the protein production system, in blood cells, the circulatory system, and the nerves.

Eggs, poultry, and seafood contain sizable amounts of zinc, as do organ meats. Excellent vegetable sources include peas, soybeans, mushrooms, whole grains, most nuts, and seeds, especially pumpkin.

Lack of taste or smell is a sign of zinc deficiency. Skin problems also may indicate zinc deficiencies. Stretch marks are an indication that elastin, the fibers that make your skin springy and smooth, are not incorporating enough zinc to keep your skin healthy. Acne and psoriasis can result from zinc deficiency, as can an abnormal wearing away of tooth enamel. Other signs of zinc deficiency include opaque fingernails, brittle hair, and bleeding gums. The daily zinc requirement for adults is 20 to 25 mg. By including sesame, sunflower, and pumpkin seeds in our diet, we can obtain a good portion of this daily.

7

Water, Air, Enzymes, and Antioxidants

The environment from which we gain sustenance can also have an adverse effect on us. Consider the life-giving and life-supporting elements of the world around us. Although it comprises 50 to 70 percent of our body weight, water is too often overlooked or taken for granted when we consider amounts of water needed and proper balance of nutrients necessary for good health. Similarly, we too often pay little attention to the quality of air we breathe and the very activity of breathing itself. By not taking seriously the impact of our environment on the enzymes and antioxidants in our bodies, we place our health in danger. We must be as aware of the air we breathe and the water we drink as we are of the food we eat.

Water

You can go days without food, but only a few days without water, the sixth of the major nutrients. Of all the components necessary for life, water is second only to oxygen in importance. It is present in all tissues, including teeth, fat, bone, and muscle. It is the medium of all body fluids, such as blood, digestive juices, lymph, urine, and perspiration. It is a lubricant for the saliva, the mucous membranes, and the fluid that bathes the joints. And it regulates body temperature. Water also prevents dehydration, flushes out toxins and wastes, supplies the body with oxygen and nutrients, and aids muscle cells in producing energy.

The average body contains 40 to 50 quarts of water, with 40 percent of that water inside your cells. Lean persons have a higher percentage of body water than fat persons; men have a higher percentage than women, and children have a higher percentage than adults. Water is your life's blood. Indeed, 83 percent of your blood is water. With a loss of 5 percent of your body water, your skin shrinks and muscles become weak. The loss of less than a fifth of your body water is fatal.

How Much Water Do You Need?

Although water occurs naturally in most foods, it must be consciously included in our daily diets. Include 8 glasses, 8 to 10 ounces each, every day. To rehydrate after exercise, drink one glass of water every 20 minutes for the first hour, then one glass for several hours afterward. Your body will determine how much it needs; it will absorb water at a particular rate and eliminate whatever is excess.

Eating a high-protein diet results in the body eliminating water. If you are not a vegetarian, it's especially crucial for you to keep careful track of water consumption to replenish the water lost in the excretion of animal-protein wastes. If you are concerned or uncertain about pollutants in your tap water, buy pure spring water, not distilled water. Be sure to read the label, even on spring water jugs.

Despite popular theories and practices to the contrary, fruit juice, soda pop, and Gatorade-type drinks—ones that mix sugar and water—will not aid in athletic performance. A Rube Goldberg-type series of reactions occur instead. The sugar in these drinks triggers insulin to be released into the blood. The insulin inhibits epinephrine, which is needed to release free fatty acids, substances you will need for fuel. The insulin also lowers blood sugar levels, which causes glycogen stored in the muscles to leave the muscles and enter the blood. This reduces the store of energy you need to exercise. Drinking such sugar drinks 30 to 60 minutes before exercise, therefore, has a negative effect on athletic performance. Also, concentrations of too much sugar force the body to tap water from other cells to help dilute and digest the sugar. This activity will lead toward dehydration.

It's best to avoid beer, wine, and other alcoholic beverages, although some recent studies support extremely moderate amounts (one glass per day) for cardiovascular health. In general, though, they cause fatigue and dehydration through their diuretic actions. Avoid caffeine drinks like coffee and iced tea. They also act as diuretics, resulting in dehydration.

Drinking during meals, in a sense, can "drown" your enzymes, reducing their strength. When foods are dry, it is better to allow extra salivation prior to swallowing, to moisten them, rather than washing them down with liquids. Eating green and succulent vegetables with a meal also will help provide natural water or lubricate dry foods.

Breathing

The first and last thing we do on this planet is breathe. But too often we go through life almost ignoring this vital process. Oxygen enters the body through the food we eat and the water we drink as well as the air we breathe. Our bodies have elaborately designed mechanisms for taking in, absorbing, distributing, and utilizing this oxygen.

Disciplined breathing exercises, such as those performed in yoga, are designed to control the vital energy represented by our breath. Some people believe you can tune into the larger energies of the universe by working on proper breathing techniques. Breath and thought are integrally related: calm one and you calm the other. It is known that deep breathing can reduce stress and tension and regularize body rhythms.

It is not within the scope of this book to provide a comprehensive discussion of proper breathing—a subject worthy of several volumes. But it is important to note here that attention should and must be paid to proper breathing in everyday life, even as we eat. This is an important key to success, as we try to relieve stress and relax.

Enzymes

Enzymes are natural substances that stimulate some of the internal reactions necessary for life. Your body contains more than 700 types of enzymes, each one responsible for a different task. A shortage of even one type can dramatically affect health. Enzymes are found throughout the body, with the most vital ones in the salivary glands, pancreas, stomach walls, intestines, and liver.

Without enzymes, food could not be digested. Enzymes help transform food products into muscles, nerves, bones, and glands. They assist in storing excess nutrients in the muscles and liver for future access, help create urea to be excreted in the urine, and facilitate the departure of carbon dioxide from the lungs. Enzymes also help stop bleeding and serve to decompose poisonous hydrogen peroxide to liberate needed oxygen. They help you breathe and attack poisons in the blood.

Enzymes are abundant in fresh, raw foods. However, they cannot survive at temperatures higher than 122 degrees F, which means that they won't exist in cooked foods. The best sources of enzymes are fresh fruits and vegetables, which should be eaten in season and fresh. When cooking vegetables, use as little water as possible to conserve the enzyme content as well as the vitamin content. Cook vegetables only until tender, in a tightly covered pot. Do not soak most fresh foods; the water can destroy enzymes.

The enzyme that begins the entire digestive process is found in the saliva. Proper chewing is necessary to make that enzyme best perform its work. Food that is not chewed well enters the digestive canal only partially prepared; digestion is therefore less nutritious.

Mental strain or worry also has a deleterious effect on enzyme actions. It is better to avoid large meals during such times, since stressful situations tend to inhibit the flow of enzymes and interfere with the actions of the digestive tract.

In order to perform their life-sustaining tasks, enzymes must be continually replaced. Unnatural components of our environment, such as pollution, artificial additives in foods, and stress, all negatively affect the makeup of your cells and increase your need for health-promoting enzymes. To get enough of these fragile chemicals, it would be better to avoid processed, refined foods as much as possible, looking to natural foods for nourishment instead.

Antioxidants

Antioxidants, which oppose oxidation or the burning of substances within the body, have been identified as important factors in helping us live longer, fight heart disease and lung problems, and combat carcinogen formation. They accomplish these, in part, by battling the degenerative processes associated with free radicals.

Free radicals are substances released by your body when certain fats are broken down in specific ways. Radiation exposure—either accidental or intended—can cause the release of free radicals. They are also released by a variety of other inopportune circumstances—from the presence of chemical pollutants found in water, air, food, tobacco smoke, and in many cancer-causing agents.

Antioxidants can save us from these free radicals, trapping them and preventing the degenerative processes associated with their reactions with unsaturated fatty acids to form the molecules that ultimately cause harmful disruptions in our cells.

Free radicals also have been linked to certain symptoms of aging. It is with some degree of logic then that scientists believe antioxidants, which can slow down the destructive processes of free radicals, can also help reduce some of the effects of the aging process. Vitamin E is the most common antioxidant. It is known to have some effect, for example, on preventing or delaying the brown pigmentation of skin caused by the aging process—so-called liver spots. Vitamins A, C, and D are less powerful antioxidants, as are selenium and sulfur-containing amino acids.

Pollution can have a serious effect on a variety of body processes. Environmental pollution, for example, seems to defeat or otherwise interfere with the beneficial effects of antioxidants. In the face of such environmental obstacles, it is therefore necessary to take nutrients that will contribute to their formation.

Pollution poses a variety of challenges for those seeking healthful nutrition. Much of our fish comes from rivers, lakes, and waterways poisoned by sewage, chemicals, and a host of other pollutants. Shellfish, particularly, are prone to feed on this sewage and absorb it into their bodies. Fatty fish, as well, are more prone to absorb chemical pollutants and then pass them on to the humans who eat them.

In addition to all the obvious stresses environmental pollution causes, it also depletes our vitamin E supplies. A deficiency in vitamin E can put the urban or suburban dweller at even greater risk from pollution in the air we breathe, the water we drink, or the food we eat. Vitamin E is our major hedge against environmental stress. It helps dilute the harmful effects of drinking water that may have lead in it, an excess of minerals like sodium in it, or an otherwise unbalanced mineral content. Vitamin E as an antioxidant protects us from many types of contaminants simply by impeding the formation of compounds that lead to cellular destruction.

The urban or suburban dweller faced with these challenges should stock up on vitamin E. Wheat germ and wheat germ oil are superior sources of vitamin E. All whole grains, unrefined cereals, whole grain baked goods, seeds, nuts, bran, and organic eggs are also excellent sources. Vegetable oils like safflower oil are likely to have vitamin E if they have been refined only minimally. The best source for such scarcely refined oils—so-called cold-pressed oils—are to be found in natural foods from health food stores.

The active chemical ingredient in vitamin E is pure alphatocopherol. If you're seeking a supplement, get natural vitamin E. There is some indication that the natural form is more active and therefore more useful than the synthetic variety.

Since environmental pollution and other factors seem to have a negative effect on antioxidants, it may be necessary to supplement your intake of nutrients to help you make more antioxidants for possible use.

8

Diet and Digestion

The digestive system is composed of intricately interconnected parts which set into motion the incredibly complicated process of digestion. Every time you put food into your mouth, you unleash a nearly infinite number of clockworklike reactions and interactions. Although it is possible to track and understand this process to some extent, many aspects remain a mystery. Digestion and absorption of nutrients occur harmoniously and simultaneously.

How Foods Are Broken Down

The digestive system begins with the mouth and runs some 30 feet to the anus. It is essentially a long, hollow canal that mechanically chops, grinds, and transports food mass while chemically breaking it down into molecules fit for absorption into the blood and cells. The teeth and various internal muscular systems provide the mechanical action. The pancreas and liver are the major contributors of the digestive juices necessary for chemical processing.

All foods are broken down into four elements. Three of them—carbon, hydrogen, and oxygen—are derived from foods containing fats and carbohydrates. The fourth—nitrogen—is obtained from foods containing protein. These four units are metabolized through different body tissues and are made available for the body's maintenance and physiological functioning at the cellular level.

Chewing constitutes the first stage of digestion. The way you masticate food is critical to the sort of nutritional benefit you will receive from the food you ingest. If you do not chew slowly to break down food thoroughly, the saliva secreted in your mouth will not mix sufficiently with the food. Improper chewing also leaves food in chunks that are too large to pass easily through the esophagus and into the stomach for the next stage of digestion.

When food reaches the stomach improperly broken down, it will create an excess secretion of digestive enzymes. Extra stomach acids such as hydrochloric acid (HCl) must be produced to break down oversized food particles. This means subjecting the inner wall linings of the stomach and intestinal tract to a higher and more sustained acid level. Over the long term, this can be quite damaging since digestive acids are extremely corrosive, can aggravate ulcers, and may cause heartburn and indigestion. Most important, it upsets the digestive process and internal chemical balance, leaving you susceptible to virtually every disease state.

Another problem is that when food is not broken down into small enough bits, it can enter the bloodstream as oversized particles. These particles cannot be utilized at the cellular level, and so they are carried along until they eventually pass out through the kidneys. But during their prolonged stay in the blood they are likely to elicit an immune response through the activation of antibodies that do not recognize them as being compatible with the body's needs. Thus, improper chewing can lead to heightened levels of stomach acid and overstimulation of the allergic response.

Fluids do not require chewing, but they have a significant impact on the digestive process. Drinking large amounts of fluids while you eat can create another problem. Fluids dilute both saliva and digestive acids, interfering with their ability to break down food. To make matters worse, drinking while eating encourages gulping down food chunks that you would otherwise have to chew more thoroughly. You may tend to do this if you are in a hurry or if you are impatient with the chewing required by certain foods. "Washing food down" with liquids not only hampers digestion, it is also dangerous. It makes it too easy to get large chunks of food stuck in the throat, and so, "choking down" food may lead to just that—choking.

Foods That Work With Your Body, Not Against It

In selecting food, make sure to choose foods which facilitate digestion and thereby work with your body, and not against it. These include (1) foods that do not cause allergic reactions or sensitivities; (2) wholesome and natural foods instead of processed, chemically altered, or denatured foods; and (3) foods that contain bulk and have a low density or no fat content. Basically this means that you will be selecting many more complex carbohydrates—potatoes, rice, and vegetables—rather than fats and proteins along with mostly nonanimal products, in order to avoid heavy concentrations of fat and protein.

Among prepared foods, get those which are as close as possible to their natural state. Frozen peas, for instance, are much closer to the natural, raw state than peas that have been boiled and canned. Avoid irradiated produce; while it does not spoil as quickly as raw produce, its essential chemical structure has been so altered that it is hardly the same food anymore.

Produce often is doused with pesticides and chemicals or is dirty. Some has been waxed. Wash these foods thoroughly or even peel them. Better yet, don't buy them unless they have been organically grown, that is, grown without pesticides and potentially poisonous chemical fertilizers. You don't need to load your body with any more chemical pollutants than it gets from everyday living in today's society. No amount of washing and scrubbing will completely rid tainted foods of waxes and chemicals. It will cost more money for food of this quality, but consider the money spent as a contribution to your health. Eating right means eating to enhance your vitality. Ingesting pesticide-ridden and waxed produce is not much better than eating processed items filled with chemical preservatives, artificial colorings and flavorings, and other additives.

In preparing foods, try to maximize their digestibility without altering their essential integrity and cellular structure, since these things are critical to facilitating digestion and keeping the colon and upper gastrointestinal track clear of food mass and toxic buildup. For instance, plant foods with a lot of cellulose (the cellular structure of plants) need to be softened for easier digestion so that the benefits received from the cellulose can be optimized. Celery can be soaked; cauliflower, carrots, and even sprouts can be steamed; and beans and corn can be mashed.

Take care not to overcook your food. Much of the fibrous structure, can be lost, which aids in digestion as well as nutritional benefits in the form of its vitamin and mineral contents. Steaming is generally preferable to boiling, boiling in 1 inch of water may be better than boiling in 6 inches, and boiling for 5 minutes is usually preferable to boiling for 20 minutes.

Stress is another integral part of the digestive process. Don't eat when you are tense, upset, or in a hurry. Wait until you have relaxed. If you come home from work and are worried about something that happened at the office or if you are upset because a friend is sick, take some time to get your emotions in order before you eat. Otherwise you will not digest your food properly. The digestive mechanism is interrupted by stress, and if you are nervous or anxious or hurried, you may not chew your food well to begin with. Digestive enzymes are not properly secreted because your stressful condition has affected normal enzyme production, and you will get little benefit from the meal. If you make a habit of eating on the run or eating while under stress, you are setting yourself up for chronic digestive problems.

If you select, prepare, and masticate your food properly, you will have pretty much done the best possible job. After the food is swallowed, the digestive system for the most part takes over.

The Process of Digestion

Many different chemicals and chemical processes are involved in digestion. The most important substance in saliva is protein, including many free-state proteins and amino acids. Besides digesting starch, saliva keeps the mucous membrane of the mouth moist, and its constant flow helps keep teeth and gums clean and free of food particles. Without adequate salivation, you will have dryness of the mouth, bacterial overgrowth, a buildup of food particles and dead cells, and a loss of the ability to taste, leading to appetite loss.

Enzymes are complex organic compounds, usually proteins, that are task-specific: that is, they work in a specific manner on particular foods. Enzymes that catalyze reactions leading to the breakdown of carbohydrates, for instance, have no effect on fat or protein digestion. Complementary sets of enzymes ensure that the cells get sufficient amounts of the specific foods on which they act.

Carbohydrate digestion is the most important in relation to the energy requirements of the body. Plants, grains, legumes, vegetables, fruits, nuts, and seeds—all carbohydrates—offer the greatest source of energy for proper physiological functioning.

All carbohydrates are broken down into one type of sugar or another. In fact, carbohydrates are composed primarily of sugars, but also fiber, essential fatty acids, and amino acids. They are classified according to how many glucose or sugar units are present in each molecule. Glucose, which produces most of the complex sugars, is the main form of carbohydrate that goes into the bloodstream and enters the cells in the presence of insulin. It plays a critical role in normal brain functioning and is the chief source of energy for the nervous system.

Carbohydrates may contain either complex or simple sugars. Glucose and fructose are monosaccharides or single-unit, simple sugars. Starch is a polysaccharide, or complex sugar. Some carbohydrates are indigestible and merely pass through the digestive system to be excreted with other waste products in their original, unaltered state. These are the fibers, and even though they are not digested, their action while passing through the digestive system is extremely important. They stimulate peristalsis—the wavelike alternating contractions that move food and waste through the digestion and elimination systems. They further enhance the elimination of toxic wastes by absorbing excess water and joining with other residue to create bulk matter which passes more readily out of the system. Fiber, then, while indigestible and containing no nutrients, plays a major role in digestion through its stimulating, cleansing, and detoxifying action.

The carbohydrates that are digestible go through various processes. The simple sugars can enter the blood system almost immediately upon ingestion, even before they are swallowed. The multiple-unit sugars are partially digested in the mouth by salivary enzymes. They are moved along until they reach the stomach, where they are passed into the large intestine. This is where the greatest amount of carbohydrate digestion takes place. The sugars are broken down into glucose in the small intestine and are finally ready to pass into the blood in that form. Once in the blood, they are absorbed into the cells and used as a form of energy for the brain and the nervous system.

Different classes of foods are digested differently. For example, proteins are far more complicated than carbohydrates, and they vary greatly in their function. All proteins are made up of chains of amino acids, the so-called building blocks of life, which make up part of every living cell in the body; they can be enzymes, hormones, or antibodies.

While there is a great deal that is not known about protein digestion, it is known that proteins are far more difficult to digest than carbohydrates. In order to be reduced, proteins must have their bonding peptide linkages broken down by the gastric juices.

Some peptides are more difficult to reduce than others. Those with a lot of fat surrounding them, such as those in meat, are difficult to digest, but not nearly as difficult as deep-fried or charcoal-broiled foods, which form strongly bound molecules that are extremely difficult to separate. When proteins that are hard to digest (e.g., meats) are made even more resistant (e.g., by deep frying), they remain undigested longer. In trying to digest them, the body continues to produce gastric juices so highly acidic that if not properly buffered, they can eat a hole (a penetrating ulcer) through the stomach lining.

Digesting proteins is obviously quite different from digesting carbohydrates. Of course, both proteins and carbohydrates provide the body with essential nutrients, and both are sources of energy. There is a substantial difference in the kinds of energy they produce. It is often thought that proteins are synonymous with high energy, and for that reason hypoglycemics (people with low blood sugar and therefore low energy levels) are frequently fed high-protein diets. But if one looks at the way these two types of foods are digested, one sees that a high-protein diet may not be what the hypoglycemic needs.

If a hypoglycemic feels weak because of low blood sugar and eats a piece of fruit, 30 or 40 minutes later the fruit is digested and glucose enters that person's bloodstream to restore energy. If the hypoglycemic person eats a lean steak instead, he or she will have to wait one to four hours for the meal to leave the stomach, depending upon how much is eaten, how it was prepared, and the state of his or her digestive system. It will take even longer for the amino acids derived from the meat to be translated into usable energy. The protein meal will feel satisfying because of its saturated, high-density fat, which is very slow to digest and therefore delays the hunger mechanism for a long time. In comparison, a carbohydrate meal—fruits, vegetables, pastas, etc.—will pass through all the stages of digestion quickly, and the person may be hungry again an hour later. But carbohydrates deliver the required energy rapidly and efficiently, while protein not only takes longer in getting energy into the cells but even saps energy in the process in order to keep the gastric juices flowing and the whole digestive system working overtime to break down the complex, high-calorie piece of beef.

The Right Diet for You

It is difficult to separate the fats from the proteins from the carbohydrates. You may be eating too much of one to get some of the other, or you may be cutting down on one to reduce the other. Understanding a little about why you do and don't need each one will help you formulate a sensible diet for your particular needs.

Diets should be individual matters. Not everybody requires the same amounts or proportions of proteins, fats, or carbohydrates. Your body chemistry or lifestyle may indicate that you need to slant your diet a little bit toward this or away from that. What's good for your friend may not be the best for you. Men, women, and children have different requirements. Adults at different ages have varying dietary needs. Don't eat what everyone around you is eating or what a book or article suggests. Tailor your diet to your specific needs, which may include your particular health problems. It is best to work with a nutritionist or a physician who is knowledgeable about nutrition in drafting the right program.

PART TWO

Taking Charge of Your Health

9

Detoxification

We are surrounded in our world by toxic substances in the air, water, soil, and food. Food that is manufactured or processed is usually treated with chemical preservatives, dyes, and food additives. A healthy body can usually eliminate these potentially toxic or harmful substances through the liver and other organs. But a diet that is too high in fats, processed proteins, sodium, refined sugars, and other refined foods, reduces this natural capacity to rid the body of these toxins. When that happens, the toxins in the body can accumulate.

Why Detoxification is Necessary

Toxins in food may not all be poisons in the classic sense. They often do their damage more insidiously, inhibiting the actions of enzymes in our bodies. Many things can go wrong if enzymes don't properly do their work. Since enzymes are important activators of almost every digestive or energy-producing activity in the body, our digestive systems can become sluggish and slow down if they are adversely affected by toxins, with the result that fat digestion can become difficult and protein digestion inefficient. Our kidneys and liver then become overloaded and fat may be deposited in arteries. Cardiovascular illness and other degenerative diseases can result.

Foods that are commercially fertilized may also be denuded of their proper mineral levels. Potassium, for example—our most important activator or catalyst of enzyme actions in the body—is one of the most vital minerals to be lost in this way. Without the right amounts of this mineral, the natural chemicals and enzymes that make our digestion efficient could not function. Yet potassium is reduced—and sodium added—in many of our processed foods, and toxins will often deplete potassium supplies. This changes our basic metabolic balance, opening the door for a host of potential problems. The detoxification process will often depend on rebuilding potassium supplies in the body by including fresh fruits and vegetables in our daily diet.

Toxic substances may severely depress the immune system. It is only in the past half-century, with the increase in environmental pollution and dependence on processed foods, that we have seen a rapid increase in diseases like cancer, heart disease, arthritis, and legionnaires' disease—maladies, unknown not too long ago, that a healthy, normal immune system would be able to fight off.

While those who live in polluted urban or suburban areas may say they have little control over many toxic substances—like air pollution—there are things we all can do. People can stop smoking, drinking liquor, using drugs, and eating processed foods. These are all toxic substances. What we need to do instead is to start using fresh, untreated foods, raw foods, and fresh juices, whose actual nutrients are more easily available to the body than packaged foods. They can help restore and reactivate our depressed immune systems and eliminate many toxins.

The solution to this problem is to offer the body the right nutrients. Allow the body to open up the eliminative processes, in which the liver and digestive tract play key roles. Start to detoxify by getting used to natural juices, natural mineral sources, and other organic substances, sometimes supplemented by enema or medically supervised, short-duration fasts. The process may be a slow one at the start. When toxins have had so long to build up, their breakdown also will take time.

Finding Out What's Wrong through Proper Testing

Once you have decided to make a change in your diet and lifestyle, you may want to undergo some simple inexpensive tests to ascertain whether there are specific aspects of your health that should be taken into consideration in your diet. According to Dr. Martin Feldman, a preventive medicine physician, some of the most useful standard testing options include: the glucose tolerance test (also called the GTT or blood-sugar test), a hair analysis (which detects toxins), and the SMA-24 blood test (Sequential Multiple Analyzer, a multiple blood-chemistry screening test), and the complete blood count (CBC), which includes tests of the red blood cell sedimentation rate (also called the ESR or sed rate), and thyroid function. These tests are particularly appropriate if your decision to be tested is prompted by health problems or health complaints, such as generalized fatigue, that you already have. But very often a state of imbalance may be present long before symptoms appear. The best care is prevention, correcting the imbalance nutritionally before it has developed into a symptomatic disease state.

PERSONAL MEDICAL HISTORY Every individual is biologically unique. This should be reflected in the health profile. Testing should always be preceded by a proper medical history, taken by a physician. If you ever go to a medical facility and they don't take your medical history—thoroughly—then there is something wrong with that group of physicians. By taking a history, symptoms begin to stand out. Some of these symptoms are early warning signals of what later may become a toxic or imbalanced state.

Some types of symptoms that will appear during a personal history have not always been duly appreciated by physicians as indicators of an imbalanced or toxic state. For example, problems on the surface of the skin may signify underlying toxicities requiring attention and treatments. The skin, after all, is not just a covering on the body like a coat. It is a living, breathing part of our bodies. It is, in fact, our largest organ and has a great deal to do with our internal health. If the body is harboring toxins, one of the routes to eliminate poisons, besides the kidney, the liver, and the lungs, is the skin. Many early warnings of toxicities often appear as minor skin problems, even as simple blemishes on the face. Acne, for example, is a manifestation of an internal hormonal toxicity. Red, blotchy skin, may provide an early warning that the liver, kidneys, or lungs are malfunctioning by not eliminating toxins. Headaches also can provide clues. Many headaches are responses to stress or tension. But other headaches may instead signal a toxic condition. Generalized fatigue may also be caused by a toxic state. Pre-menstrual syndrome (PMS) in women may reflect a state of hormonal toxicity; cystic breasts may also reflect an imbalance; osteoarthritis may reflect a calcium imbalance associated with toxicity. These are a small sampling of conditions that may come up when the personal history is taken. While many physicians will accept these conditions without identifying a specific, treatable cause, these symptoms may in fact stem from correctable toxic states.

THE GLUCOSE TOLERANCE TEST The glucose tolerance test (also called the GTT, blood-sugar, or glucose test) measures the blood level of glucose, the most important sugar in the body. Glucose is usually maintained at a constant level by means of insulin and other hormones so that, for example, when a person fasts, the body produces glucose from its stores of fat and protein. Normally, blood glucose is obtained from the digestion of carbohydrates in the diet.

There are certain imbalanced states, however, where the glucose level is either too high or too low. Symptoms of lethargy, dizziness, or irritability may be caused by an abnormally low blood-sugar level, or hypoglycemia. It can occur without a clearly identifiable cause, or as the result of excessive use of alcohol or strenuous exercise. At the other extreme, an abnormally high glucose level may cause frequent urination and chronic infections.

The glucose tolerance test requires that you eat adequate carbohydrates for several days prior to being tested, and then fast 12 hours immediately beforehand. Blood and urine samples are taken prior, during, and at the termination of the test, during which glucose is administered, either orally as a syrup or intravenously.

Other tests to measure glucose in the blood include the hemoglobin, A1C test, also called the glycosylated hemoglobin test. This measures the glucose in the red blood cells and may be performed during routine blood tests. It measures average glucose levels over many weeks, rather than the minute-to-minute glucose levels measured by the glucose tolerance test.

Tests of pancreatic function, adrenal gland function, and liver function may also be used to measure the glucose levels since, ultimately, glucose is controlled by those three parts of the body. The pancreas, for example, is in charge of insulin production. If the pancreas does not create enough insulin, high glucose levels result. If insulin is excessive, low glucose levels appear. Chromium levels are also important in any glucose test, since they control how cells actually absorb or use glucose. The presence of chromium can be determined via hair analysis or blood analysis methods, which are inexpensive.

HAIR ANALYSIS Hair analysis as a valid scientific measurement is often criticized and maligned. Yet, there is a specific advantage of hair analysis: When you examine just three inches of hair, you're observing growth over a period of three to four months. You therefore can obtain the average level of the body's status over a several-month period. As the hair grows each day, the mineral status of the body is reflected in the growth of the hair on that day. When examining hair, you're looking at a relatively stable part of the body—almost like examining a fossil—as opposed to the blood, which is constantly in flux.

In the case of exposure to mercury through a silver amalgam mercury filling that you received from your dentist, for example, the blood level of the mercury may rise for about 12 to 24 hours after you were exposed. After a day or so, the mercury leaves the bloodstream. But hair analysis will show mercury's impact over days, weeks, or months. This is true of other minerals as well. Lead is another good example. In the case of exposure to lead in a work environment, blood levels rise during the exposure, but 12 to 24 hours afterward, the lead level in the blood will be nondetectable. Hair analysis, however, will continue to show evidence of the change.

The cost of hair analysis is relatively modest compared to other tests. The most problematic aspect is in the proper interpretation of the results. Many labs overinterpret by overemphasizing data of minor importance. The hair has two major strengths in analysis. First, it is useful in showing when the body is not absorbing particular minerals efficiently and an imbalance has occurred due to this malabsorption, particularly of minerals like calcium, magnesium, zinc, manganese, and chromium. Second, the hair reveals the presence of toxic metals very well, including lead, mercury, cadmium, arsenic, and aluminum.

THE CLASSIC BLOOD TEST—SMA-24 The standard blood test gives us a lot of data, some of which can serve as an early warning, and some of which, unfortunately, is already a late warning. Commonly called the SMA-24, or the SMA-12 when abridged, the test is relatively complete, reasonably inexpensive, and provides a lot of data for the money. It should be performed as part of a six-month or yearly examination.

A patient should always be tested on an empty stomach, that is after not having eaten for six to eight hours. No food, no juice, no coffee, no tea. Water only. If you've eaten within four hours before the test, this makes it very difficult to interpret the glucose and triglyceride levels on the blood specimen that is drawn.

The first item on an SMA-24 is the *glucose level*. Glucose, if a body has been fasting, should be at a level roughly between 75 and 100. A glucose below 75 is evidence of a possible hypoglycemic (low blood sugar) tendency.

Above 100 is too high. Does that mean you have diabetes? The answer is maybe in time. A high glucose level serves as an early warning sign. The next step is to look into whether the cause is a glucose "thermostat" imbalance or a malfunctioning of the pancreas, the adrenal glands, or the liver. Chromium levels should be considered as a related aspect. A glucose imbalance may mean that something is going to go wrong in the future and is deserving of more attention now.

Next on the SMA-24 are the *sodium levels*. Occasionally sodium is too low. An important aspect rarely appreciated by traditional physicians is that low sodium may indicate an adrenal malfunction. The adrenal gland may be sluggish, not making enough aldosterone, which is the sodium-retaining hormone.

Potassium is a potential problem if it is too low. This may happen when people take blood pressure medicines, and the body is asked to remove salt. One can remove too much potassium.

Carbon dioxide is usually tested on the SMA-24. An elevation of the carbon dioxide is a reflection of an alkaline state. The most common cause of an excessively alkaline state is a diminished flow or amount of stomach acids.

Next is *blood urea/nitrogen*. If the urea/nitrogen levels are elevated, the body is experiencing urea toxicity. One should then look at whether the kidneys are working properly, or whether one is protein toxic. Too much protein can eventually lead to excessive urea.

Creatinine is a kidney-related enzyme. Its elevation is kidney related, so one has to go beyond the blood levels themselves.

Blood calcium may be normal and appear normal on the test, even if a person's true calcium status is not. Here's an example where one has to intelligently analyze the blood and not assume that the calcium level overall is correctly balanced, just because the blood level is. In about one person in five with a severe calcium imbalance, the blood will show too-low calcium levels. On the other hand, in four out of five people, the calcium may be off without the imbalance appearing on the blood test.

Phosphorous. When phosphorous is too high, it can adversely affect calcium levels.

Uric acid. Elevation of uric acid indicates a gout condition. Many people have gout early on. Even then, uric acid levels may not appear over the upper end of the range. But high uric acid can be a warning of gout that will develop later on, so one has to monitor the uric acid level. In such cases, the physician may also need to take a family history to determine whether gout runs in the family.

Alkaline phosphatase is a complex part of the blood. If elevated, it may reflect a liver imbalance or bone problem.

The *total protein* in the blood may occasionally be low and may indicate a malabsorption of protein.

Albumin in the blood relates to its protein component as do *globulin* levels.

The measurement of *SGOT and SGPT* in most SMA-24's are measures of liver-related enzymes. Elevation of either may indicate that the liver is out of balance. If the liver is even slightly off balance, it can cause a variety of health problems. Such an imbalance should be dealt with nutritionally.

Bilirubin levels also are potentially liver related. Elevation of bilirubin may also have other meanings that require further testing.

The *cholesterol* in the blood should be looked at. One also has to look at the HDL (high density lipoproteins, or "good" cholesterol) verses the total serum cholesterol levels. Ratios of four to one (of total cholesterol to HDL) or better are desirable.

For almost all people with cholesterol levels above 225, the liver is sluggish or out of balance. This problem plays a major role in cholesterol elevation.

One should always also ask for a *triglyceride level* as part of their SMA-24 test results. Triglyceride levels are almost as important as cholesterol levels. An elevated level is usually due to malfunctioning of either the liver or the pancreas. Triglycerides are dangerous because they are blood fats and may play some part in clogging our arteries with harmful plaque.

These are the primary items of importance that can be tested with the SMA-24.

THE COMPLETE BLOOD COUNT (CBC) In the CBC, we look both at the white blood cell components and the red blood cell components.

WHITE BLOOD CELLS

You could have a white blood count (WBC) as low as 4.8, or as high as 10.8, and still be within the normal range. If you fall below 4.8 WBC, it probably indicates that your immune system is not working properly. Even just slightly below the 4.8 level is an early warning sign that your immunity is not at 100 percent. The CBC is very inexpensive; at the same time it provides a lot of valuable information.

Occasionally the white blood count may be very high (counts in the range of 9, 10, or 11). This is usually indicative of an internal infection. The elevation of the white blood cells represents the body's attempt to deal with the invasion of a foreign substance or agent. The white blood cells are the soldiers that the body mobilizes to do battle. When the enemy has entered it, the body will, if it can, make many more white blood cells. The elevation that appears on the CBC is an indication that there is some kind of internal battle raging.

Conversely, when the body, even at rest, is not making enough white blood cells (in the case of a low WBC), it means there aren't enough soldiers around to do battle in case the need arises.

It is also important to go beyond the total number of the white cells, to look at the different types of white blood cells. The basic types of white blood cells are the neutrophils or the polymorphonuclear white blood cells, the lymphocytes, the monocytes, the eosinophils, and the basophils.

The neutrophils or polys tend to make up between 50 and 70 percent of the total white cells. We have more neutrophils or polys than any other type. That's normal. That's the way the body is set up. The lymphocytes comprise between 20 and 40 percent of our white blood cells. There are fewer eosinophils, monocytes, and basophils.

If there are more lymphocytes than neutrophils, an inversion of the usual ratio, most doctors would not even mention it to the patient. They may not even notice it, or if they notice, they may take no action. But it should be examined. It's a potential early warning that the body's immune mechanism for making white blood cells is really not up to par. If there were a viral illness, however, either recently or at the time when the test was taken, that may explain the imbalance. During a viral illness, the body will make more lymphocytes because lymphocytes tend to be the main soldiers against viruses. In the absence of a viral problem or an infection, when lymphocytes still outnumber polys, the possibility of an immune system imbalance should be examined further.

RED BLOOD CELLS

There is basically one issue which concerns red blood cells—anemia. Occasionally there's an excess of red blood cells, but that's a rare state. Most of the time the question is "are there too few?" A decreased red blood cell count indicates anemia.

There are two types of anemia, depending on the size of the red blood cells. If the cells are too small, small-cell or iron deficiency anemia may be the cause. This condition is almost always related to an iron deficiency, where the body doesn't have enough iron or isn't properly handling the iron it does have. Since the body can't make enough cells without the necessary quantities of iron, it produces smaller and fewer cells.

In the second type of anemia, the cells are too large. The most common reason for this abnormality is a vitamin B_{12} deficient anemia. Treatment is different for each specific type of anemia. (See chapter 34.)

TESTS OF SEDIMENTATION RATES AND THYROID FUNCTION People should also be tested on a routine basis to determine sedimentation rates and thyroid function.

The sedimentation rate is a very inexpensive test. In women, if the sedimentation rate is above 20, there is an indication that some inflammatory process exists or is developing. If there is no cold, sore throat, or other obvious infection, one has to seek out other possible causes. In men, a sedimentation rate above 15 is considered an abnormal elevation.

Thyroid testing can involve special difficulties. For example, thyroxin is the hormone that allows the thyroid gland to carry out its function. You can have normal thyroxin levels and normal blood iodine levels at the same time as a food sensitivity to the thyroid gland is causing your metabolism to slow down, so that you gain weight at an abnormal rate. Chronic fatigue may also be caused by malfunctioning of the thyroid gland.

A standard blood test for thyroxin would not detect either the food sensitivity or the chronic fatigue.

Detoxification Techniques

There are a variety of detoxification techniques available. Several that can be used in combination to improve your well-being and increase your self-awareness are described below.

Maintaining Intestinal Fortitude

It is estimated that nearly half of all illnesses originate in the intestinal tract—the receptor of the foods we eat, the water we drink, and the air we breathe. Anything that passes through the intestines will impact, positively or negatively, on your health. Cleansing the intestines will help free the body of some hazardous toxic substances.

Certain organisms proliferate in the colon, depending on what we eat and what foods go through it. One of those organisms is the *Candida albicans* organism, which causes candidiasis or yeast in the intestine. Another is the E. coli bacteria. Still, other bacterial flora help maintain a healthy balance in the colon. If we eat the right types of food that can be digested quickly, transit time in the colon should also be fast. This helps keep bacteria in balance and diminishes harmful bacterial activity. However, if we eat animal proteins such as meat and hard cheeses, food transit time in the colon slows down. Everything begins to clog up, and the trouble begins.

Another concern in keeping the colon healthy is the sometimes deleterious effect of antibiotics on the digestive system. Most antibiotics destroy the friendly bacterial flora in the colon in a short time. This allows the proliferation of two harmful organisms, the E. coli and the *Candida albicans*.

We are exposed to antibiotics in many ways. We may take them as medication to cure infections, but we also get them in the meat we eat. The antibiotics, tranquilizers, and hormones that animals have been fed before slaughter remain in the meat. Some believe that we also are being flooded by the animal's adrenaline, which it produces just prior to being killed.

In any case, there are a number of nutritional experts who urge people to consult with specialists on ways to cleanse the colon of these harmful substances—either by having a yearly cooling irrigation, where water is used to clean out the colon, or by using a variety of different types of enemas.

Yeast Infection Control

Successfully combating candida or common yeast infections may require changing the diet. But cleansing of the colon will also help. One reason these infections affect large numbers of people is that many of the foods we eat have molds in them. Mushrooms and wheat are prime examples.

To fight candida, people can go on a special diet. For their new diet, they should first go off wheat, breads and cereals, yeast, vinegar, cured or processed meats, and all sugars. They should include garlic, vitamin C, B_6, pau d'arco, and acidophilus—as daily supplements. Fresh vegetable juices and some fresh fruit juices also are important in any cleansing program because they provide needed vitamins and minerals, and they help specifically to cleanse the colon.

In particular, papaya and watermelon juices both have useful cleansing and therapeutic properties. Carrot juice, celery juice, and cucumber juice, mixed in a one to one ratio, are sometimes useful for intestinal cleansing. Adding kelp to carrot, celery, parsley, and spinach juice results in a combination quite rich in potassium and calcium. And small quantities of fresh garlic juice helps us to get rid of some intestinal parasites. (For a complete discussion of candida, see chapter 53.)

Detoxification with Herbs

Detoxification with herbs can be another key approach to renewed health. Two authorities in this area are Dr. Paul Lee, one of America's leading spokespersons on the health properties of herbs, and Jeanne Rose, author of *Herbal Guides to Inner Health* and *The Herbal Body Book*.

Both experts point to specific herbs that are excellent detoxifiers, primarily because they stimulate macrophage activity. Macrophages are parts of our immune system that attack, engulf, and digest toxins and other substances that cause us to be ill. (See chapter 15 for a full discussion of the healing properties of herbs.)

10

Weight Management

There are virtually hundreds of diet programs available today. Most are based on high-protein, low-calorie regimens, or involve products that are supposed to melt away fat, change the metabolism, or stimulate muscle development. Before embarking upon any of these, first examine the notion of what is proper weight, making sure your perception of what constitutes your ideal weight is not mistaken.

The Scope of the Problem

You may not realize it, but it requires from two to four years of being overfat before you become overweight. Excess fat will first infiltrate the muscle tissue before it spills out as subcutaneous tissue, that which you can see underneath the folds of skin. By the time the fat is visible on your arms and face, the problem has already reached the advanced stages and the buttocks, thighs, belly, upper arms, and back have already been saturated. To assume that a crash diet based on fasting or calorie restriction is going to reverse this process can be a dangerous assumption to make. The end result of easy solutions may only be repeated failures. The key to weight management, and ideal weight control, is not diet alone but exercise in combination with diet.

Exercise is more important in maintaining proper weight than counting calories. You may have heard that for every 3,500 calories in excess of your body's metabolic requirements you will gain a pound, while for every 3,500 calories under that requirement you will lose a pound. These are both cumulative figures. So that, for example, if you were eating one extra slice of bread per day, you would have gained over 10 pounds by the year's end, at the rate of 70 extra calories per slice, 490 calories per week. But this represents a gross misunderstanding of how our bodies work. Diets based on such a seemingly rational, log-

---

ical, though mechanistic view of the body sounds simple. Yet they don't work—because the body does not work that way—so rationally, logically, and, worst of all, so mechanically. Look at all the thin people who eat great quantities of food and never gain an ounce. Look at all the fat people who just have to think about food, or smell food, and gain pounds.

We need to determine what causes weight problems and treat the causes, not the symptoms. The way to do this is to understand how the body works, and then use its own natural mechanisms to produce the desired results. Exercise is the key.

The Setpoint: Your Body's "Fat Thermostat"

Primitive man gorged when food was available and starved when there was none. His body had built-in survival mechanisms that stored fat when he gorged and then conserved energy when food was scarce. The conservation mechanism slowed down his metabolism, making use only of enough energy to keep him alive and functioning. That mechanism is still with us and still working. Decreasing your caloric intake, skipping a meal, or even eating irregularly may trigger the starvation mechanism. Your body's protective response is to go into its conservation mode—to conserve energy and preserve the fat, just in case starvation is really imminent. When the body gets food, it puts it in a "band," to ensure against any possible further deprivation. Each of our bodies seems to have a certain natural level, or setpoint, that it strives to maintain to keep itself functioning.

Researchers are now looking at how the body gains and retains weight and are redefining their understanding of weight control. What are the causes of weight control. What are the causes of weight gain? The answer seems to lie in a weight-regulating mechanism located in a control center in the brain called the hypothalamus. It determines the level of fat that it considers ideal for the body. It proceeds to maintain that level, come what may. That level, selected by the weight-regulating mechanism, then becomes the setpoint. The setpoint is analogous to a thermostat. A thermostat set at 70 degrees kicks off and activates the heating system when the temperature falls below 70 degrees. Similarly, a setpoint of 140 pounds activates the weight-regulating mechanism to store more fat if the body weight falls below that 140-pound level. In its effort to maintain the setpoint, the weight-regulating mechanism works in two ways: It controls the appetite, and it regulates our metabolism and the storage of energy.

First, appetite control determines when you feel hungry. It sends you a message to eat. You may have no control over the urge to eat—the hypothalamus makes sure of that—but you do have complete control over your response. You can choose when and how to respond. What you eat and how much you eat are totally up to you. The hypothalamus will continue to stimulate the feeding mechanism and decrease satiety, you will continue to feel hungry and eat, until the desired setpoint level is achieved, and your weight is back to where it was.

Second, a weight-regulating mechanism signals the body when to conserve energy and store it, or when to use it up. If you eat a large amount of food, it increases the rate at which the body burns calories. If you eat a small amount, the body decreases the rate. In each case, the goal is to preserve the setpoint. This explains why people on diets may lose weight temporarily, but ultimately regain it, and then keep their weight closer to the former, albeit unsatisfactory level. It's called the yo-yo syndrome, and every dieter is familiar with it. Usually one's weight has been typical for them for many years. It is their setpoint. The body is accustomed to it, feels safe and secure at that level, and consequently does what it can to maintain it. People who are overweight commonly observe that they don't really eat that much. Indeed, studies have confirmed that under-weight people commonly eat more than overweight people.

What we distill from this is that overweight people may have a body chemistry geared to making fat even from a low-calorie diet. It seems that they are just better at storing fat than at burning fat. Their bodies are programmed to make fat and protect their setpoints. This also explains why some other people never seem to gain weight. Their setpoints are low, their ability to use energy is efficient, and so they don't store fat. You can, however, change the setpoint, but only through aerobic exercise.

The Aging Factor

From the age of 30 on, your metabolism decelerates about 5 percent every 7 years. In other words, if you were eating the same number of calories at 50 years of age that you ate at 30, you would be gaining several pounds every year. But weight itself is not an indication of optimal body health. A person weighing 200 pounds, who lifts weights and exercises, may have only 3 to 4 percent body fat. Many football players, for example, would fall into this category. But if these individuals stopped all their physical activity, and a year later they weighed the same, their entire body structure would be different. They would look and feel obese, because their muscle would have turned to fat. Muscle that is not used atrophies. Weight itself should not be taken as the primary indicator of health. What is important is the percentage of lean muscle tissue and the percentage of fat to total body mass. Ideally, most men should be approximately 15 percent body fat, most women no more than 18 to 20 percent. However, studies indicate that most men are between 22 and 24 percent, most women between 26 and 34 percent.

Reprogramming the Setpoint through Aerobic Exercise

Lean body mass increases when intramuscular fat is replaced with muscle. Muscles have special enzymes that burn calories during exercise. The more muscle you have, the more enzymes you have that burn calories. As the amount of muscle increases, the amount of fat decreases, and the capacity for burning more calories is further enhanced. So when muscles move, they burn calories and increase lean body mass. It's a new cycle, but this time it's not vicious!

Although there are probably genetic tendencies that predetermine that one of us will have a low setpoint and be thin, or a high setpoint and be overweight, it is still possible for most people to "reset" their fat thermostat. The key to reprogramming your setpoint lies in understanding and acting on the relationship between the kind and amount of exercise you do (your energy output) and the kind and amount of food you eat (your energy input). The trick lies in changing from a fat cycle to a fit cycle.

Running and other aerobic exercises can help you enter the fit cycle. Aerobic exercises uses large muscles in a repetitive rhythmic pattern.

To measure the effect of aerobic exercise on your body you will need to "watch"—or more appropriately "feel"—your heart rate, by measuring your pulse. There are three different heart rates to monitor.

RESTING HEART RATE The resting heart rate is the rate at which your heart has been pumping after you sit quietly for at least 15 minutes. It is usually 5–10 beats per minute slower than your "normal" heart rate.

Measure by taking your pulse for 10 or 20 seconds and then multiplying the result by 6 or 3, respectively. The average resting heart rate for men is 72–78 beats per minute, for women it's faster: 78–84. The better your aerobic circulation, the lower this rate will be.

Studies seem to indicate that people with resting heart rates above 70 have a greater risk of heart attack. By beating fewer times per minute, an efficient heart has more time to rest between beats. Hence, at each contraction or beat, it may be pumping more oxygen to the body's cells.

TARGET HEART RATE To produce a beneficial cardiovascular effort during exercise, you should elevate your heart rate sufficiently to strengthen heart muscles while at the same time avoiding any damage to the heart or cardiovascular system.

Take your pulse throughout your aerobic workout to make sure you are neither under- nor over-exerting yourself. Generally, your target rate is determined by taking 220 and subtracting your age and then multiplying the result by 70 percent.

Whatever you do you should not exceed 140 beats per minute when you're just starting an aerobic exercise program.

RECOVERY HEART RATE This rate records your heart beat 5 minutes after you've stopped exercising. It gives you some indication about whether you have gone 1 or more beats too far. If this rate is 120 beats per minute (150 in those over 50 years old), you need to cut back during your next workout.

To achieve a training effect on cardiovascular functioning or to lower your setpoint toward "thinness," you must do the exercise continuously for 20 to 60 minutes at your target heart rate at least three times a week.

During aerobic exercise, the body uses free fatty acids primarily and glycogen secondarily as fuel. While exercising, you do not use many calories. For example, you would have to walk 11½ miles to burn up 3,500 calories or 1 pound. Weight loss is the effect of a cumulative process in which calories are being used on a more regular and frequent basis. This cumulative use of calories produces ongoing changes in the body's chemistry, lowering the setpoint, increasing the lean muscle mass with its fat-burning enzymes, and increasing the metabolism so the body burns calories at a higher rate. For hours following the exercise period, the body continues to burn calories at a higher rate. The effects of exercise on the body last long after the exercise period has ended. This will be true as long as you continue to do aerobic exercise at least three days a week. Remember, duration is more important than distance or intensity.

Although many people may intellectually recognize the need for and benefit of aerobic exercise, too often they would rather spend their time doing other things, or hope to take a pill to reduce their weight because it requires no particular effort or ongoing commitment. Making a change in your lifestyle to accommodate exercise does require effort and commitment. Your health and well-being are worth the price.

Exercise increases muscle, which has fat-burning enzymes. The more you exercise and develop muscles, the more lean body mass and less fat you will have. All this will happen in addition to the much heralded cardiovascular and psychological advantages of aerobic exercise. Lowering the setpoint is a bonus.

Your individual exercise program will start the same way whether your goal is overall fitness or weight management. If you step on the scale after a few weeks of exercising, you may notice an increase in pounds. Don't be dismayed. That is a good sign. It means you are increasing muscle in relation to intramuscular fat (muscle weighs more than fat). Interpret the increase as getting better and stronger, not heavier. Then throw away the scale. Pounds do not measure fitness. Your tape measure and your clothes are better indicators of changes in your body. You will lose inches, usually in the "right" places.

Eating Plans

Counting calories is not as important as thoughtfully choosing the kinds and amounts of food you eat. The typical American diet needs to be adjusted to include more complex carbohydrates, fewer proteins, and less fat. Begin your new eating plan by eliminating the three whites from your diet: white sugar, white flour, and salt. Then eliminate processed food including most canned, frozen, or prepared convenience foods. Read labels and do not eat anything you can't pronounce.

There is one point that most books on dieting fail to mention. That is the importance of getting in touch with your appetite thermostat. Your body tells you when to eat and when to stop, and you don't always hear it or listen to it.

The best eating plan is to eat more frequently—smaller meals, every four to six hours, so that both hunger and satiety can be experienced. Do eat breakfast, just keep down fat and sugar consumption. More people who skip breakfast are overweight than underweight. Get in touch with your eating drives. Keep lunch light, preferably eating complex carbohydrates, which are low in calories and high in satiety. Soup is a satisfying lunch, especially a water-based soup full of vegetables, grains, and legumes. Salads are good for lunch, but after eating one you could feel hungry again quite soon. Add whole grain bread to complement it. Beware of salad dressings; most are high in fat, sugar, and calories. Eat enough breakfast and lunch to take away the strong hunger drive, but not enough to feel full. If you are hungry before the next meal, have a snack. Eat only in response to hunger, not for entertainment.

Another divergence from traditional diets, but designed to pay attention to your body's natural eating drive, is to eat one meal a day to complete satiety, until you do not want to eat anymore. The evening meal is preferred, so it will hold you through the evening until bedtime. This is the most difficult time to avoid snacks.

BEWARE: The weight you eventually reach may not necessarily be the weight you desire. Be realistic and be philosophical. The genetic determinants of your setpoint may limit what you can realistically accomplish. If you follow the principles of exercise and diet for a reasonable period of time, and your weight stabilizes at a point higher than your fantasy weight, accept it and enjoy being yourself, as you are.

If you continue to exercise aerobically and eat a healthful diet, your weight-regulating mechanism will stabilize your weight and keep it at the new setpoint. Eating and exercising in this way will soon become a natural way of living for you. You won't need a maintenance diet or some other interim discipline to follow. Once you've set your own course, there will be no other course to follow and no need for fad approaches to dieting.

The Egg Project

More than a dozen years ago, I reviewed the available literature on protein requirements for human beings and found that there was as inconsistency between the prevalent beliefs of the scientific community as stated in the medical literature and the personal experience of many individuals. The people who should have been feeling healthy because they were getting more than adequate amounts of protein in their diets were frequently not receiving the healthful benefits from the protein. There was an escalating incidence of kidney disease in America that had no apparent cause. The prevailing myth stated that all of the protein from animal sources was complete, meaning that it contains all the essential amino acids, and, furthermore, that all other amino acids, those from plant foods, are incomplete—capable of sustaining life, but not of promoting optimum growth and maturation. Plant food diets were considered to be both faddist and dangerous. Clearly, this view had to be challenged.

I, along with Dr. Hillard Fitsky, who has a background in computer sciences, and my brother Steven, did a computer-assisted analysis of the 110 or so most commonly consumed vegetarian foods. We matched each one of the amino acids in the given food against the food source that is considered to contain the most complete protein, the chicken egg.

As the research progressed, it became clear that many of the assumptions concerning protein and our selection of foods were grossly in error. First, we found that not all animal protein is high quality and complete. Generally, only 40 percent is high quality. Second, we confirmed that not all vegetarian foods are incomplete. To the contrary, the vast majority of vegetarian foods are complete, containing all of the essential amino acids. The bean or legume family in particular tended to have protein in large quantities and of a high quality. This made it easier to understand how the Asian and Indian cultures have been able to sustain themselves and demonstrate remarkable longevity on a limited vegetarian diet.

Taking this logic one step further, I reasoned that if single foods in the grain, legume, and sea vegetable families tended to have remarkably high-quality protein, what would be the result of combining two or three of these together? What I found was that the overall quality of the protein tended to increase tremendously. Not only did I find specific combinations that approximated the completeness of the egg, but some that actually exceeded the egg in terms of the amounts of complete, usable protein they provided.

Of the 5,000 combinations that I was able to compute over a five-year period, all offered protein of a quality nearer to the egg than the closest animal protein food source, milk. Other animal protein foods, including fish, hamburger, veal, chicken, and cheese all proved to offer far less complete and less usable protein than that available in the right combinations of vegetarian foods. Of course, the plant foods had far less calories, none of the cholesterol, the high saturated fat, the toxic growth-stimulating hormones, or the antibiotic residues such as penicillin that you would find in the animal products. They offered instead quality protein, abundant fiber, plentiful B vitamins, vitamin A, vitamin C, minerals, and the full spectrum of other nutrients. In other words, the concept of protein complementation allowed the acknowledged benefits of the vegetarian foods to be viewed alongside an appreciation of their demonstrable protein value even when compared to meat. In effect, it was time to virtually rewrite in a revolutionary way the whole notion of how we perceive protein. Even vegetarians, we found, are generally receiving between two and three times more protein than they require.

In the diets described in the next chapter, and a later chapter on vegetarianism, the principles of food combining and food rotation are observed.

11

A Beginner's Weight Management Diet

H ave you ever wanted to start a diet plan but kept finding reasons to put it off? Or perhaps you've tried quick weight-loss programs, only to gain back what you've lost and then some. You can lose that weight and keep it off.

This chapter will explore how you can break the cycle of overeating and crash dieting with a program that's appetizing, nutritionally sound, and designed to last a lifetime.

In this program, you'll learn how to detoxify your body—how to get rid of the poisons accumulated from years of poor eating habits. You will gain tips on how to determine your individual nutritional needs, and how to satisfy them. And you'll learn about food rotation: why it's important, what kinds of foods to eat, and when. This chapter will outline a 14-day plan for you, so you can rebuild your health, lose that weight, and never have to worry about gaining it back.

This chapter is organized around the experiences of a group of average, overweight Americans whom I gathered together so that their real diet experiences might serve to help others beginning on the road to improved health.

Begin with Detoxification

I've been on every ridiculous diet that one can think of. At my age, or any other age, it's not healthy to be doing that. It worries me that I weigh so much. I am really serious about learning to diet right, and I am determined to lose the weight. But where do I start?—Joyce, age 55

There is no need to upset your whole system and your life in the process of losing weight.

In our society, most people don't really eat right for total health. Are you like most Americans? Do you tend to eat too much of foods that undermine your health: animal proteins, saturated fats, fried foods, overly spicy foods, and foods made of refined carbohydrates, such as pizzas, french fries, and different types of confections? Do you indulge, all too often, in bagels, donuts, white bread products, and preserved, pickled or processed foods? These foods have been denatured. That is, much of their vitamins and minerals have been destroyed.

Once you have done all that to yourself, your body, in effect, has become a toxic waste dumpsite. Thousands of man-made chemicals end up in your lean muscle and fat tissues. They don't belong there. They can't be utilized for energy, for repair or growth of your body. On the contrary, they disrupt your normal biochemical processes.

One byproduct of this disrupted biochemistry is a malfunctioning metabolism. Your metabolism—the way in which your body burns foods—is the process that allows you to have energy when operating normally, or lack energy when it is out of balance; to gain weight properly; or to gain it excessively. You may be overweight because your body's biochemistry is out of balance.

Yet you don't have to be a biochemist or an endocrinologist to understand the basic rules of proper eating. If you drink a lot of alcohol, you can't compensate by taking a vitamin B_1 tablet. Your body doesn't work that way.

The first step toward proper eating is to detoxify and rebalance your body so you can start afresh. A Taj Mahal built on quicksand would soon sink. You don't have a strong foundation until you get rid of the debris that litters that foundation. You can't just repaint an old house whose wood is rotted and deteriorated. You first have to repair it; otherwise the decay continues, hidden under that fresh coat of paint.

The single most important thing anyone who wants to change his or her diet can do is to detoxify by getting rid of the pollution in the body.

The rewards will be substantial. You will feel better, have more energy, feel lighter, and have an easier time maintaining a normal weight. You will find you have more endurance. Your body will no longer feel sluggish, and you will probably find you need less sleep.

Detoxifying need not be harsh upon either the mind or body. To begin though, you have to know your relative state of health. Each of us is biologically unique; we all have particular needs and wants. Any diet doctor, who says everyone should have 5 mg of B_2, and 10 mg of B_6 is wrong, because no other person has the same biochemistry as you. Even two people who are the same age, the same sex, the same height, and the same weight, even identical twins, will have different biochemical needs.

That's why faddish popular diets, in general, don't work. Too often, they try to provide specific information for a general audience, as if everyone were the same. *We're not all the same.* There is no message I could share with you that would be more important, no specific counsel I could give you, no recipe I could offer, that would have the significance of this statement.

You will maximize your health, normalize your weight, lose weight, and feel good when you understand what your own nutritional requirements are. They have nothing to do with anyone else's.

The Importance of Proper Testing

For as long as I can remember I've been about 10 to 15 pounds overweight. Nothing I do seems to get rid of that excess weight. I can lose weight temporarily, but I've tried everything from grapefruit to horseradish, and nothing really seems to help me get my weight down and keep it down. How do I find out what my own nutritional requirements are?"—Steve, age 40

The answer to Steve's concern begins with a basic blood chemistry test that evaluates the different components of your blood (the SMA-12, or SMA-24; see chapter 9). It measures a variety of vitamin, triglyceride, cholesterol, and mineral levels. Steve should also have a hair analysis done to determine whether there are toxic levels of different minerals in his system—harmful metals like cadmium, mercury, and lead. An excess of lead or cadmium can come from smoking cigarettes. These metals will directly affect the mechanism in the brain that determines the appetite and satiety levels.

When you get your blood chemistry results back, you may find that your individual biochemical profile indicates a need for some nutritional support and detoxification. What other tests can help you determine your nutritional and health needs?

Everybody should also have a musculoskeletal examination. An osteopath or a chiropractor can make this diagnosis for you, checking to see whether your muscular system is functioning properly. Frequently, the posture is so poor that there are blocked energy pathways. When you use certain muscle groups improperly, other muscle groups overreact in the body. For example, if you lean on one side while watching television, then the muscles on the opposite side of your body pull in the opposite direction. The result may be a sore back, sore arms and legs, hunched shoulders, or a hunched back.

We are a nation of people who sit, stand, and walk with poor posture. Posture can make an enormous difference in your energy levels and how you feel.

To summarize the way to begin: Step one is to cleanse out the old debris. It is necessary to eliminate the toxic metals, pesticides, herbicides, fungicides, and other synthetic substances from your system. Then you want to determine your own biological nature. What do you need—how much vitamin C, how much vitamin B_1? You don't want to put excessive amounts in your system, and yet you don't want to be deficient.

Numerous studies show that as a nation we are deficient in vitamin C, selenium, calcium, magnesium, and vitamin A. Those are easily obtainable from food in the diet. If you're eating what would be considered the average American diet, you're still almost certainly eating poorly.

Building Good Health

I've always been about 25 to 20 pounds overweight. A couple of times in my life I've gone on crash diets. I've lost all the weight I wanted to and felt great for two weeks. But I also have these terrible junk food habits with midnight binges. I think I'm ready to change my entire way of looking at the way I eat food, because what I've been doing is obviously not helping me. I've taken the tests and I've gotten back the results. What do I do now?—Barbara, age 25

A detoxification program will show Barbara and you which foods and nutrients to take on a daily basis, to help take away some of the negative effects of eating a high-sugar, high-calorie, high-fat, animal protein diet. You should then go on to a special 14-day eating program. First you detoxify, then rebuild health by losing weight, and then continue to eat right.

What are some good foods for building good health? At the top of the list is a group of foods called sprouts. Sprouts are the knockouts of nutrition. The sprout, quite simply, is one of the most nutrient-rich, powerful, health-building foods in nature. You just cannot find anything healthier. They will help cleanse and rebuild your entire system.

What kind of sprouts should you try? Don't stop with just common sprouts like alfalfa or mung beans. Expand your cuisine. Try high-protein buckwheat sprouts; the sweet sunflower sprout; the aromatic fenugreek sprout; clover sprout; and for a little bite and pinch, try a radish sprout. A mustard sprout will turn your tongue twice around your mouth. It tastes as good as mustard, and yet it has that nice salad feel to it.

Over 15 different seeds for sprouting are available commercially. They're inexpensive and versatile. You can make salads out of them, put them into pita bread, use them in casseroles, and put them in soups.

Next, add miso to the list of detoxifying and rebuilding foods. For over 3,000 years, this nutritionally superior food has been helping people to better health. Miso is a fermented product. Like yogurt, its bacteria work well in your intestines. After all, the health of the intestine determines the health of your body. Remember that miso is to be used sparingly, however, because it does have a high sodium content.

Vegetable juices are a third health-giving detoxifier. Generally speaking, take no more than one glass of carrot juice per day. Beta carotene is a precursor of vitamin A in the body. If you drink too much carrot juice, you'll be overloading the liver with vitamin A and your skin may turn yellow. One glass a day is fine. You will get the beneficial effects of vitamin A, which has been shown to be an antiviral vitamin; it protects against viruses.

Add to carrot juice: celery, cabbage, parsley, sprouts, or cucumber for a variety of delicious juices. For people who've never really enjoyed vegetables, juices are another way to get good-tasting, high-quality nutrition into your diet.

Grains are another group of foods that help the body cleanse itself and rebuild its strength. It is unfortunate that most Americans, unbelievably, never taste whole grain. They taste refined carbohydrates in white bread, or white rice, but never eat brown rice or whole grain bread. Yet these are inexpensive and readily available, even in supermarkets.

Whole grains are loaded with far more nutrition than their refined counterparts. The grain family includes rice, corn, buckwheat, rye, oats, and millet, as well as less well-known, newly available grains like triticale, amaranth, and quinoa (pronounced keen-wa), a light, fast-cooking grain from South America now available in some health food stores.

The next group of foods to include as part of your health-rebuilding program is the sea family of vegetables. These include hijiki, a form of seaweed that tastes salty like fish. You can buy seaweed dry and store it for months. There are many types, including kombu, wakami, and nori. To cook them, place a small piece in cold water. After five minutes, replace the water with fresh water; after five more minutes, replace the water again. You now have rinsed the seaweed and it's ready for cooking. You can cut it into pieces, flake it, or put it into casseroles or soups. Include seaweed in your miso soup to increase its nutritional value. You can wrap up seaweed like grape leaves. Seaweed is so versatile that entire books are devoted to its use in cookery.

Seaweed is loaded with minerals. In fact, there is 10 times more available calcium in hijiki, by dry weight, than in cow's milk.

Rethinking the Myths

At this point, we can answer a question raised by Joyce, who speaks for many when she says she's "been told for years that starchy vegetables such as potatoes and yams are fattening." She asks, "but are they?"

These foods are low in calories and rich in minerals and vitamins. It's what you put on them that makes them high in calories. A potato alone has only about 80 calories. But people often put about 150 calories' worth of butter or margarine on it. In fact, potatoes are an excellent source of vitamin C, in quantities comparable to that found in oranges.

Another benefit of eating starchy, high-fiber foods is that, because they digest rather slowly, you benefit from the natural sugars they contain over a period of several hours. Unlike that quick jolt of energy that you get from sugar when you have a soft drink, or a dessert, that makes you very high and then very low quickly, potatoes and other complex carbohydrates provide sustained energy.

There's one last group of healthy, detoxifying foods although, too often, Americans deliberately stay away from them. These are the beans, or legumes.

Why do people leave the room when Aunt Gertrude helps herself to beans? We have kept ourselves away from one of nature's most important sources of vitamins, minerals, and fiber, because we have never really understood how to cook them. Most people, and most restaurants, do not soak beans overnight. Because beans are not soaked overnight, when our body finally digests them, gas is formed in the colon, causing indigestion and flatulence. That uncomfortable feeling needn't be. All you have to do is soak beans overnight and then boil them for one to two hours. That usually takes care of most gas-producing properties. Then be sure to combine them with the right foods: Don't eat fruit or sugary foods with a bean meal.

Beans have more protein than grains or seeds. They are an excellent source of protein, as good in protein quality as animal proteins, yet also high in fiber.

Try adding legumes to your diet. Legumes include black-eyed peas, red beans, kidney beans, great northern beans, lentils, garbanzo beans, alfalfa, lima beans, and split peas, among others. There are over 60 different legumes.

Beans are a great way to help your body. They are low in calories, and high in protein, minerals, and complex carbohydrates.

If you eat this way, you're not going to have a problem with weight. You will be able to lose the extra weight that you are carrying, while you cleanse your body. You won't be taking toxic materials into your body and will meet the body's nutritional needs for proteins, vitamins, essential fatty acids, and minerals. And you will spend less on food. A detoxifying diet is exciting eating. And it's the basis of good health. The foundation is where we start.

The Four-Day Rotation Diet

Now let's look at what we can do to incorporate all this into a 14-day eating program. Keep in mind that the 14 days could be 1,400 days, 14 years, or the rest of your life. But here is a menu for two weeks to help get you started. Let's begin on Monday. We're going to take this on a 4-day rotational basis. I'll explain why later in the chapter.

DAY 1

BREAKFAST: Monday morning, start your day with a hot cereal breakfast. Today the hot cereal can be oatmeal.

SNACK: For a midmorning snack you can have a piece of fruit if you are not hypoglycemic or severely diabetic. If you are, you may want to have a food such as non-dairy cottage cheese or yogurt.

Take only small quantities of each food. On this eating program, you won't be eating until you're full, but only approximately 3 to 4 ounces of a given food. Thus, you may have as many as 12 to 14 ounces of total food in a given meal. The idea is to space your food over the day rather than eat a lot at one time.

By spacing your food, you will provide your body with energy, protein, carbohydrates, vitamins, and minerals throughout the day. After all, your body needs them 24 hours a day. People who skip breakfast, skimp on lunch, and then have the entire kitchen sink for dinner are only—after all is said and done—utilizing about 12 ounces of the food they eat. They're only able to use a small percentage of the protein they're taking in; the rest becomes fat. When you eat small amounts of food, several times throughout the day, very little becomes fat because your body is using it for energy throughout the day. This is a very important lesson if you want to lose weight and stay healthy.

LUNCH: For Monday lunch, help yourself to a sardine salad, an egg salad, or a tofu salad. Or, you can have a regular salad with a side order of any vegetables you like. You can choose steamed or stir-fried vegetables, and eat them with a grain, such as brown rice. If you are eating a salad, you might want to try serving your rice cold, the way the Japanese sometimes do. But remember—brown rice is preferable to white.

SNACK: For your midafternoon break, let's say between 2:00 and 4:00, have a juice, a fruit, or perhaps some marinated vegetable sticks. If you marinate them the night before in a vinaigrette sauce, you will find that your vegetables have a nice tangy quality to them.

DINNER: For dinner, you can start off with a soup. Try, for example, split pea soup with an appetizer of seaweed. There are many recipes for either cold or warm seaweed.

As a main entree, have a soy food over rice. In this way you combine a grain (rice) with a legume, soy beans in this case, in the form of either tofu or tempeh. By the way, if you like the taste of chicken and want to give it up, tempeh is a great alternative. It contains no cholesterol and is made from soy beans. It tastes like chicken, has as much protein, is low in calories, and high in calcium. It is, in fact, one of the best foods, nutritionally.

Finally, you can enjoy a salad at dinner. It should be a sprout salad on Monday. Make yourself a dressing, one without oil. There are many recipes for oil-less dressings. There are also already-prepared mixes to which you need only add water, vinegar, or lemon juice.

BEFORE BEDTIME: If you feel hungry before bed, drink some carbonated water with a pinch of lime or lemon in it.

Let's take a look at what Monday's foods will do for you. You will have eaten foods that are low on the food chain, meaning they contain lower concentrations of pesticides and other chemicals than animal protein. You've eaten plenty of fiber. Not only are high-fiber foods low in calories, they will also improve your digestion. You have eaten plenty of calcium and moderate amounts of protein. You've consumed no refined sugar or starch. You've eaten modest amounts of foods that are easily digested, therefore ones that don't overtax your digestive systems, taking away the oxygen and blood that you need in your brain. You've eaten foods from which nutrients are readily and easily available for absorption. Also, because so much chewing is necessary with these foods, you've been helping your jaws and lowering your appetite. The more you chew, the more quickly your appetite is satisfied. Chewing each bite well prevents you from gorging. A short list of foods for the day—oats, rice tofu, split peas, sprouts, seaweeds, and, if you wish, sardines or eggs—have accomplished so much to help detoxify and rebuild your health!

DAY 2

Hopefully, you are starting off your day with exercise. Fifteen minutes of aerobic exercise will improve your metabolism and stimulate the cells to burn more fatty acids, reducing overall body fat content and improving muscle tone as well as your overall sense of well-being.

BREAKFAST: For breakfast, begin with a glass of fruit juice. Fresh fruit juice is preferable to frozen or canned juices. Try making yourself fresh-squeezed grape juice. If you do, dilute it with some water, because grape juice is sweet.

Then, enjoy a different hot cereal. Today, try an alkalinizing cereal, millet. With the millet, you can puree in a banana, adding a sprinkle of cinnamon or nutmeg. Add just a little soy milk, fruit juice, or regular milk.

SNACK: For a midmorning snack, I generally carry a little extra millet with me in a plastic container, and eat four or five tablespoons when I get hungry. If I tell myself I'm going to have five tablespoons and no more, I count them out, and that's all I have, as a way of controlling the urge to overeat.

LUNCH: For lunch today, try a three-bean salad of black beans, kidney beans, and lentils. These beans supply protein, fiber, vitamins, and minerals galore. Also, try a salad of vegetables different from those eaten on Monday. For instance, if on Monday, you ate watercress, arugula and spinach, then on Tuesday, take chicory, romaine, or Boston lettuce. You might have a soup as well. This would be a good opportunity for a black bean soup with a slice of whole grain bread. No butter, no margarine. Just moist, chewy whole grain bread.

SNACK: For a midafternoon snack, have a piece of fruit, perhaps with another piece of whole grain bread. Whole grain bread only has around 100 calories and plenty of fiber in it. Therefore, it will be easily and quickly digested.

DINNER: For dinner on Tuesday, you might have hot millet, stir fried. Again, I like to make extra millet in the morning and have it all day long. Cooking it is just a matter of heating it up. Add a salad, and a different soup: kidney bean soup or a great northern bean soup.

For your main dish, eat fish. Salmon is a good choice. Fish not only gives you quality protein, but also essential fatty acids that your body needs. Omega-3 fatty acids—the kind found in many fish—have been shown to help the heart by lowering cholesterol levels.

SNACK: Later on, you can have your dessert. Never eat your dessert right after your meal: That's improper food combining. You do not want to combine a protein food, such as fish, which may take one to three hours to digest, with a simple sugar food that might have honey or fruit in it and may take only a half hour to digest. Combining sugary foods with protein or fat in the same meal leads to acid indigestion.

Wait till later in the evening and then have a banana. Try freezing it and then putting it into a blender or food processor. Whip it up, and it tastes like banana custard. For a special treat, take frozen cherries and frozen bananas and whip them together in a blender. You will be rewarded with a delicious, nutritious, and tasty dessert, low in calories, and high in complex carbohydrates, vitamins, and minerals. It is also very filling.

Thanks to your banana dessert late in the evening, and your fish, salad, soup, and millet earlier, you will feel full without having consumed too many calories. That's eating right for total health.

DAY 3

BREAKFAST: On Wednesday, begin your day with a hot rye cereal. Add to the rye cereal a fruit of your choice. Make it a fruit you have not eaten on either Monday or Tuesday. Take your cereal with some juice, rice milk, or soy milk.

SNACK: Later in the morning, eat a bit more of the morning cereal cold.

LUNCH: For lunch, enjoy a salad. Make it with different vegetables or different sprouts than Monday's or Tuesday's. Toss a handful of garbanzo beans into the salad today. Garbanzo beans are loaded with protein and are very nutritious. Mix some black-eyed peas or great northern beans in with the garbanzo beans to enhance the protein value of the beans.

Then, enjoy a soup made from any legume you didn't already eat on Monday or Tuesday. For example, you might want an aduki bean soup for lunch today.

SNACK: Later in the day, have some fruit or a vegetable if you still feel you need a snack.

DINNER: For dinner, start with miso soup. Then, try a guacamole, or avocado salad, made with mashed avocado, tomatoes, and lemon. Avocado is the fattiest fruit, so use only a quarter of an avocado for your guacamole. If you don't want guacamole, try another nutritious appetizer, babaganoush. This is a dish made from eggplant, garlic, and lemon juice. Anyone who's enjoyed Middle Eastern foods knows the joy of babaganoush.

For your main course, turn again to fish, this time filet of sole. You can also have a side dish of vegetables, such as peas and kale. In the salad, try such vegetables as marinated asparagus tips, broccoli, and cauliflower. That gives you a lot to eat, and you'll feel full, but not filled out, having kept your calories low but nutrients high.

DAY 4

BREAKFAST: Start off your day with a juice as before—a different fruit juice than the other days this week. For example, if one day you drank orange juice, you shouldn't repeat orange juice for another four days. Instead, you should have apple juice, prune juice, or grapefruit juice.

Then, enjoy a steaming bowl of wheatena or cream of wheat. These cereals are available everywhere. They are loaded with nutrition and high in fiber. But, to get more fiber into your system, to help cleanse your system, eat a bran muffin as well and be sure it's unsweetened.

SNACK: For a midmorning snack, have another bran muffin, since it contains only 70 calories. The muffin will help fill you up, but will also pass easily through your system.

LUNCH: For lunch, start off with some navy bean soup. Have salad, this time a marinated salad, like a cold salad or a seaweed salad. For your main entree have eggs, sardines, or tuna, whichever you didn't have on Monday.

SNACK: For later in the day, enjoy any type of fruit or vegetable, one that you haven't eaten on other days.

DINNER: For dinner, begin with a vegetable soup. Then, enjoy a tabouli salad, made with wheat and chopped parsley. As your main entree, try either sea bass or blue fish, served with hot seaweed. For your vegetable, have some red potatoes. This meal supplies complex carbohydrates, complete proteins, and plenty of fiber, along with chlorophyll, vitamins and minerals.

SNACK: Later at night, you could have a piece of frozen fruit or juice, if you feel the need.

The Rewards of Rotation

What was just described was an eating program for the first four days of your diet. This will form the pattern for the subsequent days. The basic concept is a four-day rotational diet.

Why a rotational diet? Because, very often, people's headaches, mood swings (going from a pleasant to an angry disposition), fatigue, musculoskeletal aches and pains, indigestion, postnasal drip, puffy eyes, and many other symptoms of not-quite-perfect health are exacerbated or caused by food sensitivities. We can become sensitive or allergic to any food we eat too frequently, including wheat, dairy, beef, chicken, corn, citrus fruits, peanuts, chocolate, soy, or any other food.

If you generally eat one or all these foods every day, you are likely to be food sensitive. This list includes the foods that clinical ecologists and allergists have found most likely to cause allergic reactions, as they predominate in the typical American diet.

Most people are familiar with the kind of allergies in which a person gets a skin rash immediately after eating, for example, strawberries. But there are other kinds of allergies that can be at fault when a child can't pay attention in class, or when an adult feels so tired after eating that he or she just wants to lay down and sleep. The allergies that cause these symptoms are very often caused by food sensitivities and can also lead to unnecessary pounds.

Studies have shown that when we are allergic to a food, we frequently have a faulty metabolism and gain weight above normal.

One of the fastest ways, then, to lose weight healthfully is to go on a four-day rotational diet and eliminate those foods to which we are allergic, or rotate them so that we don't have any one of them more frequently than every fourth day.

For example, if on Monday we ate oats, rice, split peas, the seaweed hijiki, and soy foods such as tofu or miso, we wouldn't have them again until Friday.

On Tuesday, if we ate millet, black-eyed peas, lentils, and kidney beans, we wouldn't have those again until Saturday. On Wednesday, if we ate rye, garbanzo beans, adzuki beans, sole, broccoli, asparagus and cauliflower, we wouldn't eat those foods again until Sunday. If on Thursday, we ate cream of wheat, navy beans, blue fish or sea bass, and red potatoes, we wouldn't consume those foods again until Monday.

Thus, we are creating a four-day rotational diet plan. Virtually all of the environmental medicine experts (also known as clinical ecologists) believe that our bodies need four days to recuperate after exposure to a food to which we are sensitive.

By now it should be clear how to turn a 4-day rotation into a 14-day eating program. You simply continue the same eating plan for 14 days. In other words, every fourth day you would start from the beginning. You can change your recipes, adding any vegetables or fish you haven't eaten for at least 4 days or longer. Give yourself two weeks to see the effects of combining exercise with a rotational eating plan, 14 days of eating wholesome, nourishing foods. If you've been allergic to foods, weaning yourself off them will frequently assist weight loss. You will also feel much better, and this will help inspire you to eat right from then on. The rotational diet can be used as the basis for a maintenance dietary program. It's easy, it's inexpensive, and the rewards of eating right for a lifetime will pay off a thousandfold.

This program doesn't just address the problem of weight loss. Excess weight is a symptom of a larger problem, one that can't be solved by going on a crash diet, even if you do lose 10 pounds in one week. This program is not an instant solution, but it offers you the chance to revitalize yourself in many areas of health. Weight loss is only one benefit. If you follow these guidelines, you'll feel more energetic and less stressed, and you'll probably live longer. In short, the quality of your life will improve.

If this diet seems to work for you after two weeks, try moving on to a vegetarian food diet (see chapter 13). Begin by extending your original 14-day program into a 21-day program, using only vegetarian foods during the final week. Then try staying on the vegetarian diet alone.

12

Vegetarianism

I s it possible to eat without partaking of the poisoned fruits of technology? A natural food diet, which relies on unrefined grains, legumes, seeds, nuts, and fresh produce, and steers clear of unnatural additives (including sugar and salt), is a step in the right direction. A diet that cuts down or eliminates meat is even closer to an unadulterated, healthful ideal.

There is abundant scientific evidence that proves the adequacy and, in fact, the superiority of a vegetarian diet. The medical literature is filled with studies indicating the protective qualities plant foods possess against many common degenerative diseases currently sweeping the Western world. More importantly, modern medicine is discovering that many of these diseases are directly linked to animal products consumption.

Being a vegetarian offers a wide variety of benefits, but to fully understand this dietary option it is useful to understand that there are a number of diets included under the broad term "vegetarianism."

Types of Vegetarians

VEGANS, the strictest of the vegetarians, thrive solely on plant foods, specifically vegetables, fruits, nuts, seeds, grains, and legumes. This regimen omits all animal foods, including meat, poultry, fish, eggs, dairy products, and honey.

LACTO-VEGETARIANS eat milk and milk products in addition to vegetable foods.

LACTO-OVO-VEGETARIANS consume eggs along with milk products and vegetables. This basically is a nonflesh diet.

PESCOVEGETARIANS eat fish in addition to the plant sources. In Asia, hundreds of millions of people follow this type of diet, living on staples of rice and fish.

POLLOVEGETARIANS omit red meat from their diets, but eat poultry in conjunction with plant sources.

All of the vegetarian diets include an abundance of complex carbohydrates, naturally occurring vitamins and minerals, polyunsaturated fats, fiber, and easily digestible quantities of protein. A statistical analysis shows that they closely resemble the diet recommended in the "Dietary Goals for the U.S." set by the Senate Select Committee on Nutrition and Human Needs.

Man, The Herbivore

Underlying any scientific evaluation of vegetarianism is evidence that humans are not biochemically suited to eat meat. Indeed, we possess all of the features of a strictly herbivorous animal. Our flat teeth are not sharp enough to tear through hide or bone. Our lengthy digestive tract resembles that of the classic herbivore. Most carnivores are anatomically constructed to quickly get rid of the meat they eat before it putrefies, and to eliminate the majority of their dietary cholesterol. We aren't. Our digestion begins in the mouth as the salivary glands secrete an enzyme designed to break down the complex plant cells. Carnivores don't have this enzyme. They secrete an enzyme called uricase that breaks down the uric acid in meat.

The Dangers of Meat

Although designed to subsist on vegetarian foods, man has perverted his dietary habits to accept the food of the carnivore, and thus has increased the risks of developing a number of disorders and diseases.

For instance, saturated fat and cholesterol, which are found in high amounts in many meats and other animal fats, increase the risk of hardening of the arteries and heart disease.

The leading cause of death in America, heart disease, is three times more likely to occur in meat eaters than vegetarians. Consuming meat doubles your chances for colon and rectal cancer, while tripling them for breast cancer. The high-protein intake of beef eaters places undue stress on the liver and kidneys, two important organs of detoxification. It may deplete your calcium supply, leading to osteoporosis, and the uric acid it contains can settle in the joints, inducing painful gouty arthritis.

In addition, there are hidden poisons in meat and poultry that, when eaten, place undue stress on our digestive systems. These include hormones, antibiotics, tranquilizers, additives, preservatives, and pesticides that are added to the meat in breeding and processing the animals. Such long-term bodily pollution creates a vast overall negative effect on our health, making us susceptible to a host of pathological abnormalities. Health benefits commonly noticed by vegetarians include improved digestion and decreased gastrointestinal disturbances, including less gas and constipation.

If meat is so bad for our health, how has it become the principle staple of the American diet? Alex Hershart, of the Vegetarian Information Service, was asked that question at a Senate Subcommittee on Health and Scientific Research. He replied: "The answer goes to the very heart of what's wrong with the decision-making machinery of the federal government, where issues are decided less on the basis of their scientific merit than of their economic and political consequences. Few politicians are willing to face up to the $35 billion meat industry and to the several million farmers who make their living from raising animals for food."

Time after time, the public is warned against the nutritional deficiencies of "ill-planned vegetarian diets," or we read that "most nutritionists agree that vegetarian diets can be adequate, if sufficient care is taken in planning them."

The fact is that any ill-planned diet should be avoided, no matter what foods are eaten. Sufficient care should be taken in the planning and preparation of all meals—vegetarian and nonvegetarian alike.

The misguided meat eater reading the warnings that surround vegetarianism by rivals of that diet, such as the American Dairy Association, will incorrectly assume that as long as they are healthy, they don't have to give up anything in their diets—even pork, fat, or sugar. We have blindly assumed for too long that so-called "healthy" foods cannot hurt us and that meat is magical. These, quite simply, are myths that have been fabricated and propagated by the meat and dairy industries.

No one food is indispensable or magical. Animal flesh, for instance, is nearly void of carbohydrates, has little or no fiber, and is a poor source of calcium and vitamin C. It is naturally high in saturated fats and cholesterol. Meat eaters derive their complex carbohydrates, dietary fiber, and other nutrients from the same source as vegetarians—vegetables. When meat is omitted, you sacrifice all the harmful ingredients it has while still being able to acquire needed protein from plant sources. Lacto-vegetarians, for example, eat dairy products as sources of calcium and B_{12}. While one cup of whole milk contains 288 mg of calcium, thiamin, iron, and trace minerals, nuts and other seeds contribute fat, protein, B vitamins, and iron. Dark green, leafy vegetables are sources of calcium, riboflavin, and carotene and should be eaten in generous amounts.

Depending not on variety but on meat instead for one's nutritional requirements can lead to a variety of health problems. We maintain a false sense of security because meat provides an adequate amount of high-quality protein. But amino acids, the component parts of protein, are only one of the things that make us thrive.

Vegetarians can dispense with animal products because a varied diet of whole grains, nuts, seeds, vegetables, and fruits will automatically provide all nine essential amino acids (the eight essential amino acids plus one, histamine, which is essential for children) in a quality and quantity equal to or sometimes surpassing the "incredible edible egg," nature's most complete protein food.

The Vegetarian Spectrum

When we sit down to a freshly mixed salad filled with dark green, leafy vegetables, a variety of sprouts and carrots, millet with tahini-oat gravy, and sautéed tempeh with garlic, we are receiving complex carbohydrates, essential fatty acids, complete protein, various B complex vitamins, calcium, iron, and a host of other nutrients. A variety of colorful, wholesome, unprocessed foods encompassing a flavorful spectrum provides the greatest nutritional package.

Americans have a number of misguided ideas about vegetarianism and how it might affect their health. Some, for instance, fear that a vegetarian diet is fattening. This would, of course, be true if one exceeded one's proper caloric needs, no matter what foods are eaten. People think of certain vegetarian foods as especially fattening, and they're often wrong. The biggest victim of this misconception is the potato. A medium-sized plain potato has only about 70 calories, and is packed with essential amino acids and vitamin C. Excess calories come only from the garnishes that usually accompany the potato, from the globs of butter, sour cream, or oil, to chili, cheddar cheese, and bacon.

A nonflesh diet will, in the long run, lower your risk of developing many diseases and raise your chances of maintaining good health. Vegetarian diets are especially health promoting during periods of physiological of physical stress in which more nutrients are needed than at other times. These include pregnancy, lactation, periods of rapid growth as during childhood and adolescence, and times of illness and convalescence. Everyone from the very young to the very old can probably benefit from such a diet.

Reasons for Choosing Vegetarianism

Although health improvement is the primary reason why an increasing number of people are giving up meat, there are a number of other reasons for adopting a vegetarian diet.

ECONOMICS. The rising cost of living in general and of meat in particular has forced many people to adopt a vegetarian meal plan. Ounce for ounce, plant foods are more economical than other foods. They supply more fiber and a wider variety of vitamins and minerals. The same amount of protein costs one-fifth as much when obtained from plant sources as from animal sources.

In addition, agribusiness—huge agricultural companies—has dominated the animal food industry; its high technology and centralization have created unemployment and forced many small farmers out of business. Many people choose not to support these companies by not buying meat. The switch to a no- or low-meat vegetarian diet can benefit the individual without disrupting the overall economic structure by tending to support small farmers rather than giant agribusiness conglomerates.

NATURAL RESOURCES. The production and processing of animal products demands an enormous amount of land, water, energy, and raw materials. The rapid depletion of these precious, finite resources is of great concern. The grim reality of the fragility of our ecosystem encourages responsible vegetarian lifestyles, which do not involve wasting more resources than they use, as does the meat industry.

FOOD RESOURCES. The idea of eating simply so that everyone may eat is supported by the animal-free diet. Our land is capable of supplying food for nearly 14 times as many people when it is used for human food crops as when it is being used to feed livestock, as animals are a grossly inefficient source of nutrition. They need to consume approximately 26 pounds of grain in order to yield one pound of flesh. It has been estimated that our current supply of plant foods could nourish more than double the world population if we managed it better. This substantial waste of protein, calories, and other essential nutrients contributes to global imbalances and starvation. Ultimately, our demand for meat must be drastically curtailed if we are to positively affect the worldwide hunger problem.

REVERENCE FOR LIFE. Many people are now refusing a dietary style that supports the cruel treatment and wanton slaughter of millions of animals. Since every person who consumes animal products perpetuates the unnecessary and agonizing existence and brutal death of these innocent creatures, these vegetarians actively defy the harsh reality of this inhumane treatment by adhering to plant food diets.

RELIGIOUS BELIEFS. There are various contemporary and ancient faiths that advocate abstinence from meat. Some favor spiritual awareness and reincarnation, others emphasize ethical considerations and health benefits. In the East, these faiths include the Hindus and Buddhists; in the West, they include the Seventh Day Adventists.

PERSONAL TASTE. Meat consumption is an acquired habit, not an organic necessity. It starts in childhood for most people, backed by the encouragement of generations of misinformed parents. Our natural taste is actually for the full-flavored, wholesome taste of vegetarian cuisine. This is shown by the fact that most people lose their taste for flesh once it is omitted from their diet. Innumerable culinary delights can be concocted from a wide variety of plant foods, including herbs and spices, and these delicious dishes prove that the only limitations that exist are man-made.

There are numerous reasons why more people than ever before are adopting the vegetarian diet. Such a simple change in our individual style of eating not only enhances our health and well-being, but also strongly influences our economic, political, and environmental systems. The dietary regimen we follow is an important aspect of our existence, making a statement for each of us that either supports or attacks the earthly sphere and natural order in which we dwell. The choice is ours.

A Guide to Vegetarian Foods

Being a vegetarian means more than subsisting on lettuce. A variety of wholesome food combinations are possible within this dietary option. Creative preparation can yield an infinite array of culinary delights.

WHOLE GRAINS To the vegetarian, grains are a particularly important food staple. Use a variety of them; each has a rich flavor to impart. But to enjoy these grains' true taste, choose those grown free of chemical fertilizers and sprays. Also, the less whole grains are processed, the greater their nutritional value.

Whole grains contain everything needed to nurture themselves, from germ stage to sprout to mature plant. Plant a whole kernel of any grain and, given the right combination of earth, water, and air, it will naturally sprout and grow to maturity. Not so with refined grains. Bury a milled kernel and cultivate it as much as you like; nothing will grow because the kernel is already dead.

Milling the root of whole grains only refines away a wide range of trace minerals and vitamins in the outer layers, resulting in grains that are bulkier and less healthy. Refined grains, robbed of the minerals and vitamins found in the discarded outer layers, strain the body's delicate mechanism of digestion. Nearly all of the B vitamins, vitamins E, unsaturated fatty acids, and quality proteins are found in whole grains, but refining removes most of these nutrients. Even in so-called enriched foods, only a few B vitamins and iron are replaced; the remaining B vitamins, as well as a rich variety of minerals and proteins, are "refined" out.

There are three ways to prepare whole grains for eating: sprouting, soaking, and cooking until tender. All grains can be sprouted in two to three days, or until the sprout reaches the same length as the original seeds. You can reconstitute some semiprocessed grains, such as bulgar wheat, by soaking them overnight or pouring boiling water over them and allowing them to fluff up.

When you cook grains, first rinse them in a colander or strainer, then pour the grain into a pot of water, and swirl it with your hands, removing the hulls and bits of dirt that may float to the surface. Drain the grain through a strainer, dry pan-fry it in a heavy skillet, and add two parts boiling water. Cover the skillet, reduce the heat, and let the grain simmer for about a half hour (time varies with the grain).

When preparing grains in a pressure cooker, the proportion of water to grain is roughly 2½ parts water for each part of grain. Add grain and water to the cooker and bring them rapidly up to full pressure. When the regulator on the lid makes a juggling sound, the cooker has reached full pressure; reduce the heat to simmer and maintain the same pressure throughout the cooking. Allow the pressure to return to normal before loosening the lid, then open the pot and gently stir the grains, mixing the kernels toward the bottom with those at the top. Let them sit for a few minutes, then mix again.

Most grains at least double in size from their dry to cooked states. This means that one cup of cooked grain can feed two or three enthusiastic grain eaters or three to four people eating grain along with other foods. To achieve a sweeter flavor and crunchier texture, try dry-toasting the grain or sautéing it before cooking. To dry-toast, start with a cold skillet, preferably cast iron. To sauté, you must first heat the skillet and then quickly, evenly, coat it with oil. (If the oil smokes, it's too hot.) Whether dry-toasting or sautéing, stir the grain until a few kernels pop and a delicious aroma begins to rise.

BARLEY

Barley has much to offer as a solo grain dish. Some of the best barley in the world—consistently high in protein and minerals—comes from the rich soil of the Red River Valley of North Dakota and Minnesota.

Since unhulled barley is almost impossible to cook, practically all barley available in food stores has been "pearled" so as to remove its tenacious hull. The factor to consider here is just how much pearling has taken place; too much results in a whiter product robbed of the nutrients in its outer layer. Look for the darker barley available in most natural food stores.

Allow 30 to 35 minutes to cook simmered barley using 2⅓ parts liquid (water, stock, etc.) to 1 part grain. The barley can also be browned before adding it to the boiling liquid. Pressure cooking (2 parts water to 1 part grain) takes approximately 20 minutes. If the resulting grain seems too chewy, simply add ¼ cup more water, cover, and simmer until soft. You might also try cooking barley with other grains, such as brown rice and wheat berries.

Barley can be sprouted, but first it has to be hulled (try seed houses and grain suppliers). Harvest the sprout when it's about the same size as the grain. Barley flour can be obtained already milled or ground fresh from the pearled grain. It is often pan-roasted before being used in breads, muffins, and cakes. Recently, researchers have found that barley, eaten daily, is successful in lowering cholesterol levels by 25 percent.

BUCKWHEAT

Buckwheat is actually not a true grain but a grass seed related to rhubarb. When raised commercially as a grain crop, buckwheat is unlikely to have been fertilized or sprayed. Fertilization encourages too much leaf growth; spraying stops the bees from pollinating. The best buy is whole, hulled, unroasted (white) buckwheat grains, known as groats. Roasted (brown) and cut groats are less nutritious, and the roasting can easily be done just before cooking without disturbing the flavor or the B vitamins.

Buckwheat cooks quickly, so it is rarely pressure cooked. Simmer for 15 to 20 minutes in the same saucepan or skillet you first roasted it in, using two parts water to one part buckwheat. If you prefer a porridgelike consistency, use three parts water. Cooked buckwheat can serve as a stuffing for everything from cabbage leaves and collard greens to knishes. Buckwheat flour combined variously with whole wheat, unbleached white, and soy flours is a delight to pancake lovers. Whole grain buckwheat flour is always dark; light-colored buckwheat flour is made from sifted flour rather than from unroasted groats. A Japanese pasta called soba (containing anywhere from 30 to 100 percent buckwheat flour) is now readily available in natural food stores and in Asian markets. Its subtle flavor and light effect on the stomach should encourage pasta enthusiasts to give it a try. It needs no heavy sauces; try a simple garlic or onion and oil topping.

You can prepare a buckwheat cream for morning cereal from buckwheat flour sautéed in oil in a heavy skillet. Allow it to cool and then return it to the heat, gradually adding water and bringing it to a boil. This mixture is then stirred and simmered about 10 minutes or until it reaches the desired consistency.

Sprout buckwheat from the unhulled groats in half an inch of soil on wet paper toweling and allow it to reach a height of three to four inches. The sprouts or young grass, called buckwheat lettuce, can then be juiced or chewed. The bioflavonoid rutin, which is reported to speed the coagulation of blood, helping to stop bleeding, is very high in sprouted buckwheat.

CORN

Corn, a staple food for thousands of years, has changed from a small shrub with only a few kernels to today's hybrid varieties with six-foot stalks bearing several ears that contain over a hundred kernels apiece. Both white and yellow varieties of dried corn are readily available, but in the American Southwest the blue and varicolored older types of corn are still grown. "Sweet" corn is normally boiled or steamed in water; field corn is likely to be ground into meals and flours. Field corn is allowed to dry out completely, which changes the simple sugars of the grain into starches.

Yellow cornmeal contains about 10 percent protein and is higher in vitamin A than the white variety. The only difference between a meal and a flour from yellow corn is its degree of coarseness. The germ of cornmeal starts deteriorating in a matter of hours, so you should grind your own meal or flour as you use it for cornbreads, muffins, Southern spoon bread, johnnycakes, or whatever. You can fry it in a pan and then cook it with five to six parts water as a hearty "mush". Adding cornmeal to whole wheat flour in a tempura batter gives it a delicious crunchiness.

Another favorite form of this versatile grain is creamed corn. You can make creamed corn by cutting off the kernels just far enough down to allow the milky, sugary liquid to flow. Pour in enough water or milk to cover, a dash of salt, and cook the mixture gently for a few minutes. Corn flour can also be used in small amounts in whole grain pastas. A variety of Texas Deaf Smith County sweet corn can be sprouted successfully until the sprout is about a half-inch long.

MILLET

The many virtues of millet are often overlooked because of its reputation as "the poor person's rice". Being the only grain that forms alkaline, millet is the most easily digestible. It is also an intestinal lubricant. Its amino acid structure is well balanced, providing a low-gluten protein, and it is high in calcium, riboflavin, and lecithin.

Millet is cooked the same way as most grains, with two parts water or stock to one part grain. Preroasting releases a lovely aroma and adds texture to the cooked grain. Leftover cooked millet is a highly versatile stuffing for anything from hollowed-out zucchini halves to mushroom caps.

Millet meal and millet flour are quality protein additions to any bread recipe. Millet meal also makes a good hot cereal. Sprouted millet makes an excellent base for morning cereal; just harvest the sprout when the shoot is the same size as the grain.

OATS

Oats must be hulled before they can be eaten; after hulling they are cracked or rolled into the familiar cereal forms. Rolled oats are shot with steam for a number of seconds and then passed through rollers; thus some nutrients are lost. Rolled oats will cook faster than whole oat groats, but whole oat groats are the most beneficial. Known variously as Irish oatmeal, Scotch oats, or steel-cut oats, whole-oat groats are soaked overnight before being cooked as porridge. (None of these or any other cereals or porridges should ever be prepared in a pressure cooker; they tend to clog the vent on the lid of the cooker.) Whole oats are wonderful in soups. You can add both rolled and whole groats to all sorts of breads and patties.

Oat flour, available at most natural food stores, can be used in equal proportions with whole wheat flour to bake up a tasty batch of muffins. Oat sprouts can be used in soups, salads, and baked goods; just harvest the sprout when it is as long as the groat.

RICE

Rice, from a nutritional point of view, means brown rice—whole grain rice which, unlike white rice, has not had its bran, and with it much of its nutrition, removed. Brown rice is available in short, medium, and long grain varieties, the difference being largely aesthetic. The shorter the grain, the more gluten, which means that short grain rice cooks up stickier and long grain comes out fluffier. There's even a sweet rice grain, the most glutinous of all. Excellent quality long- and medium-grain brown rice comes from southeast Texas and Louisiana; this rice is hulled by a special process that protects the bran layer.

Rice is traditionally simmered, the proportions of water to grain being as follows: short grain—2½ to 1; medium grain—2 to 1; and long grain—1½ to 1. All three varieties take from 25 to 35 minutes to cook fully. Stir regularly to prevent the grains that are on the bottom from scorching.

For pressure cooking, the proportion of water to grain is different: short grain—2 to 1; medium grain—1½ to 1; long grain—1¼ to 1. When the rice is cooked, allow the pressure to return slowly to normal. Some of the cooling steam will add moisture to the grain.

Brown rice is a versatile grain aside from its variety of lengths. Rice cream is made commercially by a dry-roasting method, after which the grain is stone ground to a consistency somewhat coarser than rice flour. You can prepare it as a porridge from the whole grain itself, or from prepacked rice-cream powder. Combine the rice with four cups of lightly salted boiling water and stir constantly over a low heat to prevent lumping. Rice flour is used extensively in baking, especially by those on gluten-restricted diets. Rice flakes make quick additions to soups or casserole bases when no other leftovers are available.

The flaking process for grains and beans was originally developed to improve animal nutrition. The grains are cooked for 15 to 20 seconds under dry radiant heat and then are dropped onto rollers and flattened into whole grain flakes. Since no wet methods of processing are used, there is only very minimal leaching and modifying of nutrients. And flaked grains and beans cook in half the usual time. You can add them to breads and casseroles for protein, texture, or taste. In chili, wheat flakes serve to complete the protein of the bean.

A rice-based grain milk called kokoh is available prepacked at natural food outlets. This mixture of roasted and ground rice, sweet rice, soybeans, sesame seeds and oatmeal is good as a morning cereal or tea.

But be careful about your source of brown rice. Commercially produced rice is among the most heavily chemically-treated food crops.

RYE

Rye is mostly known in its flour form, used in bread loaves often flavored with caraway seeds. Especially in its sprouted form, rye is rich in vitamin E, phosphorus, magnesium, and silicon. Like wheat sprouts, rye sprouts sweeten as they lengthen because the natural starches turn to sugar. For salad purposes, use the rye sprout when it's the same size as the grain; allow it to lengthen up to one inch for a sweeter intestinal-cleansing sprout and for cooking. Rye can also be harvested as a grass and chewed for its juice.

The whole rye berry is a good grain, adding chewiness and nutritious value, to combine with rice (use about one part rye to two parts rice). Rye flakes can be added to soups and stews, or used as a cereal if soaked overnight. Rye flakes, like wheat and oat flakes, make good homemade granolas. For cream of rye, somewhat coarser in texture than rye flour, add four parts water to one part grain and simmer it over a low heat for about 15 minutes.

TRITICALE

Triticale, a highly nutritious grain with a relatively high protein content (approximately 17 percent) and a good balance of amino acids, can be cooked whole in combination with other grains, especially rice (two parts water to one part triticale). Sprouted, it can be used in salads or breads; flaked, in granolas and casseroles. Triticale flour has become a favorite of vegetarians because of its unusually nutty sweetness and high protein content. As a flour it must be mixed with other flours containing higher gluten contents, since its own protein has a low gluten content.

WHOLE WHEAT

Today, whole wheat holds a pre-eminent position among grains because of its versatility and high nutritive qualities. Containing anywhere from 6 to 20 percent protein, wheat is also a source of vitamin E and large amounts of nitrates. These nutrients are distributed throughout the three main parts of the wheat kernel or berry. The outer layers of the kernel are known collectively as the bran; there is relatively little protein here, but it is of high quality and rich in the amino acid lysine. The dietary fiber of wheat bran is also the site of about half of the 11 B vitamins found in wheat, as well as the greater portion of the trace minerals zinc, copper, and iodine. Next comes the endosperm, the white starchy central mass of wheat kernel, which contains some 70 percent of the kernel's total protein, as well as its calorie-providing starch. Finally, there is the small germ found at the base of the kernel, which, in addition to containing the same B vitamins and trace minerals as the bran, is the home of vitamin E and the unsaturated fatty acids.

If you use the wheat berry in conjunction with other grains such as rice, you get the entire nutritive value of the grain. Try pan-roasting ⅓ cup of wheat berries with ⅔ cup rice and then simmering them with 2 cups water for 25 to 30 minutes until both grains are tender. You can also eat whole wheat as wheat flakes, cracked wheat, bulgur, couscous, sprouts, and flours (both hard and pastry). The flaking process preserves most of the nutrients of the original form.

Wheat flakes lend themselves especially well to chili dishes, where their addition to the beans provides a completed protein. If added dry to vegetarian chili about 20 minutes before serving, they will break down into tiny pieces to satisfy the appetites of even the most ardent chili con carne aficionados. Cracked wheat (simple coarse-ground wheat) is most often used as a morning cereal cooked with about three cups salted water to one cup wheat; it is often added cooked to uncooked to breads and muffins.

Bulgur is a variety of whole grain wheat that is parboiled, dried (often in the sun), and then coarsely cracked. This Near and Middle Eastern staple has found its way to America in a distinctive salad called tabouli. Bulgar does not require cooking but is simply reconstituted by spreading the grain an inch deep in a shallow pan and pouring enough boiling water over it to leave about half an inch of standing water; once the water is absorbed, stir the grain several times with a fork until it's cool. It can then be chilled, combined with greens such as parsley, fresh mint, and watercress, and marinated in a dressing of sesame oil, lemon juice, and tamari.

Couscous is a form of soft, refined durum wheat flour ("semolina") that has been steamed, cracked and dried. It can be prepared for eating by adding one cup of couscous to two cups of boiling salted water with a teaspoon of butter or margarine if desired, reducing the heat and stirring constantly until most of the moisture is gone. Remove the couscous from the heat and let it stand covered about 15 minutes, fluffing it up several times with a fork.

Wheat also makes an excellent sprout, containing substantially larger amounts of all the vitamins and minerals found in the dormant kernel. The sprout, which sweetens as it lengthens, can be used in desserts.

Whole wheat flour can be made from hard wheat (high protein, high gluten) or soft wheat (lower protein and gluten, high starch), or from spring or winter wheats. Hard wheats are excellent for making bread. The spring wheat contains a higher gluten content than the winter wheat. Soft wheat, either spring or winter, is known as pastry wheat because it yields a fine, starchy flour. Wheat flours are available at natural food stores in many pasta forms—from alphabets to ziti—often combined with other flours such as buckwheat, corn, rice, soy, and Jerusalem artichoke.

Whole grain flours can become rancid. Rancidity occurs when the unsaturated fats in the flour are exposed to the oxygen in the air. The vitamin E in the whole wheat flour acts as a natural preservative, but within three months it is exhausted. This problem can best be handled by storing the flour in a cool dry place immediately after milling. There are a number of small natural food companies that mill and distribute their fresh-ground flour. Home grinding machines are now available at many natural food stores.

STANDARD WHITE FLOUR

Standard white flour is purely endosperm, with most of the bran and germ removed, which means a loss of up to 70 percent of the essential nutrients of wheat. In addition, white flour may be bleached by chlorine dioxide, which completely destroys the vitamin E. "Enriched" flours are actually attempts at making up for these losses; but only four nutrients—compounds of thiamine, niacin, riboflavin (vitamin B2), and iron—are replaced. Most unbleached white flour has had much of its bran removed, but at least it has not been bleached. Soft wheat pastry flour, which can be substituted for unbleached white flour in any recipe, is a nutritionally superior, whole, refined flour.

WHEAT GLUTEN

Wheat gluten (kofu, in Japanese cookery) has long been a popular vegetarian source of protein in many places around the world. It is prepared by mixing whole wheat flour and water in a 2½ to 1 ratio and kneading it into a stiff dough. This dough is then covered with cold water and kneaded underwater; as the water clouds up with starch sediment, it is replaced and the procedure is repeated about five or six times until the water remains clear. Then the remaining gluten dough is steamed or cooked in a double boiler for 30 minutes. Kofu may be eaten as is, flavored with soy sauce, or baked in casserole loaves combined with other grains, such as rice and beans.

AMARANTH AND QUINOA

Amaranth and Quinoa are two grains new to the American diet that have recently come on the market.

Amaranth is a native grain. It has been cultivated in the American Southwest for hundreds of years. The plant yields a tiny seed that should be prepared similarly to rice. When cooked, it has a very soft, nutlike consistency.

Quinoa, a staple of the Inca Indians, is a delicate, light-textured, high-protein grain that resembles tiny granules of tabouli or couscous. Known as "the mother grain," it is high in complete protein, cooks in 10 to 15 minutes, and approximately triples its volume when cooked, somewhat mitigating its current high price in health food stores.

BEANS (LEGUMES) The members of the bean family are important, inexpensive sources of protein, minerals and vitamins. Legumes can be cooked whole, flaked like grains, sprouted, ground into flours, even transformed into a variety of "dairy" products.

As a general rule, 1 cup of dry beans will make about 2½ cups of cooked beans, enough for four servings. Some beans should be soaked, preferably overnight; these include adzuki beans, black beans, chick-peas (garbanzos), and soybeans. As an alternative to overnight soaking, you can bring the beans (1 cup) and water (3 to 4 cups) to a boil, remove the pot from the stove and cover, let the beans sit for an hour, then cook the beans by simmering after first bringing them to a boil, or by putting them in a pressure cooker.

When using beans for a soup dish, allow five times as much water as beans at the beginning of the cooking process. Don't salt the water until the beans are soft (or after the pressure in the cooker has come down), because the salt will draw the moisture out of the beans.

ADZUKI

Adzuki are small red beans that have a special place in Japanese cuisine as well as in traditional Japanese medicine, where they are used as a remedy for kidney ailments (when combined with a small pumpkin called hokkaido). Very high in B vitamins and trace minerals, adzukis should never be pressure-cooked because it makes them bitter.

After overnight soaking, simmer adzukis with a strip of kombu (a kind of kelp) for about 1 to 1½ hours until tender, with four to five cups of water to each cup of beans. One favorite preparation: add one cup each of sautéed onions and celery to the tender beans and then puree them together in a blender. The resulting thick, creamy soup can be thinned with water or bean juice and flavored with a dash of lime juice, tamari, and mild curry.

BLACK BEANS AND TURTLE BEANS

Black beans and their close relative, turtle beans, have served as major food sources in the Caribbean, Mexico, and the American Southwest for many years. These beans should not be prepared in a pressure cooker since their skins fall off easily and may clog the valve. A smooth, rich black bean soup, a specialty of Cuba, is made by cooking the soaked beans until tender, adding sautéed garlic, onions, and celery, and then pressing the mixture through a colander (or, more easily, quickly blending it in an electric blender). A small amount of lime juice may be added to lighten the taste.

BLACK-EYED PEAS

Black-eyed peas, a Southern favorite, provide a delicious complete protein-balanced meal. Among the quickest-cooking beans, they become tender in 45 minutes to an hour. Eating this bean on New Year's Day is said to bring good luck throughout the year.

CHICK-PEAS (GARBANZOS)

Chick-peas, or garbanzos, are so versatile that they have been the subject of entire cookbooks. High in protein, they are also good sources of calcium, iron, potassium, and B vitamins. They can be roasted, like peanuts, or boiled. After a very thorough roasting, chick-peas can even be ground and used as a coffee substitute. Hummus is a thick paste that combines mashed chick-peas, hulled sesame-seed tahini, garlic, and lemon juice. Bean patés using chick-peas as a base offer many creative opportunities for creating complete proteins, by combining different beans. Cooked grains, ground seeds and nuts, raw vegetables, herbs, and miso may all be combined with the cooked beans to produce a sophisticated and appealing paté or paste.

GREAT NORTHERN BEANS AND NAVY BEANS

Great northern beans and their small counterpart, navy beans, cook in less than an hour and require no presoaking. They are often used for hearty soups. Cook the beans with five to six parts water or stock to one part dry beans. Firmer vegetables, such as carrots, rutabagas, or turnips should be added one-half hour before the soup is finished; other vegetables, such as onions, celery and peppers, should be added 15 minutes later, either sautéed or raw.

KIDNEY BEANS

Kidney beans, standard in all sorts of chilis, will cook in about an hour, after having been soaked overnight. The fragrant brown bean juice produced in cooking the beans makes the addition of tomato virtually unnecessary. Once the beans are tender, try dicing onions, garlic, and red and green peppers; sauté them lightly in sesame oil until the onions are translucent, then add them to the beans. Season them to taste. Rich Mexican chili powder seems to lend more flavor to the beans than does a scorching Indian one. Tamari, a dash of blackstrap molasses, or fresh-grated ginger root can further enhance the beans. For a perfect final texture, add dry wheat flakes to the chili about 20 minutes before serving; this allows time for the flakes to cook and disintegrate, thickening the dish while complementing the protein of the beans.

LENTILS

Lentils come in a rainbow of colors, but generally only the green, brown, and red varieties are available in the United States. All are inexpensive and nutritious sources of iron, cellulose, and B vitamins. Lentils require no presoaking and disintegrate when cooked, leaving a smooth base to which you can add fresh or sautéed vegetables (including carrots, turnips, onions, and peppers). They sprout well in combination with other seeds and produce large quantities. The flavor of the uncooked sprout is similar to that of fresh ground pepper on salad; when cooked it has a more nutlike taste. The sprouts should be harvested when the shoot is as long as the seed.

MUNG BEANS

Mung beans are probably best known in their sprout form, eaten raw or lightly sautéed with other vegetables. They can be cooked as a dry bean, using three times as much water as beans, and then pureed in an electric blender into a smooth soup. The result is rather bland and benefits from the addition of tamari and fresh or dried basil. But as sprouts, mung beans really come into their own. Mung sprouts are rich in vitamins A and C and contain high amounts of calcium, phosphorus, and iron. The hulls are easily digestible and rich in minerals. Mung sprouts can be harvested any time from the second day, when the shoot has just appeared, to the third or fourth day when the shoot is about four inches long. Mung beans make a good first choice for beginning sprouters.

PEANUTS

Peanuts, though commonly grouped with seeds and nuts, are actually members of the legume family. Their high protein content is well known. In the United States eating peanut butter is virtually a national pastime. Peanut butter can— and should—contain 100 percent peanuts; sugars, colorings, stabilizers, and preservatives are neither necessary nor desirable. A single grinding under pressure extracts enough oil from the nut meal to give the peanuts a creamy texture.

PINTO BEANS

Pinto beans are popular in American Southwest dishes and lend themselves especially well to baking. Naturally sweet in flavor, they adapt to many types of seasonings, and once cooked tender, they can be used in casseroles. Pinto flakes cook quickly and reconstitute themselves into tender round beans in about 40 minutes (two parts water to one part dry flakes). Cumin blends nicely with these beans, if used sparingly.

SOYBEANS

Soybeans, unquestionably the most nutritious of all the beans, have been the major source of protein in Asian diets for centuries. They are increasingly being viewed as the most realistic source of high-quality, low-cost protein available today on a large enough scale to meet worldwide needs. In addition to high-quality protein, soybeans contain large amounts of B vitamins, minerals, and unsaturated fatty acids in the form of lecithin that help the body emulsify cholesterol.

Thanks to their bland flavor after cooking and their high concentration of nutrients, soybeans can be made into an amazingly diverse array of foods. Western technology in recent years has focused on creating a wide range of synthetic soybean foods. There are protein concentrates in the form of soy powder containing from 70 to 90 percent moisture-free protein, isolates (defatted flakes and flours used to make simulated dairy products and frozen deserts), spun protein fibers (isolates dissolved in alkali solutions for use in simulated meat products), and textured vegetable proteins (made from soy flour and used in simulated meat products and infant foods). Most Western cooks also have come across soybeans in the form of full-fat soy flour, soy granules, and defatted soy flour and grits—all of which are available in natural food stores. Full-fat soy flour, which contains about 40 percent protein and 20 percent naturally occurring oils, makes a fine addition to many forms of baked goods. Soy granules contain about 50 percent protein, as do defatted soy flour and soy grits, which are basically byproducts of the extraction of soy oil. Both are used in breakfast cereals, simulated meats, and desserts. Soybeans are also processed into flakes which, unlike raw soybeans, require no presoaking and only about 1½ hours of cooking.

The soybean can be enjoyed in many ways, as tofu (see below), or as a fresh green summer vegetable, simmered or steamed in the pod. Roasted soybeans are now available in many varieties: dry-roasted, oil-roasted, salted, unsalted, and with garlic or barbecue flavors. They contain up to 47 percent protein and can either be eaten as a snack or added to casseroles for texture.

When cooking whole dry soybeans, a pressure cooker can save a great deal of time. Use 2½ to 3 cups of water over a low flame for each cup of dry soybeans. Once the right pressure has been reached, cook until tender—about 90 minutes. Before cooking soybeans by the ordinary simmering method, soak them overnight in 4 cups of water. Bring them to a boil in 4 more cups of liquid and simmer about 3 hours, adding more water whenever necessary.

An interesting soybean preparation called *tempeh* is made from cooked, hulled soybean halves, to which a Rhizipus mold is introduced. The inoculated bean cakes are then fermented overnight, during which time the white mycelium mold partially digests the beans and effectively deactivates the trypsin enzyme, which could inhibit digestion. The soybeans have, by this time, become fragrant cakes bound together by the mold; you can then either deep-fry or bake them into a dish that tastes remarkably like veal or chicken. Tempeh is rich in protein (from 18 to 48 percent) and highly digestible. In addition, like the other fermented soy products and sea vegetables, it is one of the few nonmeat sources of vitamin B_{12}. Tempeh can be made easily in any kitchen. The tempeh starter (*Rhizopus oligosporus*, mold spores) is available from the Department of Agriculture, complete with an enthusiastic brochure on its use.

A further use of this "queen of the beans" is as a sprout. Significant amounts of vitamin C, not found in the dried bean, are released in the sprouts, which are also rich in vitamins A, E, and the B complex, as well as minerals. The yellow soybean does well for sprouting, and the black variety can also sprout prolifically.

Rinse the sprouts two to three times a day and harvest them when the shoot is from ¼ to 1½ inches long. As a matter of taste, you may or may not prefer to remove the outer husk before using the sprout. Steaming or boiling the soybean sprouts lightly before eating will destroy the urease and antitrypsin enzymes that interfere with digestion. The sprouts can be ground and used in sandwiches and salad dressings, and they make a fine addition to any sauté of crisp Chinese-style vegetables.

TOFU

Tofu (soy curd or soy cheese) is among the traditional East Asian soy products. Tofu is a remarkable food. It is very inexpensive when purchased at Oriental markets or natural food shops and even more so if made at home. Two other related products, tamari soy sauce and miso (fermented soy paste), will be discussed later in this chapter.

You can make your own tofu by grinding soaked soybeans, cooking them with water, pouring the resulting mixture into a pressing sack, and collecting the "milk" underneath by squeezing as much liquid as possible from the sack, leaving the bean fiber behind. The soy milk is then simmered and curdled in a solution containing sea-water brine (called nigari), lemon juice, or vinegar. Any of these three solidifiers will work well, although commercial nigari is most often used for this coagulation process.

After the white soy curds curdle and float in a yellowish whey liquid, they are ladled into a settling box, covered and weighted, and allowed to press into a solid cake, which is then ready for immediate use as is—or for further transformation into a virtually unlimited variety of tofu products. Tofu is high in quality protein and is excellent for creating complete protein, especially when combined with grains. Tofu contains an abundance of lysine, an essential amino acid in which many grains are deficient; on the other hand, grains such as rice are high in the sulfur that contains methionine and cystine, amino acids that are absent in soybeans. These soy and grain proteins complement each other naturally.

Tofu is easy to digest, low in calories, saturated fats, and cholesterol. When solidified with calcium chloride or calcium sulfate—as in most commercial American tofu—tofu contains more calcium by weight than dairy milk; it's also a good source of other minerals such as iron, phosphorus, and potassium.

Since it's made from soybeans, tofu is free of chemical toxins. Soybeans are an important feed crop for the beef and dairy industries and the spraying is therefore carefully monitored by the Food and Drug Administration.

SPLIT PEAS

Split peas, both green and yellow, make a simple soup filled with protein and minerals. They do not require soaking. Start with one part dry peas and five to six cups water and cook about 45 minutes. Once the peas are cooked, the soup will continue to thicken; this leftover paste can be diluted several times in the following days for a quick hot soup. Sautéed onions, tamari, and ½ stick of soy margarine complete the soup.

NUTS AND SEEDS Nuts and seeds are fine sources of protein, minerals (especially magnesium), some B vitamins, and unsaturated fatty acids. They can be eaten as snack foods or used with other foods to add interesting flavors, textures, and nutritional values.

A general sprouting procedure for seeds and nuts: soak the dried seeds for about eight hours (approximately four parts water to one part seed). Don't throw away the soaking water; use it as a cooking liquid, or water your houseplants with it. Rinse the seeds with cool water and place them in a sprouter.

Keys to successful sprouting include keeping the sprouts moist but never soaked, keeping them moderately warm, rinsing them as often as possible, and giving them enough room so that air can freely circulate around them. Actually, only about five minutes a day is needed for growing a successful sprout garden. Use the sprouts as soon as possible. They have a refrigerator life of 7 to 10 days. Sprouts can also be dried easily for use in beverages, nut butter, and spreads. Place the sprouts on cookie sheets for a few hours in a warm room, or keep them in a warm oven until they're dry. Then grind them in a blender and store this nutritious food concentrate in a jar and refrigerate.

ALFALFA

Many people think of alfalfa as a barnyard grass, which it is. Because its roots penetrate deep underground to seek out the elements it craves, alfalfa is one of the best possible fodders. But the fresh, mineral-laden leaves of this plant are especially nutritious for humans when juiced. Alfalfa seeds purchased at a natural food store may seem expensive, but a few of them go a long way—½ teaspoon of dry seeds yields an entire trayful of sprouts. The sprouts have a light sweet taste and are particularly rich in vitamin C, as well as in chlorophyll (when allowed to develop in light). They also have high mineral values, containing phosphorus, chlorine, silicon, aluminum, calcium, magnesium, sulfur, sodium, and potassium. Alfalfa seeds sprout well in combination with other seeds and have a high germination rate. They can also be used when dried.

ALMONDS

Almonds will sprout only from the fresh unhulled nut after soaking overnight; they must be kept very moist until their sprouts reach a length of about one inch (four days). They can then be used to make almond milk: a combination of one cup of almond sprouts (or merely almonds soaked overnight) blended with four times as much water or apple juice. Almonds, which have an exceptionally high mineral content, are delicious raw or roasted with tamari. The raw nut can be sliced, slivered, or chopped, and even can be ground into almond butter.

BRAZIL NUTS

Brazil nuts, like other seeds and nuts, have a high fat content. But because they are also high in protein, they are actually not much higher in calories per gram of usable protein than are whole grains. They also offer unusually high amounts of the sulfur-containing amino acids. For this reason, you can serve them to good advantage as a chopped garnish for fresh vegetables, such as brussels sprouts, cauliflower, green peas, and lima beans. These vegetables are all deficient in the sulfur-containing amino acids but high in the amino acid isoleucine lacking in Brazil nuts.

CASHEWS

Cashews are also popular nuts that can be added to many dishes. Use them as a layer in a casserole, or simply roast them lightly and toss them in a bowl of steamed snow peas. Cashew butter, from both raw and roasted nuts, is growing in popularity and is well-suited for use in sauces, where it can be diluted with water and miso paste. You can mix it yourself in a nutritious soy "milkshake." Blend two cups of plain or sweetened soy milk with ½ cup of cashew butter; add two tablespoons of carob powder, a pinch of salt, and a dash of vanilla extract and nutmeg.

CHIA SEEDS

Chia seeds, now available in natural food stores, have long been a staple in Mexican and American Indian diets, where they were traditionally used to increase endurance on long hunts and migrations. Although a member of the mint family, chia seeds have a mild flaxlike taste. They can be chewed raw or sprinkled into hot or cold cereals. Since they are in a class of seeds called mucilaginous, which become sticky when soaked in water, their sprouting procedure is slightly different. Sprinkle the seeds over a saucer filled with water and allow to stand overnight. By morning, the seeds, having absorbed all the water, will stick to the saucer. Gently rinse and drain them, using a sieve if possible. Then, as with other seeds, rinse twice daily. Also try sprouting the seeds in a flat, covered container lined with damp paper towels. Harvest the chia seeds when the shoot is one inch long.

CLOVER

The red variety of clover makes a delicious sprout similar in taste to alfalfa. In its sprout form, this forage plant can be an excellent source of chlorophyll; when the primary leaves are about one inch in length, spread them out in a nonmetallic tray and dampen them. They should be covered with clear plastic to hold in moisture and placed in a sunny spot for one to two hours.

CRESS SEEDS

Cress seeds are tiny members of the mustard family. They add a zesty taste to salads when used in their sprout form. They are also mucilaginous seeds and so are sprouted in the same way as chia seeds. Harvest the sprouts at about one inch long and use them in sandwiches instead of lettuce.

FENUGREEK SEEDS

Fenugreek seeds were first used to brew tea by the ancient Greeks. This strong tea is an excellent mouthwash, as well as a tasty and nutritious addition to soy or nut milk. The ground dry seed is one of the components of curry powder. When sprouted, fenugreek can be added to soups, salads, and grain dishes. The sprout should be harvested once it is ¼ inch long, for it will become very bitter soon afterward.

FILBERTS (HAZELNUTS)

Filberts or hazelnuts are tasty nuts that, once chopped, make a delicious garnish for both greens and creamy tofu pudding. These nuts, however, contain an excess amount of calories for the amount of protein they provide.

FLAX (LINSEED)

Flax, also known as linseed, is a versatile plant. The fiber of the mature plant is used to make linen and pressed to extract its oil. As a sprout, flax has been used for centuries; it is recorded that at Greek and Roman banquets, flax sprouts were served between courses for their mild laxative effect. Though flax is sprouted as a mucilaginous seed, its sprouts work well in conjunction with wheat and rye kernels. Harvest when the shoots are about an inch long and serve as a breakfast salad. Taken on an empty stomach, this sprout mixture cleanses and lubricates the colon.

MUSTARD

The small seeds of the common black mustard plant will sprout quite readily and are usually available at herb and spice stores. Small amounts of these sprouts add a spicy flavor to salads and sandwiches. Harvest when shoots are about an inch long.

PECANS

Pecans are nuts that are cultivated organically in Texas and New Mexico. Though high in potassium and B vitamins, pecans are not good sources of protein; like filberts, they contain too many calories for the amount of protein they offer. Pecans are delicious as tamari-roasted nuts: dry-roast in a heavy skillet and, when they begin to emit a pleasing fragrance, remove to a plate and sprinkle lightly with tamari.

PIGNOLIAS (PINE NUTS)

Pignolias, or pine nuts, have an unusual flavor, but are a poor source of protein. Pignolias, found in the cones of the small pinon pine, which grows in the American Southwest, have been used by many Indian tribes as a food staple. Most of the pignolias consumed in the United States, however, come from Portugal. Pan-roasted pine nuts are delicious with green vegetables like peas and beans, and are also tasty in bread stuffings.

PISTACHIO NUTS

Pistachio nuts are familiar to many as an Italian ice cream flavor. For snacking purposes, use the naturally grown pistachio rather than the dyed varieties. Like other nuts, pistachios should be consumed only in small quantities, since they are high in calories.

PUMPKIN SEEDS, PEPITAS, AND SQUASH SEEDS

Pumpkin seeds, pepitas, and squash seeds are delicious seeds rich in minerals that can be eaten as snacks or ground into a meal for use in baking and cooking. Eastern Europeans, who eat many more pumpkin seeds than do Americans, use them to help prevent prostate disorders. Save the seeds from a pumpkin or squash and sprout them. Harvest when the shoot is just beginning to show (after three or four days); if allowed to lengthen any further, the sprouts will taste bitter.

RADISH SEEDS

Radish seeds, both black and red, make wonderfully tangy sprouts. They sprout easily and work well when combined with alfalfa and clover seeds. They're relatively expensive compared to most sprouting seeds, but you don't need many of these peppery-tasting sprouts to perk up a salad. Harvest these shoots when they're about an inch long.

SESAME SEEDS (BENNE)

Sesame seeds, or benne, are popular around the world because of their taste and high nutritive content. Most sesame seeds available in the United States are grown in southern Mexico, where few sprays are used, and they are available hulled or unhulled. The unhulled variety is nutritionally superior since most of the mineral value is found in the hull.

The seeds are an excellent source of protein, unsaturated fatty acids, calcium, magnesium, niacin, and vitamins A and E. The protein in sesame seeds effectively complements the protein of legumes, because both contain high amounts of each other's deficient amino acids. Therefore, an especially good addition to a soy milk shake is tahini, or sesame butter.

Used extensively as the whole seed in breads and other baked foods, in grain dishes, and on vegetables, the unhulled seeds can also be toasted and ground into sesame butter, which has a stronger taste and higher mineral content than sesame tahini. Tahini, made from toasted and hulled seeds, is a mild, sweet butter. Tahini is used extensively in the Middle East, where the oil that separates from the butter is used as a cooking oil. Tahini is an excellent base for salad dressing and acts as a perfect thickener for all sorts of sauces.

The unhulled seed must be used when sprouting. The sprouts can be used, like the whole seed, in cooked foods or blended into beverages. Harvest when the shoot reaches 1/16 inch in length (usually within two days). At this stage the sprouts are sweet, but become bitter with further growth.

SUNFLOWER SEEDS

Sunflower seeds are sun-energized, nutritional powerhouses rich in protein (about 30 percent), unsaturated fatty acids, phosphorus, calcium, iron, fluorine, iodine, potassium, magnesium, zinc, several B vitamins, vitamin E, and vitamin D (one of the few vegetable sources of this vitamin). Their high mineral content is the result of the sunflower's extensive root system, which penetrates deep into the subsoil seeking nutrients; their vitamin D content is partially due to the flower's tendency to follow and face the sun as it moves across the sky.

Sunflowers were cultivated extensively by American Indians as a food crop. In their raw state, sunflower seeds can be enjoyed as snacks or included in everything from breads to salads. The seeds are also available in a toasted, salted nut butter.

Sprouted sunflower seeds should be eaten when barely budded or they will taste very bitter. However, it usually takes four to five days for the shoot to appear. Unhulled seeds, or special hulled sprouting seeds, are used when sprouting, but the husk should be removed before eating.

WALNUTS

Walnuts are a good source of protein and iron. Black walnuts contain about 40 percent more protein than English walnuts (also known as California walnuts in the United States). Walnuts will keep fresh much longer when purchased in the shell. This is true of all nuts. It also brings down the price considerably.

SEAWEEDS Seaweeds rank high as sources for the basic essential minerals, as do green vegetables such as dandelions and watercress. They all contain calcium, magnesium, phosphorus, potassium, iron, iodine, and sodium. Most Westerners dislike the idea of eating seaweed. If they were to sample what they're missing, though, they'd find a new world of taste and high-quality nutrients—especially trace minerals—in the six varieties of sea vegetables available in most natural food stores and food co-ops.

AGAR

Agar, or agar-agar (called *kantan* in Japanese, and also known as Ceylonese moss) is a translucent, almost weightless seaweed product found in stick, flake, or powdered form. You can use it like gelatin to thicken fruit juices or purees. Agar also can be used to make aspics and clear molds of fruit juices, fruits, or vegetables. If you tear 1 to 1½ sticks into small pieces and dissolve them in one quart of liquid, you will produce a puddinglike consistency. More agar can be used to achieve a jellied texture. When used in stick form, agar should be simmered in liquid for 10 to 15 minutes, to ensure that all the pieces have dissolved. This simmering isn't necessary when using the flaked or powdered varieties.

DULSE

Dulse is the only commercial sea vegetable that comes from the Atlantic Ocean (specifically, the Canadian Maritime Provinces). This ready-to-eat seaweed can be chewed in its tough dry state, but a short soaking to rinse it and to remove any small, clinging shells is worthwhile. Dulse can be added to miso soup.

HIJIKI (HIZIKI)

Another Japanese seaweed is the jet-black hijiki or hiziki. This stringy, hairlike seaweed contains 57 percent more calcium by weight than dry milk and has high levels of iron as well. Dried hiziki should be soaked in several cups of water for about 20 minutes, then strained in a colander and lightly pressed to squeeze out excess moisture. Once reconstituted, hiziki is best when sautéed together with other vegetables—especially onion and leeks—or cooked with beans and grains.

KOMBU (KELP)

Kombu is the Japanese term for several species of brown algae. In English, these are usually referred to collectively as kelp. Kombu is especially rich in iodine, vitamin B2, and calcium. When using the dried form of kombu, rinse it once and soak for 10 to 15 minutes.

Note that all dried seaweeds increase greatly in size when reconstituted. For example, ¼ cup of dried hiziki would yield 1 cup when soaked. Save the water in which the seaweeds are soaked and use it as soup stock. Reconstituted kombu strips can be used whole in the cooking water for beans and grains, or can be cut into thin strips or diced for use in soups and salads.

NORI (LAVER)

Nori is the most popular Japanese seaweed, also known as dried purple laver. It is sold in the form of paper-thin purplish sheets, with 8 to 10 sheets per package. Laver has been used a food by many peoples. The Japanese and Koreans are, however, the only people to cultivate these plants and dry and press the mature leaves into sheets.

The nori sheets are toasted over a flame until crisp, during which their color changes from black or purple to green. They are then crumbled or slivered and used as a condiment for noodles, grains, beans, and soups. Remarkably rich in protein, nori is also high in vitamins A, B_2, B_{12}, D, and niacin.

WAKAME

Wakame is a long seaweed with symmetrical and fluted fronds growing from both sides of an edible midrib. Although generally used fresh in Japan, it is only available dried in the West. It is reconstituted in the same manner as kombu: rinsed once, soaked, and pressed of excess moisture. If the midrib is particularly tough, it can be removed. When used in soups, wakame should be cooked for no more than a few minutes and should therefore be one of the last ingredients added to miso soup. This delicious vegetable is rich in protein and niacin, and contains, in its dried state, almost 50 percent more calcium than dry milk.

FERMENTED FOODS: MISO AND TAMARI Miso and tamari, derived from soybeans and grain, deserve special consideration in any sensible vegetarian diet. The fermentation process in the healthy human intestine isn't that different from what occurs in the production of fermented soy foods. For example, in our digestive tract, maltose and glucose are broken down to form lactic acid, ethyl alcohol, and organic acids. The microorganic cultures responsible for these syntheses enter our own bodies when we digest them in fermented foods and help us to assimilate the nutrients we need.

Miso, a fermented soybean paste, has long been a staple seasoning in the Oriental kitchen. It is produced by combining cooked soybeans, salt, and various grains. Barley miso is made with barley and soybeans. Rice miso is made with both hulled and unhulled rice plus soybeans, and soybeans alone are used to make hatcho miso. These cooked and salted combinations are dusted with a fungus mold, koji, which produces the enzymes that start to digest the bean-and-grain mixture.

Tamari is naturally fermented soy sauce. Originally considered excess liquid, it was drained off miso that had finished fermenting. Today it is a product in its own right and is made from a natural fermentation process of whole soybeans, natural sea salt, well water, roasted cracked wheat, and koji spores, all aged for 12 to 18 months. Tamari, like miso, has a range of colors, textures, and aromas as wide and varied as that of wines and cheeses.

Miso and tamari contain between 9 and 18 percent complete protein; the higher the soybean content, the higher the protein. The protein in these products is "predigested": it is already broken down into 17 amino acids, which makes for easy digestion. Also, the digestion-inhibiting enzyme present in raw or poorly cooked soybeans is destroyed by their fermentations. During the microorganic synthesis of miso and tamari, the amounts of B vitamins, riboflavin, and niacin increase. In addition, miso and tamari are among the few vegetable sources of vitamin B_{12}, which is actually manufactured by fungi and bacteria in the fermenting mixtures just as it is synthesized in the human intestine.

Miso and tamari are useful in all cuisines, but because of their high salt content—11 percent for the saltiest of hatcho miso and 18 percent for tamari—they should be used sparingly. Miso diluted with water can be used as a base for a sauce made with tahini; a dash of tamari brings out new flavors in familiar grains. Miso also makes a wonderful soup base to which tofu, mushrooms, seaweeds, and many fresh or cooked vegetables can be added.

All of the natural miso and tamari available in the United States today comes from Japan. If a package of miso you purchase has started to expand, you can be assured its contents have not been pasteurized and that the microorganisms are still alive and producing carbon dioxide gas. Get rid of it.

In the future, the United States may begin producing its own fermented soybean foods. A lively market now exists and many people are acquiring the necessary technical know-how. Organic farmers are already producing soybeans, wheat, barley, and rice; the koji starter and engineering skills are always available from Asia. As fermented soy foods play a larger role in American diets, we may start to develop and adapt our own distinctive varieties.

SALT: SOME ALTERNATIVE SOURCES A controversy continues about the virtues and dangers of salt. Some people consume large quantities of salt. Many others attempt to get their salt from the juices of celery, spinach, beets, or carrots; very little sodium, however, is derived from these supposedly sodium-rich foods. Still other people decide upon, or are prescribed, low-sodium or even "salt-free" diets. People on low-sodium diets have often been suffering from hypertension or kidney problems. Overconsumption of salt will lead to hypertension: The salt draws water out of blood cells and vessels, which in turn causes dehydration of the tissues and forces the heart to pump much too strenuously. Overconsumption of salt also clogs the kidneys and creates an excess of water that cannot be properly eliminated from the body.

On the other hand, moderate and intelligent consumption of salt helps the body retain heat by slightly contracting the blood vessels, which is why we tend to consume more salt in cold months. Sodium also helps maintain intestinal muscle tone. You should evaluate your own salt needs according to your physical activity, climate, water intake, and—above all—diet. People in meat-eating cultures seldom need extra salt per se, because they get all they need from the blood and flesh of the animals they eat; vegetarian or agricultural peoples, however, tend to have a high regard for salt and use it to cook, pickle, and preserve foods.

If you want to eat salt, you should use the natural sun- or kiln-dried variety, which still contains important trace minerals. Refined "table" salt is made fine by high heats and flash-cooling, and then combined with such additives as sodium silico aluminate to keep it "free-flowing." Kosher salt is an exception; it has larger crystals due to its milder processing, and nothing is added to the better brands. Natural salt—rock salt or sea salt—is not free-flowing, but some brands add calcium carbonate, a natural compound, to prevent caking. All salt is or once was sea salt, so differences between salt obtained from inland rock deposits or from the sea are minor and unimportant.

No natural salt contains iodine, which is far too volatile a substance to remain stable for long without numerous additives. But there is an excellent source of iodine from the ocean: sea vegetables, the most common being kelp. These contain a natural, sugar-stabilized iodine—as well as about 4 to 8 percent salt. They are harvested, roasted, ground up, and marketed as salt alternatives.

Another healthful way of adding salt to your diet is to use sesame salt, sold as gomasio. This versatile condiment can be used in place of ordinary salt on cooked greens, grains and raw salads. Gomasio can be purchased in most natural food stores, but the serious cook should grind his or her own.

The ridged, ceramic grinding bowl called a suribachi is needed to make sesame salt. A proportion of 15 parts sesame seeds (unhulled) to 1 part salt is recommended by Lima Ohsawa in her cookbook, *The Art of Just Cooking*. She suggests that this formula should be adjusted to fit the individual taste and climate and advises a milder salt content for children. Start with one cup of sesame seeds, wash them in a fine strainer, and set aside to drain. Roast one level teaspoon of salt in a heavy skillet until the strong odor of chlorine is no longer released. Then transfer the salt to the suribachi and pulverize it with the wooden pestle.

Roast the drained sesame seeds in the skillet over moderate heat, constantly stirring until they are light brown in color and they begin to release their characteristic aroma. Transfer these browned seeds to the suribachi and grind lightly with salt until about 80 percent of the seeds are crushed. Store the mixture until needed in an airtight container. Making gomasio becomes a beautiful ritual well worth the effort.

Another alternative is salted umeboshi plums. These small Japanese plums are known for the high quality and quantity of citric acid they contain. The citric acid in plums allegedly helps neutralize and eliminate some of the excess lactic acid in the body, helping to restore a natural balance. An excess of lactic acid in the body is caused by excessive consumption of sugar; if not converted to body energy, the sugar turns into lactic acid and combines with protein to contribute to ailments like headaches, fatigue, and high blood pressure.

In Japan, these organically grown plums are available in a variety of preservative-free forms—from concentrates to salted plums. In most American natural food stores, only the salted plums are available. These are potent alkaline sources, excellent to aid indigestion, colds, and fatigue. Umeboshi also have many culinary uses. Use them to salt the water in which grains will be cooked or use several in tofu salad dressings instead of tamari or sea salt.

SWEETENERS Carbohydrate sugar is unquestionably essential to life, but try to get it in as unadulterated a form as possible. Common table sugar has been processed to 99.9 percent sucrose, devoid of the vitamins and minerals found in sugar cane or sugar beets. This refined sucrose taxes the body's digestive system and depletes its core of minerals and enzymes as the sugar is metabolized. For this reason and others, white sugar has earned a bad reputation and the label, "empty food."

Carbohydrates include many sugars. The best known is sucrose, or white table sugar, which breaks down in the body into simpler sugars, glucose and fructose. There are also starches in whole cereals (together with their own component enzymes, vitamins, minerals, and proteins) that break down uniformly in the body into simple glucose molecules once they have been cooked, chewed, and digested. Compared with these refined starches, refined sugars tend to overstrain the body's digestive system. So, it would seem wiser to get the sugars you need from abundant natural stores in cereals, vegetables, and fruits. Eaten in moderate amounts, starches are not fattening, contrary to public opinion.

When cooking with natural foods, you should simply replace refined sugars with the richer flavors of naturally occurring sugars. Maple syrup, for example, or honey or fruit juice can substitute for sugar in almost any home recipe. Maple sugar is expensive and very sweet, so use it in moderation. Use ½ cup of maple syrup instead of 1 cup of sugar and either reduce the other liquids in the recipe or increase the dry ingredients accordingly. Maple syrup is believed by some to be a source of the trace mineral zinc. But be sure that the maple syrup you buy has not been extracted with formaldehyde.

All honeys are basically the fruit sugar fructose, which consists of varying amounts of dextrose, levulose, maltose, and other simple sugars. The flavor of honey depends on the source of the bees' nectar. All honey you use should be unheated and unfiltered so that its natural enzymes and vitamins are still intact. When cooking with honey in a recipe originally calling for refined sugar, divide the amount of sugar called for in half and adjust the recipe with less liquid or more dry ingredients.

In fact, not too much sugar of any kind should be used in cooking or baking, because heat can be destructive to protein in the presence of sugar. This is especially true when using honey or a refined glucose such as corn syrup. Try using fruit juices or purees made from soaked dried fruits to sweeten dishes; a little of these natural sugars will go a long way.

Granulated date sugar, available in many natural food stores, is indispensable when your recipe specifically calls for a granulated dry sugar. This sugar has the distinctive flavor of whole dry dates. Another dry sweetener is carob, or St.-Johns bread. This powder comes from the dried pods of the carob tree and can be purchased roasted or unroasted. Use the unroasted variety and toast it yourself for a fresher taste. In addition to its natural sugars, carob is rich in trace minerals and low in fats. Not much of this strong sweetener is necessary; either mix with the dry ingredients or dissolve in a little water or soy milk before adding to the other liquids. Carob is also available as a syrup. If you are using carob as a substitute for cocoa or chocolate, the equivalent of one square of chocolate is three tablespoons of carob plus two tablespoons of water or soy milk.

From the starches, two grain sweeteners are available: barley malt (also made from other grains and containing the sugar maltose) and a rice syrup called *ame* in Japanese. These grain syrups are produced by combining the cooked grains, rice in this instance, with fresh sprouts from whole oats, barley, or wheat. This combination is allowed to stand for several hours until it has reached the sweet stage, when the liquid is squeezed off through cheesecloth, lightly salted, and cooked to the desired consistency. This thick, pale-amber syrup works well in pastries and sauces. Its semisolid state can be softened by beating it to the consistency of thick honey. It is also sold in health food stores in the West as a chewy taffy.

For those who use dairy products, noninstant dry milk powder is a versatile natural sweetener containing the milk-sugar lactose.

So-called raw sugar, or turbinado, is available in many stores, but is only slightly more nutritious than white sugar. It is 96 percent sucrose, compared with the 99.9 percent sucrose in white sugar. The only refining step to which it has not been subjected is a final acid bath that whitens the sugar and removes the final calcium and magnesium salts. This "pure" sugar was, as a juice from either sugar beets or sugar cane, only 15 percent sucrose; in its final form, all natural goodness has been lost.

Several sweeteners produced in the intermediate stages of sugar refining can be used somewhat more nutritionally than white table sugar. Once the cane or beet juice has been extracted, clarified to a syrup form, and crystallized, it is then spun in a centrifuge where more crystals are separated from the liquid. This remaining liquid is molasses, which is then repeatedly treated and centrifuged to extract more and more crystal until the final "blackstrap" form contains about 35 percent sucrose. Blackstrap molasses also contains iron, calcium, and B vitamins. Another variety of molasses is known as barbados. This milder, dark-brown syrup is extracted from the processes described earlier, resulting in a lighter-tasting product with a higher sucrose content. Sorghum molasses is produced by a similar process, but uses as raw material the cane from the sorghum plant. It has a distinctive, rather cloying, taste and is best used in baking, especially cookies.

UNREFINED OILS For a healthful diet, you should obtain necessary unsaturated fatty acids primarily from unrefined vegetable oils. Like other unrefined foods, these oils still contain all the nutrients present in the grains, beans, or seeds from which they were derived.

Nearly all cooking oils are made by first heating the grains, beans, or seeds; then, to produce "unrefined" oils, they are pressed with a centrifuge and expelled without the use of chemicals or solvents. No further processing occurs, but some firms do filter their "unrefined" oils to remove the remaining particles of the germ. It is better, of course, to purchase unfiltered, unrefined oils with some sediment left in the bottle; too much filtering removes nutrients. Commercial processing also results in the loss of vitamin E, which is found naturally in the oil and is essential for the proper utilization of important unsaturated fatty acids. You therefore benefit very little form refined oils, since they are a poor source of unsaturated fatty acids.

Refined oils also lack the natural odors and flavors that are noticeable in all unrefined oils. The mildest of the unrefined oils are safflower and sunflower. Unrefined sesame oil imparts a unique nutty taste to sautéed foods, while unrefined corn-germ oil gives a buttery taste to baked goods. Everyone has appreciated the full-bodied flavor of unrefined olive oil in salad dressings. Peanut and soybean oil are stronger in flavor and can be better utilized in sautéing, which reduces the intensity of their taste. Unrefined coconut and palm oil are also available in natural food stores; these partially saturated oils are used extensively by Southern cultures for all types of cooking (and in many processed foods).

Another reason for using unrefined oils is that at high temperatures the chemical makeup of an oil is altered and possibly becomes detrimental to health. Many advertisements praise refined oils for their ability to be used at extremely high temperatures, but these high heats are neither necessary nor desirable. Unrefined safflower oil can be used for deep-frying at about 400 degrees, and can withstand higher temperatures than most other oils. Cooking temperatures above this simply aren't necessary. Overheating of unrefined, unfiltered oil causes the germ to scorch and most nutrients to be lost. When substituting unrefined oils for solid fats in recipes, reduce the amounts of other liquids slightly or increase the dry ingredients.

OTHER USEFUL FOODS Bancha tea is high in calcium. It is a coarse, undyed green tea. The leaves, which must have remained on the bush for three years, should be roasted in the oven until browned. Bancha twig tea, known as kukicha, consists of the twigs of the tea bush and is generally available. One spare teaspoon of kukicha should be used for each cup of tea, which is prepared by simmering the twigs for about 15 to 20 minutes.

Baking powders are used to make "quick breads" that can usually be put together and baked in less than half an hour and that rise by virtue of the baking powder included. It's best not to use too many quick breads, but they occasionally do lend themselves well to the use of concentrated nutrients such as seeds and nuts, and they can contain a mixture of flours such as whole wheat with fresh ground corn, millet, triticale, and soy flour. Never use sodium bicarbonate in making quick breads; its action is not only unnecessary but potentially unhealthy, destroying vitamin C and some B vitamins. Instead, the baking powder you choose should be low-sodium and aluminum-free; aluminum is known to be toxic. Potassium bicarbonate does not destroy vitamin D in the body. Most natural food stores carry this type of low-sodium baking powder, but you can make your own by using one part potassium bicarbonate, two parts cream of tartar (potassium bitartrate) and two parts arrowroot powder. It may be necessary to obtain potassium bicarbonate through a chemical company because it is not generally available at pharmacies.

Nutritional yeast is a natural treasurehouse of proteins, vitamins, and minerals that can be used as a dietary supplement when added to juices or included in cooked dishes. Often called brewer's yeast because at one time it was a byproduct of the brewing industry, nutritional yeast is the tiniest of cultivated plants. The minuscule plants are grown on herbaceous grains and hops under carefully controlled temperature conditions. The yeast plant grows at an astoundingly fast rate. Once it has multiplied many times and matured, it is harvested and dried in a way that preserves all its nutrients. These yeast "flakes" are one of the most economical sources of the B vitamin complexes. In addition to these vitamins, yeast flakes contain minerals such as calcium, phosphorus, iron, sodium, potassium, and many of the amino acids, all of which work in conjunction with the B vitamins.

Many people take several tablespoons of yeast daily. If yeast is to be used in a beverage such as a vegetable juice, the flakes should first be mixed with a small amount of the liquid and stirred into a paste, then added to the rest of the liquid and thoroughly mixed again. A blender will simplify this method of preparation. Yeast flakes also may be added to baked foods such as breads and casseroles or mixed in small amounts with nut butter or bean-paste sandwich spreads.

Thickeners for smooth soups and sauces are usually based on a finely ground starch or flour, the most widely-used being whole wheat, rice, and whole wheat pastry. The thickness of a flour-based sauce is determined by the ratio of flour to liquid. One tablespoon of flour to one cup liquid yields a thin sauce; up to three tablespoons flour to one cup liquid, a thick sauce. Cornstarch, corn flour in its finest version, is used in the same way to thicken sauces. Arrowroot powder, or flour made from the arrowroot plant, produces a finer sauce than cornstarch. The arrowroot starch should be dissolved in cold water before being added to hot foods to prevent lumping. Once the arrowroot has been added, simmer the thickened sauce to allow all the flavors to merge.

Kudzu is another high-quality but rather expensive thickening agent. The kudzu plant grows wild in the United States as well as in Japan, where it has long been used in folk medicine, often prescribed for diarrhea and head colds. The crumbly white chunks should first be dissolved in cold water before being added to hot sauces to prevent lumping.

If vinegar is called for in a recipe, never use the white distilled or wine varieties; use an apple cider vinegar made from whole, unsprayed apples, undiluted and naturally aged. Refined, distilled vinegar has few of the naturally occurring nutrients (such as potassium) and virtually none of the indefinable subtle flavors of slowly-aged cider vinegar. Because of the predominance of acetic acid in white distilled and wine vinegars, use them sparingly. Apple cider vinegar, on the other hand, contains a predominance of malic acid, which when wisely used is a constructive acid, naturally involved in the digestive system. Besides its culinary uses for preparing salad dressings and preserving foods, vinegar has long been useful as an antiseptic and blood coagulant. Rice vinegar is also available at natural food stores and in Oriental markets. It has a distinctive aroma and taste; so use it with utmost discretion in pickling and salad dressings. Thanks to its natural fermentation, it contains none of the problematical properties of commercial distilled vinegars.

13

A Vegetarian Rotation Diet and Recipes

The recipes in this chapter have benefited from years of research and experimentation. They have been designed to fit easily into a four-day rotational diet plan in which specific foods such as brown rice, soy beans, or wheat are eaten only once every four days. On any one day, a food may be eaten several times in relatively small quantities.

Additionally, the recipes included here have been devised according to the principles of proper food combining in order to allow for optimal digestibility, absorption, assimilation, and elimination. Following a diet using these recipes will provide all the protein and fiber that you need, as well as a full spectrum of vitamins and minerals.

At first, the idea of avoiding animal products in your regular diet may seem foreign. But perhaps you have heard the warnings of the American Heart Association, which link excessive consumption of red meat and dairy products to heart disease, or those of the American Cancer Society linking breast, colon, and prostate cancer to these products. Or you may have heard of the statement issued by the National Academy of Sciences containing evidence that the ideal human diet is essentially a vegetarian one, high in fresh fruits, vegetables, and grains, while low in animal proteins, fats, and refined foods. You may have grown curious about the benefits of a vegetarian diet as you've become aware of the risks associated with a diet high in animal protein foods, but still you hesitate. Don't worry, you are not alone.

The habit of eating meat may be fixed in a number of popular beliefs with a strong hold on many of us. First among these is the myth that you have to eat meat to get sufficient amounts of protein. Other fixed ideas include the belief that milk is our best source of calcium, and that only meat and animal products provide vitamin B_{12}. Meat is commonly associated with sexual potency and virility. On the other side of the coin, vegetarian cooking is commonly considered monotonous and unappetizing. Very often, there is an underlying fear of disapproval of friends and family should you become a vegetarian, and the feeling that it is simply too difficult to eat properly without meat as a mainstay.

The recipes offered in this chapter were designed specifically to dispel the myths that a vegetarian diet must be boring, unappetizing, and nutritionally inadequate. While a macrobiotic diet has been of benefit to many people, too often those who are unfamiliar with vegetarianism consider macrobiotic cuisine, as prepared in many restaurants, to be synonymous with vegetarian cuisine generally. And yet the major cuisines of the world, including those of China, India, the Middle East, and Mexico are essentially vegetarian, using meat only sparingly, as a spice rather than an entree. Vegetarian cooking can be both tasty and varied.

Being a vegetarian should not be a burden, nor should it alienate you from your friends and family. Of course, at first you may find it necessary to make a certain number of lifestyle changes. You will want to look for a good health food store that is convenient to shop in and provides the products that you need. At first you may have to spend a little more time planning and preparing your meals, but with time it will become second nature.

Two important things to remember are flexibility and gentleness. Rigidly held beliefs and dogmas will lead to an accumulation of stress that can deplete your body of essential vitamins and minerals no matter how well you eat. At the same time, as you establish your new diet, see if you can relax too. The important thing to remember is to be gentle with yourself. You are learning something new, and initially you may well make mistakes. If, for example, you go off of the diet at a party or if you go on a "binge," it will not help to beat yourself up for it. Simply chalk one up to experience and plan on doing better the next time. If you are out with friends at a restaurant that does not serve brown rice or vegetarian meals, don't panic. You will learn to see your way through such situations without feeling embarrassed or making those around you uncomfortable. For instance, you can order the baked potato instead of the rice, and a grilled piece of fish instead of red meat.

The ideal diet involves eating a number of small meals throughout the day. Eating just one large meal can interfere with the proper absorption of nutrients and place a burden on digestion. It can also add surplus calories. Generally, you should eat no more than three to four ounces of a given food at any one meal. In these quantities, you may eat the same food several times during the day, however. This approach will reduce your overall caloric intake and keep your body functioning with optimal energy. Keep in mind that it is best to meet the body's vitamin, mineral, and protein requirements throughout the day.

Reader! If you wish to prepare additional servings of these recipes, increase the amounts of main ingredients (vegetables, fruits, seeds, grains, legumes, flour, etc.) in proportions equal to the existing recipes. Condiments should only be increased by 1/8 teaspoon per additional portion.

First Cycle

DAY 1

BREAKFAST

Warm and Sweet Morning Cereal

6 oz. amaranth
3 oz. fresh pineapple, if possible;
if not, pineapple sweetened
in its own juice

3 oz. raisins
1 tbsp. honey
pinch cinnamon

In a medium saucepan, combine amaranth and water. Lower the heat when the water begins to boil. Allow to simmer for approximately 25 minutes. While the amaranth is cooking, cut the pineapple into ½ inch pieces. When the amaranth is cooked, add the pineapple and the remaining ingredients. Mix thoroughly. (Serves 1.)

LUNCH

Three-Grain Vegetable Bake

3 oz. amaranth
3 oz. basmati rice
3 oz. couscous
3 oz. carrots
1½ oz. watercress
3 oz. celery
1½ oz. pecans

2 tbsp. safflower oil
2 oz. water
¼ tsp. basil
¼ tsp. rosemary
½ tsp. fresh mustard
3 oz. golden raisins

Prepare a medium saucepan for each of the grains (amaranth, basmati rice, and couscous). Place 10 oz. of water in the saucepan with the amaranth and cook for 25 minutes. Place 10 oz. of water in the saucepan with the rice and cook for approximately 20 minutes. Place couscous in 10 oz. of water and cook for 10 minutes. Carefully wash carrots and then grate into a small bowl. Rinse watercress and chop. Clean the celery stalks and chop. In a large mixing bowl, combine all the grains and then add remaining ingredients. Mix well. Place mixture in a baking pan. Bake for 20 minutes in a 325-degree oven. (Serves 2.)

DINNER

Italian Vegetable Toss

3 oz. carrots
6 oz. zucchini
3 oz. arugula
1 oz. parsley
2 tbsp. safflower oil
1 clove garlic, chopped finely

⅓ tsp. tarragon
⅓ tsp. basil
2 red cabbage leaves
½ oz. pine nuts

Carefully clean the carrots and zucchini. Cut them into bite-sized pieces and steam in either a bamboo steamer basket or a stainless steel steamer. Steam for approximately 8 minutes. Rinse arugula and parsley, pat dry with a paper towel and tear into smaller pieces. In a separate small bowl, combine the oil and the herbs. When vegetables are steamed, allow them to cool to room temperature. Transfer them into a large bowl and toss in the arugula and parsley. Pour oil mixture into the bowl as well. Place cabbage leaves on each plate and place mixture on top. Top with pine nuts. Serve with 6 oz. of fish. (Serves 2.)

DINNER
(2ND OPTION)

Aromatic Indian Sweet Potato Bake

3 oz. sweet potato
2 oz. amaranth
3 oz. basmati rice
3 oz. zucchini
2 oz. celery
2 tbsp. safflower oil

¼ tsp. basil
⅔ tsp. salt
⅓ tsp. curry
½ tsp. tarragon
½ tsp. cumin

Place sweet potatoes in a preheated 400-degree oven for 40 minutes or until done. (You can test it by inserting a fork.) In a medium saucepan, place the amaranth in 10 oz. water. Cook for approximately 25 minutes or until done. In another saucepan, prepare the rice similarly in 10 oz. of water, and then cook for 20 minutes. While the grains are cooking, carefully wash the zucchini and celery. Cut the zucchini into ½" cubes. Slice the celery in ¼ " pieces. When the sweet potato is cooked, allow it to cool so you can handle it. Then scoop the sweet potato out of its skin and place it in a medium-sized mixing bowl with the cooked rice, amaranth and the remaining ingredients. Turn the mixture into the baking dish. Bake for 15 minutes in a preheated 375-degree oven. Serve with 6 oz. of fish. (Serves 2.)

DAY 2
BREAKFAST

Crunchy Sweet Rice

6 oz. brown rice
1½ oz. coconut,
shredded and unsweetened
1½ oz. cashews
1½ oz. dates

½ tsp. cinnamon
2 oz. water
1 oz. chopped apples
1½ oz. sunflower seeds

In a medium saucepan, cook brown rice in 14 oz. of water. Lower heat when it comes to a bowl. Cooking time is about 30 minutes. When rice is cooked, add coconut. Chop cashews and dates finely and add to rice. Add cinnamon. Take half of the mixture and puree along with 2 oz. of water for a few seconds. Then add the pureed mixture back to the rest of the rice. Sprinkle sunflower seeds and apples on top. (Serves 1.)

LUNCH

Vegetable Filbertasia

3 oz. kidney beans
3 oz. cauliflower
3 oz. asparagus
3 oz. celery
2 oz. mushrooms
2 oz. zucchini
1½ oz. filberts
2 oz. water

2 tbs. sunflower oil
¼ tsp. basil
⅔ tsp. dill
⅓ tsp. chili powder
¼ tsp. celery seed
1 garlic clove chopped
½ tsp. salt

Soak the beans in a large bowl in 16 oz. of water overnight. In the morning, rinse the beans and replace with 16 oz. of fresh water in a medium pot. Cook for 1¾ hours to 2 hours until done. Carefully rinse the cauliflower, asparagus, celery, mushrooms, and zucchini. Steam cauliflower and asparagus for 10 minutes. Chop celery, slice mushrooms and zucchini. Chop filberts medium fine. Put filberts in a blender with water, oil, spices, and salt. Place all the vegetables in a serving pan. Top with filbert/kidney bean sauce. Serve at room temperature. (Serves 2.)

DINNER

Nutty Butternut Squash

3 oz. butternut squash
1½ oz. shallots
1½ oz. peanuts

1 tsp. fresh ginger, diced
½ tsp. basil
½ tsp. salt

2 oz. water

1 garlic clove, finely diced

2 tbsp. sunflower oil

3 oz. avocado, sliced

Cut squash in half, remove the seeds and discard them. Place squash in a baking pan with ⅓" water, cut-side down. Bake for 40 minutes at 400 degrees. When squash is cool enough to handle, remove its skin and cut into 1" pieces. Place in a medium-sized mixing bowl. Chop shallots medium fine and add to the squash. Place peanuts, water, herbs, salt, and oil in a blender. Mix well. Add this sauce to the squash and the shallots. Place mixture in a greased, covered baking pan at 350 degrees for 20 minutes. When done, place avocado slices on top as garnish. Serve with 6 oz. of fish. (Serves 2.)

DAY 3
BREAKFAST

High-Protein Cinnamon Millet

6 oz. millet

1½ oz. almonds

pinch cinnamon

1½ oz. brewer's yeast

1 tsp. vanilla

1 tsp. maple syrup

In a medium saucepan, cook millet in 13 oz. of water. When the water comes to a boil, lower heat. Stir occasionally. Cooking time is approximately 30 minutes. In another saucepan, blanche the almonds by placing them in scalding water in order to remove the skins. Then chop them. Add cinnamon, brewer's yeast, vanilla, and maple syrup as well as the almonds. (Serves 1.)

LUNCH

Thick and Spicy Potato Chowder

9 oz. potato

4 c. water

3 oz. tomato

3 oz. green pepper

3 oz. carrots

3 oz. broccoli

½ tsp. cumin

½ tsp. basil

3 tbsp. sesame oil

1¼ tsp. salt

3 oz. scallions, chopped

Scrub or peel potatoes and place in 4 cups of water in a medium saucepan. Boil for approximately 15 minutes. When the potatoes are cooked, place in a blender with the water in which it was cooked, the seasonings and the oil and salt. Wash the tomatoes, pepper, carrots, and broccoli. Chop into bite-sized pieces. Transfer the potato mixture back into a saucepan. Add the chopped vegetables. Cook over a low heat for an additional 10 to 15 minutes. Top with scallions. (Yields 4 to 5 cups approximately.)

DINNER

Almost Spaghetti Squash Dinner

3 oz. spaghetti squash
3 oz. scallions
6 oz. tomato
3 oz. green pepper
1½ oz. mushrooms

2 tbsp. olive oil
¼ tsp. basil
½ tsp. Rosemary
1 tsp. fresh garlic minced
1 tsp. salt

Cut squash in half, remove the seeds and discard them. Place the halves in a baking pan with ⅓" water, cut-side down. Bake for 40 minutes at 400 degrees. When the squash is cool enough to handle, remove the pulp or "spaghetti." Carefully wash the scallions, tomato, pepper, onion, and mushrooms. Chop them medium fine. In a large skillet, add the oil and sauté the vegetables along with the seasonings and salt for 5 minutes. Combine all the ingredients in a large bowl. Mix carefully and then transfer to a serving dish. Serve with 6 oz. of fish. (Serves 2.)

DAY 4
BREAKFAST

Banana Barley

6 oz. barley
2 tbsp. barley malt

3 oz. mashed banana
2 oz. raisins

In a medium saucepan, cook barley in 14 oz. of water for 20 minutes or until done. Add barley malt, mashed banana, and raisins. Mix well. Serve hot. (Serves 1.)

LUNCH

Rainbow Vegetable Salad

3 oz. soy beans
3 oz. kale
3 oz. cauliflower
3 oz. carrots
2 oz. yellow squash
1½ oz. Brazil nuts

1½ tbsp. sow oil
⅓ tsp. garlic, minced
1½ oz. chives
¼ tsp. coriander
¼ tsp. tarragon
½ tsp. salt

In a large bowl, soak beans overnight in 16 oz. of water. In the morning, rinse the beans and transfer to a medium soup pot with 16 oz. of fresh water. Cook for 2 hours or until done. Carefully rinse kale, cauliflower, and yellow squash. Tear the kale and cut the vegetables into bite-sized pieces. Steam in a bamboo steamer basket or stainless steel steamer for 8 minutes. Chop Brazil nuts finely. Combine all ingredients in a medium-sized mixing bowl. Mix well. Serve hot or cold. (Serves 2.)

DINNER

Brazilian Broccoli Bake

3 oz. lima beans

3 oz. broccoli

3 oz. tofu

2 oz. onions

1½ oz. Brazil nuts

2 tbsp. soy oil

1 clove garlic, minced

1 tsp. coriander

1 tsp. parsley

½ tsp. salt

1 tsp. fresh mustard

In a large mixing bowl, soak lima beans overnight in 16 oz. of water. In the morning, rinse the beans and transfer them into a medium soup pot with 16 oz. of fresh water. Cook for 1½ hours or until done. Rinse broccoli and cut into ½" flowerettes. Rinse tofu and cut into ½" cubes. Peel and slice the onion. Place all ingredients in a large mixing bowl. Add half of the Brazil nuts, the oil, and seasonings. Add the mustard. Mix well. Place in a greased baking dish with lid. Top with remaining Brazil nuts. Bake for 20 minutes in a preheated 350-degree oven. Serve with 6 oz. of fish. (Serves 2.)

Second Cycle

DAY 1

BREAKFAST

Carob Gruel

6 oz. oatmeal

1½ tbsp. carob powder

pinch nutmeg

¼ tsp. cinnamon

In a medium saucepan, boil 15 oz. cold water. When water begins to boil, add oatmeal and lower heat. Stir frequently. Cooking time is approximately 10 minutes. Add remaining ingredients one minute before the oatmeal is fully cooked. Serve hot. (Serves 1.)

LUNCH

Light 'n' Easy Squash Salad

3 oz. couscous

3 oz. mushrooms

3 oz. carrots

3 oz. summer squash

1½ oz. parsley

½ clove garlic, chopped

2 tsp. thyme

½ tsp. basil

½ tsp. salt

1½ oz. pine nuts

4 cherry tomatoes for garnish

In a medium saucepan, cook couscous in 9 oz. of water for 10 minutes or until done. Wash mushrooms, carrots, and squash carefully. Slice the mushrooms, carrots, and squash into bite-sized pieces. Steam in a bamboo steamer basket or stainless steel steamer until tender but crunchy. Take into consideration that the carrots will take longer to steam than the squash and the mushrooms. Rinse parsley and chop finely. Chop garlic. Combine all ingredients in a large salad bowl. Garnish with cherry tomatoes. (Serves 2.)

DINNER
Vegetable Cornucopia Soup with Black-Eyed Peas

3 oz. black-eyed peas	2 oz. onion, chopped
3 oz. basmati rice	1 tsp. tamari
1 oz. hijiki, dry	2 garlic cloves, finely diced
1½ oz. watercress	3 tbsp. safflower oil
2 oz. parsnip	1 tsp. coriander
3 oz. carrot	1 bay leaf
2 oz. celery	1 tsp. salt

In a large bowl, soak peas overnight in 3 cups of water. In the morning, rinse well and transfer to a medium soup pot with 4 cups of fresh water. Bring beans to a boil, lower to medium heat and cover. In a medium saucepan, cook rice in 10 oz. of water for 20 minutes. Meanwhile soak hijiki in 8 oz. of water and rinse twice. Rinse the watercress and tear into smaller pieces. Clean the parsnips and carrots well and cut into bite-sized pieces. Clean celery and slice in ¼" pieces. When peas have cooked for 1½ hours, add the cooked rice and remaining ingredients. Cook over a low heat for 25 to 30 minutes or until beans are tender. (Yields 4 to 5 cups.)

Tossed Garden Salad

3 oz. red leaf lettuce	2 oz. red pepper
2 oz. endive	1 oz. alfalfa sprouts

Wash lettuce, endive and pepper. Cut into bite-sized pieces and put into a salad bowl. Top with sprouts. (Serves 2.)

DAY 2
BREAKFAST
Tropical Rice Breakfast

6 oz. brown rice	½ banana, mashed
1½ oz. raisins	2 oz. of your favorite

1½ oz. sunflower seeds
1½ oz. coconut

fruit juice, optional

In a medium saucepan, cook brown rice in 14 oz. of water. When water comes to a boil, lower heat. Cooking time is approximately 30 minutes. During the last 10 minutes of cooking, add the raisins, sunflower seeds, and coconut. When it is completely cooked, add the mashed banana. When serving, you may add the fruit juice if you wish. (Serves 1.)

LUNCH

Butternut Arugula Salad

3 oz. butternut squash
3 oz. arugula
3 oz. alfalfa sprouts
1½ oz. currants

2 tbsp. sunflower oil
½ tsp. dill
½ tsp. parsley
½ tsp. salt

Peel the butternut squash. Cut it in half and remove and discard the seeds. Place the squash cut-side down in a baking pan with ⅓" of water. Bake for 40 minutes at 400 degrees. When squash is cool enough to handle, cut it into bite-sized pieces. Place in a medium mixing bowl. Rinse arugula carefully to get all the dirt off. Tear off the stems and discard. Then add the arugula to the squash. Add the remaining ingredients. Toss gently so as not to mash the squash. Serve hot or cold. (Serves 2.)

DINNER

Herby Italian Noodles
with Rice

3 oz. brown rice
3 oz. buckwheat noodles
3 oz. avocado
3 oz. marinated artichokes
2 tbsp. sunflower oil
2 tsp. scallions, chopped

1 tsp. parsley, chopped
1 garlic clove, minced
½ tsp. basil
½ tsp. salt
1 oz. black olives, garnish

In a medium saucepan, cook brown rice in 12 oz. of water for 35 minutes or until done. Cook noodles according to directions on package. Chop the avocado and artichokes into bite-sized pieces and place in a medium mixing bowl. Add the remaining ingredients. Toss gently. When the rice and noodles are done, place them on plates. Top with the avocado mixture. Serve at room temperature. Serve with 6 oz. of fish. (Serves 2.)

DAY 3
BREAKFAST

Almond Millet

6 oz. millet   1½ oz. brewer's yeast
1 oz. dried banana   1 tbsp. maple syrup
1½ oz. almonds

Cook millet in 13 oz. of water in a medium saucepan for 30 minutes. Add dried banana. Chop almonds. Add them to the millet along with the brewer's yeast and maple syrup. Serve hot. (Serves 1.)

LUNCH

Savory Mushroom Dip

3 oz. potato   1 tsp. salt
3 oz. mushrooms   ¼ tsp. cayenne
1½ oz. onion   ¼ tsp. cumin
¼ oz. sesame seeds   ¼ tsp. coriander
3½ oz. water or broth   vegetable sticks (celery,
3 tbsp. olive oil   carrots, daikon, etc.)

Peel potatoes. Wash them. Slice approximately ¼" thick and place in a medium saucepan with enough water to cover. Cook until the potatoes are tender when you stick a fork in them. Rinse and slice mushrooms and onion. Sauté in a medium skillet until the onions are a golden brown. When the potatoes are cooked, place them in a blender with all the other ingredients. Puree well into a diplike consistency. Serve with a variety of vegetable sticks. (Yield is 12 oz.)

DINNER

Spaghetti Deluxe

3 oz. onion   3 oz. yellow pepper
1½ oz. olive oil   2 oz. zucchini
¼ tsp. basil   2 oz. tomato paste
¼ tsp. oregano   3 oz. water
¼ tsp. cumin   1 garlic clove, minced
6 oz. tomato   ½ tsp. salt
6 oz. spaghetti

Peel and slice onion. Sauté in the oil with the herbs in a 2-quart saucepan along with the tomato paste, water, garlic, and salt. Continue to cook, covered, for 15 minutes on low heat. Cook spaghetti in 20 oz. of water in another saucepan for 10 to 12 minutes or until done. Combine with vegetables in a medium mixing bowl. Serve hot with 6 oz. of fish. (Serves 2.)

DAY 4
BREAKFAST

Chock Full of Protein Drink

1½ oz. Brazil nuts	1 tbsp. carob powder
4 oz. soy milk	½ banana
1½ oz. apple cider	pinch cinnamon

Chop Brazil nuts finely. Combine all of the ingredients in a blender, including the Brazil nuts, and blend well. It tastes best when the mixture is smooth and creamy. If you like your drinks sweeter, you may use the whole banana. (Serves 1.)

LUNCH

Hearty Lentil Soup

3 oz. lentils	½ tsp. garlic powder
2 oz. carrots	½ tsp. coriander
3 oz. corn (may be fresh and	½ tsp. rosemary
removed from the husk or frozen)	½ tsp. basil
3 oz. fresh chives	¾ tsp. salt
3 tbsp. soy oil	several parsley sprigs for garnish

Cook lentils in a medium soup pot with enough water to cover. Bring to a boil and then set on medium heat with the lid on. Cooking time is approximately 1 hour. Scrub carrots and cut them into bite-sized pieces. After the lentils have cooked for approximately 20 minutes, drop the carrots into the pot along with the corn and remaining ingredients. When the mixture has cooked for an additional 30 minutes, take half of the mixture out of the pot and put it into a blender. Puree it for 15 seconds and then pour it back into the pot. Cook for an additional 10 minutes. Garnish with parsley sprigs. (Yields 4 to 5 cups.)

Nutty Bean Salad

3 oz. black beans	1 garlic clove, minced
1½ oz. walnuts	1 tsp. tarragon
2 oz. celery	½ tsp. sage
2 oz. carrots	½ tsp. salt
1½ tbsp. soy oil	

In a large bowl, soak the black beans overnight in 10 oz. of water. In the morning, rinse the beans and transfer them to a medium saucepan with 16 oz. of fresh water. Cook for 1½ hours or until done. Chop walnuts very finely. Rinse celery and scrub carrots. Cut celery and carrots into bite-sized pieces. Place oil in a wok or skillet and heat. Place all ingredients into the wok or skillet and sauté for 5 minutes. Serve at room temperature. (Serves 1.)

DINNER

Hot and Crunchy Veggie Mix

3 oz. snap green beans	½ tsp. parsley
3 oz. cauliflower	juice of ½ lemon
3 oz. brussels sprouts	pinch cayenne
1½ oz. walnuts	2 tbsp. soy oil
¼ tsp. sage	¾ tsp. salt
½ tsp. dill	2 oz. water

Wash beans and cut them into bite-sized pieces. Steam in a bamboo steam basket or stainless steel steamer for 10 minutes or until tender. Rinse cauliflower and brussels sprouts and cut into bite-sized pieces. Steam for 8 minutes. In a blender, place the steamed beans, walnuts, and the remaining ingredients. Pour sauce over the cauliflower and brussels sprouts. You may serve this dish either hot or cold. Serve with 6 oz. of fish. (Serves 2.)

Third Cycle

DAY 1
BREAKFAST

Sweet Cinnamon Couscous

6 oz. couscous	½ tbsp. honey
3 oz. apple	½ tsp. cinnamon
2 oz. raisins	3 oz. favorite fruit juice, optional

In a medium saucepan, cook couscous in 14 oz. of water. Bring to a boil, stirring often. Then lower heat. Cooking time is approximately 10 to 12 minutes. Wash and slice apples. When couscous has cooked, add apple slices and remaining ingredients. Mix well. Transfer to serving bowls. Add fruit juice if you wish. (Serves 1.)

LUNCH

Milano Bean and Vegetable Soup

3 oz. mung beans
6 oz. zucchini
4½ oz. summer squash
2 oz. Spanish onion
2 oz. carrots
1 oz. parsley

1 garlic clove, finely diced
3 tbsp. safflower oil
¾ tsp. salt
½ tsp. basil
¼ tsp. oregano

Place mung beans in a large bowl with 3 cups of water. Allow the beans to soak overnight. In the morning, rinse the beans well and transfer into a large soup pot, adding 4 cups of fresh water. Bring beans to a boil and lower to medium heat. Keep the lid on. Scrub the zucchini and summer squash, peel the onion and the carrots. Chop the vegetables into bite-sized pieces. Rinse parsley and chop finely. After the beans have been cooking for approximately one hour, add the vegetables and the remaining ingredients. Remove half of the mixture and transfer into a blender. Puree for 15 seconds. Return the puree to the rest of the soup to finish cooking for another 30 minutes. (Yields 4 to 5 cups.)

DINNER

Superb Vegetable Rice Salad

3 oz. amaranth
3 oz. basmati rice
1 oz. watercress
1 oz. dill
1½ oz. parsley
1½ oz. carrots

2 tbsp. safflower oil
juice of ½ lemon
½ tsp. salt
2 oz. water
¼ tsp. tarragon

In a medium pot, cook amaranth for 25 minutes in 10 oz. of water. In another pot, cook the rice in 10 oz. of water for 20 minutes. Rinse the watercress, dill, and parsley and chop medium fine. Scrub the carrots well and chop into bite-sized pieces. Place all the ingredients in a medium bowl and mix well. (Serves 2.)

DINNER (2ND OPTION)

Oriental Zucchini Salad

3 oz. amaranth
3 oz. hijiki seaweed
(1 oz. dry; 3 oz. soaked)
2 tbsp. safflower oil

3 oz. carrots
3 oz. zucchini
2 oz. daikon
¼ tsp. coriander

⅔ tsp. salt
¼ tsp. garlic

½ tsp. cumin
1½ oz. pecan

In a medium saucepan, cook amaranth in 10 oz. of water for 25 minutes. Rinse hijiki and soak 3 times. Scrub carrots and zucchini. Peel daikon. Cut carrots, zucchini, and daikon into bite-sized pieces and steam in a bamboo steamer basket or stainless steel steamer for 8 minutes. In a skillet or wok, sauté the hijiki with the safflower oil and the herbs for 5 minutes. Combine all the ingredients together in a medium bowl. Add the pecans. Mix well. Serve with 6 oz. of fish. (Serves 2.)

DAY 2
BREAKFAST

Fruity Rice Breakfast

6 oz. brown rice
1½ oz. coconut
1½ oz. cashews

1 tbsp. your favorite fruit
conserve (no sugar, just fruit)
1 oz. chopped figs

In a medium saucepan, cook brown rice in 14 oz. of water. When water comes to a boil, lower heat. Cooking time is approximately 30 minutes. When cooked, add the coconut and cashews. Mix well. Remove from the heat. Add the conserves and the figs. Mix again. Transfer to bowl. (Serves 1.)

LUNCH

Curried Vegetable Rice

6 oz. split peas
6 oz. brown rice
3 oz. broccoli
3 oz. carrots
3 oz. zucchini

2 oz. onions
3 tbsp. sunflower oil
½ tsp. curry powder
¾ tsp. salt

In a medium saucepan, cook split peas in enough water to cover. Bring to a boil then lower heat. In another saucepan, cook rice in 14 oz. of water for 30 minutes. Clean vegetables well and cut into bite-sized pieces. After peas have cooked for 15 minutes, add the chopped vegetables, cooked brown rice, and remaining ingredients. Cook for an additional 15 minutes. (Yields 4 to 5 cups.)

DINNER

Sunny Squash

3 oz. butternut squash
3 oz. buckwheat noodles

1 tsp. parsley
1 clove garlic, minced

3 oz. asparagus
2 oz. watercress

5 tbsp. sunflower oil
¾ tsp. salt

Cut squash in half, remove the seeds and discard them. Place the squash in a baking pan with ⅓" water, cut-side down. Bake for 40 minutes at 400 degrees. When the squash is cool enough to handle, remove the squash from the skin and set aside in a medium-sized bowl. Drop the noodles into salted boiling water and cook for 5 minutes. Set aside. Rinse the asparagus. Steam in a bamboo steamer basket or stainless steel steamer. Cut into 2" pieces. Rinse watercress and chop. Add noodles to the squash along with the asparagus, watercress, and remaining ingredients. Mix well, tossing gently. Serve with 6 oz. of fish. (Yields 4 to 5 cups.)

Basic Tossed Salad

3 oz. romaine
3 oz. carrots

2 oz. red cabbage
2 oz. tomato

Rinse vegetables and cut into bite-sized pieces. Combine everything together in a salad bowl. (Serves 2.)

DAY 3
BREAKFAST

Heart-Warming Breakfast

6 oz. cream of wheat
2 oz. chopped dates
1 oz. coconut

1½ oz. brewer's yeast
½ tsp. cinnamon

In a medium saucepan, cook cream of wheat in 12 oz. of water for 10 minutes or until done. Stir occasionally on medium heat. When cooked, add the remaining ingredients. Transfer to bowl. (Serves 1.)

LUNCH

Baked Potato Sesame

3 oz. potato
3 oz. spaghetti
1½ oz. scallions
1 tsp. dill
3 oz. tahini

1½ oz. sesame seeds
1½ tbsp. sesame oil
¼ tsp. coriander
½ tsp. salt
1 garlic clove, minced

Bake potato for 40 minutes at 400 degrees. When cool enough to handle, cut into 3/4" cubes. Cook spaghetti in a medium saucepan in 20 oz. of water for 10 minutes. Rinse scallions and chop them medium fine. Mix potato and spaghetti in a medium mixing bowl. Add the remaining ingredients. Transfer to a baking pan and bake for 15 minutes in a preheated 375-degree oven. (Serves 2.)

DINNER

Crunchy Vegetable Bean Salad

3 oz. adzuki beans
1 oz. almonds
3 oz. scallions
3 oz. red pepper
1 tsp. parsley
3 oz. tomato

2 tbsp. sesame oil
¼ tsp. oregano
1 tsp. salt
½ tsp. thyme
1 clove garlic, minced
several leaves of romaine lettuce

In a large bowl, soak beans overnight in 16 oz. of water. In the morning, rinse the beans and place them into a medium pot with 16 oz. of fresh water. Cook for 1 hour or until done. Blanch the almonds by bringing 18 oz. of water in a small saucepan to a boil and dropping the almonds into the water. Remove from the heat. Let the almonds remain in the boiling water for 5 minutes and then run cold water into the saucepan. Squeeze the skins off and let the almonds dry. Sliver the almonds. Rinse the scallions, red pepper, parsley, and tomato. Cut them into bite-sized pieces. In a medium mixing bowl, put the beans, almonds, and vegetables. Toss gently. Add the remaining ingredients and mix well. Serve cool on a bed of romaine lettuce. (Serves 2.)

DAY 4
BREAKFAST

Creamy Banana Tofu Pudding

6 oz. banana
2 oz. raisins
3 oz. tofu
4 oz. barley malt
½ oz. carob powder

1 tsp. vanilla
3 heaping tsp. Ener-G Egg Replacer
6 oz. apple juice
pinch cinnamon
pinch nutmeg

Place all ingredients in a blender. Puree until smooth and creamy. Transfer to a medium saucepan and cook over medium heat for 5 minutes, stirring frequently. Allow to chill for 45 minutes. (Yields 20 oz.)

LUNCH

Mid-Eastern Tempeh

3 oz. chick-peas
½ oz. dulse, dry
3 oz. cauliflower
3 oz. tempeh
2 oz. onion
6 oz. tomato sauce

2 tbsp. soy oil
a garlic clove, minced
¼ tsp. salt
½ tsp. basil
2 oz. water

In a medium bowl, soak the chick-peas overnight in 16 oz. of water. In the morning, rinse the chick-peas and transfer into a medium soup pot with 20 oz. of fresh water. Cook for 1 3/4 to 2 hours or until done. Rinse dulse 2 or 3 times in cold water. Rinse cauliflower and cut into flowerettes. Cut tempeh into ½" cubes and put all the ingredients together in a medium mixing bowl. Peel and slice the onion and add to the mixture. Toss gently. Add the remaining ingredients and mix well. Transfer to a greased baking pan and bake for 20 minutes in a preheated 350-degree oven. (Serves 2.)

DINNER

Double Bean Delight

3 oz. lima beans
3 oz. lentils
3 oz. okra
3 oz. cauliflower
1½ oz. brazil nut butter
1½ tbsp. corn oil

1½ oz. water
¼ tsp. tarragon
½ tsp. sage
½ tsp. salt
1 garlic clove, minced

Note: Brazil nut butter is made with a "Champion" juicer or a similar grinder

In a large bowl, soak beans overnight in 16 oz. of water. In the morning, rinse and replace with 16 oz. of fresh water in a medium soup pot. Cook for 1½ hours or until done. In another pot, cook lentils in 12 oz. of water for 25 minutes. Rinse and cut vegetables into bite-sized pieces. Steam in a bamboo steamer basket or stainless steel steamer for 8 minutes or until tender. Transfer all ingredients into a medium mixing bowl and gently toss. Add the remaining ingredients and mix well. Transfer to a baking pan and bake for 15 minutes in a 350-degree oven. (Serves 2.)

Additional Desserts

Multi-Fruit Oatmeal Pudding

3 oz. pears
3 oz. oatmeal
6 oz. pear juice
1 banana

2 heaping tsp. Ener-G-Egg
Replacer
pinch cinnamon
3 oz. apples

Place all ingredients, except for apples, in a blender. Puree. Transfer puree into small saucepan and cook over medium heat for approximately 5 minutes. Wash and cube apples. Add them to puree and stir frequently. Place in a medium mixing bowl or individual dessert dishes and allow to chill in the refrigerator for at least 45 minutes. (Yields approximately 18 oz.)

Tropical Pudding

6 oz. pineapple
6 oz. apple juice
3 tbsp. honey
2 tbsp. Ener-G-Egg Replacer

2 tbsp. coconut
pinch nutmeg
4½ oz. papaya
1½ oz. pecans

Place all ingredients, except for papaya and pecans, in a blender. Puree. Transfer puree into small saucepan and cook over medium heat for approximately 5 minutes. Peel papaya, remove seeds, and cube. Chop pecans. Add both to the puree and stir. Place in medium mixing bowl or individual dessert dishes and allow to chill in refrigerator for at least 45 minutes. (Yields approximately 16 oz.)

Mango Strawberry Canton

4 oz. mango
4 oz. strawberries
12 oz. apple juice

2 heaping tbsp. agar-agar
1 tsp. vanilla
2 oz. dates, chopped

Peel mango and remove pit. Put in the blender with 2 oz. strawberries. Add apple juice and blend. Transfer to medium saucepan and bring to a boil. Lower heat and add agar-agar. Stir and dissolve agar-agar and simmer for 5 minutes. Add vanilla and chopped dates. Transfer to mixing bowl or individual dessert dishes and place in the refrigerator until juice begins to gel (about 10 minutes). Drop in the remaining strawberries. Chill for 1 hour. (Serves 2 to 4.)

Papaya Brown Rice Pudding

3 oz. brown rice
6 oz. papaya
1½ oz. coconut
1½ oz. figs

10 oz. pineapple coconut juice
2 heaping tsp. Ener-G-Egg
Replacer
2 oz. blueberries

In a medium saucepan, cook brown rice in about 10 oz. of water for 25 minutes. When cooked, place in blender. Peel papaya and remove seeds. Add to blender along with remaining ingredients, except for blueberries. Puree until creamy and smooth. Transfer to medium saucepan and cook over medium heat for approximately 5 minutes. Stir frequently. Transfer to medium mixing bowl or individual dessert dishes and place in refrigerator to chill for 45 minutes. Serve with blueberries. (Yields approximately 15 oz.)

Blueberry Kiwi Pudding

3 oz. millet
5 oz. blueberries
2 oz. kiwi
½ banana
1½ oz. slivered almonds

6 oz. apple strawberry juice
2 heaping tsp. Ener-G-Egg
Replacer
1 tsp. lemon juice

Place millet in a small saucepan with approximately 10 oz. water and cook for 20 minutes. When cooked, put in blender with the remaining ingredients, except for almonds. Puree until smooth and creamy. Transfer puree to medium saucepan and heat for 5 minutes over medium heat, stirring frequently. Transfer to medium mixing bowl or individual dessert dishes and allow to chill in refrigerator for 45 minutes. Top with almonds. (Yields approximately 23 oz.)

Strawberry Tofu Pudding

4½ oz. strawberry
6 oz. tofu

3 tbsp. maple syrup
1 tsp. vanilla

Place all ingredients in the blender. Puree until creamy and smooth. Transfer into one medium mixing bowl or individual dessert dishes. Place in refrigerator and allow to chill for 45 minutes. (Serves 2.)

Peach Canton

6 oz. peaches
12 oz. apple blackberry juice
2 heaping tbsp. agar-agar

2 tbsp. Barbados molasses
3 oz. pitted black cherries

Wash and cut peaches into small pieces. Place half of the peaches in a blender with juice. Place mixture in a medium saucepan and bring to a boil. Lower heat and add agar-agar. Stir and dissolve agar, and simmer for 5 minutes. Add molasses. Transfer to a medium mixing bowl or individual dessert dishes and place in refrigerator until juice begins to gel (around 10 minutes). Add remaining peaches and cherries. Chill for 1 hour. (Serves 2.)

Peachy Tofu Pudding

6 oz. peaches
3 oz. barley malt

1 tsp. vanilla
6 oz. peach juice

Wash and cut peaches. Place all ingredients in blender and puree until smooth. Transfer to medium saucepan and place on medium heat for 5 minutes, stirring frequently. Transfer to medium mixing bowl or individual dessert dishes and allow to chill in refrigerator for 45 minutes. (Yields 18 oz.)

Blueberry Banana Pudding

6 oz. blueberries
1 banana
3 oz. tofu

3 oz. apple juice
4 oz. nectarines, sliced
2 oz. almonds

Place blueberries, banana, tofu, and apple juice in a blender. Puree until smooth and creamy. Transfer to medium mixing bowl or individual dessert dishes. Top with nectarine slices and almonds. (Serves 2.)

14

Exercise

We have already mentioned the critical importance of exercise not only to weight management but also to overall good health. Doing the same exercises all the time, however, develops certain of our muscles to the exclusion of others. Runners, for example, typically have very healthy internal body systems and well-developed legs, but they lack proportional upper-body strength. Combining different forms of exercise can help achieve a good balance of muscle activity throughout the body.

Any aerobic exercise should be done three or four times a week for 20 to 30 minutes each time for maximum benefit. Start slowly, increasing the amount of time and intensity by about 10 percent every two weeks. Use good quality equipment, including proper foot gear. All sports require both pre- and post-game stretching.

After completing any aerobic exercise you should:

- ♥ Check your pulse. See if you have achieved your target heart rate. If you haven't exercise a bit harder next time.
- ♥ Avoid hot showers, saunas, or whirlpools. Heat keeps the peripheral capillaries dilated, making it difficult for your blood to return to your heart right after exercise.
- ♥ Avoid strength exercises like weightlifting after doing aerobics. Weightlifting constricts blood capillaries so the blood does not return to your heart. Do them before the aerobic exercises or at another time.
- ♥ Rehydrate yourself, replacing body fluids lost doing exercise.

This chapter describes some of the most popular aerobic exercises, as well as common anaerobic ones. Anaerobic exercises, which require explosive bursts of energy followed by longer periods of lower energy output or rest, build strength, power, endurance, or the skill of specific muscles or muscle groups. The chapter also looks into the link between nutrition and exercise, and then describes a comprehensive 28-day exercise plan for the runner or anyone else serious about regular exercise.

Aerobic Exercises

WALKING Walking can be done by almost anyone, almost anywhere. For some, including the elderly, pregnant, arthritic, or those with heart disease, it is the only form of reasonable cardiovascular exercise. All you need is some comfortable old clothes, a good pair of running (walking) shoes, and a hat to protect you if the weather is hot and sunny or cold and windy.

Walking is a low-intensity exercise, so you have to do it for a longer time than a sport like running to get maximum cardiovascular conditioning. About 1½ hours of walking will give you the same aerobic effect as 30 minutes of running.

Walk with an even, rhythmic heal-to-toe gait; swing your arms from side to side in a natural way. Don't keep them pressed tightly against your body or in your pockets. Try not to carry anything since it will weigh you down and upset your balance.

Start by taking your pulse and doing the warm-up exercises. For the first two to three weeks, walk 20 to 30 minutes a day. Increase that to 1½ hours a day in 10 percent increments every two or three weeks. Begin each session by walking slowly, building up to your target heart rate, and then tapering off to a slow pace. Check your pulse every 10 minutes. If you feel tired, slow down or stop altogether until you recover. Then start slowly and build up your speed and heart rate again.

You can walk anywhere. Your first choice, and the most fun, should be outdoors on a soft surface of grass or earth. If you walk in the street, be sure to face the traffic by walking on the left side. If the weather or your health do not permit you to go outdoors, walk on a treadmill, up and down the hallway in your apartment building, or snake in and around the rooms in your home. (In chapter 30 you will find a complete walking program as well as other information on keeping your feet, legs, and whole self healthy the natural way.)

SWIMMING Swimming is an outstanding cardiovascular exercise. It is rhythmic, uses all the major muscle groups, stretches the muscles, and keeps you limber. The water's buoyancy reduces the pressure on bones and joints, pressure that can cause injuries in other sports. As a result, people unable to walk or jog because of a skeletal or structural problem often can still take up swimming.

If you are a nonswimmer, you can still take up a water sport. You can begin by taking your pulse while walking back and forth slowly in the waist-deep area of a pool. Swing your arms naturally when walking. Build up the intensity of this regime to reach and maintain your target heart rate.

If you are a swimmer, take your pulse and do warm-up exercises. Once in the pool, start slowly and easily with a restful stroke, like the breast stroke or the side stroke. Build up slowly until you reach your target heart rate. You may eventually change to more intense strokes, such as the crawl or butterfly. Aim to swim for a full 20 minutes, even if you have to swim on your back for a while.

As with other aerobic exercises, swim for 20 to 30 minutes, three to four times a week. But be careful; daily swimming can lead to strained or pulled muscles. Skip a day to allow your body to recover. Periodically, try to increase your swimming speed by sprinting for up to 30 seconds at a time. As soon as you feel yourself winded, return to your normal pace. Repeat this three to five times in a row with a 30-second recovery interval between sprints. This type of interval training can enhance your cardiovascular conditioning.

Swimming builds powerful shoulders and arm muscles, as well as rear leg muscles. After swimming, stretch your rear leg muscles. And since the back stroke uses the anterior leg muscles more, they may also require additional stretching afterwards.

Wear a comfortable suit that will stay on without constant fuss and attention. The ideal pool water temperature is 77–81 degrees. Warmer water makes it difficult for the body to eliminate heat; colder water makes it difficult to warm up muscles.

There are some drawbacks to swimming. The biggest problem may be finding a pool. If you choose swimming, choose an alternate sport as well, for those times when a pool is not available.

Another disadvantage is the possibility of getting conjunctivitis or ear infections. You can protect yourself against both by wearing goggles and either a bathing cap or ear plugs. Select only good goggles—the cheap varieties are ineffective. Be sure not to use a nose plug if your nose is inflamed in any way, since that condition actually is better served by allowing the free circulation of moisture. Some people react badly to the chlorine in the water, especially, as is often the case, if the concentration is high.

BICYCLING Bicycling is another good exercise. Whether you use a 3-speed or 10-speed bicycle does not really matter. What does matter is that the bike is sturdy, that the frame is suited to your size, and that it is kept in safe operating condition. Structurally, men's bikes are often sounder than women's, and for this reason many women buy them. Adjust the seat height so that you can pedal. Your knee should be almost straight when the pedal is closest to the ground, but even at that position, the leg should be slightly bent. Use pant clips or rubber bands to keep your pants from tangling in the chain. At night, dress so that you can be seen. A red leg light provides a moving signal of your presence on the road.

For exercising, you might want to use a bike with handlebars tilted upward, so you can sit up straight. Your bones will be in alignment, and such bikes are friendlier to your lower back than bikes with racing handles. For distance or racing, you will want to use downward-tilted handlebars.

Riding indoors on a stationary bicycle is also beneficial. The same basic principles apply. The more interesting the exercise bicycle is (for example, with built-in computers), the more the exercise will help hold your interest, reducing some of the boredom that you might otherwise experience.

Anybody who is able to ride a bicycle and at the same time read a novel or a magazine is not riding the bicycle hard enough to gain a cardiovascular benefit. Your concentration should always be on the sport itself.

If you ride a bicycle very slowly, you need more time on it to gain proper cardiovascular conditioning. At the same time, if you sprint all the time you will lose any aerobic benefit as well, so never try to ride a bicycle to the point that you are exercising at over 80 percent of your maximum heart rate. However, you can do interval training, much like swimming, while you bike ride. Ride the bicycle as fast as you can for 30 seconds at a time. Then rest for 30 seconds by riding at a normal pace. Do this three to five times in a row. Such interval training will help increase your aerobic capacity and stamina.

Remember to stretch out properly after bike riding. It is best to wear good biking shoes, since they transmit force to the pedals more efficiently. Walking and running shoes will do well, if you can't find biking shoes. You should use foot clips to secure your shoes to the pedals.

Bicycling causes less trauma to the joints and muscles than jogging or running. Still, problems can occur. In addition to collisions, the most common injuries are outer calf pain, knee pain, and chronic soreness of the hands.

ROPE JUMPING Rope jumping, or jumping without a rope, gives you cardiovascular conditioning with a bonus: you can burn more calories per minute jumping rope than running, swimming, or bike riding. Jumping rope, however, can have a disastrous effect on the legs and lower back. Never start jumping for a long period of time. In the beginning, even a few minutes can be too long.

To begin properly, run in place, or walk in place, faster and faster, until your legs are coming off the ground at a very fast rate. Stay light on your feet. Avoid pounding them into the ground. Then, for a period of 10 to 20 seconds, start to jump very lightly on both feet at the same time. It is not necessary to jump high. Just keep jumping, and then after 30 seconds (with or without a rope), start walking or jogging in place again. Do this for a minute or two. As soon as you feel your breath return, start jumping again. Spend no more than two to three minutes jumping the first day. The older or heavier you are, the less you should do the first few times.

Never jump rope on a daily basis. It can lead to a lot of serious problems, since it can just be too stressful for the body. Increase your jumping time by about 10 percent every two weeks. This will allow your bones and musculature to develop proper stress buildup, as opposed to the overstress that would likely be caused by a too rapid increase, leading not only to calf pain and lower back pain, but to stress fractures of the bones in the leg and foot. Your ultimate aim is to jump for 20 to 30 minutes continuously. Interval training can be used with jumping rope, in much the same way described for swimming or bicycling.

Remember, duration is more important than intensity.

Rope jumping can be done in a small space, like a patio or small yard. In inclement weather, it can be done in a garage, basement, or any room with a ceiling high enough for a rope to clear. A jump rope travels well; it packs easily and permits a workout almost anywhere.

OTHER AEROBIC ALTERNATIVES Other aerobic exercise alternatives include rowing (using a boat or rowing machine), roller skating, aerobic dancing, and minitrampolining (or rebound jogging). You can also get aerobic effects from tennis, handball, racquetball, squash, and basketball.

Cross-country skiing is another option. Since weather or location may make this alternative difficult, indoor cross-country machines are available and can be used year round. Some experts even think that cross-country skiing is better aerobically than running, since in cross-country skiing you use more muscles than just those in your legs. The more muscles involved in exercise, the better the aerobic effect you get.

Popular Anaerobic Exercises

WEIGHT TRAINING Start with low weights that are easy to lift. Do three sets of 8 to 12 repetitions. The last two repetitions should be difficult; your muscles strengthen only when they fatigue. The initial repetitions—or reps—result in muscle tone, the final reps give muscle strength. As soon as the last two reps become easy, it means it is time to increase the weights by a minimum of 2½ pounds to a maximum of 10 pounds.

To build muscle mass, or "beach" muscles, use heavy weights and do fewer reps, about 8 to 10. To improve tone, use light weights, and do more reps, about 12 to 15 per set.

Remember, allow a full 48 hours between weight-training sessions for the muscles to repair and heal since weight training breaks down muscle.

As a rule, weight trainers think that athletes need to eat huge amounts of protein to rebuild and repair the muscle tissue broken down by exercise. In fact, athletes typically eat too much protein and not enough complex carbohydrates (which are also excellent sources of protein).

Different forms of weight training will help increase general muscle strength. One involves the use of free weights. A second utilizes universal machines, and a third uses isokinetic, or Nautilus-type, training procedures. All three systems basically do the same thing. They help muscle become completely fatigued and so increase the size of the muscle fibers.

Free weights can be used at home as well as in an athletic club. But since it takes some time to prepare for each of the different exercises, it may seem to take a long time to get the effect you want. Free weights have to be used very carefully; they pose the most risks of all weight-training procedures. They help develop better coordination, however, than other weight-training procedures.

Weight training can provide an excellent way for the runner to maintain strength and flexibility. By increasing the strength of all your muscles, not just those in your legs, you can increase your ability to withstand the stresses of long distance running. Also body parts that are weak tend to get injured much faster.

Arm, shoulder, and anterior leg muscle exercises should be emphasized in weight training. It is important, however, not to try to build up big muscles through weight training; this will only add to the weight and exercise burden you have to carry during running. While it is important to be strong, weight training can also tighten you up. Thus, flexibility and range of motion programs as well as a good stretching program are needed to loosen you up.

RACKET SPORTS Tennis, racquetball, squash, paddleball, and handball are basically discontinuous, stop-and-go sports. Players need power for explosive bursts of energy and stamina to run around the court. They come closest to aerobic activity when there are long volleys that result in the continuous use of large muscles.

Racket sports are very popular. Indoor and outdoor courts are abundant and many are accessible year round. To begin, find a place to play, and a good instructor who will guide you on proper technique, equipment, and clothing.

Try to play with people who are at your level to avoid unnecessary tension and embarrassment. Remember, exercise is supposed to benefit you—physically and spiritually.

GOLF Golfers need good neuromuscular coordination and focused concentration. The game is characterized by short bursts of energy interspersed with longer periods of slow activity or rest. Unfortunately, a good deal of stress builds up around each shot. Your caloric expenditure will depend totally on whether you walk (how far and how fast), or ride an electric cart around the five- or six-mile golf course. If you walk briskly between holes, you can approach some aerobic conditioning for brief periods of time.

To start, find a golf instructor who will guide you to appropriate equipment and clothing. It is best to learn proper stance and movement from the beginning, rather than later having to unlearn improper techniques.

If you are playing golf for exercise and pleasure, it can give you both. If you bring your business or social problems to the court, however, you lessen these benefits. Golfing in hot or humid weather can lead to dehydration. Drinking water before, during, and after play therefore becomes essential.

Exercise and Nutrition

When you exercise regularly, your body burns a higher than normal percentage of fats, even while you sleep. To give your body an adequate supply of essential fatty acids, steer clear of animal fats and eat extra oils selected from a variety of available vegetable sources. Rely primarily on unrefined oils found in foods such as raw seeds, raw nuts, avocados, and grains. Refined oils increase your risk of consuming too many free radicals—unstable molecules that can attack your cells, speed up the aging process, and weaken your body.

Protein is an inefficient fuel that is pressed into service only after preferred fuels are depleted. It is digested slowly and tends to dehydrate your body by using lots of water for its digestion and elimination. Under normal circumstances, you can only digest and utilize three ounces of food at a time, so regulate your protein intake to avoid the taxing waste of energy that follows overconsumption. Complex carbohydrates are much more efficient and should serve as your key foods for replenishing glycogen, the energy fuel.

CARBOHYDRATE LOADING Carbohydrate loading is an eating regimen followed by some athletes in preparation for a long competition, such as a running marathon. A typical schedule for a runner begins seven days before the event with an exhausting bout of exercise, depleting the stores of glycogen in the body. To further aid the glycogen depletion, the runner eats a low-carbohydrate, high-protein, and high-fat diet. Three days before the event, he packs in as many carbohydrates as possible to replenish the glycogen, keeping protein and fat at moderate levels. The body is stressed by this deprivation of carbohydrate fuel, and it responds to that stress by overcompensating and storing extra supplies of glycogen in the muscles. Thus, the marathon runner has more energy and can run longer before tiring.

One modification of this classic loading technique is to substitute tapered rest for the exhaustive bout of exercise during the week preceding the event. Also, the last week might feature a high complex carbohydrate diet. A further modification sometimes suggested is for the runner to rest and eat a high complex carbohydrate diet 48 to 72 hours before the event.

What was just described is preparation for an extraordinary event that few of us would even participate in. For regular exercise, or competition in general, guidelines for eating are: (1) Eat enough so as not to feel hungry during the event. Eat modest amounts of complex carbohydrates up to 2½ hours before exercising. Stay away from fat and protein. Avoid salty or spicy foods, simple sugars, and unfamiliar foods that could irritate or upset you. (2) Allow time for your stomach and small intestines to empty. (3) Drink water or diluted fruit juice until one hour before the event, then continue to drink water only.

You may wonder if, after drinking so much water, a runner, walker, or biker will need to stop and urinate. The fact is that the kidneys slow down during exercise, so the body will retain fluids for use by other tissues to reduce heat buildup that comes with exercise and produce sweat. The body, in effect, turns off the water-eliminating system and turns on the water-retention system.

SUPPLEMENTS In general, a person who eats a well-balanced diet will not need vitamin or mineral supplements for their exercise needs. However, not all the vitamins and minerals naturally available in foods will be available to everyone, due to food sensitivities, poor absorption, chemical imbalances, and improper food combining. Persons affected by these factors may need supplements, even megadoses, of vitamins and minerals to bring a particular deficiency up to par or to strengthen a weak point.

Exercise stresses the body, with B complex vitamins in particular burned off by stress. It is recommended that B complex vitamins as well as vitamin A, which helps stimulate the immune system, be taken as part of an exercise regimen. The antioxidants, vitamins C and E, and selenium, are also recommended before and after exercise. Calcium and magnesium, in a 1:1 ratio, are commonly used to benefit muscles, as are coenzyme Q10 (100-200 mg) and L-carnitine (500-1,000 mg). Iron deficiency is common among women and athletes, and runners should be tested for iron deficiency before training begins.

SALT INTAKE AFTER EXERCISE A common misconception is that your body loses salt through perspiration after exercise. In fact, it loses only water, leaving the body's salt in higher concentrations than before. You need more water after exercise, not more salt, to help prevent fatigue, irritability, and exhaustion. Salt pills are not recommended.

A BIG DINNER OR A BEDTIME SNACK? If you are serious about exercise, dinner should be your smallest meal of the day. In the late afternoon or early evening, your body is in a state of recuperation and repair from exercise. Burdening it with a heavy meal hampers this process.

You shouldn't eat anything substantial for at least two hours before you go to sleep because little will leave your stomach within an hour after eating. Once you're in a prone position, whatever is in your stomach has difficulty moving into the intestine. If you are hungry late in the evening, try a very light food such as fruit, or have a liquid refreshment like an herbal tea.

POSTEXERCISE NUTRITION During exercise, you use up water and fuel. You need to replenish them—in that order. Water, the recommended beverage, helps alleviate feelings of exhaustion. Give your body an opportunity to return to normal before eating.

Even if you are not consciously thirsty, drink an 8- to 10-ounce glass of water after exercising, and again at 20-minute intervals for the next hour. You cannot restore the water you lost in exercise simply by drinking a lot at one time. Your body's tissues, after all, can only absorb water at a certain rate; the rest is eliminated. The average water consumption per day for a healthy adult who exercises is eight 8- to 10-ounce glasses. What you do not use, the body will eliminate.

If you are ravenous after exercising, it may mean you have run out of fuel. You have depleted your supply of glucose and/or glycogen and your body wants to start replenishing it immediately. In this case, pay attention to eating more as a part of your regular diet to build up glycogen levels.

While pre-exercise nutrition should consist of a high complex-carbohydrate diet, postexercise meals should include protein as well, since you will need protein to rebuild or repair muscles and other tissues.

A 28-Day Exercise Plan for Runners and Other Serious Exercisers

This comprehensive exercise program is designed for the runner or anyone serious about regular exercise who wants to develop and maintain good health. But for it to work, you must be willing to make a commitment to incorporate this gentle, realistic, exercise routine into your lifestyle. Exercise should be viewed in the same way as brushing your teeth, something to develop as a daily habit whose importance you recognize. Don't regard it as something extra you'll do if you have time after you do everything else. Exercise is part of everything else. Yet also understand you won't die if you miss a day.

The Basic 28-Day Exercise Plan calls for your choice of running or some other aerobic exercise on Days 1, 3, and 5. For the first four weeks, do the exercise for 20 minutes. Increase the duration by 10 percent every two weeks if you are under 35 years of age and have no history of heart disease. Increase the duration by 10 percent every four weeks if you are over 35 or have a history of heart disease.

These exercise plans are designed in one-week cycles, since most people plan their time that way. Day 1 of the exercise plan may be any day of the week. The sequence is what matters.

Your exercise program, to be viable, needs to reflect your goals, attitudes, strengths, weaknesses, and lifestyle. Use these suggested plans as guidelines; feel free to alter them to suit your individual requirements.

When choosing aerobic alternatives, use both sides of your brain. Use the left side to choose activities that will enable you to get and keep your body functioning at your target heart rate for 20 to 30 minutes at least three days a week. Also be realistic in your expectations. So use the right side of your brain to evaluate activities that appeal to you.

Different exercises affect different muscles. You can combine two complementary exercises in your total program and rotate them according to whim or weather. You could have one indoor and one outdoor choice. For example, skiing and biking build up the anterior leg muscles while providing good aerobic conditioning. If you run outdoors and use a stationary bicycle indoors, you have come up with a set of complementary exercises good for all seasons. Either one could also be combined with swimming. There are outdoor and indoor pools. Weight training is a beneficial form of anaerobic exercise that augments any aerobic exercise. It can be done with free weights or an isokinetic machine, like Nautilus equipment.

When you purchase equipment, choose sturdy, safe, well-built, quality equipment. Junk breaks down quickly. Appropriate clothes and foot gear are also important. Be particular about your running shoes. Perfect fit is critical.

BEFORE YOU BEGIN Prior to starting any serious exercise or conditioning program, most people should have a complete physical exam, including a stress test. A cardiovascular stress test entails hooking you up to an electrocardiograph, which monitors your heart and blood pressure as you walk or run on a treadmill. The workload is increased at regular intervals. The results can indicate hidden or small conditions that could lead to trouble. Stress tests are done in various centers, hospitals, and some cardiologists' offices. If you are under 35 years of age, not overweight, and have no family history of heart disease, you probably do not need a stress test. A routine physical examination will do.

If for some reason you cannot or do not wish to have such an exam, it is important to start and proceed very slowly. If any unusual signs manifest themselves, stop right away and check them out immediately with your doctor.

What time of day is best to exercise? If you guessed either morning, noon or night, you'd be right. There are three more facts to consider:

Most people are more flexible and looser (also more fatigued after a day's work) at about 6 p.m. So exercising in late afternoon takes advantage of the flexibility, pumps up energy to revitalize a tired body, and reduces the tensions of the day. Exercising in early morning, on the other hand, takes advantage of a well-rested and fresh state of mind.

Each person needs to be in tune with his or her own body, following the monthly rhythms that seem to affect our intellect, mood, and physical energy levels. Do it when it feels good.

The right time for exercise is any time you manage to find in your busy schedule, It is best to plan your exercise.

If you feel exhausted, reduce the intensity and duration of any exercise by 50 percent. Your body is talking to you. Listen to it. That's good preventive sports medicine. The only legitimate reason for skipping your exercise is illness. Business is the worst excuse. You probably could use exercise most when you are under stress from work.

Relaxation, warm-ups and cool-down exercise should be used with all types of exercise: physical activity, aerobic, anaerobic, and all those in between. They maintain flexibility in muscles, tendons, ligaments, and joints, and help to prevent injury.

Too much, too fast, or too soon are the most common reasons for sport injuries. DO NOT OVERDO. Less is better—at the beginning—at least until your body adapts. Be in touch with your body to avoid injury and disillusionment because of some bad, though probably avoidable experience. Test yourself to see what affects your body. If you overdo, you will lose your sensitivity to the small clues your body will provide.

The Basic 28-Day Plan is a one-size-fits-all plan, and it is good for the rest of your life. The exercises will work for you as long as you do them. There is a variation of the Basic Plan presented here if you wish to go beyond good health toward excellence, or have special fitness goals. Option A provides an opportunity for anaerobic exercise or sports. Option B adds interval training to aerobic exercise.

Steps 1 through 5 are the warm-up sequence: Relaxation, Nonspecific Warm-Up, Joint Warm-Up, Pre-sport Stretching, Specific Warm-Up. Together with *Steps 7 and 8*, the cool-down sequence (Post-sport Stretching and Cool-Down), they should be done every single day of your life to maintain good flexibility, circulation, balance, and a sense of well-being.

Step 6 is the slot in which you should put your running or chosen aerobic alternative. It is the one part of the sequence that will change from day to day, or from time to time, as your needs and goals change.

The Basic 28-Day Plan

(WEEKS 1–4)

DAY	STEPS	TIME
1	warm-ups (#1–5)	20 min.
	choice of aerobic exercise (#6)	
	cool-downs (#7-8)	
2	#1–5 & #7–8	
3	#1–8	
4	#1–5 & #7–8	
5	#1–8	
6	#1–5 & #7–8	
7	#1–5 & #7–8	

Repeat the 7-day sequence four times for a total of 28 days. Beginning on Day 1 of the fifth week (roughly the beginning of the second month), increase the time you exercise by 10 percent. Instead of 20 minutes, exercise aerobically for 22 minutes. Follow the increment schedule as described above until you reach the time limits listed below:

EXERCISE	TIME LIMIT
Walking	1½ hours
Running	30 minutes (unless you want to compete)
Swimming	45 minutes to 1 hour
Bicycling	30 minutes (unless you want to compete)
Jumping	30 minutes (due to high intensity of jumping, it is detrimental to go beyond this limit)

Monitor your pulse to be certain you are exercising within your target heart range. As you become more fit, and your body handles the stress of exercise more efficiently, you will have to work harder to get up to and stay at your target heart rate. Do this first by increasing duration until you reach the defined time limit, then by increasing intensity as measured by your heart rate.

This is a lifetime exercise plan. As such, it accommodates itself to you each year. On your birthday, recalculate your target heart range. The formula is 220 minus your age times 70 percent.

If, for reasons of your own, you desire a more demanding schedule, do Step 6, your aerobic exercise, a fourth time during each week. A good choice is Day 6 or Day 7. If you decide to train for a marathon, you could train three days, rest one, train three days, and then rest one.

OPTION A The 28-Day Plan's Option A suggests you choose an anaerobic exercise or sport to alternate with your aerobic exercise. Step 6 will be an aerobic exercise or sport one day a week. Option A is designed for persons who enjoy a particular sport, like tennis or golf, and want to incorporate it into their exercise regimen. It will also appeal to persons who want to develop stronger and more balanced musculature through weight training or calisthenics.

If you are enthusiastic about your sport and want to play twice a week, below is a suggested schedule to accommodate that. Remember, you need to space bouts of anaerobic exercise at least 48 hours apart. The intensity of such exercise breaks down tissue and it takes two full days to repair and recover from that stress.

The Basic Plan is sufficient to achieve and maintain optimal conditioning. Option A is only for those who want more.

Option A suggests an anaerobic exercise or sport on Days 2 and 5 (or only one day if you prefer). This allows you to include tennis or any other racket sport, golf, weight training, etc. You may choose to do calisthenics: (1) push-ups for the arms, shoulders, back, stomach and most of the body; (2) bent-knee sit-ups for the abdominal muscles; and (3) jumping jacks for the legs and shoulders. Start with a few of each and build up. Use proper form and technique with every repetition. If you get sloppy, you will get tired and then quit.

For the first four weeks of Option A, follow the Basic Plan. Begin here on Day 1 of Week 5. Notice that on Days 2 and 5, Step 6 is anaerobic. On Days 1 and 3 continue your usual aerobic exercise—this time for 22 minutes each session.

OPTION A
(WEEK 5)

DAY	STEPS	TIME
1	warm-ups (#1–5)	22 mins.
	choice of aerobic exercise (#6)	
	cool-downs (#7–8)	
2	#1–8	
	#6 anaerobic	
3	#1–8	
	#6 anaerobic	
4	#1–5 & #7–8	
5	#1–8	
	#6 anaerobic	
6	#1–5 & #7–8	
7	#1–5 & #7–8	

(WEEK 6)

8	#1–8 aerobic	22 min.
9	#1–8 anaerobic	
10	#1–8 aerobic	
11	#1–5 & 7–8	
12	#1–8 anaerobic	
13	#1–5 & 7–8	
14	#1–5 & 7–8	

During weeks 7 and 8, increase the sessions by 10 percent if you are under 35 and have had no heart condition. The Step 6 aerobic exercises on Days 2, 5, 9, and 12 will be performed for 24 minutes. Repeat Days 1–14 for week 7 and 8 (Days 15–28).

At the beginning of week 9, increase the time again by 10 percent to 26 minutes of aerobic exercise if you are under 35 and do not have a heart condition; or 24 minutes of aerobic exercise if you are over 35 or have a history of heart problems.

If you feel like having a heavy workout, you may do your aerobic exercise AFTER your anaerobic exercise or sport. For example, you may want to swim after tennis. That's fine. But do not do anaerobic after aerobic. If interferes with the body's ability to recover properly.

If you reach a plateau, or a point in your regimen you cannot get past, yet you feel you have not reached your physiological limit, seek professional guidance. Something you are doing (or not doing properly) could be imposing a limitation. You could be getting in your own way. Or it may just be that your body can't work any harder.

OPTION B This option adds interval training one or two days a week to the aerobic exercise in Step 6 of the Basic 28-Day Plan. This option is for those who strive for excellence in cardiovascular fitness, beyond what it takes to stay in good physical condition. This is not training for marathoners, but for those who want to do a bit more to improve their stamina, endurance, and conditioning.

Interval training can be done with any aerobic exercise. For example, if you were running, you would run at your target heart rate for 10 minutes. Then run to get your pulse to beat as close to your maximum heart rate as possible (220 minus age times 85 percent) for 30 seconds. Next, run at your target heart rate (220 minus age times 70 percent) for 30 seconds. Repeat four consecutive times during one exercise period. Increase by one repetition every month to a limit of 10 times.

There are cautions to be observed in interval training. The high-intensity nature of this kind of training can lead to injury, and it is not recommended for persons who have heart disease or other serious medical problems unless they have a doctor's approval.

Interval training is anaerobic, so the cautions regarding anaerobic exercise hold. A full 48 hours is required between anaerobic exercise periods to allow for recovery from the stress it causes.

Once a week this kind of conditioning is recommended. If you have specific fitness goals, you may choose to do interval training twice a week. The plan schedules it twice to demonstrate the ideal spacing. Four sets are enough to fatigue most people. A set consists of a 30-second sprint plus a 30-second rest.

Do not attempt to combine the Basic Plan with Option A and Option B. It is too much to add both anaerobic and interval training to aerobic exercise without professional guidance.

OPTION B
(WEEK 5)

DAY	STEPS	TIME
1	warm-ups (#1–5)	22 mins.
	choice of aerobic exercise (#6)	
	cool-downs (#7–8)	
2	#1–5 & #7–8	
3	#1–8 with interval	
4	#1–5 & #7–8	
5	#1–8 without interval	
6	#1–8 without interval	
7	#1–5 & #7–8	

Repeat above for Days 8–14 (week 6).

Thereafter increase time by 10 percent every two weeks until you reach the time limit for that particular exercise as listed under the Basic Plan.

Running a Marathon

If you are really serious about exercise and about running in particular, you may someday go the final distance—like the ancient Greek Olympic athletes—and train to run a marathon. Here are a few sensible and practical tips for those who want to go that extra distance.

Top marathon runners seem to follow training routines in which they run 110–150 miles a week. This does not constitute normal training. If the average runner attempted this kind of regimen, it would probably end up totally wrecking his or her body.

The best way to train for a marathon is to do it gradually. Start with 3 miles, five days a week for the first month. Increase it 1 mile a day for the next three months, taking off one day and adding a longer run on Sunday. Increase until you are able to do 6 miles a day, let's say, Tuesday, Wednesday, Thursday, and Friday; then, rest Saturday, and do 12 miles on Sunday, for 36 miles a week. When you run 24 miles during the week and 22 miles on Sunday, you have a total of 46 miles a week. If one of the days during the week is for interval training (faster training), you will get both speed and endurance.

Consistency is very important when you train. So is getting enough rest. If you run seven days a week, your body never gets a chance to recuperate. If, on the other hand, you do a 20-mile run on Sunday, rest on Monday, loosen up with 4 miles on Tuesday, do 8 miles on Wednesday, skip Thursday, run 10 miles on Friday, and skip Saturday, you would be doing the same mileage with three day's rest. You should definitely rest the day before a marathon. Remember you will also need about one day of rest for every mile after you race.

It's also important to keep a diary while you train. There are many factors that will impact your performance, including biorhythms and circadian rhythms, and keeping track of the way you feel can help you understand these subtle cycles.

PACING Try to focus in on your pacing. Keep a stopwatch so that you know, within two or three seconds every mile, how well you're doing. Shifting pace throughout a long race can be very stressful on the body. If you start out slower and get faster in six-mile increments, you will be doing much better. Because of changes in blood and brain chemistry, proper pacing will improve the way you feel during a long run.

A marathon is tricky. You may feel like you have energy right up to the 23rd mile, and then suddenly, it's gone. Your muscles are tight, and you feel lucky even to be able to walk. Suddenly at the 24-mile mark, your legs might say, "I quit," and then you find yourself, with thousands of others, starting to walk. It happens because those people, in all likelihood, didn't do one or some of the following: They didn't eat properly; they didn't properly pace themselves in their training; they started their exercise program too vigorously; or they peaked weeks before the race.

WATER It is crucial to properly hydrate yourself before, during, and after a marathon. Drink at least a pint of water before the race. During a marathon, you need to have water every mile.

The best thing to do is have a plastic water container with a sipper in it. When you pick it up, you can sip it as you run for a mile. People who run races in areas where they have friends generally have two or three people throughout the course of the race helping them with water.

Diluted grape juice in your water gives you extra glucose, so that you're delaying the time that your body will have to rely upon the extra glycogen it has stored up. In effect, you're always keeping your reserve in reserve. When other people hit the 20-mile mark and their glycogen and glucose are gone, they're out of energy. You don't want this to happen to you.

FORM Keep your head high, breathe through your mouth, and keep your shoulders loose. Your hands and arms should not be swinging; the wristbone should be at the level of the hipbone. If you hold your arms higher, you'll cause a muscle contraction that will cause fatigue in that muscle group. When muscle fatigue in the shoulders causes the arms to be raised higher, the shoulders slump forward, the neck drops down, and you'll get less air and your cells will get less oxygen. Try to keep your feet close to the ground, almost in a shuffle motion, with your knees slightly bent. You don't want to be running stiff-legged because that can jar the knees. Your body should be slightly bent forward at the waist. When you're running uphill, elbows should be elevated slightly behind you; run more toward the ball of the foot and take shorter steps. Again, your knees should be bent. Your shoulders should be forward to take advantage of the momentum you'll get coming down.

GEAR Most runners tend to wear a pair of running shoes for a time longer than shoes are able to provide good support. Run-down heels can lead to the displacement of musculoskeletal structure and subsequent hip problems, tendinitis, and strains. Yet they are not the only sign of the end of a shoe's serviceability. A good athletic supply store can help determine the condition of your running shoes.

Make sure that the back lip of the shoe, where the heel is, has been cut off. It serves no purpose, and it can actually dig into the Achilles tendon every time you move, bruising it.

Make sure you wear tight, thin socks. Heavy socks tend to bunch up because of sweat, giving you blisters. Improperly worn socks, more then anything else, also will give you blisters. Put Vaseline around all your toes, around the ball of your foot, and around the heel. Also put Vaseline in your crotch, around your breasts, under your armpits.

In cold weather, it's important to avoid overdressing, because trapped perspiration can lead to severe chills.

In warmer weather, wear clothes that permit free perspiration. Never wear sweat suits.

DIET On the sixth, fifth, and fourth days before a marathon, you should eat only protein, three times a day. Animal protein is not recommended. You could have soybean powder, or protein powder, or tofu—in other words, a high-quality protein.

On the three days immediately prior to the race, you should have no protein, just complex carbohydrates. On the day before the race, cut out fruits and salads. Try to eat something that will be only partially through your intestines during the race.

That night, have something about an hour before you go to sleep. Try to retire around midnight. This will be a major meal because you want to really saturate your body with glycogen. You could have buckwheat pasta, or brown rice, and if you're not allergic to wheat, you could have whole grain pasta or whole grain bread. Avoid greasy, highly-seasoned, and sugary foods.

In the morning, if it's at least four hours before the race, you could blend two bananas with grape juice. This will give you additional carbohydrates that will help you through the race. Eat no solid food before the race. Your body's system will be too nervous. When you're nervous and anxious, your body doesn't digest food normally. Electrolyte replacers are very important. Try to have two of the electrolytes (like potassium or magnesium) prior to a marathon, one every five miles during the race, and two at the end.

BEFORE AND AFTER Try to have a full-body massage, a Shiatsu massage, or a reflexology massage the day before the marathon. It's also important to float, if possible. Do an isolation tank float one or two days during the week before the marathon, preferably the day before, along with guided imagery.

When you've finished your race, don't just stop running and walk. Take at least 12 minutes to cool down by going from your running pace to a jog, a slower jog, and then a brisk walk. Never go directly into a sauna, hot tub, hot bath, or hot shower.

Always enjoy what you're doing and what you've accomplished.

15

Bringing Herbs into Your Daily Life

A Brief History of Herbalism

Herbs have been used for healing for as far back as we can trace the existence of man. In a Neanderthal grave in Iraq some 60,000 years old, scientists found pollens belonging to eight plants, seven of which are still used medicinally by people in that area. The Chinese Shennong Herbal lists 365 herbal drugs; it has been historically dated back to 200 B.C., but legend credits it to the emperor Shennong, of around 2700 B.C. Herbalism was not limited to the East. It reached a peak in England in 1653, when Nicholas Culpeper published his Complete Herbal, the first and greatest herbal work in the English language.

Yet, soon after that time, the pendulum swung away from the use of herbs, which had become inextricably tangled with magic, myth, and astrology. The Church of Rome objected to these pagan practices; and, in the 16th century, the Swiss physician Paracelsus began to use inorganic cures like mercury and antimony instead of herbals, heralding the near-monopoly of chemical-based medicine which would last until today.

The first determined effort in the modern Western world to break this pharmaceutical monopoly came from America in the 18th century. Samuel Thomson, the son of a farmer, lived during a time of great yellow fever epidemics; the accepted medical practice in curing this (and almost any other) ailment was a liberal use of bleeding and mercury, which a healthy patient would be lucky to live through. Thomson instead used herbs and steaming—with great success—but was met with hostility from the orthodox medical establishment, and even imprisoned briefly.

In the 19th century, herbal medicine made a popular comeback. So broad and exaggerated were the claims made for various tinctures, potions, "patent" medicines, and favorite cure-alls like mandrake root, however, that this popularity only contributed to a medical bias against herbal remedies. Modern science's success in synthesizing powerful drugs and the advent of highly rational double-blind testing procedures has confirmed this bias further.

Recently there has been another rebirth of popular interest in herbal remedies. A facsimile edition of Culpeper's *Complete Herbal* is one of a number of herbal health books that have been successfully published in the last decade. Yet the government has been indifferent or actively hostile to new studies which suggest that ancient beliefs about the healing powers of herbs have scientific foundation.

The antipathy of the medical orthodoxy, the American Medical Association (AMA), and government bodies like the Food and Drug Administration (FDA) to herbs as medicine or even as nutrition has grounds in several factors. In the age of double-blind testing and standard doses, herbs are difficult to quantify or analyze. Sometimes a single chemical component can be isolated and purified or synthesized. Digitalin, used to treat heart disease, was isolated from the foxglove plant; quinine from the bark of the quinoa tree; salicylic acid (aspirin) from willow bark; and on and on.

But herbal medicine is by nature an inexact, individualized science. Herbs may work differently on different people; the conditions under which a plant has grown, the time at which it is harvested, or the form which its preparation takes may all modify its effect. And despite successes such as aspirin and quinine, the "scientific" method of isolating, analyzing, and extracting the active ingredient in a plant often doesn't work very well. A chemical which might be isolated as the active component in an herb may in fact be modified by other, less obvious constituents which make it more powerful or moderate its side effects. And sometimes, even with rigorous research, the ways in which a plant affects the body can remain stubbornly mysterious; though there are many theories about ginseng, for example, it is not clear exactly how it boosts resistance to stress.

A second, no less powerful reason for the particular hostility of the AMA toward herbal remedies is the threat which they present to the vastly powerful, multibillion-dollar pharmaceutical industry. Herbal remedies can not be standardized, packaged, and marketed like drugs; they can usually be grown and prepared by anyone, and cannot be patented; in many cases they cut into the consumption of over-the-counter and prescription medicines. The pharmaceutical companies underwrite the very existence of the AMA. The pressure of the AMA and the pharmaceutical industry has dictated that herbs may be treated as food additives but not in any way as medications; the law forbids labeling any herb in connection with a specific affliction.

Other modern countries have no such hostility to the complementary use of herbal remedies within an orthodox medical framework. In 1958 Chairman Mao urged that China's traditional sciences of herbal medicine and acupuncture should not be abandoned; China's goal now is to develop a medicine which combines both the ancient and the new. For instance, herbal tonics are often used to strengthen a patient's ability to cope with modern chemotherapy. Russia has been committed to research on herbs, carrying out hundreds on Siberian ginseng alone, which has even been used to combat stress on Russian cosmonauts. Even in Britain, the National Institute of Medical Herbalist (created in 1864 as the National Association of Medical Herbalists) is a flourishing—and scientifically respected—body.

The Practical Use of Herbs

You don't have to be an herbalist, know complicated formulas, study the chemistry of plants, or learn the Chinese philosophies of herbal medicine to enjoy the benefits that herbs can bring into your life. If you are a novice in the world of herbs, go to a bookstore or library for books in their health and diet sections. Start small, with perhaps five herbs—some good ones to try first might be garlic, rosemary, comfrey, echinacea, and thyme. (Some herbs and their benefits, along with recommendations for the forms and quantities that they can be taken in, are listed below.)

The best way to begin to use herbs is the simplest; incorporate them into your cooking in progressively increasing amounts, or make a tea of one or more herbs. Cookbooks already often recommend the kinds of herbs that go well with different foods, but make your own experiments. Just put a few pinches in the stew pot, sprinkle them over a salad, or mix a little with a sandwich spread. Also, start reading the labels on the herbal tea boxes at the supermarket. Pick out a tea you think would taste good. Add an herbal tincture to your shampoo, your skin lotion or massage oil, or your bath tub. Within a short period of time, you will have incorporated a number of different herbs into your life. And you should start feeling better naturally.

Remember, though, not all herbs are equal. How they are grown, harvested, stored, and prepared will effect their potency and usefulness. Fresh and homegrown is always best, because you know the conditions under which herbs have been planted, monitored, fertilized, and cared for. Many nurseries sell not only herb seedlings but kits that can be used to conveniently grow herbs on the windowsills of city apartments. Investment in a full-spectrum light tube will even allow you to grow herbs on the kitchen counter. If you live in the country and you really know which plants you are looking for, some herbs can be collected wild. Be careful, though; some toxic plants can look very like useful herbs. It would be best to have someone with an expert knowledge of wild plants in your area along at first. A city dweller should not pick herbs that are just growing in the streets. With people, animals, and traffic circulating around them, such herbs can actually become quite toxic.

When buying herbs form a store, especially in bulk, make sure you use your senses of smell and sight. The herb shouldn't seem dusty or have a moldy aroma. If it looks more brown than green, then it will definitely have reduced effectiveness. Consumers ought to insist on fresh herbs if they're buying in bulk in herbal stores. The more information you can get about where the herb was grown, how it was cultivated, and when it was harvested, the better. Stay away from potent dried herbs in powder or capsule form. They generally have not been tested for safety or efficacy and are all too often a rip-off. It is almost impossible to determine what the actual ingredients are of a powder inside a capsule; you have no way of telling the age of such a preparation, or even if it is made from the herb it claims to be.

Also, some people may have allergic reactions or other problems with specific herbs. To test those sensitivities, use one herb at a time at first. Try them out; see what they're like; taste and smell them. If one causes no problem, add another.

As well as fresh herbs and dried herbs, there are several other forms in which herbal medicines can be taken. Often the form in which an herbal remedy is prepared is as important in therapeutic terms as which herb is used. *Infusions* and *decoctions*, two of the simpler forms, are both made with boiling water. Infusions are made by pouring boiling water over dried or fresh herbs, while roots and barks are boiled in water and left to steep as they cool. Distilled or spring water is preferable; the traditional proportion is about one ounce of dried herb to a pint of water. The pot or cup should be covered to prevent the escape of volatile oils; it should not be made of aluminum, which can enter the preparation in minute amounts.

Tinctures are made by macerating herbs in a mixture of water and alcohol for at least two weeks. Water extracts many constituents of plants, but oils, gums, and resins are most efficiently extracted in alcohol, which also preserves the preparation. The strength of the alcohol varies; vodka or brandy can be used to make tinctures at home. Some herb liqueurs, such as Chartreuse, were originally a kind of therapeutic remedy in the tradition of the monks who made them, although they no longer have these properties. *Ointments*, which are useful to treat some skin conditions, can be made with herbs and oils.

Herbs and the Immune System

One area in which herbs can play a vital role in our day-to-day lives is by stimulating our immune systems. Many people find that their health seems to be sapped by recurring or chronic colds and viruses; synthetic drugs, far from being a solution, seem to be merely encouraging new, more resistant strains of bacteria and viruses. Those people with more serious immune problems, like

AIDS and cancer, too, can help their systems to fight back as much as possible by using herbs to stimulate a healthy immune system.

Dr. Paul Lee, the founder of the Platonic Academy in Santa Cruz, California, is one of America's leading authorities on the use of herbs for immune-system health and overall well-being. Dr. Lee links herbology, immunology, and molecular biology together in his theory that there is an herbal code in our immune system memory which is carried by our DNA. One of the most phenomenal aspects of our immune system is this immune memory, genetically transmitted from our ancestors, which records their own struggle against illness and disease. When the Spanish conquistadors brought smallpox into Mexico, three and a half million Mexican Indians died; they had no such genetic immunization to ward it off.

Few in the world die from smallpox today, because the World Health Organization has effectively eliminated it. But despite all our triumphs in conquering diseases, it seems that cancer and other immune system diseases have taken their place. Dr. Lee believes that our generation is suffering from a kind of immune system amnesia. We have become detached from the botanical basis of health care and the medicinal herbs which are the natural agents of our immunity.

The body's ancient natural response to herbs is evident to anyone who has grown them. The aroma of specific herbs brings a unique and clear reaction. Anyone with any familiarity with herb gardening would never mistake thyme for oregano or oregano for rosemary, even with their eyes closed. The recent development of aromatherapy is a recognition of the power of our genetic memory of certain herbal substances, which even responds to just the smell of them.

Most humans in the modern world have lost the ancient talent for "intuitive herbalism" that ancient cultures recognized, and that animals still possess. Dogs and cats will nibble certain grasses when they feel ill. More startling is an observation of African chimpanzees recorded in the *International Herald Tribune* in 1986, showing that sick chimps methodically seek out the leaves from a bush called Aspilia, keep them in their mouths for about 15 seconds, and then swallow them whole. Analysis showed that the Aspilia leaves contain a powerful antibiotic chemical. Humans, however, have largely forgotten how to select herbs that they need to keep their immune responses healthy. Certain herbs can augment immunity because we're coded or programmed for them; this needs to be reactivated in our generation because one of the worst health problems that faces Americans today is a collective deterioration of the immune system. If we could restore a botanical emphasis to health care in a widespread way, it would make a great contribution to public health.

Rather than just concentrating on a better immune system, however, look at your system as a whole. As much as possible, consider the elements which contribute to your condition: lifestyle, stress, clinical and subclinical infection, toxins, and anything else that would divert the immune system from functioning properly. Then, with all this in mind, examine the herbs that can help you in these areas.

What to Use for Specific Types of Disorders

Although it is important to try to treat the body as a whole for almost any disorder, some herbs can be suggested as specifics for weakness or disorder in one system of organ. (More information on each herb is contained in the Glossary of Herbs below.) A few suggestions follow:

ANTIBIOTICS: Dandelion, garlic, goldenseal, marigold, myrrh, and thyme.

ARTHRITIC DISORDERS: Alfalfa, cayenne and feverfew for pain relief, and sarsaparilla.

BLOOD-CLOTTING: Cinnamon helps mild, passive hemorrhaging.

CIRCULATION/HEART TONICS: Barberry, blackberry, and, especially, hawthorn.

CHOLESTEROL REDUCTION: Cayenne, ginger, and garlic.

CLEANSING AND DETOXIFICATION: Barberry, blackberry leaves and fruit, celery, chaparral, goldenseal, rosemary, and seaweeds.

COLDS AND FLUS: Cayenne, chaparral, garlic, osha, and thyme.

DIGESTIVE SYSTEM: Alfalfa, barberry, celery, chamomile, cinnamon, comfrey, and marigold.

DIURETICS: Dandelion and celery.

IMMUNE ENHANCEMENT: Astragalus, echinacea, garlic, ginseng, goldenseal, marigold, pau d'arco, suma, turmeric (especially for allergies), and wild indigo root.

LIVER TONICS: Dandelion and milk thistle.

NERVOUS SYSTEM/BRAIN TONICS: Avena, chamomile, ginseng, and rosemary.

PAIN REDUCTION: Cayenne and feverfew.

RESPIRATORY TRACT: Cayenne, garlic, and milk thistle.

A Glossary of Herbs

ALFALFA (*Medicago sativa*), used as a tea or eaten whole as sprouts in a salad, is rich in a variety of vitamins and minerals, as its roots can reach as far as 30 feet into the ground to gather up essential minerals. Alfalfa is also plentifully stocked with enzymes that can help in the digestive process. Alfalfa is used as a tonic to increase vitality, appetite, and weight—interestingly, it is fed to horses for the same reason. The root of tooth-leaved clover, a close relative of alfalfa (which, in fact, is given the same name—*mu xu*—as alfalfa by the Chinese), was found to be very successful in curing night blindness in a 1960 study in China. Alfalfa also has a reputation for healing peptic ulcers and is an old folk remedy for arthritic conditions. It may work by cleansing the bowels.

Alfalfa grows wild throughout America and is also cultivated as live stock food and for other commercial purposes; it is a major raw source in the manufacture of chlorophyll. Extracts of alfalfa are used commercially to flavor beverages and food products. It is easy to grow alfalfa sprouts at home for use in salads. Some caution should be observed in using alfalfa, however. Some individuals may be allergic to alfalfa; in addition, it is difficult to tell if powdered alfalfa sold in health foods in capsule form is pure, or, indeed, if it is really alfalfa at all.

ASTRAGALUS, a Chinese herb, is only now gaining popularity in this country although it has been used for thousands of years in China as the basis of an immune-enhancing therapy called *fuchang therapy*. The immune system is basic to the Chinese approach to health, which is concerned with bringing the body back into balance. Dr. Sun Yan, who came from China to a research program at the University of Texas Medical School, Houston, works with astragalus and ligustrum, another traditional Chinese remedy, which are routinely used in China to protect the immune systems of cancer patients undergoing chemotherapy and radiation treatment.

This root is a staple of traditional Chinese medicine and can be found easily at herbal markets. It is best prepared in a decoction, simmering the root for 10 to 15 minutes, then straining while still hot.

AVENA has been a folk remedy for several hundred years as a general nerve tonic, for nervous exhaustion and certain kinds of mental disease, in the form of the fresh, undried oat plant—*Avena sativa*—harvested at the milky stage (a seed will give off a drop of milky juice when squeezed). Ayurvedic medicine in India uses avena—oat plant extract—for opium addiction, as did the eclectic physicians in the U.S. at the turn of the century. Evidence from studies in Scotland suggests that avena also helps with nicotine addiction, and it may prove effective in treating such addictions as alcoholism or even heroin addiction. Several companies have now come out with commercial oat extracts.

This extract from the oat plant can be mixed into porridge or baked into cakes or cookies.

BARBERRY, a common shrub, is of interest to the herbalist primarily because of its bark, although the Japanese barberry's berries were once used to make jellies and relishes. Like goldenseal and yellow dock, barberry bark is yellow because it contains berberine, an antibacterial and antiviral alkyloid. Barberry bark is a tonic to almost every organ in the body. It has excellent bitters, much preferable to those of the marigold, which makes it a good digestive. It stimulates the liver and the gallbladder, aiding not only digestion but the cleansing of toxins from the body through the eliminative functions. It is also a tonic to the spleen, which strengthens the immune system. As a laxative, it again plays a role in detoxification. Finally, it increases the circulation.

The bark can be infused into teas or tinctures. To make a tincture, crush about eight ounces of the bark and add it to a screw-top jar filled with six to eight cups of a clear spirit, such as gin or vodka. Store the tincture in a warm, dark place and shake the jar twice a day to thoroughly mix. After two weeks, strain the tincture through a cheesecloth, draining well. Keep in tightly sealed bottles. Instead of alcohol, you could use a sweet cider vinegar.

BLACKBERRY LEAVES are an astringent; and infusion is considered an effective blood cleanser and may be useful for improving the circulation of the blood. Blackberry fruit is useful as a cleansing food to help correct diarrhea. It can also be used as a gargle for throat inflammation or in douching to help with irregular vaginal discharges.

A tablespoon or two of dried leaves can be brewed in tea.

CAYENNE shares with ginger an ability to help the body metabolize cholesterol. Studies in Mysore, India, found that it depresses the liver's production of cholesterol and triglycerides, countering the effect of cholesterol-rich foods. It also seems to have a host of other benefits. Chili peppers and other spicy foods act as expectorants in the bronchial passages, benefiting patients with chronic bronchitis and emphysema. Swedish research has indicated that capsaicin—the ingredient that makes a chili hot—desensitizes the lungs to irritants like cigarette smoke. A common cold can be temporarily relieved with a gargle of a little chili sauce in water.

Surprisingly enough, the capsaicin that stings your mouth in food is also an effective pain suppressant, inhibiting the relay of pain signals to the central nervous system.

In 1965 German researchers discovered that chili peppers seemed to dissolve blood clots. Further research in Thailand has confirmed this finding; after eating hot peppers the blood-clot-dissolving activity increases almost immediately. The effect is short-term, lasting about half an hour, but frequent consumption of chilis in food can prevent clots from building up.

Finally, chili peppers have an effect on the brain; the burning they cause in the mouth provokes the release of endorphins, the body's natural morphine which blocks pain and induces a sensation of pleasure related to "runner's high."

A pinch of finely-chopped fresh cayenne peppers added to a curry or chili is perfect for the most benefits. Cayenne is the active ingredient in Tabasco sauce and a few dashes in anything from tomato juice to brown rice adds a healthy jolt.

CELERY has a cleansing diuretic effect, whether it is taken as a tea or as juice, which can be combined with the juice of other vegetables like carrots. Carrot juice is a good complement to celery as it contains a different kind of pectin from that in apples. Celery's alkalinity also makes it soothing to the digestive system.

A handful of chopped celery can be added to salads, but it is best when a few stalks are juiced along with carrots or other vegetables. An aromatic tea can be made from steeping a tablespoon of seeds in a cup of boiling water for three to five minutes.

CHAMOMILE is an herb that can be used as a tea or a tincture. Chamomile has a slightly alkalinizing affect on the blood; it helps to stimulate digestion and acts as a nerve tonic. Folk wisdom has aptly given chamomile a reputation as a calming herb. It can be taken at night as a mild sedative. In a bath or as a decoction, chamomile soothes the skin, and it brightens blond hair when added to shampoo. It is antispasmodic when taken internally.

Tea made from a tablespoon of dried leaves should be taken before bedtime to help fall asleep. For swelling or pain in the joints, chamomile oil can be applied. To make the oil, use about one ounce of fresh or dried flowers and combine with a half cup of olive oil. Crush the flowers in the oil and let them steep for 24 hours. Strain the flowers out and rub the oil on the affected areas.

CINNAMON is a very effective diarrhea remedy. It can be made into a tea, with just a pinch or two in a cup of hot water; an old-time variant is apple sauce with cinnamon, doubly effective since apple pectin is very soothing to the intestinal tract, as well as delicious.

Cinnamon was also used by the Eclectics—a school of 19th century American herbalists devoted to the specific, proven use of herbal remedies—as a first aid remedy to treat mild, passive hemorrhaging, such as blood in the urine or sputum. Many midwives swear by cinnamon for postpartum hemorrhaging. Of course, never attempt to treat any serious bleeding in this way without consulting a doctor first.

COMFREY (*Symphytum officinale*) is an ancient healing herb. It has a soothing effect on the stomach lining. A British study showed that comfrey activates local hormones called prostaglandins, which protect the stomach lining from inflammation. Comfrey root contains mucilage—a slimy or gelatinous form of sugar which is soothing to digestive tract mucous membranes. Comfrey also contains allantoin, a natural cell healer; it is one of the few plant sources of vitamin B_{12}.

A tablespoon of dried leaves steeped in hot water for three to five minutes makes a gentle tea. Fresh leaves can be chopped and added to salad.

DANDELION is an unlikely healer to most of us who know it as a lawn pest, but in fact the entire dandelion plant is a valuable herbal source. Dandelion is rich in potassium, which makes it an ideal diuretic as it does not leach potassium form the body as diuretics tend to do. Dandelion greens are also very rich in vitamin A, and are an excellent salad ingredient. Dandelion root has been used for centuries as a laxative, tonic, and diuretic, and in treating liver, gallbladder, and kidney conditions. Its extracts are used in modern pharmaceutical preparations for these properties. Recent Chinese research has shown that the juice of the dandelion fights certain bacteria; it is particularly efficient in treating upper respiratory tract infections, bronchitis, pneumonia, appendicitis, mastitis, and dermatitis. It creates fewer side effects than modern antibiotics, and these disappear as soon as treatment is discontinued.

A handful of tender, fresh leaves can be a delicious addition to a salad. Dandelion juice can be easily extracted by putting a few leaves in the juicer with carrots or other vegetables.

ECHINACEA, commonly known as the purple coneflower, is the most popular herbal immune stimulant in America today, although serious research of its properties in this country only began in recent years. Dr. Edward Alstadt, a naturopathic physician in Portland, Oregon, is one of the leading experts on echinacea. Echinacea is indigenous to the United States alone, where the American Indians have used it for over a recorded 150 years. In the 1930s the German scientific community began to research this herb. It was a New York doctor who provided the first written documentation of it, however; he reported that it caused an increase in leukocyte formation, resulting in a greater ability to attack bacteria and a general immune system stimulation.

Nevertheless, echinacea was relegated to the realms of folk medicine until the 1960s, when renewed in-vitro studies focused on its stimulation of leukocytes. It was found that echinacea also inhibits hyaluronidase, an enzyme which pathogenic organisms use to break down our body tissues to make way for their own spread, and strengthens the tissues against this enzyme by stimulating the production of hyaluronic acid, the base of the cell membrane in most body tissues. Finally, echinacea helps the body to regenerate new tissue by stimulating fibrocytes.

Many researchers see a similarity between echinacea and cortisone; a 1953 study by Koch and Heugel demonstrated that echinacea was more effective than cortisone in stopping streptococcus in rats. Echinacea stimulates the adrenal cortex, the area where the corticosteroids—which have a cortisonelike action—are released within our own body.

The most prominent researcher on echinacea is Dr. Wagner, at the University of Munich Institute for Pharmaceutical Biology. His studies have indicated that echinacea's effect is due to polysaccharides, or sugar molecules, which fool the body into believing that they're pathogens even though they're perfectly benign and nontoxic. Thus, they boost the body's natural immune reaction, giving it a jump start on fighting colds and infections.

At the first symptoms of cold or flu, echinacea taken immediately, and regularly, every two to three hours for about 10 days, will stop the cold or flu before it has a chance to get hold.

Only the root of echinacea is used. There are two kinds of echinacea: *Echinacea angustifolia* and *Echinacea purpurea*. Most research has involved the angustifolia, which seems much more effective. Because echinacea is expensive, the consumer should be aware of forms which have been adulterated or substituted for by purpurea.

The root of echinacea can be steeped in boiling water for 15 minutes. The tea should be taken every two or three hours up to six cups a day until symptoms of cold or flu have begun to subside.

FEVERFEW (*Chrysanthemum parthenium*) is an immune enhancer that lowers inflammation. Its name is due to its ability to reduce fever. It's good for arthritis because of its anti-inflammatory properties.

Attention was first focused on feverfew in England when a miner gave the wife of a medical officer of the National Coal Board a cutting of the plant to cure her migraines. Dr. Stuart Johnson, intrigued by this report, carried out clinical trials in which feverfew completely cured the migraines of a third of migraine patients; 7 out of 10 noticed some improvement.

The dried or fresh leaves can be steeped in boiling water for a therapeutic tea.

GARLIC has always had a down-home folk reputation as a restorative; how many grandmothers swear by chicken soup with plenty of garlic for a cold? And this reputation has a history almost as long as written history itself. Jean Carper notes in her recent best seller, *The Food Pharmacy*, that 22 garlic prescriptions "for such complaints as headache, throat disorders, and physical weakness" were found on an Egyptian medical papyrus dating from around 1500 B.C. The confidence the Egyptians had in garlic is demonstrated by the fact that they reportedly used it to strengthen the workers who built the pyramids. Pliny recommended garlic for 61 maladies in his *Historia Naturalis*; Hippocrates recommended it as a laxative, diuretic, and cure for tumors of the uterus. Garlic has been used to treat high blood pressure for centuries in China and Japan. In first-century India, garlic and onion were thought to prevent heart disease and rheumatism. Garlic even had a reputation as an aphrodisiac in Shakespearean England. It is probable that only the smell of garlic has prevented it form becoming as omnipresent a cure-all as aspirin.

Garlic's distinctive odor is due to its sulfur-containing compounds—the most important being allicin—which also are responsible for many of its therapeutic effects. Allicin is a powerful inhibitor of bacterial growth with an extremely broad spectrum; hundreds of studies have confirmed its effectiveness over as many as 72 separate infectious agents. Not only does garlic directly attack microbes, but it also seems to boost the body's own immune powers. A 1987 study found that the immune system's killer cells from people who had consumed large quantities of garlic destroyed half again as many cancer cells in a culture.

Studies also show that garlic lowers cholesterol and thins the blood, lowering the chances of dangerous blood clots. If this was not enough, it is a hypertensive; Bulgarian studies have demonstrated that it produces dramatic blood-pressure drops in humans. Finally, garlic is an effective decongestant for common colds and can prevent or ease chronic bronchitis.

The best way to get garlic is to grow your own or buy bulbs that are as fresh as possible. Raw garlic is most effective, especially in antibacterial activity; but garlic in cooking retains many of its therapeutic benefits. The garlic sold in health food stores as capsules, pills, and deodorized preparation, however, may have relatively little power. It is the smelly part of garlic that is the most therapeutic. Japanese Kyolic paste is one commercial garlic preparation that may approach the value of fresh garlic, but is certainly no better. The best approach is the most simple and natural. If you can't stomach eating garlic cloves raw, cook with it; use it in salad dressings, soups, and garlic bread.

A teaspoon or two of freshly chopped garlic is a healthful addition to all menus. An infusion of two cloves of mashed garlic to an ⅛ cup of room temperature water can be dripped into each nostril to clear sinuses.

GINGER is useful for upset stomachs or motion sickness. A double-blind study published in the *Journal of the American Medical Association* compared the effects of ginger and Dramamine, a common over-the-counter motion sickness drug, and found that ginger was actually more effective. In addition, ginger had none of the side effects—such as drowsiness—of the commercial drug.

Ginger is an even more effective anticoagulant than garlic or onions; gingerol, one of its compounds, has a structure very much like that of aspirin, which also thins the blood. Ginger is a folk remedy for menstrual cramps. It reduces blood pressure and cholesterol, stimulates the heart, and has blocked mutations leading to cancer in mice.

Ginger can be taken in capsules, used fresh in cooking, or as a tea. Caution should be taken, especially with powdered ginger, which can burn the esophagus.

A slice of fresh ginger should be taken to avoid motion sickness. A few tablespoons of grated fresh or powdered ginger can be used in cooking to add some excitement to your meal.

GINSENG (*Panax ginseng* is Latin for the Chinese variety; the species native to North America is *Panax qinquefolium*), considered the master herb by the Chinese, is probably the most researched herb in the world. It is highly valued in China; in fact, the fist diplomatic liaison between the U.S. and China was a trade agreement for selling ginseng. Ginseng was used as far back as 3100 B.C. in China; around 2597 B.C. it was discussed as a medicine in a scroll. At one time, only the imperial family was allowed to grow or own ginseng.

Wild ginseng, which has been left to grow for 30, 40, or even up to 100 years, is extremely expensive, if it can be obtained at all, and is highly prized. Cultivated ginseng may be uprooted anywhere from the age of 2 to 6 years. Preferably it should be at least 6 years old for optimum pharmacological quality. Interestingly, the soil from which a 6-year-old ginseng root has been pulled is permitted to lie fallow for 10 years to recover its nutrients—an indication of ginseng's ability to pull nutrients into itself. In America, ginseng is grown extensively in the Wisconsin-Michigan area of the Midwest, but most of this crop is exported to the Orient.

Ginseng does not only improve physical efficiency and stamina. Experiments with proofreaders found a 12 to 54 percent reduction in misreadings when ginseng was used. It is thought that this results from an improvement of oxygenation of the brain cells. One of the elements found in ginseng, germanium, is a chelator—that is, it can pull heavy metals, such as mercury, lead, or cadmium, out of tissues. Experiments in animals have found that the concentration of mercury in tissue was reduced after the administration of ginseng. Germanium also seems to rid the cells of excess hydrogen; in consequence there is a higher proportion of oxygen, and more efficient energy production.

One of the most fascinating properties of ginseng is its apparent ability to protect the bone marrow against radioactivity. A study given at the Third International Symposium on Ginseng in Seoul, Korea, showed that mice pretreated with ginseng survived intensive x-ray irradiation at a rate some 82.5 percent better than the control group. The damage done to the bone marrow—an important factor, because this is where the red blood cells are synthesized—was significantly less in these mice.

Siberian ginseng (*Eleutherococcus senticosus*) has been the subject of more than 400 studies in Russia. Discovered as a result of a search for an indigenous substitute for Chinese ginseng, it was found to make mice able to swim half again as far as those without it before becoming exhausted. Another study was done on several thousand carefully monitored telegraph operators, a group in which it was easy to quantify efficiency, for two decades. Not only was the work efficiency of those who had taken the ginseng greater, but they also had fewer sick days, less cancer, less heart disease, and less diabetes. In 1962, Siberian ginseng was added to the official Russian pharmacopoeia. So convinced are the Russians of the therapeutic value of *Eleutherococcus* that it is used by their athletes and cosmonauts.

Ginseng's powers to help the body cope with stress are so dramatic and far-ranging that a new term, "adaptogen," has been defined by Dr. I. I. Brekhman, a Russian physician who oversaw many of the studies on Siberian ginseng, to describe it. Both Panax and Siberian ginseng function as adaptogens. An adaptogen works as a balancing mechanism: it raises low blood pressure but also brings high blood pressure down, for example. An adaptogen has nonspecific properties that enable animals to cope with both physical and mental stress more efficiently, to be more resilient, and to maintain a balance, or homeostasis, under widely varying conditions. As an adaptogen, ginseng helps the body to balance itself under a wide variety of stress factors.

Steep one ounce of the macerated root in boiling water for 15 minutes and strain. Also try concocting a tincture of two ounces of ginseng with two pints of rice wine.

GOLDENSEAL (*Hydrastis canadensis*) has been much misunderstood, and used as a panacea for many ailments. This root is quite powerful, and should be used sparingly and for limited periods of time; the consumer should also be wary, as goldenseal is expensive and may be sold in adulterated preparations.

Goldenseal contains alkyloids which are strong antiseptic and antiviral compounds. One of these, berberine, has been used to treat malaria when quinine is not available; berberine gives goldenseal its yellow color. Goldenseal is effective on the mucous membranes of the gastrointestinal tract, activating the stationary immune system through a cleansing of the lymphatic tissue of the gastrointestinal system. It reduces inflammation throughout the body. Goldenseal also indirectly stimulates the immune system by helping to build up the glandular system, rather than directly attacking microbes as its alkyloids do. Goldenseal also acts as a mild laxative and, as such, detoxifies the system.

It is best to chew goldenseal, or, if preferred, drink it as a tea with one-tenth to one-quarter of a teaspoon per cup. If it is self-prescribed, begin with a very small amount, perhaps one-tenth of a teaspoon, slowly increasing to a quarter teaspoon.

An infusion made with one-quarter ounce of goldenseal has been shown to help sinusitis. Also a gargle prepared with a tincture of goldenseal in warm water can soothe a sore throat.

HAWTHORN (*Crataegus oxyacanthoides*), the familiar red-berried tree, is used extensively throughout Europe as a heart tonic. In this country digitalis, or foxglove, is used for this purpose, but it is highly toxic; hawthorn, on the other hand, has none of this toxicity. Hawthorn berries, leaves, and flowers are all excellent for the arterial and peripheral circulation.

Use the leaves to brew a stimulating tea. The berries can be preserved in a tincture and used as needed.

MARIGOLD especially the flowerhead, is a very effective herb. The marigold flowerhead is antibacterial, antiviral, and antiseptic. It also enhances the function of the lymphatic system, which in turn aids both the acquired and fixed immune system. The flowerhead is useful in treating superficial wounds.

Most of the benefits of the marigold flowerhead come from its volatile oil. This oil, when extracted, has shown to promote blood clotting and the formation of granulomatous tissue, the first stage of healing in wounds. It also contains salicylic acid, which in itself is helpful in reducing the inflammation.

Both the leaves and flowerhead of the marigold contain bitters, which trigger beneficial gastrointestinal responses, boosting the production of hydrochloric acid and enzymes in the stomach. Chefs often use marigold flowers in salads for color, as well as the greens. Do not underestimate the marigold; it is not only beneficial but very gentle. The flowerheads are so light that there is no need to worry about dosage. Sprinkle a few freshly chopped leaves in a mixed green salad.

MILK THISTLE (*Salybum marianum*), a noxious weed to farmers, is effective in treating liver disorders, helping the liver properly process toxins and poisons. Milk thistle contains tyramine, which stimulates mucous secretions. Thus, milk thistle tea can be used to help stimulate congested lungs to discharge their excess fluids and mucous, especially in the winter. Milk thistle is available in tinctures.

MYRRH, a resin extracted from the myrrh tree, is packaged in its solid form, looking somewhat like rock candy. Myrrh is used in a number of consumer products because of its antiseptic qualities; for example, it is often an ingredient in natural toothpaste. Myrrh is also antifungal and antiviral. Clinical tests have shown it to fight staphylococcus and E. coli bacteria, for which reason it has been used clinically in hospitals in Egypt and India. Myrrh seems most effective in local application, but should not be ruled out for systemic use.

Myrrh is not easily used because of its market preparation; it must first be caramelized—liquified with water over heat—and tends to become a gummy mass when stored in water. The recommended internal dosage is about one-half teaspoon.

Dissolve a small portion, about an ounce, of the gummy resin in warm water and use as a refreshing mouthwash. Also, sip the liquid as a cure for a stomach ache.

OSHA, an herb native to Rocky Mountain area of the United States, is used extensively in that area for colds, flus, coughs, sore throats, and urinary tract infections.

PAU D'ARCO (as it is known in Brazil; known as *La Pacho* in Argentina), is a native of South America that has attracted a lot of attention with evidence of its strong antiviral, antitumor, antifungal, and antibacterial action since it was introduced in the U.S. in 1980.

Grind the root into a powder, then fill gelatin capsules. Take one capsule twice a day.

PECTIN is not an herb, but rather a substance found in some plants. The most well-known source of pectin is apples; carrots contain a different variety. Pectin is soluble fiber; it is used commercially to make Jello. It is a well known depressor of cholesterol levels. A more recent discovery is that pectin helps to absorb and remove some toxic metals that can accumulate in our tissues, and may increase our ability to withstand irradiation.

Increase your apple consumption for the best quality pectin. Try apple sauce or baked apples for variety.

ROSEMARY has been gaining publicity recently as an antioxidant, helping to counter the destructive effects of modern industrial toxins and pollutants in the air. Traditionally it has been used as a preservative, especially to keep meats and fats from going rancid; chemicals extracted from rosemary are used in the modern food industry for this purpose. The folk history of rosemary has been as a brain or memory tonic; this may have something to do with its antioxidant properties. Scientists have found that rosemary promotes menstrual discharge in women and hair growth.

Rosemary oil is used widely in cosmetics such as soaps, creams, and lotions. Infusions of rosemary are used externally for wounds, sores, bruises, eczema, and rheumatism.

Crush the dried leaves and sprinkle in soups or salads.

SARSAPARILLA ROOT (*Smilax ornata*) is an adaptogen (see the entry for *ginseng* for a definition of adaptogens) which has been around for centuries. It was first introduced to Europe in the Middle Ages as a treatment for syphilis—though there is no evidence that it can cure syphilis, it may relieve its symptoms. Chemically, sarsaparilla falls into the class of phytosterols. Phyto is from the Latin for "plant," and sterol is related to the adrenal hormones called steroids, so phytosterols are plant analogues of steroid hormones. Claims have been made that sarsaparilla contains testosterone, the male sex hormone. There is no evidence for this, and the related claim that sarsaparilla increases the production of male testosterone, especially in older men, has been suggested by new evidence but not proven. However, sarsaparilla has been touted as a male sex tonic for centuries, all over the world. Interestingly, it is also used as an anti-inflammatory; and it is chemically similar to the clinical steroids used in modern medicine to treat inflammation.

Several major pharmaceutical companies in Germany make a product for psoriasis using sarsaparilla extract; it is also effective in alleviating eczema and other skin diseases, as well as arthritis.

Steep the leaves and berries in hot water for an aromatic tea. The root was once used with wintergreen and sassafras to flavor root beer.

SEAWEEDS contain virtually all the vitamins and minerals needed in a diet. *Algae* and the sea plants such as *hijiki, kombu, wakame, nori,* and *arame* combine with toxins in the body, enabling them to be more easily excreted. Seaweeds also contain above-average amounts of iodine, which helps stimulate the thyroid gland.

Sprinkle steamed hijiki on salads. Roll your own vegetable sushi with sheets of nori and steamed rice.

THYME (*Thymus vulgaris*) is mentioned here together with oregano because they are both high in a chemical known as thymol. Thymol is used throughout the pharmaceutical industry; in fact, it's a main ingredient in Listerine. It is a strong antiseptic, effective as an antibacterial and antifungal. Interestingly, thyme's Latin name is the same as that of the thymus gland, the central organ of the immune system.

Thyme can be used to make a mouthwash, a bath oil, or a deodorant. I strongly recommend oregano and thyme tea for the common cold and mild infections—most people have it around and like the taste of it. As a strong tea it is a good wash for minor cuts and scratches. Also use to flavor soups or salads. Crush the dried leaves and sprinkle on these foods.

TURMERIC, a vivid yellow spice made of ground roots, gives curry powder (and mustard) its classic color. Studies in China and Russia in recent decades have found that in tests on animals, turmeric promotes bile secretion, lowers blood pressure, stimulates the appetite, alleviates pain, and reduces inflammation. A recent study in China showed extracts of turmeric to prevent 100 percent of pregnancies in rats. It also seems to have antibiotic properties.

This powdered spice has a subtle taste, but helps support the stronger spices in curries, and prepared mustard. Use a teaspoon along with other aromatic spices.

Turmeric has been getting a lot of attention lately from evidence of its ability to stabilize mast cells, which line our trachea and intestinal tract and serve as a first line of defense for the immune system. Healthy mast cells have a tight weave that can keep out deviant material from our bloodstream—bacteria, pollen, and protein which has not been properly broken down. Turmeric contains corsitin, a bioflavonoid which can strengthen the mast cells over time.

Many doctors use turmeric for allergies. You might think of the lining of your trachea or sinuses as fabric; tears or holes in this fabric, or a loose weave, allows things like pollen to enter the bloodstream, where they trigger an exaggerated response in the immune system, leading to inflammation and all the symptoms of allergy. Turmeric heals the cracks and tightens the weave, providing greater resistance to allergens. In the same way, food allergies can be lessened by strengthening the mast cell tissue in the intestinal tract.

Although it should not be taken as a panacea, turmeric is very safe and is already used in many foods. It can also be taken in capsule form or made as a tea.

WILD INDIGO ROOT is not a very popular herb, but it is valuable for its direct antimicrobial activity, which helps fight infections throughout the body and particularly upper respiratory infections. More importantly, wild indigo root is a gastrointestinal tract stimulant, maintaining its levels of hydrochloric acid. This is the first line of defense in the immune system; without an adequate level of hydrochloric acid in the stomach, microorganisms which enter with the ingestion of food may pass through the stomach and enter the lymphatic or blood systems. Wild indigo root is also a liver tonic, helping to detoxify the body.

The strength of wild indigo root lies somewhere between that of echinacea and goldenseal. A self-prescribed dose should be no more than half a teaspoon in a daily cup of tea, and should not be continued for more than a month.

The root can also be used in prepared ointments to help soothe the inflammation of arthritis. Macerate about two ounces of the root and leave for 24 hours in a well sealed jar filled with two cups of olive oil. Shake frequently. Then strain and apply as needed.

Herbs, Regulation, and the Government

In recent years, millions of Americans have been trying the herbal remedies commonly found in health food stores as cures for specific diseases. People take them with the expectation of being cured of their condition, often at great expense. I have contacted a number of the companies producing and marketing these herbal remedies and could not find one that had performed scientific tests to confirm the efficacy or safety of the cure as proclaimed on the labels. In my opinion, this is clearly an unethical policy.

As Dr. Paul Lee notes, the problem of regulatory control is a burden to the herbal industry. Because herbs are neither food nor drugs, they are extremely difficult to define and hence hard to regulate. When the use is medicinal, they can be considered as drugs; when the use is culinary, they can be considered as spices; but it is not always easy to draw the line. The regulations of the Food and Drug Administration (FDA) stipulate that a product that is being sold as a food or a nutritional supplement is limited as to the health benefits that can be claimed to result from its use. On the other hand, the cost of testing drugs, which tends to be in the millions or tens of millions of dollars, is prohibitive for herb companies, which tend to be relatively small as compared to the huge pharmaceutical conglomerates. This puts herb companies in a bind. Some, aware that the FDA usually takes several years before it will catch up with a company, choose to go ahead without scientific proof of the efficacy of their product.

If the mainstream health industry were to consider the health properties of herbs more seriously, this would not be a problem. Traditional Western medicine in this country has long been prejudiced against herbs. In no other country is this the case to such an extreme. In one recent case, for example, an internationally renowned scientist, Dr. Bruce Halstead, was sentenced to eight years in prison for prescribing an unapproved drug when he recommended herbal teas that enhance the immune system to his cancer patients. In less industrialized, less wealthy nations, there tends to be a greater acceptance of medicinal herbs. In part, this is simply due to economics. In many countries, if you are poor, your health care will depend largely on medicinal herbs because industrial medicine is only for those who can afford it.

Recently, one of China's leading cancer researchers, Dr. Sun Yan, was invited to the University of Texas to perform a three-year study of two prominent Chinese herbs that enhance the immune system. Both are used in China to help bolster the immune systems of patients that have undergone chemotherapy and radiation therapy. Perhaps the willingness to test the herbs is a sign that the attitude in this country is changing. But there are few other signs. And it is all too characteristic that while America is one of the world's foremost producers of the renowned herb ginseng, 98 percent of the American crop is exported to the Orient, and in this country its properties remain relatively unknown.

Were conventional health practitioners to include herbal medicine in their training and delivery of health care, a significant improvement could occur almost immediately in the quality of medicine available to patients. In particular, the problem of iatrogenic (doctor-induced) illness would be substantially reduced. The side effects of synthetic drugs are often substantial: the medicines we take frequently make us sicker. In many patient care situations, if medicinal herbs were used, there would be little or no side effects.

PART THREE

Mental Health and Psychological Well-Being

We have been led to believe that we are a nation with a mental illness epidemic. The National Institute of Mental Health estimates that more than 40 million Americans may be suffering from mental and emotional problems severe enough to restrict or limit the quality of their lives. These include depression, obsessive-compulsive disorder, and schizophrenia, as well as other conditions, which, while they may not fall strictly under the rubric of "mental illness," have a mental component. These include insomnia, attention deficit disorder, eating disorders, and alcoholism. When you consider that probably an additional 50 million people suffer from intermittent bouts of one or a number of these conditions, then you can see that close to one third of the entire American population is personally grappling with mental health concerns.

Yet despite the extent of mental disorders, the American medical establishment has paid little attention to causes, so intent are they on obtaining the relief of the symptoms of these conditions. Take alcoholism, for instance. There are dozens of studies showing that alcoholics are chronically deficient in certain essential nutrients. Other studies show that when these nutrients are given at optimal levels, the chemical imbalances that precipitate the craving for alcohol are diminished or eliminated, thus biochemically breaking the addictive response. One would think that the medical establishment would at least attempt to address the ramifications of these studies in the approaches to treatment that are currently favored. But they have not done so. Currently, many tens of billions of dollars are being spent yearly on drug and alcohol treatments, of which the vast majority ignore nutrition-based approaches. Since few of the now-prevalent approaches have been shown to be successful, it is worrisome that nutrition-based approaches continue to be relegated to the margins. We need to look at the fact that when biochemical imbalances are corrected and chemical sensitivities addressed, the treatments work, and with a lack of relapse. This is the kind of cause-and-prevention oriented approach we should be encouraging, for alcoholism and other problems.

In the following chapters, we compare the traditional and alternative approaches to mental health in general, and then look more specifically at the various disorders.

16

Orthomolecular Psychiatry: An Alternative Approach to Mental Health

Traditional treatments of mental disorders since Sigmund Freud invented his "talking cure" have included psychoanalysis, various other psychotherapies, and more recently, drug-induced behavior modification.

In psychoanalysis, the therapist helps the patient retrace his or her past in order to attain an understanding of the cause of the patient's irrational behavior. Whether this insight actually helps patients overcome such behavior, however, remains controversial, and a wide variety of psychotherapies have developed that claim greater effectiveness than traditional psychoanalysis. Psychiatry is concerned not so much with having patients explore the roots of their behavior as with directly intervening with pharmaceutical aids to render the behavior more socially acceptable. While psychotropic drugs can be dramatically effective in some cases of depression, psychosis, and anxiety, some patients are not helped, some require long-term treatment with drugs that have serious side effects, and others become addicted to mood-alternating medications.

Historical Roots

The psychiatric profession's control over the manner in which mental disorders are treated in this country is undeniably very strong but by no means goes unchallenged. Discouraged by the results and opposed to the invasive and toxic nature of the treatments utilized by mainstream practitioners, certain physicians specializing in mental health began to look for alternatives to the excesses of the traditional approach. These physicians, many of whom were themselves psychiatrists, studied the effects of food allergies, nutrition, vitamins, minerals, and amino acids in the treatment of such conditions as schizophrenia, depression, anxiety, hyperactivity, and autism.

One of these alternative approaches is orthomolecular psychiatry. The term "orthomolecular" was coined by Nobel Prize laureate Linus Pauling in an article written for *Science* magazine in 1968 and refers to the preservation of good health and the treatment of disease by supplying optimal concentrations of substances that are required for good health and are normally present in the body. The term stems from the Greek *ortho* meaning "to correct." As used by Dr. Pauling, it refers to the correction of imbalances within the body through the use of vitamins, minerals, amino acids, and other naturally occurring nutrients. Orthomolecular physicians believe that with these substances there is less of a chance of harmful side effects and a greater potential for cure.

Dr. Michael Lesser, an orthomolecular psychiatrist, contends that orthomolecular medicine is more in keeping with the type of therapeutic care associated with Hippocrates, the Greek physician whom many regard as "the father of medicine." He notes that Hippocrates believed in treating illnesses by using their opposites. In other words, if your affliction is caused by too much stress, you should be taught relaxation techniques. Your depression or memory loss may be caused by a copper excess, which can be offset by increasing your level of zinc. Orthomolecular medicine involves balancing the nutrients in the body.

If you are in need of professional care for mental health, keep in mind some of the main differences between orthomolecular and traditional medicine. Orthomolecular practitioners identify and treat the root cause of a disease. Their objective is to rebalance and rebuild the whole body, not merely to mask or suppress symptoms. To do this, they try to establish an equilibrium among the essential nutrients that may be lacking, may be present in excess, or are being poorly absorbed by the body. The imbalance of minerals, vitamins, or amino acids may be the cause of your psychiatric problems.

An example of orthomolecular care is provided by a patient treated by Dr. José A. Yaryura-Tobias. He describes one of his patients "who was very depressed, somnolent, and anxious and who had lost interest in life." His previous physician had put him on antidepressant medication, but it had not really helped. The patient had also been seen for psychological problems and had undergone talk therapy. The results were equivocal and did not make that person feel well and functional.

"When I examined the patient, I observed that he had poor dietary habits, skipped meals, did not sleep well at night, suffered from nocturnal sweats, and was often fidgety and restless around noontime. Given these symptoms, the first thing I did was have the patient take the five-hour glucose tolerance test in order to see how glucose was being metabolized in his body. When the results came back, they confirmed that the patient was suffering from a functional hypoglycemia, meaning that he had important drops in blood sugar. These shifts in levels of blood sugar can easily interfere with the normal biochemical and electric activity of the brain, which in turn can cause not only physical but also mental problems. When I corrected this disturbance with the proper diet, the patient improved dramatically. He reported that he was happier and feeling better and that life looked brighter. This is a case where depression was, in part at least, related to something as basic as sugar metabolism. Sugar may not be the only factor. Illness may, for instance, reflect an amino acid problem of some kind. The point is that by correcting the underlying cause or causes of an illness, it is possible to correct the illness. In this case, there was no need whatsoever for antidepressant medication."

How Orthomolecular Psychiatry Differs from Traditional Psychiatry

The whole-body approach to treatment used by orthomolecular psychiatrists also makes their diagnostic techniques differ substantially from those of traditional psychiatry. Traditional psychiatry approaches diagnosis from a purely symptomatic point of view. If a "cause" is identified, this usually occurs not through an individualized analysis of the patient's biochemistry but rather by means of an implied causation. In other words, traditional psychiatry does recognize that certain biochemical imbalances or "organic" factors may be the cause of certain mental conditions.

Traditional psychiatrists also assume that a given mental illness involves a biochemical imbalance. Depression, for instance, is treated with antidepressants designed to operate on the supply or metabolism of neurotransmitters. However, the traditional psychiatrist usually will not conduct tests to confirm that a patient with a given illness has the specific biochemical imbalance which psychiatry deems causative in that illness. The treatment is usually more of a guessing game in which one neurotransmitter, say, serotonin, may be supplemented and then the doctor and patient wait to see whether an improvement results. Even if the patient is found to have that specific biochemical imbalance, the diagnosis ordinarily stops with this discovery and the doctor does not look into the factors which may have triggered the imbalance to begin with.

With the orthomolecular approach, while a patient may present the classic symptoms of a mental disorder, this presentation forms only a minor part of the diagnosis. The orthomolecular psychiatrist will look at diet, glandular functions, glucose metabolism, and a host of other biochemical factors which may play a role in the patient's mental health. Without such a thorough diagnosis, it is impossible to design a good treatment. A diagnosis that does not take the whole individual into account cannot provide long-term relief. It may lead to suppression of symptoms, but it is not curative.

"First Do No Harm": Drugs as a Last Resort

Another difference between traditional and orthomolecular psychiatry is the attitude of each toward the use of drugs. While traditional medicine uses drugs as the treatment of preference, in most cases the orthomolecular approach is to use drugs only as a last resort or in an emergency. Dr. Robert Atkins, author of *Dr. Atkins' New Diet Revolution* (Avon, 1998) and a leading proponent of orthomolecular medicine, maintains that using harmless substances such as vitamins and nutrients first, and having recourse to drugs only after safer and less toxic treatments have proved ineffectual, is another way in which orthomolecular medicine is in keeping with the Hippocratic oath, which states, "First do no harm."

Dr. Bernard Rimland, a research psychologist, explains orthomolecular medicine by contrasting it with what he calls "toximolecular medicine." Dr. Rimland states:

"The two parts of the definition of orthomolecular medicine are not difficult to understand. Everyone can grasp the idea of obtaining optimal concentrations of nutrients. But the other part, the idea of trying to attain health by avoiding unnatural substances—chemicals that are not normally found in the body—is quite new to most people."

Dr. Rimland compares this approach with that of traditional medicine, which uses "sublethal doses of toxic substances" to try to restore health. He points out that if all the contraindications, side effects, and adverse reactions of drugs were deleted from the *Physicians' Desk Reference* (PDR), this comprehensive drug index which is about three inches thick would be reduced to about one-quarter inch. Drugs used in the treatment of mental disorders are particularly good examples. The adverse reactions and contraindications for the major tranquilizer Thorazine (chlorpromazine) alone takes up two pages of fine print in the PDR. This is one of the primary reasons why orthomolecular practitioners began to question the propriety of using these drugs before safer and less toxic avenues of treatment had been exhausted.

The use of drugs can be effective, of course. Antidepressant drugs, for instance, are helpful insofar as they raise serotonin levels in the brain. But nutrients can also do this, and since they are more compatible with the body's natural chemistry, they should be tried first. Why cure a malady with substances so foreign to the body that they may create new problems? This sort of chemical approach may be appropriate when nutrients have not been successful, but it should be seen as a last resort, not a first-line treatment.

Dr. Michael Lesser talks about a patient who was suffering from apparent melancholy. "She was severely depressed to the point where she wanted to give up her affairs and her finances to her children. She was in the hospital and was put on lithium, which did not seem to help her. She came to see me, and I did something that a traditional psychiatrist would probably not do, which was simply to have her get a blood test. I do a comprehensive blood-testing procedure in cases of severe depression, and in her case I found that she was suffering from megaloblastic anemia, which is a form of pernicious anemia. This anemia can and often does cause mental illness as a side effect of the general anemia picture because it is due to a deficiency of certain important nutrients, in particular vitamin B_{12} and perhaps folic acid.

"So, with a series of vitamin B_{12} injections, this woman is now up and about, no longer depressed at all, and perfectly capable of taking care of her financial affairs. There is a good chance that this would have been missed by traditional psychiatrists because they would not have thought to look at the body in this way. It is not part of the routine testing of traditional psychiatry."

Addressing Nutritional Deficiencies

Dr. Abram Hoffer, one of the world's most distinguished orthomolecular psychiatrists and research scientists, and author of *Putting it All Together: The New Orthomolecular Nutrition* (Keats, 1996), pioneered the use of nutrition-based therapies for mental illness nearly 50 years ago. In his judgment, the most common causes of depression and anxiety are nutritional deficiencies.

"In fact," he says, "the first symptom of almost any vitamin deficiency is depression. Second, we have allergies, and one of the most common villains is sugar. You would be amazed at how many people are depressed because they consume huge quantities of sugar. Some of my best recoveries have occurred when a patient has agreed to go off sugar. This can also apply to common foods which generally are okay, but which can cause depression if you happen to be allergic to them. I've estimated that at least 65 percent of all depression is probably caused by food allergies."

Dr. Hoffer, therefore, begins by determining if there's a problem with nutrition. "If there is, one corrects this by taking the junk out of one's diet and also determining what foods the patient is allergic to and how to get rid of them. We also have to use vitamins because the neuroreceptors, which have a lot to do with the way we see, think, and feel, have to have vitamins in large quantities before they can perform properly. So we find that many of the vitamins are helpful, not just one...."

"We have also begun to explore the healing properties of the amino acids. Some extremely interesting work is currently being done showing that the use of pyracine in the morning and tryptophan at night can be a very fine substitute for some of the common antidepressants. And tryptophan is also coming in as a treatment for manic depression or bipolar disorder...."

"The orthomolecular approach to mood disorders consists of a comprehensive program. Of course, our treatment has to be administered by a physician who understands what these patients are going through, who can deal with them and provide support, because there is nothing worse than a deep depression. I don't know of any condition that's more devastating than this. And unless the doctor understands what is going on, he will not help his patients sufficiently."

Focus on the Individual

Mental illness can be as diverse as the people who suffer from these disorders, and so the most appropriate treatment for any given person will depend entirely on that person's particular symptoms. If the person is treated orthomolecularly, the treatment will depend on any causative factors which may be discerned. Dr. Michael Lesser gives an example of a patient suffering from a combination of anxiety and depression to illustrate the importance of an individualized approach to treatment:

"I saw a man who was quite upset. He was a very frightened and frightening man—sort of a backwoods hippie type who was referred to me by another doctor who didn't know what to do with him because the patient was very angry and very upset. When I first saw him, he was on the lawn of my yard tearing up the grass, screaming in a very loud guttural voice. I was really frightened by him.

"I managed to talk to him long enough to get a history of a very severe depression and fearfulness approaching paranoia. When we did the blood tests, we found out that he had a low vitamin B_{12} level. I always check the vitamin panel in severe cases like this. He also had a pernicious anemia picture in the bloodstream—the megaloblastic anemia where one gets abnormally large blood cells, which is generally due to a deficiency of vitamin B_{12} and/or folic acid. We put him on vitamin B_{12} injections. Because he lived some distance from my office, I trained him to give himself the shots. A person has to have a series of these injections; usually one or two won't cure the problem. With these injections, he became considerably better."

Orthomolecular Psychiatry Today

It appears that today there is an increased acceptance of the ideas and therapies of orthomolecular psychiatry. Many orthodox physicians are beginning to react favorably, something which occurred only rarely 10 years ago. There are probably between 500 and 1,000 orthomolecular physicians currently practicing in the United States and Canada. That's approximately 500 out of 500,000—one-tenth of 1 percent—of practicing physicians, so there's a lot more that needs to be done to make more doctors aware of this approach.

If you're suffering from mental or emotional disorders, you should certainly explore orthomolecular psychiatry before starting years of unduly expensive and often fruitless psychoanalysis or psychotherapy, or subjecting yourself to the potentially harmful mind-altering drugs employed by psychiatrists that can exacerbate rather than alleviate your problems. It makes sense to find out whether your "emotional" problems have a physical cause before proceeding with an analysis of your history or psyche!

17

Depression

D epression is a major health problem that can leave an otherwise healthy person unable to cope with the even the simplest, everyday situations. It affects roughly 10 percent of the American population—perhaps 25 or 30 million people. This does not include the many individuals who function normally for the most part despite frequently finding themselves in low moods. Two-thirds of those who suffer from true depression are never treated and live their lives in misery without being recognized as sufferers of mental illness.

Causes of Depression

BIOCHEMICAL FACTORS For the past 30 years psychiatry has been aware that certain biochemical changes which take place in the brain can both influence and reflect fluctuations in people's moods. A change in the delicate biochemistry of the brain is capable of governing how a person feels at any given moment. A physical deficiency in any of the chemicals responsible for maintaining "good moods" may lead to depression, just as a psychologically stressing factor in a person's life may manifest itself in the body by altering the sensitive chemical balance in the brain, thereby also causing depression or low moods.

While psychiatry has recognized this mind-body connection in general terms for the past three decades, it is only in the last 10 to 15 years that it has actually isolated some of the specific brain chemicals involved. Especially important among these chemicals are substances called neurotransmitters, which are released at the nerve endings in the brain and allow messages to be relayed throughout the rest of the brain and the body. Perhaps the most commonly known neurotransmitter is endorphin. It is responsible for pain relief within the body and is thought to be the chemical responsible for the "high" that runners experience after exercise.

Mood swings can be traced to a similar mind-body relationship. Scientists have found that a large number of depressed people have significant deficiencies of the neurotransmitters norepinephrine and serotonin. These neurotransmitters belong to a chemical group called the amines which are responsible for the control of emotions, sleep, pain, and many involuntary bodily functions such as digestion. Almost 90 percent of these amines are found deep in the brain; because of their importance, the normally functioning body has developed a recycling system, called reuptake, by which the nerve cell takes back 85 percent of the neurotransmitter for future use once the chemical reaction has been completed. Only the remaining 15 percent is destroyed by enzymes.

The metabolism of the neurotransmitters is intricate, and deficiencies can occur for many reasons. Dr. Priscilla Slagle, a board-certified orthomolecular psychiatrist practicing in southern California, states that age or genetics may cause a person to use up amines more rapidly than someone else might. She also points out that a defective receiving cell or reuptake mechanism, or a deficiency of the amino acids, vitamins, and minerals that make up amines, may be the culprit here. The nutrient deficiencies involved may result from excessive intake of caffeine, sugar, alcohol, or tobacco. Sugar and coffee can destroy the B vitamins and the minerals magnesium and iron, all of which figure significantly in neurotransmitter formation. Alcohol and tobacco also deplete almost all the B vitamins, vitamin C, zinc, magnesium, manganese, and tyrosine. These nutrients are essential to maintaining a good mood.

STRESS Stress is another factor which can contribute to depression. Most people tend to associate depression with what are called major stressors, such as the loss of a loved one, being fired from a job, or another circumstance which upsets one's life in a very significant way. However, even the stress associated with everyday living can directly deplete the vitamins, minerals, and amino acids that are so important in maintaining a good mood. Dr. Slagle explains:

"We have found very high levels of the hormone cortisol, which is secreted by the adrenal glands, in severely depressed patients. Indeed, scientists have devised a test which measures the levels of this hormone in the body to determine the degree of depression present. When people are depressed and highly stressed, their adrenal glands may secrete higher levels of cortisol, triggering certain enzymes in the body that destroy tyrosine and tryptophan. One would think that under extreme stress the body would compensate for this breakdown by facilitating the survival of these important amino acids. Instead, for whatever reason, these amino acids are used up. I believe that high cortisol levels induce depression in certain people."

SIDE EFFECTS OF MEDICATIONS Another observation noted by Dr. Slagle is the prevalence of depression as a side effect of many prescription medications. The list of these medications is quite extensive, including antibiotics, antiarthritis pills, antihistamines, blood pressure medication, birth control pills, tranquilizers, and even aspirin. When people are given these medications, they often are not warned that they may experience depression as a side effect. Dr. Slagle, together with most other orthomolecular psychiatrists, believes that rather than ignoring these side expects or waiting for them to appear, whenever a prescription drug is given that has a side effect such as depression listed in the Physician's Desk Reference (PDR), a nutritional program should accompany the prescription in order to replenish the particular vitamins and amino acids which may be depleted by the medication.

ENVIRONMENTAL FACTORS It is common for depressed people to have a family history of depression. In addition to the genetic factor, such family histories may also be due to common environmental factors, shared experiences in depressed families, and poor eating habits that are passed on from one generation to another.

Environmental factors may play multiple roles among the causes of depression. For example, being raised in a family in which one or more people are depressed may often be associated with poor nutrition. As Dr. William J. Goldwag reminds us, "Just being exposed to depressed people can be an influence, since children learn how to behave by imitation. Also, family members are eating the same food, and if, for instance, the mother is depressed and cooking and serving her family, that food is apt to be sparse in nutrients since she is interested in just getting the meal over with and has difficulty finding enough energy to prepare it."

Being abused physically or verbally can be another factor that inhibits children of depressed parents. As a way of handling abuse, the child may withdraw and become depressed and inactive as a defense against very harsh treatment from the parent.

Dr. Doris Rapp, a board-certified pediatric allergist and specialist in environmental medicine, adds that mood disorders often lead to battering of family members and intimates: "Husbands batter wives, wives batter husbands, they both batter the children, and boyfriends batter their girlfriends. Mother battering, I might add, is very common. Many of the children I treat beat, kick, bruise, bite, and pinch their mothers. When some individuals have typical allergies and environmental illness, if they have a mood problem, they can become nasty and irritable and angry. All I ask is, 'What did you eat, touch, and smell?'

"To help find the cause I try to discover whether the change in behavior occurs inside or outside, after eating, or after smelling a chemical. It might be a food, dust, mold, pollens, or chemicals, which not only affect the brain, but discrete areas of the brain. As a result, the allergen or food or chemical exposure might make you tired or, if it affects the frontal lobes, it might make you behave in an inappropriate way. It could affect the speech center of the brain so that you speak too rapidly, or unclearly, or stutter, or don't speak intelligently. It's just potluck as to what area of the brain or body will be affected when you are exposed to something to which you are allergic."

MAGNESIUM DEFICIENCY According to Dr. Lendon Smith, a specialist in nutrition-based therapies and author of many books on the topic, including *Feed Your Body Right: Understanding Your Individual Body Chemistry for Proper Nutrition Without Guesswork* (McEvans, 1995) craving chocolate is also a sign of depression." It usually means that people need magnesium, because there's magnesium in chocolate. Women, the day before their menstrual period, often find themselves searching through the cupboards for chocolate. They find a big canister of Hershey's and drink it down before feeling better from the magnesium.

"I often had the delightful experience of giving an intravenous mixture of vitamin C, calcium, magnesium, and B vitamins," Dr. Smith says. "Usually it has more magnesium than calcium. Afterwards I asked patients whether they would like some chocolate and they told me they didn't need it. It really is connected.

"Women in the sixth month of pregnancy will often send their husbands out for ice cream because the baby is starting to grow fast. The woman has a conscious need for dairy products because she knows they will bring her the calcium she needs, but she also says, 'Don't forget the pickles.' She knows, somehow, that she needs to acidify that calcium source for the baby. She will not get much out of it and she will suffer from leg cramps.

"The chemist I work with in Spokane discovered something about GGT, a liver and gallbladder enzyme called gamma glutamil transpeptidase. The range that the lab has is anywhere from 0 to 40. They find these values all over the place. The mean would be about 20.

"What we've found is that if their level is below 20, they're more likely to have some of these magnesium deficiency symptoms—short attention span, trouble relaxing or sleeping, little muscle cramps in the feet and legs, and a craving for chocolate. Most of these people don't like to be touched. They may be a little crabby. Those symptoms go with low magnesium."

Dr. Smith explains that once food has been processed, magnesium is one of the first minerals to disappear. "Magnesium is also one of the first minerals to leave the body when there is stress, which accounts for how many women behave a day or so before their periods. They feel stressed because they're losing their magnesium.

"We need to supply magnesium to these people. We can determine who needs it by the blood test and by the sense of smell. If people smell a bottle of pure magnesium salt—magnesium chloride is a good one—and it smells good or if there's no smell, then the person needs it. The blood test we usually use is the 24 chem. screen, the standard blood test.

"Many symptoms of depression, hyperactivity, headaches, loss of weight, and other conditions are related to genetic tendencies. If there is a tendency to be depressed in the family, a magnesium deficiency will allow that tendency to show up. If there's alcoholism, diabetes, or obesity in the family, then low magnesium may allow those things to show up in a person. There are reasons to explain all these things and nutrition is basic to this. The patients don't have an antidepressant pill deficiency; they usually have a magnesium deficiency."

The first thing Dr. Smith does when he sees patients is ask what they're eating. "If I find that they're eating a lot of dairy products, and that as a child they had their tonsils taken out, and that they had a lot of strep throat and ear infections, then I know they're allergic to milk and they're looking for calcium. Sure enough, the blood tests will show this. That's the first thing they have to stop. Whatever they love is probably causing the trouble because food sensitivities can cause low blood sugar."

TOBACCO Orthomolecular psychiatrist Dr. Abram Hoffer tells the story of a classic case of a misdiagnosis corrected, enabling one man to start anew after his previous life had already been ruined. "A high school teacher and principal of about 45 developed a severe depression. In fact, I believe he was misdiagnosed as a schizophrenic. He exhibited what we call a straightforward, deep-seated, endogenous depression. He was in a mental hospital for about a year or two, and then discharged. He was so depressed that no one could live with him. His wife divorced him and eventually he was living with his aunt, who looked after him as if he were a child. As a last resort, he was referred to me.

"When he came to see me, which was many years ago, I had just started looking into the question of allergies. At that time, I wasn't very familiar with food allergies, but I thought he was a very interesting case and I said to myself, 'He is a classic case of a depression, maybe schizophrenic. He'd be the last person in the world who would respond to this antiallergy approach.' At that time I was using—and I still do—a four-day water fast. This is a way of determining whether or not these allergies are present. He agreed that he would do the fast, which also involved refraining from any smoking or consuming of alcohol; he had to drink about eight glasses of water a day and nothing else. His aunt said she would help make sure he complied. When he came back to see me two weeks later, he and his aunt explained that, at the end of the four-day fast, he was normal. All of the depression was gone.

"This same man then began to get tested for food allergies and he found that not a single food made him sick. But now he began to smoke again. Within a day after he resumed smoking, he was back in his deep depression. The ironic thing was that he had a brother who was a tobacco company executive, who kept sending him free cartons of cigarettes. Now when we made the connection to his cigarette smoking, he stopped smoking. Thirty days later, after he had been depressed for four years and hadn't been able to work, he was back in school teaching. And I remember this clearly because the insurance company that was then paying his monthly pension was so astounded at this dramatic response that they sent one of their agents to see me, to find out what the magic wand was that I had waved to get this patient off their rolls. This is a classic case of an allergy to tobacco that was causing this man's depression."

Diagnosing the Problem

Traditional psychiatry diagnoses depression according to the criteria set forth in the DSM-IV (Diagnostic and Statistical Manual of Mental Disorders, 4th edition), which essentially defines it as a condition that includes at least five of the following symptoms during the same two-week period:

1. Depressed mood
2. Markedly diminished interest or pleasure in all or almost all activities
3. Significant weight loss or gain (when not dieting)
4. Insomnia (a constant inability to sleep) or hypersomnia
5. Psychomotor agitation (a hyperanxious state) or retardation
6. Fatigue or loss of energy
7. Feelings of worthlessness or excessive or inappropriate guilt
8. Diminished ability to think or concentrate or indecisiveness
9. Recurrent thoughts of death

While orthomolecular psychiatrists may use this definition as a starting point, they do not confine the diagnosis to these criteria. Orthomolecular psychiatry views depression or any other illness as a unique and individual condition. While there may be certain guidelines, such as those set forth in the DSM-IV, a diagnosis which rigidly adheres to these criteria can arrive at a wrong conclusion either by missing the diagnosis altogether because the person's symptoms are not those normally associated with depression, or by falsely diagnosing a person as being depressed simply because he or she has the text-book symptoms.

Often the depressed patient is not aware of the condition, especially when it is complicated by associated physical symptoms. If you suffered from chronic back pain, indigestion, or neck stiffness, would you immediately think that you might be manifesting symptoms of depression? Probably not. You might go to several doctors in search of relief, and there would be a very good chance that none of them would ever consider depression as the root of your problem. Even if someone were to ask whether you were depressed, you might quickly protest if, as Dr. Priscilla Slagle puts it, you "have 'somatized,' that is, put [your] emotional feelings into the body, thereby inducing bodily symptoms."

Sometimes a patient may develop responses to medication that are misinterpreted as purely physical. "For example," Dr. Slagle says, "an acquaintance of mine who lost her daughter through death a year ago became so anxious that her doctor started her on tranquilizers. Although she was on tranquilizers for six months, she became worse and worse. When I visited her, it was readily apparent to me that she had severe depression. It was difficult to convince her of this because she could only relate to the anxiety and the insomnia she was having. I started her on a nutrient program, and she improved dramatically in two to three weeks. Of course, I tapered her off the tranquilizers, because if they are stopped abruptly, one can have withdrawal symptoms which can aggravate the anxiety."

Traditional Treatments

Orthodox treatments for depression range from counseling and psychotherapy to medication and electroshock therapy. However, when a traditional psychiatrist arrives at a diagnosis of depression, more likely than not the next step will be to put the patient on antidepressant medication. Some of the most common of these medications are Elavil (amitriptyline), Sinequan (doxepin), Tofranil (imipramine), and Nardil (phenelzine). They are all designed to increase in one way or another the concentration of the neurotransmitters, thereby prolonging their biochemical reaction. Although the manufacturers claim that there is no evidence of addiction to most of these drugs, they are not without serious side effects. The PDR entry for one of these, for instance, mentions many contraindications, warnings, precautions, and adverse reactions, including severe convulsions and possibly death if this drug is used improperly with other drugs, complications in patients with impaired liver function, hypertension, stroke, disorientation, delusions, hallucinations, excitement, tremors, seizures, blurred vision, dizziness, fatigue, baldness, and elevation and lowering of blood-sugar levels.

Because suicidal tendencies are a frequent characteristic of depression, perhaps one of the most serious problems associated with antidepressants is the potential for drug overdose. The potential for suicide caused by the very medication prescribed to prevent it is further enhanced by the synergistic interaction of the antidepressives with alcohol, barbiturates, and other central nervous system depressants. A glance through the PDR indicates that the quantity and the magnitude of the dangers associated with Elavil are equally present with the other antidepressants.

Alternative Therapies

DIET AND NUTRITION It is surprising how often diet and nutrition are factors in depression, and how effective enhanced or improved nutrition can be in helping someone suffering from depression to improve his or her mood. According to Dr. William J. Goldwag, "Often the quality of the diet suffers in depressed people. If the depression is profound, the individual doesn't even feel like eating. Depressed people who live alone or who are major providers or cooks in the house may not feel like preparing meals or even shopping. They're apt to restrict their nutrition to fast food or anything just to get eating over with." In many cases, weight loss is a symptom of severe depression. In many other cases, there is substantial weight gain.

Dr. Goldwag notes that significant weight loss is likely to bring about "marked deprivation of the essential nutrients, including the amino acids needed to manufacture the proper proteins, as well as a deficiency in many vitamins and minerals. That in itself can then aggravate the depression."

Dr. Goldwag suggests straightforward solutions to at least some of the challenges associated with depression: "There are some simple ways to prepare food in advance so that the food has to be prepared less often. I recommend preparing a raw salad once a week. Certain fresh vegetables can be stored for quite a period in a refrigerator and will keep quite well. There are a whole variety to choose from: carrots, celery, radishes, cauliflower, broccoli, peppers, red cabbage, green onions, snow peas, string beans. These can all be cut up and mixed together. They can be stored in a plastic bag or sealed container. When mealtime comes, a person can take a handful of these vegetables and then perhaps add some other ones that don't keep as well, such as tomatoes or sprouts. You then have a fresh salad that is already prepared with a lot of important nutrients. This is just one way of having food prepared in advance. It's good for people who are depressed and don't have the energy to make a whole meal."

Dr. Goldwag believes that the B-complex vitamins are especially important. "One of the major groups of vitamins to incorporate are from the B complex family. Years and years ago, when people suffered from severe vitamin deficiencies, some of the resultant diseases like pellagra and so forth were characterized by accompanying psychotic reactions. That is, the thinking process was the most obvious one to be affected by the vitamin deficiency. Simply providing the proper vitamin, in this case vitamin B_3 or niacin, was the treatment. It cleared up the psychosis.

"There's no doubt that brain function is very dependent upon nutrients like niacin and others, because when they're absent there is apt to be some very disturbed thinking. Depression is one of the symptoms that can occur with this.

"It is important to get all the B-complex vitamins, since they work together. Thiamine, B_1, is important, as is riboflavin to a lesser extent. Another important one is B_6, pyridoxine. B_{12} is still another one that can affect the mental processes.

"Niacin is often used in much higher doses than the others in order to accomplish some of these changes. Niacin is a ubiquitous vitamin. It is being used greatly to help reduce cholesterol levels, to improve the good cholesterol and reduce the bad. The dosages being used are much greater than those used to simply overcome a deficiency."

At the same time, there are plenty of foods that should be avoided. Fast foods can affect mental symptoms by causing blood-sugar abnormalities. People who tend to hypoglycemia or low blood-sugar patterns should avoid eating too many simple carbohydrates, such as candy bars, which are converted very rapidly to sugar in the blood. As Dr. Goldwag says, "Simple carbohydrate foods temporarily raise the blood sugar, but then they drop it to a very low level several hours later, resulting in depression. This encourages the individual to repeat the cycle of taking sugar or some simple carbohydrate that's converted to sugar in order to feel that high again. This constant seesaw from high to low mood can account for many episodes of depression in individuals."

Both alcoholics and chronic dieters often have depressive tendencies. Alcoholics often suffer from symptoms of low mood, and although alcohol may appear at first as a stimulant and mood enhancer, it is in fact a depressant and substantially decreases the ability of the body to extract nutrients from the food we eat. Dieters tend to eat very few B-complex-containing foods, and they often suffer from depression as well.

AMINO ACIDS A leading authority on the treatment of depression with amino acids and nutritional therapy, Dr. Priscilla Slagle became interested in the treatment of mood disorders as a result of her own depression, which lasted for many years and did not respond to traditional psychoanalysis or psychotherapeutic treatment. Disinclined to use antidepressant medications because of the adverse reactions which so commonly accompany them, Dr. Slagle discovered that "there are natural food substances that will create the same end-effects, that is, elevate mood in the same way without causing side effects or toxicity. I started myself on [a program using certain single amino acids to control mood] and achieved very dramatic results. Although I have had tremendous stress over the past 10 years, particularly the past year, I have not had one day of a low mood. This has been a marvelous reprieve, since I have had and therefore understand the pain that low moods can create for many people."

In her book, *The Way Up from Down* (Random House, 1987, and St. Martin's Press, 1988, 1991), Dr. Slagle outlines a safe and easily implemented program of treatment for depression using amino acids and other precursors required for the production of norepinephrine and serotonin. She is careful to emphasize that people should follow the program under the supervision of a physician. For those already on antidepressant medication, it is not advisable to stop abruptly since they may experience withdrawal symptoms.

Dr. Slagle explains the basis of the program: "It consists of taking an amino acid called tyrosine, which in the presence of certain B-complex vitamins, minerals, and vitamin C will convert into norepinephrine in the brain. This neurotransmitter not only sustains positive moods but also helps our concentration, learning, memory, drive, ambition, motivation, and other equally important qualities. Additionally, it helps to regulate food and sexual appetite functions. Thus it is a very important chemical. The other amino acid used in the program is tryptophan, which forms serotonin in the brain, provided that the requisite cofactors—the B vitamins, minerals, and vitamin C—are present. In addition to sustaining mood, tryptophan also has other functions such as controlling sleep and levels of aggression. People who are quite aggressive, irritable, or angry are often suffering from a marked deficiency in serotonin. Indeed, very low levels of serotonin have been found in the brain of suicide victims at autopsy.

"With these two amino acids, a good multivitamin-mineral preparation is taken to provide all the nutrients necessary to catalyze or promote the conversion of the amino acids into the neurotransmitters."

Dr. Slagle provides the following dosage for the two amino acids: around 500–3,000 mg of tyrosine taken twice daily and about 500–2,000 mg of tryptophan, an amino acid nutritional supplement. Public sale of tryptophan was banned by the Food and Drug Administration (FDA) in March of 1990, a ban still in effect today, but the supplement is now again available by prescription through most compounding pharmacies. Dr. Slagle recommends that the tyrosine be taken first thing in the morning on an empty stomach and then also some time in the mid-morning or mid-afternoon. The tryptophan, because of its sleep-inducing effects, is taken before bed. Any amino acids used therapeutically must be taken separately from other protein foods, because protein interferes with their utilization. Dr. Slagle also specifies that the amino acids be taken in capsules (tablets can pass through the body undigested) and in the "free form," a preparation in which the amino acids are ready for absorption by the body, thus avoiding pre-existing problems with digestion.

OTHER SUPPLEMENTS Nutrients that enhance brain function, such as the ones listed below, can improve mental and emotional states:

ACETYL-L-CARNITINE. This nutrient crosses the blood brain barrier and provides the brain with more energy. This is a gentle, not jittery, energy, and it is especially important for older people, who tend to lose brain cells due to a lack of energy. Between 500 and 1,500 mg should be taken on an empty stomach.

LIQUID ZINC. Dr. Alexander Schauss, clinical psychologist, certified eating disorder specialist, and author of *Anorexia & Bulimia* (Keats, 1997), describes his studies with liquid zinc: "In our eating disorder studies, we used a multidimensional design, and evaluated the affective or mood state of our patients for five years. One of the first things to improve in patients treated with liquid zinc was the degree of depression that they were experiencing based on psychometric instruments such as the Beck Depression Scale, the profile of mood scales, and other depressive indices. This suggests that we might consider using zinc as an antidepressant. There is a growing concern among many patients, and even therapists, that antidepressant drugs, such as Prozac, might not be safe, and we are looking at viable alternatives. We have discovered this antidepressive effect and have documented it in patients under blind conditions."

PHOSPHATITYL SERINE. This nutrient is produced by the body but lessens with age. Taking 200 to 500 mg improves the ability of brain cell membranes to receive signals and function better. That, in turn, can elevate mood levels, help overcome winter depression, and enhance short-term memory.

HERBS

St. John's wort extract is an herbal remedy for depression that has made it into the mainstream media in recent years. Other plants containing chemicals with antidepressant properties include:

Pastinaca sativa (parsnip)
Myrciaria dubia (camu-camu)
Malpighia glabra (acerola)
Lactuca sativa (lettuce)
Amaranthus sp. (pigweed)
Portulaca oleracea (purslane)
Nasturtium officinale (berro)
Chenopodium album (lamb's-quarters)
Cichorium endivia (endive)
Spinacia oleracea (spinach)
Brassica chinensis (Chinese cabbage)
Brassica oleracea (broccoli)
Lycopersicon esculentum (tomato)
Avena sativa (oats)
Raphanus sativus (radish)
Anethum graveolens (dill)
Phaseolus vulgaris (black bean)
Cucurbita foetidissima (buffalo gourd)
Corchorus olitorius (Jew's mallow)

HOMEOPATHY Homeopathic remedies can be quite effective in lifting depression. Dr. Gennaro Locurcioas, a homeopathic physician, says that while money does not create happiness, the king of remedies for treating depression is gold—also known as *aurum metallicum*. Here he describes this and other remedies for treating depression in women; men certainly can benefit as well:

AURUM METALLICUM. This is for the perfectionist woman who has set high goals for herself but is unable to meet them. At first, she will become irritable, a state that can last for several months. She feels as if she has lost the love of those around her and that it is her fault. This leads to feelings of frustration, accompanied by a strong sense of guilt, which may push her to suicide in extreme cases. Dr. Locurcioas observes, "At first sight, this woman appears perfect and polished. When we start talking to her, we get the idea that there is an abnormal focus on career and achievement. Being a workaholic just covers up the emptiness inside."

ARSENICUM. This remedy is for depression accompanied by anxiety. The woman is restless day and night. She is constantly on the phone, calling her friends, for fear of being alone. She wakes up at night and walks around the room thinking about her fears and anxieties. She is afraid of a poverty-filled future and of death. "*Arsenicum* is from arsenic," says Dr. Locurcioas. "If we give that to a person, they die. But giving homeopathic arsenic to a person is completely safe and better than Xanax."

IGNATIA. This helps depression associated with grief. A woman has lost her child or her mother, or has been disappointed by a romantic relationship. The patient may exhibit physical characteristics, such as a tic on the face, numbness, a lump in the throat, or sighing. "According to the homeopathic literature, if the patient says that she gets aggravated when she eats sweets, and she improves by traveling, these are signs that *ignatia* is indicated," notes Dr. Locurcioas.

SEPIA is a good example of how homeopathic remedies use substances that relate to a person's symptoms: "This remedy is made from a black mollusk that emits a black ink. Black is the ink from which the remedy is prepared. And black is the color the depressed woman sees around herself. She sees black in her future. This little sea creature, at some point in its life, will deposit about 300 eggs, which are incredibly big for the size of this little animal, and then it will die. This is the housewife who had a job, and had to come home and prepare dinner for the husband and children. For years, she gives the best of her energy to her family and children. Now she is 40, 45, or 50. The children are gone, and she feels as if her mission in life is over. She sees no purpose in her life anymore. She does not hate her husband, but feels indifferent toward him. She does not want to be touched sexually, and cries many times during the day without knowing why. Inside she feels despair and isolation. Physically, she has a dull, inexpressive face, and the muscles of the body have lost their tone. The woman has varicose veins, constipation. Sepia is a remedy for the exhausted housewife."

ACUPUNCTURE Acupuncture frees blocked energy, and in so doing naturally lifts depression. Look at what one woman has to say about her experience: "When I was in my twenties, just after finishing college, I would go into a depression whenever I was about to get my period. It came on so suddenly that it was frightening. I went to see a doctor about it and was given a referral to an acupuncturist.

"After being in treatment for six months, my practitioner and I sat down to talk about how I was feeling. I realized then that the depression was gone.

"That was 12 years ago. I've stayed in treatment, although not as regularly as when I first started. It's my primary form of health care. My eating habits and sleeping patterns have become totally regulated. I have been able to lose 40 pounds and to maintain my weight without dieting. I also quit smoking without ever trying. I never get sick anymore. I never get colds or flus. In general, I'm much more balanced.

"The whole experience of being brought into harmony keeps me from going to extremes. I don't work too hard, I don't play too hard, I don't rest too hard. I manage to stay pretty much in the center of my life. It's a huge improvement. I often wonder how people live without going through a treatment process like I did."

EXERCISE Physical exercise is another key to lifting depression, especially when accompanied by a nutritious diet, meditation, and vitamin and mineral supplementation. According to Dr. William J. Goldwag, exercise is one of the most profound aids in the treatment of depression: "One of the major errors in the thinking of patients and therapists is the notion that in order to be active, you have to feel better. This is exactly contrary to our approach.

"We recommend that you *do* first, and then the feeling comes later. In other words, you must do what you have to do regardless of how you feel. This aids in feeling better. You can't wait until you feel good to do something, because in depression that may take days, weeks, months, or even years. You want to accelerate the process.

"Those of us who exercise regularly have had days when they just didn't feel like it. That's the way depressed people feel about everything. They just don't feel like it. They don't have the energy, the motivation, the stimulation to go and do even the ordinary things. When it's severe, you may not even have the will or desire to get out of bed in the morning.

"The exercise may consist of very, very simple things, like just getting out and walking, getting up and doing some simple movements, some mild calisthenics, any kind of physical movement that gets the body in action. For some people just getting out of bed and getting dressed is a big accomplishment. That may be the first step.

"Another benefit of exercise is a feeling of accomplishment. Even doing a little bit of exercise will make you feel more energized later on. Finishing an exercise routine, even one that's fatiguing, after a brief period of rest will give you a feeling of revitalization, of energy, and a psychological feeling of accomplishment. It gives a feeling of, 'I've done it. It's completed.'"

YOGA AND MEDITATION Dr. Michele Galante, a complementary physician in Suffern, New York, overcame depression in adolescence by learning how to center energy using yoga and meditation: "When I was in my late teens, I went through a period of depression, where my energy was low. My whole being was unhappy. My parents and others I loved thought I should try seeing a psychiatrist for a while. I went a few times, but that wasn't satisfying to me. I thought nutrition might help so I started drinking raw vegetable juices and became veg-etarian. I started eating to detoxify myself and to get myself back to feeling stronger again.

"Then I got into meditation and kundalini yoga. I learned about energy centers and started to learn how inner energy flows through the system. I began to sense blockages, and to identify emotions and limiting thoughts that were holding me back. Through practice, I was able to center energy into the emo-tional center in the chest and into the abdomen where stabilizing rootedness can occur. That started to awaken inner energies and to strengthen me.

"The important thing is to not get too hung up in the head, where we have all these conflicts. Our center is the lower abdomen, where a baby grows in a woman. The Japanese call this the *hara*. In Zen we concentrate the mind and the whole being there. That's the hub of the wheel. The mind can be clearer when you do that, and you don't get hung up living in the realm of thought.

"Set aside 10 to 20 minutes daily to quiet the mind, to let tensions drain, to open up, and to resonate with the environment. Everyone does it in a different way. You can do it with meditation or biofeedback. You can do it with music, yoga, a hobby, it doesn't matter what. Anything that takes you to a creative, quiet place, allows you to recharge. Learn to take the time to express your inner needs.

"I like to ask my patients the question, 'Why do we have a physical body?' My answer is always that we exist as a physical entity to carry around our minds and our hearts, in a sense our spirits, so that we can fulfill ourselves. We can then learn and grow and do what we need to do in life. We are nothing with-out our emotions. Yet we neglect and suppress our feelings. We don't consider nourishing ourselves in a spiritual way. We need some sort of daily practice.

"We have a lot of outward pressures. We have rules made by corporations which are fulfilling needs of profits and ruining resources. There is a huge lack of wisdom across the board. The only thing that can make you happy is look-ing inwardly. Bring your mind and energies inside. Sometimes, when you start out, all you see is unhappiness and tension. But if you keep at it, sitting down, breathing quietly, not moving, and slowly bringing the mind inside, you will start to feel a sense of peace, relaxation and buoyancy. That is recharging your battery. That is the most profound thing you can do to bring your energy up."

Patient Story

Depression and anxiety are very difficult. You get up and do the things you feel you have to do. But you don't feel like you are in the flow of life. My con-ditions were probably not that apparent to the rest of the world, but I experi-enced them as very uncomfortable, and they took away from my quality of life. I felt stressed much of the time. And I had difficulty concentrating. At times I would forget things. Someone would ask me to do something, and I would forget to do it. I knew there wasn't something wrong with my mind. I felt my lack of focus was due more to my being so hyped up and tense.

I felt overwhelmed by ordinary, everyday demands, and I felt exhausted by the end of the day. Many times, after lunch, I would feel really tired, almost like I needed to have a nap. Anxiety and depression seemed to gobble up my energy very quickly. By the end of the day, I was not in the mood for recreational activities. Work wore me out. I would just go home and bug out in front of the boob tube. And I wanted more than that.

Once in a while, I would have a drink and notice a difference; I would be able to focus much better. The reason was that the drink helped me to relax. But I didn't want to relax that way. I wanted to find an alternative that would really work for me and help me to feel more joy in my everyday experience.

I went to several physicians, and they prescribed various medications for me. But I couldn't take medicines. They had all kinds of strange side effects, which were just as bad as the anxiety or the depression. The drugs masked my conditions, but underneath they were still there. All they did was make me feel very sleepy much of the time. I would be sitting at a meeting, dozing off, and I couldn't afford to do that. So I only took medications briefly.

I was looking for help when I happened to hear a Gary Null lecture at the Learning Annex. I was very impressed with some of the things I heard about limiting belief systems, and how difficult it is to see beyond them. I liked the talk on vegetarianism as well. As a result, I went to see Dolores Perri and was very impressed.

Dolores went over my history and concerns. I really enjoyed talking to Dolores because, unlike most physicians that I've encountered, she was very relaxed. I didn't get a sense that we were limited by time; we were done when we were done. Basically, I asked my questions and expressed my concerns. It was a very good experience. After we talked, she recommended certain foods, herbs, and supplements.

I have been following a nutritional routine for about two and a half months now, and I have definitely noticed a very dramatic shift. In particular, my hypoglycemia has disappeared. That's mostly from getting rid of refined sugars and processed foods. I used to feel very restless and nervous if I didn't eat. That's been stabilized, and I feel much calmer now.

My energy level is much, much better with a vegetarian regime, supplements, and herbs. The aloe I've been using is outstanding at perking me up at the beginning of the day.

I feel clearer as well. There are subtle differences in my ability to concentrate. And when I go through the day, I feel much calmer. A couple of days ago, I was late for a meeting, through no fault of my own. I had to be late for something I thought was very important. Normally, I would be a complete wreck about it. But because of my new regime, I was calm and centered, and

I didn't run up the stairs. I just walked in, explained what had happened, sat down, and joined in.

In the past, I would have been practically shaking from anxiety. This is a real departure, which I attribute largely to my change in diet as well as to my holistic orientation.

I think it's important to know that it's not only a shift in diet that has helped me. I became involved in meditation to clear my mind and help me reach that stillness. I do that in the morning before anything else. In addition, I take a greater interest in the holistic world and participate in seminars. All these different elements help to enhance my well-being—Maria

18

Alcoholism

Alcoholism is a pervasive problem today, affecting people of all ages from all walks of life. Traditional medicine views it as a disease that can be managed with drugs, counseling, and social support. The alternative community has other notions. For example, complementary physician Dr. Robert Atkins says that alcoholism is so tied in with carbohydrate metabolism that it is fair to say they are "genetically superimposable." In other words, it is possible to understand alcoholism in terms of carbohydrate metabolism alone. This is an extremely radical assertion, but one that lends important insight into a problem that plagues our society.

Alcoholics and "Sugarholics"

"I have seen families in which half of the members were alcoholics and the other half were sugarholics," Dr. Atkins explains. "And you could switch them over. You could probably make alcoholics of the people that were addicted to sugar, and it is well known that when alcoholics go through a psychologically-based program, and not a biochemically-based program, they have a tendency to become sugar addicts."

In fact, it is unusual for ex-alcoholics *not* to become sugar addicts. More commonly, individuals replace one addiction for the other. As Dr. Atkins notes: "Unless people get the clue that there is a connection between alcoholism and sugar addiction, they will just go from one to another and will not feel any better. The phrase 'dry drunks' refers to what happens to alcoholics that start switching to sugar instead of getting on a diet in which all the simple sugars are eliminated."

Nutritional Awareness and Support

Clearly, in such situations nutritional awareness can make all the difference. Dr. Atkins considers it a necessary component of any successful alcoholism program: "Of course, nutritional support is also important. Minerals, such as chromium, zinc, and manganese, are all very important in regulating this sort of problem."

Orthomolecular psychiatrist Dr. Abram Hoffer also believes in the nutritional approach: "The general regimen that orthomolecular medicine uses for alcohol addiction (as with depression, schizophrenia, and a number of other mental disorders) is to pay careful attention to nutrition and the use of the right supplements.

Dietary Modifications

"The first order of business," Dr. Hoffer continues, "is to make sure that the individual's basic diet is optimal. We do that by trying to take away most of the additives in food he or she eats on a daily basis. It is impossible to get them all out, but we try to do the best we can. One of the best simple rules is to put the patient on a sugar-free diet, because almost all foods that contain sugar contain a large variety of other chemicals. By avoiding sugar you will cut out most additives, by about 80 or 90 percent. Since we are all individuals, and many of us have food allergies and can't tolerate large quantities of carbohydrates or protein, for example, each one of us has to develop a diet that is optimal for ourselves.

Supplements

"Second, we add in the supplements that are right for this particular individual. Many of us have been so deprived of these proper supplements over our lifetime that, even with a very good diet, we cannot regain our health. That's why we need supplements. This is where the treatment differs markedly from person to person (and depending upon whether someone is being treated for alcoholism, or a mental illness, such as depression or schizophrenia). So while the dietary regimen is largely the same for all—avoid sugar and any foods that make you sick—supplements are determined on a case-by-case basis.

Alcoholics Anonymous (AA)

"For alcoholism the basic treatment starts with Alcoholics Anonymous. Bill W., the cofounder of Alcoholics Anonymous, first showed that when you added niacin to the treatment of alcoholism you got a major response that you did not see before. Today, there are a large number of very good alcoholism treatment programs in the United States, where they depend primarily on a combination of the type of nutrition that I have just referred to, make use of the right supplements, and implement AA and other social aids to help these patients get well."

Patient Story

I am a recovered alcoholic. It's been about seven years that I've been off alcohol. At first, I ate a lot of sugar in cakes and things like that. One of the psychological-emotional components of my behavior was that I always had a very difficult time getting started in the morning. The first thing I would think about when I got up was what I was going to eat, which usually included cereal with sugar, a pastry, and sugar-laden coffee. There has been a slow, progressive bettering of my diet, but there has still always been the sugar craving. Sometimes I would be able to get away from it for a week or two weeks, but it would always creep back in.

Recently, I completed a seven-day fast and a colonic cleansing and I found that after that cleansing process the craving pretty much disappeared. Also, I wake up in the morning feeling rather alert, and I don't have this compulsion to eat sweets. I think that because I am staying away from sugar, I generally am having better days psychologically—Bob

19

Anxiety Disorders

A nxiety can be due to many different causes. Practically any nutritional deficiency that affects the mind (and almost all do in one way or another) can cause anxiety as a symptom. The most common type of anxiety is called neurosis, neurotic anxiety, or anxiety neurosis.

Orthomolecular treatment of this disorder involves approaches that would rarely be thought of in traditional psychiatry. These include metabolic studies, digestive analyses, diet modifications, and stress-reduction techniques.

How Metabolism Affects Anxiety

A glucose tolerance test is important in determining whether sugar is being properly metabolized. Anxiety attacks can occur when sugar levels get too low, as in hypoglycemia. Hypoglycemia can also cause a rebound effect when adrenaline is secreted to raise blood-sugar levels. This adrenaline rush also causes anxiety. Orthomolecular psychiatrist Dr. Michael Lesser checks out sugar tolerance "rather than getting involved immediately in looking for...Oedipal or pre-Oedipal fantasies," because in a recent review of his cases he found that 92 percent of people with neuroses had abnormalities in the glucose tolerance test.

Dietary recommendations based on the results of a glucose tolerance test may help the patient far more effectively, quickly, and safely than either psychotherapy or drug treatment. The main objective is to create stability so that sugar levels neither drop nor rise too sharply or rapidly. For the hypoglycemic, a high-protein diet is recommended by Dr. Lesser, because it digests very slowly, sending just a small trickle of sugar into the bloodstream, so that the blood sugar is kept stable for a long period of time. Then, when the patient eats frequently, the blood sugar remains stable. "I have these patients eat six or seven times a day, small snacks so as not to put on weight," he reports. "Actually, they can handle more calories than they could if they were eating one, two, or three large meals a day because the body is set up to metabolize the small meals frequently. When you have a large meal, you cannot metabolize all that nutrition, and the body turns a portion of that into fat."

The Role of Digestion

Dr. Walt Stoll, a board-certified family practitioner who combines his traditional Western (allopathic) training with holistic healing practices, has found that anxiety disorders are often linked to the inability to completely break down proteins, during the digestive process, into their amino acids.

"Just three or four amino acids still hooked together (peptides), if they get through the intestinal lining, can stimulate the immune system to make antibodies against them. Since our body is also made up of peptides, hooked together to make proteins, these antibodies can attack us. To an antibody, a peptide is a peptide. It frequently doesn't matter whether the peptide came from outside the body or is a part of the body. Many of the chronic diseases, which presently are so baffling to the allopathic disease philosophy of conventional Western medicine, are now being found to be related to autoimmune processes.

"In addition," Dr. Stoll adds, "some of these peptides have been found to be identical to certain brain hormones (endorphins) that are associated with panic attacks, depression, manic depression, schizophrenia, and other conditions. In these cases—with more certain to be discovered—there is no need for the immune system to be involved; the effect is direct. The two first examples to be discovered were peptides from imperfectly digested casein (milk protein) and gluten (wheat protein). Of course, these are the two most commonly eaten foods in our culture!"

Dr. Stoll usually sees patients after they have tried a number of different therapies. "These patients come with stacks and stacks of records documenting that nothing seems to have worked in spite of every imaginable test having been done and every imaginable treatment having been tried. Psychoactive drugs have either worked poorly or have even caused the problem to worsen due to the side effects exceeding the benefits.

"Since every other conceivable cause has been ruled out by the time I get to see them, I am free to look for the things that have not been evaluated. One of the first things I look for is how well the lining of their intestinal tract protects them from their environment. I frequently find that either they don't have the normal bacterial balance in the colon or that they have gone beyond that stage to having candidiasis. Candida can only escape from our control if the normal bacteria are not in control. If candida has converted from the normal yeast form into the disease-causing fungal form, it further damages the lining so that the leakage of peptides is much greater. (See chapter 53.)

"The greater the amount of peptide leakage, the more likely it is that the brain will interpret these protein particles as being identical to the endorphins it produces during panic attacks, depression, etc. This same leakage is responsible for the increasing sensitivities we see in patients who are sensitive to environmental substances other than foods. It is much simpler, in most cases, to correct the leakage than it is to eliminate the substance. But why not do both?"

According to Dr. Stoll, dramatic improvement is often seen once the reason for the leakage is corrected. "The antibodies involved only last for 72 hours. Once the leakage is stopped completely, symptoms lessen substantially in just a few days; and just reduction of the leakage helps. There are many patients today that have had that kind of experience. Not everyone's mental symptoms are caused by poorly digested food playing tricks on the brain. However, in my experience, it is the most commonly missed diagnosis and one that is relatively easy to resolve."

Diet and Nutritional Remedies

Dr. Michael Lesser stresses the fact that good nutrition is also important, since junk foods can spur anxiety. Simple, processed carbohydrates, such as white sugar and white flour products, may give a quick lift to the hypoglycemic, but this is followed by excessive insulin secretion that drives the blood sugar down again, only to be pumped up once again by an adrenaline rush. This episode leaves a person with cold hands, jitters, anxiety, and panic.

Special nutrients can help alleviate this problem, especially chromium—also called the glucose tolerance factor—which helps normalize blood sugar. Zinc and the B vitamins, especially thiamine and vitamin B_1, are also beneficial. Vitamin B_3, or niacin, has also been identified as an antistress factor. It lowers cholesterol and triglyceride levels, which are increased by anxiety, and affects the brain in ways that are similar to the effects of tranquilizers. Dr. Lesser is convinced of the efficacy of this nutritional approach, but emphasizes the need to be patient when looking for results.

It may take months for the condition to begin to clear because "the body has been often run-down for a number of months or years, and you have to gradually repair all the cells in the body. The old cells have to die off and be replaced by new ones that are better nourished. The natural life span of cells varies throughout the body. Some, such as blood cells, live 120 days, so you cannot really expect sudden dramatic improvement unless the condition has come on suddenly and you have caught it early."

According to Dr. Allan Spreen, a specialist in nutrition-based medicine, anxiety disorders will respond to treatment by certain natural substances. The advantages of treatment with natural substances can be numerous and substantial: by freeing people from having to take more toxic medication, the holistic approach can also spare the patient the medication's side effects, as well as the extra expense.

"Some amino acids, when given individually," says Dr. Spreen, "can be very effective in calming down the symptoms of anxiety disorders and panic attacks." For example, tryptophan, which has been banned from public sale as a nutritional supplement, "was used as a sleeping agent, until there was a problem with some batches of it being contaminated, which caused a syndrome that wasn't related to the tryptophan but to the contaminant. Some doctors use tyrosine for depression and anxiety. The 'DL' form of phenylalanine is often used on a short-term basis for depression and can be very effective if given correctly. It can lessen anxiety and depression in people by giving them more of an 'up' mood. Phenylalanine is also an appetite suppressant for many people. If they're given correctly, there seems to be no toxicity associated with amino acids, and they're much cheaper than antidepressants or antianxiety prescription medications."

Stress Reduction

Besides diet modifications and nutrient supplements, anxiety may be ameliorated by relaxation techniques, yoga, massage, exercise, and stress management. An orthomolecular psychiatrist will often suggest these approaches before turning to drugs. Drugs, unlike nutrients or stress-reduction techniques, often become addictive. If you suffer from anxiety and then develop an addiction to drugs that were intended to help that problem, you will only have augmented the agony you were trying to eliminate. In addition, the direct side effects that drugs often have may leave you less capable of living a normal, healthy life than when you first underwent treatment.

Orthomolecular psychiatry also puts psychotherapy on the back burner. The shortcoming of psychotherapy, according to Dr. Michael Lesser, "is that most people who suffer from anxiety have only a limited capacity to deal with it through insight psychotherapy. There is a real risk and danger that an individual, by concentrating on his or her pathology—phobias and anxiety—and by delving deep into his or her childhood and looking for trauma, will become 'fixed' on the idea of his or her pathology. Rather than becoming more able and competent, that person will become fixed in his or her neurosis and in some cases will become even more anxious as a result of exploring the so-called unconscious. I have seen many cases—I am not saying this occurs in every case; perhaps I am seeing only the failed cases—of individuals who have been in psychotherapy for 4, 6, 8 or even 12 years with no apparent improvement. It seems to me that when a case goes on that long, someone should think about the possibility of using another approach."

20

Eating Disorders

A norexia nervosa and bulimia are pernicious conditions that are pervasive in our consumption-centered society, affecting women in particular, especially younger women and teenagers. Anorexia is signaled by muscle wasting, body image problems, an exaggerated fear of becoming fat, and loss of menstrual periods in women. Bulimia is characterized by compulsive eating and forced vomiting or the use of laxatives or diuretics to eliminate much of the calories that are consumed during binge episodes.

Obesity is an enormous increase in the ratio of fat to muscle. A common dual diagnosis is depression.

Causes

Research shows that the eating disorders anorexia nervosa, bulimia, and obesity may be the result of a zinc deficiency. Clinical psychologist and eating disorder specialist Dr. Alexander Schauss reports that science has long been aware of this connection. "We've known, from at least the 1930s, that when animals were experimentally placed on diets deficient in zinc, those animals would develop anorexia. Our interest in eating disorders in relationship to zinc has to do with the observation that when humans are placed on zinc-deficient diets, they too develop eating disorders.

"By characterizing three of the most common eating disorders," Dr. Schauss continues, "you can see how vital zinc is. In morbid obesity, when people are significantly overweight in such a way that it could shorten their life span or increase their risk of disease, we know that there is an inverse relation-

---

ship between the level of obesity and the level of zinc, meaning that the more obese they are, the less zinc they have in the body. We don't know yet whether this is cause or effect, but it is a very important observation because at the other end of the continuum, with anorexia nervosa, self-induced starvation, we also have individuals who are generally always zinc-deficient. We believe there is strong evidence today, from studies done at the University of Kentucky School of Medicine, at Stanford University, and the University of California at Davis, in addition to our research institute's work, that the lower the zinc status, the more likely it is that the patient will not recover from any treatment plan to resolve their anorexia."

Stress is commonly associated with the onset and continuation of eating disorders, and can also be understood in terms of zinc loss, since constant mental stress results in the depletion of this mineral. In 1975 it was reported that between ages 15 and 20, zinc loss due to stress is at its lifetime peak. Women are more prone to stress-related zinc loss than males, and therefore more likely to have eating disorders.

Dr. Schauss explains: "The answer may lie in the fact that males have prostate glands and women do not. Zinc is highly concentrated in the prostate in males; it provides a mineral that is essential for the development, motility, viability, and quantity of sperm. If a man is under psychological stress, he can catabolize or seek out storages of zinc in the prostate. Since women don't have a prostate, they will catabolize the zinc from other tissue.

"In women, the richest source of zinc is found in muscle tissue and bone. A common feature of anorexia is muscle wasting and an increased risk of osteoporosis. Anorexics actually catabolize or eat their own tissue as a way of releasing nutrients that they are not getting in the diet. The last muscle, and one that only contains about 1 percent zinc, is the heart muscle. When the body starts to scavenge zinc out of heart muscle tissue, it can interfere with the heart's function, which contributes to bradycardia, tachycardia, arrhythmia, and eventual heart failure. It is particularly dangerous when patients with damaged hearts are in recovery. As they put on weight, they add extra pressure to the heart. That is what killed the singer Karen Carpenter, for example."

Zinc Therapy

Liquid zinc has a positive effect in the treatment of eating disorders, as it is directly absorbed into the blood. Powders, tablets, and capsules, which must first be broken down by the stomach and absorbed by the small intestine, do not work as well because many eating disorder patients are unable to digest nutrients properly.

While results are not usually immediate, taking from several days to weeks, once liquid zinc takes effect, its benefits are long-lasting. According to Dr.

Schauss, "In 15 years, I worked with hundreds of eating disorder patients. Until I saw this treatment, my colleagues and I felt that the best we could expect in long-term outcome, in treating patients with either bulimia or anorexia, was maybe a 20–30 percent recovery. In our 5-year study, we found that bulimics had a 64.1 percent success rate after recovery on the liquid zinc treatment. In anorexic patients, our 5-year follow-up study found an 85 percent recovery rate. These are extraordinarily high recovery rates for a condition that is considered difficult to treat and insidious."

Besides being highly effective, liquid zinc is inexpensive. This makes it a first-choice treatment for eating disorders, especially when you consider the options. "Within 20 years of initial diagnosis, a British study found, 38 percent of patients with severe eating disorders are dead," says Dr. Schauss. "Many times the families have spent enormous amounts of money keeping their children alive, as the average institutional cost is about $650 a day."

Another favorable finding is that liquid zinc can lift the depression that is usually associated with eating disorders, Dr. Schauss reports.

Cognitive Therapy

Dr. José Yaryura-Tobias finds that due to the life-threatening severity of a condition like anorexia nervosa, any nutritional approach must be preceded by a program of cognitive therapy. "Anorexia nervosa, from our perspective, is an obsessive-compulsive disorder that is related to self-image, the way that we perceive ourselves. Basically, anorexia nervosa is the process by which a human being self-starves. Thirty percent of the population who self-starve eventually die.

"In the vast majority of cases, when patients come for a consultation they are already very emaciated. The chemistry we can measure is very altered. From the biochemical viewpoint, we know that there is a groove related to an area of the brain called the limbic system. This is the hypothalamic area, which regulates sugar, thirst, appetite, and so forth. This information can help us classify some of these patients, but does not tell us how to manage and eventually cure the problem. The rest of the problem, we feel, has to do with body-image perception, the way that these patients see their own bodies. They feel too fat. They have different perspectives than the rest of us.

"How do we treat this condition? Basically we use a nutritional approach after the patient has undertaken a behavioral program with cognitive therapy. Cognitive therapy is important because the idea is to educate the person about their problems and to discuss with them how many false beliefs they have about who they are, why they think this way, why their body looks the way it does for them, and so forth. So false-belief modification is an important part of treatment."

Breaking the Cycle of Food Addiction

As I have said and written for many years, food cravings and food addictions often mask food allergies to the very same foods we crave.

Dr. Hyla Cass, a holistic psychiatrist who integrates psychotherapy and nutritional medicine, describes her experience treating patients suffering from food addiction as follows: "Some time ago, a psychologist who specializes in eating disorders began to send her clients to me because she had heard that antidepressant medications worked for these patients. I had shifted to a more holistic way of looking at things, so I told the psychologist that before I did anything with antidepressants I would try some other things. With certain eating disorders, such as food cravings, the underlying problem is a food allergy. We often crave the very foods to which we are allergic. Typically, it's the very things we want to eat that are the most damaging, that create the symptoms. In fact, it's like an addiction to alcohol: As you abstain from the foods you're addicted to, you begin to have withdrawal symptoms and crave those foods even more.

"In order to break the cycle in cases of food addiction, just as when breaking the cycle with drinking (alcoholics are actually allergic to alcohol), you need to supply the body with the appropriate nutrients. When we correct the deficiencies and restore body balance, the food cravings and allergy symptoms will often be relieved. Rather than having to rely strictly on 'willpower,' it is possible for individuals to break addictive cycles by achieving metabolic balance, through avoiding the offending foods and supporting the body with a balanced nutritional program of vitamins, minerals, and amino acids. Often, the cravings will then simply go away. It's quite remarkable: With a good vitamin and mineral product, you can often put a stop to the food allergy and its accompanying symptoms.

"I may order a plasma amino acid analysis, a blood test to determine which amino acids—especially among the essential ones which the body cannot synthesize by itself—are low. The amino acid glutamine, in a dosage of 500–1,000 mg, is particularly useful for reducing cravings, including alcohol cravings.

"There are other things to do for food allergies as well," Dr. Cass adds. "Addictions and allergies are often related to magnesium deficiency and can be corrected by supplementation. There are also techniques that can actually eliminate food allergies through the use of acupuncture and acupressure. As we can see," Dr. Cass concludes, "there are many ways, other than psychotherapy and medication, to approach what at first seems like a psychological problem."

Dr. Doris Rapp, pediatric allergist and environmental medicine specialist, brings us more detail concerning the connection between food cravings and allergies: "In my experience, eating disorders and alcoholism can be related to allergies. Frequently, eating disorders are food addictions. When you have a food sensitivity, there is a certain phase of it that makes you really crave that food. And if you happen to be addicted to wheat or baked goods, for example, you can never get enough of them, with the result that you may become obese. To give another example, men who are addicted to corn may drink a lot of beer and they can become alcoholics. They're sensitive to and addicted to the beer, but it's the corn—or sometimes some other component—in the beer that is causing the problem. Sometimes, for those with an allergy to grains, they may feel 'drunk' after eating cereal or certain types of baked goods."

Patient Story

Dr. Alexander Schauss gives the following account of one patient's recovery from an eating disorder:

We were doing blind studies, which means that neither I nor the patient were aware of whether they were receiving a placebo or liquid zinc. One of the women in the study was 47 years old. She was a psychotherapist who had been treating patients with eating disorders for the last 15 years, and who herself had bulimia, involving about five binge/purge episodes per day for the last 34 years. She could hardly recount a single day in the last 34 years when she did not engage in bulimic activity. We have a protocol in which we give a small amount of liquid zinc, about 5 or 10 ml, which is less than a tablespoon. We ask a person to swirl it around in his or her mouth for a few seconds and to tell us what he or she tastes. Zinc has a strong metallic taste. If the person can't taste the solution, it's evidence of a systemic zinc deficiency. This has to do with a zinc-dependent polypeptide known as gustin, which helps us to distinguish metallic tastes.

The zinc tasted like water to this woman. Since she couldn't taste anything, she thought that she was receiving a placebo. She followed the protocol, taking about 120 ml of the zinc solution spaced out through the day, about 30 or 40 ml each time on an empty stomach.

Four days later, she called back saying that she couldn't explain why, but she had no desire to binge or purge that day. That was the first day she could recall feeling that way in 34 years. This is very similar to the experience that we have had with hundreds of bulimics that we've studied.

We were intrigued as to how a simple nutrient, like zinc, could cause a major change in the way the brain functions and in the perceptions of the individual. When you've done something for 34 years, whether it's cigarette smoking, nail biting, or engaging in bulimia, you have to wonder how it is possible for that obsessive/compulsive type of behavior to disappear in just four or five days.

It has now been five years since that day, and she has never gone back to bingeing/purging. More importantly in terms of the study, she received no psychotherapy, nor did she have any contact with me personally. The protocol was given to her by a staff member. So we're quite convinced, in this case and in hundreds of others, that it was the liquid zinc that was effective, rather than some tangential treatment.

On the Research Front

Studies have found that dieting may produce alterations in the brain in women (and not in men), which in turn may produce brain deficiencies of, for example, L-tryptophan. This may partially explain the higher prevalence of eating disorders in women. Supplementation with tryptophan with pyridoxine has been shown to improve both eating behavior and feelings about eating. In women whose bulimia worsens in winter, light therapy has proven helpful. In the treatment of bulimia, zinc has proven helpful through its action on thyroid hormone conversion.

Obesity has been associated with low thyroid function in a substantial number of cases. Chromium supplementation, which can help speed up metabolism and stabilize blood sugar levels (reducing the desire to eat) has also proven helpful. Evening primrose oil has been shown to reduce appetite and contribute to weight loss in obese patients, as has ascorbic acid supplementation. Green tea has proven to be a much better weight-loss aid than amphetamines.

21

Insomnia

Although we spend roughly a third of our lives sleeping, the essential nature of what sleep is still isn't fully understood. Insomnia is a very common symptom of many of the disorders discussed elsewhere in this book, ranging from depression to anxiety to schizophrenia and including various other mood disorders. Typically, anxiety makes it more difficult to go to sleep, and depression can cause early waking.

Causes

Insomnia can also result directly from physical symptoms, such as pain or indigestion, or as a side effect of drug medication. A major cause of insomnia, especially if it's chronic, is reactive hypoglycemia. This is frequently exacerbated by eating late at night, especially if you eat foods with a high glucose level, such as pastries, candy, or even fruit juice. Such foods cause your blood-sugar level to go up and then plummet, a fluctuation that can contribute to insomnia. Also, overindulging late at night in highly fatty foods can cause sleeplessness. That's because foods with a lot of fat take four to five times longer to empty from the stomach and be digested than simple or complex carbohydrates do.

Another big factor in insomnia is intake of stimulants, such as the caffeine in coffee, tea, chocolate, and even colas, which people consume at all hours without much thought as to the stimulant effects. Alcohol, although generally considered a depressant, can have stimulant effects in some cases. In addition to food and drink, certain medications as well can be culprits in insomnia. Drugs that interfere with the natural sleep cycle include Prozac, the newer drugs related to it, and Xanax.

Exercising in the evening is another possible bane for the insomnia-prone in that it can overstimulate adrenal levels and excite the musculoskeletal system, resulting in difficulty getting to sleep. Likewise, overstimulating the mind by thinking about unresolved conflicts can be a problem when the goal is sleep.

Herbal Remedies

Herbs that are nontoxic and have no contraindications can be a real help to those challenged by insomnia. Unlike sleeping pills, herbs won't leave you in a fog in the morning, or feeling like you haven't really slept. Passionflower is an important relaxant herb popular in much of Europe. Other possibilities include valerian root, a natural calmative used by orthomolecular psychiatrists for people who tend to be anxious, and hops.

Supplements

Dr. Robert Atkins points out the efficacy of tryptophan, which has been banned from public sale in the U.S., in the treatment of insomnia: "Tryptophan is very valuable for sleep disorders because serotonin is the sleep chemical. If you take it right when you are ready to go to bed, when your serotonin level is on the upswing anyway, you are really fitting in physiologically with your body's chemical rhythms."

Other things to try: foods with naturally occurring tryptophan in high amounts; calcium citrate and magnesium citrate—1,200 mg of each taken any time after dinner; 50 mg of the B complex; and 200 mg of inositol. Also, 200 mcg of chromium in the evening will help stabilize your blood-sugar level.

Other Natural Therapies

For those with a partner, a gentle neck and head massage for 15 minutes may do the trick in conquering insomnia, and 15 minutes in a warm bath may be helpful as well (no partner required).

Along the lines of positive affirmation, writing in a diary shortly before bedtime can be extraordinarily beneficial. It can be a way of really seeing what you've done that's affirmed your mental, spiritual, and physical health, as well as any deeds you've done that have had positive effects on others. If a person spends some time at the end of each day reflecting on what they've done in the past 24 hours that's been positive, and on plans for the next day, he or she gains a sense of completeness about the day. In a sense, then, diary-writing legitimizes going to bed; it's as if you can now see that you really deserve the good night's sleep you' re about to get.

22

Obsessive-Compulsive Disorders

Obsessive-compulsive disorders affect an estimated six million Americans. They are characterized by repetitive thinking and the inability to control or put a stop to this thinking process. As Dr. José Yaryura-Tobias explains, these thoughts become urges that are so extremely demanding that they appear to have to be carried out. Two of the main compulsions are double-checking and hand washing.

Behavioral Characteristics

Dr. Yaryura-Tobias tells us some of the peculiar characteristics of obsessive-compulsive behavior: "It usually takes about seven years or so for a patient to come in for a consultation, which tells us that the condition tends to occur gradually, becoming a part of the patient's behavioral system in a very, very slow manner. It occurs with equal frequency in males and females. Fifty percent of obsessive-compulsive patients manifest their sickness during childhood or adolescence. Later on—primarily after the age of 40—it fades away, and it becomes very rare after the age of 50.

"As to why this condition exists at all, we don't have a sure answer to that question. The behavior may result from a learning process that takes hold during childhood...[It may relate] to changes in neurotransmitters—the chemical substances in the brain that build bridges between neurons in the nervous cells so that they can transmit signals from the outside into our system or, in the reverse direction, have us act to affect the outside world. The key neurotransmitter that is being studied in this regard is serotonin."

Conventional Treatment

According to Dr. Robert Atkins, there is some common ground between conventional Western medicine and more holistic approaches such as orthomolecular psychiatry, or what he refers to as "complementary" medicine. "Both orthodox medicine and complementary medicine, which is the nutrition-based alternative to orthodox medicine, recognize that if a certain neurotransmitter is in short supply, certain syndromes will result. A classic example is that the serotonin-deficient person will often be an obsessive-compulsive. These are the people who can't get out of the house because they've got to make sure the light switches are off or the gas jet isn't on—the people who have to wash their hands 20 times a day, and whose desks have to be perfectly neat. These same people are serotonin-deficient."

The difference between the conventional and the alternative medical communities lies in how they address the problem. Dr. Atkins describes the conventional approach: "Now there are drugs that block the degradation of serotonin and allow the serotonin level to lift, but these drugs do a lot of other things: They poison a lot of enzyme systems and that's why so many people got into trouble with Prozac and drugs like that."

Behavioral Therapy

To treat obsessive-compulsive disorders, Dr. Yaryura-Tobias uses behavioral therapy and an amino-acid approach, such as the use of L-tryptophan, along with some other nutrients.

"We basically treat with behavioral therapy. We try to use thought-stopping, exposure (flooding), and response prevention to prevent the brain from repeating the same thought. That is difficult, so we also use cognitive therapy to explain the reasons we think the things we do, and try to modify the thought.

"Compulsions are the area where behavioral therapy is most effective. We expose the patient, either in reality or in his or her imagination, to face what he is afraid of. If you have fears of AIDS or of blood, you are exposed to blood or taken to the hospital where there might be patients with AIDS. Or you will read articles on the condition.

"If it is contamination from dirt the patient is afraid of, we teach the person how to touch objects and not to be afraid of them. Then we prevent the patient from washing their hands; in other words, they must remain unclean for awhile. I'm talking about patients who, when they are seriously ill, might completely use up one or two bars of soap per day. They might engage in rituals of washing for many hours. They may wash their hands sometimes a hundred or more times a day. Some of these patients, in addition, will clean their hands with alcohol or other substances. Sometimes their skin becomes extremely raw. I've seen cases where patients require plastic surgery.

"Overall, the treatment takes about six months. With medication there is improvement up to 60 or 70 percent of the time."

Amino Acids and Other Nutrients

People with obsessive-compulsive and anxiety disorders often improve on the amino acid tryptophan. But, as Dr. Robert Atkins explains, "since the FDA [Food and Drug Administration] ban on tryptophan, pure tryptophan has not been available in the United States, even by prescription. However, some pharmacies will compound capsules of 5-hydroxy tryptophan. This compound is an intermediary between tryptophan and 5-hydroxy-tryptamine, which is serotonin, the neurotransmitter you are trying to build up. The whole idea of supplying a precursor to build up a neurotransmitter that is in short supply is a fruitful approach to treating psychiatric disorders and should, in my opinion, be considered before the use of nonphysiologic psychotropic drugs, which have more potential for toxicity."

Dr. Yaryura-Tobias adds, "My colleagues and I were the first to use tryptophan and with it we were able to reduce and almost eliminate completely the use of drugs for this condition, and we obtained very good results...We were using between 3,000 and 9,000 mg per day.

"Then we used vitamin B_6, 100 mg, three times a day. Vitamin B_6, pyridoxine phosphate, is a vitamin that is very important for the breakdown of tryptophan into serotonin. The idea behind this was that either these patients didn't have enough serotonin in their brains, were very dependent on serotonin, or that the normal conversion of tryptophan into serotonin was not occurring.

"When we found by measuring that there was a lack of serotonin, this could be reversed by the administration of L-tryptophan with niacin and vitamin B_6. Some medications also accomplish this result, but with medications we face many types of side effects.

"About 30 percent of patients do not respond to any form of therapy. But it is not a closed chapter for these patients either. An investigation has to be conducted. Now that we have brain imaging, we are able to visualize the brain. We can measure, for instance, the metabolism of sugar in the brain. We find, for instance, the frontal and temporal lobes and the basal ganglia, that are related to Parkinson's disease, disrupted. We see the metabolism of the breakdown of sugar and also images of an abnormal brain. The same can be seen with some electrophysiological measurements of brain wave tests and so forth.

"Interestingly," Dr. Yaryura-Tobias concludes, "work has been going on using pure behavioral therapy before and after measuring serotonin. With just behavioral therapy, we were able to modify the levels of serotonin in the body.

In other words, we may not need medication to change or challenge the presence of a neurotransmitter such as serotonin. Simply the mere interaction of behavioral technique may have an effect."

23

Schizophrenia

Schizophrenia is a group of illnesses of unknown origin that involve disorders of perception and emotion. Schizophrenic illnesses are classified as paranoid or nonparanoid, and they are termed either chronic or acute. According to Dr. Garry Vickar, an orthomolecular psychiatrist, "schizophrenic illnesses as a group are among the most serious biochemical disorders there are; it can be said that schizophrenia is to psychiatry what cancers are to general medicine. The bulk of the lost revenue to society, the bulk of psychiatric expense, and the sheer horror to the families, which is not easily quantifiable, are unfortunately all consequences associated with the diagnosis of schizophrenia."

Thought Disturbance and Other Symptoms

Among the most disturbing aspects of schizophrenia is the disturbance of thought. Dr. Vickar explains: "These patients may have vague symptoms, go through periods of what German psychiatrists used to call 'stage fright,' and then something happens and they start to believe that their disordered perceptions represent true events. Their strong belief in these disordered perceptions transforms them into delusions, which are simply fixed, false beliefs. Patients will start to believe their delusions and then start to believe their misinterpretation of a perceptual nature. They may hear a voice and believe that the voice is real and represents some real event or real person. They'll act on that. An example would be, if I hear somebody calling my name, if I don't think it's my thought anymore but that there really is somebody calling my name, I will act accordingly. If I think that people are looking at me and making faces, I might think there is something very wrong with me and feel bad or upset about it. If

I'm eating my meal and there's a piece of moldy cheese, I might think I've been poisoned and that someone did it to me purposefully. The process starts to escalate and snowball.

"The most diabolical part of the illness is the loss of insight, loss of the ability to reality-test. For instance, if you're driving down the street at night and it's dark and hard to see, and you see something at the side of the road, you might slow down to be cautious, thinking that somebody is going to cross the street. Then you get close enough and see that it's really just shrubs or a mailbox or just part of the normal landscape, and you say, I'm glad I was cautious. If instead, however, you start to distort the original perception and really believe that there's someone who might jump out on the road or that somebody is trying to hurt you and can get in the way of your vehicle, you might take evasive action. In the process, you could have an accident or cause somebody else to have one. You start to distort things without realizing that you are distorting them. That's similar to what happens when the really disastrous part of the illness takes over.

"When you become paranoid and don't know why, you begin to wonder, 'What is it about me that's so bad? Why are people saying bad things about me?' It can become very serious. I had a patient who believed that then-President Reagan was making comments about him—about this individual—and he felt compelled to call the White House and protest to the FBI that he was being hounded by President Reagan. He firmly believed it. When he recovered he didn't believe it, but when he was delusional be firmly believed that the President was, in fact, personally interfering with his life. Such paranoid delusions can become all-consuming and unfortunately very painful."

Early Work in Orthomolecular Psychiatry

Some of the earliest work in orthomolecular psychiatry involved the treatment of schizophrenia. As early as 1952, Drs. Abram Hoffer and Humphrey Osmond, pioneers in the field, conducted a double-blind study on the effects of megadoses of vitamin B3 (in the form of niacin or niacinamide) on schizophrenic patients. This was the first such double-blind study performed in the field of psychiatry.

They found that schizophrenia is not purely a behavioral or mental disorder but that it also has a basis in biochemical imbalance, particularly a deficiency of niacin. Schizophrenia is among the most difficult psychiatric conditions to treat. But Hoffer and Osmond had good results with the niacin treatment they offered to half a dozen schizophrenics in 1952. One patient—an overactive, delusional, and hallucinating 17-year-old boy—was nearly normal after just 10 days on this treatment and was reported well 10 years later. Encouraged by these results, they then set up a double-blind experiment with 30 schizophrenic patients. Those given niacin treatments did far better than those given only the placebo.

By 1960, they had completed five double-blind controlled experiments, all yielding similar recovery rates. The two-year cure rate was around 75 percent, twice that achieved by placebo. Since then Dr. Hoffer has concluded that 90 percent of early schizophrenics will recover if they receive at least one year of orthomolecular therapy. He treats about 500 chronic patients in Victoria, British Columbia, Canada, and its environs. A sample study of 27 of those who remained on therapy for 10 years shows that about 60 percent have become well. One example is a woman who burned her house down in response to the voices she heard. After recovering on megavitamin therapy, she started her own business, and now supervises several dozen employees.

Vitamin B₃ Therapy

"The treatment for the schizophrenic patient is really relatively simple," Dr. Hoffer explains. "It's a combination of the best of modern psychiatry, which includes the proper use of tranquilizers, antidepressants, or other drugs, with proper attention to diet and the use of nutrients. The main nutrient is vitamin B3, which has to be given in large quantities. It's not enough to give the tiny amount present in food. One will have to give many thousands of times as much in the standard dose.

"For the patients I work with, I give 3,000 mg per day of either nicotinic acid or nicotinamide, which are both forms of vitamin B_3. I also use vitamin C at the same dose level and sometimes a lot more because vitamin C is a very good water-soluble antioxidant. It is considered the foremost, the most active water-soluble antioxidant present in the human body. That's extremely important.

"In many cases," Dr. Hoffer continues, "we use vitamin B_6 as well for a particular group of schizophrenic patients. This is combined with an overall nutritional approach that may also include the use of a very important mineral, zinc. Zinc and B_6 function together and are extremely important.

"Finally, we use manganese to protect our patients against developing tardive dyskinesia. This is a condition which afflicts chronic schizophrenic patients who are placed upon large quantities of tranquilizers. According to Dr. Richard Kunin, founder and past president of the Orthomolecular Medical Society, when you take tranquilizers for a long period of time you take manganese out of the body, which is the reason patients develop tardive dyskinesia. When you give them back the manganese this condition goes away in most cases.

"I put my patients on a diet that is junk-free. I exclude any of the prepared foods that contain additives, including sugar. I also pay attention to patients' allergies, because 50 or 60 percent of all schizophrenics have major food allergies. If these are not detected and eliminated, the patients are not going to get any better.

"This is essentially the treatment for schizophrenia, although there is one more important variable—the patients themselves. You have to take a lot of time dealing with schizophrenic patients."

CLINICAL EXPERIENCE Following are other examples of the results Dr. Abram Hoffer has attained with vitamin B$_3$ therapy:

EXAMPLE 1: "This was a patient I knew very well. She was admitted to a mental hospital in 1939 and was in that hospital continuously until 1952. During that time she received every treatment known to psychiatry. Eventually they had to give her a series of shock treatments every six months. In 1952, as part of our research program, I took her into my home, where she began to work for us. I started her on niacin, vitamin B$_3$. Since she had not left the hospital for so long, she had to be reeducated in terms of how to use the telephone, how to get into her car, and how to shake hands. She had to be completely resocialized. She was with us for about two years, during which time she improved dramatically. In 1955 she got a job at the university hospital on the cleaning staff, and recently she retired.

"She used to come to Victoria for her holidays every 2 or 3 years. During the summer of 1996, I called her. She was still well, happily living with her partner, and planned on saving some money from her retirement pension to visit Victoria once more. Every schizophrenic patient not treated, or treated with orthodox treatment only, will cost the state two million dollars over their lifetime. This woman had been in a chronic mental hospital for 13 years and after, as a result of alternative treatment, became a useful, productive member of society. Her recovery has saved the province of Saskatchewan at least one million dollars in costs."

EXAMPLE 2: "This is an especially good case because the patient was not even mine; I did not treat him. This was a young patient who, when he was 13, was examined in a West Coast university psychiatric department. There, he was declared to be a hopeless, chronically ill schizophrenic. His father was advised to send him to a mental hospital and forget him. The father, who was a professional person—a doctor—would not accept this advice. He read the literature, ran across our work, and called me. I advised him what to do—that is, to start the boy on vitamin B$_3$—and he did it.

"He began by feeding the vitamin B$_3$ to his son in jam sandwiches because the psychiatric department would not let him give the boy the vitamin. He would go to the hospital every day to take his son out for a walk, and while they were walking he would feed him jam sandwiches with B$_3$. After 6 weeks, the boy said, 'Daddy, I want to go home.' His father took him home. This boy remained well and finished in the fifth percentile in his twelfth-grade exams. After he had been on the vitamin for 18 months, in consultation with me, the father took him off to see if he still needed it. The boy had a relapse; he was put back on the therapy again and remained well. Since that time he has become a research psychiatrist and has recently published a very fine paper in the psychiatric literature."

Not every patient can tolerate niacin. They then have a choice of using niacinamide, which is almost as effective, or of using inositol niacinate. The latter product is an excellent niacin preparation which provides two important vitamins, vitamin B_3 and inositol. So far, in over 40 years of practice, Dr. Hoffer has not run across a patient who was intolerant of all three preparations.

Potential Side Effects of Vitamin B₃ Therapy

The side effects of this megavitamin therapy are very minor compared with those of traditional treatment. Remember, the aim of this therapy is to supply optimal amounts of substances normally present in the body and required for good health. As little as 5 mg of vitamin B3 a day is sufficient to prevent the disease pellagra, which only 70 years ago caused hundreds of thousands of people to suffer what was referred to as the four D's: diarrhea, dermatitis, dementia, and death. On the other hand, relatively massive doses of the vitamin can be administered with only minor side effects which disappear as soon as the dose is decreased or the vitamin is temporarily discontinued. The side effects include a tingling or numbness in the extremities and most commonly "flushing," in which parts of the body may become red and sensitive. Dr. Michael Lesser reports that a buffered or time-release form of niacin taken with food and cold liquids has been shown to diminish this problem by helping the stomach handle large doses of niacin. The chemical niacinamide, by contrast, is potentially dangerous in high doses and can cause liver ailments.

Because the B vitamins appear as a complex in nature, a large dose of one of them can over time cause a deficiency to develop in the other members of the complex. Accordingly, during a megavitamin program involving the augmentation of a specific B vitamin, such as niacin, the other B vitamins should also be increased in the form of a B-complex supplement.

Additional Alternative Approaches

Dr. Garry Vickar emphasizes the holistic foundation of the treatment approach he prefers. "I think in any chronic illness, such as schizophrenia, you have to maximize the person's whole functioning. You want to make them as healthy as possible. You don't want to have an imbalance where your left arm is really maximally in shape because you're a pitcher, but the rest of you is flab. You have to have the whole organism as healthy as possible...

"With the schizophrenic patient I use niacinamide or niacin (more frequently niacinamide because most patients won't tolerate niacin). I tend to use much of what Abram Hoffer has come up with. I look for a minimum of 3,000 mg of niacinamide a day with an equal amount of vitamin C. I recommend a B complex with 50 to 150 mg of the entire B-complex, mineral balance, depending upon zinc and copper levels. We try to titrate a dose until we reach a level of improvement with the least amount of medicine and the amount of vitamin and mineral supplements that the patient can tolerate."

Dr. Vickar continues, expressing the broad philosophy of his treatment of schizophrenic patients: "I have patients who have been diagnosed as having schizophrenia, and while I don't argue with the diagnosis, it hasn't captured the whole essence of what is going on with that patient. I prefer to see it as an incomplete diagnosis, rather than as a misdiagnosis. Very often the goal, in the schizophrenic diagnosis, is just to subdue behavior. When people are in such states of distress that their behavior is inappropriate, or agitated, or out of control, the goal is primarily to treat that behavior. I think that there is more we can do. We have to try to understand why the patient is doing what he or she is doing—not necessarily psychologically, but in some way biochemically.

"We don't know what the ultimate causes of schizophrenia are. Each new drug that comes along throws the current theory into such disarray that it doesn't apply anymore, because the new drug doesn't work the way that those preceding it did. So I don't think that anybody knows the causes, but there is one thing that we are sure of: We can make a big difference in how a schizophrenic is doing by applying two basic principles, as Dr. Hoffer has indicated: good, sound nutrition and vitamin supplements.

"These are not synonymous. Nutrition has to be the floor upon which the treatment is built. Then, after that, you have to start looking at other factors—whether it be smoking, coexisting alcohol-related problems, dietary disturbances, or absorption difficulties. Also, the patient may not be doing well because what they have been given is, in fact, creating more problems. So we have to be sensitive to such reactions to treatment and continue to modify the treatment all the way along. And again, the approach I find to be most useful is that schizophrenia is not so much a missed diagnosis as it is an incomplete one."

Dr. Philip Hodes, who has spent more than three decades researching, writing, and speaking about holistic health, detoxification, and orthomolecular medicine, describes some additional approaches to the treatment of schizophrenia.

"In the 1970s, Dr. Alan Cott went to Russia and brought back the practice of fasting, and helped to detoxify many of the brains of schizophrenics who had not responded to any other kind of treatment. He helped them clear their brains so that they became rational and normal.

"Today we live in a state of environmental pollution. There are over 90,000 chemicals in the external environment that we ingest through what we eat, drink, and breathe. Contaminants are in the soil, water, air, and food supply. The particles which are toxic penetrate and leak through the blood brain barrier over time and get into the brain. This process also happens with several of the heavy toxic metals, such as lead, cadmium, copper, iron, arsenic, mercury, and aluminum. These chemicals and heavy metals, by affecting brain chemistry, affect the mind and behavior, so they must be removed. They need to be chelated out.

"In the Science Section of *The New York Times*, on April 27, 1993, an article stated, 'New suspect in bacterial resistance, amalgam. The mercury in dental fillings may spur resistance to antibiotics.' Dr. Hal Huggins has shown that the silver mercury dental amalgams are very harmful; when you chew, the mercury is released, causing immune suppression and brain poisoning. Many of the people who have developed so-called 'mental illnesses' are suffering from things like mercury, lead, copper, iron, and aluminum poisonings. These toxic metals affect one's thinking and behavior. People can develop bizarre behavior and distorted thinking, along with warped perceptions, as a result of these toxic metals. Add to this toxic stew all the insecticides, pesticides, and herbicides that we ingest daily.

"The orthomolecular approach to schizophrenics is to detoxify them, change their diets, and remove foods that are chemically treated, or that contain a lot of sugar and refined carbohydrates, or that have been laced with pesticides. Then these patients are placed on the optimal doses of nutrients for their individual bodies. The nutrients used include vitamin B complex—especially thiamine, niacin, pyridoxine (B_6), and B_{12}.

"The late Dr. Henry (Hank) Newbold demonstrated that many of his schizophrenic psychiatric patients were suffering from a vitamin B_{12} 'dependency' and that they needed large amounts in order to feel well and sane again. Then, as the years went by, orthomolecular doctors discovered that the essential minerals—macro minerals such as calcium and magnesium, as well as the trace-mineral elements zinc, manganese, chromium, and selenium—also helped balance the cerebral chemistry of schizophrenics. Dr. Priscilla Slagle published her research in a book, *Up From Depression*, showing the important role of amino acids in the brain, and in the treatment of manic depressives and schizophrenics.

"You also have to look at the water supply. Many water supplies contain chemicals, such as iron, silicone, aluminum, fluoride, and chlorine. We ingest all of these things and once they hit the blood stream, they are rushed to all of the 64 to 67 trillion cells in the body. These toxins block out the opportunity for the vital nutrients to be absorbed.

"The basic constituents of the human body are proteins, amino acids (the building blocks of proteins), carbohydrates, fats, vitamins, minerals, oxygen, enzymes, nucleic acids, water, and electromagnetic and biomagnetic energy forms. If any of these are unbalanced or deficient, and there are nutritional deficiencies, different conditions and diseases can arise. Our diet is not really a healthy diet: the soil our food is grown in has been overworked; there have been artificial fertilizers added; and the foods are refined, processed, and sprayed with all kinds of chemicals and inundated with all kinds of food coloring and dyes.

"When we eat these foods we become both malnourished and toxic. In answer to those who say, 'Oh, you don't need vitamins. Just eat a well-balanced diet,' I say you can't get a well-balanced diet and you do need extra nutrients to help stave off the deleterious effects of all the chemical pollutants in the environment. With orthomolecular therapy," Dr. Hodes concludes, "many people feel a lot better when they get more nutrients than their diet gives them."

Schizophrenia and Alcoholism

Dr. Abram Hoffer estimates that about 10 percent of all schizophrenic patients are also alcoholic. "It's not a big figure," he adds, "if you remember that 10 percent of all adults in North America are probably alcoholic. In other words, the same proportion is present in schizophrenics. If you start the other way, a certain percentage of alcoholics are, in fact, also schizophrenic. There is an overlap.

"It has been acknowledged for many years that this particular group that have both problems is very tough to treat. The first person to really show that you can help them was Dr. David Hawkins, who was then practicing on Long Island. He found that when he placed his alcoholic schizophrenic patients on the proper vitamin treatment, including mostly niacin and vitamin C, he began to see a fantastic number of recoveries.

"I have seen some recoveries, but not as many as he has. I can attest to the fact that patients do a lot better if they are treated for both conditions. This treatment includes niacin or niacinic acid and the other vitamins that I use for the treatment of these conditions.

"I think that whether or not they are alcoholic they have to be treated the same way. If they're alcoholic it's vital that they stop drinking. The best way to achieve that is to try to get them to join Alcoholics Anonymous." (See chapter 18.)

A Final Note

If schizophrenic patients are treated with traditional medicine, they most likely are put on tranquilizers to make them more subdued and manageable. Perhaps psychotherapy sessions complement the drug therapy. Nutrient deficiencies or malabsorption and allergies to common foods—notably wheat in the case of schizophrenia—are almost certainly disregarded. In an attempt to mask the symptoms of the disorder, the traditional physician or psychiatrist is likely to overmedicate the patient, leaving the patient calmer but virtually nonfunctional while completely ignoring the actual cause of the problem.

The orthomolecular psychiatrist, by directly addressing nutritional deficiencies and imbalances from the start, might find a simple biochemical cause for what a traditional psychiatrist would deem a complex and perplexing problem. Mental illness can indeed result from nutritional deficiency, but certainly, as Dr. Michael Lesser points out, "no one has ever claimed that mental illness is caused by a deficiency in Thorazine." Moreover, even if no nutritional cause for the malady is found, such patients can only be made better off by improving their nutrient intake and absorption. Failure to do this can lead to further complications of the mental illness.

Dr. José Yaryura-Tobias points out that some of the more severe cases of schizophrenia—those in which the patient manifests paranoid delusions—are very difficult to treat. While some patients may respond to the administration of certain vitamins or amino acids or to a correction of certain biochemical imbalances, others may not. However, he says, recent studies have indicated that patients who are given Haldol (haloperidol), an antipsychotic drug, appear to have better results when the drug is given in conjunction with vitamin C, which is an important coenzyme in some of the sophisticated functions of the brain. This is an example of how orthomolecular psychiatry can function as an adjunct to conventional treatment.

24

Behavioral, Affective, and Mental Disorders in Children

During the past 10 to 15 years there has been a significant increase in the number of American children who are diagnosed with mental disorders and who, as a consequence, are put on drugs to treat their "disease." To what is this increase attributable? Are our kids really more troubled than they were 10 years ago? And if they are, is drug therapy the best way to treat mental disorders in children? The following example will address the first two of these questions, namely, how the treatment of childhood mental disorders came to be a major area of modern-day psychiatry. Later we will contrast the traditional approach to these disorders with that of orthomolecular psychiatrists and other health care practitioners in order to provide insights into the many different alternatives to drug therapy available in the treatment of children with mental problems.

> *Bobby is six years old and has just started the first grade. He is precocious and has been reading and writing for at least a year. He is an only child, has been somewhat spoiled at home, and is used to being the center of attention. He is extremely active and often plays from morning until night. Sometimes his activity gets on his mother's nerves, but on the whole, she and everyone else who knows Bobby find him to be a normal, healthy child who is usually well mannered and considerate.*
>
> *From the very start, Bobby hits it off poorly with his first-grade teacher. Because he is used to being active, he usually starts to fidget 15 minutes into the class. Often when the teacher asks a question, Bobby blurts out the answer without being called on. The teacher, Ms. Thomas, has admonished him a*

number of times, and he does try to control himself. Since he already knows what Ms. Thomas is teaching and is not called upon to answer questions, Bobby often becomes bored and restless and is apt to become absorbed by things going on outside the classroom window to the point where he often does not hear what Ms. Thomas is saying.

Bobby's teacher finds him to be a disruptive influence and believes that he is hyperactive. She sends him to the school psychologist with a report stating that she suspects that Bobby is suffering from what is technically called attention-deficit hyperactivity disorder. A copy of the report is sent to Bobby's parents, who immediately become alarmed that something may be wrong with their son. The psychologist examines Bobby, notices nothing out of the ordinary, and sends him back to class with a note to both the teacher and Bobby's parents telling them about his conclusions and asking them to keep an eye on Bobby so that they can alert him if anything new occurs.

A month or so later the teacher files another report. This time, after the psychologist again examines Bobby and fails to notice any aberrant behavior, Bobby's parents are advised that he should be seen by a psychiatrist. After reading the teacher's report and examining Bobby, the psychiatrist concludes that Bobby is in fact suffering from attention-deficit hyperactivity disorder and prescribes Ritalin (methylphenidate).

Bobby's parents are somewhat bewildered by this and ask the doctor what the drug is and whether it is really necessary. The doctor explains that while he has not noticed any particular signs of the disorder, symptoms are not necessarily present when the child is having a one-on-one exchange or is in a new setting, such as his office. "Typically," the doctor says, "symptoms worsen in situations requiring sustained attention, such as listening to a teacher in a classroom or doing class assignments." This is why Ms. Thomas has been in the best position to notice and report the disease. The doctor tells the parents that he suspects that Bobby is suffering from a chemical imbalance in his brain which, if uncorrected, could start to affect his performance at school and that bad grades could ruin the rest of Bobby's life. He adds that although scientists do not yet know how it works, Ritalin seems to stabilize children who have this disorder.

At first Bobby's parents are so confused by the diagnosis, and so alarmed that their child is so ill as to require medication for an indefinite period of time, that they simply go along with it. However, shortly after Bobby starts taking the medication, his parents notice that he has become very nervous and complains that he cannot sleep at night. He also shows a marked decrease in appetite and begins to lose weight. They decide to look into the drug more fully and discover that Ritalin is an addictive appetite-suppressing drug of the amphetamine family with numerous side effects, including those already experienced by Bobby: insomnia, loss of appetite, weight loss, and nervousness. When they discuss this with the psychiatrist, he tells them that the side effects are minimal compared with the damage that the boy could sustain if he

*stopped taking it and that furthermore, Ms. Thomas does not want him back
in her class unless she is assured that he is taking the medication.*

This example is hypothetical, but it is by no means exaggerated. Every year children like Bobby are diagnosed with nebulously defined "mental disorders" and receive treatment with Ritalin or other even more potent drugs such as Haldol and Thorazine. Since the "diseases" for which these drugs are prescribed first came into vogue in the 1960s, literally millions of American children, about three-quarters of whom are boys, have been labeled and drugged in order to tone down their conduct and make it more acceptable to those with whom their energy and activity may collide. But a bored and/or restless child does not deserve to be turned into a virtual zombie with sedating drugs that have numerous side effects.

The Traditional View

During the 1960s and 1970s many of these "disorders" were lumped together under the rubric of minimal brain dysfunction (MBD). The history of MBD and how it suddenly became a childhood disorder provides us with an opportunity to more clearly see into the nature and purpose of much of psychiatric diagnosis and treatment.

The term "minimal brain dysfunction" has been around in medical literature since the 1920s. In its original sense, the term was used to describe learning and behavioral problems that result from identifiable damage to the brain, such as those which sometimes occur at birth or through head injuries. The key is that actual physical brain damage existed which was impairing the child's or adult's ability to do certain things according to fairly objective standards. In 1963, however, all of this changed following a conference held by the U.S. Public Health Service and the National Easter Seal Society for Crippled Children and Adults, which convened to discuss the issue of MBD. A report issued after the conference essentially claimed that the cause of the disease was organic (of a physical origin within the body) and redefined the term so broadly as to include almost any imaginable form of behavior. According to the head of the Public Health Service at that time, Dr. Richard Maseland [quoting from Richard Hughes and Robert Brewin, *The Tranquilizing of America*, (Harcourt, Brace, Jovanovich, New York, 1979)], the intent was to single out "that group of children whose dysfunction does not produce gross motor or sensory deficit or generalized impairment of intellect, but who exhibit *limited alterations of behavior or intellectual functioning.*" (Emphasis added.)

The new definition of MBD was drafted by a special task force led by a psychologist at the University of Arkansas Medical School. It included a list of 99 criteria which were so vague and all-encompassing that the definition would have been laughable had it not become the basis for the psychiatric labeling and drugging of millions of American children. In *The Tranquilizing of America*, Brewin and Hughes synopsize some of the "symptoms" contained in the MBD definition and comment on its impact:

"It would be difficult to write a more all-inclusive definition for this new disorder subsequently used to label millions of children, but the task force didn't stop there, offering 99 symptoms to help doctors and teachers spot these otherwise normal children. The symptoms include hyperkinesis (too active) and hypokinesis (not active enough); hyperactivity and hypoactivity (activity opposites of a milder nature); 'rage reactions and tantrums' and being 'sweet and even tempered, cooperative and friendly'; 'easy acceptance of others alternating with withdrawal and shyness'; being 'overly gullible and easily led' and being 'socially bold and aggressive'; being 'very sensitive to others' and having 'excessive need to touch, cling and hold on to others'; and 'sleeping abnormally lightly or abnormally deeply....'

"It's unlikely that any child, no matter how normal or healthy, could escape classification under such a hodgepodge of 'signs' pointing to an MBD child in need of treatment."

According to Brewin and Hughes, notwithstanding this basically meaningless cornucopia of definitions, the concept of MBD was enthusiastically welcomed by the psychiatric community, governmental health agencies, educators, and pharmaceutical companies.

Brewin and Hughes continue: "There is no way to get an accurate fix on the number of children drugged with Ritalin or other stimulants or tranquilizers since the MBD phenomenon began to flourish in the late 1960s, but it is safe to estimate conservatively that 3 to 4 million children have been chemically harnessed for MBD or various MBD symptoms, ranging from hyperkinesis to fidgeting, in the past decade. Ciba-Geigy continues to identify a substantial number of children as candidates for an MBD diagnosis and Ritalin therapy. The company estimates that '1 out of every 20 schoolchildren has MBD—three-quarters of them boys.' This means an MBD target population of 1.6 million children—some 1.2 million of them boys—between the ages of 5 and 13. With the federal government estimating the number of children with learning disabilities at 10 percent of the grammar school population of 32 million, there is an even greater potential for indiscriminate drugging of youngsters...."

The drug companies have focused their promotional efforts not only on advertising their medications but also on convincing the public that MBD is a bona fide disease. Amphetamines became so highly esteemed in the educational community that many schools would not allow children diagnosed with MBD (often by their teachers) to continue in attendance unless they were on drugs. "By the early 1970s," Brewin and Hughes remark, "Ritalin had become so widely used that it was referred to as the 'smart pill' in playground talk, and some cynics referred to the three R's as 'reading, 'riting, and Ritalin.'"

How Children are Classified

While the term "MBD" is no longer used in the psychiatric jargon, the concept has by no means been abandoned, nor has the use of amphetamines in its treatment. The DSM-IV (*Diagnostic and Statistical Manual of Mental Disorders*—the official diagnostic guide for psychiatrists) has an entire section devoted to "Disorders Usually First Diagnosed in Infancy, Childhood, or Adolescence." This class includes developmental disorders such as "Mental Retardation," and "Pervasive Developmental Disorders" (including autistic disorder, among others), as well as the "Attention-Deficit and Disruptive Behavior Disorders," such as attention-deficit/hyperactivity disorder not otherwise specified, conduct disorder, and oppositional defiant disorder. If your child is diagnosed with any of these disorders, Ritalin will most likely be an integral part of the treatment the child will receive from traditional psychiatrists.

Nowhere is the DSM-IV more vague or subjective than in the sections concerning and defining childhood disorders. While some of the developmental disorders do contain somewhat more objective criteria, the diagnoses of the "behavior" disorders are very subjective and the symptoms are so broad-ranging that many healthy children could easily fall within their ambit.

A major problem with definitions such as these is that they purport to establish a scientific basis for a medical diagnosis when in fact the diagnosis is totally subjective and has no scientific rationale whatsoever. The DSM-IV does specify that a criterion should be considered satisfied only if a given behavior is considerably more frequent than that of most people of the same mental age, but rather than clarifying or objectifying the criteria, this condition only serves to introduce a further element of subjectivity into the definition. What is considerably more frequent? Once a week? Once a day? Many times a day?

The determination of what constitutes normal behavior and what does not is often made by people who have an interest in labeling such things as restlessness and the blurting out of answers to questions as pathological. In other words, implicit in many DSM definitions is a belief that certain behavior should be controlled and suppressed simply because those in a position of authority may find it troublesome. Even a cursory examination of these definitions reveal that they are primarily directed at a child's behavior at school. Ultimately, then, it is in the school rather than the doctor's office that learning and mental disabilities are first diagnosed.

The Citizen's Commission on Human Rights (CCHR), a nonprofit organization investigating psychiatric violations of human rights, comments:

"Presumably, there is a 'disease,' and teachers, practicing medicine without a license, and not the parents of the children, are the final and proper judges of which children have it."

According to a quote from a CCHR booklet, "How Psychiatry Is Making Drug Addicts Out of America's School Children" (1987), "It is the teacher's consideration of who is a 'normal' child which sets the standard for all other children. The psychiatrists (clinicians) don't have to see [the 'disease'] but can treat (cash in on) it, based on the teacher's 'diagnosis.' We're not to believe anyone who doesn't see the 'symptoms' of this mental disease because it's apparently invisible or at least disappears when the child is being seen by a new or perhaps impartial person in a 'one-to-one-situation,' including the parents when they disagree with the teacher."

It should be clear by now that the diagnosis of many childhood disorders is far from a scientific endeavor. Symptoms can inexplicably appear and disappear, teachers with no medical or psychiatric training are given the power to diagnose the disorder, and the definition of the disorder is based on subjective criteria which depend more on the temperament of the person doing the diagnosing than on the actual mental health of the child being diagnosed.

This is not to say that children do not suffer from emotional and behavior problems which can dramatically affect the quality of their lives. Many doctors treating children for these problems report that such children are often aware of not acting like everyone else and are very disturbed and upset by this realization. Few would deny the importance to these children, and to society as a whole, of diagnosis and treatment aimed at getting at the root of their problems and designed to help them live a happy and fulfilling life. However, the treatment of legitimately ill children with safe, caring, and effective therapies is not what we have been talking about here.

ALTERNATIVE APPROACHES TO CHILDHOOD DISORDERS

There are a number of alternative approaches to childhood disorders which you may want to explore before letting a doctor put your child on drugs.

Treating Food and Environmental Allergies

One physician who has had considerable success in the treatment of children with emotional and behavior problems is Dr. Doris Rapp, author of *Is This Your Child?* (William Morrow & Co., 1992), *Is This Your Child's World?* (Bantam Doubleday Dell, 1996), and the companion video *Environmentally Sick Schools*. Dr. Rapp practices a branch of medicine called environmental medicine which looks at the role that the environment plays in people's overall health and well-being. In particular, doctors such as Dr. Rapp are concerned with environmental allergies, which they believe are responses a particular individual may have to substances in the environment that are tolerated by most people.

Dr. Rapp explains that most emotional and learning disorders can be caused by allergies in both children and adults. Children can become moody, depressed, or even suicidal, hyperactive, agitated, or panicky—all for no apparent reason. They may suddenly cry, spit, or kick or hurt others or themselves.

Dr. Rapp has "observed that almost any emotional expression imaginable can occur as a result of an adverse reaction or sensitivity to substances in the environment. It sometimes happens in relation to ingesting certain foods or being exposed to certain chemical odors (such as tobacco or perfume), lawn herbicides, chemicals, or pollens and molds. Any of these can cause problems in some individuals at certain times."

Dr. Rapp offered the following observation during a radio interview: "In my office I have seen and documented many patients, young children, who have acted in a very bizarre manner when they have been exposed to something that is unusual. For example, I had one little girl, about five or six years of age, who became very depressed and wished she was dead on days when it was damp and moldy. When she came into our office and we skin tested her for molds, she became very depressed, pulled her hair over her face, and became untouchable. When her mother walked toward her, she would pull away and scream; she wouldn't let anybody touch her. Then, when we gave her the correct dilution of mold allergy extract, on her own, she walked over to her mother, sat in her lap, gave her a hug and a kiss, and said, 'Mommy, I love you.'

"I had another little boy, about nine years old, who never smiled. His mother brought in pictures of him at Easter, Christmas, at birthday parties and things like that, and he always looked very dour; he just didn't look happy at all. When we placed him on a diet that merely excluded highly allergenic foods, his mother said that she was really amazed because at the end of 1 week, he was smiling and happy for the first time in his life. When I talked to him, he said that he felt much better on the diet; he said that he didn't want to take Mikey's knife and put it right here, and he showed me where he thought his heart was. He was going to put a friend's knife right into his chest."

WHEN TO SUSPECT ALLERGIES According to Dr. Rapp, if a child is having behavioral or emotional problems, the parents should consider the potential role of allergies in these problems if the family has a history of allergies. She says:

"If your parents had hay fever and asthma or any of your children have these conditions, and you have one child who is having behavior and personality problems, you might consider the fact that the dust or the milk that is causing the asthma in one child may be causing bed-wetting or hyperactivity or aggression in the other. If a patient has an allergic history or typical allergies such as asthma or hives, this particular patient may also be having brain allergies—allergic reactions within the brain—that may be affecting his or her behavior or emotions."

Dr. Rapp also states that children or adults who suffer from allergies often have a characteristic look. They frequently have bags or dark circles under their eyes, and many have bright red cheeks and earlobes when they are reacting. Many children with allergic reactions affecting the brain tend to wiggle their legs, fidget constantly, and have trouble remaining seated. Dr. Rapp has also noticed that very often the handwriting and drawings of children will vary significantly when they are reacting. She explains: "The child who is exuberant and all over the place writes in a very large manner. However, the writing may be upside down or backward or in mirror image. But the child who is depressed and goes into the corner frequently writes in extremely small letters. The writing will be as small as it can be, or the child will just write his or her name as a dot. Then, when you treat the child with the correct dilution of the stock allergy extract, he or she can write, and can act in a normal manner.

"I recently saw one eight year old, for example, who becomes depressed and suicidal each year during the tree pollen season. Last year when she came in, she drew pictures which were very unhappy with sad faces. Then, after we treated her for tree pollen, she drew a smiling face of a youngster who was very happy."

Dr. Rapp describes a nine-year-old boy who became very vulgar whenever he ate certain foods or was exposed to molds. His mother found that he was particularly offensive when he went to a particular school. Dr. Rapp explains: "'We went to the school with an air pump, collected samples, and then bubbled this air through a saline solution. We took the youngster, who was sensible and normal at the time, and made him vulgar simply by placing a drop of his school air allergy extract under his tongue. He became vulgar in both his speech and his actions. In addition, he jumped on the furniture and scribbled on walls. He threatened to pee on his mother's leg and do very strange things. When we gave him the correct dilution of the school air, he came right back to normal."

Dr. Rapp says that before this boy is given the allergy extract, he is "a very nice intelligent youngster who draws very complicated pictures of fish, and if you just inject a drop of the school air extract in his arm, within a short period of time he is vulgar and abusive, writing on the walls and giving everyone the finger. If you ask him to draw at that time, he draws a note which says somebody 'sucks royal.' He uses all the four-letter words, and he is just terrible.

"After he is given the correct dilution, within a few minutes he is drawing a fish again. On one occasion I said, 'C'mon, I'd like to hear you say some dirty words now.' He looked at me somewhat startled and said, 'Why do you want me to do that? I don't feel like it.' Finally, with a lot of prodding, he said a couple of dirty words, but he didn't say it as if he meant it, whereas before he was having a great time and was amused by his actions."

Dr. William Philpott, a leader in the field of environmental medicine and author of *Brain Allergies: The Psychonutrient Connection* (Keats, 1987), provides other examples of how allergic reactions can affect children:

> "*A 12-year-old boy diagnosed as hyperkinetic had the following symptoms on testing for spinach: he became overtalkative and physically violent, had excessive saliva, was very hot, developed a severe stomachache, and cried for a long time. Watermelon made him irritable and depressed, cantaloupe made him*

aggressively tease other patients. Once he avoided the incriminating substances in his diet, his hyperkinesis symptoms diminished dramatically."

"A four-year-old boy diagnosed as hyperkinetic had a variety of reactions. String beans made him hyperactive, and he wanted to fight with everyone. Celery gave him a severe stomachache, after which he cried and became grouchy. Strawberries made him angry and hyperactive and caused a great deal of coughing. Unrefined cane sugar caused him to be irritable, after which he coughed and developed a stuffy nose."

"A 12-year-old boy became listless and depressed, and cried when tested for bananas. Then he became aggressive and picked up a stick as if to hit another patient. When he ate oranges, he sang at first but then became very tired, impatient, and eventually wild and aggressive. Rice caused him to experience a sensation of heat, followed by rebellious hyperactivity."

As can be seen from these examples, it is not necessarily unhealthy or "junk" foods which can be the worst offenders. Virtually any food can cause problems in a given individual. In fact, one of the major characteristics of allergy is that it is an individualized reaction to substances that ordinarily are well tolerated by other people.

Dr. Theron Randolph, considered by many the founder of environmental medicine (formerly called clinical ecology), estimates that as many as 60 to 70 percent of symptoms commonly diagnosed as mental are actually caused by allergic-type reactions. Many emotionally disturbed people, especially those with psychoses, develop major symptoms when exposed to foods and chemicals that they frequently consume. Wheat, corn, milk, tobacco, and petrochemical hydrocarbons are some of the more common substances that trigger these allergic responses, which may include delusions and suicide attempts.

ELIMINATION DIET There are a few tools that environmental medical specialists use in treating children with allergy-related behavioral problems. The first is an elimination diet, which usually is recommended after the first visit with the physician. In certain severe cases the diet may take the form of a total fast for four to five days, but usually it eliminates only the specific foods the doctor suspects are a problem for the particular patient. The targeted foods are those which are common allergens (provoke allergies in many people), such as chocolate, dairy products, wheat, and cane and beet sugars, as well as foods which the patient has a tendency to "abuse."

Environmental medical specialists have found that people are often especially allergic to the foods which they eat most often. Sometimes the frequent consumption can even lead to a sort of addictive-allergic reaction where one craves the very food that is making one ill. As food residues can remain in the body up to four or five days, the object of the elimination diet is to clear the body completely of foods which may be causing problems. If allergy is at the root of the problem and the correct foods have been eliminated, the symptoms will clear at the end of the five-day period. Dr. William Philpott gives an example of how this can work:

"Henry, 17 years-old, had been mentally ill for 3 years. Prior use of tranquilizers, psychotherapy, and electric shock had not succeeded in helping him appreciably. He believed that people were out to kill him, and he often had to be placed under restraint because of his attacks on innocent children and adults. He was placed on a fast from all foods and given spring water only. He remained mentally ill until the fourth day, at which time his symptoms cleared; he was released from his restraints. He telephoned his parents, saying, 'I love you. Please come and see me.' On the fifth day of the fast he was fed a meal of wheat only. Within an hour, he began to feel strange and unreal; within an hour and a half, he thought people were going to kill him. He telephoned his parents again, saying, 'I hate you. You caused my illness. I don't want to ever see you again.' Further testing confirmed the fact that when specific foods were withheld, his symptoms cleared, and when he was given wheat, the same paranoid reaction occurred consistently."

The body is particularly susceptible to allergens, particularly after the elimination diet. A small drop of an extract of the substance placed under the patient's tongue can reduplicate symptoms, sometimes very dramatically. This procedure of testing for allergies by placing a drop of extract under the tongue or injecting it subcutaneously is called provocative testing, and it is one of the major diagnostic techniques used by environmental medical specialists.

Once the allergies are determined, a technique known as neutralization dose therapy is often used to eliminate the symptoms. In this procedure the physician uses increasingly diluted extracts of the particular substance until a dilution is found that reverses the patient's symptoms. This is the neutralizing dose. If you find this confusing don't worry. It is paradoxical, and science cannot explain how a diluted substance can have a more potent effect in relieving symptoms than a stronger solution of the same substance. Because neutralization therapy often is based on very weak dilutions of things such as wheat, milk, and corn, it is an extremely safe and nontoxic form of treatment providing a food doesn't cause a life-threatening medical emergency. It is particularly useful for people who have a moderate allergic reaction whenever they eat a particular food. For example, where chocolate invariably provokes hyperactivity in a child if the child eats birthday cake or inadvertently eats something containing chocolate, the symptoms can be "neutralized" by placing a few drops of the properly diluted extract under the child's tongue. The following example, provided by Dr. Rapp, shows how neutralization dose therapy helped both a mother and her child:

"There is one woman I've tested three times for sugar allergies. She is about 40 years old, and when she is tested for sugar, she develops a catatonic state. She will be talking and kidding and joking, and you can give her an injection of a saline solution, and she stays fine; she doesn't know what you are testing her for. Then you can give her another injection of the saline, and she continues to write her name and act normally. But when you give her an injection of a weak allergy extract of sugar, within 10 minutes she is staring into space and unable to talk, her fists begin to clench, and she does not respond at all—she is totally unconscious. At that point, if she does write, she doesn't write her name as 'Catherine,' as she did before, but instead writes 'Cathy.' She seems to regress at that point and act much younger, more immature than she is. If you continue to give her weaker dilutions of the sugar allergy extract every seven minutes, or faster if she doesn't look well, her hands will loosen up and her eyes will open. When you give her the right dilution of sugar, she comes completely back to normal and acts as if nothing had happened.

"We repeated the test three times on her and drew blood samples each time before as well as during the tests, when she had contracted her body into a tight little knot and was nonresponsive, and again when she was back to normal. We can show that there are changes in the neurotransmitter at the time when she is reacting. We also found something rather unusual in this patient: Her sedimentation rate changed. That is another study on the blood serum that usually is not altered by this kind of reaction, but it certainly was in this individual. If she eats sugar at home, the same thing happens to her that happened in the office.

"With this patient we were able to show that what we did is reproducible. We showed that she could not write her name when she was reacting, and then her handwriting went back to normal. We showed that there were changes in her blood each time we tested her, and showed that we could treat her so that if she made a mistake and ate something with sugar in it she did not have this kind of bizarre reaction.

"I might add that she has a son who became unconscious when he ate cherries from a cherry tree in the backyard, and when we gave him the correct dilution, he came back to normal. We also tested her for cherry, and she became unconscious again and had the tight fists."

FOUR-DAY ROTATIONAL DIET Another treatment commonly used by environmental medical specialists is the four-day rotational diet. It is especially useful for patients who are not allergic per se to a given food but become "sensitized" to it when they abuse it or eat it frequently. In this diet almost all foods are rotated so that they are not eaten more than once every four days. This way the patient not only avoids the food to which he or she may be sensitive but also decreases the possibility of becoming sensitive to other foods which might have been overconsumed to compensate for the decreased consumption of the "abused" food. (See chapter 11 for more on the four-day rotational diet.)

Megadose Vitamin Therapy

Dr. Bernard Rimland, a research psychologist, has also done extensive work in childhood disorders. While recognizing the role that load allergies can play in many of these disorders, Dr. Rimland has also focused on the role that vitamins in "megadoses" can play in such conditions as autism and hyperactivity. Dr. Rimland focused his research particularly on autism, a condition that manifests before the age of three. Three-quarters of the victims are male. They look normal but are not responsive to their environment. They can hear perfectly well yet do not look at or appear to hear people when they are spoken to. It is as if they lived in a different world. While this was once thought to be purely a mental problem, it is now clear that autism has a basis in biological and neurological disorders.

Dr. Rimland's research, which has been confirmed by researchers in France and around the world, indicates that autistic children have deficiencies in certain nutrients, in particular vitamin B_6, and that for some unexplained reason their bodies require these nutrients in much larger amounts—up to 50 mg a day more—than do ordinary individuals, who require only 10 to 15 mg daily. To maximize the effectiveness of this B_6 supplementation program, magnesium is also given. It is a very important mineral here because it can dramatically enhance the effectiveness of B_6. In addition, Dr. Rimland gives the rest of the B-complex, zinc, and other complementary minerals. "If that is done," he explains, "the individual's body has the maximum chance of using the vitamin effectively when it is given in large amounts to correct the metabolic error it is prescribed to correct."

Dr. Rimland's studies indicate that between 30 and 50 percent of children treated with vitamin B_6 and other nutrients show significant improvement. Not only do they improve behaviorally, his studies have shown that their objective tests improve as well. Urine tests run on autistic children indicate that they have much higher concentrations of a phenol called homovanillic acid (HVA). When autistic children are given vitamin B_6, their HVA levels often normalize along with their behavior. Additionally, certain abnormal brain waves which have been measured in autistic children also tend to normalize after the treatment. "So," says Dr. Rimland, "the B_6 and magnesium treatment has been shown to improve autism behaviorally, electrophysiologically, and biochemically."

A study published in 1979 by a doctor in Washington, D.C., showed that vitamin B_6 is at least as effective as Ritalin in ameliorating hyperactivity in children. The B_6 was found to be safer and cheaper, and its beneficial effects lasted longer. Even though this was a well-documented, carefully controlled double-blind study published in a reputable medical journal (*Biological Psychiatry*) it could not shake most medical professionals from their bias against nutritional approaches to mental and behavioral disorders. "Pediatricians, psychiatrists, and other physicians," observed Dr. Rimland, "continue to give kids Ritalin instead of B_6 to control their hyperactivity."

Amino Acids, Herbs, and Other Nutrients

Dr. Ray Wonderlick, who has a background in pediatrics, explains his approach to treating children with learning disorders or behavior problems: "We try not to give them Ritalin or amphetamines when they have hyperactivity or attention-deficit disorders. Instead we look at their basic quality of life and their lifestyle. Are they troubled by any infections? Do they have allergies? Do they have nutritional deficiencies? Do they have chemical toxicities? Are they having some kind of nutritional disorder that is underlying the problem? We are directly opposed to the conventional approach, which relies primarily on just treating the symptom by the use of medication. We've determined that very rarely is it necessary to use prescription drugs for these children. The drugs may be needed on a temporary basis while you're testing the patient or while the family is discovering how to reform the diet, for example, or deciding which vitamin and mineral supplements to use. However, in the vast majority of cases—90 percent, I would say—we were able to manage the problem, whether behavioral or academic, without the use of drugs."

Five million children are now using Ritalin, which does nothing to cure the child, and may actually mask the real nature of the problem. Dr. Wonderlick believes that if you use the drug, and you get a "good" response, everybody thinks everything's okay. They couldn't be more wrong. The child sails along, but without growing well, without eating well, and the actual nutritional problem may be compounded. His approach, by contrast, utilizes amino acids, herbs and other nutrients:

"We assess the child's-amino acid pattern through a plasma amino acid test or a 24-hour urine test to spot the amino acid deficiencies and imbalances. We often find that the essential amino acids are not being received by the child. It could be because the diet is so poor, or it could be that the child's digestion and absorption are inadequate, so that the child, while eating well, isn't achieving the amino-acid levels that he needs. We address that issue with supplements to correct either the inadequate input of food or the digestive, malabsorption problem.

"We use herbs in the detoxification process initially. Many of these children are toxic—their bodies react adversely to other elements to which they're exposed. Sometimes, if you give these children vitamins for example, they are unable to take them. The same applies to adults. And when you see that, you know that there is a high level of toxicity in the body and you have to go to some kind of detoxification process. Herbs are very safe and a very convenient way to do that. You get a good response and the family often will see the difference in the child and will then listen more openly to the nutritional message.

"These herbs are given under professional guidance. It is not something that individuals should do themselves. Some of the herbs we use are red clover, goldenseal, black walnut, and acansosyanicide—acansosyans come from blueberries and from pine bark. They strengthen the blood/brain barrier and that enables us to protect the child whose brain is more or less on fire—hyper-reactive because of reactions to foods, indigenous chemicals or exogenous toxins. These herbs have been a great help in protecting the brain until we can get the diet changed or the environment cleared up so that it isn't suffering such a toxic assault.

"As far as amino acids are concerned, in some children you have to use just a general, across-the-board supplement including all 8 or 10 of the essential amino acids. In others, we use tryacine, cellalonine, tryptophan, cysteine—particularly the sulphur bearing amino acids—glutamic acids and, of course, the branch-chain of amino acids, particularly in individuals who have an absorption problem.

"Typically we see the most dramatic improvement in the child's use of his or her intellectual ability. It's like putting an engine into gear. The child is better able to listen in class, respond in a communicative way, participate in a dialogue, handle visual tasks—this is enormously important because auditory/visual functioning are linked in learning, and control of eye movement in focusing is a big factor in how well one learns. In many cases, the special lenses which optometrists sometimes prescribe for children with learning difficulties can be discarded several months after these nutrients have been added."

PART FOUR

Musculoskeletal Fitness

25

Arthritis

I t is estimated that more than 40 million Americans suffer from some form of arthritis. More than 250,000 children have the disease, and its prevalence is rapidly increasing. We know the kind of discomfort this can mean: swollen joints and excruciating pain. It can be so bad it prevents a person from having a quality life.

There is evidence from various disciplines that the westernization of culture worldwide is responsible for the rapid global increase of arthritis and other degenerative diseases. The underlying causes of these diseases include the nutritional deficiencies of commercially grown, processed foods; the presence of pesticides and other toxins in the environment; and the quality of the soil in which food is grown.

The mainstream medical community has done the best it can, giving immediate relief but seldom sustaining it or, even less often, offering a cure. But are there techniques that have a different view of cure and treatment? Is it possible, by radical modification of lifestyle and by acquiring knowledge of detoxification, perhaps by working with acupuncture, reconstructive therapy, herbs, physical therapy, chiropractic and other alternative methodologies, to actually prevent and reverse arthritis?

What is Arthritis?

The word arthritis means pain and swelling of the joints. A joint is the place where two bones meet. Cartilage covers the end of each bone and prevents the bones from rubbing together. The joint capsule surrounds the joint and protects it. Special membranes surround the joint and make a fluid that lubricates.

Muscles and ligaments around the joint provide support and make it move. When all these parts are working right, the joint moves smoothly and easily, but when something is wrong with the joint, arthritis may develop. In osteoarthritis, the cartilage is worn away so the joints rub against each other. When the cartilage breaks down, the joint may lose its shape. The ends of the bone may thicken and form spurs. In rheumatoid arthritis, the lining of the joint becomes inflamed, swollen, and feels warm, tender, and puffy. Eventually the bone and cartilage may be destroyed.

Besides these two types of arthritis, there are over 100 other diseases that affect the area around the joint, including lupus, fibromyalgia, polymyalgia, gout, scleroderma, juvenile arthritis, and ankylosing spondylitis.

The Arthritis Industry

In the mid-1980s, *The New York Times* ran an article on arthritis in its Sunday business section. The title, "Arthritis: Building an Industry on Pain" (August 18, 1985), together with its placement in the business section (as opposed to the health, lifestyle, or human interest sections), gave the article a uniquely realistic point of view. For many people arthritis is seen not as a health issue, per se, but rather as a very lucrative growth industry. Though the article is nearly 15 years old, this view is just as prevalent today, if not more so. Using the example of Ann, a fairly typical arthritis sufferer, the article reveals how the symptomatic approach to arthritis of traditional medicine offers little in the way of health benefits while providing tremendous profit-making opportunities for those involved in the arthritis industry.

Ann began to suffer from arthritis at age 28. She was walking downstairs when her knees suddenly gave out, followed by a sharp burning pain. Ann's doctors diagnosed her as having rheumatoid arthritis and started her on an arduous and expensive journey through the maze of treatments used to battle arthritis in the United States. According to *The Times*, Ann spent more than $200 a year on medication (this is probably a very conservative estimate compared with the amount most arthritis sufferers spent on antiarthritics during this time period, and of course, medical costs have increased since 1985). This included a daily dosage of 8 to 10 Ecotrin (aspirin) tablets, a prescription pain reliever, and 5 mg of the steroid prednisone. She visited the doctor at least once a month, at $20 to $50 a visit. Even with all this medication and regular medical attention, Ann was physically incapacitated. She found it necessary to acquire a number of new arthritic devices designed to replace her ever-decreasing mobility: $35 for a walker, $25 for a set of canes, $15 for a reacher to get objects from shelves or retrieve them from the floor, and $130 for a padded bathtub seat. Ann also had four of her joints replaced at a cost of $15,000 per joint. "And so," the article concluded. "Ann is one of the nearly 40 million consumers of the arthritis industry. It may sound odd to label arthritis as an industry, but in fact any disease—cancer, diabetes, AIDS—is not only an affliction, it is an employer. For thousands of people and scores of companies, battling arthritis is a livelihood."

The Times estimated that arthritis costs this nation $8 to $10 billion annually in medical bills and adds to those figures another $7 billion in lost wages and taxes resulting from absenteeism.

Arthritis medications are one of the pharmaceutical industry's biggest and most lucrative products. In 1982, *The Times* estimated in another article (also in the business section) that the projected $717 million in industry sales that year for prescription arthritis drugs would continue to increase at a phenomenal 20 percent annually. Additionally, according to *The Times*:

"Drug company estimates suggest that arthritis relief accounts for anywhere from one-third to one-half of the $900 million in annual aspirin sales.

"Some arthritis sufferers gulp down as many as 10,000 aspirin tablets a year, 30 a day. The extra-big bottles, with as many as 1,000 tablets, are earmarked for arthritis sufferers.

"It is hard to pinpoint how much drug-makers earn from arthritis because antiarthritis products also are taken for headaches, trick knees, and the many other guises of pain. But when one considers all the drugs that find use in fighting arthritis, the market bulges to something close to $3 billion in retail sales, according to analysts. Over-the-counter sales make up more than half of that total, but the swiftest growth comes from prescription drugs."

According to the 1985 article, a spokesman for Upjohn, the manufacturer of Motrin (ibuprofen), one of the best-selling prescription antiarthritics, says about the market for arthritis products: "Every new drug that comes out seems to expand it. Since no one has a cure for arthritis and it's such a debilitating disease, people seek everything that comes along, hoping and praying that this may be the ticket."

Even now, a decade and a half later, one reason the arthritis industry is still so lucrative is precisely because so many people still share this attitude. According to the Arthritis Foundation, the estimated annual cost of arthritis to the economy is some $72 billion in medical care and a whopping $77 billion due to indirect costs such as lost wages. Additionally, according to the Foundation, individuals with rheumatic disease average eight doctor visits per year, twice the average number of visits for persons with other conditions.

The arthritis establishment, which includes the pharmaceutical companies, special interest organizations such as the Arthritis Foundation, and specialized medical personnel such as rheumatologists, physical therapists, and surgeons, has consistently maintained that arthritis is an incurable disease. Therapeutically, this translates into the possible need for physical therapy, ad hoc surgical intervention to replace joints, and a lifetime of medication which, even if it is effective at relieving pain, does nothing to address the cause or arrest the progression of the disease. Economically, addressing arthritis as an incurable disease is a prescription for steady long-term profits.

Traditional Diagnosis and Treatment

Typically, arthritis is diagnosed on the basis of a patient's symptoms, which most commonly include pain or swelling in the joint areas or some limitation of movement. There are some diagnostic tests, and x-rays may show abnormalities in the joints, but often these tests are not accurate. Thus the patient's symptoms are the central factor in determining the diagnosis.

Because medical students have been taught that there is no cure for arthritis, as doctors, they do not look for the cause of the disease but rather focus on alleviating the symptoms. This approach can be very dangerous because many of the drugs used to counteract pain and swelling can have serious side effects. Even aspirin, which is ordinarily considered one of the least toxic medications and normally constitutes the first line of attack in the traditional treatment of arthritis, is not without side effects. In the treatment of arthritis, aspirin is given in large doses on a constant basis. Consequently, arthritis patients have consistently high levels of aspirin in their systems; this can result in dizziness, ringing in the ears, intestinal tract bleeding, and kidney damage.

When aspirin does not work, or an arthritis sufferer develops adverse reactions to it, other medications called nonsteroidal anti-inflammatory drugs (NSAIDs), such as the widely advertised Motrin, are used to control inflammation. Since these drugs are nonsteroidal (i.e., do not contain cortisone), they are less toxic than some medications commonly used to combat inflammation, but they nevertheless have side effects.

The NSAIDs came onto the market as effective alternatives to aspirin, which had caused internal bleeding in many long-term users. Ironically, while the NSAIDs are less effective than aspirin as anti-inflammatories, they also have side effects which include gastrointestinal bleeding, and peptic ulcers. Other side effects include dizziness, nervousness, nausea, vomiting, and ringing in the ears. If these drugs are unsuccessful, doctors will often prescribe cortisone-derived drugs such as prednisone. These drugs are notorious for their severe toxicity. They interfere with the immune system, leaving the patient defenseless against infection and other diseases. Cortisone-type drugs also interfere with the body's healing ability, and it is not uncommon for a person taking these drugs to have bone fractures or wounds that do not heal for long periods of time.

Some rheumatologists, or doctors who treat arthritis patients, use gold injections. This method of treatment was abandoned years ago because it was considered too dangerous, but today gold treatments are finding their way back into the medical establishment. Another technique finding acceptance among arthritis doctors, despite its tragic consequences, is the use of chemotherapy drugs. The theory behind this drastic measure is that when a patient's immune system is knocked out, the patient's body is no longer able to form the antibodies which may be causing the inflammation in his or her joints. Other expensive and highly dangerous techniques include radiation therapy in the area of the inflammation, again with the intent of destroying the patient's immune response; and plasmapheresis, a procedure by which a patient's blood is drained out, filtered to remove antibodies, and then reinjected into the patient.

While the traditional medical approach to arthritis is undeniably becoming more sophisticated, it also appears to be totally missing the mark. Not only do these treatments fail to get at the cause of the disease, they are becoming more expensive, invasive, and toxic, and lead to the inevitable question, Do the ends justify the means? When traditional medicine begins to turn to anticancer therapies to treat arthritis—therapies which often are cancer-causing themselves and result in such radical side effects as nausea, hair and weight loss, and total devastation of the immune system—this question becomes even more pressing.

Dr. Warren Levin, of Physicians for Complementary Medicine, recalls that a couple of years ago the American Medical Association (AMA) put out a series of videotapes instructing physicians on how to take care of and diagnose rheumatoid arthritis. The lecturer on the tape was adamant that nutrition had nothing to do with arthritis. "His whole face filled the screen and he said, 'Nutrition has no place in the treatment of arthritis. We can use drugs.' That is the AMA way. They have not come to Physicians for Complementary Medicine to see what success we have with our methods and how the vast majority of our patients dramatically improve without the use of the toxic drugs that characterize American medicine's treatment of arthritis."

Alternative Treatments

"The way I treat arthritis is probably quite different from the approach of most physicians," says Dr. Peter D'Adano, a naturopathic physician. "As a naturopath, I was taught we should not always think about treating a disease, but about treating a person. Arthritis is a very good example of a disease which is highly individualized. Not only are there different types of arthritis, but people get it and express it in different manners."

It's a good idea to try to listen to the body and realize it has an intelligence. In other words, if you are following a certain lifestyle and your problems are the result of this lifestyle, then possibly a change in lifestyle will change the illness.

People say that as the body gets older, the most natural thing in the world is for it to get decrepit. But give the body credit for the intelligence it has. When the body tells you something, if you will listen and follow what it says, you will improve.

What is arthritis? It's pain. Why is it painful? Well, what have you been eating? Maybe you say, "I have a very good diet. I have pancakes in the morning with sausages. Then orange juice. I use saccharine"—precisely a diet loaded with substances that will bring complaints from the body. So we must think of detoxification. Our air is noxious, our oceans are polluted and so is the body. So we have to help the body heal itself first by cleansing.

DIET AND NUTRITION Dr. Peter Agho of the Healing Center says, "I do diet. Not just for arthritis. The thing about the whole diet is this. Change the diet, and the arthritis—along with obesity, high blood pressure, and other problems—will get better. The diet should include fresh fruit, including fresh fruit juice, and vegetables. You should eliminate animal fats and cut high fat foods."

Dr. Howard Robins outlines his treatment: "We use a complete vegetarian diet, including a lot of green, leafy vegetables. These are important because of all the phytochemicals and phytoestrogens that help in all the chemical processes that are necessary to being well again. We give them juices, six to eight fresh green juices a day—the best way to take in these chemicals."

Dr. Luke Bucci, author of *Pain Free: The Definitive Guide to Healing Arthritis*, notes that part of the reason people get arthritis is because of the lack of essential nutrients in a highly processed, refined diet. Sure you get plenty of calories, protein, and fat—usually the wrong kind of fat. What you do not get is just as important—the minerals: magnesium, zinc, copper, manganese, boron. Many people are not aware of boron as a nutrient, but boron might turn out to be essential to our joints' health. These are what you do not get with our current, typical American diet. We lack the substances that prevent the joints from repairing themselves from the damage they get. That is why you want to start eating a whole food diet, rich in organic vegetables, fruits, and nuts.

Dr. Rich Ribner tells this story: "Recently, a woman came to the clinic with a terrible case of arthritis. She was in terrible pain and had been taking anti-inflammatory medication and tranquilizers. She was miserable. She said she thought about killing herself. I said, 'Stop this nonsense. I'm going to ask you to do something. You may not even want to do it.' She said, 'Anything.' So, I said, 'Between now and next week, I want you to drink six to eight glasses of water a day, but it has to be distilled or spring water. And eat nothing but brown rice, just brown rice.' 'But, but...' she began. 'Wait,' I said, 'You were talking about killing yourself. So, listen, I'll add a few green vegetables to that.'

"You have to make sure there is a cleansing. Make sure they drink the water. Have a bowel movement daily.

"Well, this woman was so desperate that she stayed on the diet one week. When she came back there was marked improvement. She still had a long way to go, but there was a change."

SUPPLEMENTS Dr. Bucci believes that special nutrients can help prevent rheumatoid arthritis, and the most important substance for healing arthritis is glucosamine. There are several types of this. For glucosamine sulfate, you should take 1,500 mg a day in divided doses; glucosamine hydrochlorides work quite well also.

They "convince" your joint tissues to repair the damage. If the situation is not too far gone and you still have cartilage, you can rebuild it greatly which may mean being pain free.

Another very important nutrient is chondroitin sulfate. Chondroitin is synthesized to glucosamine in your joints. Chondroitin is one of the molecular "cements" or "glues" that holds together cartilage and lets the collagen protein be laid down, forming the actual tissue.

Another interesting finding has been the value of our friend vitamin C. This should be taken as 4,000 mg/day in two or three doses with meals. We have thought about using C for many other problems, but is it also a very important nutrient for the joints. Along with glucosamine, it is the only other substance that can stimulate the cartilage to repair itself. Drugs have not been able to do this.

Another substance of value is vitamin E. Take 400 IU/day in one pill. It helps reduce pain, as has been shown in human clinical trials. Also useful is vitamin B_3 (niacinamide). This should be taken in 150–200 mg dose three to four times a day. It will not kill pain right away—it takes time, maybe up to one or two years. But you'll see a gradual improvement, as range and function of the joint are bettered.

Magnesium and the obscure mineral boron are valuable. Areas of the world where they have low soil levels of boron show more osteoarthritis. Several human studies have been done that show that a very minor dose of boron, some 3 to 6 mg a day, can reverse the symptoms of osteoarthritis. This is very promising and exciting. I think boron is related to another mineral, magnesium, which has not had as much clinical trial. But we know it is extremely important for every healing process in the body. So there is a very definite link between boron and magnesium.

Interestingly, if you do not eat your fruits and vegetables, it is almost impossible to get a dietary intake of boron, since it comes almost exclusively from vegetables and fruits.

"One of the questions I get as I go around the country," Dr. Luke Bucci continues, "trying to spread this message of the connection of nutrition and arthritis is: 'Where is the evidence? No one's heard of glucosamine.'

"Well, I'm not the one who thought this up, though I may have rediscovered it. There is valid, strong scientific research and human clinical trials on this substance, millions of man hours of use of glucosamine sulfate by doctors, mostly in Europe. Others in Europe are using substances they extracted from the cartilage itself, such as the chondroitin sulfate.

"There is a very large body of literature on the topic, with dozens of human studies and even more with animals. We know how and why these substances work because this is how the body heals itself. So I answer their question about where are the studies with my own question: 'Where's everybody been?' Why have people not read the prodigious literature available? Why don't people just open up their eyes and read?"

AVOIDING CERTAIN FOODS AND CHEMICALS Dr. Warren Levin points out that another important aspect to look at is allergies to foods and chemicals. Removing the offending substance from the patient's environment—whether internally with food, externally with chemicals—we see dramatic changes over and above what we see with just vitamins and minerals.

Some doctors believe that the most apparent cause of arthritis is common foods, what the patient eats all the time.

Dr. Morton Teich elaborates that the food the patient wants the most is the problem, like milk, for example. He cites a study by Richard Pettish (*Arthritis and Rheumatism*, February 1986, "Food induced arthritis. Inflammatory arthritis exacerbated by milk") that shows that milk can cause severe allergies and arthritis.

Many studies indicate that food definitely causes problems; the nightshades, for instance—the family including potatoes, tomatoes, tobacco, coffee—bring on allergies. They also crossreact with ragweed.

Dr. Teich warns, also, of the glycoproteins in milk, wheat, corn, and cinnamon, as well as inhalants such as dust, mold, or pollen. Chemicals are also vitally important in causing allergies, as are additives in foods.

HERBS Letha Hadady, an herbalist, says that an important thing to remember about arthritis is that it is essential to eliminate the underlying problems that make it possible. Killing the pain is not enough, you need to eliminate the toxins that result from poor digestion and poor circulation.

She shares some of her herbal secrets for total health—using produce and herbal remedies, substances you can find in the grocery store, the health food store, or through mail order.

In dealing with arthritis, one thing you must have every day is alfalfa. You could chew 10 tablets a day with a little water to eliminate much of the uric acid that could build up to create joint pain. Rhubarb also eliminates acid. It is a laxative but it also breaks apart the crystals that form around your joints which give you pain.

Dandelion greens are full of vitamins and minerals. In fact anything green will be a rich source of calcium. Dandelions break down pain-giving acid, too.

Star fruit is a sweet, delicious fruit you can find in your grocery store or vegetable stand. Juice it. Add a cup and a half of cold water. Drunk three times a day, it will eliminate inflammatory joint pain, bleeding hemorrhoids, and burning urine—it is cooling and cleansing.

It is important to realize that not everyone's arthritic pain is the same. Do you wake up in the morning with your joints feeling stiff and sore? Do they feel better after you move them around and after you exercise? If so, you need to take warming, tonic herbs that build vitality, increase circulation, and warm joints. Adding a pinch of turmeric to your stews will do this. Turmeric and cinnamon are a good combination for achy shoulders. If you have rheumatism that gets worse in cold weather, add a quarter of a teaspoon of turmeric and cinnamon to a little water and drink it as a tea.

Asafoetida is a spice available in Indian stores. A little added to cooking beans or other hard-to-digest foods will help cleanse the body and warm the joints.

One other thing you can use is the resin myrrh; a few drops added to your tea makes your joints feel warm and your blood move, bettering circulation.

Hadady says Asian medicine uses many herbs that can be added to cooking. For example, Tang Kuei increases circulation and warms joints. Another very safe and classic Chinese remedy is Du Huo Jisheng Wan, one that Chinese doctors have used for generations, which makes arthritis in all parts of your body feel better.

Her favorite, Guan Jie Yan Wan, is translated as "walk as smoothly as a tiger." This remedy brings blood circulation exactly where you need it—your hips, legs, and joints.

The wonder of Asian remedies is that a combination of herbs take the painkiller where it needs to go. There are so many, including Raw Tienchi ginseng, Efficacious Corydalis, Tien ma, Three Snakes Formula, Mobility 3, Clematis 19, Eucommia 18, Leigong Ten Pian, and Rinchen Dragjor-Rilnag Chenmo.

THE FIRST RULE TO HEALTH: GOOD HYGIENE, PERSONAL AND INTERNAL To understand the nature of the treatment, you have to understand that the first rule to health is good hygiene, personal and internal.

What does that mean? Well, a lot of Americans are eating fairly good diets some of the time, but not all of the time. Whenever you eat something bad for yourself, you undo whatever a good diet was accomplishing.

Not all diets are the same. I say get a good diet. But what does that mean? Does it mean eat hamburgers and cheeseburgers? No! It means keep a diet that is rich in live food. Does live food mean raw food? Not necessarily. It means nutrient-rich food loaded with life-supporting live enzymes. Give up meat, yes. Caffeine, absolutely. Sugar, yes. And give up chicken. Eat fish: the ones that are rich in the Omega fatty acids that help lubricate joints and will help your heart. Mackerel, cod, salmon, and sardines are the most important fish for a good diet that helps prevent arthritis.

Take six glasses—and I'm talking about 12 to 14 ounce glasses—of fresh, organic juice. These juices should be aloe vera, cabbage, cucumber, celery, apple, and carrot. These are the mainstays, the primary beverages. (The aloe vera should be taken from the bottle, not as a plant which has diarrheal properties.) Concentrate on these unless you are hyperglycemic or diabetic, in which case you will have to stay away from carrot and apple because they make your blood-sugar level too high. Add such things as dandelions and a small amount of mint. Almost all the other vegetables can be juiced, and these are outrageously good, particularly for arthritis.

Make sure you are getting the right nutrients—to find out, you can check your blood. Make sure you get folic acid, niacinamide, pantothenic acid, vitamin D, and vitamin E (400 units/day). You can take from 2,000 to 20,000 mg/day of vitamin C, adjusting what you need each day, depending, for example, on how much stress you are under. Under stress, increase your dose. If you have a disease such as cancer or chronic fatigue syndrome, increase your dose even more. The necessary nutrients are vitamin B_{12} (1,000 mcg), vitamin B_6 (50 mg/day), vitamin B_2 (50 mg/day), vitamin B_1 (25-50 mg/day), vitamin A, a lot of which you'll get from the juices and fish oils (25,000 units/day), and MaxEPA (1,000 mg/day).

The minerals we need are calcium-magnesium (1,200 mg per day), iodine, and sea vegetables, which are wakame, kombu, nori, and hijiki. One 4-ounce serving of these vegetables a day is good for the trace minerals. Also take phosphorous (700 mg), potassium (500 mg), sulfur, which can be found in garlic (2,000 mg), onions—an onion a day keeps the heart and blood circulation in good order—and manganese (25 mg). There are also the more esoteric minerals such as evening primrose oil (200 mg/day), superoxide dismutase, coenzyme Q10 (100-200 mg/day), silicon extract, boron (5 mg), copper lysinate (2 mg), methionine, and selenium.

Selenium, by the way, is not in our soils. And if it is not in the soil, it is not in the plant and so it will not get in our bodies.

Methionine is an amino acid found in soy. Take enzymes. People with arthritis often have deficiencies in liver enzymes. Rebuild the intestine, the liver, the pancreas. Take the plant-based enzymes which are the primary nutrients.

Here is what it comes down to. You must eliminate milk, red meat, sugar products, green peppers, eggplant, tomato, tobacco, alcohol, salt, deep fried foods, preservatives. Then you have made a major step in re-balancing the body chemistry.

You are doing two things: detoxifying, so you do not have those triggers going off and damaging your body, and fortifying your body with those green vegetables, supplements, minerals, phytochemicals. You are exercising and doing other good things; in total, something has to work.

I know it sounds complex, but look at the benefits.

The average person with arthritis does none of the above. He will try simply to take a drug and hope for a miracle. But the miracle does not come. Who are you going to blame. The doctor? No. The pharmaceutical company? No. It is our expectation that something outside of ourself is better equipped to help us than our own innate healing capacity.

CHIROPRACTIC Many arthritis sufferers we interviewed for this chapter said of all the things they tried to eliminate the pain, going to a chiropractor helped the most.

Dr. Mitchell Proffman, a chiropractor at the Healing Center, showed me two x-rays. The first showed bones nice and clean and square in shape; the second showed degeneration of the bones.

He showed what arthritis looks like in the human body; thinned disks and a little lip or spur, the body's defense mechanism to heal or shore up the area so it does not totally disintegrate. He said to think a person has a pinched nerve somewhere in his or her body, in the neck, for example meaning it is out of alignment. He administers a gentle push with his hand, which is not painful, to move the bone back into position. The nerve energy comes through and the joint can start to heal.

RECONSTRUCTIVE THERAPY Noted physician Dr. Arnold Blank has used reconstructive therapy as an important means of treating arthritis. He mentions that thousands of patients complain to doctors each year of chronic pain and of joint, muscle, tendon, and ligament dysfunction. Frequently, the doctors aim to relieve the symptoms but do not deal with the cause of the illness. People take pills, anti-inflammatory drugs, steroids, even use surgical procedures. Many times, they're worse off after the treatment than they were when it started.

Reconstructive therapy, created in the 1920s by osteopathic physicians Gedney and Schumann, is a healing approach that works by stimulating the body's ability to heal itself. Their design was to help stimulate the body's ability to heal ligaments, tendons, and cartilage. The doctors found that by injecting substances that caused a slight irritation to these tissues, they would help the blood vessels grow into the region, thus bringing more oxygen, vitamins, and minerals, as well as the fibroblast growth factor, into the cartilage, promoting tissue growth.

Dr. Blank introduced me to one of his patients. "George has had an injury to his shoulder due to chronic overuse. I have been injecting into the ligaments in and around his shoulder joint.

"This therapy works best when the patients are in an optimal nutritional state. Vitamin and mineral levels are important in our healing response and ability.

"The injection consists of a variety of different liquids. Primary liquids I use are calcium, lydicaine, and saline. They take a moment and really aren't painful.

"The majority of patients feel improvement after the first three or four treatments, developing some strength and feeling less pain, even increasing the range of movement.

"The nutrients we may use, natural ones, include ones that have an anti-inflammatory effect, such as vitamin C, shark cartilage, sea cucumber, glutathione, and glucosamine sulfate.

"All of these substances are used once reconstructive therapy has begun because the new blood vessels going to the tissues will enhance healing. These nutrients may not work well when there are no blood vessels going into the area, so they should be administered after the therapy has begun its work."

Another male patient recounts his experience:

"I injured my back and didn't realize it until I started getting aches in the back of my leg. I had heard about reconstructive therapy so I started on my back, had so many treatments, then I went to the hip, knee, and shoulder. They all feel great at present."

ACUPUNCTURE Acupuncture has been used by countless people throughout the world to help alleviate the pain and suffering of arthritis. Dr. Yuan Yang of the Healing Center reminds us that arthritis around the joints causes much pain. "We put the needle around the joint to create circulation, taking the pain away. There may be cold, blocked blood and low energy, so I apply the needle for smooth blood. Moving blocked energy takes the pain out."

I asked her, "Are you saying that putting acupuncture needles around the joints where they are swollen will stimulate better blood flow and help relieve the symptoms?"

"Yes," she responded, "then we have to do energy points. We must find the whole body energy points. Maybe we will work with the spleen point, the meridian and kidney points. These points will help circulation anywhere in the body and will make for better circulation and digestion."

PHYSICAL THERAPY Shmuel Tatz works at Medical Arts at Carnegie Hall with an exercise physiologist doing mostly hands-on treatment, going directly to the problem, to the arthritis. He typically works with people who have arthritic problems from overuse syndromes or accidents.

They go directly to the joints. For example, working with a pianist who has problems with the hands they will try to move the bones, separating the joints to make more space.

"Today in physical therapy we use many modalities. One of these is magnetic pulse therapy. We know of the positive effects of magnetism on the body. Scientists have developed a machine with different programs so that we can make adjustment for every different situation.

"We put electrodes on the body. For example, on the hip joint. Here it stays for 15 to 20 minutes. Usually, patients report a very mild relaxing sensation and the pain decreases.

"Many people with pain from osteoarthritis are afraid to be touched. People with a swollen knee, for instance, can do reflexo therapy. For the knee we touch an acupuncture point on the ear which gives relief."

Once this manipulation has had an effect, they start to exercise the knee by putting the legs in slings, relieving the pressure on the joint, making it easier for the patient to move the body. By trying to open the joint and make more space around the bones, it allows for better circulation.

The same can be done for every part of the body—for the shoulder, neck, and so on—movement is very important for people suffering with arthritis.

One patient, Lori, speaks about her improvement:

"Here at Medical Arts, I was able to receive physical therapy, which has enabled me to avoid surgery and has greatly improved the quality of my life. I'm still dancing."

YOGA Molly McBride, a yoga instructor, believes you do not have to stop working on your health simply because you may have some physical limitations. You will see how easy it is, even working with something as simple as a chair, to stay fit and help yourself with the problems of arthritis.

The basis of yoga is breath and breathing practices, she says, which helps circulation and also helps flush the body out by collecting toxins to exhale them. Breath is the foundation of all the yoga stretches.

We start with just taking a simple breath; the basic beginning exercise is a three-part breath. Let the air fill the abdomen, then the ribcage, then the upper chest. Exhale, letting the breath exit the upper chest, then ribcage and then abdomen. Inhale, exhale.

It is important to take time everyday to do these breathing exercises. A really good time to do them is first thing in the morning when your stomach is empty or, if you have eaten, wait a few hours before you start the practices. These breathing exercises can be combined with some simple joint lubrication exercises. To regenerate the body and increase the flow of oxygen through the whole system, to help relieve all of the toxins that get built up in the muscles and the protective cartilage around the joints, try simple yoga exercises.

Specific Treatment Approaches

In the following pages, we discuss some specific alternative approaches to treating arthritis. These include Dr. Robert Liefman's balanced hormonal treatment for arthritis; Dr. Marshall Mandell's allergy-related approach; Dana Ullman's homeopathic treatments for arthritis and fibromyalgia; and the nutritional approaches of Betty Lee Morales, who has helped many people overcome arthritis and other degenerative diseases through the use of whole foods, and Dr. Laurie Aesoph, a naturopathic physician who uses a special diet to help prevent and treat arthritis. Dr. David Steenblock's approach, which focuses on the correlation between arthritis and atherosclerosis, also is discussed. Although there are many other approaches, these have had a consistently high success rate, are not toxic or expensive, and in some cases may actually get to the cause of the disease rather than merely masking its symptoms.

Dr. Robert Liefman: Holistic Balanced Treatment

Holistic balanced treatment (HBT) is derived from the work of the physician Dr. Robert Liefman (1920–1973). Dr. Liefman first used this treatment in 1961, after 20 years of research. Since that time more than 30,000 arthritis sufferers have received the treatment, and many of them are living pain-free, normal lives.

HBT is based on the results of Dr. Liefman's research, which showed that many arthritis sufferers, especially those with rheumatoid arthritis, have specific hormonal imbalances. Within the body there are naturally occurring hormones called glucocorticoids whose role is to reduce inflammation and raise the level of simple sugars in the blood. One of the ways these hormones raise blood-sugar levels is by converting nonglucose molecules such as protein into glucose. If unchecked, these glucocorticoids can be responsible for the collagen breakdown of cartilage in joints, which may be a contributing factor in the development of arthritis. The glucocorticoids are balanced within the body by other hormones such as testosterone and the feminizing hormones, which include estradiol; these hormones induce tissue building, and hence balance the tissue-wasting effects of the glucocorticoids. If the body is not regulating these hormones, there are therapies to correct these imbalances. Dr. Liefman developed formulas consisting of varying amounts of three basic ingredients: (1) prednisone, an anti-inflammatory steroid, (2) estradiol, an estrogenic hormone, and (3) testosterone.

According to the proponents of HBT, the anti-inflammatory property of the steroid prednisone and the healing properties of sex hormones can be used to treat arthritic conditions with minimal side effects because of the balancing action between the different components. The anabolic, or building, quality of the sex hormones acts to control the catabolic, or devastating, effects of the steroidal drug therapy (these include infection, decreased immunity, improper healing, suppression of pituitary and adrenal gland function, and fluid retention). On the other hand, the feminizing and androgenic activities of sex hormones are kept in check both by the catabolic nature of the glucocorticoids and by careful adjustment of the concentration of the sex hormones in accordance with the specific requirements of the individual patient during treatment.

EARLY RESEARCH

Dr. Liefman, an American married to a Canadian, graduated from McGill Medical School in Montreal, Canada. During World War II he was drafted into the U.S. Army. A doctor in the medical corps, he was left relatively free to do research on endocrinology. After the war Dr. Liefman continued his research in endocrinology, focusing in particular on the hormones estrogen and progesterone. Around that time cortisone was being researched and developed at the

Mayo Clinic by Dr. Philip Hench, who won the Nobel Prize in physiology and medicine in 1950 for his work on this wonder drug. In the early stages of research, cortisone was hailed as the miracle for arthritis for which scientists had been searching for many years. This fanfare caused many to begin funneling grant money into research on cortisone; accordingly, Dr. Liefman also began to explore its potential uses and effects.

Early on, it became apparent that cortisone produces dangerous side effects when used alone. Dr. Hench and his associates continued their work to see how they could counteract the effects of cortisone. Even as early as the 1950s, Dr. Hench and his associates observed that there were fewer side effects when the drug was used concurrently with estrone (the estrogens include estradiol, estrone, and estriol) and that side effects were almost nonexistent when testosterone was used with the cortisone. It is unclear why Dr. Hench apparently discontinued his research into the benefits of combining hormones with cortisone to minimize potential side effects. However, around this time both Dr. Liefman and another American physician, Dr. W. K. Ishmael, and his colleagues were conducting similar work which essentially confirmed the finding of Dr. Hench, namely, that the side effects of cortisone could be reduced greatly when it was administered in conjunction with the proper balance of sex hormones.

Parenthetically, 30 years later, in November 1975, another group of researchers would confirm these results in a paper presented at the Southern Medical Association's 69th Annual Scientific Meeting in Miami Beach, which followed the direction of the work done earlier by Drs. Hench, Liefman, and Ishmael. In their study the researchers measured the responses of 14 women with severe rheumatoid arthritis who were given estrogen and progesterone in amounts similar to those present in pregnant women. (In 1948, Dr. Hench had observed the effect of pregnancies on 34 women. In 30 of the 34 pregnancies, the women experienced substantial or total relief from arthritic symptoms during pregnancy. He also noted that the disease rarely began during pregnancy.) In the 1975 study researchers found that the response to the hormones was often very rapid and dramatic. Not only were decreases in pain and swelling noted, together with increases in mobility and strength, but objective test results also improved. The degree of inflammation decreased, and 6 of the 14 patients had normal sedimentation rates (which indicate the extent of inflammation) at the time the paper was presented. Before treatment, 12 patients had been moderately anemic; after the hormonal treatment, their blood tested normal. Also, x-rays indicated a lessening of soft tissue and bone softening (osteoporosis) and increased calcification of bones.

THE TREATMENT When, in the 1950s, he received an offer from the Arthritis Hospital in Sweden to apply the results of his work, Dr. Liefman decided to leave Montreal. For a year he was given carte blanche to put to clinical use the research he had done on balancing the body's hormonal system. Much to his surprise, almost all the rheumatoid arthritis patients he treated showed great, if not total, improvement. A paper he wrote on his work was published in one of the leading medical journals in Sweden. Quite naively, Dr. Liefman expected that when he returned to North America he would be acclaimed for the fine work he had done. He was sorely disappointed when his medical professors and colleagues were not interested in his findings. He attempted to sell his treatment to one pharmaceutical giant after another, but no one was interested because his hormone compounds could not be patented and hence could not generate the type of profits to which the drug companies were accustomed. These companies told Dr. Liefman that instead of bothering them he should give away his medication to the government. He went to the Veteran's Administration (VA) and offered to treat the veterans with his hormonally balanced formulas, but the VA rejected his offer because this medication had not been approved by the Food and Drug Administration.

Knowing the value of his treatment, Dr. Liefman began quietly treating patients in his home in Montreal. His first patient was a doctor who suffered from rheumatoid arthritis. After several days on the hormonally-balanced treatment, all the doctor's crippling symptoms disappeared. The doctor in turn sent a child who was suffering from juvenile rheumatoid arthritis, and the same thing occurred. Word began to spread, and before long Montreal newspapers were running stories on this "miraculous" new treatment for arthritis discovered by a local resident.

The news of miracle cure for an "incurable" disease was met with considerable skepticism in the United States. *Look* magazine even sent two investigative journalists to Montreal to "expose" this "quack" doctor who had bamboozled the Canadian press into believing that he could treat arthritis successfully. The journalists spent a week or so outside Dr. Liefman's home, where they observed people entering in wheelchairs and on crutches. After spending a few days there, many of those people left without their wheelchairs or crutches. Based on the personal observations of these journalists, *Look* presented a very favorable report on Dr. Liefman's work which explained his method of treatment and told of the high degree of success he was having. Following that article, people from all over the United States and Canada flocked to Dr. Liefman for treatment. With this mass migration came the wrath of the medical establishment, which was outraged that an individual doctor could succeed where they had failed.

Over his lifetime, and notwithstanding persistent harassment by the medical establishment, Dr. Liefman treated over 20,000 arthritis patients with a very high level of success. They were, for the most part, people who had tried orthodox medical treatment to no avail and had been essentially abandoned by the medical establishment as hopeless. Professor Henry Rothblatt, an attorney and a close friend of Dr. Liefman who was to defend Liefman throughout the many legal battles waged against him, recounts how they met:

"I came to know about Dr. Liefman from a woman physician who learned about his treatment through *Look* magazine and went up to see him. She was literally left to die by her colleagues. She had been rheumatoid for 25 years. She had been in one of the leading hospitals in New York, and her colleagues said, 'Doctor, we have done everything that medical science can do for you. You are just going to have to suffer your last few years and make the best of it.' Well, she decided not to suffer. She went up to see Dr. Liefman, and within one week her crippling symptoms came to an end. She became one of his biggest fans and one of his most zealous disciples. It was through her that I met Dr. Liefman at a time when the Canadian bureaucracy finally decided to go to work on him...."

The persecution of Dr. Liefman was unfortunate since his treatment has been so effective for an illness that affects so many people. The fact that it is innovative and unconventional is probably the main reason for its unpopularity within the medical establishment.

THE SUCCESS OF HBT In contrast to the symptom-suppressing approach taken by the traditional medical establishment, HBT is designed to address the causes of arthritis. It does this first by restoring a positive protein-building balance within the body through the administration of the trihormonal formulas described above, which at the same time works to stop pain and inflammation. Secondly, according to Dr. Henry Rothblatt, "HBT is never administered without considering the particular need of the individual patient. The medication is adjusted for every patient so that the proper tissue-building and healing response can be obtained. Respect for the uniqueness and the unique need of the individual patient is one of the essential principles of the holistic approach to medicine."

Dr. Liefman developed four basic formulas to account for the different requirements of each individual using HBT: (1) White Cap, which contains prednisone, testosterone, and estradiol, (2) Black Cap, which has only prednisone and estradiol, (3) Red Cap, which contains prednisone and testosterone, and (4) Green Cap, which contains only prednisone, and is used only to allow women to shed the endometrium proliferation caused by the intake of the estrogen-containing preparations. In turn, the proportions of these different compounds may vary from individual to individual and may also be altered for the same person during the course of treatment. If, for example, a female patient begins to exhibit an adverse reaction to the treatment, such as the growth of excess body hair, the testosterone level in the medication will be reduced to eliminate these reactions. The same holds true for men who experience breast development or other sex-related changes as a result of the medication's estrogen content. Patients who exhibit some of the typical side effects of cortisone-type drugs will have the amounts of prednisone in their medication decreased, or appropriate increases in one of the sex hormones will be made to counterbalance the wasting effect of the steroids. Generally, the adverse reactions to any of the elements in the compounds disappear within a short time once the proper balance among the hormones has been attained.

In addition to the importance of balancing the anti-inflammatory hormones with the sex hormones to establish a healthy protein-rebuilding environment, Dr. Liefman explored other biochemical interactions within the body which play important healing roles in arthritis. For example, he discovered that a growth hormone, which is produced in the pituitary gland, reacts synergistically with estradiol and testosterone to stimulate bone growth. He looked at the health of the pancreas to determine whether adequate insulin was being produced to ensure the efficient breakdown of sugar within the body, because without proper sugar metabolism, the body lacks sufficient energy to build and repair bones.

HBT also incorporates principles of nutrition and stresses the importance of regular exercise. The diet recommended in HBT eliminates junk foods, such as sugar and sugar products, and salty and processed foods such as luncheon meats, canned goods, and fried and refined foods. The diet is essentially moderate in protein and emphasizes high-fiber complex carbohydrates in the form of fresh fruits and vegetables, whole grains, and legumes. Vitamin and mineral supplements are used to bolster the patient's immune system and enhance the body's natural healing abilities. For instance, vitamin D is important for strong and healthy bones because it regulates the absorption of calcium from the stomach into the bloodstream, which carries it to bone tissue. Vitamins C and A are important for the maintenance and repair of collagen, the gluelike substance that holds the tissues together and is essential for joint and muscle stability. Vitamin E and B-complex vitamins are important for bone growth. Among the minerals, adequate supply and absorption of calcium, phosphorous, and magnesium are essential for the formation of healthy bones, while zinc and selenium are important immune-system nutrients.

Exercise is also an important adjunct to HBT and is recommended to restore joint and muscle mobility and function as well as muscle mass lost during periods of inactivity. However, patients are generally told not to exercise until they are free of pain, swelling, and stiffness and feel confident enough to engage in it. Walking may be the first exercise; then, as patients improve, they can be given specialized exercises for the hands, knees, fingers, shoulders, and other areas which may have been affected by arthritis.

The medical establishment has basically ignored, attacked, or criticized HBT therapy, even though its basis is drugs already widely used by the medical establishment. All Dr. Liefman did was combine certain commonly prescribed drugs so as to maximize the benefits and minimize the side effects of each component drug. The balanced hormonal approach to arthritis did, however, do one unorthodox thing: It challenged the rigidly held position of the medical establishment that arthritis is an incurable disease. Was it for this reason alone that, before his death in October 1973, Dr. Liefman faced considerable opposition from the American arthritis community and was actively prosecuted by the FDA?

THE PATIENTS The following are some examples of the results arthritis patients have had over the years from using HBT:

EXAMPLE 1. Malcolm had his first attack of arthritis when he was 21 years old. By time he was 44, the pain had become constant. Deformities started to appear in the joints of his shoulders, hips, knees, upper and lower spine, and breast bone. He was diagnosed with Strumpell-Marie disease (spondylitis), a form of arthritis which causes such deformities in the spine that the patient is literally doubled over.

Malcolm also had severe iritis, an inflammation of the eyes which is not uncommon in rheumatoid arthritis patients, and later extensive retinal hemorrhages were found in both eyes. During the year before his treatment with HBT, he was taking 12 to 14 aspirin tablets daily, received cortisone injections in his knee once a week, and had tried another medication which had no effect.

Malcolm began treatment with HBT in August 1962 after reading the aforementioned *Look* magazine article in May. He experienced almost immediate relief. According to his physician, his arthritis had almost disappeared and his eyes were normal. When he was unable to get his medication in 1968, his symptoms began to return, but they subsided upon resumption of the HBT. About his treatment, Malcolm wrote years later:

"In August 1962, when I started the medication, I weighed 149 pounds and was using a cane. I could not turn my head and could do no physical work. Today I weigh 190 pounds (I am 5 feet 11 inches tall), show absolutely no sign of arthritis, and maintain an active schedule seven days a week. I have had my blood checked three times, and each time I have been pronounced to be in top physical condition.

"I would like to add that in 1961 I was in the hospital for tests and observation. X-rays showed that my hips were so clouded with calcium that the joints could not be seen and five vertebrae in my back were fused. I was told that in about five years I would be so bent I would not be able to sit in a wheelchair. About five years ago, for my own information, I had a set of x-rays taken and was told that my back and hips were in better condition than the average person's."

EXAMPLE 2: At age 19, Cynthia began to experience the symptoms of rheumatoid arthritis. Initially the arthritis was confined to her jaw and elbows, but over a period of 2½ years, while she was undergoing treatment by a traditional physician, the arthritis spread to nearly every part of her body. Five years later Cynthia was so crippled with pain and stiffness that it took her a half hour to get out of bed in the morning. The morning after she started HBT, her pain had almost disappeared except for some stiffness and soreness, which also went away during the following three days. About her condition and her subsequent treatment at the Arthritis Medical Center in Fort Lauderdale, which administers HBT, Cynthia said:

"I was getting worse and worse. When I first went to my doctor, I had it just in my jaw and elbows. After 2½ years, I had it in just about every place except my hips and knees. l couldn't turn my head at all.

"The doctor actually told me once that he felt really bad, that he had tried everything and didn't know what else to do, and that I had better go to the crippled children's center in Palm Beach. To tell a young woman that ... I just wanted to drive off a bridge. But I thank him for saying it because if he hadn't, I don't think I ever would have tried this place. I did it in desperation."

At the time Cynthia started HBT, she was taking 30 aspirin tablets a day, which were causing headaches, ringing in her ears, and ulcers. She was spending approximately $1,000 a month on painkillers alone. While Cynthia found that she bruised and bled more easily after starting HBT, she notes that she had the same symptoms while taking large doses of aspirin. On the other hand, while the aspirin and other treatments did nothing to arrest the progression of Cynthia's arthritis, a day after she started treatment with HBT, her pain virtually disappeared and returned only when she forgot to take her medication. At present Cynthia is pain-free and works out three times a week at a health spa. She continues on her medication, but in much smaller dosages than when she started treatment with HBT.

EXAMPLE 3: June also suffered from severe crippling arthritis for two years before starting treatment with HBT. Over that two-year period, June received almost every form of traditional arthritis treatment available: gold injections, penicillamine, Butazolidin (phenylbutazone), small doses of prednisone, and 16 aspirins daily. June says that she was spending over $100 a week for medication alone. In the meantime she kept getting worse, and when she started HBT, she says, "I was immobile in my hands and shoulders. It was at the point that I thought, 'What's the use of living?' I couldn't even turn my head." Additionally, her liver, stomach and kidneys were damaged by the large doses of medication. She was forced to give up her business because she was too weak and in too much pain to work. Her medical bills were ruining her financially. The second day after June received HBT, her pain disappeared. June says about her progress with HBT:

"I woke up and I could move my ankles, I could move my hands and my feet. When I stood up, the pain wasn't there. I said to [my husband], 'My God, there's been a miracle.' It got better and better, and I guess within two months I didn't even know I had rheumatoid arthritis. I got a bicycle and I started dancing again and going to the beach again. It used to be if I lay on the sand, I couldn't get up again."

June continues to be pain-free, leading a normal life, and her medication has been reduced by more than half the initial amount.

Dr. Theron Randolph and Dr. Marshall Mandell: Environmental Allergies

Environmental medicine, also called clinical ecology, was developed by Dr. Theron Randolph in the 1940s and 1950s when he observed early in his medical career that food allergies and sensitivities to environmental chemicals were a major contributing factor in a wide range of diseases, including arthritis. Dr. Randolph also noted that the causal relationship of allergy to disease was a very individualized phenomenon: One person could eat beef every day and never have an adverse reaction, while another patient could develop a food allergy to beef even when consuming it only on rare occasions. Similarly, people with an allergy to the same product did not necessarily manifest the same symptoms. One might break out with hives while another developed depression and still another became arthritic. Dr. Randolph also found that seemingly innocuous chemicals found in the home, workplace, or school could, in certain individuals, trigger symptoms ranging from mental problems to aching joints to chronic fatigue.

The work of Dr. Randolph was applied to arthritis by Dr. Marshall Mandell, a board-certified physician from Connecticut, and one of the country's leading environmental medical specialists. He has found that a considerable number of patients who come to him with arthritis or arthritislike symptoms are in fact suffering from a form of environmental allergy such as the ones outlined by Dr. Randolph. According to Dr. Mandell, "The basic process that underlies many cases of arthritis is a completely unrecognized or unsuspected allergy or allergylike sensitivity to substances that are part of daily life, including the food we eat, the liquids we drink, including the water supply, the chemicals that are deliberately or accidentally introduced into a diet, and the various forms of chemical pollutants in the indoor and outdoor air that get into our bodies." From his clinical experience, Dr. Mandell has found that more than half the patients he treats who would, by standard medical diagnostic techniques, be confirmed arthritics can be helped by means of simple dietary or environmental changes.

THE TREATMENT "My approach and that of my colleagues in the field of environmental medicine and clinical ecology, supplemented by the benefits of nutritional therapy, begins by looking at the person who is predisposed to having arthritis to see if there are identifiable substances in the diet and environment which can trigger or cause the episode of illness," says Dr. Mandell. "We deal with demonstrable cause and effect relationships. What we do is study the patient.

"First, we take a carefully formulated history which is designed to help identify people who have problems with foods, with various chemicals, with pollutants, and perhaps with seasonal airborne substances. From this, we are able to get a fairly good idea of what we're dealing with."

Before patients are actually tested for food or environmental allergies, Dr. Mandell often will have them fast or go on a restricted diet for four days to one week to rid the body of any residue of substances suspected to be responsible for the symptoms.

"Next," says Dr. Mandell, "we test these people using a technique known as 'provocative testing,' to determine their response to extracts prepared from all the foods in their diet. The most commonly ingested foods are often the culprits, so it shouldn't come as any surprise that wheat, corn products, milk, beef, tomatoes, potatoes, and soy are leading offenders.

"The most common technique used for provocative testing is to place a few drops of the test substance under the tongue of the patient, where it is almost immediately absorbed. This is called 'sublingual' provocative testing. When we test in this manner, only small doses are used, so the effect is brief but since the solution enters the bloodstream, the entire body is exposed. Symptoms can show up in the joints, muscles, brain, skin, or any other part of the body.

"If we are able to produce joint pain, stiffness or swelling or redness within a few minutes after placing the solution under the tongue for absorption into the bloodstream we know that we've found something that must be important, because we have flared up the patient's familiar symptoms—we have actually precipitated an attack of the patient's own illness.

"Many people will have what we call 'polysymptomatic illness,' meaning that many bodily structures, organs, or systems can be involved at the same time. The arthritic person's whole body may be sensitive, and this is why such patients may have a headache or fatigue or asthma or colitis, although they may not actually have any of the well-known allergies such as hay fever, eczema, or hives.

"We also find that many people react to chemicals. We have some people whose arthritis may be due in part or exclusively to the chlorine that is in the water supply, or perhaps to an artificial flavoring or coloring which is used very frequently, or perhaps to a preservative. We have people who have trouble because they are inhaling fumes such as tobacco smoke. We have people who, in heavy traffic, have trouble because the exhaust fumes will travel, along with the oxygen, through the walls of the lung, into the circulation; once again, the whole body is exposed."

After Dr. Mandell determines the substances in the patient's overall environment which he suspects are responsible for arthritic symptoms, he double-checks with test meals of the specific substances.

"I confirm the results of our testing in the office with feeding tests," he says. "Three foods can be tested during the course of a day; however, for the test to be accurate, the food to be tested must be out of the person's system for at least five days. Sometimes we can get away with it for four days, but it is even better if that food has been completely omitted from the diet, in all forms, for five, six, or seven days. We give patients a single food as the test meal; since we want to test the food all by itself, we don't put any ketchup, pepper, mustard, sauce, or anything else on the food. Instead of a usual portion, we allow patients to consume as much of the single food as they can comfortably eat as an entire meal....

"Then we observe them for at least four hours. If we're able to reproduce that patient's specific symptoms, if we can actually turn the symptoms on and off like a switch we know that we have nailed it down, because we have demonstrated a cause and effect relationship that can't be questioned. Should food be the primary causative factor, we will design a diet that eliminates all of those foods. Then, depending on how well they follow the diet, the patients will be either well or sick."

THE PATIENTS Dr. Mandell provides some examples of how allergic reactions can result in arthritis or arthritislike symptoms:

EXAMPLE 1: Sarah was a rabbi's wife who began to have arthritis in her hands, but the flare-ups would take place only on Saturday mornings and then disappear during the course of the day. Using Saturday as a starting point, Dr. Mandell began to explore the possible sources of Sarah's "Saturday arthritis."

"Since she woke up with the arthritis in the morning," Dr. Mandell explains, "we knew it was not caused by something she was doing in the morning. So we went back 24 hours to explore Friday. What did she do on Friday? What did she eat? Drink? Breathe? What came into her system? Could it be, perhaps, the paraffin fumes from the candles on the table which were lit ceremonially every Friday night? Or could it be something they ate? Was it caused by something she was exposed to when she went to temple on Friday night, perhaps from clothing just taken out of the dry cleaner's? Or was it hair spray, perfume, cologne, or men with after-shave lotion? Was it that the temple perhaps had had the rug shampooed the day before the services or that the furniture was polished? I had no way of knowing, but I retraced all her activities, and then I tested her systematically.

"This actually turned out to be an easy one, and it was humorous, because the great 'Jewish penicillin,' chicken soup, was the thing that was undoing her. When I placed a few drops of chicken extract under her tongue, within minutes the knuckles that were affected by arthritis swelled up and became painful and red. I did this on a few occasions, and so we were able to demonstrate this. It is rare to find a patient in whom a single substance is the factor, but it does happen now and then. So here is a rabbi's wife with chicken and chicken soup arthritis—Friday night ingestion, Saturday morning appearance of arthritis."

EXAMPLE 2: Dr. Randolph treated a surgeon who became so incapacitated by arthritis that he had to stop performing surgery and had to restrict his medical practice to office consultations. He had developed severe arthritis primarily in the hips, knees, shoulders, and hands, and had had traditional treatment for 10 years. While he derived some relief from the treatment, he still was incapacitated. He had to walk downstairs backwards, he no longer had the strength or dexterity in his hands to perform surgery, and he lacked the physical strength even to stand at the operating table.

The surgeon went to Chicago to see Dr. Randolph, who admitted him to the hospital and immediately put him on a pure spring water fast, free of chlorine and fluoride; and without any of the contamination that affects city water supplies. Additionally, he was placed in a special room where the environment was controlled. There were no air fresheners or disinfectants and no bleaches, the floor was not waxed or polished, and the personnel were not permitted to smoke or wear perfume.

Within five days the surgeon was free of pain. He regained some dexterity in his hands and reported that if he was a little stronger, he felt he could return to the operating room and resume his normal work. Then he was given single-food feeding tests, and Dr. Randolph discovered that when he was tested with corn (cornmeal with some corn syrup), within a matter of hours he became miserably uncomfortable with severe pains in the shoulders and hips. He had so much pain it felt as if he had been kicked by a mule. A few days later he was tested with chicken extract, and the effect was different. While he did not experience pain right away, the chicken affected his brain. He became so sleepy that he actually dozed off. When he awoke, he was in such severe pain that he was actually crying.

The surgeon found that as long as he avoided corn and chicken, he was virtually pain-free and could resume his regular daily life.

EXAMPLE 3: This example not only documents the dramatic effects which can often be achieved by eliminating an offending food from an arthritic person's diet, it also shows the degree of resistance orthodox arthritis doctors have to accepting this even when it has been unequivocally demonstrated.

Back in the mid-1970s Dr. Mandell sent out a mailing to rheumatologists in the northeastern part of the country, indicating that he was studying the relationship between food allergies and arthritis and that he was interested in studying some of their patients free of charge. Out of 90 letters, he received six responses, of which three said yes and three said no. Through one of the doctors who agreed to send patients, Janet eventually saw Dr. Mandell. He discusses her testing and the results:

"I want to emphasize that we never tell the patient what the test material is, so we completely eliminate suggestion. When we tested her with pork, she had pain almost immediately in one finger on her right hand, and this was her arthritis joint. We caused the joint to swell up and become red and painful.

"This test was repeated three times, once a week, and after the last test I told her to stay off pork for at least a week and then have a large portion of it one morning as a feeding test. Once again the same thing happened. However, when she told her rheumatologist, the man who was willing to have her come to me, he said he didn't believe it because we didn't have any controls. This is…more than pathetic, it's almost a medical crime! Here the patient had her symptom reproduced…and the doctor says he doesn't believe what has happened to her."

The ironic thing about this skepticism by the orthodox medical establishment is that many of the treatments that it prescribes for arthritis have never been proved either safe or effective. Gold injections are a good example. This treatment is extremely costly, has very high toxicity, and is only rarely of benefit to arthritis sufferers. Furthermore, in cases where gold does provide some relief, rheumatologists are unable to offer a scientific explanation of how it operates within the body. Nevertheless, gold continues to be endorsed by the arthritis establishment while something as simple as eliminating a food from a patient's diet, even if that food has been demonstrated to cause the patient's symptoms, is totally ignored or criticized as being unscientific.

EXAMPLE 4: Dr. Mandell has a friend, Dr. Bullock, whose wife suffered from arthritis. Dr. Bullock had noticed something strange about his wife's condition. When she would go to the hospital for testing and treatment, her arthritis would improve, but the moment she returned home, the symptoms would flare up again. Her rheumatologist told Mrs. Bullock that he felt that it was all psychological; the "protective environment" of the hospital made her relax, and this in turn had a beneficial effect on her arthritis. The rheumatologist concluded that something was "emotionally" wrong with Mrs. Bullock's home and that she should seek psychiatric help to discover what it was.

Her husband was skeptical about this, and after talking with Dr. Mandell he began to look at possible environmental and dietary changes which could have been responsible for his wife's improvement in the hospital. Mrs. Bullock's problem, it turned out, was very simple. At home, she ate a very limited southern diet which included certain favorite foods eaten either daily or very frequently. When she was in the hospital, however, and was presented with a long list of foods from which to choose, it was like being in a hotel or a restaurant, and she ate an extremely varied diet. For Mrs. Bullock, varying her menu made all the difference in the world. Her husband created a diet that eliminated the major offending foods and rotated a wide variety of foods so that no one food had a chance to building up in her system. Her condition improved enormously.

Dana Ullman's Homeopathy for Arthritis and Fibromyalgia

Homeopathy is based on the idea that the cure to an illness is similar to its cause. As a result, treatment consists of administering small doses of a very diluted natural substance that would cause the symptoms of the condition being treated if it was taken in larger amounts.

Dana Ullman is the president of the Foundation for Homeopathic Education and Research, and is a board member of the National Center for Homeopathy. He is the author of five books on homeopathy, including *The*

Consumer's Guide to Homeopathy: The Definitive Resource for Understanding Homeopathic Medicine and Making it Work For You (J. P. Tarcher, 1996), and *Discovering Homeopathy: Medicine for the 21st Century* (North Atlantic Books, 1991). Ullman describes the positive role that homeopathy can play in treating this crippling condition, explaining how the homeopathic remedies are selected and what they're made up of:

"There are estimated to be 200 types of arthritis. I'm glad that [the medical establishment has] increased that number from before. [In the past], it's been... about 10 or 20. From the homeopathic point of view, every person with arthritis has their own species of arthritis, so that homeopaths see disease as a syndrome. Just like a woman experiences premenstrual syndrome, which not only includes a certain degree of bloating and cramping, and emotional changes, in homeopathy, we see people with all diseases have a syndrome, and it's a body/mind constellation of symptoms. Before rushing into the practical stuff, I also do want to make a note about the research behind homeopathy, and specifically in light of arthritis. The *British Journal of Clinical Pharmacology*, a major pharmacology journal, published a double-blind placebo-controlled study on the homeopathic treatment of rheumatoid arthritis; this was way back in 1980. This study showed that 82 percent of the patients given an individualized homeopathic medicine got some degree of relief with the homeopathic medicine, whereas those given a placebo, only 21 percent got that similar degree of relief.

"Rheumatoid arthritis, as many people out there know, is an autoimmune disease. It's not simply a disease of the joints. That's where it manifests in terms of pain and dysfunction, but the bottom line is that medicine today sees rheumatoid arthritis as a systemic disease. From a homeopathic point of view, conventional medicine is finally catching up with homeopathy... [in recognizing that] all disease is systemic, that you cannot even have just a disease in the joint. You cannot have just kidney or liver disease. Every manifestation of disease, that's only its most external source, and there's a complex of symptoms and syndromes that we all experience. All too often, in conventional medicine, they're unable to deal with the complexity and simply prescribe different treatments for different symptoms, not recognizing the unitary system that we are.

"There are several key approaches that homeopaths and the general public can use in order to make the best use of these homeopathic remedies to treat their own health problems of a musculoskeletal nature. One approach is the use of single remedies to treat the acute exacerbation of the problem. Acute exacerbation of the problem means the immediate problem of a short-term nature, like a flare-up of some sort. Homeopathy and homeopathic remedies can be used to allay and relieve some of the pain and discomfort that a person's having.

"A better approach, however, is using the single remedy prescribed by a professional homeopath. What this provides is what would be called constitutional care. It's a more highly individualized remedy, not just for the acute flare-up, but for the person's overall genetic health and their entire health history. For the homeopath to do this, it requires a detailed interview, lasting at least one to sometimes two hours. And sometimes a homeopathy doesn't prescribe on that first interview, but needs more information. This type of care is probably, in my estimation, one of the more profound ways to augment the body's own immunity defense system, to not just relieve a person's condition, but to really initiate a healing and curative process.

"This is so important. We shouldn't just suppress our symptoms. Nor is it always adequate just to relieve them. Of course, relief is better than just living with it. We all have to be compassionate with all of us, including ourselves, as we experience pain and discomfort, and look for ways—ideally, natural ways, first—to relieve our pain and discomfort. But ultimately, the real goal of a physician-healer has to be real cure... not only temporary relief but getting underneath what's happening, and initiating a curative process."

FIBROMYALGIA To explain in specific terms how homeopathy can be effectively utilized, Ullman uses the treatment of fibromyalgia as an example, describing the condition itself, some of its primary causes that may be preventable, and the treatments of choice:

"Fibromyalgia's also called fibrocytis. For some people who aren't familiar with it, it's a somewhat newly-defined disease. At first, it was controversial as to whether it existed or not, but now there's basic acceptance that it is a condition. It's not officially arthritis, although it is thought to be a type of rheumatism, where the person experiences pain and discomfort in the joints. But they can, and will experience a variety of, and once again, a syndrome of symptoms. And they can be extremely diverse. Also, it can and will include fatigue, and even emotional and mental changes, such as poor concentration, anxiety, and irritability. It might have with it irritable bowel, headaches, and cramps. These syndromes come on in exacerbations. The person may be fine at one point, and then all of a sudden have all of these symptoms and syndromes.

"What's interesting is that a study was done in the *British Medical Journal* on fibromyalgia. What the researchers did was they only admitted into the study those patients that fit the most popular remedy, using homeopathy to treat fibromyalgia for the acute stages of fibromyalgia, and it's a remedy called rhus tox. That is poison ivy, believe it or not. [With] poison ivy, not only [does] an overdose cause skin eruptions, but if taken internally, and I don't recommend it, at least in crude dose, it can and will have effects upon connective tissue in a way that it makes the person feel extremely stiff, and recreates many of the symptoms that people experience when they have, not only fibromyalgia, but even many types of arthritis.

"They found that 42 percent of the people they interviewed fit this typology. So, they admitted these people into this study. In the first half of the study, half the people got a placebo and half the people got the real remedy. Then halfway through the study they switched, and the people who got the placebo now got the real remedy, and the people who began with the remedy got the placebo. The researchers found, and they published in the *British Medical Journal*, that when people began the real remedy, the homeopathic medicine, that's when relief began. And this type of study, which is not only a double-blind placebo... controlled and crossover is what it's called... the researcher is comparing a patient with themselves. It's the most sophisticated type of research presently available, presently done. It cannot always be done because these crossover effects, which we notice in homeopathy, are problematic because often homeopathic remedies have effects even after the person stops taking the remedy. So, when they begin taking the placebo, they're still feeling better. That sort of muddies the water. But this study did show, real clearly, that whenever people started to take the remedy, rhus tox, they began experiencing relief. So, one of the things I want to recommend to people out there that maybe even before going to a professional homeopath, you can try rhus tox.

SPECIFIC REMEDIES "Rhus tox is also used in many, many musculoskeletal problems. For arthritis, it is one of the leading remedies. It is a leading remedy also for carpal tunnel. It's a leading remedy for lower back pain. Rhus tox is known for alleviating the type of pain syndrome in the joints which is worse on initial motion. In other words, when the person just begins moving that particular part of the body. But then once they begin moving it more frequently, they loosen up and it doesn't hurt as much. Once they sit or lie down or sleep for any period of time, that's when they experience this rusty-gate syndrome again. So, if you happen to have this type of rusty-gate syndrome, one of the remedies you need to think about is rhus tox. The people who need rhus tox also tend to have an exacerbation of their symptoms from cold and wet weather. Many people with various types of rheumatic conditions are hypersensitive to cold and wet weather.

"One of the nice things about homeopathy is that you can talk about this broad field of musculoskeletal problems. Although initially I was talking about fibromyalgia, these remedies can be used for many of these conditions. Another remedy that comes to mind is called bryonia. Bryonia is an herb called wild hops. This is not the same hops that you drink in a beer. It's a different botanical substance entirely. This is for people with various types of musculoskeletal problems, where any type of motion exacerbates it, whereas people who benefit from rhus tox have this rusty gate syndrome where they only feel worse on initial motion, and then they loosen up and limber up. People who need bryonia, the more they move the worse they are. Here is a real obvious difference. That's one of the unique and nice things about homeopathy. We can be quite precise in finding a remedy that fits each person because the bottom line is that we are all biologically individual. We don't have the same type of joint disease or headache or depression or fatigue. We all have our own unique constellation, our own pattern of symptoms, and homeopathy is an exclusively effective, individualized approach to using these substances from the plant, mineral, or animal kingdom to augment the body's own defenses.

"One of the other remedies that immediately comes to mind too [is] for various types of musculoskeletal types of problems, including fibromyalgia and arthritis, and also some carpal tunnel and repetitive strain disorder syndromes when people are aggravated by heat or hot weather or hot applications. There is a medicine called *apis mellifica*, or simply apis. What *apis mellifica* is is the honey bee. For those of us who have ever been stung by a honey bee, or at least we know what it's like, is that, one, it's a burning and stinging type of pain, and it's somewhat sharp. If you've ever had a bee sting, you also know that if you put ice on the bee sting, it provides some relief. But if you get near heat or you apply heat to it, it worsens the pain syndrome. Likewise, people who will benefit from homeopathic doses of bee or apis will have joint pain. First of all, with the swelling, much like a bee might cause, because the bee not only causes that burning stinging pain, but also causes that inflammatory redness and heat. So, there will be swelling that will be increased by cold applications and aggravated by heat.

"One of the interesting things, one of the known parts of folklore, is that bee keepers do not seem to get arthritis very often. Part of the reason why they don't is that they occasionally do get stung, though they don't react anymore in the same type of way that the rest of us do because they become more immune to it. Their body has developed more sophisticated histamine responses so that when there is any type of sting, the body just deals with it very rapidly and easily. And there's something about that sting that also provides protective effects. It's although you're taking, if you will, a homeopathic medicine. You're taking something that will cause a similar syndrome as to what that substance causes. Although I don't recommend bee-venom therapy, usually. I don't recommend that a person with arthritis be stung multiple times by a bee. Not that I discourage it, I [just] think there are safer, easier ways, like taking homeopathic doses of bee venom, which is, once again, this medicine *apis mellifica*.

DOSAGES AND STRENGTHS OF HOMEOPATHIC MEDICINES "I do want to mention something about the dosage in homeopathy, and the strength of the homeopathic medicines. Don't be fooled by these extremely small doses. Don't think that just because we use small doses that then you need to take more frequent repetitions of the remedy. During acute exacerbations, you do need to repeat them approximately every two hours in intense types of syndromes, and every four hours in less intense syndromes, but the idea of homeopathy is to take as few doses as possible, but as much as necessary. It's a fine balance. In other words, at times, you might take it more frequently, but then as pain and discomfort diminish, you reduce the frequency of taking the remedy.

"If you look in a health food store or pharmacy, it will list the name of the medicine, usually in Latin, because all homeopathic manufacturers have to be really precise on the source and species of the plant, mineral, animal or chemical that we're using. But next to it will be a number, like 6x or 30c. Well, x refers to the number of times that particular substance has been diluted one to ten. X is a roman numeral which stands for 10. So 6x means it was diluted 1 to 10 six times. C is the Roman numeral for 100. [If it says 30c], that means it was diluted 1 to 100 thirty times. So, the C potencies are a little more dilute because they're diluted 1 to 100. But both these potencies are widely sold, widely effective, and generally, we recommend that people who are not professionals in homeopathy should not use medicines higher than the 30th potency. The 6th potency, the 12th, and the 30th are quite fine, quite effective. Although the 200th and the 1,000th are even more effective, the way those work is that you have to be more knowledgeable of these remedies because the higher potency used, the more precise the prescription has to be.

"One of the other choices that people have is not just the use of single remedies, but various combination homeopathic remedies or formulas. These are mixtures of homeopathic medicines, usually two to eight of the most common remedies for a specific ailment, like arthritic pain, back pain, PMS, allergies, sinusitis, and headaches. You see these in health food stores and pharmacies these days. Although these are not part of what would be called classical homeopathy, and although they are not as precise as prescriptions, they are a user friendly and quite effective means of providing help to people and relief to people, akin to using a single remedy for acute care.

"These formulas do not provide constitutional treatment. They do not really cure a person of the underlying problem that they have. But they do provide wonderful relief. So, I do recommend that people consider using formulas when they cannot find the single remedy that they need or do not know how to find the single remedy that they need. Or if they do know how to find the remedy, but it is not immediately available, as is often the problem.

"There is a place for both single remedy homeopathy, professional homeopathy, and formula homeopathy. In fact, in speaking of formula homeopathy, in terms of some injuries and trauma, I personally believe that people will experience—and I have observed this myself—even more rapid relief of an injury from using a formula of some sort. Because when you have an injury, you often need to give the person arnica. But at some other point, you need to give the person another remedy for the specific ailment. If it's a nerve injury, you give hypericum; if it's a connective tissue injury, you might give rhus tox or ruta. The bottom line here is that eventually, anyone involved in homeopathy will need to give several remedies to the person. And I say, well, why not give several remedies together? A fellow colleague of mine is a homeopath and a podiatrist. Every other day or so, he conducts surgery on patients with various types of foot disorders, and he always gives a combination of homeopathic remedies, and he has systematically observed that people heal from the surgery better from a combination rather than just a single medicine given sequentially. Once again, I do want to acknowledge that there is some controversy to these formulas, but as far as I'm concerned the controversy should be null and void."

Betty Lee Morales' Nutritional Approach

Many practitioners of alternative health care who address degenerative diseases (e.g., cancer, diabetes, heart disease, atherosclerosis, and arthritis) in their practice agree that most of these diseases stem from a buildup of toxins in various parts in the body, which in turn result in metabolic dysfunction and eventually in the manifestation of the symptom typifying the particular disease. As to how these toxins begin to accumulate in the body, Ms. Betty Lee Morales, a long-time advocate of a natural approach to health and disease prevention, contributing editor of *Let's Live* magazine, and member of the National Health Federation, comments that this follows directly from modern lifestyles and realities.

"The pesticide sprays, the poisons that are getting into the air, soil, and water," she says, only worsen the conditions that she calls nutritional deficiencies. All these things have a negative impact on what she describes as the weakest link, genetic inborn metabolic errors. "In short," she continues, "the proliferation of processed and refined foods, drugs and man-made chemicals [are] really at the root of this rapid increase in all degenerative diseases.

"Although it is frightening, it is well to stop and think that there has been no advancement in the treatment or correction or prevention of degenerative diseases in the last 100 years."

EFFECTS OF PESTICIDES, FERTILIZERS, AND DEFICIENT SOIL ON FOOD One of the specific sources of this problem is the manner in which food is produced and soil is treated in this country today. Dr. Max Gerson, one of the first physicians to take an environmental approach to the treatment of cancer (for more on Dr. Gerson's cancer therapy, see chapter 42) and other degenerative diseases, referred to the soil as our "external metabolism." Even at the outset of his career as a medical doctor more than 60 years ago and long before the soil was depleted and stripped to the degree that it is today, Dr. Gerson was a strong proponent of organically grown, unprocessed foods.

According to Dr. Gerson, chemical pesticides and fertilizers essentially poison and denature fruits and vegetables by altering their chemical composition. For instance, he found that chemical fertilizers often cause the sodium content to rise in certain foods while decreasing their potassium levels. As chronically ill patients are very often chemically imbalanced, with excesses of sodium and deficiencies of potassium, the effects of the fertilizers were exactly opposite to what was required by these patients to begin to recuperate and served to exacerbate their metabolic imbalances. In other words, even patients who had the willpower and determination to follow a strict regimen in which, among other things, salt and sodium were restricted and potassium was supplemented could find their efforts undermined simply by eating foods grown in chemically treated soil.

Additionally, says Ms. Morales, "When foods are grown in deficient soil, deficient plants result, and then the farmer poisons them with pesticides in order to bring them to harvest and to market. We must get back to taking care of the soil and regenerating it. It is not possible to keep taking from something without ever replacing it. It's just like a bank account; if you kept writing checks and didn't put more money into the bank, you would be bankrupt—and our soil is bankrupt. Through bankrupt raw materials and food, bankrupt animals and their byproducts, we are producing nutritionally-bankrupt people from the standpoint of health and nutrition. The United States probably leads the world in excessive consumption of overly-processed, overly-refined carbohydrates and sugars."

Because of today's agricultural and manufacturing practices, foods once full of vitamins, minerals, protein, and fiber have indeed become bankrupt. Not only does refining wheat and other grains strip them of their fiber, the wheat grown on today's soils contains only a fraction of the protein content it once had. But this is not the only adverse consequence of modern-day food production. Even with thorough washing, many of these chemicals (pesticides, herbicides, etc.) are not removed. They penetrate the skin of fruits and vegetables and poison the body's systems.

If you eat meat, poultry, or dairy products, you are ingesting even higher amounts of toxic chemicals with your food. Meat production in the United States is big business, and the bottom line is maximizing profits, not consumer health. American cattle are fed a myriad of drugs, ranging from antibiotics to steroids, are given feed contaminated with feces and sprayed with pesticides, and are themselves sprayed with pesticides. All these chemicals remain as residues in the meat when it is consumed. As meat takes an especially long time to digest and is essentially fiberless, these chemicals are not easily eliminated and can accumulate to cause all sorts of toxic reactions within the body.

SUSCEPTIBILITY OF JOINTS TO TOXIC MATERIAL Because of the specific physiology of the joints, they are especially susceptible to the buildup of toxic material which can over time result in arthritis.

Joints are surrounded by the synovial membrane, which is responsible for the production of synovial fluid. This fluid allows for smooth and efficient movement. Between the blood vessels and the inner portions of the joint, the only thing that keeps the blood from the inner surface of the joint is the synovial tissue; there is no structural barrier in this tissue which prevents toxic material from passing from the blood into the joint space. Usually the blood vessels have a surface called a basement membrane, a structural barrier that keeps the toxins in the blood and out of the tissues. In the synovial tissues that structure is not present, and this allows any toxic material from the blood to pass into the joint space. Once it is in the joint space, this toxic material can scratch and irritate the joint.

According to Ms. Morales, "All these things ending in 'itis,' which simply means 'inflammation of,' such as arthritis, neuritis, and bursitis, are really just new and fancy terms for old-fashioned rheumatism. The new names make them appear to be different diseases when they really are not. Among 16 million osteoarthritics, the most common form of arthritis is called the 'wear and tear' disease of degeneration of the joint cartilage. There is much we can do to prevent that. If it has already taken us over, there is a great deal we can do to reverse it."

THE TREATMENT Ms. Morales gives an example of how detoxification of the body and rebuilding of health with an improved diet can be used to prevent and treat arthritis.

"I work with people who are ready to do almost anything just to get a little relief," she says. "They don't even expect reversal, but sometimes they do experience it. One of my sisters was married to a professor at a leading university who was very skeptical of anything to do with diet and nutrition. When my sister developed rheumatoid arthritis...she also had five other diagnosed diseases including high blood pressure, elevated cholesterol, and heart trouble. Her husband took her all over the world; they went everywhere looking for a magic cure. After they had spent over $40,000 she not only failed to get better, she was actually worse. They returned home and got a practical nurse to come in. She could not even wait on herself.

"Finally, when she reached the bottom of the barrel, she called me one day and said, 'Well, I would like to try the natural-methods way to see if I can get some relief.' At that time, she was on about five or six prescribed drugs and obviously had many problems from them: digestion, assimilation, constipation, etc. I said that I would be very glad to help her. Then she said 'I'll take these things, but I don't want my husband to know.' I said, 'Hey, back up a minute.' Although it broke my heart, I told her that I could not help her until she had suffered enough and was willing to do whatever she needed to do, especially since not all of it was going to be pleasant. I explained that she was going to have to examine her life closely and detoxify from years of faulty diet.

"Detoxification is a very important part of regaining health and maintaining it. I also told her that she could not do this on the sly without her husband knowing about it because it becomes a way of life. It begins with what you eat, the way you live, even the way you think, and you certainly cannot do it living in a house with another person and not have that person know what you are doing. 'In fact,' I said, 'he should be doing it too.' Then she got hysterical and said, 'Well, he's not open to it.' But I had to tell her that I couldn't help her by telling her to take these things, which are not drugs. The first thing you need to do is to start educating yourself. I sent her a few books, and I said, 'When you've read some of this and you are willing to say that you will really try anything, I'll give you three months. Then I will be happy to help.'

"She reached that point when she was in bed and could not go to the bathroom alone, could not hold a glass of water or a cup of tea. She called for me, and I went over. They live in a beautiful home, and there is no problem with money, but when I outlined the things that were needed, both she and her husband said, 'Does it really cost that much?' I requested that they buy a juicer, the kind that grinds and presses, because it gives the maximum nutrition. I also wanted to bring in a practical nurse who was trained in this type of thing. I told them to think it over.

"They talked it over and decided that they would try it so I sent over a juicer and 25 pounds of organically grown carrots. I gave instructions to practical nurse to throw out everything in the cupboard that was opened and was refined or processed. Anything that was in cans or closed containers was to be given to Goodwill. I made it very clear that nothing was to go into that home that I didn't send in. I got rid of all the salt and sugar and all the easy-mix stuff—this was all a trauma to them because it costs money and nobody likes to throw away money. But I told her that she had to go the whole way or not at all.

"We put her on a seven-day detoxification to cleanse the small intestines and the bowel. She had coffee enemas every day for about a week. She had nothing but the juices, the potassium broth, and water and herb tea—no solid food for seven days. We broke the fast carefully. She had a massage every day and I made sure she was taken outdoors at least once a day. I also had the nurse read different things to her every day so she would understand what her body was going through.

"Before she started the treatment, I sent her to a laboratory to have complete blood tests, and then after the cleansing, I had her do the same tests again....Not that it was necessary in this case, but I knew that if she didn't see the results confirmed by a medical laboratory, she wouldn't believe them. Her cholesterol count was 535, which is incredibly high. Her doctor had told her that she was a walking time bomb. He was keeping her on drugs, but the cholesterol did not go down, although her liver problems increased.

"Three weeks later on this program—remember, this is a woman who could not get out of bed alone—she got up one day, went out to her own car, and drove down to the city to have her hair done. That's very typical of women and probably of men. As soon as they start to feel better, the first thing they want to do is look better. She wanted to have her hair done, and a facial and a manicure. It was a great morale booster. When her husband came home from the university, he did not know his own wife, because she was up, was beginning to start to fix a juice cocktail, and they were so delighted that I never had more arguments or problems out of them. But she also felt so well that she decided not to wait the full six weeks to have the other tests done; it had only been three weeks. She went back to the medical lab and asked to have all the tests done over. She wanted to send her doctor a copy because she still was under the care of a medical doctor who had told her 'these health food things won't hurt you, but they won't help you. It will only cost you some money, but you can afford it, so go ahead and do it.'

"When she had the second batch of lab tests [which showed substantial improvement] done and sent to him, he wrote her a letter in which he said, 'If you are going to pursue these quack remedies, I can no longer be responsible for your health, and I am dismissing you as a patient.' She called me up crying and said, 'I don't even have a doctor in case I need one.' She was still laboring under the horrible fear that this doctor had laid on her by saying that she could have a stroke or heart attack at any minute.

"We continued with the program. Within a total of three months, she was able to go on a South Pacific cruise with her husband. Today, you won't meet two people who are better advocates of the nutritional way of living. They have gone 90 to 95 percent holistic and no longer feel that they have to be under the wing of a doctor who does not recognize nutrition.

"One of the positive offshoots of this is that my brother-in-law, who was a professor for 50 years at one of the most prestigious universities and a staunch opponent of the nutritional approach to healing, also turned 180 degrees around. He too had been taking quite a few medications for high blood pressure. He had what is called a Dupuytren's contracture, where the fingers curl down toward the palm and cannot be straightened—this is a classic vitamin E deficiency. After seeing what it had done for his wife, he said that he was ready to go on an intensive program and see what it could do for his fingers. His brother also had this condition and had had his tendons cut, so it obviously ran in the family. Fortunately, my brother-in-law was willing to try the nutritional program first. Today—he has just turned 80—he's in better health than he has ever been in his life. He is vital and virile and active and full of the joy of life, and the two of them are enjoying their life together so much when they could have been crippled and bedridden."

Dr. Laurie Aesoph's Six-Step Nutritional Approach

Dr. Laurie Aesoph is a naturopathic physician, as well as a medical writer. She has authored more than 200 articles on topics ranging from nutrition and herbs and homeopathy, and she also is a senior editor of the *Journal of Naturopathic Medicine*.

Dr. Aesoph relates what she sees as the role between arthritis prevention and treatment, and which foods may help treat this ailment and why:

"People with arthritis don't need to give up hope. Diet and nutrition is… the foundation of good health anyway, and can be used specifically to treat the more than 100 different types of arthritis that there are.

RESTORATIVE FOODS "What many, many studies tell us is that what I call restorative foods, which merely is the good food that we should be eating anyway, [such as] whole grains, and fruits, and vegetables... are what we need to insert in our diet. What the studies show is not only do good diets help out with arthritis, but specific, different types of food seem to have healing qualities. For example, the oils from different fish have an anti-inflammatory and pain relieving benefit for arthritis patients. Many fruits, vegetables, and even spices double as herbs. You can use those specifically for different arthritis symptoms.

"In an article printed in the *Lancet*, which is a British medical journal, in 1991, the researchers there put their patients on a cleansing diet. But eventually what they did is switch them over to a lacto-ovo-vegetarian diet, in different stages, and they had a group that was their control, their placebo, where they just ate as normal. They found that even on the lacto-ovo, where people are eating vegetarian diets, but also eating eggs and dairy, that the benefits continued throughout that year and at the end of the year. So, here's evidence where we know that diet is helping.

"Even the Arthritis Foundation is admitting to this. There are enough studies that they are taking notice. They have always said that, of course, if you're overweight, that the stress on the joints... so, if you have something like osteoarthritis or what we call degenerative joint disease, that's going to aggravate and wear out your joints. But they are also looking at studies involving food allergies and cleansing and the fish oil that I mentioned earlier, and, of course, the purines are involved with gout. And diet has always been a large part of treating gout.

STRESSOR FOODS "I've talked about restorative foods a little bit, but one other thing that I [want to] mention is what I call the stressor foods. Basically the stressor foods are what kind of set the stage for joint degeneration and breakdown to occur. And just to give you an example of what these foods are, basically, if you look at the fat category, and I want to remind [people] that fats per se are not bad. In fact they're essential, and there's something called essential fatty acids that we need to have and the fish oils fit into that category. But the trans fatty acids—hydrogenated vegetable oils, for example, and margarine—[contain] too much saturated fat. Those are the sorts of things that should be stressor foods, and that we should be avoiding. Alcohol doesn't do us any good, nor does caffeine. Refined carbohydrates, like sugars, flour, white rice, the different sweeteners, the artificial sweeteners, like aspartame and saccharine, processed foods, of course, and the additives and chemicals that are added to our foods are other things that we should also be avoiding.

"When you eat stressor foods, a lot of them are really deplete in the different nutrients: vitamins, minerals, and all the other phytochemicals and nutrients that we're discovering that are in our foods. These, of course, are essential for general body function. Now arthritis isn't just restricted to the joints, but what we've discovered is there is a link between the joints and different body systems, so the immune system is involved, and we'll find out about rheumatoid arthritis is actually what we call an autoimmune disease, where basically the immune or defense system of your body is attacking yourself. So, if you don't have the vitamins and minerals, your immune system isn't going to function as well as it can. Also, with regard to our intestinal tract, it's also vital that it is functioning properly for all sorts of different conditions. When that isn't functioning right, it will aggravate an arthritic condition. I mentioned that if you are overweight that will stress the joint. If you tend to eat stressor-type foods, that tends to play into or add to conditions of obesity. Also, we talk about stress in our lives, and I really believe as the label says, stressor foods, that foods that are not complete in nutrition and aren't as whole as they should be are a stress on the body. So, that doesn't help your body function any better.

"Also, if you are eating a lot of cooked or processed foods, they tend to be lower in enzymes that help us digest our foods. There have been numerous studies done where when people eat a diet that is largely comprised of cooked foods, then their digestive systems, the pancreas, different organs that contribute digestive enzymes to the gut have to work a little harder, and it makes it harder to digest, and then that adds to your gut being a little thicker than it should be, and then that aggravates the arthritis down the road. So, you can see that there are direct and indirect effects that these stressor foods have.

"When you use natural medicine and conventional medicine, it doesn't need to be an either/or situation. You can also use nutrition to cut back on the medication that you're using. So, you can take a compromised view, and perhaps gradually get away from the drugs. Also, if you happen to be on steroids, [such as] prednisone, if you plan to cut back and use nutritional means, you need to work with your doctor on that. That's something you don't want to cut out cold turkey. The nonsteroidal anti-inflammatory drugs are not as much of a problem. But when going off any prescription drug or steroids, talk to your doctor about that first."

THE PROGRAM Dr. Aesoph outlines her six-step nutritional program to overcome arthritis:

(1) Cutting out all the stressor foods from your diet. You want to eliminate anything that is harming your body or undermining your body's functions, and really setting the stage for joint problems to happen. These foods not only weaken the joints, but they really impinge their ability to repair themselves as well. These are also the foods that add to excess weight which can overburden the joints. Some of these foods are also high in purines, which tend to aggravate gout.

(2) Cleansing the body with a real whole-foods diet, and start to add the restorative foods. This helps repair the gastrointestinal tract, which is an imper-

ative part of healing arthritis. At this point, you should be starting to learn how to incorporate healthy eating habits, and what foods to choose.

(3) Testing for and then beginning to cut out allergy foods.

(4) Rebuilding the damaged joints and overall health again by starting to refine your choice of restorative foods. Sea cucumber at 1,000 mg may help, as can manganese at 25 mg, and the bioflavonoid complex. Glucosamine sulfate and chondroital sulfate, both at 500 mg, can also produce phenomenal results. Flax at 1,000 mg from the omega-three fatty-acid group re-establishes normal fluid and osmotic pressure, the synovial fluid in those joints. Taking an alpha lipoic acid, your best all-around intracellular antioxidant, actually fights free-radical damage inside the cell. Then you have a very powerful healing mechanism to get your joints circulating nutrients and oxygen, and expelling carbon dioxide and waste products as they should.

There are many supplements and minerals and vitamins and herbs. Other ones that you can add are ginger, cumin, and cayenne. Cayenne cream can be rubbed on arthritic joints because they deplete substance p, which decreases pain.

(5) Decreasing weight, if that's a problem, because it is a stress on the joints.

(6) Eliminating any stress by learning to eat properly, such as by chewing your food properly and eating in a relaxed way.

Dr. David Steenblock: Arthritis and Atherosclerosis

Because of the susceptibility of the joints to the accumulation of toxic material which can scratch and irritate the inner linings, leading to the pain and inflammation characterizing arthritis, an analogy has been made between arthritis and atherosclerosis (degeneration of the arteries). In both diseases corrosive substances scratch the inner linings of the body part involved, causing irritation which can lead to degeneration. These substances can come from toxic material in the bowel which gets into the bloodstream. They can also come from food. In the case of atherosclerosis, these substances include cholesterol, fats, and fried foods, which, when they get into the blood, scratch and irritate the very sensitive inner linings of the blood vessels. The same substances can also pass from the blood into the joint space and irritate the inner linings of the joints.

According to Dr. David Steenblock, a physician specializing in the relationship of diet, nutrition, and arthritis, this correlation between arthritis and atherosclerosis is one of the reasons why a low-fat, low-cholesterol high-fiber diet has been useful in treating arthritis. "Many patients on this type of diet," says Dr. Steenblock, "show substantial improvement because the fiber cleanses the colon and removes much of the toxic bacterial waste products, which frees up the blood system and makes it more pure. This in turn allows for the toxic materials to be eliminated from the joints, and so the joints themselves can begin to heal."

HIGH-FIBER DIET Dr. Steenblock also explains how a diet which eliminates processed foods and focuses on the consumption of high-fiber natural grains, fruits, and vegetables works specifically in the treatment of arthritis:

"We want to eliminate white sugar and white flour products and processed foods and foods which contain food additives because these processed foods cause abnormalities in the state of health of the intestine. When you eat processed foods with little fiber, the bacterial content of the colon changes from the so-called good bacteria, which are lactobacillus vivitus and acidophilus, to organisms which are anaerobic such as anerococci and streptococci and organisms which generally are not healthy and produce many toxic substances themselves. When these toxic substances are present as a result of eating a diet high in refined food and lacking fiber, these toxins pass through the bowel into the blood. Also, refined foods, because they are so easily digestible and do not require work by the intestine, cause the muscle wall of the intestine to atrophy or become thinner. This thinness of the wall allows more toxic material to pass through the bowel into the blood. Once it is in the blood, it can pass easily into the joints and cause more problems.

"The use of the high-fiber, natural diet goes against this trend because the fiber changes the bacterial content of the colon back to normal, and this eliminates many of the toxic materials, the carcinogens, and the mutagens which are formed otherwise, which are well-documented causes not only of osteoarthritis but also of cancer of the colon and atherosclerosis. The fiber also strengthens the bowel wall, making it thicker and healthier, and this creates more of a mucosal barrier between the colon's interior and the blood. Thus the diet should be more of a natural and raw foods diet if you want to get a good result."

Dr. Steenblock does warn, however, that people who have spent an entire lifetime eating refined, fiberless foods must approach a change to a raw, high-fiber diet with caution (excess dietary fiber can, for instance, cause calcium and zinc to be washed through the system so that calcium and zinc deficiencies result) in order to give their intestinal tract time to strengthen. A good physician with a solid background in nutritional therapy should be consulted before any drastic dietary changes are made.

CHELATION THERAPY While atherosclerosis and arthritis often serve to exacerbate each other, treatments other than diet which are directed at one condition often are beneficial in treating the other. For example, Dr. Steenblock discusses how chelation therapy, an intravenous chemical treatment (discussed more fully in chapter 33) commonly used for atherosclerosis and heart disease, can also benefit arthritic patients:

"One of the problems with osteoarthritis is that the capillaries of the synovium have become rigidified, or more rigid than they should be as a consequence of the aging process and of atherosclerosis. This limits the blood flow through these joints; therefore, the heat that is produced when the joint is put in motion cannot be taken away because the circulation is poor. As a result pain occurs when you exercise, and conversely, when you are resting, the blood flow through that tissue is poor and toxic materials accumulate and can cause pain. Anything that increases the diameter and the blood flow through these capillaries will aid in the restoration process. This is where chelation therapy is very valuable because it actually gets into these small blood vessels and capillaries and removes the cross-linkage of the collagen and elastin. This makes these small blood vessels more pliable and elastic, gives them more diameter so that more blood can pass through them, and thus helps in the healing process."

SUPPLEMENTS Different vitamins, minerals, and nutritive substances can play important roles in the treatment and prevention of arthritis. There is some evidence that the essential fatty acids furnished by substances such as cod liver oil, linoleic acid, and marine lipids, by replacing missing fatty substances in the synovial fluid, can be important in treating arthritis. The synovial fluid consists primarily of mucin with some albumin, fat, epithelium, and leukocytes. When the joint surfaces become irritated and undergo degeneration, some of the fat from the joint itself is lost. This fat acts as a lubricant and keeps the joint surfaces apart so that the cartilage-covered bone ends are protected and can move smoothly. When a person takes extra cod liver oil or other essential fatty acids, the oil goes to the joints and provides more lubrication.

Vitamin A, which is found in large quantities in cod liver oil, is also important for the maintenance of the mucous membranes of the body, which manufacture mucous in order to cleanse the body of infectious bacteria and toxins. Without adequate supplies of vitamin A, infection and accumulation of toxic materials can set in around the joints. Furthermore, a vitamin A deficiency can lead to the insufficient production of synovial fluid; when this occurs, the joints lack proper lubrication, the cartilage becomes subject to drying and cracking, and movement becomes difficult and painful.

Because lubrication is vital to the smooth functioning of the joints, vitamin E, whose primary role is to protect against the destruction of the essential fatty acids by oxidation, is also an important antiarthritic nutrient. Both vitamins E and C, which generally act as free-radical scavengers within the body, can be especially important in the treatment as they can "clinch" the free radicals present at the site of inflamed or irritated joints, thereby decreasing pain, swelling, and inflammation. According to Ms. Betty Lee Morales, university studies have also suggested that vitamin E can play an important role in neutralizing toxic substances in the air. Furthermore, Ms. Morales notes:

"Many women are stricken about the time of menopause, which suggests that arthritis has something to do with a falling production of hormones within the body. Men go through menopause, but about 10 years later than women. If women would take extra vitamin E and make sure that they eat the hormone-precursor foods so that their bodies are fortified, then they would also be taking a step forward in preventing the diseases that are related to a hormonal deficiency. Hormone-precursor foods include the unrefined whole grains and pollen, which has all 22 free amino acids and is a great hormone-precursor food for both sexes."

Many symptoms of arthritis are alleviated by establishing a proper balance of calcium and phosphorus in the body, since these are the two minerals most responsible for bone formation and healing. This can be one of the most confusing aspects of arthritis because x-rays of arthritic joints often show excessive calcification. Afraid of further calcification, patients mistakenly believe that they must avoid calcium-rich foods. Actually, the calcification is not due to an excess of calcium but rather to malabsorption of existing supplies caused by an imbalance in the calcium-to-phosphorus ratio. This imbalance is caused by two major factors: (1) excessive consumption of foods containing high levels of phosphorus such as meat, dairy products, and soft drinks and (2) the process of joint degeneration, which releases high levels of phosphates. This excess phosphorus at the joint site binds with calcium and results in calcification. Taking extra calcium orally does not contribute to this localized calcification. Rather, by increasing calcium levels in the blood, it draws the excess phosphorus away from the joints to bind with the blood calcium so that both are eliminated; this in turn inhibits calcification around the joints.

It should be noted here that soft drinks are the number one source of phosphorus in the American diet today. These drinks contain more phosphorus than the average food or beverage, and the typical American consumes nearly 500 gallons of them a year. According to Dr. Steenblock, excess phosphorus is one of the major contributing factors to the development of osteoarthritis. He says, "We see this clinically in many people, who come with osteoarthritis in their early 40s, who are large consumers of soft drinks, who also consume excess quantities of meats and other high-phosphorus foods, and who do not eat enough of the green, leafy vegetables which contain calcium." The other problem associated with soft drinks is that most of them contain citric acids, which bind calcium and cause it to be excreted. "So," says Dr. Steenblock, "not only is there extra phosphorus in the soft drinks, they contain the material that takes calcium out of the body. If you want to develop osteoarthritis, that's a very good way of doing it."

PROTEOGLYCANS Another therapy for arthritis entails the use of naturally occurring substances called proteoglycans, which are molecules made up of approximately 10 percent proteins and 90 percent carbohydrates. There has been very promising research in other countries on these substances, but to date little has been done in the United States. Dr. Steenblock explains this therapy:

"What we are talking about is a particular substance called chondroitin sulfate, which is a type of proteoglycan. In the person with osteoarthritis these substances gradually diminish in concentration in the joint as the joint becomes worn. If the chondroitin sulfate could be put back into the joint, this would allow for an inhibition of the calcification process and also smooth out and seal the irregularities, the cracks, and the irritations which have occurred through time with wear and tear.

"Over the past 10 years or so, chondroitin sulfate has been used in both Europe and Japan for the treatment of osteoarthritis, rheumatoid arthritis, and also atherosclerosis. Again, there is a great similarity between osteoarthritis and atherosclerosis in the sense that both result from the wear and tear caused by irritative substances in the body. We need to protect these collagen surfaces from the irritative substances which circulate in the blood and ultimately get into the joint...

"Chondroitin sulfate appears to be one of the best treatments for both arthritis and vascular disease. When you take it orally, it actually enters into the body through the intestinal tract and will selectively go to the joints and all the areas of damage in the blood vessels. It not only acts preventively but also will help reverse the diseases that are present. This substance is now available in this country in health food stores.

"There are a few companies which are making it from an extract of the trachea called 'mucopolysaccharides.' That is having very good results. Research in Europe and Japan is showing that this substance is probably the best form of therapy that there has been and probably will be for a long time in treating of arthritis and vascular disease. The treatment is not, however, the sort of miracle drug type of treatment where you give the person one pill and get immediate results. What we are dealing with is a natural substance, and it takes time for these natural substances to create the result we are looking for, namely, healing of the injured areas. When you take these mucopolysaccharides, you have to take them for anywhere from two to four months in order to achieve results. Patents who are sticking with them are having very positive results and report upwards of 80 percent relief of pain and also a stoppage of the degeneration.

"There is another substance, which is derived from the New Zealand green lip mussel. There are a number of trade names for it. This substance is also a mucopolysaccharide, and it is effective in treating osteoarthritis as well as rheumatoid arthritis. This material is available in most health food stores.

"These mucopolysaccharides can also be used preventively to heal the small nicks and irritations that occur routinely in the blood vessels and joints. These substances immediately seal these little cracks and crevices so that they do not get larger. Our bodies are not really capable of doing that on their own, and we need to help them along with a little bit of these substances all the time so that these joints and arteries that we have are protected."

26

Osteoporosis

O steoporosis (the word means "porous bones") is a serious problem in which the skeletal system weakens and fractures easily. It may be accompanied by pain, especially lower back pain, loss in height, and body deformity. More females than males become afflicted, with postmenopausal women being at greatest risk. Osteoporosis is attributed to the gradual loss of calcium. In women, this loss begins in the mid-30s at a rate of 1 to 2 percent a year, and can increase during menopause to a rate of 4 to 5 percent a year.

Causes

According to naturopathic physician Dr. Jane Guiltinan, the most likely candidates for osteoporosis share a number of characteristics:
- Northern European ethnic origin
- Small frame
- Family history of osteoporosis
- Diet high in meat, caffeine, sugar, refined carbohydrates, and phosphates (found in sodas and processed foods)
- Cigarette smoking
- Alcohol use
- Sedentary lifestyle

It may surprise some people to learn that dairy foods, while rich sources of calcium, can also contribute to the condition of osteoporosis. Registered nurse and acupuncturist Abigail Rist-Podrecca notes, "When I was in China, we noticed that no dairy was used. We expected to see a high incidence of osteoporosis, rickets, and other bone problems. In fact, we saw the lowest incidence. In the West, dairy is used a lot and osteoporosis is rampant. Something is not quite right here." Two main factors responsible for the Chinese not getting osteoporosis, she learned, are diet, weight-bearing exercise, and acupuncture.

Conventional Approach to Treatment

Synthetic estrogen is the traditional drug of choice for postmenopausal osteoporosis prevention, but controversy surrounds its safety and effectiveness.

Diet and Nutritional Alternatives

The first step in osteoporosis prevention is noting whether or not you are at high risk for the condition, says Dr. Jane Guiltinan. Obviously, certain risk factors cannot be changed, but many can be addressed, and will prevent the destructive effects of the disease.

A diet that is low in animal products and high in plant foods promotes bone growth and repair. Green, leafy vegetables contain vitamin K, beta carotene, vitamin C, fiber, calcium, and magnesium, which enhance the bones. Other calcium-rich foods include broccoli, milk, nuts, and seeds. Sesame seeds have high calcium content. The Chinese, who as mentioned earlier have low rates of osteoporosis, use sesame often in their foods, and cook with sesame seed oil.

Foods to avoid include sugar, caffeine, carbonated sodas, and alcohol, as these contribute to bone loss. Too much protein from chicken, fish, eggs, and meat are also contraindicated. These are high in the amino acid methionine, which the body converts into homocysteine, a substance that causes both osteoporosis and atherosclerosis.

Women over 25 need adequate calcium, approximately 1,000 mg in supplement form, and an additional 500–1,000 mg from the diet. After 40, 1,500–2,000 mg is needed. Women on estrogen replacement therapy require between 1,200 and 1,500 mg.

In addition to calcium, the following nutrients are critical for keeping bones strong:

Magnesium (800–1,200 mg in citrate form)
Vitamin D (400 IU)
Vitamin C (1,000 mg)
Vitamin K (100 mcg)
Beta carotene
Selenium (75–150 mcg)
Boron (3 mg)
Manganese (5 mg)
Strontium
Folic acid (1 mg)

Silica

Copper

Zinc

A balanced vitamin/mineral supplement will provide most of these nutrients. It is best to take zinc separately, however; otherwise, it can have an adverse effect on vitamin and mineral absorption.

Research indicates that natural progesterone from wild yams is safer and more effective than estrogen in that it builds strong bones and has no harmful side effects. Dr. Jane Guiltinan notes that "Estrogen minimizes calcium loss from bones, but progesterone can actually put calcium back into bones." Natural progesterone can be taken in pill form. It also comes in a cream form. Half a teaspoon should be rubbed into the skin over soft tissue and the spine, twice a day, for two weeks out of every month.

DHEA, a precursor to estrogen and testosterone, is important in the prevention of numerous chronic conditions associated with aging. As we get older, there is often a drop in DHEA. If blood levels are low, 5 mg a day can safely be taken as a supplement.

Exercise and Yoga

Dr. Howard Robins, former director of the Healing Center in New York City and coauthor of *Ultimate Training* and *How to Keep Your Feet & Legs Healthy for a Lifetime*, stresses the importance of weight-bearing aerobic and weight-lifting exercises for osteoporosis prevention.

Aerobic exercises use major muscle groups in a rhythmic, continuous manner. Weight-bearing aerobic exercises such as brisk walking, jogging, stair climbing, and dancing produce mechanical stress on the skeletal system, which drives calcium into the long bones. Non-weight-bearing aerobic exercises such as biking, rowing, and swimming are not as helpful in osteoporosis prevention, but they do promote flexibility, which is useful for people prone to arthritis.

People "need to perform aerobic exercises anywhere from three to five or six times a week," says Dr. Robins. "You need a day off every third or fourth day so that the body can heal and re-energize."

"Most women stay away from weight training because they are afraid of developing huge muscles like Arnold Schwarzenegger," says Dr. Robins. "The good news is, that won't happen. No matter how hard you train, you will never get huge muscles as a woman unless you take steroids to alter your body's metabolism."

Not only is weight training safe, it is important for preventing osteoporosis. As muscles are pulled directly against the bone, with gravity working against it, calcium is driven back into the bones. It also stimulates the manufacture of new bone. This adds up to a decrease in the effects of osteoporosis by 50 to 80 percent. People need to do weight training two to three times per week for 15 to 30 minutes. All the different muscle groups should be worked on. Twenty-four hours should lapse between sessions to rest muscles. For best results, an exercise program should be started long before the onset of menopause.

A complete routine is more than aerobic and weight training exercises only. It incorporates warm-ups at the beginning and cool-downs at the end of a routine. Warm-ups are not to be confused with stretches. Rather, they are gentle exercises that produce heat by getting blood to flow into the muscles. To warm up leg muscles, for example, one could lie down on one's back and move the legs like a bicycle, or walk gently in place. Moving the arms and joints gently in all their ranges of motion will warm up the upper body. Warming up the body helps prevent injuries.

After exercise, when the body is loosest, stretching is performed. Stretches are long, continuous pulls, not bounces. Bouncing only tightens the muscles and can lead to injury. Dr. Robins's book *Ultimate Training* describes a holistic workout in detail. Aromatherapist Ann Berwick adds that essential oils enhance a warm-up and cool-down routine. "Before exercise, use warming and stimulating oils, such as black pepper, rosemary, ginger, and sage. Additionally, eucalyptus helps to deepen breathing. After exercise, you can apply a blend of lemon, rosemary, and juniper. These help to carry away waste products and to ease any stiffness."

YOGA Yoga prevents osteoporosis in four ways: it builds and fortifies bone mass; it keeps muscles strong and flexible; it improves posture; and it helps balance and coordination. Physical therapist and yoga teacher Bonnie Millen explains why this is important: "With yoga, the old adage 'Use it or lose it' applies. Building and maintaining bone mass is most important for preventing osteoporosis. Remember, bone is alive. Yoga is unique in that it incorporates weight bearing on the upper extremities. This is important because many wrist, forearm, and upper arm fractures occur when people reach forward with outstretched arms as they are falling.

"Also important is building and maintaining muscle strength and flexibility. Let's keep the muscles strong so that they can receive the stress before the fracture happens. Also if the body is strong and flexible, it can cushion falls when they occur.

"Good posture improves overall functioning and prevents osteoporotic fractures of the spine. I teach yoga to a lot of older women who tell me they are afraid of getting a dowager's hump. This is where the body slouches forward and there is a hump on the back. Just take a moment to get into that posture where your chest caves in and your shoulders slump forward, with your head looking down toward the floor. Try to raise one arm up as if you wanted to touch the ceiling, and see how high the arm comes up. Now let the arm down and come into a nice seated posture, as if someone were going to take your picture. Sitting very tall, raise your arm up and see how high it goes. You can see from that little exercise that the slouched posture really decreases your range of motion. That makes it difficult to function. This is why you want to keep a good posture.

"By placing great pressure on the spinal vertebrae, the dowager's hump often leads to compression fractures of the spinal column. This is very painful, as you can well imagine, and you do not have to do anything special for it to happen. Just going up and down stairs or taking a step can cause breakage.

"The fourth way yoga helps is by improving balance and coordination. When you are balanced and coordinated, there is less chance of your falling in the first place. You are quicker to respond. And that can help prevent fractures."

Bonnie Millen points out that there are several styles of yoga but that all systems have foundation poses that address the above needs. Here she outlines a few basic postures:

DOWNWARD-FACING DOG. This posture strengthens bone mass in the wrists and arms. In this pose, you stand and bring your hands to the floor so that the space beneath you is triangular. One part of the triangle is from your hands to your hips, and the other part is from your hips to your heels. The space on the floor between your hands and your feet is the third part. As you hold the position, you will feel that you are bearing weight on your arms.

WARRIOR POSES. These poses increase muscle strength and flexibility, as well as balance. Here you are standing with your legs three to four feet apart, depending on your height. With your legs apart, you work at the hip to turn one leg out to the side. The other leg is turned slightly inward. That really works the hip muscles, which is important in helping to prevent the all-too-common osteoporotic hip fracture. The arms are either held out to the side or up over the head, depending upon which warrior posture it is.

COBRA. This is a back-bending pose that helps posture and gives flexibilityand strength to the paraspinals, the muscles of the back of the spine. To begin, lie face down on the floor. Using the back muscles, sequentially lift the head and chest away from the floor.

SIMPLE STRETCH FOR CHEST MUSCLES. This is another exercise for improving posture that is especially helpful for women who tend to slouch forward. Take a blanket and fold it to resemble a box of long-stemmed roses. Lie down on this bolster, making sure that your head and your entire spine are completely supported. Place your arms out to the side or up to form a V-shaped position with the palms facing up toward the ceiling. Just allow gravity to relax the shoulders down to the floor (Shoulders should not be on the blanket). Breathe deeply. That will expand the intercostals, the muscles between the ribs. This is important because the intercostals become constricted with slouching. That, in turn, decreases lung capacity and causes all the organs to become compressed. This is a wonderful pose where you don't have to actually do anything. You just allow gravity to work for you and your breath to move through you.

Millen says that the best time to begin yoga is before osteoporosis sets in: "The time to begin a yoga practice, or any exercise, is not when you've gotten to menopause, and all of a sudden you realize, 'Oh my gosh! I'm at risk for osteoporosis.' You need to build bone mass throughout your whole life so that you have bone stored up. It's like preparing for retirement. You build up bone mass through exercise, you eat right, you maintain a healthy lifestyle. Then, when you reach your menopausal years, you've got a good store of bone mass to help protect you."

Other Alternative Therapies

ACUPUNCTURE As mentioned earlier, in China, osteoporosis is the exception rather than the norm. When it does manifest, acupuncture is used. Acupuncturist Abigail Rist-Podrecca explains how this works: "The Chinese use an electrical stimulus along the spine. The electrical impulse actually helps the bone-stem cells, which are the reproductive cells of the bone, to reproduce, thereby strengthening the bone mass. It was very exciting to see this because we have some Western studies proving that peripheral stimulation by electricity, especially in the long bones in the leg, help this process also." She adds that women low in calcium need to take this supplement so that the body has the raw materials for making bones denser. When weight-bearing exercises are added, the benefits are remarkable.

HOMEOPATHY Homeopathy can be used as an adjunct to the nutritional and lifestyle factors discussed above. These are some remedies to consider:

CALCAREA PHOSPHORIC. This may help where the bones are weak, soft, curved, and brittle. It can be given for a long period of time.

CORTICOID. Homeopathic corticoid is for painful posttraumatic osteoporosis, especially when it affects the hip. Consider this remedy for an elderly person who has fractured her hip because of osteoporosis.

PARATHYROID. For diffuse pain in the bones, especially the long bones. Walking is very painful. Often, there is pain in the ankles, hips, and knees. Regarding potencies, homeopathic physician Dr. Ken Korins says, "For acute conditions, meaning they come on suddenly, and they are very intense, use a 200c potency. That is a very dilute potency, but energetically speaking, it is very powerful. For more chronic conditions, where you will be giving the remedy for a longer period of time, you might want to start with 12c or 30c. In general, the remedies should be taken as three to four pellets placed under the tongue. Take them on an empty stomach. Wait 15 to 20 minutes before or after eating. Avoid coffee and aromatic substances, such as mints, perfumes, and camphors, which can interfere with their effectiveness. Also, it is a good idea not to touch remedies with your hands because any residues from perfumes or other substances can interfere with their energy properties."

27

Temporomandibular Joint (TMJ) Dysfunction

The temporomandibular joint (TMJ) is a hinged joint that opens and closes the mouth. The jaw is part of a wider system, the craniosacral system, which lies along the center of the body. It begins with the feet, moves up to the knees, the pelvis, the shoulders, and then to the head and jaw. Disruption at any level can result in TMJ pain. The problem may originate with the TMJ itself, or it might start in the feet or with neck tension, for example.

The two most common causes of TMJ problems are poor bite and stress. Poor bite may be the result of new dental work that affects tooth alignment. Sometimes braces shift the palate, which affects the jaw. In recent years, more adults have been undergoing this procedure, hence, increasing numbers of TMJ disorders. Dentists who specialize in TMJ can diagnose the condition.

TMJ dysfunction affects larger numbers of females than males due to stresses brought on by hormonal changes. Dr. Deborah Kleinman, a chiropractor who works with TMJ patients, explains: "There are various stress factors we can talk about that are specific to women. First, we have pre-menstrual tension. This further weakens an already weakened system. I know women who only have a problem with their jaw three days before their period. As soon as their period comes, their pain goes away. This tells me that there is a weakness in the system and that hormones push the body past the point of being able to compensate for it.

"These hormonal changes also occur during pregnancy and menopause. In addition to hormonal changes and added stress, pregnancy creates structural changes through weight gain and the loosening of ligaments. Hormones loosen the pelvis so that the woman is more flexible during delivery. These changes can further aggravate TMJ dysfunction.

"With nursing, postural changes can play a big role. Nursing places stress on the upper back muscles, especially if the woman doesn't use the proper pillows or if she gets lazy and slumps over while feeding her baby. These upper back muscles insert into the occiput, which is part of this craniosacral system. The occiput is the bone at the bottom of the skull. Tightening or pulling on the occiput can affect the head, neck, and TMJ."

Symptoms

Pain can be isolated in the joint itself or it can radiate to the face, neck, ear, and shoulder. Headaches may be a part of the picture. There may be a nagging toothache, even though the tooth is healthy. There can also be difficulty with opening the mouth all the way. If the muscles around the joint become inflamed, they may spasm and lock open. Clicking, grinding, or popping noises may accompany chewing or movement of the joint.

Craniosacral Therapy

Cranio means skull and *sacral* refers to the sacrum, which is a part of the pelvis. This therapy is founded on an understanding of the relationship between these structures and several points in between, including the TMJ. Dr. Deborah Kleinman, who uses a specific form of craniosacral therapy called sacro-occipital technique, explains: "A chiropractor like myself who uses this technique understands that there is a balance between the nervous system and the musculoskeletal system, and a relationship between the pelvis and the sacrum and then the head and the cranium. Between both structures rests the spine, the shoulders, the neck. All of these structures react to shifts in the pelvis and the cranium. The TMJ is part of that." She adds that a stable pelvis balances the body and works in harmony with the cranium. This allows information to flow to the brain smoothly.

A doctor performs a series of tests to determine whether structural stresses exist, and, if so, where. Once this is known, treatment can begin. Dr. Kleinman explains: "We place wedges or blocks under the pelvis. The muscles will relax and contract around these levers in an unforced way, based upon what these levers tell the brain. Then we incorporate breathing techniques to assist the brain in making musculoskeletal changes. This reestablishes the proper craniosacral flow." Sometimes secondary manipulations are necessary to readjust parts of the spine that lie between the pelvis and cranium that get knotted up as a result of compensating for the pelvis and the cranium. Cranial adjustments, made specifically to the temporomandibular joint, also help to re-establish proper balance.

Other Physical Therapies

Regularly done isotonic exercise can help some cases of TMJ dysfunction. In addition to jaw exercise, self-treatment for TMJ problems may include jaw awareness, in which the patient tries to notice and avoid clenching and grinding the teeth, as well as biting on gum, ice, or fingernails. Eating soft foods and avoiding resting or sleeping on the stomach can also help, as can learning to rest the jaw and to adopt proper jaw posture. Other potentially helpful techniques include self-massage; relaxed rhythmic opening and closing of the jaw; alternating moist heat (15 minutes) with ice (2–3 minutes) to increase circulation; cool spray/cryotherapy; bite guards; and splints. Surgery should be a last resort when dealing with TMJ problems.

Nutritional Supplements

Nutritional supplements may help in treating TMJ problems. Some of the most useful:

CALCIUM AND MAGNESIUM. These minerals are essential for proper muscular function and have a sedative effect.

B-COMPLEX VITAMINS. Take 100 mg, 3 times a day.

PANTOTHENIC ACID. 100 mg, twice daily. B-complex vitamins and pantothenic acid are essential for combating stress.

COENZYME Q10. This is another stress fighter.

L-TYROSINE AND VITAMINS B6 AND C. These will improve sleep quality and alleviate anxiety and depression.

MULTIVITAMIN AND MINERAL COMPLEX.

On the Research Front

Additional therapies that have proven helpful in relieving temporomandibular joint dysfunction in studies are acupuncture; biofeedback in combination with intraoral appliances; progressive relaxation training; and isokinetic exercise. Another natural remedy is Euphytose, a mixture of plant extracts, including *Passiflora incarnata*, *Valeriana officialis*, and *Cola nitida*.

28

Chiropractic

I t is no secret that some members of the medical establishment in this country have been trying to eliminate the chiropractic alternative ever since it emerged as a major healing modality and increasingly since it became the chief rival of traditional medical care. Chiropractic is second only to orthodox medicine as the preferred provider of primary health care. Threatened by what it perceived to be a challenge to its professional exclusivity, established medicine determined to get rid of this menace or at least keep it as far away from mainstream health care institutions as possible.

Despite these concentrated, tightly organized, and well-funded efforts to malign and discredit chiropractic, it continues to thrive. During an 11-year court battle with the American Medical Association (AMA) that began in 1976 and was finally settled on August 28, 1987 (more information about the case appears later on in this chapter), it was argued that chiropractic is not an unscientific cult but rather is a drug-free, surgery-free health care system based on the hypothesis that disease can be caused by displacements (which chiropractors call subluxations) of the spinal vertebrae. These subluxations can impinge on the nerves and disrupt their normal functioning. The court decision affirmed that chiropractors are fully qualified to adjust the skeletal system.

Currently, between 50,000 and 65,000 chiropractors in the United States are treating an estimated 20 to 30 million patients a year, about 30 percent of the population as a whole. The government's statistics on worker's compensation cases show that chiropractic medicine offers the best care for back and neck injuries. Chiropractors get their patients back on the job twice as fast as medical doctors on average. Chiropractors can help with most musculoskeletal disorders involving mechanical dysfunction.

Besides describing chiropractic treatment, this chapter includes a look at the politics of the AMA's court-documented war against chiropractic care.

How Chiropractic Works

Chiropractic treatment involves the manual manipulation of vertebrae that become misaligned, causing nerve pressure and energy blocks to various organs. This manipulation is called an adjustment. It involves the chiropractor's gentle and painless application of direct pressure to the spine and joints. The chiropractor may squeeze or twist the torso, pull or twist the limbs, or wrench the head or back. What the chiropractor is doing is readjusting the spinal column to restore the normal relationship of one vertebra to another. This eliminates the body's energy blocks and keeps life-sustaining energy flowing freely to the vital organs.

Chiropractic is effective in dealing with pain and as a preventive treatment because it relieves nerve pressure as the spine is properly adjusted. The buildup of this pressure is cumulative in its erosion of the health and integrity of specific body organs or regions. If one vertebra is out of relationship to the one next to it, a state of disrelationship is said to exist. This disrelationship throws off that vertebra's environment, that is, the blood supply and detoxifying lymphatic drainage surrounding it. When this occurs, a congestion of blood, toxins, and energy creates pressure that upsets both local and systemic homeostasis, or balance.

Tissues all need normal nerve functioning in order to transport required nutrients to the cells. Insofar as the vertebrae are misaligned, the blood becomes congested and slow in its delivery, creating the absence of this nutrient supply. The cell's normal activity is thereby hindered, and it becomes irritated. Moreover, once the cell's metabolic processing is interfered with, its waste-removing lymphatic servicing to that area is diminished. This leads to toxic buildup that causes further irritation and inflammation. The chiropractor is concerned with alleviating all these problems.

The Battle Against Chiropractic

Despite the success that chiropractic has had in relieving pain and chronic disorders, for more than a quarter of a century the medical establishment has bullied this licensed profession into having to defend itself as if it were a subversive activity. The main reason for this attack appears to have been the desire to ensure the traditional medical doctor the top spot on the ladder of licensed healing professionals. Chiropractors pose a serious threat to this coveted role since, as a federal court judge pointed out, the leaders of established medicine were well "aware that some medical physicians believed chiropractic to be effective and that chiropractors were better trained to deal with musculoskeletal problems than most medical physicians." This is especially scary to medical doctors since they know very little about the musculoskeletal system even though it constitutes nearly two-thirds of the human body.

Unfortunately, this long-standing attempt to inhibit free competition in health care has left countless numbers of people who could be relieved of pain confused and therefore hesitant about going to doctors of chiropractic. Moreover, because chiropractic care often is not covered by major health insurance companies, it looms as a financial burden to many. Even though it is far cheaper, it is frequently not covered by insurance policies, and so the final out-of-pocket expense to the consumer tends to be higher than the cost of far more expensive traditional medical care which is covered by insurance carriers. The administrative law judge of the Federal Trade Commission (FTC) ruled in 1982 that the AMA—the largest medical trade association in the nation, representing the interests of half the 660,000 medical doctors—had created "a formidable impediment to competition in the delivery of health care services by physicians in this country. That barrier has served to deprive consumers of the free flow of information about the availability of health care services, to deter the offering of innovative forms of health care and to stifle the rise of almost every type of health care delivery that could potentially pose a threat to the income of fee-for-service physicians in private practice. The costs to the public in terms of less expensive or even, perhaps, more improved forms of medical service are great."

This chapter will give some of the basic information about chiropractic care that has been withheld from the public, but first it is necessary to review the rocky road that chiropractic has had to travel in order to be recognized as the highly effective health care provider that it is.

HOW IT BEGAN The AMA was so bent on destroying the reputation of the doctor of chiropractic that in 1963 it formed its own Committee on Quackery almost exclusively toward that end. Shortly thereafter a flood of press releases hit the media; their goal was the total condemnation of chiropractic. *In the Public Interest*, anonymously published in 1972, contained an alleged AMA document which outlined the Committee on Quackery's chief goal: to contain and eliminate chiropractic. Since this attitude and the actions issuing from it were clearly intent on the blatant restraint of trade, a small group of chiropractors decided to fight back. They formed the National Chiropractic Antitrust Committee to fund litigation to help expose this conspiracy. It will be shown later in this chapter how such a legal action was initiated in the United States District Court in Chicago in 1976.

Meanwhile, the AMA maintained its assault on chiropractic by working to deny state-licensed doctors of chiropractic the same hospital privileges that medical doctors enjoyed, and by trying everything feasible to keep chiropractic colleges from being accredited by state medical organizations, while campaigning actively against the inclusion of chiropractic programs in accredited colleges and universities.

A major complaint against chiropractic is that chiropractors rarely research and publish their findings as medical doctors do. Publishing often entails presenting one's findings at a conference of peers to open dialogue and invite constructive criticism, but chiropractors were denied the right to convene with medical doctors on a professional basis in associations or to present research or clinical findings at cooperative meetings. A case in point is a seminar that was arranged by the workmen's compensation board in Oregon. The purpose was to entertain different ideas from health care providers that might help reduce the pain and discomfort of industrial accident victims while accelerating their return to work. Those in attendance were assured by the sponsoring medical societies that they would receive educational credit toward mandated license renewal.

When it was learned that the board had invited a chiropractor to speak, the Multnomah County Medical Society and the Oregon State Medical Society, the sponsors of the event, reneged on their support. They spread the word that attendees would not get education credit after all. Why? Because a single representative from a licensed profession known for years to offer the most effective treatment for industrial injuries was invited to share his experience on the subject.

In a similar situation, Dr. Philip R. Weinstein, a neurologist practicing in California, was pressured into ceasing his efforts to cooperate with doctors of chiropractic for the benefit of both professions as well as that of patients suffering from spinal disorders. Dr. Weinstein had frequently lectured to chiropractors on the diagnosis of such ailments before he came to realize that the AMA was strongly opposed to such cooperative action. He decided to back off from lecturing to chiropractors, explaining to one such group that "this late cancellation [of a scheduled lecture] is due to circumstances beyond our control. We were unaware that delivering medical lectures to your [organization] was prohibited." (Null, "The War Against Chiropractic," *Penthouse*, October, 1986.)

ATTACKS AGAINST THE EDUCATIONAL BASE OF CHIROPRACTIC The AMA's attempt to destroy the educational base of chiropractic went much deeper than this sort of harassment. In 1962 attorney Robert Throckmorton authored a master plan eventually put into action by the AMA, representing its general approach to "the chiropractic menace." The plan proposed attacking chiropractic on many fronts. Referring to the chiropractic schools, it states: "To the extent that [the schools'] financial problems continue to multiply, and to the extent that the schools are unsuccessful in their recruiting programs, the chiropractic menace of the future will be reduced and possibly eliminated."

To ensure that chiropractic's financial and recruiting problems multiplied, the AMA tried to keep the government from granting student loans to prospective chiropractors and research-teaching grants to faculty members. It also fought to keep chiropractic schools from receiving accreditation. It bitterly complained that chiropractic schools were being operated without proper accreditation while at the same time vehemently opposing the creation of proper state accrediting bodies. To its dismay, national accreditation finally came in 1974 when the U.S. Health, Education and Welfare Department sanctioned the Council on Chiropractic Education to meet this need.

The AMA also fought to keep chiropractic programs out of universities. The idea here was to keep chiropractic in isolation, away from mainstream educational health care institutions. The AMA could then point a finger at chiropractic as being substandard because of its lack of affiliation with these same institutions.

In the early 1970s, when C. W. Post University entertained notions of teaching prechiropractic students, pressure was brought to bear. Dr. Ernest R. Jaffe, acting dean of Albert Einstein College of Medicine of Yeshiva University, wrote to the school: "I urge you to take all appropriate measures to terminate any relationship with the Lincoln College of Chiropractic. It can only bring discredit to your university." C. W. Post backed off and refused to offer chiropractic instruction. Even today, chiropractic instruction is not available at C.W. Post.

The University of Illinois was urged to discriminate against students and state-licensed doctors of chiropractic by the chairman of the board of trustees of the Illinois State Medical Society. In January 1974 he wrote to the executive dean of the University of Illinois College of Medicine about the AMA's displeasure at learning that the college had collaborated with the National College of Chiropractic on an educational television program. He warned: "Any time chiropractors can gain a foothold by reporting on collaboration with the Medical Center, it will give them status. It might be wise to prohibit any contact of any kind at any time by persons at the Medical Center with any chiropractor. You might wish to discuss this with others who have been involved in this problem."

DENIAL OF HOSPITAL PRIVILEGES To further deny status to chiropractors, the AMA has fought bitterly over the last 30 or so years to keep them out of hospitals. If chiropractors were given hospital privileges, and if they could operate programs within universities, how could the AMA continue to argue that their educational and professional status was substandard?

The late Dr. Irvine Hendryson, an orthopedic surgeon and onetime professor of surgery at the University of Colorado, had been a trustee of the AMA. He was concerned with the mechanical problems that give women such pain and discomfort in the final stages of pregnancy and during childbirth. These problems are often caused by the dislocation of vertebrae resulting from the heavy burden of carrying the fetus and the strain involved in delivering it. In a report that was ultimately suppressed by the Committee on Quackery, Dr. Hendryson wrote:

"It is commonly known that in the third trimester of pregnancy, unrelenting, unmitigated back pain is one of the prices that is paid for perpetuation of the race. I have learned from personal experience that general manipulations of backs in this particular condition have given these women a great deal of physical relief and has permitted them to go on to term and deliver without having to be bedridden during the latter term of pregnancy.

"I would not for an instant indicate that it is manipulation alone that permits these women to go on and carry on normally, for at the present time we are giving them manipulation to relieve them of their acute symptoms and also fitting them with support, which is well recognized in medical practice. However, I must say that I am impressed by the many cases who are able to go on to term, to manage their households, to lead a comparatively comfortable third trimester without having to be hospitalized or given traction, heat, support, and all the rest of it."

Because this information would lend status and credibility and possibly even give hospital privileges to chiropractors, it was withheld. The AMA took control of hospital policy toward chiropractic through its power over the Joint Committee on Accreditation of Hospitals (JCAH). Without accreditation, a hospital stands to lose its "internship and residency programs, its nursing affiliations, and its automatic check-off for direct insurance payments. Its malpractice insurance rates would soar, and the interest on its financial bonds for building would probably increase."

The threat of withholding or "reviewing" accreditation became an effective means of limiting chiropractic presence in hospitals. This is clearly illustrated in a letter of August 1974 from the JCAH to a hospital administrator: "Any arrangement you would make with chiropractors and your hospital would be unacceptable to the Joint Commission. This would be in violation of the Principles of Medical Ethics published by the American Medical Association that is also a requirement of the Joint Commission on Accreditation of Hospitals." Even more blatantly, in January 1973 the JCAH supplied this information to a hospital in Silver City, New Mexico: "This is an answer to your letter of December 18 referring to a bill which may be passed in New Mexico that hospitals must accept chiropractors as members of the medical staff. You are absolutely correct—the unfortunate results of this most ill-advised legislation would be that the Joint Commission could withdraw and refuse accreditation of the hospital that had chiropractors on its medical staff."

CHIROPRACTORS FIGHT BACK In an effort to return health care to the public and take it out of the clutches of the AMA and the medical physicians, litigation was finally initiated on October 12, 1976. Five chiropractors filed a 38-page complaint in the United States District Court in Chicago. They charged among other things that the AMA had masterminded a years-long conspiracy aimed at isolating, containing, and eliminating its chief health care rival—chiropractic. This conspiracy included fostering a general boycott of chiropractors, discriminating against them in public institutions such as hospitals and universities, manipulating government studies on the efficacy of their practice, and directly pressuring insurance companies to deny chiropractic patients coverage similar to that offered for health care sanctioned by the AMA.

The case was a costly one for the plaintiffs, involving travel, legal expenses, and many hours away from their practices. It took over four years to gather evidence before the trial finally began on December 8, 1980. But as the evidence was presented it became clear that the AMA had operated for years in restraint of trade. It had even manipulated Congress. For instance, a 1967 "impartial" congressional study to determine whether chiropractic should be covered by Medicare was tainted by the ever-present influence of the AMA, a clearly biased party. Doyle Taylor, secretary to the AMA Committee on Quackery, wrote to Dr. Samuel Sherman, the AMA representative on the congressional committee, "I am sure you agree that the AMA hand must not 'show' at this stage of the proposed chiropractic study." Five months before the study even began, Dr. Sherman already was reporting to Taylor on the nature of its results. "Dear Doyle," he wrote in March 1968, "There was complete acceptance of the concept of preparing the decision on the basis of lack of scientific merit."

After reviewing the evidence in detail, the court finally rendered its decision in August 1987. Judge Susan Getzendanner ruled that the AMA and its co-conspirators, the American College of Surgeons and the American College of Radiology, had conspired to isolate and eliminate the profession of chiropractic and that in the process they had violated the Sherman Antitrust Law. The American Academy of Orthopedic Surgeons was found to have been a part of the conspiracy until 1986, when it backed away. The American Hospital Association, the Illinois State Medical Society, the American Osteopathic Association, and the American Academy of Physical Medicine and Rehabilitation all settled with the chiropractors before the case ended by agreeing to cease their harassment of chiropractic. However, it was ruled that there was insufficient evidence to convict the JCAH or the ACP.

Judge Getzendanner, in her decision, offered this opinion:

"I conclude that an injunction is necessary in this case. There are lingering effects of the conspiracy: the AMA has never acknowledged the lawlessness of its past conduct and in fact to this day maintains that it has always been in compliance with the antitrust laws; there has never been an affirmative statement by the AMA that it is ethical to associate with chiropractors; there has never been a public statement to AMA members of the admissions made in this court about the improved nature of chiropractic despite the fact that the AMA today claims that it made changes in its policy in recognition of the change and improvement in chiropractic; there has never been public retraction of articles such as "The Right and Duty of Hospitals to Deny Chiropractor Access to Hospitals"; a medical physician has to very carefully read the current AMA Judicial Council Opinions to realize that there has been a change in the treatment of chiropractors and the court cannot assume that members of the AMA pore over these opinions; and finally, the systematic, long-term wrong-doing and the long-term intent to destroy a licensed profession suggests that an injunction is appropriate in this case. When all of these factors are considered in the context of this 'private attorney general' antitrust suit, a proper exercise of the court's discretion permits, and in my judgment requires, an injunction."

VICTORY FOR THE PUBLIC AS WELL AS THE PROFESSION The plaintiffs in the case saw the decision as a victory for the American public as well as for the chiropractic profession. Dr. Patricia Arthur, for instance, believes that the extraordinary cost of health care is due largely to a lack of fair competition in the health care industry. She says, "The nation is headed toward a $1.4 trillion annual health care budget. Each person in the country will be expending more than $3,900 per year on health care costs. Chiropractic is a low-cost substitute for certain segments of medical care. That is the result of a monopoly in the health care field centered around the AMA."

Another plaintiff, Dr. Chester A. Wilk, thought the decision long overdue: "Eleven years of litigation have demonstrated the folly of allowing the AMA, whose primary purpose for existence is the economic interest of medical physicians, to sit in judgment on control of any other licensed health care provider...Every sick person and every taxpayer in this country has suffered because of the actions of the AMA."

J. F. McAndrews, D.C., former president of the largest chiropractic college in the United States, agreed that this decision was long overdue, and that its delay caused unnecessary suffering: "As an educator and administrator I spent almost 25 years combating the despicable actions of the AMA now declared to be illegal by the court. How many students, patients, and professionals have had to suffer from the AMA's folly? Perhaps now the government will listen when we point out the corrupt power exercised by the AMA. Perhaps now the people of the United States can get cooperative care from all segments of the health care spectrum."

CURRENT STATUS OF CHIROPRACTIC While chiropractic is still far from being accepted as a part of standard health care, it attracts more patients now than ever before and is more accepted than ever before by the mainstream medical community. There are now about 20 chiropractic colleges nationwide and chiropractors can get licensed in all 50 states. Some liberal arts colleges offer undergraduate degrees in chiropractic, and additionally, some facilities at member hospitals of the American Hospital Association have been opened to chiropractors. Now that chiropractic care finally seems to be on the verge of much broader acceptance than it has ever enjoyed in the United States, it is appropriate to consider more carefully how it can help in the treatment and prevention of various human ailments.

Types of Chiropractic Treatment

There are two basic types of chiropractors: the "straight" chiropractors, who employ chiefly manipulation of the spinal vertebrae in treating disorders, and the "mixers," who in addition to this counsel their patients on different aspects of diet, stress control, and exercise as it pertains to particular problems and to the overall health profile.

Chiropractic considers the body to be a whole, natural organism that possesses its own healing capabilities. These capabilities may be interfered with when the spine is out of place. The movement or shifting of vertebrae creates local nerve pressure, which in turn may block the energy going throughout the system and the organs that correspond to particular vertebrae. The energy interference resulting from improper spinal alignment throws off the whole body. It upsets the body's balance and harmony, or what is called its homeostasis. When one body part begins to malfunction, it is compensated for automatically by another body part, but this compensating body part may then become overstressed. For instance, a weakness in the heart may cause an overstress of the lungs, which are forced to work overtime to bring in extra oxygen to make up for the oxygen loss from the reduced circulation resulting from the heart's weakness. This can cause a chain reaction effect which can continue indefinitely until the entire body system becomes unbalanced, weak, and prone to further degenerative diseases.

It is good that the body is an interrelated organism, because one part can come to the aid of another as when the lungs help the liver. However, this compensatory feature of whole-body mechanics also means that meticulous care must be taken to make sure that every part is in prime condition to avoid a damaging drain on other parts. The longer a person learns to tolerate nerve dysfunction instead of relieving it, the more problems will accumulate that will begin to impinge on one region after another. Morton Jacobs, D.C., who has been practicing for over a quarter of a century, notes that "if you can minimize or eliminate any type of nerve pressure in your body, you can eliminate any type of body dysfunctions, and therefore you can maintain a higher function, a higher level of adaptability of health and function in your body. That's why chiropractic adjustments are very good for preventive care."

Besides its use as preventive treatment, chiropractic care can also be very helpful in relieving acute pain as well as chronic disorders. Dr. Jacobs states that this is possible because chiropractic does not overwhelm the body as drugs and other methods may. It simply and naturally restores the body's natural ability to heal itself.

Treating Bursitis

A condition with which chiropractors have had considerable success is bursitis, a chronic pain that is actually an inflammation of the bursal sac which cushions every body joint. It can cause severe, ongoing pain in the neck, shoulders, hip, and lower back. The inflammation can be caused by a physical trauma to the joint, as when a person lifts something too heavy or too quickly. It may also result from a bacterial infection or an allergy. Whatever the cause, the site of the irritation becomes extremely painful since the bursal sac has many tiny nerve endings.

The most common place bursitis appears is in the neck and shoulders. The chiropractor will try to locate a pinched nerve in this area and then apply ice to it to reduce the blood congestion and swelling resulting from poor circulation and deficient lymphatic drainage in that location. This will enhance circulation and lymphatic drainage. According to Dr. Jacobs, the ice is followed by the application of moist heat to relax and expand constricted muscles, allowing better blood supply into the area and helping to "regulate the environment of that tissue so it has the ability to start repairing." It should be mentioned here that dry heat should not be used since it creates a thickening and congesting of the blood; this may cause a condition known as hyperemia, or blood blockage.

Rest and exercise follow the ice and heat treatments. Rest gives the joint time and the relaxed environment it needs to repair itself. Exercise, including joint exercise or "cracking" (as in cracking the knuckles), stimulates circulation into the joints while relaxing congestion, fixations (misalignments of the vertebrae causing trauma and/or spasm), and energy blockages.

Treating Arthritis

Arthritis is another condition with which chiropractors have had good success. This condition is often brought on by some sort of allergy, which in turn stimulates the creation of an inflammatory agent that causes swelling, tightness, and pain in the joints. Chiropractic adjustments help stimulate the body's enzymatic, metabolic, and nervous systems. This gives the body the ability to deal better with the allergen and to begin repairing the damage that has already been done.

The tissue or joint directly affected by arthritis is treated in much the same way as bursitis; ice, moist heat, and exercise. Additionally, soft tissue manipulation, or "milking," may force out toxins and wastes while stimulating better blood supply to the joint. Milking also increases joint movement and rotation.

This again represents a nontoxic intervention that can help the body re-establish a homeostatic balance without the side effects of drugs. While they may help reduce blood pressure and swelling and help manage pain, the drugs commonly used for arthritis do not treat the condition at its source. They also adversely affect the body's essential functions and processes in several ways. They may, for instance, interfere with vitamin and mineral absorption, so that a whole new set of physical problems will eventually arise from this situation.

Managing Stress

Stress is a major contributor to most of the ailments a chiropractor is able to treat. The treatment is done partly by helping the patient release this stress. Pinched nerves or energy blockage from pressure brought to bear on nerve areas may be the direct result of stress. It is important to understand why this is so and what a chiropractor can do about it.

The autonomic nervous system, which controls involuntary body functions and mechanics, is divided into the sympathetic and parasympathetic systems. The autonomic nervous system is important because all the vital functions and overall state of health are under its control. Heartbeat, the rate of blood flow, breathing, hormone and enzyme secretion, and so forth are all managed without conscious input by the autonomic nervous system.

The parasympathetic nervous system represents the normal, well-coordinated, balanced functioning of these vital processes. The sympathetic nervous system, though, is called into play when this harmony has been disrupted and special bodily reactions are required to meet specific situations. The sympathetic nervous system can be described by what is called the fight-or-flight syndrome; when an organism perceives a direct threat to its existence, it must temporarily and spontaneously interrupt all other body functions so that the crisis may be met by all the body's available resources. It must actively resist this danger (the fight response), or it must do everything possible to avoid it (the flight response). Either way, the integrity and harmony of the organism may be restored and the parasympathetic nervous system may resume its normal ordering of those physiological processes which ordinarily sustain life as the sympathetic system retires from the arena.

However, if the sympathetic nervous system is called into action too frequently, the body may suffer from a chronic depletion of its vital energies, and its effort to maintain a state of homeostasis will be negated. Stress is a primary engager of the sympathetic mechanism. Feelings such as fear, anger, jealousy, and extreme emotional episodes call the sympathetic system, which normally is not needed, into play. When these stressors become chronic reactions or coping mechanisms, stress syndromes may evolve. In this case, certain target organs are most likely to be fatigued and exhausted as a result of the overactivity of excessively stimulated glands, usually the adrenal, thymus, and digestive glands.

Even when stress is not chronic, the body's internal harmony is disrupted spontaneously by hyperactive emotions and responses to circumstances and events. If you are angered by a nuisance phone call, for instance, your heart rate is immediately altered, your blood pressure rises as the vascular system constricts, and your normal digestion may cease, allowing stomach acids to harm the inner stomach wall. If you are always angry, these occurrences will become common or even regular as you begin to suffer from a chronically-imbalanced body mechanism.

A chiropractor may release stress centers and sites of energy blockage for temporary relief, but more important is a review and modification of the patient's overall lifestyle. The chiropractor may suggest such things as yoga, transcendental meditation, and regular exercise as ways to learn to mellow one's reactions to daily problems and confrontations. Meanwhile, the chiropractor can help the body with regular adjustments to keep it in relative harmony, with a free energy flow. This will, in effect, defuse the sympathetic nervous response and allow the parasympathetic mechanism to resume its task of maintaining the body's vital functions and harmony.

Treating Musculoskeletal Disorders

In general, chiropractic is most helpful in treating musculoskeletal disorders. Back pain may be caused by emotional stress, while curvature of the spine may result from physical stress. In either case, the stressor creates nerve pressure that throws off first the spinal alignment and eventually specific bodily functions. Adjustments are helpful here, especially when combined with stress-management counseling and exercise programs.

Exercise to keep the muscles strong and resilient is critical because muscles move bones and thus protect the skeletal system and afford it mobility and ease of activity. Physical or emotional stress in turn may render the muscular system fatigued, spastic, and tight. When this happens, joints—specifically the spinal vertebrae—are more readily misaligned and a disrelationship results.

Muscles must be kept strong through exercise to support the skeletal system against the negative gravitational pull everyone lives with. This is why weakened muscles will lead to poor body posture. This structural attitude will ultimately have an impact on the internal organs, putting undue weight and physical pressure on them. Exercise, then, counters fatigue. It stimulates such vital functions as elimination and respiration, both of which require ease and fluidity of internal body movement and function. Since stress and exercise are so tightly interwoven, the chiropractor will do a thorough stress evaluation before giving the patient a specific exercise program. If it is not done properly, and in conjunction with one's general health and state of mind, exercise can lead to chronic and debilitating injury. Done right, it will promote the establishment of a healthy metabolism, burn intramuscular fat, and slow the body's aging process.

Choosing a Chiropractor

There are things to be mindful of when selecting chiropractic care. Chiropractic manipulation is not indicated as a primary treatment for degenerative diseases, although it can be a valuable adjunct to more direct therapies. Fractures and degenerative lesions such as joint or bone cancer may be exacerbated by chiropractic treatment, and such treatment should be avoided in these instances. Acute trauma, such as whiplash, may also contraindicate chiropractic treatment.

When chiropractic care is to be employed, take notice of the following: What type of chiropractor are you choosing? A straight chiropractor may be fine for a disorder such as an injury requiring only manipulative adjustment. A mixer may be preferred for an internal problem that can also benefit from lifestyle, stress, dietary, and exercise counseling.

Whichever type of chiropractor you choose, be sure you are not put through needless, extensive, and expensive batteries of tests. Blood tests, hair analysis, x-rays, cytotoxic tests, allergy tests, and other diagnostic procedures may be needed, but they should be decided upon only after a full, thorough medical history has been taken. The history should include a survey of subjective attitudes, exercise and dietary habits, and a full symptomatic report. Once this background has been established, the chiropractor may prudently offer the patient selective testing based on what seems to be needed.

Chiropractic care has been available for nearly a century, but its potential as a primary and adjunctive health care modality is only beginning to be understood. The recent court ruling showing that chiropractic has for years been maligned and conspired against by the AMA and others should also help pave the way for placing this type of treatment in a better perspective. Chiropractic care is not right for every condition, but it is very effective for many. As a preventive, it may be among the best types of health care available.

29

Pain Management

E very day tens of millions of Americans wake up knowing they are going to contend with pain, whether it be from arthritis, musculoskeletal problems, or a variety of other aches. Many do not realize that there are varied ways of treating pain naturally.

In this country we need a different approach to acute and chronic pain. We need to go from treating just the symptoms to treating the sufferer holistically through a mind/body approach.

Getting the proper nutrition through sensible eating and ingesting natural supplements, such as minerals and herbs, are key ways of treating pain, though other methods, such as the Trager technique, shiatsu and acupuncture also have a part to play. In this chapter, we survey a broad range of healing strategies that can be used by anyone suffering from chronic or occasional pain.

Herbal Remedies

Herbs eliminate pain by dealing with the underlying causes. In chapter 15, we spoke at length on the way herbs can be used to deal with different health problems. We stressed how herbs help stimulate the immune system. We mentioned the theory that our DNA may carry an immunological memory, grounded in our inherited knowledge of the efficacy of plants. In this section, we will add a little to what we have said so far by suggesting some uses of herbs to lessen or do away with pain.

There are different types of pain. Some are inflammatory, hot and pounding. Some are due to toxins in the body that need to be cleansed. Proper herbal treatment can assist the body to do away with both the pain and the causes of this pain.

For women, herbalist Letha Hadady offers the following recommendations: We must approach the pain of PMS (pre-menstrual syndrome) from both the emotional and physical sides. Emotionally, there are two types of PMS. One is the angry type. Aloe root is recommended for this. It cleans the system and cleanses the liver. It may taste a little bitter, but it is easy to take when added to a little apple juice.

A stronger gall bladder and liver cleanser that lessens the impact of menstrual pains is the Chinese preparation *Lung Tanxieganwan*—20 percent ginseng, it aids digestion and reduces anger. It also calms and quiets headaches and other pains.

The second type of PMS is weepy. It comes from sadness and excess phlegm, brought on by eating foods that are too rich, too sweet, and too oily, or by drinking too much milk. Eating radishes, parsley, or barley soup will cut down on the phlegm. A remedy for this type of pain is homeopathic Pulsatilla.

To treat the pain of both types of menstruation, warming herbs like cinnamon and myrrh are invaluable. Capsules or drops taken in tea will increase blood circulation and clean the uterus, inducing a more complete period; one that does not start too early, stay too long, or finish early only to begin prematurely. A warming and cooling remedy for the pain is as follows:

½ cup aloe vera gel

10 drops or one capsule myrrh

apple juice

This combines the cleaning action of myrrh with the cooling of aloe.

Vitamins, Minerals, and Other Supplements

Previously in this book, we discussed how minerals are essential for building up the body, maintaining the body's fluid balance and helping with many chemical reactions. Now, we look more narrowly at how minerals and vitamins have proved effective in treating pain.

Dr. Luke Bucci, author of *Pain Free: The Definitive Guide to Healing Arthritis*, states that for handling spinal column disorder, carpal tunnel syndrome, or arthritis, an antidepressant may prove helpful. Carpal tunnel syndrome occurs when, because of repetitive tasks, the tendons in the wrist are inflamed, which squeezes the nerves, which then tingle and go numb. About one third of the cases of this syndrome can be cured by the administration of B_6 (100 mg/day) to which can be added B_2 (50 mg/day). To deal with the pain of the condition, one should take St. John's wort (*hypericum perforatum*). This substance has a molecule that works like a pharmaceutical drug without any of the drawbacks or side effects.

Magnesium salts are also useful for those facing pain from torso or joint aches. Many people are already deficient in magnesium. It is a calmative mineral, obtained from nuts and seeds that are raw and unroasted. Nuts are also beneficial in that they contain essential oils, including the omega-3 fatty acids, which also have mild anti-inflammatory properties that help reduce pain.

For torso and joint problems, the dosage of magnesium (citrate) salts should be 400 mg/day, divided into doses of 100 to 200 mg each.

Sound sleep is an essential part of good health. For those people who have trouble sleeping due to headaches or other pains, there are a number of useful supplements. Valerian can be used or hops (the same element found in beer), skullcap, or passion flower. These supplements, which can be mixed, should be taken one half hour before sleep, in either capsule or tincture form, in a dosage of one or two capsules. One might also try taking 1 mg of melatonin before sleep.

For the pain arising from PMS, GLA (gamma linolenic acid) is valuable. It can be obtained from evening primrose oil, black currant seed oil, or borrage oil. The sufferer should take three to six pills per day. As an adjunct to GLA, vitamin E is helpful. Also to be taken is B_6 (100 mg/day) and magnesium, which smoothes muscle contractions.

Here, as with all vitamin therapy, the patient must be consistent, following through on taking the supplements for two or three months to be assured of the effects.

The pain of sciatica, or pinched nerve, can be reduced by lowering the inflammation at the nerve root. Here one should try a proteolytic enzyme, such as bromolone, papain, trypsin, or chymotrypsin to support the body's natural healing properties.

Muscular skeletal pain, which may be due to too much lactic acid, can be removed by a number of substances. L-carnitine allows the body to burn fats and soak up excess lactate. Also helpful with muscles are the methyl donors, such as DMG (di-methyl glycine) and TMG (tri-methyl glycerin), taken at a rate of 100 mg/day.

To reduce the soreness after exercise, one should take vitamin E (400-800 IU/day), which prevents the leakage of enzymes from the muscles.

A final way to approach pain is to modify the way the brain perceives it. DLPA (D.L. Phenylalanine), which is a synthetic form of amino acid, slows down endorphins, making the ones you have work better. Taken in a dosage of 500 mg/three times a day, it reduces chronic pain while getting the sufferer off analgesics.

Thus, there are many ways to nutritionally enhance the body without using pharmaceuticals that overwhelm the receptors.

Shiatsu

Shiatsu is based on the principle that a vital energy, called *qi* (chi), flows through the body. The primary cause of pain is imbalance of this energy. The goal of the healer is to balance the client's energy so pain and discomfort do not manifest or, if they do appear, will be relieved.

As Thomas Claire, a body work practitioner, explains, in performing shiatsu, he use thumbs, fingers, palms, forearms, elbows, and even knees to apply pressure to specified points in the body to modulate the flow of energy. During a shiatsu treatment, the client lies on the floor on a comfortable padded surface, such as a futon, fully clothed or undressed to his or her level of comfort. What the client feels is pressure, which can be gentle or deeper at the places where the practitioner is working. As the pressure continues, the patient will generally feel relaxed and energized at the same time.

Shiatsu is good for treating a variety of different pains. It is especially beneficial in combating chronic pain that may be found in the back, neck, or shoulders but it has also proved effective in treating whiplash, herniated disk, and nervous problems, such as Bell's palsy.

The shiatsu healer concentrates work on certain pressure points that have metaphoric names that tell us something of what they do or how they are to be worked with.

The first point of interest is on the ankle and called Spleen 6. It is at the meeting of three yin meridians and is the most powerful point for tonifying the feminine energy in the body. It can be located by placing the little finger on the border of your inside ankle and counting up four fingers. At the very top of these fingers, and at the center, is Spleen 6. To modulate the energy, you can put pressure on this point with your thumb, pushing three times in succession for 7 to 10 seconds each time. This pressure will stimulate the feminine energy, helping a woman control PMS and irregular cycles. Moreover, since all of us have feminine and masculine sides, use of this point can also be beneficial to men and can help with sexual problems such as impotence.

The corresponding point for male tonification is called Stomach 36. To locate this point, find the indentation just outside the kneecap. Put one finger at this indentation and go down four fingers. There you'll find Stomach 36, which is also known as Leg 3 Mile. This second name is given since, it is said, if you have a strong Stomach 36, you can walk three miles with no trouble due to your strong stamina. Manipulation of this point can lead to a tonification of masculine energy as well as the whole body. For women, this point can be used to ease childbirth and labor pains.

A third important point, located at the middle of the web of the hand, is Large Intestine 4, also called Meeting Mountains. This latter denomination comes from the "mountain of flesh" found jutting up between the thumb and index finger when you close your hand. To locate this point, find the highest point on that protruding flesh, then open your hand. This point should also be pressed three times running for 7 to 10 seconds in order to tonify the upper body. Pressing this point can also help with nausea, vomiting, colds, and constipation.

Pericardium 6, or the Inner Gate, is found on the forearm. If you flex your hand, you'll find two tendons that pop up on the inside of your wrist. Go up these tendons and press. This point is particularly good for controlling nausea (such as that from morning sickness or motion sickness).

Another valuable point is found right in the middle of the palm. Pressing it can relieve tension like that arising from a stressful work environment or relationship.

Runny nose, allergy, colds, and sinus infections can be treated by pressure on the point called Welcome Smell, so named since nearly any smell is welcome to a person whose nasal passages have been blocked. To approach this point, take the index finger and bring it in at a 45 degree angle to the crease under the nose. This pressure can be applied on either side of the nose though it is not recommended that both sides be touched simultaneously, which might block breathing.

In fact, all these pressures can be applied to either side of the body, since the meridians are bilateral and bring the same energies to each side of the body.

Acupuncture

Like shiatsu, acupuncture sees pain as derived from blocked energy or *qi* (chi). In treating this blockage, the practitioner has to determine whether it stems from an overabundance or deficiency in energy, so the treatment can be adjusted depending on whether it is necessary to strengthen or decrease qi.

The acupuncturist first records the patient's medical history in the manner of a conventional doctor. Then, with the patient lying down or seated, depending on the area to be treated, fine-gauge, stainless steel needles are inserted into significant points and meridians to exert different physiological effects on the body and induce both relaxation and energization. The patient will remain in this position from 20 to 30 minutes, though an appointment with an acupuncturist may last up to an hour, since part of the time will be spent consulting about the employment of other traditional and herbal treatments that might be recommended. Body work and massage might also be included in the session.

Dr. Christopher Trahan notes that the treatment will have analgesic and anesthetic effects, will block pain, and accelerate recovery from motor nerve injury. Moreover, it enhances the immune system, can have a sedative effect, help with muscular spasms or neurological problems, have a homeostatic effect so as to balance blood pressure, and have psychological effects, acting directly on brain chemistry.

If we look specifically at what acupuncture treats, we would have to mention muscular, skeletal and structural problems of the body, arthritis, TMJ, carpal tunnel syndrome, insomnia, asthma, headaches, digestive problems, such as ulcers and irritable bowels, menstrual cramps, and pleurisy.

Trager Technique

The Trager technique is a way of working with the mind and body simultaneously. According to the philosophy backing up this technique, pain comes from the accumulated action of the patient frequently tightening his or her movements and posture. To correct it, the practitioner uses gentle motions to increase the patient's pleasure in the quality of the tissues and decrease the restriction and the sense of holding. The practice works by reaching into the functional subconscious with particular qualities of movement, posture, and sensation. Gentleness is emphasized so that no message will be sent to the body alerting it that pain is on the way or causing the patient to tighten in on him or herself. The movement reaches into the central nervous system with a motion at once pleasurable, lengthening, softening and opening, conveying this sensation to the tissues and joints. The movements can be very small and internal or at the peripheries of the body in the limbs. In the latter case, the limbs are used as handles to reach the core.

Roger Tolle, a Trager practitioner, says some clients will feel results immediately as the touching allows them to release pain. In other cases, it takes a repetition of the information into the body/mind, which will gradually allow the client to relearn how to go about daily activity with a different quality of motion.

The Trager method works with the kind of pain we see in the neck and upper back, in migraines and sciatica, in holding patterns in the lower back, in the pelvic rotation muscles, in TMJ, and carpal tunnel syndrome, also with pains due to repetitive motion of a constrictive kind.

Rolfing

According to the practitioners of rolfing, pain is due to chronic shortenings in the tissue. Correction of this pain can be accomplished by soft tissue manipulation. This manipulation acts to create order in the body so the client stands tall and free of restriction.

David Frome, a physical therapist, states that rolfing is done in a 10-session series, designed to address all the shortenings in the structure systematically. Each session works in a different area. In the first hour, for instance, concentration is on the trunk, shoulders, and hips. The second hour works on the back and lower leg. Going through the complete series allows the therapist to work through all the body's shortenings. During a session, a patient may experience a tingling sensation and a sense of release. The patient should strive to draw the deepest possible breath to aid in the treatment.

The major goal of the treatment is not pain relief per se but it has been found to help with TMJ, frozen shoulder, tennis elbow, carpal tunnel syndrome, chronic hip problems, sciatica, cervical neuropathies, and knee, foot, and ankle problems.

Craniosacral Therapy

The sacral region is that at the top of the spine. Between it and the head there should be a balanced rhythmic motion maintained for the health of the organism. When pain arises, it may be due to a restriction that disturbs the harmony between these two regions or between them and the rest of the body.

In craniosacral therapy, the practitioner places his or her hands on the client's body in such a way as to try and bring the cranium and sacrum back into alignment with a natural rhythm re-established. Charles A. Kaplan, the founder and director of the Center for Pain Management, points out that this hands-on technique is usually centered on touching the head or lower back but can be done anywhere, such as on the fingers or toes. Some patients will go through a first treatment and not feel anything, but most will leave the treatment table feeling very relaxed and stress free.

Craniosacral therapy is recommended for dealing with muscular and skeletal pain, headaches, pains in the back and neck, sports injuries, sciatica, and nerve pain. It can also be beneficial to those recovering from pneumonia or bronchitis, helping by loosening the ribcage. This treatment is a tremendous stress reducer, while it can eliminate back pain and improve the immune system.

Magnet Therapy

With an ancestry as old as that of acupuncture and shiatsu, magnet therapy, like them, acts to influence the body's energy.

Jim Joseph mentions that the healing power of magnets was known in 2200 B.C. China. Such ancient fathers of medicine as Galen and Aristotle discussed magnets as did Paracelsus, one of the founders of chemistry. The value of magnet therapy was a belief of Mesmer and others in the 19th century and is still being developed and practiced today.

Down through history, magnets have been used to deal with the causes of various ailments. As Dr. Joseph remarks, "Pain is a messenger. We don't want to kill the messenger but find the cause."

When there is pain in the body, it can be because positive energy is being drawn to the site of injury. To bring about this transfer, the brain sends out a negative signal. Using the negative side of a magnet can augment and assist that reaction. Furthermore, around an injury there will be an acidic buildup. The negative side of the magnet is an alkalizing force that can help alleviate the pain accompanying this acidity.

A second source of pain arises when a person is overworked or suffering from undue stress. The individual cells of the person become distorted, overly positively charged. Putting a negative magnet on a weakened area will repolarize the cells, bringing them back to balance.

The distortion of the cells' polarity and resultant pain may also be caused by our technological environment. We are swamped with positive electromagnetic pulses coming from TVs, radios, electric clocks, and all the other electrical devices around us. The pulses of their fields are not congruent with the one found in our body and so can throw us into disharmony and disease.

Magnets can be obtained in a plastiform that can be molded and shaped for a particular area. They last indefinitely and are low priced. A medium-sized magnet may cost $20. Available healing magnets are color coded with the negative pole green and the positive red. The positive side of the magnet is active, sun oriented; while the negative side is relaxing, and earth oriented. All of the treatments to be discussed utilize the negative pole. One must be careful with the positive pole since positive magnetism causes growth to any biological system, even the growth of cancer when it is present. Treatment should last from 20 minutes to overnight. The magnet's power should be from 1,000 to 6,000 gauss.

A magnet can be wrapped on the area to be covered with Velcro. Special wraps in which the magnets are inlaid in the Velcro are available. These wraps can be placed on most parts of the body, though they should not be used on the eyes. Since negative magnetism pulls fluids and gases, placed near the eyes, the magnet would draw out its fluids. If work is to be done on the eyes, the magnet can be placed off to the side. From this position, magnetism can be exerted on cataracts to reduce oxidation and free radical development. The magnet's value in reducing oxidation is due to the fact that oxygen is paramagnetic. When you breathe, you are pulling negative energy from the earth into your body.

To deal with edema, a magnet is placed on the body, not at the site of the problem, but near it and directed toward the heart so as to pull the edema away from its place of occurrence. If you have edema in the calf, for instance, place the magnet above the knee to draw the fluid up from the site of the disturbance to the kidney from which it can be excreted.

For the pain of menstrual cramps, a magnet should be placed on the lower abdomen, two inches below the belly button. This placement should not be used, though, for one or one-and-a-half hours after eating since it will interfere with peristalsis. Also, a magnet should never be used by a person using a Pacemaker or implants of any metal.

The negative side of the magnet is also good against parasites, who will stop eating when hit by the negative energy.

At night, it is useful to lie on a magnetic bed pad and put magnets behind the head where they will bathe the pineal gland in energy. This usage will induce a restful night's sleep. By using a magnet, one could sleep less than one's normal night's sleep and feel even more rested than one did with the greater time. The magnet has also been known to increase sexual abilities.

The magnet can help with shoulder pain, that of the rotator cuff, as with aches in the back and lumbar regions. Magnets can be attached to the head or neck to deal with hypothyroidism, depression, migraine headaches, and problems with the vestibular system. For depression, the magnet should be placed near the occipital lobe.

Mind/Body Connection

Lastly, some therapists have recommended a more eclectic approach, one that looks for and relies on the often overlooked synergies that flow between the mind and body. One physician, Dr. Ron Dushkins, brings up a number of points to consider when dealing with pain. He notes, first, the importance of relaxation, which will quiet and calm the nervous system. Remember that when we feel pain, we also are feeling a layer of stress on top of that pain. If the layer of stress is relieved, then the pain will diminish significantly.

Human touch can also play a part in relieving pain. As babies we like to be touched and as adults we still find this important.

A third overlooked factor in healing is humor. The writer Norman Cousins tells the story of how he was hospitalized with a critical health problem. As he saw it, a lot of his physical deterioration was due to stress and negative thoughts from that stress. He reasoned if we can create disease by stress then by alleviating stress, through means such as humor, we can cure disease. He had a movie projector brought into his hospital room and began showing Marx Brothers' films and other comedies. Soon his room became a place of congregation for other patients who wanted to enjoy the shows. It got rather chaotic because so many people were coming into this room and laughing. You're not supposed to laugh in a hospital. Some people were scandalized. Cousins said doctors would give him blood tests before and after he had been laughing at a humorous film and they would find an improvement. He had less pain after laughing.

Guided imagery is also an element of the mind/body connection. With this technique, a sufferer will place a hand over the injured area and invite the other cells in the body to go to the aid of this damaged area. After all, the body's cells always work together and this is one way to encourage their interplay.

All of the methods mentioned as part of the mind/body connection get the patient to take charge of personal recovery. Many people are strong in many areas of their life, in career, in forming relationships, in playing sports, but when it comes to their own health, they cede all control to a doctor. To really escape pain, the patient must take a big part in the recovery process.

This could be said to inform all the strategies for dealing with pain we have encountered in this chapter. Whether you are taking appropriate herbs or mineral supplements to reduce suffering or selecting a nontraditional, natural healer to help you redirect your energy or repolarize your cell, in each case, you have studied, meditated, and selected the natural way to diminish pain.

PART FIVE
Foot and Leg Care

The film *Raise the Red Lantern* concerns the problems of a bride who marries into a polygamous household in early 20th century China. Although it is basically a tragic story of rivalry between the husband's four wives, it does have a few lighter moments. The newest wife, played by Gong Li, learns that whichever wife the husband temporarily favors receives more gratifications than the others, such as better food, more attention from servants, and so on. This includes, as one of the most prized features, the right to a foot massage. Of course, the reprehensible ancient Chinese practice of foot binding probably accounts for some of the respect given to foot massage. However, Western audiences see nothing but humor in the sensuous pleasure Li obtains from the massage, not recognizing, as this section will show, the value of massage, which should be part of the regimen of anyone who wants to have and maintain healthy feet and legs.

Massage is just one way to have healthy feet and legs. It is also necessary to choose good shoes, exercise properly, and have the right attitude toward your extremities. After discussing the components of keeping your feet and legs in good health, this section will look at some of the typical injuries and disease conditions that attack our lower extremities—and suggest remedies. We also include a special focus on sports injuries.

30

Healthy Feet and Legs For a Lifetime

In the modern world, our feet are at a disadvantage. Long ago we used our feet, along with our hands, to swing from trees. Our toenails were helpful for maintaining a strong grip on the bark of trees. When our feet weren't taking us through the treetops, they were taking us along the ground—with our hands doing the other half of the work. Through many generations our feet gradually adapted to carrying our weight alone and walking miles across soft, grassy earth.

Even now, our feet have not fully adapted to bearing our entire body weight, and they are far from adapted to walking on hard surfaces like concrete. They are still evolving, growing longer and wider, in response to the hard surfaces we pound them on. The bigger the area of the foot, the more the weight of our bodies and the pressure of the concrete is dispersed, and the less trauma to the foot. This evolutionary change is happening rapidly: Each new generation has feet larger than those of their parents. You can even see the change reflected in the sample shoe sizes displayed in stores. Where the ladies' sample size used to be a five or six, it is now more likely to be a seven or even an eight.

Because our feet have not completely evolved into organs for walking on hard surfaces, many problems develop merely out of the trauma of hitting concrete. We have to take up the slack that remains between where our feet are from an evolutionary point of view and what we do with them, which is something they aren't quite ready to handle.

How can we help our feet? First, keep in mind our feet are not quite up to the harsh treatment we give them. Second, provide the best possible conditions for them to take that treatment.

Getting Familiar With Your Feet

If you were shown pictures of 10 pairs of feet, including your own, could you pick yours out? Many people couldn't. If you want to pamper your feet, you first have to recognize their features and be aware of the changes they go through at different periods of life.

Let's start with the foot's "normal" shape. (Don't worry about normality too much, though. Nature offers wide variations and what my be "abnormal" for some is perfectly normal for others.)

Take a look at the line of your foot. Does your foot appear to be twisted, or is it straight? If you trace your foot on paper, you may find it easier to see. Look at your toes. The first should be nearly straight, the second through fifth curving slightly. The shape of the normal foot is smooth, with no lumps or bumps. Is your heel well-rounded and smooth without bumps? Are your arch and instep high or low? If you notice your arch is dropping, then you know something is changing, and you should have it checked. If you have smooth heels now but later see a bump on one of them, you know something unusual is happening. This is significant: If you know what the normal shape of your foot is now, then you'll be alert to any changes that are taking place.

What about size? Don't just go by your shoe size. Some people are wearing the wrong size shoes! If you ever have problems with your shoes, it advisable to have your feet measured by a professional.

Does your skin look and feel normal? Is it soft, supple, and evenly colored? Skin color should be uniform, with no red marks. What is the texture of the skin? Do you normally have hair on your toes or not? A minute detail like a disappearance of hair from your toes can alert you to a circulation problem.

Now with a full-length mirror, watch yourself walk. What is your normal posture? Is your head erect and your shoulders straight? If your head and shoulders are slumped too far forward or held back too rigidly, the rest of your body will be thrown out of line. Your chest should be slightly out, stomach slightly in. Look at the upper body as a unit. It should be held squarely over the pelvis, which should be in line with your legs. Do you throw your hips or your upper body forward when you walk? Too much of a forward thrust can create an imbalance, which can cause back, hip, knee, ankle, or foot problems.

Look at your feet as you walk. Each foot should strike the ground on the heel, just slightly to the heel's outside, then twist slightly in. At that point, the foot should start to twist up again until "toe-off" occurs. This may sound complicated, but if you walk slowly and mindfully for a minute, you can determine your normal pattern.

You can heighten your awareness even further by observing what is normal for other people in walking. If you think you have posture problems, it would be worthwhile to consult a professional to help you diagnose, correct and control any difficulties. Professional treatment can help you return to or maintain your normal gait, which can prevent foot and leg problems further down the line.

Feet From Infancy to Old Age

As we age, what is normal for our feet and where difficulties are likely to occur will change. So, along with knowing what is normal now, it's important to know how our feet are going to change as they move through time.

INFANTS Be as familiar with your infant's feet as you are with your own. You are in intimate daily contact with your baby, so you can observe the changes in his or her body. If you see something unusual in your baby's feet, consult your pediatrician, or even a podiatrist.

Here are guidelines for your observations.

The rotated-out positioning of a baby's legs stems from the thigh bone's outward rotation. The rest of the leg and foot structure follows suit. Babies' feet are supposed to point outward. This is a reason that Charlie Chaplin's walk, that mimics this quality, is so endearing. Dr. Howard Robins, my consultant for this chapter, often sees worried parents who say, "My baby's feet are twisted out. How will he walk?" Out-toeing should correct itself naturally, normally disappearing by the time the child is two. But in-toeing, pigeon-toedness, is not normal and will not correct itself.

In-toeing is easy to spot in adults: Feet point toward each other as the person walks. It's harder to check for in-toeing in a baby who is not yet walking. If you notice your baby's feet turn in rather than out, ask your pediatrician to take a look. The younger the child is when you spot such a problem, the easier it will be to correct.

What about the baby's hips? An easy way to check for normal hip placement is to turn the baby over on his or her stomach, face down, and look at the creases behind the thighs. Do they line up evenly from side to side or are they out of line with one another? If they seem significantly off, the pediatrician should be consulted. Also check the "anchor sign." This is the double curve running from the crack down the baby's buttocks and through the two highest creases on the top of the thighs. It should be well formed with the line straight down the middle and evenly curved on each side. As in the case of in-toeing, any hip dislocation should be treated immediately.

If you know how the skin on your baby's feet and legs normally looks and feels, then discoloration, inelasticity, or dryness will alert you to the need for care. At any sign of inelasticity or dryness, give your baby a foot massage with oil. If the condition hasn't cleared up after a couple of days, consult your doctor.

What do your baby's toes look like? Toes that overlap or underlap are not unusual—many babies are born with one or both conditions—but they should be corrected early. You can do this yourself with a piece of tape or a small pad of 2x2 gauze, opened to its full length and then folded lengthwise. Snake the tape or gauze through the baby's toes by lifting underlapping toes and putting the gauze under them and depressing overlapped toes and placing it over them. When you finish, your baby's toes should be lying straight and flat.

Become familiar with your baby's toenails. Though nail infections and ingrown toenails are rare in infants, they can be simply treated with homestyle remedies. If you notice some redness around one of the baby's nails, wrap the toe in gauze that has been soaked in Herbal Solution One. (The directions for preparing this solution are given at the end of chapter 31.) More simply, you can try warm water, which had been brought to a boil, on the gauze. Allow the gauze to dry completely then repeat. This remedy acts as a poultice: The evaporation of the liquid draws out the inflammation.

Besides knowing what is normal for your infant's feet, you also have to respect their feet by using good hygiene. Proper footwear is necessary for good hygiene. Since babies don't walk, shoes are not needed. In fact, chances are that if your baby develops a toenail problem, it's because he or she has been wearing the wrong kind of footwear. If you want to keep your child's feet warm, use booties or socks.

Proper foot hygiene includes washing and massaging baby's feet, as well as clipping toenails. It may surprise you to hear that no soaps should be used on baby's feet and legs unless they are dirty. Otherwise, only warm water on a daily basis is necessary, since your baby is hardly likely to get dirty enough to need a soap bath, which dries the skin. In the bath, make sure to clean between the toes as well as washing the baby's feet. When you dry, gently pat over the whole foot rather than rubbing vigorously.

Babies love massage and their feet and legs can benefit from it. After drying the baby's feet and legs, gently rub in a little sunflower, safflower, or soy oil, using the same technique you would use on your own body. (Later, we will describe adult massage.) Massaging is especially useful for dark skinned babies whose skins tend to be drier than those with lighter skins.

Clipping a baby's toenails once or twice a week is also part of good hygiene. Invest in a tiny nail clipper that is made for infants. Clip straight across, never digging in on the sides. If it's impossible to clip straightly because the infant's nails are curving, ask your doctor for advice on correct clipping.

TODDLERS Once your baby starts to walk, it is as important as ever to observe his or her feet and legs. By this time, the outside edge of the child's foot should be almost straight. If you notice it turning in, have his or her feet checked.

A simple exercise can complement a physician's treatment toward correcting this condition. Sit in front of your child while the child is lying on his or her back. Grasping the baby's heel in one hand, place your thumb and index finger on each side of the foot along the borders of the sole, so the toes lie between these fingers. Very gently place pressure on the outer side of the foot to straighten it. Hold the stretch for 15 to 20 seconds. Doing this exercise five or six times in a row, twice a day, can help move the bone structure back into the proper position, avoiding later problems.

The out-toed effect should have disappeared by the time the child has begun to walk. If out-toeing persists after age two, bring it to the notice of your doctor.

As your child begins to walk, you may notice he or she has flat feet. This should not cause worry since your child's foot structure will be developing over the years and that includes developing the arch that is right for the child's weight and body type.

You also might worry if it seems your toddler is not toddling as early as the children of other parents. Your child will walk, when, and not until, the musculature in his or her feet and legs is ready to do the job. There is certainly no rush, and trying to make your baby walk before his or her time is foolish. Nationally, the average age for the first step is 16 months. However, to see a child beginning to walk at 20 or even 24 months is not unusual.

At this point, foot hygiene will become more complex in that, since the children are walking, they will need to have shoes. Feet get dirty, so washing with soap is necessary. Clipping the toenails is still a necessity, although the frequency of the procedure can be reduced to once every three or four weeks.

As far as selecting the child's shoes, remember the "rule of half thumb." There should be at least a half thumbnail's length—an eighth to a quarter of an inch—from the end of the child's longest toe to the end of the shoe. Toddler's shoes should be flexible so they respond to the movements of the foot. The shoe should actually bend with the ball of the foot, so he or she can "toe-off" properly. As for socks, cotton is best because it allows the toddler's feet to breathe and is less likely to irritate the skin than a synthetic.

Shoes and socks are important to wear. Even in the house, the child should wear socks or slippers. Even a tiny hair can penetrate a child's delicate skin, causing pain, redness and infection.

OLDER CHILDREN Children between 8 and 12 are more active than their younger brothers and sisters so there is more to look out for.

You might notice that your child seems either knock-kneed (with legs too close together) or its opposite, bow-legged. Both conditions can occur within "normal" development but if either condition seems to hamper your child's movement, then see your doctor.

Keep an eye on the skin of your child's feet and legs. If it becomes dry, give an oil or skin cream massage for a night or two after bathing. By now the toes should be lying straight, and there should not be any new twists or bends. The arch should be fully developed. For any irregularities or if the child's skin irritation persists, don't be afraid to bring it to the attention of your doctor.

Daily bathing is still important for the child's feet, though by this time it will be the child's own responsibility. Invest in a good cotton cloth so that the feet can be gently but thoroughly cleaned, especially between the toes.

Clipping the toenails only has to be done once a month at this age. A straight-across clip is still the idea, though as the corners of the nails begin to curve inward, they should be clipped at a slight curve.

Going barefoot results in one of the biggest foot problems for children: picking up foreign bodies that penetrate the skin. It's best to discourage going barefoot. But, if the child is not barefoot, what should he or she have on? Because an older child tends to be very active, a running shoe is highly recommended. However, if your child is involved in many different sports, you would be wise to purchase basketball or baseball shoes, since running shoes are made for unidirectional activity, and they may trip up a child who is making quick turns and darting off in all directions. In any case, most children this age have little use for a leather-soled dress shoe. They need the adequate support, easy movement, and protection found in a lightweight canvas or nylon shoe.

TEENAGERS By the age of 13, few children are going to want your observation of their bodies. If you have adequately prepared them, they will know the normal state of their feet and be quick to discern any unusual changes. Moreover, teenagers can take responsibility for their foot hygiene. Thorough cleaning once a week is enough unless the teenager is heavily involved in athletics.

Now foot massage has increasing importance. The feet and legs have to bear more stress, while athletics is taking its toll. The daily massage program described later is not a bad routine to start.

There is one place where your intervention around the teenager's foot care may be called for. Teenagers encounter enormous peer pressure to wear fashionable, but physically horrendous, shoes. It is your duty to help your teenager recognize shoes should be chosen for fit, suitability, and comfort, not as status symbols or part of a fashion statement. Those last considerations can enter secondarily into the selection, but only after comfort and reliability have been used as the primary qualities guiding choice.

ADULTS We will consider adult foot care in the sections immediately following, but it is appropriate to make a few comments.

In caring for your feet, observation is key. Learn what is normal about your feet and legs, so that when you notice any deviations, you can take preventive measures. Maintenance is equally important. This means good hygiene, exercise, regular massage, good nutrition—all on a daily basis. Appropriate footwear is also crucial, and we have many pages on the topic coming up.

THE ELDERLY If you are over 60, observation and maintenance are more important than ever. At this stage any change in your feet or legs can point to a larger problem. For instance, swelling in the feet can indicate general edema. Since your feet are at the far end of the circulatory system, they can give you signals as to what is happening in your system as no other organ can.

Good hygiene is central. Daily bathing is no longer imperative, particularly since you may be susceptible to dry skin. Because of the dryness, moisturizing should be stepped up to twice a day, morning and evening, with the same oils we recommended for infants. You might want to massage your feet twice a day when you moisturize because it stimulates circulation. Later we describe the Ten Minute Morning Massage, which is applicable here.

Before Your Exercise

Along with eating sensibly, getting proper rest, and having a positive outlook on life, exercising is essential to living in optimal health. Although we cover exercise in other parts of this book, in this chapter our focus will be on the proper care of the feet in situations ranging from formal exercise programs and sports to plain old fun on the beach. We will also outline a walking program.

A little later in this chapter, we will talk about sports injuries, but at this juncture let us look at preventive measures. In playing sports and in training, it is important to be in touch with your body. Your body is always giving you feedback. Any lack of awareness of this feedback can leave you prone to injury.

Proper warm-up and stretching before beginning any type of workout is crucial for preventing injuries to the legs and feet. The best way to warm up the leg muscles is with the Robins Six Step Exercise.

WARMING UP: THE ROBINS SIX STEP EXERCISE Lie down on the ground with your legs straight in front of you. This exercise is to be done with a slow, rhythmic, continuous movement. Counting with a beat, such as "and-a-one, and-a-two," and so on will give you the proper rhythm for the exercise. It is to be repeated five or six times in a row on each leg. Do not alternate legs but do one at a time.

STEP ONE: Slowly bring your heel toward you

STEP TWO: Bring your knee to your chest, without using your hands

STEP THREE: Straighten your leg up in the air so the knee is straight (even if this means lowering the leg slightly)

STEP FOUR: Lower the straight leg about halfway to the ground

STEP FIVE: Slowly let your heel come down to the ground

STEP SIX: Straighten your leg out again on the ground

This exercise will get the heart rate up slowly and gradually increase circulation to the muscles.

To prevent rear leg muscle injuries, use two gentle stretches. First, while you're lying on the ground on your back, taking one leg at a time, bring a knee under your leg and help pull your leg and knee into your chest. Never put your hands in front of the knee as the hands may slide up and cause the kneecap to jam into the thigh. When you pull the knee to your chest, it should be a long, slow pull, never letting it bounce outward. After 20 seconds, allow the leg to go straight out again. Then repeat the exercise. Do this three to five times per leg. This stretches the hamstring and gluteal muscles of your upper leg.

The second exercise is for the calf muscles. This is done by sitting up and a grabbing a towel or belt and slinging it around the bottom of your foot. Grab one end of the belt with each hand. Sit with your back and head straight and your arms straight in front of you. Do not let the arms bend at the elbow joints. Lean backward and allow your body weight to pull your foot toward you. Next, let go of the towel with one hand and your foot should flop forward to where the other foot is resting since you aren't using muscle power to pull the foot. Do this exercise three to five times per leg.

After completing your workout, there are two valuable active stretches you can do to help wind down. For both, face the wall, standing as close as you can get, with feet and legs a shoulder-width apart and palms placed flat on the wall at face level. Take a step back, keeping both feet pointed perpendicular to the wall. In the first of the two stretches that use this stance, the rear leg is kept straight. As you stretch, try to keep your rear leg, knee, hip, and shoulder all in a straight line and do not allow your heel to come off the ground. Lean toward the wall and support yourself with your entire arm and forearm. Hold the position for 20 seconds. You should feel the stretch from behind the knee all the way down to the heel. After the allotted time, push out from the wall to relax.

In the second wall stretch, allow the rear leg to bend slightly forward at the knee. This will work another portion of the rear leg muscles. You will feel this stretch more in the belly of the calf muscles and behind the heelbone. This should be done three to five times per leg, not alternating but taking one leg at a time.

We also have to stretch the upper rear leg muscles, the hamstrings. For this stretch, place your foot on a stool, chair, or table. Straighten your leg, then pull your foot forcefully toward your body, and hold it that way. Keep your back straight and arms straight out in front of you. Let your fingertips lift as you lean forward gently. By lifting your fingers and arms up as you lean, you will find that your back stays straight so it is unstressed. Pulling your foot toward you has created a strong stretch on the rear leg muscles.

The iliotibial band of muscles extends from the hip to the thigh. To stretch these muscles, stand with shoulder against a wall, then step away from the wall with both feet. Gently let your hip lean in toward the wall. This causes your body to move in the shape of the letter C, gently stretching the iliotibial band muscles. Do this stretch three to five times. It is not necessary to do this stretch often unless you have problems with these muscles.

Remember although stretching is designed to gradually warm up the muscles to prevent injury, overstretching can also lead to injury. A stretch should be slow and continuous, lasting from 10 to 30 seconds. A stretch that is too long or overextends the muscle or that involves choppy, bumpy motion can lead to injury.

Recreation for the Nonathlete

For those who are not athletes, we have plenty of good advice for when you find yourself playing outdoors.

AT THE BEACH In general, walking or running after a proper warm-up is beneficial. Surprisingly, though, there is one place where running is not recommended—the beach. Of course, it's exhilarating to run in sand under a hot sun, but injury can result. Sand, especially deep, thick sand, will allow the foot to move in any direction. Running through the sand, your feet may twist inward or outward, throwing off your whole leg and possibly your lower back as well.

What if you run on the wetter sand near the water? Your foot will not twist here, because the sand is firmer. However, the problem is here you are running on an incline. One leg actually acts as if it were shorter than the other because the limb and pelvis are raised on one side. This also can cause injury. So unless you find a near ideal coastline, where the wet sand is level, be wary of running even on wet sand.

What you should be doing at the beach is swimming. Even if you can't swim, just walking waist deep into the water and jumping up and down as the waves roll in is an excellent way to strengthen leg muscles. Ideally, spend at least 20 minutes swimming or jumping.

Also remember at the beach to apply sunscreen not only to your upper body and legs but to your poor feet. Get that sunscreen on the tops and bottoms of your feet, since when you lie down, the bottoms will be exposed. Keep in mind, that as you walk up and down the shoreline, the water will reflect a great deal of light onto your lower legs so they must be adequately protected.

It's great fun to walk along barefoot, but the fun will be short-lived if you get a splinter, sharp shell, or piece of glass jabbed into you. So wear sandals while beachcombing. They protect the feet from puncture as well as from getting burned from hot sand.

When you return from the beach, treat your legs and feet to moisture. The sun will dry your skin, cooking the skin's elastin. If you don't apply oil, you'll lose some of your skin's suppleness which protects you against cuts, bruises, and other injuries.

IN THE COUNTRY Aside from walking on the beach, in the warmer seasons many people like to exercise by taking a walk in the country. If that's what you enjoy, remember don't spend all your time looking for red-breasted tanagers in the trees, also be aware of what's on the ground, so you don't start stumbling over logs or into poison ivy.

Dress properly. Don't wear shorts since you don't want to be exposing your bare legs to the poison ivy you may be stumbling through. Wear good cotton socks and maybe even bring a change of socks along to keep your feet dry.

When we discuss shoes, we will have more to say about which shoes are most appropriate for different sports and exercise.

Walking as Exercise: The Elements of a Good Walking Program

Only recently has walking been recognized as an excellent exercise for every-one. What we want to spend a few minutes talking about is not the walking to the store each of us does every day, but a walking exercise program. To condi-tion our hearts and circulation, tone up our muscles, and generally keep our body systems functioning at optimum capacity, walking has to be undertaken systematically and conscientiously. It must be done daily. If you're elderly or out of shape, however, you might start by walking for three or four days in a row, then taking a day off to let your body rest.

BUILDING UP A WALKING PROGRAM As with any other route you take in exercis-ing, embark on walking in a gradual, controlled way. You'll need to build up the length of time you walk, from perhaps 10 minutes a day at the beginning to per-haps 30 minutes to an hour when you're in shape.

A big help when you start out is to keep a notebook of your physical signs. As with other aerobic exercise, progress is to be measured by pulse rate. First you'll have to establish what your optimum heart rate for exercise should be. Subtract your age from the number 220. Multiply the result by 60 to 75 per-cent, which gives you the range of heartbeat you should be able to reach as the goal of your walking program. Then take your pulse rate when you are sitting down. The best place to take your pulse is at your wrist or temple. If you take the pulse at your wrist, use the lesser fingertips to feel the pulse, not your thumb since it has an artery whose pulse can interfere with your reading. The fingertips are placed on either side of the two grooves found on the underside of the wrist near the outer edges. You may take your pulse for a minute or for as little as 10 seconds, multiplying by six to obtain the beats per minute. Record your pulse rate in your notebook.

As you walk, stop every 5 or 10 minutes to take down your pulse rate. This will give you an idea of the effect the exercise is having on your heartbeat and cir-culation and how close you are getting to your target pulse rate. When you get home, record the highest pulse rate reached during exercise in your notebook.

An important aspect of your walking program is that you not only increase the length of your daily walk systematically, but increase the pace of your walk.

Why? With increased exercise, your heart rate will tend to decrease. Therefore, to reach your desired goal, you must exert yourself to increase the challenge to your heart and circulation. If you are elderly or disabled, you may be unable to do this. In that case, compensate by increasing the length of time you walk. The longer and faster you walk, the more conditioning you get.

Build up slowly in terms of time and pace to a peak program. If you're using time as your guide, add about 10 percent more to the time you walk every two weeks. For instance, if you start by walking 20 minutes a day, after two weeks, add 2 minutes more. If distance is your guide, increase by the same 10 percent each two weeks. This allows safe stress buildup in the bones and muscles and lets the heart adapt to the stress that's being placed on it.

GETTING READY Wear a comfortable shoe that fits so as to cushion and protect your foot. A running shoe is ideal since it is made for the same unidirectional motion as walking. What you don't wear is as important as what you do. Don't carry anything—not even a purse. Any weight at all can throw your posture off. Wear clothing that allows heat buildup to dissipate quickly. Cotton undergarments are good because they allow the moisture on your body to evaporate.

Running shirts and jogging pants are good to walk in as long as they are constructed from materials that will absorb and dissipate perspiration. In the winter your outer clothing should be made of wool, which breathes while keeping you warm, while the clothing next to your skin should be cotton or polypropylene. Also wear something to keep your face warm as well as gloves and mittens.

It's best to walk on a somewhat empty stomach. Try not to eat for two or three hours before walking, just so your body won't be burdened by trying to digest and walk at the same time. However, you should be completely hydrated. Drink 8 to 10 ounces of water every hour before you go. This measure ensures your body won't overheat as fast while you're walking.

A warm-up is essential. Start by relaxing your mind and body. Try to let any tension and stress go. This paves the way for loosening your muscles. Once you've relaxed, stretch for 5 or 10 minutes, utilizing some of the stretches we outlined earlier. After the stretches, loosen up. Move all your joints, from the neck down. After shaking your body, spend a minute on each foot, massaging it, kneading it, flexing all the joints by hand. This prepares the feet for a good walk.

Plan your route before you leave. Decide where you are going to be walking, what terrain you will be traveling over. Try to avoid areas of rough terrain. You don't want to fall down a pothole while you are concentrating on your stride.

GOOD WALKING STYLE So, you've started a walk. The first thing to be aware of is your posture. You should be erect, with head up, shoulders back, chest out, stomach in. Avoid being slumped, stoop-shouldered or hunchbacked. Don't look straight down at the ground.

Walk with a regular cadence. Walking at a slower rate to begin helps you warm up your body. After 5 or 10 minutes of walking slowly, you can work up gradually to the actual speed you want to maintain. There's no need to take big, long steps, which can actually throw off your balance. Instead, to increase your heart rate, increase the cadence, that is, the number of steps you take in a given interval.

At the beginning of your walk, as you are building up to your optimum pace, you will have lots of energy. However, if you get winded or tired, feel free to slow down. Easing off helps build up your wind, restoring your tissues by getting more fresh blood into them to wash away waste products and increase the energy flow. When you feel stronger, you can go back to a quicker cadence. At that point, you will be able to maintain your faster speed for a longer period of time. Again, remember to make a record of your walk in your notebook so you can see the progress you are making.

As you walk, a natural swing of the arms from front to back is important. Not too tight, not too loose, is the rule. For example, never hold your hand in a tight fist, but don't let it fall totally slack at your side either. Just hold your fingers lightly together, with the thumb resting on top of the index finger. If your arms are swinging the way we described, your shoulders will be relaxed as well.

As far as the lower half of your body goes, you should be swinging your legs from the hips forward, allowing the heel to strike the ground before the ball of the foot, slightly on the outside. If you find yourself bouncing up and down and walking on your toes, your rear leg muscles probably need to stretch. It will be better, though, to do that after you walk rather than before or during the exercise.

The way you breathe is as important as the way you walk. Abdominal breathing is best. Breathe through your nose and let the breath go out through your mouth. Take long, deep breaths that fill up the upper and lower portions of your lungs. This type of breathing naturally forces your stomach to expand when you inhale. Breathing this way gets the most oxygen possible into your system quickly, increasing your strength and stamina during the walk.

If you start to get winded and need to breathe faster, do so. If you get too winded, stop and take a few deep, cleansing breaths to reoxygenate your tissues. Then continue your walk.

What if you develop cramps in your legs? Stop. Massage the muscle and let the cramp dissipate. Then continue. If you feel the cramp starting again. Stop again. Cramps may be caused by waste products building up in your tissues when not enough blood and oxygen are getting to them. By massaging the ailing tissue, you break up some of the spasm in the muscle tissue and increase circulation. This helps wash away the waste products, re-energizing the tissue.

AFTER THE WALK After your daily walk, the most important muscles you will want to stretch are those in the front of your leg since they may actually be weakened by walking. Now's the time for the belt or towel exercise and the two against-the-wall stretches we touched on earlier to relax the rear muscles before working on the ones in front.

Here's how to work on the front muscles. Sit on a countertop or firm tabletop. Slowly extend your foot until the leg is perfectly straight. You should be in an L shape with your back straight. Hold that for 10 seconds and let your leg come back to a bent knee position. Repeat this from 10 to 20 times for each leg.

After your walk, rehydrate your body by drinking plenty of fluids. You may want to eat a light meal after your pulse rate is normal.

THE BENEFITS OF YOUR WALKING PROGRAM By walking in this way, consciously and with discipline, not only are you benefiting the entire muscular system, you are burning excess fat and reducing overall body weight while gaining balance, stamina, strength, and endurance. Moreover, you'll be improving your ability to relax emotionally. The extra oxygen coursing through your brain raises the levels of serotonin and endorphin, morphinelike but natural substances that allow a state of relaxation to occur.

This is a program well suited to dieters. Recent studies have determined that if you are exercising at 70 or 75 percent of your maximum heart rate (as indicated according to the calculation described earlier), you are taking in enough oxygen to burn fat rapidly. Your body will turn to the fat for fuel to supply the energy needed for your walk, using it for about 70 percent of that supply. If you are walking above 75 percent of your top heart rate, your body will turn to the glycogen (starch) stored in the muscles and tissues and burn that as well. So if you want to lose weight, shoot for getting your heart rate into the 70–75 percent range.

footwear Basics

Whether you are embarking on a walking program, participating in sports, or just trekking to the subway on the way to work, you need to have the right shoes. In this section, we will look at what criteria to use in buying your shoes, which shoes are the best for different sports, and which are a must to avoid. In general, what we have to look at in every shoe is fit, material, and style.

IF THE SHOE FITS... Just as before you begin a walk, you should have your itinerary in mind, so before you shop for shoes, think about what they will be worn for. There's nothing wrong with even the most fashionable shoe, if you don't plan to do much walking in it.

First remember the "rule of thumb." For infants, a half thumb was sufficient, but for adults there should be a thumbnail's length between the end of your longest toes and the end of the shoe. This ensures adequate toe room. Your foot slides forward from an eighth to a quarter of an inch each time you take a step, so the rule of thumb is important. You don't want to jam those toes with every step.

Next, the width. The foot width is usually measured across the ball of the foot. If you want to tell whether a shoe you are trying on is the proper width, first, stand up. Take your thumb and roll it across the leather on the top, across the ball from one side to the other. You should be able to see the leather wave, almost as if you could pinch it between your thumb and forefinger. That's adequate width. If your big or little toe joints press out on the shoe when you're standing up, it's too tight.

Next check the width at the heel. Good shoes are wider up front and narrower in the heel. Are you getting adequate height in the front? The top of the shoe shouldn't rub against toes that are higher than others. If the shoe rubs, you're inviting corns. Also be sure that, if the shoe is leather (and that is preferable), the leather is soft enough to flex and bend with your foot.

MATERIALS AND CONSTRUCTION For the upper part of the shoe, the best material is leather, which will let your foot breathe, allowing perspiration to escape and letting the shoe dry overnight. As far as insole and inner materials go, the more natural, the better. Synthetic materials cause your feet to heat up, leading to a buildup of sweat which can cause problems for your feet as well as accelerate the breakdown of your shoes.

While leather soles were once considered ideal, with the hard surfaces we are forced to walk on today, thick rubber soles or ones made of a synthetic material are best. They save wear and tear on your feet in a way that leather simply can't.

The back part of the upper shoe, which surrounds the heel and comes along the side of the foot about midway forward, is called the "counter." The counter is usually made of a rigid material, often some form of plastic. For dress shoes as well as regular walking shoes look for a firm counter because your feet need that support.

Heels should never be totally flat. A heel height of approximately one inch, with a slight wedge construction, gives the average person the best prevention against leg, foot, and lower-back problems. Whether the heel is rubber or leather does not make much difference. A rubber heel has the slight advantage of absorbing more stress when the heel strikes the ground.

STYLE CONSIDERATIONS For dresswear, it is best to choose slip-on shoes. For walking around, however, you will do better with strap and lace shoes, which don't allow the foot to move around in the shoe quite so much. If you walk a lot on the job, you'd be better off in an oxford than in a slip-on.

If you want the ideal shoe for everyday life, for walking and standing still, choose running shoes. This applies to everyone, whether runners or not. Running shoes are more shock-absorbing than the average leather shoe or any other kind of sports shoe. They were built with a wedge. The wide-flared heel gives good ankle and knee stability by preventing the foot from moving around inside the shoe. Running shoes not only shock-absorb the forefoot but the heel-strike as well, reducing the amount of pressure that will go through to the foot and leg.

"NO-NOS"

HIGH HEELS: These can lead to high hell on your feet by shortening the calf muscles, hamstrings, and buttocks, which will often lead to lower-back, knee, and ankle trouble. Women, if you have to wear them, do proper stretching exercises after you wear them to compensate for the stress caused those muscles.

BOOTS: Boots are not made for walking on concrete. They are suited for farmers or wranglers who spend their time on soft earth. They do not hold the foot securely. The movement they allow can lead to instability. If you wear them, for dress, for instance, choose a pair with a little less than the thumbnail you would allow plain shoes. Too much room will allow too much slippage and the possibility of blisters. On the other hand, don't give yourself too little room or you will end up with corns on your toes. Try for a happy medium.

SANDALS: Wear them on the beach not on the block. The same goes for moccasins and deck shoes. In the city, with their thin soles, they just transmit huge amounts of stress and force into your feet that can end up really hurting them.

RUBBER THONGS: Unlike sandals, my recommendation for these is that they shouldn't even be worn at the beach. The synthetics in them can cause skin irritation when they react with the perspiration on your feet. At the beach, they may catch in the sand and you end up with a twisted ankle. The thongs between your toes can cause blisters.

Special Considerations for Sport Shoes

Having looked at what considerations should go into choosing a shoe for everyday life, let's look at more specialized uses that footwear is put to when it is worn for different sports.

Three factors determine what shoes are right for your sport: the motion it requires of your feet; the surface you will be playing on; and the shape, flexibility, and other idiosyncrasies of your feet and legs. Finding the right shoes, after having pondered these three factors, is largely a matter of trial and error. Safety depends on the comfort and fit of your shoes—so keep trying pairs until you find a make and model that works.

The point of this section is not to recommend particular shoes, which change season by season as the manufacturer incorporates improvement and a new understanding of what works best for individual sports. The best source of this type of concrete consumer rating is probably the magazines devoted to particular sports. They usually review new shoe models. Another potential reservoir for information is the salespeople in the stores that cater to customers who practice the sport in which you are involved.

RUNNING, JOGGING, AND WALKING As we have noted in passing, a running shoe is suited to the few sports, such as running, jogging, and walking, in which an athlete sets out in one direction—forward. Where most other sports require players to move in all directions, the runner always goes straight ahead. The runner's shoe must be one that keeps the foot and leg facing forward, so the runner doesn't twist the knee or ankle and has a cushioned landing. This is taken care of in running shoes by a flared heel. The heel helps control your rear foot and knee as they leave the ground, keeping the leg's unidirectional movement stable.

At the same time, the width of the heel absorbs the impact of your foot against the ground. This is crucial, since with each step you take your heel may have to endure three to four times the force of your body's weight as it hits. Running shoes have a special shock-absorbing wedge, called a midsole, between the rubber bottoms and the upper of the shoe. You can see the sides of this midsole when you look at a good running shoe. It's usually a lighter colored wedge of material that gives the bottom added thickness. Some of these midsoles are firm, others emphasize compressibility. In general, if you have fairly rigid feet with high arches, you need maximum flexibility together with high compressibility and shock absorption. If your feet are softer, you can tolerate a more rigid shoe, since your feet already are designed to absorb some shock.

If you are using the highly compressible, impact-absorbing midsoled shoes, there is one thing to be aware of. These shoes lose their compression ability rather quickly, which may be gone before the sole shows any real signs of wear. If you have high arched feet that demand this type of shoe, you'll have to buy running shoes more frequently than your less arched competitors. To be specific, if you are a serious runner, covering 10 to 20 miles a day, your shoes will lose their compressibility after six weeks. You may hate to toss what look like still new shoes, but giving your feet the protection of zippy new sneakers as soon as the old ones lose their bounce is your best insurance you have to keep your feet and legs healthy.

Running shoes shouldn't cost an arm and a leg, but don't buy the cheapest available either. Usually, within the $40 to $60 range you can get a decent pair. Another tip. Don't try to buy your running shoes in a regular shoe store. Go to a good running-wear store that specializes in footgear and equipment, and carries a wide variety of shoes, up to the top of the line. That way you can try on the best and compare them. Furthermore, the salespeople will understand you are comparison shopping, not to save a few pennies, but because you are searching for the shoe most fitting to your needs. Most of these stores will let you walk around for a decent period in the shoes you think you like best. Gary Murke, winner of the first New York Marathon, and now owner of Super Runner's Shop in Manhattan, even lets customers jog up and down on the sidewalk in front of his store to see how the shoes feel. He knows how frustrating it is to buy shoes without knowing whether you will feel good running in them.

As far as fit goes, remember the points already made in this section about the rule of thumb and checking width. Note also, that you shouldn't be trapped into thinking that you wear a certain size and that's it. In a running shoe, you may need a half to a size and a half larger than your street shoes.

Do you have unusually wide or narrow feet? Unfortunately, only a few companies manufacture running shoes to meet your needs. For very wide feet, try shoes from New Balance of Boston, Van's of California, and Saucony of Massachusetts. If your feet are narrow, see if you can find shoes made by Brook's, New Balance, or Van's.

RACQUET SPORTS For racquetball, tennis, squash, paddleball, and other racquet sports, another factor comes into play in selecting your shoes. Because you need to be able to twist and turn when necessary, you should avoid the flared heel of the running shoe, as it will trip you up when you try to move to the side. You want simple shoes that conform to the shape of your foot and are adequate for the terrain on which you will play.

For tennis, especially when you are playing on a concrete court, an impact-absorbing, padded sole wouldn't hurt. As opposed to running, where most of the weight falls on the heels, in racquet sports you have to be on your toes, literally, since it's the ball of your foot and toes that take most of the floor shock. Unfortunately, most tennis and racquetball shoes sold today are not as good for the feet as they should be. The soles are thin and the shoes offer little in the way of compressibility. However, a few manufacturers are starting to adopt a wedge construction that incorporates a layer of impact-absorbing material. If you play often, it would be worth your while to shop around until you found these shock-absorbing shoes.

As in running, if you have very wide or very narrow feet, you may have trouble finding shoes you can wear. However, New Balance has brought out wide widths for racquet sport shoes and, hopefully, other companies will follow this lead.

BASKETBALL Traditional basketball sneakers, which many players still prefer, lace all the way up the ankle. Researchers have found the canvas "high-top" ankle section is actually too flimsy to give the support most players need. For most people involved in this sport, we recommend a regular, low-cut sneaker. You can buy sneakers that are specially designed for basketball, but, in truth, any sneaker designed for multidirectional movement will do the job.

BASEBALL For baseball, too, normal sneakers will do. Some players feel, because baseball is played outdoors, they play best with a rubber spike, which can dig into the earth, giving them added traction. If you want to wear spikes, that's fine, but avoid shoes with long, thick spikes or metal-tipped cleats. Wearing long or metal spikes in a game in which players frequently collide is courting disaster, since they can cause serious injury to other players.

ROLLER SKATING Roller-skate boots are designed for balance and the ability to shift weight evenly from one edge of the boot to the other for ease in steering and turning. What's needed here is a rigid leg so the ankle won't wobble and distort the shifts in weight.

The most important part of the skate boot, therefore, is the counter, which is designed to keep the ankle in place. Make sure yours is strong, and if it gets worn out, replace it.

If you're using your skates for trick skating or disco dancing, you'll need extra shock absorption, though not so much as to mar your ability to transmit degrees of pressure to the wheel edges. Pick up some shock-absorbing insoles made particularly for roller skates.

Make sure the laces fit your feet comfortably. They should be neither too tight to restrict circulation nor so loose that you lose ankle stability.

CYCLING Some people swear by the special cycling shoes now manufactured.

They say these shoes are superior because they fit well into the toeclips (which are on the pedals to keep your feet from slipping off) and they transfer force more readily to the pedals.

In my opinion, unless you're a serious competitor, just about any flat-bottomed shoe will do, such as tennis or racquetball sneakers. You can even wear running shoes, since the flared heel is of no disadvantage to a cyclist, who uses no sideways motion. Though, it is worth remembering that in running the main force falls on the heel, whereas in cycling force falls on the forefoot, so a shoe with added forefront shock-absorbing qualities would be preferable.

As with other shoes, make sure your foot fits comfortably, but, in this case, also be careful that the shoe tip fits in the toeclips firmly, but not too tightly.

GOLF The metal cleats of golf shoes don't carry the same risks as those worn on baseball shoes, since you don't slide into other players on the putting green. The only risk these cleats pose the wearer, a real risk, is that the player may get caught in a pothole walking between shots. The cleats on golf shoes are not for efficient walking but so that the golfer has traction and stability when swinging the club. It might be a good idea to clean your cleats between shots so you don't slip or trip as you walk the fairway.

As an alternative to golf shoes, you can wear almost any athletic shoe, though you should avoid running footwear, which would limit rotary movement of the feet and ankles.

Socks for Sports

It may sound silly, but the socks you're wearing can make all the difference between enjoying yourself and playing your best, and being uncomfortable, cranky, and off your game. In sports and exercise, even little things count, and that means you should pay attention to even things that seem insignificant, like socks.

The primary purpose of socks is to keep your feet comfortable and as dry as possible. Socks that are too tight bind your feet. Socks that are too large bunch up, causing blisters and skin irritations.

The best socks for most sports are made of cotton or cotton/Orlon. These materials are good because they act like the wick of a candle (hence the attribute of these socks called "wicking"), which draws perspiration up and away from your feet, leaving them relatively dry and sweet-smelling while you work up a sweat. Synthetics, especially nylon, do the opposite. They insulate your feet, leaving them sticky, sweaty, hot, and, most likely, smelly. Smelly feet are not just to be avoided because they bother your locker room partners. Smelly feet are a sure sign that large numbers of microorganisms are breeding on the surfaces and in the warm, moist crevices of your skin. The best preventative is not to wear synthetic socks, though a thin band of nylon elastic to hold up the socks is acceptable.

In winter, for sports such as ice skating, skiing, and hockey, you will want the warmth of wool, but you also need something with the ability of cotton to wick away perspiration. So wear two pairs of socks: a thin undersock of cotton and a warm outer sock of wool.

Year-round, the best color for socks is white. Why white? Colored socks contain synthetic dyes. If your sweat mixes with and dissolves the dye from your socks, you may not only find your skin is tinged with the color of the socks, but that it itches and smarts because your skin has reacted adversely to the dye.

Change your socks at least once a day. If you perspire a lot, change whenever your socks get wet. Whatever you do, never wear a pair of socks twice in a row, without having washed them. Fungus and bacteria grow at an alarming rate in sweaty socks.

Massage

We have already talked about the high value Mainland Chinese place on foot massage. I want to show you such a valuation is well placed and that you should incorporate massage in your daily or, at least weekly, routine. After going a little further into the value of the massage, I will outline foot and leg massage procedures that you will find helpful.

Massage can be used to treat injuries as well as to reduce the tension that causes back pain, muscular tenderness and tightness, headaches, swelling in the legs and feet, and weakening of the immune system. Regular massage from one to three times a week, can help prevent as well as safely treat these problems, as well as reduce the strains of athletic performance.

To understand how massage accomplishes these things we must think about what happens when our muscles or tendons are injured or overtightened. First, the muscle and tendon fibers contract. They become brittle and inelastic, and hence easy to tear. This tightness causes electrochemical changes in the salts found within and outside each muscle-tendon cell. As a result, fluid gathers around the cells, and trapped protein molecules cluster and grind together. A swelling forms around the cells made up of lymph and protein molecules. The return flow of lymph throughout the lymphatic circulatory system is blocked. This disruption puts pressure on the nerve endings, causing pain in the muscle.

Massage reverses this process. It breaks up the clusters of protein cells that block the flow of lymph fluids. Electrochemical balance is restored. Finally, the muscle-tendon fibers relax. When these fibers are relaxed, energy is consumed and utilized more effectively. High blood pressure caused by constriction of arteries from tight muscles is often reduced. The circulation to injured cells returns to normal, bringing in nutrients and removing toxins and waste products. As muscles relax, tension and anxiety are reduced.

By now you are probably wondering why so few people have availed themselves of this wonderful healing and energy-enhancing therapy. The answer may be found in our increasingly complex society, where simple and beneficial methods of healing are overlooked in favor of more complex, frequently dangerous or toxic methods. Modern traditional medicine thrives on complexity and toxicity, choosing to overlook or minimize the benefits of older, proven healing methods

Try self massage or, even better, have someone you love give you a massage. Frequently, people will say they don't know how to give a good massage—but any massage is good. Just do what feels natural and pleasing. Still, there are some basic principles and techniques that will help you get the most out of massage. Following are two massage routines. The first, designed to take from 6 to 10 minutes, is easy to do by yourself. It is an ideal wake-up tonic for your feet and legs in the morning or to soothe them after a long day. The second, more in-depth massage will take between 30 minutes and an hour. It is best administered by a friend and is meant for maximal therapeutic benefit.

THE 10-MINUTE MORNING MASSAGE The best preparation for any foot massage is relaxation. Take a nice hot bath to relax your muscles or, if you don't have time for that, just lie down on the floor, close your eyes, and "let yourself go" by taking long, slow, deep breaths for three to five minutes. Open your eyes slowly. Now that you are relaxed, you can start the massage. It helps to have an oil like sunflower, safflower or soy oil—which moisturizes the skin at the same time—on hand. If you are fortunate enough to have someone massage your foot and leg, the best position is to be lying on your back. If you must do it yourself, sit up with your back supported against a wall or firm chair. This will prevent back strain. Start at the toes and work your way back to the heel and then up the leg. First, manipulate all of the joints in your toes. Flex them one at a time in each of the toes—the metatarsal joints, the bunion joints, and the ones further back. Then flex the ankle joint by rotating your foot in a circle to loosen the whole area up.

The best way to rotate your foot is to cross your legs, hold the leg of the crossed one just above the ankle bones, and relax the foot completely. The point here is not to use the muscles of your foot to rotate it—that wouldn't be very relaxing—but to use your hands and let your foot just flop. Just take the front portion of your foot and slowly turn the whole thing in small, slow circles. Go first in one direction, then in the other. Alternate directions for at least a minute. This loosens up and lubricates your ankle joint with synovial fluid, a clear liquid manufactured in your joints to lubricate the cartilage. Synovial fluid also softens your ligaments—those panels of tissue that make your joints stable—and keeps them pliable. So, getting the fluid into the joints on a regular basis is a good way to prevent sprains. As we age, the natural production of synovial fluid lessens, making it especially important to lubricate the joints.

After you've rotated each foot for a minute, gently massage the musculature of each foot, top and bottom. You can use your fingertips to knead the feet with varying pressure. Move them in circles. Use the heels of your hands, or your whole hand, to gently squeeze and knead the muscles. Don't be afraid to use pressure, unless you are very sensitive.

Massage should start with the toes and work all the way up the leg to the thigh. To do it properly spend at least three to five minutes on each leg. That may seem like a long time, but it's really not very much time for preventing injury to your feet and legs by keeping them pliable.

IN-DEPTH FOOT AND LEG MASSAGE A complete massage of the legs and feet will take between 15 and 30 minutes per side. Put aside the time. Why rush such a pleasant experience? Missing any section of tissue or point of energy blockage may minimize the positive effects of the effort. So take your time. Always be in touch with your body's sensations, and communicate them to the person massaging. This will allow the person to concentrate on areas and points that need it most.

A quiet room with dim lighting will be most relaxing. A noisy, bright room will tend to work against the stress-reducing benefits of the massage. The room temperature should be warm enough to prevent a chill. While scented massage oils are generally available, cold-pressed safflower or sunflower oil is less costly and will usually work as well. You may add your own fragrance if you wish.

Massage is best performed in five simple stages: *Stage One* is performed with short, fast, light strokes. *Stage Two* is characterized by long, firm strokes. *Stage Three* is a form of acupressure, like shiatsu, which works on energy points. *Stage Four* uses firm, fast pressure across the muscle and tendon fibers. *Stage Five* is a repeat of the first stage, with short fast, light strokes.

In each stage, begin with the tip of the toes and work up. This will encourage proper lymph circulation and energy flow. Never start with the legs and work toward the toes, as this can block flow.

All five stages have equal importance. While each stage we will describe seems slightly more important than the preceding one, all are equal. Each enhances the preceding stage, and brings with it a new benefit.

STAGE ONE breaks up swelling in the muscles and tendons and encourages fluids to flow out of the muscle fibers and into the lymph channels. This is accomplished by short, fast, light stroking of the fibers toward the heart. When muscle fibers are sore or tender, this stroke may hurt slightly. After only 20 or 30 seconds, however, the discomfort will probably diminish. Much of the pain is caused by trapped fluid between muscle cells. This stroke should be repeated for up to one minute along the whole length of the muscle. Begin at the bottom of the foot and work back toward the heel. Next go to the top of the foot and work from the toes to the ankles. Continue this process from the ankles to the knee both in front and in back of the lower leg. Next work from the knee to the hip. This process directs the flow of the extra lymph fluid toward the major collection area in the groin. If a particular areas hurts more to the touch spend more time on it, but always be very gentle.

STAGE TWO uses very firm, long, slow strokes. As in Stage One, begin at the toes and stroke first toward the ankle, both on the top and bottom of the feet. Next stroke from the ankle to the knee, and finally from the knee to the hip. Use the palm of your hand and the area between your thumb and index finger. It is very important to add more and more pressure with each stroke to help force out the extra fluid from the muscle fibers. If a particular area is very painful, go back to Stage One for that area before continuing. At this stage lotions or creams will allow the hand to slide easily over the skin. If no lubricant is used, the skin may begin to feel tender and irritated. The smooth sliding action is important to help relax the muscle fibers, and can help reduce anxiety and general tension. This stage may take from 5 to 15 minutes per leg to complete.

STAGE THREE requires slow, careful pressure applied to each point on the foot and leg, beginning at the toes and again working toward the hip. You may use your thumbs, fingertips, or both. Press down gently and feel for a firm, small lump of tissue (often the size of a pea) under the skin, deep in the muscle or tendon, as well as around it. The pressure should be straight down. These points follow the patterns of acupuncture points called meridians. Not all the places along these lines will be painful. If there is no pain or discomfort, move to the next place on the skin. As you come closer to active points, discomfort will mount, often changing to pain when you are over an active point. It is important to breathe deeply. Shallow breathing blocks lymph flow, while deep breaths pump fluids up to the center of the chest as well as reduce the pain the acupressure may cause.

Press for 10 to 30 seconds over each very painful point. Press for only 1 or 2 seconds over nonpainful points. Press each painful point three times, trying to go deeper each time. Picture each painful, firm spot as a balloon that you are trying to pop. When the point is broken, it will no longer feel firm, though it may still feel painful to the touch. People are often surprised to feel these points as they had no idea that they were there.

Charts are not necessary. Discomfort and pain will lead you to the correct places as a Geiger counter leads to radioactive material. The vast majority of points will be found on the bottom of the feet, including in the toes, as well as on the calf and rear thigh. Few exist on the top of the foot and the front of the leg, so don't waste too much time there.

STAGE FOUR is performed by rubbing transversely—across the muscles or tendon fibers—with very fast, short strokes. Increase the pressure gradually. This stroke can help break up adhesions, a form of internal scar tissue on an injured or overused muscle or tendon. Breaking up adhesions returns normal elasticity and a normal range of motion to the muscle or tendon. Spend more time over the most painful areas or points, using your fingertips as well as the palm of your hand. The time it takes to complete this stage varies depending on individual need. Begin with the toes and work your way up to the hip.

The amount of time spent massaging your feet and legs is determined by several factors. If your muscles are tight, injured, or lack adequate blood circulation for any reason, more time should be devoted to massage. How much time will be determined by such factors as who is massaging you, how much free time you have available, the cost if done professionally (the charge is usually by the hour), and the patience, perseverance, and fatigue of the massager. A maximal therapeutic effect is probably obtained somewhere between 15 and 30 minutes per foot and leg, or 30 to 60 minutes total.

STAGE FIVE repeats Stage One, completing the circle of massage therapy.

31

Common Foot and Leg Problems

In the previous chapter, we outlined the way to maintain your feet and legs in the best possible health. Preventing problems by being aware of your extremities, eating right, exercising, purchasing the right footgear, getting enough rest, utilizing massage, and living with as little stress as possible will keep you as fit as humanly possible.

Nonetheless, even the healthiest individual can be injured playing a sport, be infected by bacteria, or hurt him- or herself. This chapter will look at some of the common problems that occur in the foot and leg area, beginning with those that affect everyone and then moving to sports injuries particularly. (Arthritis will not be discussed here since it is the subject of an entire chapter—chapter 25—in this book.)

Dry Skin

Dry skin on the feet is very common, especially among elderly people, whose circulation is often poor. If your circulation is bad, that means there is a reduction in fat secretion by the feet's sweat glands, which in turn leaves the skin dry. The decrease in blood flow to the feet also leads to dryness.

Dark-skinned people tend to have dry skin. If you have dark skin, avoid using any soap on your feet at all. If you must use soap, make it one of the super-fatted ones—soaps with added oils that are low in alkalis. Among soaps of this type are ones made by Dove, Neutrogena, and Alpha Keri. It's still best, though, to use warm water without soap.

If dry skin is a problem, take the time after your bath to give your feet an oil rub, using soy, sunflower, or safflower oil. Let your skin have a minute or two to absorb the oil while you rub. Then wipe off the excess. If your skin is really dry, try Herbal Salve One (described at the end of this chapter), two or three times a day. At the same time, make a point of avoiding irritating chemicals.

Besides the dry skin oil treatments, try increasing the circulation of your feet by undertaking a cardiovascular exercise program such as the walking routine described in chapter 30. Vitamins, especially A, D, C, E, and chelated zinc, are helpful in controlling any skin inflammation or problem such as dry skin.

Blisters

Anybody who has ever taken a long hike in the wrong shoes knows all about blisters. When the skin gets irritated, it gets inflamed. To soothe the inflamed area, a natural healing fluid, lymph, flows into the tissues. The fluid puts pressure on the nerves, which can be painful.

The best treatment for blisters is prevention. With good hygiene, proper exercise and appropriate footgear, blisters will never develop.

If you already have a blister, use the following procedure. First gently wash the area with soap and water. Next, wipe it liberally with rubbing alcohol. Clean an ordinary needle by allowing it to soak in alcohol for at least 15 minutes. When the skin and blisters are prepared, remove the needle from the alcohol and use it to create an opening near an edge of the blister. Allow the fluid to drain by gently pressing the blister with a gauze pad. Apply Herbal Salve One over the entire blister and cover it with a sterile gauze pad. Never rub the salve into the blister. If the blister refills, repeat the process.

Calluses and Corns

A callus is a thickening of the skin on the bottom of the feet, usually in a pressure area like the heel or the ball. It is never "normal" and should not be ignored. If you have a normal foot structure, the fat pad that is under your foot should prevent callus formation by acting as an impact absorber. But if the bone structure of your foot is moved out of position, more pressure is placed on dropped metatarsal heads, causing calluses to form across, for example, the balls of your feet. (The metatarsals are five long bones that run on the top of the foot to the toes and correspond to the bones on the back of the hands.) If your heel strikes the ground at an improper angle or if you just happen to be heavy, calluses can also form.

Calluses are easy to treat by taking a warm-to-hot foot bath every night. Don't use soap, which dries the skin. When you're finished, use pumice stone or an emery board to gently scrape the skin smoother. Then, rub oil into the skin, until you can see it is absorbed. You might also invest in impact-absorbing insoles to reduce pressure. If these methods don't decrease calluses, consult your doctor.

"Corn" is such an innocent name for those hard, round yellow lumps that sometimes grow on people's feet. Corns, which may form either on the tops of your toes, at the tips of your toes, on the sides of your feet, where the bunion joint is located, or even inside a callus, are a symptom of intermittent rubbing. They might be caused by extra extensions of bone—calcium deposits—pressing on your skin from the inside of your shoe or from the ground pressing on your skin from the outside. They can even be traced to a bed sheet tucked too tightly. Indeed, patients in nursing homes often develop corns and calluses from this pressure. The delicate skin on your feet can't take too much pressure and so it thickens, growing a protective lump at the point of pressure.

If the corn grows too large, and the source of the pressure has not been relieved, it becomes part of the problem your body was attempting to solve in the first place.

The simplest treatment for corns is to reduce the pressure from the outside. You can do this by wrapping lambswool around high-pressure areas or by using shock-absorbing insoles. You can also work on your corns by pumicing them down after a long bath. But steer clear of over-the-counter corn removers, which have the same danger of burning your healthy skin as do wart removers. You may need a doctor's advice if the corns are persistent.

Skin Infections and Inflammations

FUNGUS INFECTIONS Athlete's foot, the most common fungus infection of the foot, develops as a result of excessive perspiration and the ensuing sensitivity to a fungus that is actually always present on the skin. That should lay to rest the idea that you pick up athlete's foot from the floor of the shower or locker room, left there by other infected individuals. No, not at all, the fungus is already on your feet, it just suddenly gets out of control.

So, the next question is why does it get out of control? The skin of our feet is the habitat for thousands of microscopic creatures, whose mutual war for food and space keeps each one reined in. However, when there is excess warmth and moisture, as when you put your socks on without properly drying your feet, the fungus gets out of control. The fungus, then, is likely to affect anyone who repeatedly forgets to dry his or her feet carefully.

The most common place for fungus infections to grow is between the toes. Along the bottoms of the feet and the soles are other typical locations.

These infections can be chronic, acute, or subacute. The chronic infection looks like dry skin. You may notice the skin is actually peeling. Sometimes it itches, sometimes it doesn't. In a subacute infection, there may be a breakout of little water blisters, and in the more acute infection, there are also breaks in the skin that can become secondarily infected by bacteria. An infection this acute is usually extremely itchy.

While fungus infections are not contagious, they can spread on your own foot until the entire sole is covered.

For an acute fungus infection, the best treatment is to wrap the foot lightly in a gauze bandage, elevate the foot and leg, and use a wet-dressing treatment with Herbal Solution One (explained at the end of the chapter). Pour the solution onto the gauze and let it dry completely. Then wet it again. This treatment should dry out the inflammation. Follow this procedure for 24 to 48 hours. If the acute stage has not subsided by then, consult a professional.

If what you have is a subacute fungal infection, you do not need the evaporative dressings. Instead you should use Herbal Salve One (also explained at the end of the chapter) three or four times a day. Rub a small amount in until it disappears, wiping away any excess. If there are fissures in your skin, protect them by wrapping them lightly in a cotton gauze bandage. Keep your feet as cool and dry as possible during the treatment. The subacute stage should be resolved in three to five days.

The chronic fungus infection is the hardest to treat. For one thing, people don't recognize dry skin as a fungus infection at all. To heal a chronic infection, use the herbal salve three or four times a day. If the condition has not cleared up in six to eight weeks, you will need to talk to a physician.

While you are treating your infection, it might be helpful to apply powder to the skin on your feet. However, do not apply powder to the insides of your shoes, because the perspiration from your feet will cause it to cake and become a new medium for fungus to grow in.

It's always a good idea, but particularly when you have a fungus infection, to change your socks several times a day. That will keep your feet dry. You can use vitamins and minerals to help with the healing. A good program for that includes 1,200 IU of vitamin E, 10,000 IU each of vitamins A and D, 50 milligrams of chelated zinc, and 5,000 to 10,000 milligrams of vitamin C, all taken orally. If you've ever had a fungus infection, taking vitamins and minerals daily is as good a preventative measure as any.

FUNGUS NAILS Nails, too, are part of the skin and can suffer a fungus reaction, which causes them to blacken or thicken. There is no lotion, salve, or other outside chemicals to treat this condition.

One treatment that will help is vitamin therapy. Vitamin E taken orally and applied topically to the skin around the nails can improve the quality of your nails. Never apply the vitamins directly to nails themselves. Put it them lightly around the nail on the skin and wipe off any excess.

The only nonsurgical way to get rid of fungus nails is through a drug, griseofulvin, prescribed by a doctor. This drug must be taken for years and produces side effects. It is important to try to avoid getting this condition in the first place, by keeping your nails filed thinly with an emery board.

WARTS It is quite common to get warts on the bottoms of your feet. A wart is a virus that gets inoculated into your system through a break in your skin. This is a problem you can pick up in the locker room.

Once this tricky virus is inside, it secretes an enzyme that prevents your immunological system from detecting it. Therefore no antibodies are produced as a defense. The body is smart enough, though, to recognize something is disturbing it, and calls up a second line of defense, surrounding the virus with skin cells to prevent it from spreading.

The majority (80 percent) of warts disappear after two years. It is not exactly understood why, but its seems your body eventually works out what is going on and develops an antibody or other means to eliminate the wart. But if a wart has existed for at least two years, then it should be treated with other means, particularly if it is causing discomfort.

There is no surefire method for eliminating this problem, but at least we can warn you about the downsides of different measures. In trying to eradicate a wart, it is important not to overuse over-the-counter remedies. Most contain acid to dissolve the wart, but this can dissolve the skin in the area as well. Professionals use these acids in a different way. They put on a little to cause a skin irritation that will awaken antibodies that will rush to the area and eventually kill the wart.

An innovation in recent professional treatment is the surgical laser. This method, while often very effective, does have drawbacks.

There is no guarantee that the wart will not return.

CONTACT DERMATITIS Contact dermatitis is another skin condition that can affect the feet. It can be caused by something as simple as a chemical in your socks. Your skin reacts to the irritation, becoming red and inflamed. Little blisters may form or the skin may crack. This problem can occur on any part of your foot.

Your first task is to find out why it is happening, that is, what is irritating your foot. Wash your socks with warm water only, using no soaps or detergents, since these contain alkalis that can irritate your skin. White cotton socks should be worn to eliminate the risk of being bothered by the chemicals in colored socks and synthetics. Change your socks regularly. If your shoes may be causing a problem, change them. Even the most natural leather has been treated with tanning agents that can irritate. The glue that holds the leather together may also be giving you problems. Orthopedic shoe stores carry hypoallergenic shoes, made without the chemicals known to irritate the feet. These may represent the answer.

While you are trying to track down the cause of your difficulty, you can start working on eliminating the problem you already have. Elevate the foot and leg, wrap the foot in gauze, and start applying the evaporating wet dressing, using Herbal Solution One. After 24 to 48 hours of this treatment, the condition should have subsided to a subacute stage. If that's happened, discontinue the wet dressings and switch to the herbal salve, applying it three or four times at day.

If you find that one of your symptoms is itching, you can get quick relief by rubbing the area with an ice cube for several minutes. Once again, if none of these methods work to control your dermatitis, consult a professional.

IMPETIGO Impetigo is one of the only truly contagious foot conditions. It is usually found in children and starts with a crack in the skin, which leads to a bacterial infection, usually around or between the toes. In the acute stage, it must be treated by a doctor.

In the milder stages, you can approach it with the following methods. Dress the foot lightly in gauze and use Herbal Solution One to draw out the infection and inflammation. The child should be kept off his or her feet as much as possible with the leg elevated. If the condition has not improved after a day or two, go to the doctor.

Related Skin Problems

PSORIASIS Psoriasis is a skin condition that commonly affects the feet and lower legs. It is not a disease, but a condition—the body's way of ridding itself of negative energy, such as tension resulting from problems at home or at work.

The symptoms of psoriasis are patches of reddened, irritated skin, with white scales. If you scratch one of these patches, it will bleed. The best treatment is Herbal Salve One four times a day, particularly if your case is mild to moderate. For a severe case, where there is a lot of thickening on the soles of the feet, it's necessary to rub the salve into the feet at night, covering them with a plastic bag to help hold the salve's moisture in all night.

While you're using the salve treatment, it's a good idea to cushion the tissue on the bottoms of your feet by wearing shock-absorbing insoles in your shoes or even flexible protective athletic shoes. Another good idea is to wear cotton socks, so as not to be bothered by the irritants found in synthetic materials.

The best ultimate treatment for psoriasis is to recognize you are taking your problems out on yourself, so you should try to relax. Change your attitude toward your problems, and loosen up.

MORTON'S NEUROMA This is a particular type of tumor. Pressure on the ball of the foot can sometimes result in pinching of the nerves that run between the metatarsal bones. The pressure that results in inflammation of the nerves will first create burning or tingling sensations in the ball of the foot, running up to the toes. If this condition is allowed to continue untreated for months, the fat around the nerves can congeal into a benign tumor, which is called Morton's neuroma. This neuroma is best treated by not allowing the pressure to create it in the first place. It can be relieved with massage and comfortable shoes. Once it has developed, however, it can only be treated by a doctor.

INGROWN TOENAILS Ingrown toenails are another common problem, especially among teenagers and young adults.

If you let an ingrown toenail go without treatment, by the time you finally see a professional, the treatment may be extremely uncomfortable because the nerves are particularly sensitive here. If treatment is sought early, surgery on the nail will be less painful. So it is important to seek professional care as soon as you realize you have an ingrown nail.

Surgical lasers offer an effective means of removing ingrown nails and permanently preventing their recurrence.

INSECT BITES Insect bites can be especially irritating to the feet. Treat them as soon as possible by rubbing the area with ice, which will prevent the release of histamines that cause swelling and itching. Rubbing the area for several minutes also prevents the toxins that were injected by the bite from spreading because it slows down circulation. Repeat the ice treatment every 10 or 15 minutes. Only if the bite might be from an insect that transmits disease do you need to seek a doctor's aid. If it's a typical bite, ice followed by an evaporating wet dressing, such as Herbal Solution One, will draw out the inflammation, and that is all that is necessary.

Circulatory Complications

Circulation is the ground of everything we have talked about so far. It feeds your bones, your muscles, every cell in your body with blood. If there isn't enough blood, your tissues will not get sufficient oxygen and nutrients to keep them healthy.

Regular aerobic exercise can prevent arterial and venous disease from getting a "foothold" in your system. Because muscular contractions assist both arteries and veins in keeping a regular blood flow, you build up the health of the conduits by using your muscles. If you don't exercise, you are contributing to the breakdown of circulation. With age, the circulation to the feet and legs becomes less efficient; therefore, the older you get, the more important it is to do some kind of exercise to aid this circulation.

Exercise is also important if you spend a lot of time sitting down. Sitting for long periods can cause a vasospasm, closing off blood vessels and diminishing the circulation. Getting up and walking around the room for 30 seconds every 15 to 20 minutes will help break up vasospasm and restart normal circulation.

The way you eat is also important. If your diet is heavy in fats and cholesterol, you are inviting fatty deposits to develop in the arteries. If you smoke you are also inviting problems. Nicotine is a vasoconstrictor. It causes the nerves to make the blood vessels contract, which stops the flow of blood in some areas.

Let's look now at some specific problems of circulation that can affect the feet and legs.

ARTERIOSCLEROSIS The arteries, which bring blood from the heart to the extremities and the rest of the body, have an elastic quality. If that elasticity is not being maintained because the artery is not getting enough oxygen or nutrients, the artery deteriorates, inviting calcium deposits. This results in hardening of the arteries, or arteriosclerosis obliterans, which keeps the artery from expanding enough to allow a sufficient flow of blood down to the feet and legs. The result of this can be pain in the legs and feet, loss of mineral content from the bones, muscle spasms, and muscle cramps.

The seriousness of arteriosclerosis in the legs and feet can be assessed by seeing how many blocks you can walk before the charley horses begin. These cramps are clinically called claudication pains.

If you suffer from this symptom, you know the only way to stop the pain is to stop walking. A rest allows your heart to pump enough blood into your feet and legs to wash away the waste products that have been clogging up the muscle and causing it to contract. Massage can help too. However, one of the only ways to overcome this problem is exercise. Exercise sends large amounts of blood into the feet and legs, forcing the arteries to open and close widely, forcing them to become more elastic.

Changing your diet can also help. If you have been heavy on the cholesterol, eating a lot of meat and dairy, fatty deposits in your arteries may be one cause of the problem. Taking at least 1,200 IU of lecithin daily is one of the best ways to nutritionally control fatty deposits, along with cutting down on the fat in your meals.

PERIPHERAL DIABETIC NEUROPATHY The arteries take the blood from the heart while the veins bring it back to the heart for another go-round. In between are the smaller capillaries, which ferry the oxygen and nutrients down into the individual cells and take the waste products out, eventually leading back into the veins.

When there is poor circulation through the capillaries to the nerves in the feet and hands, it can result in peripheral diabetic neuropathy (PDN). PDN is related to diabetes, which can bring on the condition faster than it would for a nondiabetic. One of the results of diabetes, which stems from the inability of the pancreas to produce insulin, is that there are high levels of sugar in the blood. A high level of sugar contributes to the damage of the nerves that results in PDN.

Peripheral diabetic neuropathy is often first detected by symptoms in the foot. There will be excessive sweating as well as sensations of burning, pins and needles, tingling, itching, and numbness. In the most severe cases, the skin may break down into abscesses and ulcers underneath the foot.

Keeping your blood sugar down to normal levels will minimize peripheral neuropathy and regular exercise will maintain adequate vascular circulation throughout the body. This should be aerobic exercise, which uses major muscle groups in a rhythmic and continuous way.

THROMBOANGITIS OBLITERANS Another circulatory problem that affects the feet and legs is thromboangitis obliterans (TAO). It is restricted to people who smoke tobacco. Tobacco contains nicotine, which causes the nerves that control the blood vessels to misfire, shutting them down at the wrong time. Since nicotine affects individuals differently, this condition may be minor for some but cause drastic changes, to the point of gangrene developing, for others. The obvious solution is to stop smoking.

RAYNAUD'S PHENOMENON Another condition where the sufferer's nerves are misfiring and wrongfully contracting the blood vessels is called Raynaud's phenomenon. It largely affects women and anyone who is easily stressed and deeply emotional. It results in a lack of circulation in the feet and hands. People who are extremely sensitive to the cold are also affected by it.

This phenomenon is even more difficult to treat than other circulatory problems we have mentioned because it is partly caused by psychological susceptibility and so calls for counseling to teach the sufferer how to control his or her energy by handling problems more constructively.

If you have Raynaud's, be sure to wear proper shoes and socks in the winter to keep warm and even dress warmly in the summer. You can also approach the problem nutritionally. Take vitamin E in doses of 800 IU three times a day, a half hour before you eat. Vitamin E counteracts Raynaud's phenomenon by dilating the blood vessels, which gets more blood to flow to your feet and legs. Niacin can help in the same way. Vitamin C will work to strengthen arterial walls, while lecithin helps cleanse the fatty buildups on the walls.

FROSTBITE Frostbite also works by shutting down the capillaries. The capillaries are small and those in the toes the smallest in the whole body. When the foot is very cold, it reacts by cutting off these tiny blood vessels to conserve heat. If the vessels are closed long enough, frostbite results.

Warning signs of frostbite are a painful burning sensation followed by numbness. You may notice not only that the skin on your feet and ankles is cold, but it may be mottled purple and white as well.

The first step when you've seen these warning signs is to rewarm your feet, slowly and gently, in lukewarm water of between 90 and 100 degrees. Circulation will return slowly. In a half hour, the feet will be warm enough for you to assess the damage.

If little damage has been done, applications of vitamins A, D, and E (in ointment form) would be helpful. The skin should be protected with a layer of cotton or lambswool and kept warm. If there's more extensive damage, indicated by injured skin that turns black and continued pain after rewarming, do not try to treat yourself but go to the hospital for immediate attention.

If you know you have a problem with becoming cold, try to protect yourself before you go out. Protect the skin with vitamin A and D ointment or some Vaseline in a thin, even layer all over your foot. Wear cotton undersocks and wool oversocks. An insulating insole can keep the cold from reaching your foot from the ground.

Keep moving when you are outdoors. The more you move, the more the blood circulates. It's when you stop moving that you are at risk.

VARICOSE VEINS A very common problem is varicose veins, which are the result of the improper opening and closing of the valves in the vessels that control blood flow. This makes it difficult for the blood to get back to the heart.

There are ways to help relieve varicose veins, mainly by doing what you can to keep your blood flow up, in spite of the fact that the veins are not doing their job properly. Exercise on a daily basis is one of the keys to helping this condition. By helping the blood flow, you are counteracting some of the problems due to the damaged valves. Another way to ease the problem is to sit with your feet and legs elevated, waist-level or higher, whenever you possibly can. By doing that, gravity can help the blood move back to your heart.

You can also wear support stockings. Many types are available but we recommend you buy them at a pharmacy or surgical supply store, where the items will be better quality. If you have a severe problem with varicose veins, you might look into custom-made surgical support stockings. In this country, two companies, Jobst and Sigvaris, make them. If you can't afford support stockings, sometime an Ace bandage will give you the support you need. Wrap a three- or four-inch bandage around the leg where the varicosity is a problem. This may require wrapping your legs from the toes to the groin if the problem is severe.

PHLEBITIS Phlebitis is a common adjunct to varicose veins. When the blood doesn't flow up properly because of varicosities, it starts to clot. If blood starts to clot in varicose veins, phlebitis, or inflammation of the veins, results. The overall condition is very dangerous because the clot may loosen and flow to the heart, causing a heart attack, or to the brain, where it will cause a stroke.

The phlebitic area is easy to discern because it is hotter than any other part of the body. A warm compress might prove useful. Just take a kitchen towel, soak it in warm water, wring it out, and place it on top of your elevated leg for 5 to 10 minutes. This will help dry out some of the inflammation in the veins, skin, and tissue, yet it is not hot enough to induce the clot to dislodge.

Another symptom indicating phlebitis is pain in the affected area. Also the skin in the troubled area becomes dry, itchy, and brittle. It may even crack and peel. Any superficial break in the skin over a varicose area in the leg must be treated promptly to avoid an ulcer. Apply Herbal Salve One to the spot three or four times a day, then cover it with sterile gauze.

Although the outer manifestations of the condition are not that bad, phlebitis requires great care. Total bed rest in which you stay in bed for two weeks is the best treatment. You shouldn't even get up to go to the restroom as any movement may dislodge the clot.

Sports Injuries

For athletes in any sport, the feet and legs are particularly vulnerable to injury. Here are some tips about foot and leg injuries that are common to athletes, arranged by affected area.

TOENAIL INJURIES Toenail injuries are common in athletes who wear poorly fitting footgear. No matter what sport you play, play fair with your feet by wearing shoes that fit.

If your shoes are too tight, when you run, jump, slide, dance, skid, or skate, your toenails will jam against the end of the shoe, resulting in bleeding under the nail. When the blood dries, you have a black nail. If this happens often enough or seriously enough, your toenail can even fall off.

However, if you have the right shoes and you're still plagued by black toenails, your problem may be fungus related. A fungus toenail can look a lot like one injured by being stubbed. If fungus is your problem, refer to our earlier discussion of Fungus Infections.

TOE JOINT INJURIES Toe joint injuries plague athletes of every sort. These joints are very easy to jam. All you have to do is jump onto a toe that happens to be bent under your feet. If the pressure is sudden enough, you will feel a sharp stabbing pain and hear a snapping sound.

Probably you've torn a tendon or ligament. Even if the tissue is only partially torn, it can take six weeks or longer to heal. With this kind of injury, you must stop playing immediately, get off your foot, and elevate it. Apply an icepack to keep the swelling down. Do this on and off for 24 hours. Then start moving the toes to prevent adhesions or scar tissue from forming.

When you're ready to get back to your sport, tape the injured toe with half-inch tape. Don't tape it too tightly or circulation will be impeded. Just wrap it gently so there is some compression. If it's necessary to tape a neighboring toe, do that as well. The point of taping your toe is not only to strengthen it, but to provide a built-in alarm. If your toe starts to swell again, you can feel it and will know to get off your feet before you are injured again.

But what if that snap was not a tendon or ligament pulling but an actual bone breaking? How could you tell? A broken bone doesn't just swell, it also turns black and blue. Look for black and blue marks even further up the foot than where the suspected broken toe is. When the bone breaks, so do a lot of blood vessels. If you think a bone is broken, go to a doctor.

METATARSAL JOINT INJURIES The metatarsal joints of the foot are like the knuckles of the hand. Because they are joints, they also have tendons and ligaments that will tear under stress as well as bones that will break.

You'll know the metatarsal joints are injured by the same signs you would have if you damaged your toe: sharp, stabbing pain and, perhaps, a cracking snap, and swelling. If you've broken a bone, it will likely be evident from the black and blue marks. Treatment, too, is similar to that given a toe. Use elevation, ice, and an Ace bandage or compression dressing.

A common metatarsal joint injury, injury to the joint under the big toe, is popularly know as "judo joint," since aficionados of this sport often suffer from it. Basketweave strapping of the toe can help here as a way to prevent swelling, aid the healing process, and allow for a certain amount of joint movement even though the area is taped.

A stress fracture, a complete or partial breaking of the bone, can also appear at these joints. This one is different from the type of fracture caused by sudden, intense force. You can recognize this injury by the fact that you feel intense pain from the joints when you are working out, but it disappears if you stop the exercise. This fracture will heal by itself if you decrease your workout to about half your normal time and intensity. If this doesn't work, then take a two-week break, and restart your exercising gradually.

A march fracture, so called because it frequently afflicted soldiers in World War I who marched too long, affects athletes who work out too heavily at the beginning of the season on bones that have been relatively idle. Your foot will hurt and the pain is continuous, not decreasing when you stop your workout. For this you will have to see a doctor who will set the bone and tell you to rest up a couple of months before you return to play.

ARCH INJURIES In pursuing your sport, you may notice pain under your foot along the arch. There are two common injuries to this area.

The first is a simple strain. This usually occurs in people with sharply arching feet. Flat-footed people are immune to it. They may suffer from the second problem, plantarfascitis, or inflammation of the sheet of fibrous muscle tissue that runs underneath the foot.

Both conditions call for the same treatment: extra arch support. Athletes should tape the ailing foot. Shoe inserts are not enough. Taping the foot for extra support is a temporary but useful way of relieving the pain.

Use either flexible cloth adhesive tape or elastic adhesive tape, 1½ to 2 inches wide, cut into 8 to 10 inch strips. Then reinforce the arch as follows. Place one edge of the tape about 1½ inches up on the top of the outside of the foot just in front of the outside ankle bone. Pass the tape under the foot, pulling gently on the tape as you lay it against the skin. The tape should gently lift the arch of the foot up to prevent it from flattening. The tape should end up on top of the inner side of the foot, just before the tendon which goes to the big toes. Never cover this tendon, as it will stop it from moving and could result in tendinitis. Overlap the first strip of tape with another approximately ½ inch and continue with additional strips of tape until the entire bottom of the foot in the arch area is covered with overlapped tape. It is important to protect the skin from the negative effects of prolonged taping by using a special solution sold in surgical supply stores.

HEEL INJURIES The heels are vulnerable to stress fractures when they are overused. The symptoms are the same as with metatarsal fractures: pain that increases when you exercise, decreases when you stop. Treatment is also the same. Give your heels a rest by reducing or stopping the exercise temporarily.

Heelspur syndrome, another common problem, is characterized by fluctuating pain. You feel it when you start to play, but then it goes away only to flare up a few minutes later. This condition, if untreated, will only get worse. The periods of relief will get shorter while those of pain extend.

Heelspur syndrome is caused by a bone spur, a mass of bone and calcium deposits actually growing on the heelbone and protruding from the heel. The pain comes from the irritating rub of this extra bone on the tissues surrounding it. If an athlete has all the symptoms of heelspur but an x-ray can't find a trace of it, then this may be a case of acute plantarfascitis, a condition described when we discussed arches.

In either case, your best bet is to take pressure off the heel so that the spur will not continue to grow or the muscle will heal itself. To get rid of the pressure, get some sort of padding for your shoe, either a professional orthotic device or even a simple horseshoe-shaped foam rubber pad cut to the shape of the heel.

Another simple and useful tactic to use against the pain is to stretch out your calf muscles. Sometimes your rear leg muscles tighten and contract in reaction to the spur, because they're trying to lift the heel off the ground faster than normal in reaction to the pain. If you stretch those muscles, you can break the spasm and reduce the pain in your heel.

ANKLE INJURIES Almost everyone seems to sprain ankles, the most vulnerable of joints. You're especially prone to such sprains if you turn your feet slightly inward as you take a step. You can determine if you do this by taking a look at one of your old pairs of shoes. If the insides of the heels are more worn down than the outsides, you're "pronating." When this happens, the ligaments on the outside of the ankle tend to shorten. At the same time, those on the inside are stretched to the limit. Under this situation, it only takes a little extra pressure for the ligaments to rip.

The easiest way to prevent these sprains is to stretch as part of your warm-up. Sitting down, cross one ankle over the other knee. Using the hand on the same side of your body as the ankle that's crossed, grasp your ankle just above the ankle bone and hold it steady. Then let your foot relax completely. With the other hand, slowly rotate the foot in circles, first in one direction, then in the other for at least 30 seconds each. Now gently twist the entire foot inward at the ankle. This stretches the outside ligaments. Hold it in that position for 10 or 15 seconds, then relax. Now twist the foot out for 10 to 15 seconds. Now treat your other ankle to the same stretch. Both will be limbered up and ready for your workout.

If you're prone to ankle sprains, another good preventive measure is to wear an ankle brace. A simple elastic band will give your weak ankle an extra margin of support.

However, what if, after taking all these precautions, you still get a sprain? First elevate the foot. Then wrap the ankle in an Ace bandage and apply ice. Do this for one or two days. Then begin to gently move the ankle again, while keeping up the ice applications to keep the swelling down. This way your joint will retain its normal range of motion with minimization of scars and adhesion.

ACHILLES TENDINITIS The Achilles tendon, a ropelike tendon behind the lower half of the lower leg, is formed by the two tendons that emerge from the two large muscles of the calf. It extends down the leg, inserting into the heelbone behind the ankle. It may become inflamed and can tear at any number of attachment points, both of which conditions are know as tendinitis.

To relieve this condition, put a heel lift in your shoe on the side that was injured. Try a quarter inch of felt or other shock-absorbing material. If you are careful, the tendon should be healed in about six weeks.

If this condition recurs, use the old-shoe test we discussed in the section on sprained ankles to see if you turn your ankle inward as you walk. This can complicate or even cause tendinitis. An orthotic device can help you keep your ankles from turning it. Also keep stretching your calf muscles daily.

LOWER LEG INJURIES Like the metatarsals, the lower leg bones are subject to stress fractures. Commonly this will occur in the upper or lower portions of the bones. The symptoms of the fractures are increased pain during exercise with a diminishment of that pain when you rest. Rest, ice, and elevation are suggested. Also reduce or lay off exercising for a while as the area heals. A full orthotic, made of thermoplastic, can be useful. This controls the foot from heel-strike to toe-off, allowing only normal ranges of motion, rather than the excessive ranges of motion that helped cause the fracture.

Laymen use the term "shinsplints" for any pain in the front of the lower leg. Actually this is a portmanteau term that covers a number of possible problems including "anterior compartment shinsplints," inflammation of the muscles and tendons; and "posterior compartment shinsplints," caused by the muscles pulling away from the bone. In either case, a bone scan will be needed to properly diagnose the condition.

If you suspect this condition, either in the front or rear position, use rest, elevation, and ice packs for a few days. Then do plenty of stretching and exercise for the rear leg muscles, which are partly to blame in almost every case. Before getting back into working out, check with a foot specialist to see whether you have a foot imbalance that could be corrected. Return to exercising slowly and carefully.

How to Prepare and Use Herbal Remedies

We will close by giving you the instructions for preparing and using the herbal remedies mentioned repeatedly in this section. They are only some of the tools you can use to keep your legs and feet healthy and vigorous in a natural way.

Herbal Salve One

1 qt. cold-pressed safflower, sunflower, or canola oil
½ oz. comfrey leaves
½ oz. goldenseal root
½ oz. peppermint leaves
Vitamin E (d-alpha tocopherol) capsules
Vitamin A (B-carotene) capsules
Vitamin D capsules from a vegetable source
Mason jar of the type used for preserves
Cheesecloth

Mix the oil, comfrey leaves, goldenseal root, and peppermint leaves in a large pot. An electric pot is best. Heat the mixture at a very low temperature. You must be able to test the oil by placing your finger in it without burning yourself. The oil should only be warm, never hot (at about 150 degrees Fahrenheit). Start the process early in the morning as you must allow the mixture to cook for 12 to 24 hours. The purpose of this procedure is to leach out the natural herbal-healing elements without destroying them with excessive heat. Cold-pressed oil is best because it contains vitamins, such as vitamin E, and minerals, which help in healing and can be destroyed by extraction processes that use high heat. After the oil has been cooked, strain it through clean, fresh cheesecloth, which you may want to boil first to kill bacteria. Strain it twice to remove impurities that could become abrasive to inflamed or damaged skin. Add to this the contents of the vitamin capsules.

It is wise to add at least 25,000 to 50,000 IU of each vitamin. You can pop open the capsules using a round toothpick. Mix the vitamins in well with the oil. Note that the oil will probably have taken on a green color from the herbs during the cooking process.

If the salve is kept refrigerated in the mason jar, it will last for up to six months. The vitamin E in the oil and from the capsules will help act as a natural preservative. It is a good idea to buy a small ointment jar from the pharmacy or health food store, which can hold half an ounce or one ounce of salve. Thus, a small amount can be kept at room temperature for daily use and the rest refrigerated to maintain its potency.

This salve must be used three times a day. Gently rub in a small amount. Wipe away any excess salve that doesn't absorb into the skin. Discontinue use if any skin irritation develops. This antifungal, antibacterial salve is ideal for fungus infections, cuts, scratches, bee stings, and so on. Never use it on deep wounds or cuts nor around the eyes. Yes, it is safe to eat a small quantity by mistake. You may reduce the ingredients proportionally to reduce costs.

Herbal Solution One

1 qt. boiled water
¼ oz. comfrey leaves
¼ oz. goldenseal root
¼ oz. peppermint leaves
1 qt. Mason jar
Cheesecloth

Make a tea by adding the ingredients to the boiling water. Allow the mixture to stand, covered, for 30 minutes. Carefully strain the mixture with the cheesecloth, twice to remove all the leaves. Allow the solution to cool to room temperature. Never use it boiling hot. The solution may be kept in a closed jar for 48 hours before being discarded. The amount of ingredients may be reduced proportionally.

Wrap the area to be treated with sterile gauze or bandages. Pour just enough of the solution onto the gauze to thoroughly saturate it. Allow the gauze to completely air dry. Repeat the process as often as necessary.

The solution is antifungal, antibacterial, and mildly astringent. Used as described above, it brings infection in the skin to a head, reduces itching and inflammation, and dries up oozing skin caused by abrasions, fungal infections, and so on. Be warned, however: Never soak your feet in a basin of the solution, and discontinue use if skin irritation occurs.

PART SIX

Heart, Blood, and Circulation

W.B. Yeats' poem, "The Circus Animals' Desertion," concludes, "I must lie down where all the ladders start / In the foul rag-and-bone shop of the heart." His metaphor is meant to suggest a mature person's heart that has been lacerated by romantic and political betrayals. However, given the lifestyles of many Americans, who fill their arteries around the heart with plaque and debris, we might take the poem literally. With heart disease being the number one killer, we are certainly driven to ask if there is any way to clean up our foul hearts.

A sufficient supply of blood and oxygen is critical to the body. In the case of heart attacks and angina, blood flow is severely reduced through atherosclerotic and occluded arteries leading to the heart. Strokes, which cause severe brain damage and senility, may be brought on by the inability of the oxygenated blood supply to pass freely through the arteries leading to the brain. Peripheral diseases—those affecting less vital parts of the body farther away from the heart and brain—are caused by the same mechanics. Poor blood flow through the legs can cause intermittent claudication. Patients with this problem are frequently unable to walk more than a few feet before stopping because of the pain.

Arteriosclerosis provides a sad but clear example of how cardiovascular disease is closely interwoven into the fabric of lifestyle and diet. It is estimated that by age three practically all American children have arteries that are lined with fatty deposits—the initial stage of arteriosclerosis. As this condition becomes advanced in the adult years, it can lead to associated degeneration. This may take the form of atherosclerosis and arterial occlusion, angina and heart attacks, peripheral disease of the legs, strokes, and senility, as mentioned above.

A less severe and more generalized indication of insufficient blood flow through the circulatory system is lethargy. This is fatigue that may be created by various degrees of oxygen reduction in the bloodstream. When fat-laden blood cells cannot pass through many of the tiny capillaries in remote parts of the body, the body is deprived of a portion of its required oxygen supply and feels tired and sluggish. Even a single meal of greasy meat and heavy dairy products may make the body respond with this tired, drained feeling. After one has rested sufficiently and the fat starts getting digested through the system, the blood begins to thin out and flow better. When more acceptable oxygen levels are restored, a person's energy level rises. Eating this way habitually, though, may result in a constant feeling of sluggishness—a condition of chronic fatigue.

If we ask the opinions of some of the leading doctors and nurses in the field of alternative heart disease therapies, we find reason both for hope and despair. The hope comes from the stories of dramatic reversals of coronary problems, while despair comes from pondering the persistently hard-line doctors who refuse to consider alternative approaches fly in the face of much evidence that newer therapies work. Hidebound doctors are encouraging to patients who do not want to alter their diets, exercise or do anything else to change their lives, though they are veering toward disaster.

Dr. Robert Roberti, a cardiologist, gives us hope. We have understood for the past 10 to 15 years, he relates, that these and related conditions are not irrevocable. Changing diet, reducing stress, stopping smoking, getting exercise, and other natural therapies can reverse heart and circulatory problems and put you back on the road to good health.

32

Heart Disease

Heart disease is an illness that kills more Americans than any other, one in five. In nearly every year for which we have records, heart disease has been the number one killer in the United States. The heart attack is the largest killer. In 1999, an estimated 1.1 million Americans will have a new or recurrent coronary attack. Every 33 seconds an American dies of heart disease. Heart disease accounts for 42 percent of deaths each year. Stroke is also one of the leading causes of long-term disability. On average, we have a stroke a minute and someone dies from a stroke every 3.5 minutes. In 1999, we will spend an estimated $287 billion for the nearly 60 million Americans (more than one in four) who have some form of cardiovascular disease.

Many people are confused about heart disease and the question arises: Whom do you believe? Do you believe the physician who says there is not a shred of evidence that nutrition, diet, homeopathy, and other alternative routes to dealing with the problem are valid? The physician who says this in the face of dozens of articles in peer-reviewed, respected medical journals that say these therapies work and that deficiencies in such areas of proper diet and exercise lead to heart disease while proper use of these regimens reduce the risk?

Do you believe your doctor who says you do not have to change your diet, lose weight, exercise, reduce cholesterol, even though much literature says you do have to make these changes?

Perhaps after you read this chapter, which looks at new therapies that can help with this condition, you will be in a better position to know whom to believe.

How the Heart Works

Basically, the heart is a pump composed of four chambers and works through the contraction of muscle. Blood enters the right major chamber of the heart and is then contracted to both lungs where it picks up oxygen. It then returns to the left chamber of the heart and is pumped out by the left ventricle into the arteries in order to deliver oxygenated blood to all the tissues of the body. After passing through the tissues, blood returns to the heart through the veins and the process repeats itself.

If the coronary arteries become clogged, the circulation of blood going to the heart is impaired. This is detrimental because the heart muscles need oxygen from the blood in order to contract properly. Therefore, when the circulation of blood is impaired the function of the heart is damaged as well. The heart may then have problems with electrical conductivity, which could result in abnormal heart rhythms.

Another factor important for the normal beating of the heart is magnesium. A lack of this mineral may cause the aorta or the coronary blood vessels to go into spasm. This in turn causes poor functioning because it reduces the amount of blood to the heart muscles. When the body is unable to pump as well as it might because of poor or uncoordinated muscle contraction, the body receives signals from the heart in the form of pain, called angina.

It is important to realize that the arteries are more than pipes delivering fuel to the body. Dr. Savely Yurkovsky, who specializes in cardiology, emphasizes that they are living structures with other vital functions.

"The arteries are not just some type of dead pipe whose only purpose is for something to flow through them; they are very much living structures," he says. "Their linings have about 98 different enzymatic systems, whose purpose is not only to prevent blockage buildup damage, but to allow oxygen and nutrients to permeate freely through them into the heart muscle or other tissue.

"Quite often the degree of the arterial disease present is oversimplified with an overly mechanical approach to the problem. It is simply judged by the size of the blockage in the arteries. In other words, if the blockage is big then it is said you have severe problems with the circulation and if it is moderate or if no blockage is seen, you are usually given the impression that no circulatory disease exists whatsoever. But this is not necessarily true.

Ninety-eight enzymatic systems are responsible for maintaining health in the lining of the arterial wall, and it has been found that in circulatory diseases, usually 46 out of 98 enzymatic systems are destroyed or limited. This leads to the deposition of heavy metals, calcium, and free radical pathology which further leads to the formation of insoluble complexes being deposited and injuring the intima (inner lining) of the arteries."

Dr. Yurkovsky goes on to explain that these insoluble complexes bind to lipids of the outer membrane of the arterial walls leading to an overall increase in collagen, a scar tissue, which prevents oxygen or nutrients from permeating the lining freely. This destroys the integrity of normal circulatory physiology, since the final objective of this arterial supply system is to deliver the right amount of oxygen to the cells.

If nutrients and oxygen are not delivered to the heart muscle, it will begin to degenerate. First, the metabolism of the heart muscle cells will switch from aerobic to anaerobic. The body uses this as an alarm system to try and preserve the function of the cells, like a backup mechanism. This eventually leads to a buildup of acid between the cells, in the interstitial spaces. In the long run, cells devoid of oxygen become exposed to free-radical activity, which causes them to weaken and die. Very often, accompanying this process is an increase in nerve sensitivity, and the person experiences the pain of angina.

In the early stages of this pathology, where the permeability and transport of oxygen is impaired, a patient may have classical angina symptoms suggesting blockages in the arteries but have normal angiographic studies. In other words, no coronary artery blockages are seen on the angiogram. At that point, he or she is usually told that no circulatory disease exists and that perhaps the problem is one of depression, life stress, etc.

HARDENING OF THE ARTERIES Obstruction does not occur suddenly; it is a slow, usually painless process that takes years to form through a process called arteriosclerosis, or hardening of the arteries. The cholesterols that build up in the arteries are carried by the blood in complex molecules called lipoproteins. These are combinations of fat and protein that are much larger than a normal blood cell. The LDL (low density lipoprotein) is a molecule that has a large amount of fat and a small quantity of protein. Having large amounts of LDL in the blood is a major risk factor for coronary heart disease. Another lipoprotein, HDL (high density lipoprotein), has large quantities of protein and small quantities of fat. It is thought that these help reduce the amount of cholesterol in the bloodstream.

The beginning of heart disease is thought to be in childhood. By the third decade of life, lesions (plaque) develop in the artery walls, characterized by an over-accumulation of cholesterol, other body fats, and debris which can completely shut off the blood flow in the artery. Usually the final stoppage is due to a blood clot that forms in the damaged artery, shutting off blood flow and resulting in the death of the muscle that the blood was supplying. Commonly, this is called a heart attack.

Why are Alternative Therapies Not Given a Fair Hearing?

Before beginning to discuss alternative heart treatments, it might be eye-opening to note the reasons so many doctors prefer to ignore them; traditional doctors are often enthralled by the dazzle of high technology and the promise of large financial rewards.

I asked Dr. Ronald Hoffman about this situation. Why, with so many indications that traditional therapies are not working, do not physicians, cardiologists, and other healers take a step back and see if other modalities might be in order?

Dr. Hoffman's opinion is that we have become the victims of a "medical-industrial complex" run amok. The cardiovascular unit where heart operations are performed is the crown jewel of many hospitals, a major profit center, and the source of hundreds of referrals to physicians who derive their livelihoods from hospitals. The heart unit is a high-tech wonder, very easy to develop and expand and very hard to cut back.

According to Dr. Hoffman, many respected cardiologists, professors at major universities, are decrying the current trend by saying we should get away from high-tech, expensive procedures. He thinks we should simply use medicines when necessary but handle the majority of heart cases by natural dietary modifications, sending the few remaining cases to centers of excellence scattered around the country. Unfortunately, instead, the high-tech centers are spreading like wildfire.

Diet and Heart Disease

There is not a lot of controversy over what is wrong with the American diet, with its high amount of animal proteins, saturated animal fats, dairy, deep-fried foods, and refined carbohydrates. The average American diet is 43 percent fats, 14 percent proteins, and the rest mainly carbohydrates. The average daily intake of cholesterol is 450–500 mg.

The American Heart Association recommends we cut fat intake to 30 percent and only 10 percent of this should be saturated fats (fats found particularly in land animals, palm and coconut oils, hydrogenated vegetable oils.).

(Note: We have been told that margarine, made from "polyunsaturated fats," is good for our hearts and will lower cholesterol. That is simply not true; it is loaded with the fatty acids that contribute to heart disease. Instead of margarine, use olive oil, canola oil, or other oils such as flaxseed, almond, safflower, sunflower, or soy. Of these, olive oil would be on the top of my list. But don't have margarine.)

No more than 10 percent of the oils you eat should be polyunsaturated fats, like those found in vegetable oils (such as corn and cottonseed oils). According to the American Heart Association, we should get the rest from monounsaturated fats, such as olive, and be taking in less than 300 mg of cholesterol each day.

Maybe former President Bush did not like broccoli, but perhaps if he knew some of the things that were in this marvelous vegetable, he would have changed his mind. Broccoli and other produce is the first thing to turn to for heart-benefiting foods.

We eat broccoli and all kinds of produce, seeds, legumes, and grains to get our beta carotenes and maybe the vitamin C, but they also contain important phytochemicals. This includes beta carotene, but also alpha-carotene, ascorbic acid, ash, boron, caffeic-acid, calcium, chlorophyll, chromium, citric acid, copper, glycine, iron, linoleic acid, lysine, magnesium, niacin, oleic acid, phosphorus, potassium, riboflavin, selenium, thiamin, tryptophan, and zinc, among others—there are 1,000 different phytochemicals, so important in protecting us from cancer. Among them are also the phytoestrogens, which guard against prostate, breast and lung cancer. These chemicals have all kinds of healing properties. Chlorophyll, for instance, helps purify the blood and acts as a detoxifier.

If you want to lower your blood pressure, you can do this with vegetables such as garlic, broccoli, or asparagus. Do not forget, you should have at least five servings of vegetables and three of fruits each day, raw, steamed, or juiced. Once you start, you will notice a world of difference in your overall vitality.

Other invaluable heart foods are rice and beans, complete proteins rich in fiber and B- complex vitamins.

We grow up with the pernicious myth that if it is not an animal protein, it is not a complete protein and so not really nutritious. I did studies at the Institute of Applied Biology that proved conclusively that beans, legumes, and all grains contain complete proteins just like animal proteins, without the saturated fats. They do not have the high calories, and are rich in vitamins, minerals, and essential oils.

Hence, cultures that have rice and beans as a dietary staple have been quite healthy. There are thousands of ways to prepare these foods, too. Go into a health food store and look at the different preparations along with all the other foods sold. When you see the variety, you will not feel deprived by not having steak and potatoes.

It is worth mentioning the division over the proper foods for those with heart disease. There are over 60,000 dietitians in the United States and they have been a primary source of information on what a sick person should be eating. After all, the physician has little training in nutrition, graduating medical school with only an hour or two of learning about the subject. The dietitian is well trained, yet even within the field of dietetics there is a split. A very small percentage believe the standard American diet has played a large part in causing diseases we are beset with, including heart disease.

Blood pressure medications are natural diuretics and deplete the system of magnesium, needed for heart function. Moreover, she notes, many Americans do not eat many vegetables, and it is from vegetables where you get lots of magnesium. We need to increase the magnesium content of our diets, she says, with vegetables, seeds, nuts, and beans.

Luanne Pennesi, R.N., B.S.N., a holistic nurse, also emphasizes diet as a means to deal with heart problems. She will sit down with a patient and assess his or her eating habits and lifestyle, getting patients to recognize the different facets in their lives and how they connect to their health.

The holistic nurse, she tells us, will discuss the problems with dairy in a diet and the options, such as rice milk. The nurse will tell them about the effects of raw vegetables in the diet, how many types of vegetables exist, and what the difference is between organic versus processed food. She'll mention the effect of pesticides in the soil and how they affect fruits and vegetables, having them taste the difference between organically grown and nonorganically grown produce. When we take away the stigma of organic food, the idea that it is bland and tasteless, and let patients taste it for themselves, they find it is easy to shift to organics.

Alternative Heart Therapies

CHELATION THERAPY Chelation therapy is an alternative therapy that has become especially popular since coronary bypass surgery has been pronounced ineffective for up to 65 percent of the people receiving it. Coronary bypass surgery and cardiovascular drugs and medications do offer slight though highly invasive relief of the acute complications of heart disease. However, chelation therapy, which is being administered to hundreds of thousands of heart disease patients, is proving quite successful, and it is considerably safer and substantially less expensive than bypass surgery. It is not new, having been in use for over 40 years.

Chelation therapy consists of intravenous treatment with a chemical drip solution called EDTA (ethylene diamine tetra-acetic acid), which slows or reverses some plaque formation in the arteries and thus retards the degenerative process. It does this by bonding with toxic metals such as mercury, lead, calcium, and aluminum and carrying them out of the bloodstream through the kidneys. EDTA enhances a freer flow of blood, thus permitting more essential oxygen and nutrients to circulate and be absorbed by the body.

As chelation therapy is more commonly used, chelation specialists feel that it will become the most important heart disease therapy offered in the future. This therapy is discussed in detail in the next chapter of this book.

HOMEOPATHY Dr. Ken Korins explains how his specialty, homeopathy, offers another alternative practice that seems to get results with heart disease: "Homeopathy works by giving very small doses that are extremely individualized to the person's symptoms and physical state. These doses work on a type of vibration or energy that stimulates the body much in the way that acupuncture works."

Many traditional practitioners dismiss the benefits of this technique due to a colossal ignorance of the evidence. These physicians say this therapy has never been proven by randomized, double-blind studies in the way more scientific procedures have been. Dr. Korins argues that is absolutely incorrect. He tells us that in 1993, in a British medical journal there was an article by Kleinsman, which reviewed 107 clinical studies of homeopathy. About 80 percent of them found that homeopathy had positive effects. And many of these were extremely rigorous studies. In the *Journal of Pediatrics*, for example, double-blind study showed extraordinary results from homeopathy.

What are the kinds of heart problems that improve with homeopathy? Hypertension is a big one. It will help people recovering from congestive heart failure, cervo-vascular accidents, arteriosclerotic heart disease and a very wide range of conditions.

In classical homeopathy, the specialist selects a single remedy. Korins elaborates, "For our work, we don't rely on a lot of tests and the high technology that goes with them. We prefer to look at what symptoms a person has and how they present themselves. For example, if a person is having angina, tightness, a squeezing sensation, a remedy like songea or cactus, which is extremely effective in treating angina, would be called for. Sometimes there is a congestion in the head, a hot feeling when the blood pressure goes up. The prescription there might be a remedy like gloline.

"What you are looking for is an idea of what physical state the patient is in. A particular heart patient may not have any manifestations of heart disease per se, but you are looking for the particular homeopathic remedy that will stimulate the body's healing properties. In that case, it will really be the body itself that is doing the curing and not the homeopathic remedy."

QI (CHI) ENERGY An Oriental treatment that has some success with heart patients is the manipulation of *qi* (chi) energy. Dr. Jeie Atacama, D.D.M., LaC., uses *qi* energy to accomplish healing. With this practice, one does not use needles as in acupuncture, though it does share with acupuncture the concentration on meridians of the body. In a technique he learned from his father, Dr. Atacama uses his fingers directly on the skin of patients. As Bill Moyers showed on his television reports on Oriental philosophy, such healing practices as *tai chi* and *qi gong*, depend on channeling internal qi energies to rebalance the body.

Dr. Atacama has not counted the numbers of patients he has helped, but it has been, he estimates, between 3,000 and 5,000 in 20 years of practice. Rebalancing *qi* energy can help greatly with heart disease by rebuilding the body's health and restoring its self healing powers.

This practice works exactly like acupuncture. U points are found on either side near the base of the spine. One point is connected to the large intestine, which is part of the bodily system particularly in touch with the *qi* energy, which involves all the nonliquid, biological energy that circulates through the body. The treatment should be done three times a week, lasting for as many weeks as is called for by the condition. If the problem is cramps in the leg due to poor circulation, 10 sessions would get rid of the problem.

HERBAL REMEDIES More Americans will be buying and using herbs now than they have been in the last 100 years. Dr. James A. Dukes at the U.S. Department of Agriculture (USDA) has written a major textbook and has become a major authority on the use of herbs for health. But not many doctors have caught up with Dr. Dukes. One person who has is Letha Hadady, one of the leading herbalists in the United States.

She says most Americans do not go to the doctor when they are a little sick; they wait until they are really suffering. They might have chest pains, difficulty breathing, but they generally are not going to the doctor and, of course, not to their herbalist. They say, "I'm tired; I'm under stress," and ignore it. But that is a terrible approach because some of the underlying problems of heart disease are the ones they are complaining of: fatigue, stress, and poor digestion. Poor digestion and fatigue lead to cholesterol buildup, which leads to pain and heart congestion. People try to breathe more deeply and reduce stress when they experience these early symptoms, but it does not help. But changing your diet, taking herbs and foods that reduce cholesterol, that will definitely help.

Hadady's clients often have conditions that are unrelated to heart disease, according to them; but with her special training as an herbalist, she sees a connection to the heart. Mind, body, spirit, all are interconnected and our heart is affected by all of these things. Depression, for example, is a problem connected to a weak heart. Insomnia, poor concentration and palpitations are all signs that poor circulation could be touching the heart.

Many Western doctors will say herbs, especially Oriental ones, are not tested. This is a prejudiced answer because when you go to a public library or consult a computer indexing service like Med Line, which is available to all medical students and any interested person, you will find 3,500 studies on Chinese herbs alone. The majority of the research is done in Asia and for Americans to say this research does not count is racist.

There are quite a number of these remedies available in health food stores, by mail order, or in your local Chinatown.

She points out that one of the major underlying problems associated with heart disease is fatigue. Now Chinese doctors link the heart's health to the strength of the adrenal glands, not an obvious connection. "If I had a patient complaining of fatigue and being overweight, I would suspect heart problems if not then, somewhere down the line, so I would work on the adrenals. To strengthen the adrenals, you can get the herbal preparation from Chinatown called Goldenbook. It adds to immune energy and will help with kidney and heart problems. We strengthen what is weak so the heart will not falter."

Hadady goes on to mention that clove, a spice we have at home, is a strong stimulant. A pinch in the late afternoon will act as coffee. Coffee is a major problem because it increases stuck, painful circulation in the gastrointestinal tract which will affect the whole circulation, meaning the heart will not run smoothly. A pinch of clove will replace coffee better than anything else.

Siberian ginseng, a mix of various ginsengs, is good. The ginsengs are adaptogens, that is, they will help us maintain energy as well as aid us in living under a high level of stress. They support the nervous system. Raw Tienchi ginseng, one Americans are less familiar with, comes in powdered form. When you take a little bit (½ teaspoon) in cool water every day, it will reduce cholesterol and pain around the heart.

One Chinese remedy that is especially valuable in relation to heart pain and congestion of the blood vessels is Dan Shen Wan, which combines salvia and camphor. The camphor dilates the blood vessels while the salvia increases the heart's action. Another valuable remedy is Guan Xin Su He Wan, which contains frankincense. This is mentioned in the Bible, you may recall, along with myrrh; both increase circulation. Frankincense for stuck circulation increases blood flow around the heart. You can take it once a day to prevent heart attack. It can be chewed and swallowed. Letha Hadady recommends it even if you have no heart problem symptoms. It has healthy ingredients such as liquid amber, and sandalwood, which keeps the esophagus and chest cool.

Yan Shen Jia Jiao Wan is a combination of ginseng and other herbs that work on brain circulation, freeing the circulation of the blood in the brain, so it is not just for heart difficulties, but for victims of heart attack, stroke and hemiplegia (which paralyzes and cramps on the whole side of the body). It is taken as a preventive measure when you have high cholesterol and are at high risk of heart trouble. One a day prevents problems.

Baoxin Wan is a remedy for heart attacks. If you feel faint and experience pain and weakness, you sniff it like a smelling salt. If the pain is great and you feel the onset of an attack, then take it orally. It includes ginseng and liquid amber. The ingredients are always in English or Latin on the back. It treats the congestion of the blood vessels around the heart and frees the blood vessel.

Some of the underlying problems leading to a heart attack are well countered by herbal remedies, like excess weight and cholesterol. The best way to lose weight is not to get rid of your appetite or jazz up your energy level with a stimulant, but to take a sensible diet that reduces fat as well as take some herbs that are valuable additives. One preparation with a self explanatory name is "Keep Fit, Reduce Fat" capsules. The ingredients are ginseng, hawthorn, and other herbs that are good for the heart. Hawthorn is a slightly bitter, slightly sour berry and works as a digestive. You can take a capsule of Keep Fit after meals. Cholesterol is reduced and the muscle of the heart is made stronger.

Evening primrose oil is another useful way to reduce cholesterol. Chinatown is an excellent place to purchase this remedy since the prices are apt to be considerably lower than those given for comparable items in health food stores.

Another popular remedy in Asia is green tea, which has been reported all over, including in the *New York Times*, as a very good remedy for reducing cholesterol. "This is a good alternative to other caffeine teas," Letha Hadady mentions, "because the caffeine in it is very low. It gives the satisfaction of a bitter tea while reducing cholesterol."

Bojemni slimming tea is protective of the heart. It has hawthorn in it. Also beneficial is Xiao Yo Wan, a digestive remedy that boosts circulation and combats depression. It contains ginger, mint, and other herbs, eases the flow of bile, eases the digestive process, and reduces chest congestion.

Digestive Harmony is an American-made product that uses Chinese herbs, one of many such products now on the market, sold door to door or through mail order. "This is part of a trend now," Hadady explains, "a very important trend in herbalism, of using Asian herbs manufactured with American standards. Digestive Harmony can be ordered from Oakland, California. It will ease the underlying troubles related to heart disease.

Remember depression is in part a heart problem, Hadady says. The heart is not just a digestive center, but is for our emotions. Depression is rightly associated with heart disease since it affects the heartbeat. When we are not happy and our emotions are not smooth, then we feel it in the heart.

Some remedies that combat depression come to us from China. Coschisandra strengthens the energy levels and keeps us from losing the energy we have. It is good for both the adrenals and the heart. It fights against poor memory, poor concentration and depression. Also try Anshen Bu Nao Pien, available in all the Chinatowns in the United States. It is for depression, blood deficiencies and heart-related problems such as panic and anxiety.

Also useful is Mao Dong Qing, which is the chinese name for holly, and it comes in capsule form. It is for chest pain and prevention of heart trouble. You can take several of these capsules each day as a preventive. If you already have heart problems, it reduces cholesterol, congestion and pains.

"In general," Hadady concludes, "Chinese remedies for the heart also treat emotional problems, not just pain, but sadness, anxieties and other mental suffering."

Gary Null's Top Ten Supplements for a Healthy Heart

(1) COENZYME Q10. I have seen over 100 studies, minimum, that show how important this substance can be in helping oxygenate the tissue as well as giving a great boost to the heart.

(2) VITAMIN E. I would not imagine there is a doctor in America who is not aware of the literature on this vitamin. It keeps the red blood cells in the body from clumping together. It is estimated that between 400 and 800 units are useful in preventing stroke. You may go higher, to 1,200 or 1,600 units, unless other medical conditions preclude this usage. I believe we would cut the incidence of stroke by 20 percent, saving 50,000 to 100,000 people a year, just by having everyone take this little, inexpensive supplement.

(Let me mention at this point that I remember interviewing Dr. Wilfred Shute, a man who, with his brother, had worked for 35 years on over 30,000 patients whom he treated with vitamin E. I went to see his clinic, and, while I was there, I interviewed 50 people who were his patients, including a woman who kept photos of her toes, that had been covered with giant gangrenous sores. They were going to be amputated and it was vitamin E that saved them. It all seemed too good to be true.

This was at the very beginning of my career when no one believed vitamin E had such potency. People wouldn't take it. You couldn't even find it in most vitamin pills. Today every other medical publication is extolling the antioxidants in vitamin E. Do you ever wonder about all the people that died in the interim, who did not have to die and would not have if doctors had been more progressive and flexible?

Dolores Perri points out, "The knowledge of vitamins' value was there for 25 years. I remember talking to a doctor when I was working in a nursing home and telling him about vitamin E. He said, 'There's no definitive study on that.' The doctors just wouldn't look. Many of the elderly who could have been helped, were not.")

(3) CHROMIUM PICOLINATE. A lot of people have heard about this. It has been shown to be beneficial both for the heart and blood sugar.

(4) CSA (CHONDROITIN SULFATE A), also very good.

(5) L-CARNITINE. This is one of my favorites. If every American took 500–1,000 mg/day, we could really make a dent in heart disease. When I race— and I am an American Class racewalker, holding American records in indoors, outdoors, and all distances from the 1 mile to the 40 k—and I take the L-carnitine, I find I have a greater capacity for breathing. I am not as fatigued, and my recovery is much quicker. Now you should take L-carnitine along with vitamin E, because they work synergistically together and they work terrifically.

(6) VITAMIN C. If there is one vitamin everyone needs to take every day, it is this one. If a person has a cold or flu, he or she may require 50,000 mg of C for quick recovery; we should realize for heart disease we may require substantially more. So get over that old-fashioned idea that all you need is one glass of OJ and you have got the necessary vitamin C. That idea went out with the horse and buggy. Now we have thousands of studies in the literature of the valuable properties of C, which can help with everything from cancer to heart disease and diabetes. I would take 500 to 1,000 mg/5 times a day, because vitamin C washes out of your system, so we need to take it throughout the day. By the way, two physicians, specialists in coronary heart disease, recommend their patients take vitamin C before going to bed at night because they find it helps prevent heart attacks during sleep and in the morning. This is when the majority of heart attacks occur.

(7) LECITHIN. Lecithin is made from soy. Not only does it keep our arteries strong and healthy, but it helps with the emulsification of fats, helps the brain and is good for memory as well as the heart.

(8) EVENING PRIMROSE OIL, 1,500 mg daily.

(9) VITAMIN B1. Of all the Bs, this is the most important for the heart: 25-50 mg daily.

(10) MAXEPA (EPA AND DHA). This is better know as fish oil. They are part of the omega-3 and omega-6 fatty acids that you find in salmon, sardines, and

mackerel. But many people do not eat these fish so they should be getting them in MaxEPA. They should take 500 to 1,000 mg of this supplement. It is worth noting that clinical and epidemiological experience as well as scientific studies have found that people who have a lot of fish in their diet have less heart disease than people without such a diet.

These are the 10 natural nutrients to take to prevent or treat heart disease. Taking them is not a panacea but must be done as part of an overall program.

STRESS MANAGEMENT Virtually all the authorities agree that if you are going to get a handle on heart disease, and that includes the hypertension, the high triglycerides, high cholesterol (particularly the elevated low density lipoproteins, the bad part of the cholesterol), the overweight body, and all the other conditions that frequently contribute to coronary heart problems, then you are going to have to deal with stress. Stress or distress is a major problem for the American psyche.

For a long while we have known that stress is a contributor to heart disease, but only recently have we begun to understand the physiological basis of the connection. We will look at how this occurs before turning to stress management techniques that help dissipate this problem.

Richard Friedman, Ph.D., Harvard Medical School, remarks that most of us, when we are confronted with stressful situations, try to oversolve the problem. In our society, we constantly try to fit square pegs into round holes, and when we find that is not going to work, we turn inward, brood, and look for ways to dissipate stress, frequently by acting inappropriately, such as by overeating, drinking or taking inappropriate drugs or medications, contributing to the disease process.

Dr. Friedman tells us there is a link between stress and cardiovascular disease. Very recent research supports that when we are stressed, due to a fear of physical or psychological danger, the body exhibits a fight-or-flight response, as it prepares to fight an enemy. One of the important things happening internally, as triggered by the response, is your body readying itself not to bleed if you get cut or injured, which makes a lot of sense from a biological and evolutionary perspective. However, if the threats are psychological and you have a bad diet, you may be going through stressful incidents 20 or 30 times a day, triggering the fight-or-flight response. Each time this happens, the body prepares not to bleed by making your blood platelets stickier. This internal clotting takes place every time you get angry whether on a supermarket line or in a traffic jam. As this goes on for weeks and months, this continual clotting can contribute to the plaque in the arteries. A heart attack that may occur when you are 50 years old, would not have occurred until you are 80 years old if you had undergone less of the buildup induced by platelet stickiness.

When you are exposed to a biochemical or psychological stress, a host of changes are taking place in addition to platelet stickiness. The body's ability to fight off viral and bacterial infection will be lessened by the weaknesses induced by stress. Stress compromises the immune system's ability to fight off opportunistic diseases.

There is some good news, though, about our ability to fight off the debilitating conditions leading to heart attack. Dr. Friedman notes that just as continued stress leads to a weakening of the system, there is an opposite effect, labeled by his colleague at Harvard, Dr. Herbert Benson, as the relaxation response. Eliciting this calming response on a daily basis makes it less likely you will have high blood pressure or the arteriosclerotic plaque buildup or a heart attack down the road.

The relaxation response should be combined with other behavior modifications to create a healthier response to stress and all should be combined with the best medical care. That is the way to optimize your health.

Dr. Friedman tells us how the relaxation response is engendered: Use whatever strategy you have available to let go of any muscle tension you may be experiencing. Make sure your muscles are loose and your jaw lets go. After you are feeling a bit more comfortable, focus your attention on your breathing. If you find yourself having any distracting thoughts, do not let them bother or take you away from the process. As soon as you have a distracting thought, simply say to yourself "Oh well," and return to a concentration on your breathing and to a thought or image that allows you to stay calm, peaceful, and relaxed. Become aware of the cool air coming in and the warm air going out. Keep this up till you are deeply relaxed.

SPIRITUAL HEALING Dr. Ron Scolastico, spiritual counselor and author of *Healing the Heart, Healing the Body*, believes that the process of remaining healthy involves four important elements: "The first element is our physical life, which most people know a great deal about. The second element looks at our mental life. It is becoming clearer and clearer that our thoughts promote or hinder health, and in some cases actually cause disease. The third element addresses our emotional lives. Feelings, particularly love, have a profound effect. The fourth element addresses spiritual factors. I believe those energies come from our soul, which is an incredible source of power, love, and wisdom, inside each of us."

Dr. Scolastico says that we need to draw upon each of these factors as needed. Sometimes we must take physical steps, such as seeing a doctor and taking medications or herbs, but sometimes that is not enough: "For example, one of my clients developed congestive heart failure after a painful divorce, along with pericarditis, which is an inflammation of the membrane surrounding the heart. She failed to respond to medical treatment, and her condition began to worsen. As I worked with her, she realized that she had lost touch with her soul. The divorce had wreaked such havoc in her emotional life that she could no longer feel love.

"Every day, for six months, she took an hour to connect with her soul. By doing this, she was able to regain a feeling of deep love for her body and herself. Today, she is symptom-free, and believes that without inner work, she might be dead. So many times, we need not only physical treatment but mental, emotional, or spiritual work to augment that process."

To promote health at every level, Dr. Scolastico advises the following:

CONNECT WITH YOUR SPIRITUAL NATURE. Religious or not, we need to accept the existence of some benevolent, healing force larger than our personality and physical being. Once we realize we are never alone or abandoned, amazing changes can happen.

BE MINDFUL OF YOUR THOUGHTS. We all have negative thoughts, but this alone does not cause illness. Swallowing them down and engaging them does. We must learn to release negative ideas. This work takes time, and we should not be hard on ourselves when our thoughts are less than perfect.

FOLLOW PHYSICAL PRINCIPLES OF HEALTH. Living in a healthy way includes eating the right foods, exercising, getting enough rest, play, and social activity. Giving to others has a beneficial impact on health.

CREATE LOVE IN YOUR LIFE EVERY DAY. This is perhaps most important of all. Research shows that love impacts every aspect of our being, including the physical. When we feel love, all body systems work better. The endocrine system produces beneficial hormones. Muscles relax, so that the flow of oxygen to the cells increases. Immune system function is enhanced.

When we are filled with self-love, our health is strongest and our lives improve all around. Recent studies show that teaching self-esteem improves academics, as well as promoting emotional stability and greater health.

"A powerful way to enhance self-love," advises Dr. Scolastico, "is to notice when you are creating negative thoughts and feelings about yourself. Then consciously create an experience of love for yourself right at that moment, using the power of the word to augment the process. You can say, 'I just noticed I'm creating these negative thoughts and feelings about myself. I now choose to use my imagination, my creativity, and my will to create an inner experience of love for myself right now in this minute.'"

Another way to build love into our lives is to set aside time each day for building loving energy. Dr. Scolastico says, "For at least five minutes, use your mind, open your heart, and create love in your feelings. You can do that by imagining a person you love. Let your feelings for that person fill you as you bring that loved one fully into your thoughts and feelings. Let the corners of your mouth lift up in a smile. Just let your heart swell with love. You won't need a scientific test to prove the benefits."

Equal in importance to self-love is the love we share with others. Connecting with family, friends, and community gives us a sense of belonging that is invaluable to our well-being. Recently, a link between social bonds and heart health was reported in *Natural Health*. The magazine summarized 30 years of research on the town of Rosetto, Pennsylvania, and concluded that the most important risk factor for heart disease is a lack of community and intimate relationships. In this town, people lived in three-generation households, with grandparents, parents, and children. There was a lot of interaction among families and much participation in community organizations. The incidence of heart disease was virtually nil, even though residents ate high-fat diets and did not go out of their way to exercise. In fact, there was less coronary heart disease in Rosetto than in any other population in the United States.

FULL ALTERNATIVE THERAPY PROGRAMS
Dean Ornish's Program for Reversing Heart Disease

The Ornish Program at Beth Israel, which opened in 1993, has four components:

(1) Moderate, supervised exercise.

(2) Stress management, involving stretching exercises and some yoga poses as well as the teaching of relaxation and meditation techniques.

(3) Low fat, vegetarian diet, with no animal products and no added fats.

(4) Group support sessions where patients meet to learn more about their problems and act to express themselves.

The main focus of the program is to modify risk factors known to increase the dangers of coronary disease. It is not that different from a general medical program. The goal is to reduce weight, lower cholesterol and blood pressure, control diabetes, stop smoking, and control stress.

In a study in the 1989 British medical journal *Lancet*, two groups of heart patients were studied. One group followed the Ornish guidelines, the other took the regular medical treatment for coronary disease. One year after starting this Ornish program, there was a reversal (improvement) of the coronary artery measured through an angiogram. This same group has done a follow up, five years into the program, and when they evaluated the blood flow to the heart with a PET scan (a state-of-the-art procedure), there was a significant improvement in flow even after five years of doing the program. In September 1995, the study came out in the *Journal of the American Medical Association* (*JAMA*).

"One thing we remind patients who enter this program," Deborah Matra, R.N., says, "is that they need to regard what is required as a prescription from their doctor. They need to stick with the diet and exercise, do the stress management routine daily, stay with it as they would honor their doctor's prescription."

The Healing Center: IV Vitamin and Ozone Therapy

We have been led to believe that genetics has a primary role in all diseases, and it probably does in many. We must see, however, the connected symptoms. We must see that diet and lifestyle play an enormous role and far more of a role than genetics, though genetics is a contributing factor. The Healing Center, in New York City, takes a holistic approach to healing. They use state-of-the-art, even avant-garde, techniques, vitamin C drips, dietary counseling, acupuncture, massage therapies, chelation, and body therapy, and they have had some magnificent results.

One patient, John, talks about his experience: "I'd say that I'm 95 percent responsible for my ill condition, out of sheer laziness and neglect. I weigh about 600 pounds and I realize I am apt to get various diseases because of my weight. I have already suffered some: high blood pressure, fatigue, severe viral and bacterial problems, edema of the right leg that causes cramps. I have trouble flexing the joints."

In the African-American community to which John belongs, there is, unfortunately, a high incidence of death from coronary heart disease and far too many cases of high blood pressure.

The patient mentions that much of his disease arose from faulty lifestyle habits, growing up eating too much fat, a lot of meat, drinking alcoholic beverages, all of which undermine health.

Dr. Howard Robins, formerly with the Healing Center, describes his work there in a previous interview. "We try," he says, "to let the body heal itself from all its injuries and weaknesses. We do not focus on one illness, but on the body as a whole. This is how holistic medicine was originally formulated.

"In our program, we have a medical doctor who assumes charge of the patient's medical condition, a homeopathic practitioner, a nutritionist, who does extensive nutritional counseling with each patient on vitamins, herbs, and minerals, an acupuncturist who uses this technique as well as prescribes Chinese herbal remedies to strengthen a weak organ system; and a dentist who removes mercury amalgam fillings, which cause fatigue and weaken the immune system. We also have a chiropractor who will rebalance the back structure so there will be better nerve innervations so the system won't misfire and damage the organ system. Since all the body's systems are interconnected, we need to put everything back in order."

Dr. Robins' particular specialty is to work with intravenous vitamin C and ozone therapy. He tells us that in vitamin C therapy a person is built up very rapidly to large doses, up to the 100,000 mg range and eventually to the 200,000 range. High levels of vitamin C cleanses the artery walls of calcified fatty plaques. They also use EDTA in the drip which functions by melting the calcium bonds to the walls so the plaque is freed and the EDTA and C can wash it out of the body's system. Then the solution goes on and cleanses and heals the scars left by the low density lipoproteins, healing the walls so that plaque will no longer adhere to them.

They also use ozone therapy—called major auto hemotherapy. They take out a certain amount of blood, about 300 ccs or 10 ounces, and mix in an oxygen/ozone combination. They then put the blood right back in, taking about 30 minutes. The ozone helps oxidize fatty plaques, sort of liquefying them and removing them from the walls while making the red blood cells more flexible, so they can slip through these clogged arteries. This last measure is very important in preventing the need for bypass surgery and getting rid of angina pain.

You might wonder how ozone therapy originated. Dr. Robins traces it back to World War I. It was found that men who had been burned by mustard gas or injured or shot and were kept in the back of the hospital tent, where the electric generators for the field lights were kept, were getting well. Eventually, they realized the cause of the improvement was the ozone gas created by leakage from these generators. That began the work on ozone as a means to heal and prevent the amputation of limbs with gangrene. "We've seen some miraculous results of ozone therapy at the Healing Center, for it's one thing that really does work."

Dr. Julian Whitaker: Nutrition and Education are Key

Dr. Julian Whitaker was on the medical staff at the Pritikin Center. Nathan Pritikin helped millions of people by prescribing a diet that eliminates, refined carbohydrates and animal fats and putting patients on a strict but moderate exercise regimen. In 1979, Dr. Whitaker went on to found the Whitaker Wellness Center in Newport Beach, California. He has expanded the Pritikin Program, adding special vitamin supplements and eliminating most if not all animal protein from the prescribed diet.

Dr. Whitaker runs an intensive five-day nutritional and educational clinic designed to teach people dietary and exercise guidelines that can help them prevent or overcome heart disease. Many patients attend the clinic as an alternative to major surgical procedures and/or drug therapy. They are frequently able to avoid these invasive and toxic treatments, and more importantly, in the long run, they establish or regain a healthful lifestyle and vitality that they had assumed was beyond their grasp.

Dr. Whitaker's treatment is as much a matter of education as one of actual therapeutic intervention. Patients learn what they can do about their conditions so that the responsibility becomes theirs. Once patients understand how nutrition, vitamin supplementation, and exercise can help stop and even reverse most heart conditions and cardiovascular diseases they must be resolute in applying this knowledge to their own lifestyles. They make these changes a routine part of each day.

"Heart disease," Dr. Whitaker states, "is not really as much a disease of the heart as it is a disease of the artery." The arteries carry blood to the heart at a uniform rate of flow, and if this flow is interfered with—speeded up or slowed down—the heart must adjust its activity to compensate for the change. If the arteries become clogged, the blood supply to the heart may be insufficient to the point where "the heart muscle begins to die in sections. These are what we call heart attacks when a section of the heart muscle does not receive enough oxygen and simply dies."

It is important to understand that the heart itself usually remains healthy until the arteries are damaged. The arteries, because they are too clogged or too rigid or become obstructed by clots and occlusions, are not able to get the blood supply to and from the heart at a steady, healthy rate. "Heart disease" patients must be taught first and foremost how to repair and maintain the cardiovascular system in general rather than the heart specifically.

THE PROGRAM Once patients understand these basic causes of their problems, the Newport Beach Program is geared to teach them how to deal constructively with the situation. Naturally, patients who smoke must give up the habit. Then they learn how to structure a diet that will attack the root causes of the disease as well as the symptoms. While surgical and drug remedies may relieve symptoms temporarily, they do not deal directly with the underlying causes of the disease and rarely effect an actual cure or reversal of the dysfunction. Dr. Whitaker's approach focuses on showing patients how to deal with the actual disorders; this leads ultimately to the disappearance of symptoms when the disease itself is treated effectively. This can be very exciting if you are one of the millions of people who have long suffered from cardiovascular problems that traditional physicians consider insurmountable without radical and invasive intervention.

Heart disease patients working with Dr. Whitaker are educated while being treated. They are taught about reducing fats in their diet early on. Dairy products and processed meat are the chief culprits here. Eggs especially should be avoided by those suffering from heart and cardiovascular diseases. Just like meat, eggs are directly related to elevated cholesterol levels, leading to damage and corrosion of the epithelial tissue lining the arterial walls.

ELIMINATING ANIMAL PROTEINS People who continue to consume meats, cheeses, eggs, and other animal proteins, says Dr. Whitaker, cannot seriously reduce their overall body fat. Strangely enough, even animal products such as yogurt that may have no fat or cholesterol trigger an internal reaction that treats them as if they did, simply because they are animal products. Dr. Whitaker describes a patient who could not lower his cholesterol level even though he had eliminated all meat and dairy products from his diet for four years. It was determined

UNDERSTANDING THE PROBLEM OF CARDIOVASCULAR DISEASE Many people have been helped tremendously by the program at Newport Beach. It begins by conveying an understanding of the actual causes of various cardiovascular diseases. This is something many people are lacking, yet it is critical if they are to intelligently confront or avoid heart disease. Arteriosclerosis, for example, results from damage done to the inner walls (the endothelial layer) of the arteries. This damage can be caused and/or enhanced by the presence of elevated serum cholesterol levels and by high blood pressure. Knowing this, why would a person continue dietary and lifestyle habits that result in higher cholesterol?

High blood pressure in turn may be caused by a combination of too much salt and too little potassium. Too much salt increases fluid levels because sodium attracts water. People eating a lot of processed foods—as so many Americans do—will have low levels of potassium since processed foods usually have been stripped of their potassium. Moreover, processed foods often combine deficient potassium with excess sodium. Dr. Whitaker explains, "A good example would be potato chips or French fries. The potato is very low in sodium. But when we chop it up, process it, and fry it, we take out the potassium and put in sodium. Many researchers have found that the ratio of sodium to potassium is probably more important in creating high blood pressure than is the increased sodium alone." Low calcium levels and the intake of meat products also contribute to high blood pressure, although the reasons for this are not clear, according to Dr. Whitaker.

Angina—severe chest pain—is caused by arterial blockage during exercise. This blockage is caused by the clumping together of blood platelets induced by excessive intake of fatty foods. "In the blood," Dr. Whitaker explains, "fat has a tendency to coat the red blood cells with a fatty layer. This causes a reduction in the electromagnetic charge of the blood cell. All our blood cells have to carry oxygen through the capillaries. In order to get through the capillaries, these blood cells have to go single file, because the capillary is about 7 microns—about 1/10,000 of an inch—in diameter, and the red blood cell is about [the same size]. You cannot force four or five blood cells through the capillary at the same time; that would be like trying to get seven people to go through a single doorway. When you eat fat, it causes these blood cells to clump together at the same time. When they get to the doorway of the capillary system, they can't go through. Many researchers have measured the actual oxygen uptake of heart muscle before and after a fatty meal. They have documented that there is a 15 to 30 percent drop in oxygen utilization and oxygen availability to normal heart muscle [after] a fatty meal."

than his daily nonfat, cholesterol-free yogurt was the culprit. The reason for this phenomenon is unclear, but when you are suffering from heart disease, you are not as concerned about reasons as you are about results.

Dr. Whitaker notes that by getting away from animal proteins, it is estimated that "you shift from 49 percent fat down to around 15 percent fat, and you shift your carbohydrates from 40 percent on the American diet up to maybe 65 to 75 percent. This will dramatically lower the blood cholesterol if the shift is made accurately. The drop in the cholesterol level should be anywhere between 15 and 30 percent. It will also aid in weight loss, triglyceride control, and blood pressure control.

By adding more carbohydrates to the diet, one can effectively reduce the intake of animal proteins. Dr. Whitaker explains that with animal proteins, which have only two sources of calories—fats and proteins—it is still necessary to add carbohydrates for a balanced diet. However, carbohydrates contain all three caloric sources—fats, proteins, and carbohydrates—and therefore can replace animal proteins. Instead of bacon and eggs, you might have a whole-grain cereal or bread with fruit. Pasta and rice and bean dishes such as tacos or burritos along with vegetables and a high-fiber salad with plenty of calcium-rich dark greens constitute a fine substitute for the standard meat and potatoes. There's nothing wrong with potatoes in and of themselves, but by the time they are smothered with butter, sour cream, and ketchup, they become fatty and high in cholesterol.

By turning away from meat and dairy products while increasing the proportion of fruits, vegetables, legumes, grains, breads, cereals, and pastas, the heart disease patient replaces high-fat, high-cholesterol foods with high-fiber, power-house-type foods. This switch will lower the patient's blood cholesterol levels, while the additional fiber will help clean out whatever fat and cholesterol is already clogging the system. Even foods containing significant amounts of fat, such as nuts and oils, can be used in moderation.

Olive oil, a monosaturated fat, "seems to be less deleterious to the system," Dr. Whitaker states, "than some of the polyunsaturated fats, such as corn oil and sunflower oil, which are common in our food processing. Greeks and Italians, who eat substantial amounts of olive oil, have been found to be in better [health] than, for example, Israelis, who eat a substantial amount of corn oil and sunflower oil."

In the case of nuts, some are better to consume than others. Walnuts, for example, have substantial amounts of omega-3 fatty acids, which are very beneficial for cardiovascular health. Peanuts, however, may contribute to sluggish blood flow related to serum cholesterol levels; they can be more harmful than even butter, a well-known villain in such instances. This information comes from rabbit studies conducted by Dr. Julian Whistler at the University of Chicago.

EXERCISE: GOOD BUT NOT A PANACEA Some people are under the mistaken assumption that cholesterol can be burned off by exercise and activity and that as a result, people who engage in athletic and body-building pursuits can eat more meat and eggs without suffering ill effects. There is no scientific basis for this notion. To the contrary, studies have shown that good conditioning and muscle tone do not necessarily lead a person to be in good cardiovascular condition.

Dr. Whitaker refers to "studies done on marathon runners in South Africa in which five of them died of heart attacks. These were conditioned long-distance runners. They all had cholesterol levels of 270, 290, etc. They were very fit but not very well."

Author Jim Fixx provides another case. Despite being a world-class runner and an authority on and champion of the benefits of aerobic conditioning, he died suddenly and prematurely of a massive heart attack. Many observers immediately blamed his exercise regimen, but an autopsy showed that he had vast arterial damage and blockage. This damage is not the result of too much exercise but of too much fat and cholesterol in the blood. In fact, Fixx had been advised several years earlier to lower his cholesterol count of 254. Unfortunately, he was convinced that it was of little concern to an athlete at his level at conditioning.

ESTABLISHING HEALTHY HABITS Besides the quality of the fats heart patients consume, it is crucial for them to reduce the quantity intake of all fats. Dr. Whitaker insists that "you need to reduce the fat intake by about 50 percent of what the American population is eating now to be at what I consider to be the upper limit of fat intake."

One reason why many people do not change their lifestyles sufficiently to establish good health is that they are encouraged by their doctors to maintain the average range of white blood cells, cholesterol, and triglycerides. Dr. Whitaker believes that his patients deserve better than this. He tries to get them to establish healthy, not just average, levels of these heart disease culprits. This is accomplished through exercise and socializing, proper vitamin and mineral regimens, and the reduction of animal fats in the diet, with their replacement by complex carbohydrates.

CARBOHYDRATES Carbohydrates are preferred to fats because they do not have the high cholesterol levels that fats do and do not sludge the arteries, interfere with normal blood flow, or damage the inner arterial walls. Carbohydrates are high in fiber, vitamins, and minerals, all of which promote overall cardiovascular health. They also do not convert into fat very readily, despite the fact that many people believe (partly because of misinformation from the scientific community) that carbohydrates are fattening.

Dr. Whitaker explains: "It is very difficult for carbohydrates to actually put fat weight into your system; some studies have shown that carbohydrates are not converted into fat nearly as rapidly or as efficiently as many scientists used to think. The conversion of carbohydrates into fat takes more energy than is actually present in the carbohydrate molecule trying to be converted, so the body just doesn't do it. The primary thing that really deposits fat into fat is fat itself. Often, when people add carbohydrates to their diet, they add them to an already increased fat diet. Generally, when I put people on an increased carbohydrate diet, they will almost always lose weight, and they will call begging me to give them something to stop the weight loss if they are truly following a 70 to 75 percent carbohydrate diet. Believe it or not, the high-carbohydrate diet we use causes a weight loss that creates a problem."

It should be made very clear that Dr. Whitaker does not recommend an increased intake of all carbohydrates. A lot of carbohydrates, particularly the simple and processed carbohydrates, are nothing but junk food. They are processed in such a way that their fibrous cellular structures have been broken down, and they have been robbed of much or most of their vitamin and mineral content. Cakes, jams, sugared fruit juices, baked goods, highly processed breads, and bleached flours and flour products are examples. Often the only thing left in these foods is sugar. The carbohydrates espoused in Dr. Whitaker's program are unprocessed, unrefined, and wholesome complex carbohydrates such as whole grains and fresh fruits.

VITAMIN AND MINERAL SUPPLEMENTS Vitamin and mineral supplementation is another significant part of Dr. Whitaker's treatment program for cardiovascular patients. Vitamins A, B_6, C, and E are especially important, along with the minerals selenium, calcium, magnesium, and chromium.

Between 25 and 50 mg of B_6, may be used. Some B vitamins, such as niacin, are used in large doses much like a drug. "If there is an elevated cholesterol and triglyceride level which doesn't respond adequately to our diet," Dr. Whitaker explains, "we will use niacin at a rate of 500 to 700 mg per meal." This is strictly a therapeutic dose and should be used only in conjunction with a physician's prescribed treatment.

Vitamin C is of particular significance in maintaining the sound structure of the arterial walls since it promotes strong, healthy connective tissues. Dr. Whitaker cites a Canadian study in which guinea pigs were deprived of vitamin C: "Their arteries began to corrode because the connective tissue inside the artery gave way, allowing cholesterol to go into the system."

This would probably not have happened if dogs or most other mammals had been used in the study, because these animals usually produce their own vitamin C and don't need to get it in a dietary or supplemental form. However, guinea pigs, like humans, do not manufacture their own vitamin C. When vitamin C was restored to the guinea pigs' diet, the process of arterial damage not only slowed but began to reverse. Evidence such as this has convinced Dr. Whitaker that vitamin C plays a critical role in cardiovascular health. "In my opinion," he says, "early on the most important vitamin, if there is a single one, would be vitamin C."

It is especially important that the patient's blood remain thin and free flowing, and this is where vitamin E plays a role in Dr. Whitaker's treatment. Vitamin E is an anticoagulant that keeps blood platelets from clumping together so that they can pass easily through narrow openings and small capillaries. It is also an antioxidant, protecting the arterial cells from damage which may be caused by free radicals.

Dr. Whitaker also uses MaxEPA, a blood thinner and anticoagulant that acts somewhat like vitamin E. MaxEPA, he says, "is beneficial to the patient who has an elevated level of triglycerides, plus elevated cholesterol. We use large doses of it at that stage. We will use large amounts per meal to drop the triglyceride and cholesterol level." He goes on to note that MaxEPA is ineffective in lowering cholesterol levels when very low levels of triglycerides are present. Dr. Whitaker warns that MaxEPA alone is not a "panacea for lowering the cholesterol," as some sponsors have made it out to be, but is very effective when integrated with an overall treatment program.

Mineral supplementation is equally important in the therapy. Magnesium has been found to be deficient among heart patients, up to 50 percent lower than in other noncardiac patients studied recently at the University of California. To restore the mineral to acceptable levels, Dr. Whitaker uses injectable magnesium for angina patients. Diuretics, commonly prescribed to lower blood pressure in patients with cardiovascular disorders, deplete magnesium as well as potassium. While most physicians are careful to replace the potassium lost during diuretic treatment, few replace the magnesium. This can cause further complications, especially since the loss of magnesium affects serum calcium levels. This is part of the reason Dr. Whitaker believes that "diuretics, and the way they are currently used, are making a lot of people worse instead of better."

WHY CONVENTIONAL THERAPIES ARE NOT THE ANSWER Dr. Whitaker believes that technology has been confused with science. Just because it is possible to do a coronary bypass or angioplasty does not necessarily mean that it always makes sense to undertake it. "It has been conclusively demonstrated," he states, "that bypass surgery fails to reduce mortality rates for 75 percent of heart patients who undergo the procedure." While failing to cure many heart disease victims, such surgery frequently puts the patient at needless risk, with 0.3 to 6.6 percent of such patients dying after the surgery: Still, Americans spend between $2 billion and $3 billion a year on coronary bypasses.

Angioplasty—a procedure in which a catheter is snaked through the arteries to open up blockages—has been hailed as a great technological feat. However, it has a death rate of 3.5 percent and a conversion to bypass rate of 15 percent, and the whole procedure must be repeated in more than one in three cases because it didn't work the first time.

Dr. Whitaker's treatment is not based on high technology or drastic surgical and/or drug intervention. He tries to determine what is causing the problem and decides how best to alter the patient's lifestyle to reduce the risk factors that determine whether a patient will recover. He considers the three major risk factors to be elevated cholesterol levels, elevated blood pressure, and cigarette smoking. After these factors, he looks for other high-risk factors such as obesity, diabetes, and lack of exercise. These too are important but "are not as strong or as predictive as the other three."

Dr. Whitaker is most concerned with helping his patients modify their lifestyles. "We instruct them how to eat, how to exercise, how to take vitamins and minerals, and about all the things they can do to stop the advance of cardiovascular disease and reverse the process." He notes that a condition such as arteriosclerosis "is a progressive disorder throughout life," unless patients change their lifestyle to slow it down or "become very serious about it and do what is necessary with diet and exercise to lower the cholesterol level and blood pressure. At this point the arteries which have become clogged begin to open again.

Dr. Whitaker views most of the current therapies available to heart disease patients as needless and unjustified. Most are ineffective in terms of actually stopping and/or reversing the deterioration that has begun by the time the patient seeks treatment. Catheterization, for example, has insufficient scientific basis in Dr. Whitaker's opinion, yet thousands of catheterizations are done almost routinely. Catheterizations are used to detect arterial blockages and to open them up, often in conjunction with a balloon angioplasty or a bypass. The angioplasty technique, as explained earlier, is an invasive method of trying to force open blocked spots within the arteries, while bypass surgery involves severing the artery before the blockage and rerouting the blood flow through an unblocked vein taken from the leg.

An obvious problem with this routine approach to dealing with heart disease is that the catheterization itself—sticking a catheter inside the heart—can cause harm to the body. To perform this exploration without good reason is dangerous, yet it is commonly done to patients who do not have life-threatening conditions and frequently don't even suffer from chest pains.

Moreover, the results of catheterization are not dependable. Dr. Whitaker explains: "Studies were done comparing the blockages that were found in patients who had been recently catheterized and had died from some other cause, and they did an autopsy within 30 days of the catheterization. When they looked at the arteries at the autopsy and looked at the angiogram picture of the way it was read, they found very little correlation. Even more alarming is that different doctors viewing the same catheterization had different opinions concerning the exact location of the blockage. Studies at the University of Iowa showed that blood flow measurements taken during surgery were quite different from what had been indicated by the angiogram."

Furthermore, catheterization usually leads to a series of other invasive techniques that frequently are not called for and are seldom successful in the long run. A patient may have only slight chest pain or other discomfort, symptoms that could well be stopped and reversed by means of appropriate lifestyle changes. Instead, the attending physician often finds it easier to ask that a catheterization be done "just to take a look." The dubious results may quickly lead to bypass and angioplasty. This whole chain of events, says Dr. Whitaker, "simply puts patients on a treadmill to further and further invasive techniques which then hurt the patient. We have two problems in the country today. We have heart disease and heart disease treatment. I'm not sure which is the worse problem. At least we know how to handle the heart disease with diet, exercise, and appropriate medication. But often, when you have patients who have been damaged by the treatment, there is no antidote."

A CASE IN POINT The following case provides a good example of how traditional medical treatment of cardiovascular disorders can move a patient rapidly down the road of increasingly complicated interventions that would not have been necessary if the original problem had been understood.

The patient was a prominent businessman from Denver who had developed mildly high blood pressure about five years before he visited Dr. Whitaker's clinic. According to Dr. Whitaker, this condition can be remedied with a diet regimen. However, the patient's family physician had treated him with a potent diuretic called hydrochlorothiazide which causes a drop in serum potassium, which in turn leads to cardiac arrhythmias. He was admitted to the hospital on two or three occasions because his potassium level had gone too low. He was extremely sensitive to the diuretic. Rather than stop the diuretic, his physicians prescribed another diuretic which was supposed to save potassium, and he was also given potassium supplements. For the arrhythmia, he was given two other heart medications. The diuretic elevated his blood sugar level. Rather than stop the diuretic and treat the elevation in blood sugar level with a diet and exercise regimen, the family doctor started the patient on an oral medication for diabetes and then switched him to insulin, which he later increased to 130 units. All of this occurred over a five-year period.

When he came to Dr. Whitaker, the patient was quite skeptical because he was seeing two prominent, board-certified internists and cardiologists. He did not believe that a diet and exercise regimen could improve on the kind of medical treatment he had been given.

Dr. Whitaker put him on a low-fat, high-carbohydrate diet which lowered his insulin requirements. On the first day his insulin medication was cut by half, and soon it was eliminated completely as his blood sugar remained very low. Gradually, the other medications were reduced as well, until at the end of two weeks the patient was taking no medication at all for high blood pressure, cardiac arrhythmia, or diabetes. He was taken off his 130 units of insulin as well as 17 other prescription medications. A year and a half later the man is still taking no medication, his blood sugars are normal, his blood pressure is normal, and the only problem that has lingered is a tendency to have arrhythmia, for which he is taking medication.

Several studies have indicated that physicians have a tendency to add drugs to drugs. If the diuretic, for instance, causes an elevation in uric acid, rather than stopping the diuretic, the doctor will introduce a medication to decrease the uric acid. This occurs frequently in the case of diabetes as well. A study done at Brook Army Hospital in Fort Sam Houston, Texas, found that diabetics taking insulin were also taking as many as four additional drugs for other problems, many of which altered the diabetic condition. Individuals on multiple-drug therapy must be given diet and exercise programs that address the problems for which they have been taking drugs. Only then can they begin to stop the drugs, because the lifestyle change addresses all these problems.

The preceding example also illustrates the medical community's tendency to view diseases as totally unrelated to one another. Traditional physicians often fail to see any connection between diabetes, heart disease, and high blood pressure. Doctors like to label them separately when in fact they may be related. These are generalized problems that come from general defects in lifestyle, specifically, too much fat, too much animal protein, not enough exercise, too much salt, and not enough fiber. When you address the causes of these illnesses, you can eliminate these medications quite rapidly. People should not start throwing away their medications; this should be done gradually under medical supervision of a physician who is schooled in, is interested in, and has respect for the power of diet and exercise as an alternative to these medications.

WHY DR. WHITAKER'S PROGRAM WORKS Dr. Whitaker's program works because it takes into consideration the integration of various lifestyle factors contributing to the eradication of disease. People often think that good nutrition and exercise are advisable but do not constitute actual treatment, especially in the case of advanced heart disease. The success of Dr. Whitaker's lifestyle approach, however, indicates that the healing power that comes from rebalancing one's mind and body has been vastly underestimated. Surgery and medication cannot slow the progression of arteriosclerosis, for instance, but basic lifestyle changes can accomplish this very quickly and dramatically. Lifestyle changes address the cause of heart disease and allow the body to heal itself when given the proper tools and directed by a disciplined, discriminative, and essentially positive attitude.

Dr. John McDougal: Food is the Best Medicine

Dr. John McDougall, unlike many physicians in the preventive health care field, practices what he preaches—vegetarianism. He feels that food is the best medicine; traditional therapies may be introduced in crisis situations, but the body benefits most from restoration of normal biochemical balance. The standard American diet, he feels, has lost its ability to maintain that balance. A natural diet, free of animal protein and consisting of small amounts of food eaten many times a day, can help restore it. His vegetarian diet helps not only people with heart disease but those who suffer from cancer, arthritis, and obesity.

Dr. McDougall, and others like him, offer a theoretically sound and clinically proven therapy based on such lifestyle modifications as increased exercise and restructured diet. Their success has been so profound and undeniable that their opponents, mired in the traditional hierarchy, have finally begun to adopt much of what Dr. McDougall, among others, has been espousing for years.

Today, the American Heart Association, the National Institutes of Health, and other well-established organizations are recommending moderate changes in the way people eat. Unfortunately, this so-called prudent diet does not fully address the underlying issue. If people are consuming foods or engaging in lifestyles that cause disease, suggesting that moderation be exercised is like suggesting that they try to get moderately better. To achieve more than "moderate" health, people must do something more pronounced than make token gestures: They must make drastic changes in diet and lifestyle.

DRASTIC CHANGES IN DIET AND LIFESTYLE Dr. McDougall, author of *The McDougall Program: Twelve Days to Dynamic Health* (Plume, 1991) believes that the American public needs to be informed about the best diet available, not the moderate or prudent one. He recalls a woman who complained about the severe restrictions he had placed on her husband's diet. This patient had had two bypass operations and a heart attack in three years, yet his wife thought his new diet should be more moderate. Dr. McDougall responded: "Madam, if you told me your husband had a terrible cough, was vulnerable to lung cancer, and was smoking cigarettes, what would you expect my advice to be: to cut down to half a pack of cigarettes a day, four cigarettes a day, or to quit altogether? She chose to quit. I told her that her husband was being poisoned by cholesterol. All the health associations and every reasonable scientist say that cholesterol is the cause of this disease. Then I asked her how much cholesterol and animal fat we should feed him. But she couldn't give me an answer, and there is only one answer: Cut the fat out of your diet completely."

The reasons why many physicians suggest only minimal changes in the diets of heart disease patients is that they, like their patients, do not know what the best diet is. For too many years nutrition has been given little or no attention in medical school curricula, and so few doctors know how to prescribe diets appropriate for specific conditions. They tell their patients to cut down a little on fat, add a bit of fiber, and so forth, but patients with heart disease have their lives on the line and need much more informed direction.

Dr. McDougall, like most other physicians, went through four years of medical school without learning about nutrition. He never had a course in it and rarely heard the word mentioned. In his early practice he was content to follow the standard procedures he had learned as a student and intern and prescribe for his heart patients the medications that pharmaceutical representatives suggested he push. One day a 30-year-old patient with high blood pressure came to Dr. McDougall, who administered the traditionally accepted treatment consisting mainly of blood pressure medication. However, this drug therapy proved to be inadequate. Two weeks later the patient returned, complaining that his blood pressure was just as high and that in addition his normal sexual desire and function had ceased.

Here was a young man, newly married, his health and life in disarray, who was not getting any better by popping pills. It was Dr. McDougall's job to convince this patient that despite the way he felt, he was receiving the best possible treatment and that the blood pressure pills were really helping him. Dr. McDougall couldn't deny that he was powerless to help this patient.

DIETARY HISTORIES Desperately groping for an effective way to deal with such cases, Dr. McDougall began taking dietary histories of his patients to see if he might get some clues. It was a strange experiment, since one of his greatest professional challenges had been trying to prescribe dietary regimens to his hospitalized patients. He took dietary histories of every one of his patients for the next three years and was amazed by what he found.

Practicing in rural Hawaii, he had a unique opportunity to study an isolated group through several generations. This group consisted of sugar cane plantation workers. The first, older generation was made up of Japanese, Chinese, and Filipinos who had come to Hawaii in their teens or early childhood. Their children, grandchildren, and great-grandchildren were natives of Hawaii and had a very different background in terms of lifestyle and diet.

The members of the older generation possessed far superior health to that of the second, third, and fourth generations despite the fact that they had been in the same location and the same industry for years. The members of the first generation were trim and hardy, still vital and vigorous even in old age. The younger generations, by contrast, were commonly obese or at least overweight, plagued with diseases that Dr. McDougall had been taught were primarily genetic: diabetes, colon cancer, heart disease, and high blood pressure.

Clearly, genetics was not the issue here. The only variable Dr. McDougall could clearly establish was dietary history. The members of the older generation were primarily vegetarians, consuming very few high-fat, high-cholesterol animal products such as eggs, cheese, and milk, instead eating mostly rice and vegetables. The younger generations, raised in Hawaii instead of Asia, had become accustomed to the American diet of animal products and meats, highly refined and processed food rather than whole foods, and sugar- and salt-laden snacks. Dr. McDougall came to realize that diet is a far greater factor in the incidence of degenerative disease than he and others in his field had been led to believe.

He also noted, in a broader perspective, that throughout history it was always those in the upper, rich, privileged classes who seemed to he plagued by the degenerative diseases. The royalty of past centuries were the people who had the means to enjoy rich diets replete with high fats, including dairy and meat products. The feast was a routine part of their privileged life, and gluttonous eating was a major source of socialization and entertainment. The poor peasants who tilled the earth from sunup to sunset could afford to eat only what they themselves grew—grains, vegetables and potatoes—a simple diet high in starch, complex carbohydrates, and fiber. This "poor man's diet" was largely responsible for the fact that the peasantry rarely suffered the degenerative diseases so common among the elite: heart disease, diabetes, gout, and the like. The diet rich in saturated fats, cholesterol, and salt might have been fit for a king, but it certainly did not keep the king fit.

Dr. McDougall also pondered the fact that for hundreds, even thousands, of years the general populace had not depended on high-protein foods such as meat and dairy products for their daily nutritional needs. In New Guinea and South America, whole civilizations revolved around sweet potatoes; the Indians of North America were hunters for whom meat was only an occasional treat, the main diet being primarily corn-based; for Asians, to this day, rice has been central; Europeans originally ate high concentrations of grains, breads, and later, potatoes; Africans consumed mostly grains and beans; in Mexico and Central America, rice, corn, and beans provided the main sustenance; in the Middle East, wheat, sesame seeds, and chickpeas have been the traditional mainstays of the diet. Even today in many of these parts of the world meat is consumed infrequently.

We find almost invariably that among cultures and civilizations in which starch forms the basis of the diet, there is a very low incidence of obesity, high blood pressure, and heart disease. Dr. McDougall recalls that one of his professors could remember a time when heart failure—that is, a heart attack—was a "curious disease" in Hong Kong. People would gather around the victim to witness this rare affliction. That was 33 years ago, and since the diet in Hong Kong has been westernized, the occurrence of heart attacks has risen sharply.

Wherever the traditional high-starch, high-carbohydrate diet is maintained, one finds stronger, trimmer, healthier people. On mainland China, for instance, where the traditional rice and soybean diet is still very much a part of the culture, there is very little degenerative disease. One seldom sees an overweight Chinese person. That same trim person with a strong heart and healthy cardiovascular system would quickly become obese, atherosclerotic, and hypertense if he or she came to the United States and adopted western ways of eating. Heart disease is not the only disorder resulting from the western diet. In Japan, following World War I, there were only 78 cases of prostate cancer among the entire population. In the United States today, there are thousands of prostate cancer cases every year. The incidence of breast cancer is far higher in the United States than it is in places such as China or Japan that still adhere to starch-based diets.

WHAT IS THE BEST DIET? Dr. McDougall, who had been taught nothing about nutrition in his years of medical training, came to realize how critical diet is to the likelihood of developing heart disease. He also came to comprehend that his patients would have to change their eating habits in order to control and reverse the arterial deterioration that was the root of their problems. In his search for the most effective dietary treatment, Dr. McDougall found that an abundance of supportive evidence had been accumulating for many years. He began to apply this knowledge to reshape the diets and lifestyles of his patients and has had tremendous success treating them in his clinic.

As Dr. McDougall discovered in his research, the best diet is one based on high-starch, complex carbohydrate foods containing high fiber. This includes whole grains, legumes, fruits, and vegetables. The worst diet consists of high-fat "delicacies," or what Dr. McDougall calls the feast foods, basically foods of the animal protein variety: milk, eggs, cheese, beef, pork, poultry, and even chocolate. Americans' declining health is directly correlated with the rising consumption rates of these foods.

FOCUS ON COMPLEX CARBOHYDRATES The goal of Dr. McDougall's dictate approach to coronary artery disease is to establish the best diet. He works at getting his patients off diets high in cholesterol, fat, and salt and onto diets high in fiber and starch. Dr. McDougall's complex carbohydrate diet is preferable for several reasons. For one thing, it fills the stomach with much less food more quickly. Although people eat partly to fill the stomach—to feel satisfied and relieve the pang of hunger—for many people this is the sole consideration in establishing eating patterns. However, it is important to realize that all foods are not equal in the way in which they fill people up.

Carbohydrates provide what are called low-density foods. Fats are high-density foods. The higher the density of a food, the less bulk it has. The less bulk, the more that must be consumed to fill the stomach. If you eat a small portion of low-density, high-bulk foods, you will feel just as satisfied as you would after consuming the same size portion of high-density, low-bulk foods, usually from the meat and dairy groups. Thus, you eat fewer calories to feel just as full as you would from eating far more eggs, meat, and cheese.

It is easy to see why people who eat primarily meat and dairy items are more likely to become obese. Consequently, Dr. McDougall's patients will lose 6 to 15 pounds a month eating as often as they want to but eating only the low-density starches and none of the high-density fats. They are encouraged to enjoy eating and not be afraid of it, as are so many overweight and obese people. The patients' top priority is to choose the proper types of foods.

THE PROBLEM WITH FATS Another reason Dr. McDougall's patients are taken off fats is that fats are one of the chief causes of coronary artery problems. In order to understand this it is necessary to review the nature of fats and see what they are and what they do. Fats are a fuel; they are stored energy. The body can synthesize fats; they are part of the cellular structure and are found in people's hormones, enzymes, and brains.

Essential fats are those which must be obtained through diet because the body does not produce them. The primary source of these essential fats is plants. They also come from meat, but meat is only a secondary source. The animal from which the meat (or meat and dairy products) is obtained has the essential fats because it ate plants containing them. People could choose to bypass the animal altogether and go directly to fat sources in the form of vegetables, grains, and legumes to fulfill the essential fat requirements. If you choose to eat the meat, however, you are getting a highly saturated fat that is far rougher on the cardiovascular system than are the polyunsaturated plant fats.

One of the first effects of fat in the system is to make people obese. This is why half the people in the United States are overweight and the other half are on diets and exercise programs to avoid becoming overweight. This obsession with obesity would be entirely unnecessary if people restructured their eating habits and lifestyles. People living in central New Guinea, Japan, and other places where the inhabitants primarily eat plant foods and wholesome, unprocessed carbohydrates are not concerned about their weight even though eating plays a key role in their cultures. They don't need to be, because the cause of obesity does not exist for them.

Fat makes people obese because it is easily transported to body fat tissue once it has been consumed. Carbohydrates, on the other hand, become a stored energy in the form of glycogen in the muscles and liver. Only with great difficulty does the body convert carbohydrates into fat. In victims of heart and artery disease, fat, especially animal fat, plays a sinister role by causing a sharp rise in cholesterol. The presence of excess amounts of cholesterol in the blood damages the inner walls of the arteries. The high incidence of cholesterol in the American diet is directly proportional to the epidemic of heart disease that people in this country now face.

The diet that Dr. McDougall blames for a large proportion of heart disease in this country consists of approximately 45 percent fat, mostly animal fat; 15 to 20 percent protein; and 40 percent carbohydrates, mostly processed carbohydrates and simple sugars. The American Heart Association (AHA) and other national councils have finally begun to concede that this sort of diet contributes to coronary artery disease. They now suggest that a moderate diet be adopted. By moderate, they mean a 30 percent fat intake instead of 45 percent. As noted earlier, Dr. McDougall contends that these moderate changes result in only moderate improvement in one's condition. And when one's life is at stake, one must adopt drastic alterations. He suggests a diet consisting of only 5 percent or 10 percent fat.

Many cardiologists tell their patients to eat white meat instead of red meat, but Dr. McDougall points out that this will not reduce fat and cholesterol levels significantly. Beef may be 70 percent fat, but chicken is still 40 to 50 percent fat. While eating chicken is an improvement, it will not reverse arterial blockage and heart conditions. If a patient is suffering from too much fat intake, why should that patient be told that it is all right to eat food that consists of one-third fat? Why not instead consume foods that range from 1 to 10 percent fat at the most? To get an idea of the relative fat contents of various foods, consider chocolate, a food with a 55 percent fat content, whole milk at 50 percent at solid matter, eggs at 65 percent, cheese between 70 and 90 percent, a "good steak" at 82 percent, and luncheon meats—cold cuts—up to 90 percent. Compare these high-density saturated fats with low-density, polyunsaturated vegetable fats like that of the potato, with a meager 1 percent fat, rice at 5 percent, and fruits ranging from 2 to 10 percent fat content. Realizing that these fruits and vegetables also contain high-quality fiber, which is essential to free-flowing blood and arterial health—something that is altogether lacking in meat and dairy items—it becomes clear that choosing complex carbohydrates over animal fats lays a solid foundation for recovery from heart disease. After all, the very causes of the heart disease are being eliminated almost entirely from the diet.

While the fat content of white meat may be less than that of red meat, the cholesterol levels may actually be higher. While 3½-ounce servings of beef and pork have 85 mg and 90 mg of cholesterol, respectively, turkey has 83 mg and skinned white chicken has 85 mg. Patients told by their cardiologists to switch to fish may also be victims of misinformation, since some types of fish have as much cholesterol as meat or poultry. Many people with coronary and/or vascular problems are deceived by inaccurate information into thinking they are choosing the best possible therapeutic diet when in fact they are not.

THE TRUTH ABOUT FISH OILS There has been quite a bit of discussion about the merits of fish oil in relation to heart disease in recent years. Dr. McDougall believes that the highly touted benefits of these fish oils are taken out of perspective, misleading cardiologists and patients alike. He believes only people benefiting are the drug companies that manufacture and market expensive fish oil capsules.

The fish-oil scenario seems to have its origin in the finding by researchers that Eskimos have a very low incidence of heart disease. Since they live primarily on fish, whale, walrus, and seal, it was surmised that fish oil reduces the risk of heart disease. This fish oil is a plankton fat called EPA (eicosapentaenoic acid), which stimulates hormones called prostaglandins. The prostaglandins in turn reduce the incidence of blood clotting by thinning the blood and thus preventing it from sticking, clumping, and sludging. In this way, the fish oils are indeed responsible for lowering blood pressure and serum cholesterol and for lessening the risk of heart disease.

Moreover, getting EPA from fish oil rather than directly from the plant source—the plankton—means you are getting it high on the food chain. Thus you will also get a concentration of vitamins A and D. Also, taking an excess of animal fat may increase the risk of gallbladder disease and colon cancer. However, I believe fish oil to be beneficial.

HOW THE PROGRAM WORKS Rather than look to a panacea—bypass surgery, diuretics and digitalis, or fish oil—Dr. McDougall believes people need to change their diets and lifestyles radically. This is not a simple solution, and you cannot passively sit by and expect a single substance, an operation, or a good cardiologist to cure you when everything you take into your body is harmful. You must understand the causes of coronary and vascular disturbances and actively work to avoid them.

Dr. McDougall found the earliest recorded reference to this sort of healing approach in the Bible, in the book of Daniel. Daniel's men had become sick from eating rich foods, and rather than offer them some magical cure or secret medicinal concoction, he had them ingest only vegetables and water. This high-starch, high-fiber diet helped them regain their normal health in only 10 days. At Dr. McDougall's hospital, practically everyone in the program is able to get off drugs and experience drastically reduced cholesterol, triglyceride, and blood sugar levels in a mere 12 days—the duration of the program. Their diet is similar to the one Daniel's men were given over 2,500 years ago.

There is no quick cure, however. The disorders plaguing these patients have been arrested, but true reversal and restoration of coronary and arterial health takes months to accomplish. The special diet used in the program is not a temporary one but must be continued after the patient leaves St. Helena and for as long as the patient wishes to avoid reestablishing heart disease and vascular dysfunction. In other words, the new eating habits are not really a diet but—along with a structured and progressive exercise program—constitute a whole new lifestyle.

During the 12-day live-in program at St. Helena, people with heart disease are taught how to let go of their high-fat diets and how to choose and prepare high-quality complex carbohydrate meals that are high in starch and fiber. At breakfast, coffee, ham and eggs, and white buttered toast with sugar jam might be replaced by oatmeal with strawberries. A whole-grain bread without the fat-laden butter—maybe topped with a real fruit jam instead of sugar jam or jelly—

might be paired with herbal tea or a hot beverage derived from grains rather than coffee beans.

Patients are taught to distinguish simple from complex carbohydrates. The simple sugars may be called glucose, fructose, maltose, or lactose: they are found in honey, corn syrup, milk, molasses, maple syrup, and fruit juices. They provide the body with quick-burning fuel which does little to sustain energy levels evenly or over an extended period of time. In a processed state, they do not even retain their fiber and nutrient values and become little more than highly concentrated sugars full of calories with little nutritional value. These types of carbohydrates should be avoided, but not as much as the fats and animal products.

Complex carbohydrates, on the other hand, provide a very slow burning fuel that is stored in the muscles and provides a steady energy supply throughout the day. Potatoes, rice, and vegetables such as peas, corn, and asparagus contain ideal forms of carbohydrates.

Dr. McDougall offers a variety of suggestions regarding starch-based meal planning, preparation, and variation using a carbohydrate-centered diet: "The foods we suggest are corn, pasta, rice, most vegetables, grains and all fiber-rich foods. For breakfast, you can have oatmeal or other hot whole-cereal meals, grains, waffles, and pancakes. For lunch, you can have all kinds of soups, such as lentil soup, bean soup, tomato soup, onion soup, or pea soup, as long as you make the soup yourself. Main entrees for dinner can be spaghetti with marinara sauce, curry vegetable stew, brown rice casseroles, baked potatoes, bean burritos without lard or oil, Indian curry dishes, and all kinds of Chinese and Japanese dishes. You can have all these foods as long as they are not processed in any way and are made fresh."

All the foods Dr. McDougall recommends are high in starch and fiber and have naturally balanced amounts of minerals, vitamins, and other nutrients. When these foods are eaten in the whole, natural state, they provide a highly nutritious source of calories and essential nutrients. They contribute to overall good health and a trim, easily maintained body weight. People who adhere to these dietary changes have experienced great and rapid success. According to Dr. McDougall, during his patients' brief stay at the clinic, their "blood cholesterol drops down an average of 28 points. Their triglycerides drop and blood sugars drop in a matter of 4 or 5 days. These people change from cardiac cripples who can't walk 15 or 30 feet to people who are walking 3 or 4 miles and exercising."

Dr. McDougall cites a patient who was suffering from severe restriction in the legs caused by arteriosclerosis. "He could not walk 15 feet without leg pain. He left the clinic two weeks later, and he was doing four miles on a bicycle and a mile and a half of fast walking without pain in his legs. It wasn't because he reversed his arteriosclerosis—that would take months or even years to do—but he increased the ability of the blood flow. So he dramatically increased the amount of effective circulation to his tissue. This is an example of what you can do."

TREATING HIGH BLOOD PRESSURE Besides the symptoms of their diseases, many people suffer greatly from the medications they are taking to treat those diseases. "With high blood pressure," Dr. McDougall relates, "we take people who come in on high-blood-pressure medications, and they just want to get off these medications because the side effects are so horrendous. They may even be on 10, 12, or 15 medications. It's rare that we can't get them off."

Here is an example of such a patient: "I had an accountant come into my office and state that he was on 20 drugs and wanted off them. Actually, he was on 12 high-blood-pressure pills, one diabetic pill, and several heart pills. After 4 days on a healthy diet consisting of no salt, low fat, and no cholesterol, he was off all his medication, his blood sugar, which was 235, fell to 168, and his blood pressure, which started at 190/110 became 150/70."

High blood pressure is not in itself a disease. It is a condition or symptom which may accompany a more generalized disease state, specifically, heart and arterial disease. Blood pressure rises when arteries damaged by excessive dietary fat, oil, and cholesterol begin to close up and occlude. The presence of salt attracts even more fluid into the bloodstream, and the pressure gets even greater. Decreasing the area the blood can flow through is like putting your thumb over part of the opening of a garden hose: The pressure increases, and the water squirts farther. If you increase the amount of water flow at the same time—say, by turning the faucet on higher—the pressure becomes even greater and the water squirts farther still.

To treat high blood pressure, the most obvious step is to clean out the arteries by eliminating fat, oil, and cholesterol ingestion. In other words, you take your thumb away from the hose nozzle and the pressure is reduced. Can you imagine leaving your thumb there while trying to reduce the pressure? You would be overlooking the obvious cause of the pressure buildup. Dr. McDougall says that this is exactly what happens in the traditional treatments of high blood pressure: "We treat blood pressure," he says, "by lowering it, which makes as much sense as giving aspirin to someone with an infected toe. We've lowered the fever but did not cure the infection. When there is a sign that the blood-vessel system is diseased, we use blood pressure pills to eliminate the sign, but the disease stays. What we should do is deal with the cause. So far only a half-dozen people in our program have not been able to eliminate blood pressure medications. Over the last 10 years, I have treated over 7,000 people.

"Let me tell you about a minister at the church I've gone to for several years. This young man, who is only 32 years old, had blood pressure problems for 10 years and had been taking blood pressure pills for two years before I saw him. He was recently married and was having problems with sexual function.

He was being treated by a doctor who gave him the standard line: 'You're on high-blood-pressure pills, we don't know what causes the problem, and you'll be on them for the rest of your life with no chance of getting off them.' He finally decided to see me, and when he asked what could be done for him, I told him to stop taking the blood pressure pills and told him how to do this (he was taking the kind that can't be stopped immediately). He changed his diet. This was over a year ago, and his blood pressure went down from high levels of 160/95 to 110/70 in two to three weeks. He lost 30 extra pounds he'd been carrying around since his teenage years, and he's absolutely drug-free and feels wonderful. He still sees the doctor who told him he'd never get off blood pressure pills and gloats a bit as the doctor takes his blood pressure and finds it perfectly normal. The doctor's response to all of this is, 'It was a coincidence.'"

Dr. McDougall says that this sort of "coincidence" occurs in more than 90 percent of the cases where patients have changed their diet dramatically. This is because his patients all make the required dietary changes. Frequently, people are not willing to undergo these changes. Probably the biggest obstacle to improving people's heart conditions once they have been taught how critical diet and exercise are is their reluctance to make such vast changes in their lifestyles.

THE RESULTS Dr. McDougall recalls one of his most stubborn cases, a man who only after severe debilitation finally decided to make the changes he had been told to make years earlier: "The person involved is my father and therefore is probably my most important case. I had been working on him for at least 10 to 12 years, trying to get him to change his diet. I even went to the University of Michigan to lecture to the physicians at the medical school there for four days. Since my dad respected the University of Michigan Medical School, if he saw me present this information to the doctors there, I hoped that it would make a big impression and that he would finally change his diet. Well, it did make an impression, and he did believe what I said, but he couldn't turn down Joe's kielbasa [Polish sausage]. Joe would bring down kielbasa once or twice a week, and my dad had to have a pizza on Friday nights, but otherwise he 'followed the diet strictly.' His blood pressure continued to rise and in fact went to 190/130. He gained an extra 50 to 60 pounds over what he should have weighed, he became very swollen, his cholesterol and triglyceride levels were both over 330, and he had such bad arthritis in his joints that it was difficult for him to get around. That still didn't get him to change his diet. He didn't decide it would make a difference in his life until one day when he got out of his car and tried to hobble to his office. He suddenly developed a pain in his chest which he described as feeling like there was an elephant sitting in the center of his chest. This scared him.

"I got a call from him about two hours later asking me what he should do because his physicians wanted to take an angiogram and were talking to him about bypass surgery. In this very emotional setting I told him, 'You know Dad, I've been telling you for the past eight years that you had to do something about your diet. I really think this is the way for you to go. It's your decision; it's your life, and you'll have to decide what you want to do, but you can't play around anymore.' So he decided that he didn't want a foot-and-a-half long hole in his chest and didn't want to risk the brain damage associated all too frequently with bypass surgery; he didn't want to be sick anymore. Therefore, he went home and with the help of my sister, who happened to be living with him at that time, changed his diet drastically: no kielbasa, no meats of any kind, no dairy products, and so on. He had chest pain for the first four or five days that was so bad he couldn't walk more than 10 or 15 feet. We're talking about a man who had been fully functional all 60 years of his life and who now was essentially crippled with arthritis and heart disease. Within 15 days after he changed his diet he was walking around without chest pain, and in four months he lost over 40 pounds. His cholesterol and triglycerides were below 180, a drop from 330, and his blood pressure fell from 190/130 to 110/70. This all took place over 3½ years ago. Since that time, when I go home to his farm in the fall and we load hay into the barn or do whatever else is necessary to get the farm ready for the winter, I find that this 65-year-old man can outwork me. This man who was almost dead three years ago now lifts beast bales of hay and works longer than I can."

Dr. McDougall's treatment of his father is not unusual. Most of his patients have had similarly resounding success. The attention he pays to the broader perspective of heart disease has culminated in a therapeutic approach that goes beyond the cover-up of symptoms and gets to the basic, underlying issues. When diet, exercise, and overall lifestyle are dealt with in an informed, constructive manner, coronary artery problems can be arrested and reversed rapidly. General health, outlook, and vitality improve. Not only can your life be prolonged, your enjoyment and appreciation of it and your ability to partake of it more actively will certainly be enhanced.

Dr. Eric Braverman's Approach to Hypertension

Dr. Eric Braverman has had over 60 papers published in peer review journals and is the author of numerous books including *Hypertension and Nutrition: The Amazing Way to Reverse Heart Disease Naturally* (Keats, 1996). He received his medical degree from New York University Medical School. Similar to Dr. McDougall, Dr. Braverman believes that a general wellness program that combines a proper diet, supplementation, and exercise are the best way to treat hypertension. The diet he recommends combines these elements with a special nutrient formula designed to lower high blood pressure and then help maintain good cardiovascular health.

Dr. Braverman believes that the primary causes of hypertension and heart disease are the accumulation of heavy metals such as lead, aluminum, and cadmium that produce cholesterol hardening as people age. With that hardening comes an increase in blood pressure because an aging body is no longer as flexible as it once was. This problem is compounded by the loss of hormones, and the loss of estrogen and progesterone and testosterone and DHEA, depending on your sex and the loss of growth hormone. According to Dr. Braverman, the danger of hypertension and heart disease begins at a blood pressure level that exceeds 120/80, and in some cases, the risk level may begin at 110/70.

Unsurprisingly, the first step in Dr. Braverman's approach to treating high blood pressure is a diet that supplements potassium and restricts sodium and cholesterol intake. Regarding the ongoing debate about the cholesterol content of eggs, Dr. Braverman asserts that high cholesterol usually has more to do with the other elements in the average person's diet than with eggs being the central culprit. As he puts it, "The average person is still eating white flour, junk food, and garbage essentially. So cholesterol intake will throw off cholesterol levels. But, as a rule, you're making 90 percent or more cholesterol in your body, and it's triggered by the diet. So, if you're eating a [Gary] Null diet or a Braverman style diet, then [taken in moderation] the eggs are going to be a good food for you, as long as you're not allergic."

SPECIAL NUTRIENT FORMULA Dr. Braverman also advocates the following nutrient formula to lower hypertension: 200 mg of garlic, 200 mg of taurine, 50 mg of magnesium, 10 mg of potassium, 20 mcgs of selenium, 4 mcgs of zinc, 20 mcgs of chromium, 50 mcgs of niacinimide, 50 mg of vitamin C, 50 mcgs of molybdenum, 50 mg of B_6, and 1,000 units of beta carotene. "Then," he says, "you just multiply that from about 5 to 10 to get a balance of those. Those are what I call the poor hypertensive nutrients.

"We've worked hard on a supplement called the heart or hypertensive supplement, where we put, based on the research I did, garlic, taurine, selenium, all the trace elements, B_6, zinc, chromium, all in one pill, so you could lower your blood pressure naturally with one vitamin that you could take a lot of. [However], one doesn't have to do that. There are many ways to take these supplements, but it's clear now that supplementation is one aspect of lowering your blood pressure."

OTHER PARTS OF PROGRAM However, despite the fact that supplementation is a useful tool in the lowering of high blood pressure, Dr. Braverman stresses, "The defeat of high blood pressure is a transformation of being and lifestyle." A person who exercises, keeps their weight down, generally maintains a low-fat, low-salt diet, and either gets useful supplement preferably through their diet, but alternatively from pill forms, will be better off for it in the fight against heart disease.

Other possible aspects that Dr. Braverman suggests to lower hypertension include the use of borage and fish oils; relaxation; meditation; an electrical stimulator that has been FDA-approved for anxiety; melatonin; and last but not least the revolutionary role that retreats to healing centers and wellness programs can play in people's lives when they are trying to precipitate a long-term lifestyle change. Dr. Braverman explains: "Many, many individuals can go to health retreats, go on juice fasts, go on dietary techniques, go on cleansing techniques, exercise, and they reverse their blood pressure, their weight, their blood sugar. [Even] I continue to underestimate the revolutionary nature of the wellness movement which says to the drug company and the drug managed care hospital network, no." He cites a recent example of a patient of his who had had hypertension, diabetes, and a weight problem. After going through a wellness program, all her health problems made a dramatic turn for the better.

Choosing a Therapy

Five years ago, I suggested to a leading cardiologist that use of vitamin E, stress management, exercise, dietary changes, power walking, and proper supplementation would make a vast difference in the prevention and treatment of heart disease. He looked at me and responded, "No way. It's not scientific. It won't work."

Today if you were to read *JAMA (Journal of the American Medical Association)*, *New England Journal of Medicine*, *Medical Tribune*, *Lancet*, or any other major medical journal, they recommend the same treatments disparaged five years ago. Thanks to the pioneering work of Dr. Dean Ornish and others, the concept of alternative treatment is less controversial and people are not willing to accept these treatment if they seem to offer the best possibility of health. Hopefully, in the future we will not have to reject one or the other, but accept the best features from each as they lead to better health.

Having reviewed the material in this chapter, you should know enough about the available alternatives to radical surgery and drug treatment to decide whether you prefer to seek traditional or alternative care for cardiovascular distress. Whatever sort of care you seek, you should monitor the progress you are or are not making to determine whether it may be feasible to abandon one course and embark on another. If you seek alternative treatments, you can find references in this book. In either case, select a competent physician and weigh his or her advice carefully, remembering to give serious consideration to your own observations of your response to the treatment. Don't be afraid to demand the best and most appropriate care available. When you are dealing with heart disease, your decision could be a matter of your own life or death.

33

Chelation Therapy

For the past 40 years, one of the most promising and exciting healing therapies available has been viciously attacked by the medical establishment. This treatment, called chelation therapy, could be saving hundreds of thousands of lives a year and improving the quality of life for millions more by treating heart disease, strokes, diabetes, peripheral vascular disease, memory loss, and damage due to smoking, drinking, and environmental toxic exposure to heavy metals.

Hundreds of thousands of people have undergone the therapy, more than 400 doctors now use it, and more than 4,000 scientific articles have been written on various aspects of the process. Chelation is nontoxic when properly administered, and yet it has been kept from an objective review until now because it threatens the economic stability of the multibillion dollar cardiovascular and coronary bypass industry, which profits from the very illnesses that chelation treats.

A perfect example of the difficulties involved in completing clinical studies on chelation took place some 15 years ago. During the mid-1980s, the Food and Drug Administration (FDA) approved two careful clinical studies on chelation to be conducted at the Walter Reed Hospital and Letterman Army Hospital, with the results to be published upon their completion. The studies were halted in 1991 during the Gulf War; following the war, however, the studies were never resumed due to lapses in funding and thus, were never completed. Other physicians and medical organizations attempting to acquire both approval and sufficient financing for clinical studies on chelation today have run into similar roadblocks.

Nevertheless, mainstream doctors, for the most part, still ignore the possibilities of chelation treatments despite its good track record with patients. It is the height of arrogance for physicians to decry a therapy as quackery and demean its advocates as misguided and uninformed charlatans when they have never tried the treatment on their own patients, have never attended the comprehensive seminars its practitioners offer, and have never reviewed the medical records of patients who have benefited from it.

But there are no better experts on the therapy's safety and effectiveness than the pioneering doctors who administer it and the patients who receive it. This chapter tells the story of such doctors, and of their patients, all of whom have well-documented records to prove the extent of their improvement from chelation therapy.

What Is Chelation Therapy?

Chelation therapy is a safe, easily administered alternative to drugs and surgery in the treatment of heart disease and other illnesses. The term is derived from the Greek root "chele" meaning claw, and refers to a molecule which is able to grab onto, deactivate, and remove a mineral from the body. The process involves the infusion into the bloodstream of the amino acid EDTA, which moves through the blood vessels and removes excesses of iron, copper and various other metals that are implicated in the formation of plaque. As the plaque is reduced, and through a variety of other biochemical mechanisms, blood flow all over the body improves.

When combined with a change in lifestyle, this treatment may benefit a person in other ways as well. For example, it may slow down or reverse the aging process by keeping free radicals in check. It can also strengthen oxygenation to the heart and blood vessels thereby helping major organ systems to revitalize. In addition, it can help to reverse many disease processes, like strokes, Alzheimer's, diabetes, etc., and to eliminate heavy metals which poison the body, like lead and cadmium.

In contrast to most conventional methods which address symptoms only, chelation therapy treats the basic causes of the underlying illness, thereby reversing the disease process and restoring health. Dr. Michael B. Schachter, of Suffern, New York, former president of the American College of Advancement in Medicine (ACAM), explains how this may occur:

"We know that EDTA removes metals and that it is not metabolized in the body at all. It just comes in, grabs a mineral, and goes out through the urine. In so doing, it brings about a number of profound reactions in the body that result in the therapeutic effects. For example, as people age and as disease occurs, we get an accumulation of calcium in and around the cells of the soft tissues, and the EDTA helps to remove this excess calcium from the wrong places. In other words, we like calcium in our bones but we don't like it in our arteries and our joints, and EDTA helps to get rid of that. It also helps stop excessive free-radical formation, which results in destruction of cell membranes and serves as a common pathway for diseases such as multiple sclerosis, arthritis, cancer, arteriosclerosis, and so on. So, EDTA does a number of very remarkable things in the body."

THE HISTORY OF CHELATION Chelating agents were first used by the German textile industry in 1935 to remove calcium from hard water, which was staining and ruining fabric. After considerable research, a synthetic amino acid known as ethylene diamine tetra-acetic acid (or EDTA) was found to be excellent for that purpose. So, its first use was a commercial one.

Soon afterwards it was discovered that chelation therapy could promote healing by removing heavy metals from the body. During World War II, when an antidote for poison gas was being sought, it was found that chelating agents could be helpful by chelating arsenic, an essential component of some poison gases. One chelating agent that was particularly helpful was BAL or British antilewisite. After the war, chelation therapy was used in the treatment of radiation poisoning, for heavy metals like strontium and uranium. And soon afterwards it was found that in cases of lead poisoning EDTA could effectively and quickly reverse the condition.

At the same time, an unexpected benefit of chelation was discovered. In the early 1950s, Dr. Norman Clarke, Sr. reasoned that since EDTA binds to calcium, it might benefit patients with coronary atherosclerosis. As a good scientist, he then began to explore this phenomenon, and it soon became apparent that his original hypothesis was correct. Dr. Clarke published a number of studies showing that patients with various forms of cardiovascular disease improved. In Dr. Clarke's landmark article published in the *American Journal of Cardiology* in August 1960, he stated the following:

"For several years we have been administering intravenously to patients with advanced occlusive vascular disease 3–5 grams of EDTA. An accumulative experience with several hundred patients has demonstrated that overall relief has been superior to that obtained with other methods. In occlusive vascular disease of the brain there has been uniform relief of vertigo and the signs of senility, even when advanced, have been significantly relieved. In summary, the treatment of atherosclerotic vascular complications with the chelating agent EDTA is supported by a large volume of information."

A CONTROVERSIAL TREATMENT Unfortunately, Dr. Clarke's research and future chelation work were dealt a heavy blow shortly after his article appeared, and the treatment became the object of a carefully waged and highly damaging attack from nearly all components of the medical industrial complex: physicians, their professional organizations and journals, government regulatory boards, and insurance companies.

On what is this controversy based? Is it based upon something that has been proven, or upon American Medical Association and American Heart Association propaganda, whose aim is to put chelation therapy out of business so that costly medicines, products of biotechnology, and medical procedures like coronary bypass operations can be marketed? In other words, who is being harmed by chelation therapy?

Dr. Serafina Corsello, a chelation practitioner, believes part of the problem stems from the use of cardiovascular medication being diminished and ultimately often eliminated after chelation. "Herein lies the danger. We are creating less money for the pharmaceutical industry, so why should they love us?" The precedent for this viewpoint can be traced back to 1969 when Abbott Laboratories' patent on EDTA ran out and they decided not to invest in further research on EDTA because without exclusive rights to produce the drugs there was no way that Abbott could get back the amount of money necessary to prove to the FDA's satisfaction the effectiveness of EDTA chelation therapy for cardiovascular disease.

Opponents of the procedure call chelation therapy a dangerous procedure when, in fact, there is no evidence to support this claim. All clinical research on EDTA is positive, and the only negative articles are opinions and editorials. In actuality, conventionally approved therapies like bypass surgeries are the extremely hazardous ones, especially with people 65 and older. The mortality rate from the procedure is about 5 percent a year, and a large percentage of those who do get the surgery need another bypass procedure approximately six to eight years later. Many of these people do not live longer than six or seven years from the time of their first operation. Dr. Chris Calapei comments:

"Mainstream doctors often have blinders on. They think the only thing to do for blockage of the arteries is to scoop it out and go for this high-tech procedure, but they do not realize that there are phenomenal risks to even the smallest surgical procedures when you are talking about the blood vessels and trying to remove or strip off this cemented type of plaque."

When you compare the risks from surgery to the absolutely nil possibilities of having adverse effects from chelation, it almost boggles the mind as to why doctors are constantly pushing for these surgical modalities before trying something like chelation.

Dr. John Sessions, who has given the treatment to thousands of patients in 13 years, agrees that no one has ever been harmed by the treatment when given in the proper way by a physician trained in its administration. As mentioned previously, he has used the therapy on his own father:

"I have seen some of the most astounding and gratifying results. Specifically, my father had about 10 treatments and was then able to get rid of his walker and walking cane. In 30 treatments he went back into his business, raising cattle and farming, and bought new equipment."

Bypass surgery is also more expensive than chelation therapy, which costs approximately $90 to $110 a session, or approximately $3,000 to $4,000 for a course of 30 infusions. In contrast, the average cost of bypass surgery in 1995 was nearly $45,000, with many people paying considerably more than that. In addition, coronary bypass surgery has never had a good study done on it to prove long-term benefit to its recipient. In fact, studies published in the *Journal of the American Medical Association (JAMA)* and other journals have shown that most patients getting bypass surgery should not have received it. Yet the numbers continue to increase: from 1979 to 1996, the number of bypass procedures in the U.S. soared some 425 percent.

Although discriminated against for cardiovascular disease and other degenerative conditions, in actuality, the use of chelation therapy has been approved for some period of time for the use of heavy metal detoxification. And once a drug is approved for one purpose by the FDA, physicians are permitted to use this drug for other indications provided that there is some medical justification for this unapproved use. Following this logic, there is nothing illegal about the use of chelation therapy for cardiovascular disease and other degenerative diseases. There are only some special interest groups in medicine that would like to see this fact kept secret from the general public.

Dr. Sessions believes that some of the controversy also dates back to early research done in the field when chelation was given to people without nutritional supplementation. Since chelation therapy removes many important nutritive minerals from the body, some of these early patients became deficient in zinc and other minerals during the course of treatment.

How Chelation Helps the Heart

Chelation therapy helps the heart in a number of ways. First, it cleanses the body of toxic material and moves the calcium out so that normal contractions can resume. Dr. Murray Susser of Santa Monica, California, says that according to the work of Hans Selye calcium goes to the site of an injury and acts like an internal scab. When you heal the calcium goes away, but if you keep on injuring yourself, like smokers do with cigarette smoke every day, it builds up and arteriosclerosis forms around it. EDTA can go in and take out that calcium, and when accompanied by a change in lifestyle it can reverse some of the effects of continued injury.

Another way chelation can help the heart is through the injection of magnesium along with the EDTA. More magnesium helps the coronary arteries to relax and open up so that a greater amount of blood can flow through them.

In the long term, EDTA also acts as a calcium binder. As serum calcium decreases, the body responds by secreting parathyroid hormone, which helps mobilize calcium from abnormal soft tissue sites and move it into bones where it is needed. In this way, chelation is an indirect treatment for osteoporosis.

In addition, by acting as a calcium channel blocker, EDTA may cause the blood pressure to go down 10 to 20 points and high blood pressure medications may become unnecessary over time.

Dr. Kirk Morgan, director of the Morgan Medical Clinic in Louisville, Kentucky, has been using chelation successfully on heart patients since 1982 with 90 percent or better improvement in people with hardening of the arteries. His article, "Myocardial Ischemia Treated with Nutrients in Intravenous EDTA Chelation: Report of Two Patients" documented the results of two patients with exercise induced angina pectoris treated with chelation. After the administration of less than 40 treatments, electrocardiographic heart tracings (EKGs) were taken. They showed abnormalities to become normal on repeat stress testing 15 months after beginning the treatment. Both patients demonstrated total resolution of symptoms and renal function did not deteriorate in either subject. The article concludes, "Though only two such cases are described, there is increasing evidence that chelation using EDTA is a relatively inexpensive, effective, safe, and even preferential, but often neglected technique for medical management of cardiovascular and related diseases."

Most other studies in this area show equally dramatic results. Dr. Albert Scarchilli was involved in a study of 19,187 retrospective cases of patients with peripheral vascular disease. It was revealed by thermoscan that 87.5 percent of all patients who received chelation therapy showed significant improvement.

Dr. Michael Janson of Barnstable, Massachusetts has practiced for the past 20 years using nutrition and dietary supplements in patient care and is the author of *The Vitamin Revolution in Health Care* (Arcadia Press, 1996). Dr. Janson is the president of the American Preventative Medical Association, a political group working to protect access to healthy approaches to medical care. Dr. Janson says that, almost invariably, pain from angina pectoris is relieved in 90 percent of the heart patients who are given chelation therapy. He gives an account of one patient's condition before and after treatment:

"Before treatment, this man could not walk from his golf cart to the tee to do his golfing and he told his buddies he was not going to be with them next year. He noticed some friends of his getting better and went to their doctor. He said, "Doc, I don't know what you are doing for these people but I have got to have some of it." After chelation, he is free from angina. He is golfing a full golf course and walking the course now instead of taking the cart."

Dr. Michael Schachter offers a similar success story with a patient named Tom who was first diagnosed with coronary artery disease at the age of 26. He had several angioplasties, which resulted in improvement for 1 to 18 months. By age 29, however, Tom had to have a quintuple bypass. Despite having this procedure done, four years later, shortly before becoming a patient of Dr. Schachter's in September of 1991, Tom had a heart attack. Under Dr. Schachter's care, Tom was given EDTA chelation therapy infusions consisting of specific amounts of disodium ethylene diamine tetra-acetic acid; ascorbic acid; magnesium sulfate; heparin; pantothenic acid; potassium chloride; hydroxocobalamin; pyridoxine; and sodium bicarbonate (8.4 percent). The infusions were given intravenously in 500 cc sterile water over approximately four hours. Tom was also given oral nutritional supplements, dietary recommendations, and was put on an exercise program. As of February 1996, since doing the chelation, Tom has had no heart attacks. He works full time as a police officer, where he outperforms his colleagues in physical endurance activities. According to Dr. Schachter, his stress tests keep improving rather than getting worse, as is usual with this disease.

The amount of infusions necessary to correct a cardiovascular problem varies. According to some physicians, circulatory problems due to blockages in small arteries show more rapid improvement than blockages in larger arteries, such as the aorta or the iliacs, which are the large arteries that go to the legs. Therefore, it is not uncommon to see someone with significant blockages of the big arteries to require 50 to 100 infusions before really getting better. A rough rule to apply is that the further from the heart the blockage is, the slower the response rate will be. In other words, coronaries respond the earliest, carotids second, and arteries in the legs third.

Removal of Toxic Heavy Metals

Heavy metal toxicity is a growing problem as it is present everywhere. It can get into our food if the food is grown near a polluted area. It can be found in our drinking water. Additionally, if you are breathing air with any form of metal in it, you will pick that right up as well. Dr. Murray Susser sums up the situation: "The average civilized human being now has a body burden of lead which is 1,000 times greater than primitive people had 500 years ago. We are all, to some extent, lead poisoned, some much worse than others."

As mentioned, chelation therapy is approved for the removal of these heavy metals. However, mainstream medicine would like not to see it used except when levels in the body are very, very high. The problem with this thinking is that since toxic substances, like lead, are very dangerous and have no biological function, they do not belong in the body at all and should be removed at any level.

Unfortunately, heavy metals do not show their tremendous burden to the body until a great deal of harm has already been done. Only when damage is in its acute phase will symptoms like headaches and dizziness appear. When chelation therapy is used it usually lowers the level of toxic metals in the body significantly after only 5 to 10 treatments. In one man's experience:

"I went to Dr. Yurkovsky with many complaints. I had some days where my thinking was foggy and I felt like a car with a clogged fuel filter. It was as if my brain wasn't getting enough oxygen or enough blood. And I kept losing weight.

"Dr. Savely Yurkovsky discussed the weight loss as a possible malabsorption and as a possible result of heavy metal toxicity, maybe from mercury which was suppressing pancreatic function. He asked me about my amalgam fillings and when I told him that I had a lot of them, he suggested I take them out.

"I had a chelation test where you get one treatment followed by a 24-hour urine test for heavy metals, and I was found to be high in cadmium, mercury, and lead. Then we started a program of chelation, and after 25 treatments all the metals were down within what is called a reference range. In addition, I had my amalgam fillings out. As a result I have started to gain weight and I feel much better.

"It was a good experience all around and I am continuing with the treatments even though I am below what is considered a dangerous level because my doctor has encouraged me to get all the metals out."

Other Conditions Successfully Treated with Chelation

Dr. Serafina Corsello, a chelation practitioner, notes that unlike coronary bypass operations, which work only on the heart, chelation therapy can benefit the entire circulatory system: "You often have atherosclerotic plaque of the little vessels of the kidneys even before the heart is affected and this weakens the body's cleansing process. By regulating the amount of EDTA accordingly and adding vitamin C to repair the tissues, the little vessels of the kidneys will get cleaned out. Then we can increase the amount of EDTA, and ultimately clean the whole vascular system, the heart, kidneys, liver, pancreas, and brain."

DIABETES Chelation is especially helpful to diabetics since diabetes generally involves the arteries. The blood sugar simply happens to be an indicator of how rapidly the disease is progressing. Chelation will open up insulin receptors and in some diabetic patients, may decrease the body's need for extra insulin.

STROKE Additionally, chelation improves circulation to the brain and may prevent the onset of a stroke or aid in alleviating the effects of one. A large study has indicated that an imbalance of facial circulation is indicative of those people who are prone to have strokes. Chelation softens the arteries in the neck and brain and improves the blood flow causing abnormal thermography scans (infrared scans of the face, hands, and feet) to return to normal.

ALZHEIMER'S DISEASE Some people with Alzheimer's disease also do well with this therapy. They function much better, are more alert, and are able to fit into their family setting more appropriately than in the past. In people who succumb to this disease, delicate nerve tendrils, which are responsible for allowing one part of the brain to talk to another, short out and are responsible for a loss of short-term memory. Using chelation may help the oxidative metabolism of the brain, biotron treatments, and desferroxamine, which removes aluminum from the body.

One study on the effect of chelation on the brain was performed by Dr. Edward McDonagh in which an independent psychologist tested 35 senile people with a battery of psychological tests prior to 30 treatments of EDTA chelation and 20 treatments of hyperbaric oxygen, which were given concurrently. When retested, every person showed improvement and their IQs went up about one point per bottle.

INTERMITTENT CLAUDICATION Tens of thousands of people have also been successfully treated with chelation for intermittent claudication, the name given to a type of peripheral vascular disease involving poor circulation in the legs, which may produce pain in the calf muscles upon walking. Dr. Michael Janson reports his experience with peripheral vascular disease. "We have seen dramatic results with people who have vascular disease to the legs where they had sores from diabetes or other causes. Some of them had ulcers that had not healed for up to a year. But these ulcers healed during chelation therapy."

GANGRENE Gangrene often responds as well to chelation. Over the years, Dr. John Sessions of Kirbyville, Texas, has seen people with gangrene, people who were supposed to have had their legs amputated days later, benefit from this treatment. Some of these people are still walking on their own legs.

MACULAR DEGENERATION Another disease which responds well to chelation therapy is macular degeneration, a disease of the eye which causes blindness. Dr. Martin Dayton, a board-certified practitioner of family medicine from Florida, reports that: "Although many ophthalmologists do not believe there is a treatment for this condition, chelation practitioners have found that many of these patients improve significantly and can read where they couldn't read for several years before treatments."

OTHER CONDITIONS The detoxification aspect of chelation therapy is quite remarkable and is responsible for the alleviation many other conditions, such as migraine headaches, scleroderma, hypertension, arthritis, impotence, kidney calcification, high cholesterol, and multiple sclerosis. Dr. McDonagh's Kansas City, Missouri, clinic even had success with people who had been poisoned by Agent Orange in Vietnam:

"These men were severe, tough cases. They were unable to get their wives pregnant after 10 or 15 years of marriage, and they were depressed, suicidal, and alcoholic, with all kinds of organ damage, sores on their skin, and so on. They had been treated with every kind of treatment over the years since Vietnam with no improvement, and in every case we were able to bring them back to a normal situation with an 18-month program of chelation. We think the biggest effect was not just due to an improved immune system but to detoxification that occurs when you use chelation therapy."

An Ounce of Prevention is Worth a Pound of Cure

Chelation therapy has been proven effective as a means of preventive medicine through detoxification and through stimulation of the immune system.

In one retrospective study, Dr. Walter Blumer, a Swiss physician, published a paper showing a decreased incidence of cancer death in his patients, compared to the cancer death rate of people living in the same area after they had 10 to 15 chelation treatments 18 years previously. In his practice, Dr. Edward McDonagh has noted a decreased incidence of cancer in his chelation patients as well:

"We have treated approximately 20,000 patients and of those cases we should have seen thousands of cases of cancer develop by this time compared to the national statistics. However, we have not seen them. We have probably seen three, four, or five cases total in the 28 or 29 years that I have been doing chelation therapy. I think it boils down to the fact that once you stimulate the immune system back to a normal position, the body can heal itself. The body has tremendous powers of rehabilitation even with advanced cases where people were told their conditions were hopeless."

Chelation may help prevent disease simply by removing the toxic substances that interfere with our natural physiological processes. According to Dr. Martin Dayton: "I have been doing chelation therapy for approximately 10 years now, and I have found that people who go in for treatments fare better years later. I think the reason why is that it removes toxic material and therefore helps the body repair itself and function better."

According to evidence Dr. Trowbridge of Humble, Texas, has seen, chelation helps correct the problem at the cellular level: "Calcium builds up around the little energy batteries, called mitochondria, within every cell of our body. What happens is a little change here and a little change there add up to an injury pattern. The work of Peng in 1976 showed that if you take a heart that is injured and you flush it with EDTA, calcium will get out of those energy batteries and they will work better so that you heart is stronger. This is molecular medicine, which will actually change the way people get old and die."

The treatment may also benefit those who are younger and in relatively good health as the blood vessels have to be 50 percent occluded or more before any noticeable loss of function is seen. According to Dr. McDonagh, "Young people are like a time bomb; these processes are sneaking up on them. During the Korean war, 40 percent of the autopsies done on the GIs that were killed showed significant narrowing of the arteries. We're talking 65 percent occlusion or more. After the Vietnam War it was something like 70 percent had 65 percent occlusion. So we know that this is a disease that is striking our younger people, and these people would definitely benefit from having a treatment to clean out and reverse the disease process."

As a vote of confidence, most chelating physicians utilize this treatment on themselves. For example, Dr. Serafina Corsello, who has been using chelation therapy in her practice for 10 years, says, "Chelating physicians do practice what they preach, so I utilize this on myself preventatively. My patients see me going around with the bag and pole, and when they wonder where I get all my energy and stamina in spite of the multiple things that we have to do, the answer is in chelation therapy. By *preventing* the formation of atherosclerotic plaque, I can do much better than I can do with intervention."

Toxic materials in our body cause an acceleration of free-radical activity, which quickens the aging process by causing cells to die. By pulling out excess copper, iron, lead, cadmium, and other poisons, free-radical activity is reduced and the aging process slows down and often reverses. Dr. John Sessions reports that his own father, who was white-headed before therapy, had his hair turn black and white after 30 chelation treatments.

How Effective is Chelation Therapy?

After chelation therapy most people are given functional tests to see how much their arteries have deoccluded rather than arteriograms and other tests, which can be dangerous. One of Dr. Sessions' patients had an arteriogram after bypass surgery that showed that he was still occluded in all the arteries. After chelation therapy he was able to pass a treadmill test with flying colors, which means he was getting enough circulation back to the heart muscle to carry on the strenuous activity.

Other patients elect to go back for an arteriogram to see if all the plaque is gone, with differing responses. Some will develop marked collateral circulation around the blockage, which gets the needed blood supply to the heart or other area even though all the blockage itself has not disappeared. This is because chelation therapy does not always work like a Roto-Rooter treatment. What it is doing, however, is helping the body to reestablish the proper amount of blood flow to any given area of the body.

There are other objective data on the effectiveness of chelation therapy as well. A new noninvasive MRI angiogram, done with magnetic imaging, and of superb quality, can now document the before and after results of chelation quite accurately. Other tests which can be performed involve ultrasonography, the use of ultrasound to determine the degree of opening of the arteries, and through thermography, the measurement of temperature on the surface of the skin. Temperature rises when circulation improves. In addition, changes in the color of the extremities can be seen, and one can objectively see changes in a person's ability to walk distances as well. Also, an echocardiogram may show the heart's improved ability to pump blood following chelation, and a thallium stress test can also substantiate that chelation works.

NUTRITIONAL SUPPLEMENTATION FOLLOWING CHELATION A patient undergoing chelation therapy, but on a poor diet, will not have a significant improvement with the therapy alone. It is pointless to give chelation therapy if the patient will not make other positive lifestyle changes. It is important to remember that no one modality that is so good that it can function as a cure-all and overcome the toxic onslaught so many people put their bodies through.

While the purpose of chelation is to remove toxic material from the body, the addition of various nutritional supplements can help to correct deficiencies and keep the body as healthy as possible. Therefore, chelation practitioners usually give nutritional supplements along with the therapy.

Dr. Kirk Morgan advises his patients to drink a lot of good quality water unless they happen to have inadequate kidney function. He also suggests a diet high in fiber and the avoidance of animal fats.

"I simply tell [my patients] to think of cereal for breakfast, vegetables for lunch, and beans and lentils at supper," he says. "I ask them to keep the fat down in the diet similar to what Pritikin has said and I ask them not to skip meals, particularly the overweight patients. In addition I suggest exercising. I try to teach them to count grams of fiber and grams of fat, not so that they will have to do this but so that they will get some idea of how much fiber and how much fat their various choices have."

In Dr. John Sessions' practice all patients are given an organic multivitamin that is well absorbed and well tolerated. Then a hair analysis is done, and a history and physical findings are taken into account. In this way patients can be treated on an individual basis. Some patients need more zinc, others more selenium. Only in very rare instances is a patient given copper or iron. In contrast, most conventional physicians often give an iron tablet even though it is now known that iron can accelerate the aging process. Dr. Sessions also uses fish oil supplements for improving circulation, and antioxidants to reduce free-radical activity.

In the view of Dr. Michael Janson, recent research has revealed that supplementation is essential to anyone undergoing chelation therapy. In his opinion, "Chelation is not the only answer to vascular disease. It's just an important addition to the other therapies that I think are important."

Dr. Janson goes on to emphasize, "We have to recognize that when we pull out metals from the body, we also pull out nutritional elements that are very important for health, like zinc and manganese, other minerals that we take out of the body with the chelation process. So, an important part of the approved protocol for chelation is to give certain dietary supplements along with the intravenous treatments, not at the same time, not in the IV, but as a separate oral treatment where people take these supplements to improve and enhance the effectiveness of chelation."

These oral supplements that enhance chelation are not, in themselves, chelation. Some people wrongly believe that they are being treated with "oral chelation therapy," when in fact, there is no such thing. There are some oral chelating agents that are used medicinally, but in Dr. Janson's view, they are not generally as safe as EDTA. However, the nutrients that people are incorrectly calling chelation or oral chelation have the adjuncts to chelation that are important for its safe administration. They also have some of their own benefits in that vitamins E and C, for example, can actually help to slow cardiovascular disease also, in addition to chelation therapy.

Dr. Janson, who has himself been a recipient of over 65 chelation treatments, recommends the following nutrient supplements to his patients to be taken in conjunction with chelation therapy: extra zinc, extra vitamin B_6 or pyridoxine (if there isn't enough vitamin B_6, repeated chelation treatment can cause a skin rash); and manganese, which is removed heavily by chelation.

Dr. Janson also maintains that certain nutrients, when combined with chelation, help the body's healing process along. He usually recommends at least 4,000 mg a day of vitamin C; 800–1,200 units a day of vitamin E, which helps to scavenge free radicals; 100 to 250 mg a day of coenzyme Q10, which works to reduce blood pressure in patients who have high blood pressure, works to improve the heart muscle contraction, and improves overall heart function (in more severe cases, 300 mg, and in some cases even 400 mg, may have therapeutic benefits in a number of conditions including heart problems); and 1,000 mg twice a day of taurine, a sulfur containing amino acid to improve heart failure or high blood pressure (he cautions, however that the proper dose will vary from person to person).

According to Dr. Janson, the B vitamins have been shown to lower the level of a substance in the bloodstream called homocysteine. High levels of homocysteine have been associated with increased blockage in the arteries, including the carotid arteries that go to the brain, and other arteries as well. The B vitamins that are important for dealing with this problem include B_6 or pyridoxine, folic acid, B_{12}, and another nutrient called betaine.

Dr. Janson summarizes, "Chelation is part of a comprehensive health program which includes a whole foods vegetarian diet, a low-fat diet, [which includes] the right fats, like the omega-3 and omega-6 oils that are necessary, an exercise program, and a stress management program. I think if you combine all those things together with the chelation therapy, you have done the patient a much greater service than if you just assume that these therapies can't work because the doctor who hasn't read the literature makes the assumption that they can't work."

Ultimately, it is important for the specialist in chelation therapy to be well versed in his understanding of how supplements can benefit the patient if he is not to make the patient worse than when he started.

Myths Surrounding Chelation Therapy

The most popular published myth concerning chelation is that it is going to ruin the kidneys. In truth, however, published articles substantiate the fact that chelation actually improves deficient kidney function when administered properly and that there are over 200 drugs listed in the *PDR* far more dangerous to the kidneys. Dr. Sessions confirms this in his experience with dialysis patients where at first "...the kidneys were functioning at 5 percent" and after treatments, "they were able to cut down on their dialysis to one and two times a week. In addition, their lifestyle improved to where they could go back to exercising, mowing their lawn, and having a more acceptable lifestyle."

The second thing the media and physicians against chelation promote is that this therapy makes bones weak because it takes out calcium. According to Dr. Sessions, this is a half-truth since chelation does pull out many minerals including calcium that are found in the bones. However, as mentioned previously, the lowering of serum calcium stimulate parathormone production by the parathyroid gland, which wakes up the bones and causes them to put calcium and other minerals back into the bones. The net result is that the bones are far stronger and far harder than before chelation.

Dr. Kirk Morgan feels that as we get older we tend to accumulate calcium in the soft tissues of the body, such as blood vessels, joints, muscles, and skin. This calcification contributes to the aging of the cells and tissues and interferes with their proper functioning. Chelation therapy, by helping to remove this excessive calcium in the wrong places can help to reverse this aging, degenerative trend.

EDUCATING THE PATIENTS, AND THE DOCTORS One of the prime cornerstones of a chelation therapy practice is to educate the patient, which is hard work and takes a lot of time. In Dr. John Sessions' office, every member of the staff works with these patients. "You can't just tell someone who has been eating sausage for breakfast for 50 years not to eat sausage, but if you sit down and explain to him what the fats are doing, how it is causing free-radical activity, what a free radical is, and how he is going to benefit by following our instructions, then you will get a fairly good compliance with these people. Education on a one-to-one basis is a cornerstone for being successful in getting these people to modify their diet to a low-fat, moderate protein, high unrefined carbohydrate diet.

Dr. Sessions categorizes doctors who do not use chelation therapy into three types:

First there are the pompous ones. These are the people who claim to have discovered one thing or another, and they don't want to come down from their lofty post. They are the ones responsible for some of our artery surgery.

Then there are those who are just simply ignorant. This is not faulting them in any way; they are just busy and they don't have time to learn what is new. Also, since most of the articles received on chelation and other alternative therapies are rejected by the major medical journals, these findings cannot reach the mass of doctors. All they hear is that it is dangerous and ineffective. At the same time, these people are pressured from the standard-setting bodies. If they say something good about chelation they may lose their hospital privileges and their referrals from other physicians.

Lastly, there is the group motivated by greed. If a physician is doing bypass surgery and making a million dollars a year, he probably would not want to reduce the number of coronary bypasses he does when he learns that chelation therapy is a viable alternative for many of these patients.

The Future of Chelation Therapy

Despite all the controversy surrounding chelation, there are inroads being made suggesting that this may be a more standard and accepted therapy in the near future.

One indication of this was a unanimous Florida Supreme Court decision to make chelation therapy legal without question throughout the United States. In fact, the judge in this case was very complimentary to the doctors who were persecuted by their peers, saying that their pioneering spirit was refreshing and that without people willing to take on the establishment medicine would not progress. This decision has set a precedent in the United States and, based upon this ruling, many of the state boards in different areas of the country will now think twice before persecuting doctors using chelation therapy.

CHECKS AND BALANCES: MAKING SURE CHELATION IS PROPERLY EMPLOYED Many doctors now, as well as a lot of clinics, are doing chelation therapy; unfortunately, some of these individuals are people who have no background in cardiology and are not board-certified in this area. Chelation therapy can be a valuable treatment when it is implemented properly by a physician who has been board certified. The American Board of Chelation Therapy, for example, is one organization that certifies physicians who have done the training in chelation therapy offered by the American College for Advancement in Medicine (ACAM). However, with the increasing popularity of chelation and the increased acceptance of its usage in the medical community, more and more people are getting chelation therapy from non-board certified doctors who do not use it responsibly. For example, some people may get chelation two, three, or even four times a week, without any preliminary or post-treatment testing or examination, and are told they're doing fine. Chelation should always be employed in conjunction with kidney analyses, calcium magnesium studies, a mineral balance analysis, and a general physical examination.

According to Dr. Martin Dayton, who uses chelation as part of his own practice, chelation is a serious treatment that is not to be used by someone who has not been properly trained. Administration of the technique by someone who is not board certified and does not have proper training in chelation therapy is highly irresponsible. Dr. Dayton states, "It's alarming what's going on. We have doctors that are setting up chelation clinics similar to fast food restaurants. There are 'Kentucky Fried' chelation clinics set up in numerous areas if these doctors have their way. They give lectures, speak brilliantly, and then they hire non-doctors or doctors with little experience to administer the chelation. It is very important to know all the intricacies of administering chelation because harm can be done."

Dr. Dayton emphasizes the importance of going to a chelation therapist who has board certification and explains why not finding this out can be a major risk for patients: "If the [proper] protocol is followed, that's what the board certified doctors follow. There has not been one death proven to be due to chelation in over 25 years. So, it is safe when it is done by doctors who are aware and are trained. Now, when the protocol is not followed due to either ignorance of lack of training, you can have kidney failure, you can have congestive heart failure, people can die, not from the proper treatment but from the improper treatment. It is very important to know that chelation is simply a tool that should be used in a larger scheme of things, a larger health strategy, to balance the person, to get rid of the toxic material that prevents normal function and repair, to add those things that are necessary, so we can have a person as harmonious as possible in order to obtain optimal health."

THE ISSUE OF COST AND TESTING With the increase in unqualified physicians who nevertheless administer chelation, there has also been the emergence of another potential problem for patients: inappropriate cost inflation. Unfortunately, there are always practitioners in both mainstream and alternative medicine who are more than willing to profit from their patients' ignorance of the therapies being utilized. Being well-informed is the key to avoiding this pitfall. In terms of chelation therapy, realistically, most doctors today need to charge from $90 to $110 per treatment. A physician who charges significantly more may be guilty of overcharging, and chances are, may also be non-board certified in chelation.

On a similar note, as stated previously, physicians employ chelation in conjunction with a variety of laboratory tests, such as a full spectrum blood chemistry test, a mineral analysis, and a glucose tolerance test. The total cost of these tests varies; it may cost as little as a few hundred dollars or it can extend to as high as over $1,000, depending on how detailed the doctor thinks the blood and mineral analyses should be and where the tests are done. According to Dr. Martin Feldman, the issue of cost abuse by physicians with regard to testing has more to do with whether or not the tests are being processed and analyzed within the physician's office or are being sent out to an independent laboratory for analysis. Dr. Feldman asserts that it is when the tests are done privately within a physician's office that most instances of cost inflation take place; physicians do not tend to make a profit when they send patients to an independent laboratory since the lab is usually paid directly by the patient.

As a general rule of thumb, it is helpful to know how to interview a physician before going to see him or her. You can ask questions such as, how much is my initial visit? How much time do I actually spend with the physician? Can I have these tests done anywhere else where they will cost less?

So just keep calling until you find yourself a doctor who is willing to give you what you want and to work with you. If there is a test that he or she feels is necessary, challenge the doctor by having him or her explain to you a legitimate rationale for your having the test taken.

Patient Stories

I was going through a period in life where a lot of my friends, who are in the over 50 age group, were experiencing heart attacks, angina, and associated symptoms. That prompted me to think about my own condition, so as a precautionary move I took a thallium stress test. To my surprise, they found a blocked major coronary artery. The hospital recommended at that time that I do an angioplasty. First they do a catheterization angioplasty and they open up the artery. I felt that was an invasive procedure. I discussed this with Dr. Corsello, who suggested I try chelation for a year or so. She said I could always have the angioplasty done later because it was not yet at a serious stage and I was in good condition from running. I agreed. In fact, I had wanted to take chelation therapy for another reason: as a dentist I had been exposed to a lot of heavy metals over the years.

I went through a year's chelation therapy. During that year I had a tremendous increase in my energy level. I had younger looking skin, and I felt younger, and everybody said I looked great. A year later I went back for another thallium stress test and to the doctor's surprise the blockage was no longer there. I have had two successive thallium stress tests since then with the same results. I have maintained a schedule of having chelation therapy once or twice a month since that time and my heavy metal level has decreased almost 80 percent. I feel great.

Some of my patients have used chelation and the results are equally positive. It alleviates tiredness and it restores the immune system. I have even seen people suffering from Lyme disease have equally good results. Other people who were intoxicated with heavy metals have all had very favorable experiences. We had one person with Epstein Barr who was walking around with a cane for years because nobody was able to ascertain what he had or give him a definitive treatment. He calls me up every month to thank me.—Dr. Bush

I had a blockage in the bend of my leg. My leg circulation was so bad that I could hardly walk. After running an arteriogram on me the doctor said I should take an aspirin a day. Then I went to Dr. Sessions and I have had no trouble since. I have had 95 chelation sessions and I can walk now. My legs don't hurt me like they did and I can do almost anything I want to. I believe that Dr. Sessions' chelation therapy kept me from having my leg amputated. Also, I was right on the verge of a stroke when I went to him and he straightened that out. I am over 81 years-old.—Claude

Approximately 12 years ago I suffered from diabetes, hypertension, high blood pressure (250/110), glaucoma, and kidney stones. There were weeks of time when I did not get out of bed. Evidently my condition was terrible. My kidney stones were so large that I was told they could not be removed except surgically. Dr. Sessions suggested that he might have a treatment for me and I started taking it right away. After the twentieth treatment I began to feel better and I have continued to take chelation ever since once a month. In all, I have had 300 treatments.

I am 83 years old and currently I have no kidney stones. This morning my blood pressure was 130/60 and I feel great. This afternoon I am going to go back on my ranch, take the horse, and go try to find and kill a wild pack of dogs that are attacking my calves and cows.

In addition to chelation treatments, I have changed my diet. I take vitamins and do not eat fats. I exercise as well.

If it had not been for chelation I do not believe I would be alive today. I intend to take one treatment each month for as long as I live.

I have seen many, many people come through Dr. Sessions' office, and almost everyone, including those who were facing amputation, have suffered no ill effects.

I think this is a treatment most of us need since all of us have been contaminated in some manner with lead and other chemicals that chelation removes.—Mr. Hill

Approximately two years ago, I was suffering from dizzy spells, which at times were just unbearable. I went to see a few physicians who couldn't find out the cause of my trouble. Finally, one suggested that I go to a vascular surgeon and I did. He gave me a thorough examination with all his technology and equipment and then told me that my condition was very discouraging as one carotid artery was 100 percent blocked and the other was blocked 75 percent. He said my condition was inoperable and that I would have to wait for the inevitable to happen. That was in February 1990.

I then heard of chelation therapy through a friend of the family. I have since received between 75 and 80 treatments, and as of March 1991 the results have been remarkable. My right carotid artery has gone from 100 percent to 83 percent blocked and the left one has gone from 75 to between 44 and 48 percent blocked.

All in all, I have found that this has done me a world of good as I am able to get around and do my work. I can highly recommend the treatment to anyone in the same position as myself. I am 85 years old and feel that chelation therapy has added quality to my life. In fact, I feel I would be dead today without it because they couldn't operate on me and I was going downhill at the time.—Leo

34

Anemia

Anemia is a health condition characterized by red blood cells deficient in hemoglobin, the iron-containing portion of the blood. Hemoglobin enables the blood to transport oxygen from the lungs throughout the body, and to carry away carbon dioxide; the listlessness, pallor, and shortness of breath in the anemic reflect a lack of oxygen and buildup of carbon dioxide in the tissues. It is more common in women than men.

Causes of Anemia

Dr. Dahlia Abraham, a complementary physician, describes three major causes:

"The first cause of anemia is excessive blood loss. Chronic blood loss can occur in association with menstruation, or because of conditions such as hemorrhoids or a slow, bleeding, peptic ulcer.

"The second cause of anemia is excessive red blood cell destruction. Normally, old and abnormal red blood cells are removed from circulation. If the rate of destruction exceeds that of manufacture of new cells, then anemia can result. A number of factors can cause excessive red blood cell destruction, such as defective hemoglobin synthesis, injury, or trauma within the arteries.

"The third and most common type of anemia is caused by nutritional deficiencies in iron, vitamin B_{12}, and folic acid. Of these, iron deficiency is most frequently seen. People require extra iron during growth spurts in infancy and adolescence. Pregnancy and lactation are other times when women need iron supplementation. During childbearing years, many women experience anemia caused by an iron deficiency.

"Supplementation may not solve the problem because many people have difficulty absorbing iron. They lack enough hydrochloric acid, the stomach acid that helps the body assimilate iron. This is common among the elderly, who generally produce less hydrochloric acid. Another cause of decreased iron absorption is chronic diarrhea.

"Vitamin B_{12} deficiency is most often due to a defect in absorption. B_{12} must be liberated from food via hydrochloric acid and bound to a substance called intrinsic factor, which is also secreted in the stomach. In order for B_{12} to be absorbed then, an individual must secrete enough hydrochloric acid and enough intrinsic factor. [People] with this type nemia may need to take supplements of B_{12}, hydrochloric acid, and intrinsic factor.

"Folic acid deficiency may also cause anemia. Folic acid becomes totally depleted in alcoholics. It is also commonly deficient among pregnant women because the fetus demands so much of it. Folic acid is vital for cell production in the growing fetus, and prevents birth defects, such as neural tube imperfections. This is why prenatal vitamins must contain this nutrient. In addition, a number of pharmaceutical drugs, such as anticancer drugs and oral contraceptives, can drain the body of folic acid. Women taking either of these should be supplementing their diet with folic acid, especially since this nutrient is difficult to get in foods."

Anemia in Women

Dr. Pat Gorman, an acupuncturist and educator, explains anemia and other blood disorders in women from an Asian perspective: "In women, blood has an actual cycle that rises and falls every month. There is a building phase that occurs for about a week after your period. Then there is a peak phase where the blood reaches its richest moment; that's the moment you ovulate. This is followed by a storage phase. (If you are pregnant, the blood is stored.) A week before your period, you go through a cleansing phase where your organs release toxins into the blood. That's the week before your period when you can go through a PMS hell if the toxins are not being properly released. Next is the purging of the actual period."

Using this philosophy as her framework, Dr. Gorman holds that women become anemic when they are out of touch with their monthly cycles. In our fast-paced society, one of the major reasons for this condition is that women fail to rest at the appropriate times: "Women work all the time. They show no vulnerability, and just keep on going no matter what. There is no respect for the actual rhythm of the cycle. I believe that we need to bring back the menstrual hut. When you are bleeding, you need to stop working for a day or two. I know I am saying things that sound impossible, but if you have anemia—and 60 to 70 percent of the women that I see do—you need to face the fact and work with it."

She adds that another major reason why women become anemic is that they incorrectly approach pregnancy: "There is a law called the one-month, one-year law. After a pregnancy is terminated, whether in abortion, miscarriage or birth, one month of absolute rest is needed. Women say, 'That's not possible. I just gave birth but I have other children. I have to take care of things.' The Chinese say this is a straight road to a severe anemic problem.

"The one-year aspect of this is the avoidance of pregnancy for at least another year. Women who try to conceive, and who miscarry, often frantically begin again. They need to build up the blood for an entire year's cycle before trying to conceive again. It is very difficult for me to help anxious patients relax and understand that this is the way to overcome anemia and to have a really healthy baby."

Additionally, Dr. Gorman warns that birth control pills are unhealthy because they disturb the integrity of the blood's cycle. They fool the body into believing that it is continually pregnant by locking blood into its storage phase. By eliminating the cycle of building, peaking, storing, cleansing and purging, oral contraceptives create many problems.

Diagnosis

General symptoms of anemia are weakness and a tendency to tire easily. When there is a B_{12} deficiency, the symptoms may include paleness; the tendency to tire easily; shortness of breath; sore, red, swollen tongue; diarrhea; heart palpitations; and nervous disturbances.

According to Dr. Dahlia Abraham, the treatment of anemia is dependent on proper clinical evaluation by a physician. Too often, physicians assume anemia is from an iron deficiency, but this is just one possible reason. "It is absolutely imperative that a comprehensive laboratory analysis of the blood be performed," she says. "Do not be satisfied when your physician offers a simple diagnosis of anemia," she warns. "Insist that your doctor investigate the underlying causes."

While Dr. Gorman agrees that clinical studies help confirm a diagnosis, she adds that Asian physicians are trained to accurately detect anemia and other blood disorders through observation: "In Chinese medicine, you examine the body. Look at your tongue. Is it pale? Look at your lips. Are they pale? See if the mucous membranes under the eyes are pale. These signs indicate whether or not you are anemic."

Diet and Nutritional Remedies

Green, leafy vegetables are high in iron and folic acid. It is best to purchase organic vegetables, as pesticides interfere with absorption. Eating vegetables raw or lightly cooked preserves their folic acid content. Soy or shoyu sauce, miso, and tempeh are rich sources of vitamin B_{12}.

Proteins should be eaten every day, preferably vegetarian proteins, such as from grains and legumes, like rice and beans, or oatmeal with soy milk. When animal protein is eaten, it should be from fish. Caffeine and alcohol are detrimental to healthy blood, and should be eliminated.

According to Dr. Abraham, iron, B_{12}, and folic acid should be prescribed as needed. Additionally, hydrochloric acid and intrinsic factor are often required to aid in the absorption of these nutrients.

Patient Story

I was born in Nicaragua, Central America, and I used to be a very healthy person. But in June 1993, I went to the emergency room. My hemoglobin was down to 2.8; the normal count for a woman is between 12 and 14. There I was with aplastic anemia, meaning that my bone marrow was not making any blood cells: no red cells, no white cells, no platelets. I almost had no blood. The doctor said that my sickness was idiopathic, meaning that they didn't know what caused it. They said that one possible cause was the use of an antibiotic. But the only one that I took in my life was fifteen years earlier. Another possible cause was exposure to chemicals or pesticides. A lot of towns in Nicaragua are surrounded by cotton plantations where cotton growers use a lot of pesticides to spray their crops.

In July 1993, I was referred to a bone marrow transplant unit and was put on a medication, a kind of chemotherapy. After one month of treatment, the medication failed to work. Then the doctors wanted to do a bone marrow transplant. I have seven siblings so I had donors, and one of them was a perfect match. But I had my reservations. A bone marrow transplant is very costly. Also, you get bone marrow that is working, but due to the chemotherapy or radiation, your liver, kidneys, pancreas and so forth, pay a terrible toll.

Prior to my sickness, I was following a macrobiotic diet. I was starting to use Oriental and alternative medicine, and I knew of the power of the body to heal itself. I decided to keep on my macrobiotic diet, and was able to, more or less, clean myself of the chemotherapy. During this time I did not even get a cold. I didn't sneeze through all my sickness.

I was clean, but my blood counts were still very low. I needed a transfusion every ten days. On one hand, the transfusions were very helpful, and I was grateful to be able to get them. But through transfusions I was also receiving a lot of genetic and other information completely foreign to my body. I could not control what the person who donated that blood was eating. So I was trying to clean my body of toxins and I decided to look for help.

I went to a naturopath who helped me a lot. Then I read an article on Ayurveda. That article said that Ayurveda is very specific, even with the use of grains and vegetables. There are grains and vegetables that are not appro-

priate for your body type. In early February 1994, I went to an Ayurvedic doctor. He gave me a very gentle treatment consisting of diet, aromatherapy, massage, and meditation. After three weeks of following that treatment, my blood count went up for the first time.

I keep up with this treatment still. My last checkup at the hospital showed normal white cells. Red cells were a little bit low. They were 3.83, and the normal count is four. But they are increasing day by day.

My energy level is excellent. I went back to work three months ago, and am now leading a completely normal life. I am very grateful to Ayurveda.
—Yolanda

PART SEVEN

Allergy And
Environmental Illness

35

Environmental Medicine

Environmental medicine, also known as clinical ecology, may be the fastest-growing and most exciting new field in modern medicine. This is at least in part because it represents a return to common sense. One early pioneer in environmental medicine was Dr. Walter Alvarez, a Harvard Medical School graduate, chief physician at the distinguished Mayo Clinic, medical columnist and book author in the period between the world wars. In order to complete his diagnosis, Dr. Alvarez used to listen carefully to the patient. If that didn't provide him with the necessary insight, he would talk to the patient's family. And if he still wasn't sure, he'd go to the home to observe the environment there, including things like noise levels and exposure to chemical toxins. Very often it was in the character of the patient's daily life that Dr. Alvarez found what he was looking for, in the form of immunologically or toxically driven symptoms including everything from flulike symptoms to cerebral reactions, behavioral disorders, cardiac arrhythmias, or gastrointestinal disorders. Before exploring further the field of environmental medicine, let's look back at the early research on allergies.

Early Research and Theories

Research into the nature of allergies began about a century ago. Scientists were interested in learning how people could "exempt" themselves from bacteria and pathogens by building a defense against them. They did controlled animal studies to see how injections of minute portions of offending substances might cause the body to begin defending itself. The immune system, it was discovered, can be activated by these "immunizations" to moderate its overreaction to foreign microbial "invaders." This overreaction is actually an internal reaction (intrareaction), or as it was called at the turn of the century, an allergic reaction or simply "allergy" to the pathogen.

Immunologists and allergists—the scientists who studied these phenomena—keyed in on the classical reactions, such as hives, skin rashes, and increased pulse rate. In the 1920s they determined that immunoglobulins or antibodies were produced in the blood to defend the body against the intrusion of foreign substances biologically perceived as not belonging. Immunoglobulin E (IgE) was the antibody that seemed most active in combating the antigen, or offending material, and in forming the classical reaction allergy, as the body's response to that antigen. Over the next 30 years scientists looked for ways to counter this reaction, principally by introducing small amounts of antigen into the blood so that the body would learn to recognize it and not react so violently to it.

In the 1970s this understanding of allergies began to change. Environmental medical specialists—allergists who look to a person's whole environment as having the potential to create an immune-mediated response or reaction—realized that many allergies were a major factor contributing to illnesses and diseases that traditionally had been left out of discussions of allergic responses. Migraine headaches, depression, and arthritis are just a few of the conditions that were found to be allergy-related. While clinical data have supported this work, traditional allergists and immunologists frequently believe that there is insufficient theoretical explanation of these phenomena to accept them as scientifically valid.

Types and Causes of Allergies

The type of allergies that are characterized by obvious reactions as in the case of hay fever, asthma, and various skin conditions, known as type I allergies, may be responses to inhalants or direct chemical contact. Type II allergies are also reactions to intolerable substances, but they are subtler and more insidious, as in the case of headaches and chronic gastrointestinal problems such as nausea, constipation, diarrhea, and malabsorption. These may be responses to foods to which a person is hypersensitive and therefore intolerant. The type I allergies call on IgE as their chief antibody, whereas type II allergies incite the production of immunoglobulin G (IgG).

Immunoglobulins are proteins that typically protect the body from bacteria, parasites, and pollutants. If you are subjected to a high concentration of an irritant, say pollen, your body will manufacture IgE efficiently. Then, if you directly encounter pollen, the IgE-manufacturing mechanism will be activated quickly. If you inhale pollen, you may sneeze to force it out. In the case of an actual parasite, if it contacts your skin, the IgE will attach itself to the parasite, thereby causing an itching sensation. You will then scratch your skin, and the scratching may kill the parasite. In the case of the parasite, your body's reaction protects you from potential danger. But in the case of pollen, the response is inappropriate because there are no known health hazards related to breathing in pollen. The problem arises when the body overreacts to pollen so that a whole symptomatology develops.

Inappropriate reactions to antigens are caused by the activity of the inducer or helper cells that constitute part at the T-lymphocyte system, which is responsible for scavenging and destroying unwanted substances. In general, the T-lymphocyte system is composed of both T-helper and T-suppressor cells.

The T-helper cells join the so-called B cells in encouraging antibody development, while the T-suppressor cells curb antibody reactions. If you have too much T-helper involvement, you will be allergic and hypersensitive to many things. If you have too much T-suppressor activity, your lymphocyte activity will not be sufficient to ward off truly dangerous and even life-threatening organisms and substances. Dr. Alan Levin, a board-certified physician in immunology, allergy, and pathology, uses this analogy:

The series of "inducer or helper cells can be compared to an automobile with the accelerator and brake pedals on the floor; the car isn't moving, but the engine is revving. To go from point A to point B, the brake must be removed. To modulate the car's speed as it goes from A to B, you use the brake, which is applied when point B is reached. Thus, the brake pedal is the suppressor cell and the accelerator is the helper/inducer cell. If you lose your accelerator pedal, you have AIDS, and if you lose your brake pedal, you have rheumatoid arthritis. In people with allergies, the brakes are slipping."

Since allergies are the subject here, the primary concern is with the heightened activity of T-helper cells. It is not known exactly what creates a chronic syndrome of inappropriate immune-related responses as is seen in type II allergies, but it is known that some sort of damage to the immune system is an underlying condition. Immune system damage can be caused by many things. Concentrated and/or prolonged exposures to pesticides, chemicals, toxic fumes, radiation, and broad-spectrum antibiotics are common causes. Viral damage can occur to the immune system from such ailments as herpes and the Epstein-Barr virus. Candida, a yeast which is associated with an intolerance condition, has come into focus in the last decade as being responsible for a wide range of immune system dysfunctions related to allergies, especially of the type II variety.

Sometimes people develop hormone imbalances that also impair the immune system. Hormones, which are secreted by the endocrine glands, help regulated vital physiological functions. The thyroid gland, for instance, secretes hormones T3, T4, and TSH (thyroid-stimulating hormone). In a person who suffers from hypothyroidism, or low output of these three hormones, the cellular utilization of energy and the normal activity of the immune system will be decreased. Low basal temperatures, dry skin, chronic fatigue, and weight-loss problems may ensue. All these symptoms of hypothyroidism have been cited in cases of food sensitivity.

Pancreatic enzyme production, for instance, may be impaired by specific vitamin and mineral deficiencies. These deficiencies may result from insufficient intake of foods rich in specific vitamins or minerals but can also be caused by malabsorption of the nutrients ingested.

How Environmental Medicine Differs From Traditional Medicine

Fundamentally, environmental medicine is an empirical science (meaning that it is based on direct observation and experiment), which puts it at odds with traditional Western medicine, which long ago diverged from its empirical roots. Using as an example the symptom of postnasal drip, here is the difference between the diagnostic approaches of a traditional physician and an environmental medicine specialist, or clinical ecologist. The conventional practitioner will prescribe an antihistamine, along with a cautionary mention of possible side effects. In other words, this doctor, whether an internist or a traditional allergist, is concerned primarily with two things, the symptoms and the suppression of those symptoms. Little in his education or in his practice will have taught him to go beyond this narrow minded way of seeing.

By contrast, the environmental medicine specialist will wonder why his patient's nasal mucous membranes have become more reactive. Is there a nutritional deficiency at cause, or a decrease in the ongoing repair processes of these nasal tissues due to an overload of immunologic responsiveness? A decision may be made to perform testing of delayed food and chemical sensitivity. The environmental medicine specialist in this case may also want to rule out an occupational exposure to petroleum solvent, formaldehyde, or other aromatics including tobacco. If he or she finds any such factors to be present, a decision may be made to mitigate exposure to the toxin or irritant by introducing an electrostatic precipitator or ionizer into the patient's home or work environment.

In other words, the clinical ecologist will not simply try to identify and then suppress the symptom. He or she will use the symptom as a clue and will then embark on a course of inquiry aimed at finding the underlying cause or causes. If the cause can be identified, then a program aimed directly at it can be inaugurated: e.g., providing nutritional supplementation that will help nasal tissue repair, ridding the work or home environment of a toxic chemical, improving ventilation in a work space, etc.

DEFINITION OF ALLERGIES Environmental medicine specialists define allergies much more broadly than do conventional physicians. For example, according to environmental medicine specialist Dr. Marshall Mandell, central nervous system diseases such as multiple sclerosis may have a significant relationship to food sensitivities. Mental illness is another example where allergies may play an important role. According to Dr. Mandell, as many as 80 percent of those hospitalized for mental illness could be helped by adjustments in their nutritional intake or other changes in their environment. Another example is arthritis. Dr. Mandell refers to one patient with osteoarthritis who was told by his conventional physician that he would have to have both knees replaced. The environmental medicine specialist demonstrated that this simply was not the case.

While we are used to considering an allergy as a very limited factor affecting our overall sense of well-being, environmental medicine specialists tend to view chemical or food sensitivities as a primary suspect in the presence of any symptoms of a wide range of illnesses and complaints. Environmental specialists also recognize heredity as a major factor. Children in families where both parents share a common allergy have a 75 percent chance of inheriting it. If only one parent is allergic, the risk that the child will have the same or a different allergy is reduced to roughly 50 percent. Psychological stress at work or at home is another predisposing factor which the environmental medicine specialist may consider important.

Equally important is the healthiness of a person's digestive system. The stomach must secrete sufficient hydrochloric acid, and sufficient enzymes must be released through pancreatic secretions, for protein to be broken down into much smaller units, to enable thorough absorption eventually in the bloodstream. If the digestive process is impaired anywhere along the digestive tract, any food or substance sensitivities will be intensified. Here lies one key to why the high-protein diet favored by Americans is so unhealthy. Since it takes so much longer to digest, it effectively sabotages, by means of a slow-down, the digestive process, greatly increasing the likelihood of an allergic reaction. Many types of illness prevalent in our country, such as peptic ulcers and heart disease to name just two, are relatively rare in certain less-developed countries in Africa and the Far East, which rely on a diet low in protein and high in complex carbohydrates.

As many as 70 percent of cases which physicians will diagnose as "psychosomatic" will be diagnosed by environmental medicine specialists as reactions to inhaled or ingested foods or chemicals. In other cases, as Dr. Mandell notes, clinical ecology can assist even when it cannot cure. This may be the case with individuals suffering from epileptic seizures or in patients who have multiple sclerosis (MS). Severe cases of arthritis also fall into this category. In many cases, according to Dr. Mandell, these people have nutritional needs that are not being met. And in his opinion, that goes for 80 percent of the people in mental institutions as well. Not to mention many of those among us who suffer from standard allergies like hives, eczema, or hay fever.

Natural Remedies for Allergies

While allergic reactions can be a potentially severe heath problem, there are numerous ways to keep allergic reactions under control, including the use of natural healing remedies. Dr. Frances Taylor, co-author of *The Whole Way to Allergy Relief and Prevention* (Hartley & Marks, 1996), offers examples of simple cost-effective natural remedies that can help prevent allergies from getting out of hand:

"Water is especially important for the allergic person because it helps keep nutrient insulation available for cell repair and nourishment," says Dr. Taylor. "People with allergies, the worse the allergies are, the more cell repair they need. It's necessary to flush out toxins and waste products from the cells, which reduces the total overload for the allergic person. And many allergy persons are laboring under a terrible toxic load. If they could drink a little more water, it would help flush out these toxins.

Dr. Taylor also emphasizes that people with allergies need not rely on traditional methods to keep their reactions under control. "Clearing an allergic reaction can be done simply and naturally," she says. "It isn't necessary to have an adrenaline reaction to an allergic reaction. For instance, vitamin C is marvelous for clearing allergic reactions. The form of vitamin C you take is going to depend on what your body pH does when you have an allergic reaction. For example, many people become acidic when they have an allergic reaction. You can tell this either by checking your saliva or your urine pH. Or if you're a person whose rings turn black, even expensive rings, you are acidic. People who become acidic when they have an allergic reaction need to take buffered C. Several companies make buffered C. Buffered C is ascorbic acid with calcium and magnesium carbonate and potassium bicarbonate in with the C as buffers. This helps reduce the acidity when people are having allergic reactions. And if you reduce acidity you stop the reaction."

While these over-the-counter preparations have buffering properties that can help halt an allergic reaction, many of them contain corn or corn products, so individuals who are sensitive to corn will not want to use this particular natural remedy for allergies.

Another preparation that, according to Dr. Taylor, may help stop allergic reactions by correcting and restoring pH balance in the body is a formula called "Magic Brew," which combines a teaspoon of salt and a teaspoon of baking soda (not baking powder) in a quart of water, which can be ingested hot or cold, though most people prefer it cold. People with high blood pressure may not want to use "Magic Brew," as it is high in sodium. Also effective as buffers against allergic reactions are tri-salts, which are produced by cardiovascular research, and bicarb formula. These last two items are available in many health food stores.

On the other side of the coin, some individuals have the opposite problem during an allergic reaction. Dr. Taylor explains, "Some people become alkaline when they have an allergic reaction. These people will need to take ascorbic acid, a vitamin C preparation that has nothing but vitamin C in the ascorbate acid form."

"Believe it or not," Dr. Taylor continues, "exercise will help stop an allergic reaction. When you exercise, your body produces extra adrenaline, which will turn the reaction off. And oxygen is a wonderful reaction stopper. Most people think about using oxygen when they're having trouble breathing.

However, there are more allergic reactions, which do not involve difficulty in breathing than those that do, and oxygen is wonderful for turning those off. Sometimes, just a minute or two will turn it off. Other people may require anywhere from 10 to 15 minutes to reverse the reaction. Of course, oxygen is available only with a physician's prescription."

WHERE DOES THE CLINICAL ECOLOGIST BEGIN? In many cases the clinical ecologist will begin by putting the patient on a fast which includes pure spring water and an environment completely free of cleaning agents, cigarette smoke, cosmetics, etc. Often, the patient's symptoms will disappear after three to four days. Then it is a matter of tracking back to find what it was in the patient's daily life that had been triggering the allergic sensitivity.

According Dr. Mandell, about 10 percent of his patients react adversely to chlorine. Although chlorine is necessary as a preventative measure for waterborne illness, you can buy a simple and relatively inexpensive purification system for your home that will draw out the chlorine after it comes through the faucet. It is important to be drinking pure water that is free of agricultural run-off, free of manufacturing waste, free of fluoride, and free of chlorine. All of these chemicals may be affecting people adversely without their ever suspecting. Purifying the water can be an easy way to upgrade the feeling of well-being among those around you.

Just because an environmental factor did not cause a disease, that doesn't mean it isn't important to the subsequent course of the disease and recovery. As Dr. Mandell said on my radio program, "There is absolutely no question that environmental factors play a major part in many diseases; where they do not actually start the disease, they can complicate them. Anything that makes your illness worse is important for you to know about."

In the same way that cocaine goes right from the nose of the user to the nervous system in a matter of seconds, producing a wide variety of effects, so do toxins in the food or air produce a range of effects in the systems of highly sensitive individuals. Conventional physicians and traditional allergists simply miss out on this phenomenon by recognizing only a very limited range of symptoms. If their patients aren't sneezing or itching, they will not recognize the possibility that an allergy may be present. But, logically, once a doctor recognizes that minute flecks of animal dander or pollen in the air can produce marked symptoms, is it so difficult to see that chemical toxins in meat or milk, or air pollution, among a host of other possible causes, might also have an adverse effect? Simply put, the human race has evolved over millions of years and adapted to most of the conditions on this planet. But many of the pollutants and toxins we are dealing with have arisen over the last 30 to 50 years. Our bodies just haven't had time to evolve in response to these changes in our environment. Unless we act sensibly, by at least recognizing this discrepancy, we may cause great damage to ourselves and our environment.

Whatever you breathe in enters your body along with the oxygen. If your home, work or school environment is polluted, the pollutants will travel through the walls of the lungs, into the blood vessels of the lungs and ultimately reach the heart through the pulmonary circulation. Similarly, chemicals, additives and contaminants in our food and beverages will pass through the digestive system and reach the heart. Once there, they will be pumped through the bloodstream. Every tissue in your body is exposed to what you eat, drink, and breathe. That is why so many people are sick today.

Food addiction allergies are often misdiagnosed as hypoglycemia. The patient may find that each time he or she eats the particular food, say chocolate, he or she feels fine. But what is actually happening is that the patient is having a delayed allergic reaction to the food. Ingesting the offending food is causing an allergic reaction, but only after a time delay, so that the patient never connects the food with the symptoms. Or in another case, an individual may feel better immediately after eating. He or she does not connect the foods in the meal to any chronic symptoms which may occur much later, and yet they may indeed be the cause. Dr. Mandell claims to have seen thousands of patients, previously diagnosed as having low blood sugar, who actually suffer from some form of food addiction. In extreme cases, the patients may have been diagnosed as being mentally retarded or learning disabled. According to Dr. Mandell, fasting can free them of abnormal symptoms within two weeks. Once the culprit is found and removed from the diet, the improved behavior can be permanently established. (See chapter 36 for more information on food allergies.)

FOUR CLUES TO PROPER TREATMENT Dr. Michael Schachter, also a clinical ecologist, or environmental medicine specialist, who received his medical training from the Columbia University College of Physicians and Surgeons, identifies four contributing factors which he considers to be key in his examination and in determining a course of therapy:

- the quality of nutrition generally and the identification of any nutritional deficiencies;
- infections;
- psychological stresses; and
- toxicity.

According to Dr. Schachter, the course of therapy should be determined by the condition of the patient according to these four criteria.

Dr. Schachter is also concerned with improving the oxygenation and energy utilization of the body at the cellular level. Anything we can do to improve that process is going to strengthen the immune system and thereby help reduce a person's tendency toward sensitivity and reactions. Thus Dr. Schachter encourages the use of oxidant therapies, but only up to a point, since oxygen in too high quantities can have a damaging effect. The key here, as in virtually every area of health, is balance.

Vitamins and minerals are another key component in Dr. Schachter's approach. Vitamin A is seen to be a major protective factor, guarding against both chemical sensitivities and infections. Thus cod liver oil, which parents once gave automatically to children, is indeed an excellent preventive medicine, with its high concentrations of vitamins A and D. Treating children with recurrent ear infections, Dr. Schachter has found that by simply enhancing their diet, removing most of the sugar and refined foods, and adding a spoonful of cod liver oil, the ear infections can be controlled and prevented in many cases. Other useful vitamins include vitamin C, vitamin B_{12}, and vitamin E, which is an antioxidant. Selenium and beta carotene are also important antioxidants. Vitamin B_{12} can help counteract the adverse effects in the body of pesticides in the environment. Moreover, while conventional physicians may test for B_{12} levels in the bloodstream, normal levels may be present in the blood while there are deficiencies at the cellular level.

As for oxidant therapies, the first and foremost must be aerobic exercise. Keeping in mind that oxygen is the main nutrient of the body, it is easy to understand that as we improve oxygenation, we improve the body's ability to detoxify and we enhance the immune system. Beyond exercise, a number of new nutrients are available to enhance oxygenation, such as germanium and ubiquinone, as well as a variety of traditional oxygenation techniques.

According to Dr. Schachter, infections are a key factor in going from troubled to good health. Frequently, he says infections will yield to nontoxic treatments.

Take candida, for example. There is a tendency for patients who have been exposed to repeated use of antibiotics, who include a lot of refined carbohydrates in their diet, and who may have been exposed to steroids or birth control pills, to develop a chronic overgrowth of candida, a yeastlike, funguslike organism which we all have in our bodies. In certain cases, the infection will give off toxins which may impair the immune system and produce a variety of symptoms. Some of these will be the result of food and chemical sensitivities which have been aggravated by the infection.

Dr. Schachter has found that starting the patient on special diets which exclude refined carbohydrates, especially sugars and alcohol, and include various nutrients, including certain fatty acids which inhibit candida growth, will go a long way toward controlling the infection in many cases. He also notes that garlic is a strong anticandida property.

Chronic viral syndromes are another key problem. A previously healthy individual suddenly gets a flu and instead of recovering completely, the flu is followed by frequent complaints of fatigue, exhaustion, swollen glands, sore throat, night sweats, anxiety, and loss of appetite. And yet conventional testing shows nothing definite. More sophisticated testing may show exposure to various viruses. But the main problem here may be that the person's immune system just isn't responding as it should. Dr. Schachter has obtained excellent results in patients with this kind of profile by using nutrients to bolster the immune system. Intravenous vitamin C may be used, along with germanium and a variety of other vitamins and minerals given orally. In cases of herpes virus, for example, he may use high doses of the amino acid lysine, which has antiviral effects for the herpes virus and certain other viruses. For short treatment periods, he may administer as much as 10 to 15 grams of lysine per day in these patients. (For more on these and other infections, see chapter 53.)

Psychological stress is another key factor, according to Dr. Schachter. Environmental medicine specialists, he warns, must be careful that in emphasizing the importance of the physical environment they do not underestimate the importance of psychological factors in determining the strength of an individual's immune system.

As for toxicity, Dr. Schachter feels that hydrocarbons and other chemicals are already playing a major role by damaging our immune systems. Heavy metals are also playing a role, in his opinion. He sees chelation therapy as a valid treatment to detoxify our systems of the effects of heavy metals, as well as for cardiovascular disease, where chelation therapy has shown impressive results.

In sum, in treating the allergic or chemically sensitive patient, Dr. Schachter believes it is important to look at the specific kinds of food allergens and chemical sensitivities that may be involved, employing rotation diets and neutralization diets, but also to go beyond these issues to seek any underlying factors which could be important as well, like infections, chemical pesticide poisoning, heavy metal poisoning, and stress. It is important to deal with each aspect independently and it is equally important that the program be synergistic, one which will make the patient less sensitive to his or her environment, more resilient, and healthier overall.

Keeping Your Home and Office Toxin-Free

It is no longer enough to watch what we eat or the medicines that we take; in the twentieth century environmental toxins have become an unavoidable reality, especially for those living in densely populated urban areas. The very air that we breathe, on the streets or in our homes and offices, can attack our health; noise pollution and artificial lighting add to the physical and mental stress of urban life.

The myth is that you should look for the big toxin. But it's the chronic, day-in, day-out, exposure to small toxins that does you in. It may take decades—none of these environmental toxins, even asbestos, will knock you out right away—but you may pay for your lack of awareness with lung cancer, leukemia, arthritis, or heart disease down the line. Perhaps worst are the subtle symptoms of fatigue, anxiety, and minor nagging physical problems which you come to accept as a normal part of life.

Elimination of the unseen substances that attack your system stealthily, over time, is half of health. If you never used any supplementary vitamin, mineral, or herb, but simply eliminated those factors which depreciate your health, you should be able to live to 100 years of age in a healthy way. One group of people nearly 70,000 in number, in the north of Pakistan at the base of the Himalayas, often live to 90 or 105, putting in full days of work daily until they die. It may not be possible for all of us to live in the pure atmosphere of the Himalayas—not to mention emulating the diet, activities, and social structure of these people—but we can alter our environment, realistically and functionally. A good place to start is where we live.

Dr. Alfred Zann, a fellow of the American College of Allergists and the American College of Physicians, has written a book, *Why Your House May Endanger Your Health*, which explores the relation between our homes and our well-being more thoroughly than we can here; much of the following discussion is indebted to information which he shared on the Gary Null show, as well as to Dr Richard Podell.

The Sick Building Syndrome

The "sick house" is a relatively new development. Materials and methods used to construct houses have changed considerably since World War II; an extreme example is the energy-efficient office buildings built during the energy crisis of the 1970s, about which we'll have more to say later in this chapter. But not only are houses built with more of an emphasis on energy efficiency—which means heavy insulation and minimum ventilation to the outside—but the materials of the construction itself, as well as the furnishings—carpeting, fabrics, furniture—are new, often more convenient, cheaper, lighter man-made compounds unheard of in prewar houses. The particle board which is so useful in modern house and furniture construction exacts a price for this convenience; it is a silent time bomb, giving off invisible, odorless—but no less dangerous—vapors years after it is installed.

Formaldehyde is a major culprit in the modern house or office building. Particle board, new synthetic carpets, insulation, many interior paints, and even permanent-press fabrics can give off formaldehyde. It is invisible and odorless except in high concentrations, but even quite low chronic levels can cause symptoms ranging from burning eyes and headaches to asthma or depression. New houses may be largely built of materials which vaporize formaldehyde for years; the worst culprits are mobile homes, which are, in addition, often poorly ventilated.

Another important factor in a house's potential toxicity is its source of heat. Combustion-heating appliances using natural gas, oil, coal, kerosene, or wood can all create afterburn byproducts, even if you can't see or smell them. Good ventilation can help, but makes it harder to keep a house warm. Electrical heat, though expensive, is the safest source.

What can be done about a toxic house? Some changes can be made in the furnishings, floor coverings, and ventilation and heating systems—below we'll go through a typical house room by room—but often much of the problem lies in structural components which would be expensive and difficult, if not impossible, to alter. Building your own house or having it built, with attention to all material used, is one solution if you can afford it or have the time and skill. If you are looking for a place to live, consider an older home. Prewar houses are often constructed of bricks, plaster, and hardwood, not the chemical-treated plywood, composite board, and other synthetic materials used almost universally now. If synthetic materials were used in an older house they will have had years to emit their toxins. Often a house built before the energy crisis will allow more air circulation. Ceilings are often higher, allowing fumes to rise away from the inhabitants.

There may be disadvantages in an old house, however; molds and mildews may have accumulated over the years. Old carpet is a fertile ground for mold as well as accumulated dust, animal hair, and whatever toxins have been tracked in or sprayed over the years, but it can often be pulled up to reveal a hardwood floor. Outdated heating systems can usually be replaced without too much trouble.

If moving or rebuilding your house are not options, you can still do a lot to detoxify your home. We'll go room by room, identifying weak spots. It might be best to start outside the living area.

THE GARAGE AND GARDEN An attached garage is like a toxic waste dump stuck to the side of your house. Many garages have heating and cooling systems which lead directly into the house—anything that can be absorbed through any crack or ventilation system will end up in the house. What's in the garage? The car, of course—and gasoline. Gasoline vaporizes. The afterburn fumes caused by inefficient burning of gasoline are mostly carbon dioxide, which has no odor and is invisible. Breathing these fumes results in headache, dizziness, and mood swings. (Think of people stuck in traffic jams, breathing the afterburn of all the cars around them for hours at a time.) When you park a hot car in the garage and close the door behind it, the hot oil in the engine is volatile and gets into the air. Park the car outside and wait for it to cool off before you bring it into the garage.

Other things you may keep in the garage—paint thinners and removers, and turpentine—also vaporize easily, and stay in the air for months at a time. If you smell a rag that has been used for paint thinner three months ago, you will see that it is still giving off these fumes. Try to keep down the number of these substances in your garage. If you must keep them, use a small shed or garbage can outside the garage to store them. And the garage should be ventilated out, not into the house, with a suction fan. There should be no ducts from the garage into the house.

Your garage is probably where you keep chemicals you use on your lawn and garden—pesticides, fungicides, or herbicides, for instance. In the first place, do you really need them? Look at it this way. If it's going to kill an insect, a plant, or a mouse, it's a toxin and it can affect you, your pets, and your children. If you spray a weed killer on your lawn and then walk around on it, you will repeatedly be bringing it inside on your feet. Where do you think it goes? It doesn't just go away. Think of all the things you bring in on your feet—and think, for instance of your kids playing on the carpet, perhaps putting things into their mouths that have been on it. You wouldn't let you kid rub his hand over a New York pavement and lick it, would you?

These are things we seldom think about. And, taken individually, none of them is going to kill you. But be aware that everything you spray outside is likely to be in the air you breathe or will make its way back into your house and settle there. There's no real need to run this risk: we can use diatomaceous earth, natural biological controls, or just weed without spraying.

THE BASEMENT A typical basement in a private home is often damp. People like their lawns unencumbered by debris that might wash down from the gutters of the roof through the downspout, so the downspout is kept close to the house. Thus the water runs off the roof, down the downspout, and into the ground directly by the foundation of the house. They might just as well run this water directly into the basement, since its walls are rarely waterproof. A little dampness in the basement is enough to support a healthy growth of mold, which can then permeate the house. A forced air system of ventilation in the house, which has ducts running to the basement, will create a vacuumlike effect—known as the Bernoulli effect—that will suck particles of mold into the system, to be dispersed around the house.

Many patients react to mold, whether it is eaten or inhaled—a point made obvious to anyone who begins to sneeze as soon as he or she walks into a damp basement. More insidiously, though, mold which is inhaled even in small quantities cross-reacts with mold which is ingested in food. This effect, known as concomitancy, means that a small quantity of mold inhaled—which would hardly in itself cause a noticeable reaction—will enhance sensitivity to foods which contain mold.

Any food which is made by fermentation can induce this reaction. Wine and vinegar are fermented fruit juice; cheese is fermented milk; yeast in bread ferments; and even mushrooms are in the mold family. Thus, it is easy to ingest mold three times a day, exacerbating our inability to tolerate the mold which has circulated upward form a damp basement. Obvious symptoms are sneezing and watering eyes; but allergic symptoms can also be systemic, making them harder to pin down to a specific trigger reaction. Fatigue, headaches, depression, even arthritis, can have a basis in chronic allergic irritation.

As well as water coming into the basement from the downspout, groundwater can roll down a hill toward the house, which then serves as a dam. Here it can be diverted by raising the earth around the house to encourage it to flow away from the house. If a high water table is the problem, a sump pump is needed. Thoroseal, a dense cementous material, can be applied to the outside block foundation as caulking to keep water out.

If the basement is still damp, a dehumidifier can help, but these work well only above a temperature of 50 to 60 degrees Fahrenheit. Chemicals like baking soda only serve as temporary measures. The best way to remove the mold itself is to scrub the area down with sulfur water. The basement can be hosed down and the water removed with an industrial vacuum.

THE KITCHEN What's the most dangerous toxin in most kitchens? Gas. You should always have a vent in the kitchen; it has been shown that cerebral allergies are often directly attributable to the gas burnoff of pilot lights on stoves, which leak constantly. If you often have headaches and you suspect that they are more common when you're spending time in the kitchen, try disconnecting your stove when you're not using it. If this makes a difference, you should consider replacing the gas stove with an electric one. Not only gas ovens are a health risk, though. Microwave ovens can leak; a defective microwave creates a very unhealthy environment within about eight feet of it.

What else? Frion in the condenser of the refrigerator. Freon is a highly volatile, dangerous chemical. It is a very good idea to replace refrigerators that are more 10 ten years old.

The refrigerator contributes to another seldom-considered form of pollution found especially in the kitchen: noise pollution. You should be able to tolerate background noise of about 30 to 35 decibels. Higher than 50 decibels becomes uncomfortable. Above 80, you become substantially irritated and above 100 may cause ear damage or central nervous system overstimulation. A compressor in most refrigerators is up to 60 decibels. You don't appreciate this until you turn on a refrigerator when everything else is totally quiet. But think of a kitchen with a television or a radio on, things cooking, telephone conversations—you can't even hear the refrigerator, and the noise level may be up around 100 decibels. The kitchen is one of the most stressful places because of this level of background noise. Even if you are unable to replace appliances like refrigerators and air conditioners with less noisy ones, you can cut down on the number of noisemakers you are using at the same time.

Not only the kitchen suffers from noise—street noise can be irritating in any room. This can be helped with noise-buffering double-fold drapes that keep noise down as well as insulate.

Mold and mildew are common invisible toxins in a kitchen. When was the last time you changed the water drip area of your refrigerator? There's a condenser coil and a tray under it to collect water—but it can also collect all kinds of mold. Mold spores are in the air all the time and you're inhaling them. If you're sensitive and your immune system is low, you'll feel it—your eyes will get puffy, your nose will clog, your throat will get sore. Keeping this area clean and dry could make a big difference.

Look under the sink in your kitchen; you'll be amazed at the range of toxic chemicals you keep there, so close to your food. Cleansers, for instance, especially ammonia-based products, often vaporize easily. Ammonia is very toxic, and will stay in your blood for hours when you've smelled it. When you wax the kitchen floor, the floor wax will evaporate and you will be breathing it in. Try, if you can, to install floors that will not need waxing—but if you don't want to tear up your present floors you might want to settle for a matte finish rather than a high sheen, if you have to constantly apply volatile chemicals to get that sheen. And, as with the weed-killers and insecticides in your garage, there are alternatives to chemical cleaners in the kitchen. Apple cider vinegar and hydrogen peroxide, mixed half and half in cold water, do the same job as ammonia. After you've finished with the floor, this preparation will clean windows and glassware perfectly, too.

Roach sprays are very stable. They can last for months, and vaporize constantly. A dog or cat licking the floor can pick them up directly. A safer alternative is to use boric acid—you can mix it with sugar as a bait but be sure pets and children can't reach it—and line all the counters and fittings underneath with a strip of this no thicker than a pencil. This mixture is not volatile and is safe as long as it's only put in inaccessible places. Diatomaceous earth is safe to use and works well too. Or use the roach motels which use resin that roaches get stuck on instead of poisons.

Aluminum-based cookware, when the aluminum can come into contact with the food, should not be used. Aluminum has been implicated in Alzheimer's disease. It is a heavy metal that lodges itself in the blood, brain tissue, and central nervous system where it can cause motor problems. Aluminum foil is alright for storage of cooked food but should not be used while you're cooking, when it can oxidize in microscopic amounts. You can't see this, but it can get into your food and your body. Teflon, or any of the nonstick coatings, should also be avoided. They easily scratch or flake off with age, getting into food as well as exposing it to the often inferior metal underneath.

Next time you fill up a glass with water from the kitchen tap, consider that it may contain over a thousand chemicals—those that the government puts in, like fluoride, traces of herbicides and pesticides that have leached down into the water supply from fields, and traces of metal, rust, and molds from the inside of your pipes. Most water filtration systems can only remove a portion of these; the finer particles, including toxic chemicals like pesticides, come through. If you live in a polluted area and your water supply is from underground streams, buy bottled water. I would buy plain distilled water—you get minerals from food, you don't need them from water. Since 72 to 74 percent of our bodies is water, we should be sure it is the purest possible.

THE BATHROOM One of the most common causes of allergy is what we put on our bodies—soaps, deodorants, cosmetics. We use these things day in and day out, rarely thinking about their effect on us. For example, women who wear lipstick every day and lick their lips are absorbing chemicals never meant to be eaten. Perfumes vaporize and get breathed in. Read the ingredients of your antiperspirant; most likely it contains an aluminum-based compound which can be absorbed through your skin and carries the risks of aluminum outlined above. You can minimize these sources of toxins by using natural soaps and shampoos made out of vegetable ingredients, a nonfluoride toothpaste like Dr. Bronner's or Tom's, mouthwash which you can make yourself with a little ascorbic acid in water, and natural loofa pads to scrub your self.

The bathroom is one of the wettest rooms in the house and is a likely site for mold. It's important to air out the bathroom after a shower or bath and let it dry out. A window fan to evacuate the moist air is a good idea, give the bathroom time to air and dry out. Bathrooms are too often closed up most of the time, and can be like little poison chambers trapping the perfumes, deodorants, and cleaning fluid fumes in a small space. Odor disguisers like pine- or lemon-scented aerosol sprays are worse than useless; the odor is a molecule floating around in the air that can only be removed by letting the air escape. Products that claim to take away odors only cover them up with a chemical which probably smells worse and is certainly worse for you.

The "disinfectant" cleaners so popular for bathroom tiles and tubs are virtually useless. To disinfect something you have to boil it for 20 minutes, but within 1 minute it will be covered with germs again. And those germs are not going to kill anyone, despite the fear tactics used to market these floor cleaners. Their heavy aromatic odors are often more of a problem than the germs; pine, for example, is a resinous material that is quite troublesome to allergic or sensitive people.

Never store medications in the medicine chest; it's hot and humid in the bathroom and this can cause them to go bad. Store medicine and vitamins in the refrigerator.

As with the kitchen, look around the bathroom and think about potential toxins—cleaners for the tiles and sink, toilet fresheners, and so on. Do you need all those things? Can they be substituted by natural, nontoxic products? Awareness of your environment and what you put in it is the key.

THE BEDROOM We spend a third of our lives in the bedroom; if you live 72 years, that means 23 years in bed. An ecologically ideal, safe place to spend all this time should be as free of dust as possible. Many bedrooms have wall-to-wall carpeting, which is an ecological disaster. Carpeting is toxic in your home in several ways. New synthetic-fiber carpeting contains chemicals like formaldehyde which will vaporize for a year or more. Old carpet collects dirt, yeast, fungus, and mold. Dust mites live in it. Through an electron microscope these mites look like tiny dinosaurs; their diet is chiefly composed of the shed human skin cells which are another large component of dust. House dust mites can be wafted into the air by currents and breathed into the lungs. People who are allergic to them react as if to cat or dog dander. Like dander, they can get into your eyes and make them red and puffy.

How many of you have thought about ripping up your old carpet and putting in nice hardwood floors? They're easy to maintain and nontoxic. The Japanese have never had polyvinyl fluoride or no-wax floors; they use natural resins on wood, and some of these floors are 500 years old. If you feel you must have carpets, buy wool or natural fiber, with natural dyes. Stay away from synthetic carpets. And learn to vacuum efficiently. Most people just zip the vacuum over the carpet; by the time the dust has had a chance to get up through the nap into the air the vacuum has moved on, and has only raised the dust. You've actually increased the pollution in the air. So run the vacuum very slowly over the carpet—give the dust you raise time to get into the vacuum.

You may be sleeping on foam-filled synthetic pillows, with synthetic-fiber pillowcases and sheets. Replace them with down-filled pillows and comforters and pure cotton sheets. Also be aware of what you're putting in your sheets when you wash them—bleaches and fabric softeners can be potential irritants. Many manufacturers of bedding use chemicals to fireproof the material, which many people are allergic to. The way to test for this is to sleep on bedding which is not treated to be fireproof and see if your symptoms disappear. Again, if you feel better when you are sleeping away from your house on vacation, it should alert you to the fact that something in the bedroom is causing trouble.

Sleeping on clean sheets changed frequently reduces possible reaction to dust and dust mites. When you wash bedding, it's best to keep things simple. Don't use perfumed detergents, avoid antistatics and softeners, and look for biodegradable brands. Bleach should be oxygen bleach, not chlorine, which leaves an irritating residue. Miracle White, made by Beatrice Food Company, works well. If you suspect that a pillowcase, for example, is bothering you, wash it with a simple unscented detergent, rinse it three or four times, and try it again to see if the problem goes away.

Electric blankets can affect the electromagnetic field around the body and should be avoided. It's also best not to sleep near a digital clock, which can affect the body's electromagnetic system from three feet away.

Even your closets can affect your health; moth balls emit a poisonous gas. Chicago weavers use a mixture of rosemary, mint, thyme, ginseng, and cloves instead, which has the additional advantage of smelling good.

AIR QUALITY If you ever see the sun slant into a room at a certain angle, you know how much dust and smoke is in what you thought was clear air. It's there all the time. An air purifier with a negative ionizer is the best way to eliminate airborne toxins—spores, dust, cigarette smoke, hydrocarbons and pollutants from the street, cat hairs, positive ions. The ionizer bombards the room with negative ions which attach themselves to the positive ions of pollutants, which then drop to the ground and can be filtered out by the filtration system.

Humidifiers are fine for improving air quality as well, as long as you use distilled water in them. Otherwise mineral deposits from the water will end up all over your carpet, floor, and furniture.

PLANTS One efficient and natural air-quality improver is living greenery in your house. The more plants in your environment, the better. A large number and variety of houseplants will increase the oxygen level in the air. Green, nonflowering varieties are best, as they will not issue pollen. Plants are also a great natural air pollution filtration system. New York City would hardly be bearable if it were not for Central Park. Plants help maintain humidity levels and a proper electricity balance in the air.

Plants are calming to the mind as well as good for air quality. As living things, they create an energy of their own. Not only are plants alive, but many people believe that they have a consciousness. If you've ever noticed how some people seem to have great luck with plants and others can never keep them alive, you may have thought about this. Plants don't just function as air purifiers; they create a living energy field which we can share and be invigorated and calmed by.

LIGHT Your visual environment is more important than you might realize. If you feel tired, ill, or depressed inside in the winter, especially if you live at a high latitude where the days are very short, and if you spend most of your day indoors, you may be suffering form seasonal affective disorder. In this condition the hypothalamus of your brain is deprived of full-spectrum natural sunlight—most artificial lights use only a part of the spectrum. The best solution is to allow plenty of natural light into your house; use double-glazing rather than small windows or heavy drapes if insulation is a concern. Try to spend time outdoors or arrange your activities so that you're near a window. If getting more daylight is beyond your control—the days are short, your house is dark, and you must stay indoors—the situation can be improved with full-spectrum lightbulbs. Full-spectrum incandescent lighting works on a completely different principle from that of fluorescent lighting (discussed in the section on the workplace below) and is more natural for the eyes. These bulbs are available in health stores in all sizes; using them in your office as well as in your home can make a big difference in your energy level and mental state.

HEAT In cold areas, we shut down for the winter, closing and sealing the windows to avoid ventilation from the outside. These methods contribute to the toxic state of the air inside. The air in many New York apartments in the winter would generate an official air pollution alert outside.

Oil heaters often burn inefficiently and release unburned oil fumes into the house. An afterburn catalyst, available on the market now, can recycle these, creating a clean air burn. Electric stoves are not a problem. Gas or oil space heaters are one of the worst offenders. Dry radiated heat can dry up your nose and skin. Wood-burning stoves may seem rustic and natural but can be one of the worst sources of indoor pollution.

One major problem can develop in forced air combustion heating systems, using either gas or oil; a little pinhole not infrequently develops between the heat exchanger, which is next to the combustion chamber, and the air going past it to be heated. As the air that we're going to breathe goes around that heated chamber, it sucks in the partially combusted gases. You may not even perceive this in the air, because it's at a very low level, but over a six-month period this air can produce severe illness. Therefore you must have your forced air system checked out electronically for these pinholes every year. The smell test is not satisfactory. If you don't do this, you're at risk.

THE WORKPLACE The energy crisis of the 1970s has led to a generation of very well insulated, but poorly ventilated, office buildings. People who work in these buildings often complain of fatigue, nasal congestion, dizziness, and a host of other mysterious symptoms. Yet there has been clear-cut documentation of toxic levels of pollutants in very few cases. The levels of toxins in these buildings are rarely high enough to provoke official alarm, but they are enough to cause fatigue and illness through long-term, chronic exposure. Even low levels of organic chemicals, pesticides, formaldehyde, carpet cleaners, and tobacco smoke can affect those exposed to them for long enough.

The individual pollutants can be located and reduced, but the single most important factor is ventilation. Monday is the worst day for headaches and stress, and that's at least partially because the ventilation systems have often been shut down over the weekend; you're breathing old, stale air. The ducts of your office air venting system probably haven't been cleaned in years. Dust and molds have built up inside them and are coming out into the air you breathe when the system is restarted. Ask the maintenance people to clean them; if they won't, get a heavy-duty charcoal filter and put it in the vent, with a thick white insulation pad over it. These can be bought inexpensively at any hardware store. In one week, if you look at the insulation pad it will be covered with black particles large enough to see.

If it's noisy where you work, wear ear plugs. You can also make your desk more pleasant with a small portable ionizer. This can actually fit in your pocket, and is also useful in airplanes or on the dashboard of your car.

The fluorescent lighting often used in offices flashes on and off rapidly and constantly, creating great stress on your central nervous system. Although you are not consciously aware of this very rapid flickering, your eye and nervous system are overstimulated by it—two or three hours of work under fluorescent light can have the effect of three or four cups of coffee. At a certain level of overstimulation the central nervous system will shut down, and you will find yourself deeply fatigued. Replace the fluorescent lighting at your desk with a lamp which uses incandescent bulbs, and use the natural full-spectrum light-bulbs which we described earlier. It's best to have an office with a window or skylight for true natural lighting; if you don't and can't arrange it, it's especially important to have natural—and sufficiently bright—lighting.

Stay away from the photocopier at the office as much as possible; it uses very volatile chemicals. Don't leave typewriter ink or corrector ribbons lying around open; put them in a sealed plastic bag when not in use. An exhaust fan on the ceiling will help draw away vaporizing fluids.

36

Food Allergies

t is a classic case of overreaction. Your body incorrectly senses that the food that has just been eaten is a foreign substance to be repelled. Cells begin to exhibit diseaselike symptoms as they react and over-react to the food.

Allergists conservatively estimate that up to 15 percent of the population suffers from a minimum of one allergy, frequently one that is serious enough to warrant medical attention.

Symptoms can range from a mild tension headache or irritability to criminal actions and full-blown psychotic behavior. Most common are fatigue, headache, insomnia, rapid mood swings, confusion, depression, anxiety, hyperactivity, heart palpitations, muscle aches and joint pains, bed wetting, rhinitis (nasal inflammation), urticaria (hives), shortness of breath, diarrhea, and constipation. Reactions can be immediate following exposure to the allergen or delayed for many hours after contact.

Allergic symptoms are so diverse that the reactions can occur in virtually any organ in the body. Reactions in the brain or central nervous system may lead to behavioral changes and to paranoia or depression. A response in the gastrointestinal tract may translate into bloating, diarrhea, or constipation. Different food combinations can cause multiple reactions in the same person. If a person has an allergy to wheat that manifests itself in the brain, while their gastrointestinal tract is sensitive to milk, they may experience both fatigue and irritable bowel syndrome from a breakfast of whole wheat toast and milk.

All forms of a potentially offensive food can cause an allergic reaction, not just the whole form. Corn sugars and syrup, including dextrose and glucose, for example, will cause symptoms in many corn-sensitive patients. In many instances, researchers find, corn sugars will cause a more immediate reaction than will corn starch or corn as a vegetable.

Environmental medicine experts, also known as clinical ecologists, say that one reason people are developing sensitivities to certain foods is their widespread occurrence in our diets in both the natural and processed forms. Just because you only rarely treat yourself to corn on the cob, for example, doesn't mean you're not eating corn every day. On a typical day you might eat corn flakes, a corn muffin, and processed food products containing both corn starch and corn syrup. Also, many of the daily vitamin C supplements are derived from corn.

Types of Food Allergies

The foods we eat most frequently are also the most common causes of allergies. These include milk, wheat, corn, eggs, beef, citrus fruits, potatoes, tomatoes, and coffee. Food allergies can fall into several categories:

THE FIXED FOOD ALLERGY: Each time you consume a specific food, you react. For example, whenever you eat beef, a reaction occurs.

THE CYCLIC FOOD ALLERGY: This is the most prevalent type of allergy. It occurs when you've had an abundance of a particular food. If exposure to the food can be reduced to no more than once every four days, little or no reaction occurs. The food, in other words, can be infrequently tolerated in small amounts. So, in a cyclic allergy, a person can remain symptom-free as long as he or she eats the offending food infrequently.

Of course, other factors can influence the degree of this sensitivity. Infection, emotional stress, fatigue, and overeating can increase susceptibility. The condition of the food (raw or cooked, fresh or packaged) may also be an important factor. Pollution, the presence of other environmental allergens, or marked environmental temperature change can also help trigger or subdue a reaction.

A food eaten by itself may be tolerated. But if it is combined with other foods at the same meal, an allergic response may develop. The length and severity of the symptoms will depend in part on how long the allergens remain in your body after ingestion.

THE ADDICTIVE ALLERGIC REACTION: Here the person craves the foods to which he or she is allergic. In essence, the person becomes addicted to the foods. When the individual is made to go without the food, depression and other withdrawal like effects may appear. Moreover, eating the food may momentarily alleviate the symptoms, only to aggravate them later. Over time, the symptoms of the addictive allergy may grow increasingly complex.

This type of allergy often remains hidden or masked—even to the individual who is suffering from the problem. Because of its insidious nature, the person never suspects that the foods that seem to alleviate the symptoms might contain substances to which he or she is allergic, since he or she usually feels better right after eating them.

But allergies do not always fit neatly into one of the three categories. A fixed allergy in infancy can develop into an addictive allergic reaction later in life. Milk is a good example of such a food. When first introduced to a baby, it may cause an acute reaction in the form of hives or spitting up. However, if the parents don't recognize this as an allergic reaction and continue to keep milk in the diet, the symptoms may take on a more generalized and less obvious form.

What is first experienced by the body as an acute reaction will finally—in the body's attempt to adapt by assimilating the new foreign substance—lead to more chronic symptoms such as arthritis, fatigue, depression, or headaches.

For example, if you drink milk or eat milk products every day, symptoms of allergic reactions may blur with your natural personality traits and may become an accepted, even unnoticed part of your everyday life.

Eventually, you may develop a chronic condition, like arthritis, migraines, or depression. Your daily dose of milk would never be suspect at this stage. Your body has upped its tolerance levels in trying to adapt. At the same time, milk's harmful effects have been subtly registered. You keep on with a daily dose of milk, your own substance for abuse, to keep withdrawal symptoms at bay. Acute reactions are gone—except when the milk is withdrawn completely. Chronic reactions have replaced them.

Hidden or masked food allergies, no different from allergies generally, tend to be to the very foods we eat most frequently. In the United States, dairy products, including milk and eggs, are high on the list. Corn, wheat and potatoes are also common allergens, as is beef. Yeast, which occurs in many foods, is often at cause. Finally, many people have a hidden allergy to coffee. Considering that coffee is also an addictive substance and that Americans often drink it all day long (over 100 billion cups consumed annually), it is astounding to contemplate the overall adverse health effects of this one substance alone.

Why Food Allergies Occur

IMPAIRED DIGESTION Most food allergies can be traced to an impaired digestive system. Proper digestion requires that the body secretes sufficient hydrochloric acid and pancreatic enzymes into the stomach to process foods. These substances break down large protein molecules into small molecules so they can be absorbed and utilized. When too few digestive juices or enzymes are secreted, the large protein molecules go directly into the bloodstream. The immune system reacts to these large molecules as if they were foreign invaders—the allergic response.

ENVIRONMENTAL AND EMOTIONAL STRESSES In addition, other stresses can affect a person's "allergic threshold." These include environmental stresses such as air, water, and food pollution; inhalants such as perfume, aerosol hair spray, or room freshener; and emotional stress. The less healthful the physical and mental environment, the less likely are our chances for achieving and maintaining a state of well-being.

Environmental pollution poses a particular problem. Over the past two centuries the barrage of chemicals introduced into our environment has disrupted the balance of our ecosystem. Residues of many toxic chemicals such as pesticides, herbicides, and insecticides are ingested into our bodies along with food additives and preservatives that are added during commercial food processing.

In many cases, the contamination of food is an irreversible result. Foods such as oranges, sweet potatoes, and butter can be dyed. Other processed and packaged goods like Jello, ice cream, sherbet, cookies, candy, and soda can contain large amounts of food additives.

Most of our commercially raised meats and poultry are riddled with residues of antibiotics, tranquilizers, and hormones. It is even common practice to dip certain fish in an antibiotic solution to retard their spoilage. A person allergic to these antibiotics and drugs may be unknowingly ingesting them continuously, provoking either long-term or short-term reactions or illnesses, the source of which might remain unidentified. It is estimated that more than 10 percent of all Americans are sensitive to food additives. But remember, even when a person eats only organically grown foods, they may still be food allergic.

In most cases, the more severe a person's food sensitivity becomes, the more numerous the allergens that induce it. One clinical study reported that the average person suffering from hay fever was allergic to five foods as well. A total picture of a person's allergen exposure, environment, habits, and history are vital for effective treatment.

The end result of repeated or prolonged sensitization of the body by recurrent allergic reactions is termed "breakdown"—the point at which diseaselike symptoms appear. They may be erroneously diagnosed as the onset of an illness. But the biochemical breakdown, although it manifests itself suddenly, was actually initiated years before by prolonged exposure to allergens.

GENETIC MAKEUP You can inherit allergic sensitivities. If both parents suffer from allergies, their children have at least a 75 percent chance of inheriting a predisposition to this hypersensitivity. When one parent is allergic, the chances of an inherited allergy remain as high as 50 percent. The child does not have to inherit the same allergic response. What is inherited is a genetic makeup that is more likely to have allergic reactions in general. For example, the mother may have chronic indigestion while the child's allergy manifests itself as acne. A mother may be sensitive to corn while her child is sensitive to yeast. Infants can develop allergies to the same foods as their mothers while still in the womb, through the placenta, or through breast milk after birth.

THE MECHANISMS OF FOOD ALLERGY Conventional allergists believe that the mechanism of food allergy is triggered by direct contact of the food antigens—the substances the body produces to fight the "foreign food invader"—with immune system antibodies in the gastrointestinal tract. The usually swift reaction that results is called an immune system-mediated response. This is the only kind of allergic reaction that conventional allergists recognize.

But there is a second mechanism recognized by clinical ecologists, through the absorption of the allergen from the gastrointestinal tract into the bloodstream. Circulating in the blood, allergens can react with elements other than antibodies. The resulting reaction can occur in the blood, in the nervous system, or the musculoskeletal system. Sometimes referred to as a sensitivity or intolerance, to distinguish it from a classic allergic reaction, this second mechanism can be extremely complex. However, tests to uncover these more subtle intolerances are available.

Hypersensitivity to foods can come at any time of life and continue to any age, although the onset occurs most commonly in infancy and early childhood. This is largely because the gastrointestinal systems of the very young are less efficient than in the adult. One researcher refers to the progression of allergies from childhood to adulthood as the "allergic march." Symptoms can move from one organ system to another. A child may suffer from asthma as a result of drinking milk. During teen years the allergy may take the form of pimples. Unfortunately, many people erroneously believe that they have outgrown their allergy because they no longer suffer from the original symptom. They don't consider that their current problems may have the same underlying cause. Their allergic symptoms may continue to vary throughout their lives because of an underlying imbalance that remains constant. Hyperactivity as a child may be the result of ingested food additives. In later years, these same ingredients may cause migraines and fatigue.

The Link Between Food Allergies and Chronic Disease

If food and chemical sensitivities were routinely considered in each case of chronic disease, there would be a tremendous increase in well-being in this country.

An overly analytical medical system insists instead on classifying patients into narrowly defined disease states. Environmental aspects, including a patient's diet, are considered to be nonmedical. The person's whole experience—including diet, environment, lifestyle, emotional life, and work life—may also be considered to be outside the physician's domain, although few physicians would deny that the cause of almost any patient's illness will involve one or more of these factors to some degree.

FOOD ALLERGIES AND MENTAL HEALTH It may be that up to 70 percent of symptoms diagnosed as psychosomatic are probably due to some undiagnosed reaction to foods, chemicals, or inhalants. Different allergic reactions occur. There are localized physical effects like gastrointestinal disorders, eczema, asthma, and rhinitis (nasal inflammation). There are acute systemic effects like fatigue, migraine headaches, neuralgia (nerve pain), muscle aches, joint pains, and other generalized symptoms. And there are acute mental effects such as depression, rapid mood swings, hallucinations, delusions, and other behavioral abnormalities.

It has been estimated that over 90 percent of schizophrenics have food and chemical intolerances. More specifically, 64 percent are sensitive to wheat; 51 percent to corn; 51 percent to cow's milk; 75 percent to tobacco; and 30 percent to petrochemical hydrocarbons.

Researchers now believe that food allergies may directly affect the body's nervous system by causing a noninflammatory swelling of the brain, which can trigger aggression. Despite studies at various correctional centers showing clearly the connection between diet and behavior, little is being done to change the dietary standards of correctional facilities throughout the nation. Routine screening programs for food allergies and nutritional deficiencies in chronic offenders do not exist.

While many other factors—not food alone—mitigate criminal, antisocial behavior, or mental illness, a case can be made for testing for and evaluating food sensitivities in any overall treatment, prevention, or rehabilitation program. (See part three for a full discussion of alternative approaches to mental health.)

FOOD ALLERGIES AND MIGRAINE HEADACHES Migraines are an example of a condition in which recognition and elimination of food allergens can make a tremendous difference. The trick is to recognize the possibilities.

Right now, about 25 million people who consult their physicians each year complain about bad headaches. Although there are various types of headaches, about 50 percent of these people suffer from migraines. While conventional medicine has very little to offer the migraine sufferer, clinical ecologists see migraine as a disorder frequently resulting from food allergies. The nontraditional medicine offered by the clinical ecologist may offer a unique opportunity to relieve the suffering.

Headaches due to food or chemical sensitivities often can be treated simply by eliminating the allergy, once it has been identified, with an elimination or rotary diet. Yet, as a rule, food sensitivities are not investigated in the diagnosis and treatment of headaches.

While the pain may sometimes appear immediately after eating a particular food, it may also be delayed until hours afterward. For this reason it is not unusual for a person to fail to identify the correlation between what they're eating and the onset of their headache. A food may even seem to relieve migraine symptoms temporarily—a classic example of an addictive allergic reaction.

Of course, allergic headaches typically occur as the result of combinations of factors, rather than from food allergies alone. Emotional stress, for example, may play a large role in triggering an episode. Thus, even when a food allergy is at cause, the specific food source may not produce the same symptoms on every occasion, depending on the array of associated circumstantial factors. In some individuals stress may be compounded when the allergic reaction triggers further emotional symptoms. A vicious cycle is created. Sudden changes in temperature or light may also affect one's susceptibility, as well as the presence of any other health problems.

Environmental medicine specialists have found that some of the foods that occur most frequently in the typical American diet are also the foods most commonly implicated in food allergy-related headaches. The list includes wheat, eggs, milk, chocolate, corn, pork, cinnamon, legumes (beans, peas, peanuts, and soybeans), and fish. Moreover, individuals with food allergies should avoid or limit their intake of fermented products like red wine, champagne, and aged cheese because of the presence in these foods of a substance called tyramine. Tyramine has been associated with migraine occurrence in some cases.

Too often, conventional medical practitioners tend not to look toward nutritional solutions in cases involving allergies, including allergy-related migraines. In part, this is because the medical training they have received does not extend deeply into nutrition. And yet, a preponderance of evidence continues to point to the importance of nutritional solutions for an increasingly wide range of health problems. (For more information on migraines, see chapter 47).

FOOD ALLERGIES AND FATIGUE Probably no allergic disorder is more puzzling and pervasive than "tension fatigue syndrome." Indeed, for many of us, varying daily levels of tension and fatigue are the norm; tranquillity and energy, the rare exceptions. To compensate, we choose artificial solutions for moderating energy, from the first caffeinated gulps of coffee in the morning to the quick sugar, caffeine, or drug fix during the day, and the alcoholic "equalizer" in the evening. The result is that energy levels are either depressed or falsely elevated most of the time. In many cases, these quick pick-me-ups are responses to allergic disorders with their roots in food and nutrition.

Next to headaches, tension fatigue syndrome is the most common manifestation of cerebral and nervous system allergy. Yet, too often, this far reaching malady is not even recognized by physicians or allergists. Its symptoms are usually assigned a psychiatric origin and treated with drug therapy or some other conventional modality, when in fact, a simple elimination and rotation diet is the best medicine.

There are several reasons for this all too common oversight. First, there are similarities between tension fatigue syndrome and psychiatric disorders. And second, there is the failure of standard scratch tests to identify many food and chemical reactions. The scratch tests simply have not been shown to be effective in the diagnosis of food and chemical sensitivities. And yet they continue to be used by allergists.

Of course, tension, extreme nervousness, irritability, depression, and emotional instability may be symptoms of psychological disorders in some cases. But too often this is the only possibility that is considered by conventional practitioners. In too many cases, the end result is that a psychological origin is erroneously attributed while the actual physical cause remains unrecognized and the chronic allergic reactions persist.

The allergy may be due to any number of foods, and it is only through careful testing that a definitive diagnosis can be made. In all cases where such symptoms appear, food allergies should be ruled out first—before further traditional medical sleuthing occurs. This can save an awful lot of trouble and mistaken diagnoses.

Early research has suggested that an allergic syndrome may be responsible for certain nervous symptoms in adults and children by actually irritating the central nervous system. Thus, if certain allergies act directly on the nervous system, they can cause characteristic behavioral and physical abnormalities.

Tension fatigue syndrome in a child is sometimes caused by an inhalant sensitivity; however, it is more often due to an unrecognized food intolerance. Reactions to food commonly occur along with other allergic disorders like migraine and asthma, or they can also occur alone.

SYMPTOMS

The symptoms experienced in tension fatigue syndrome can include fatigue, weakness, lack of energy and ambition, drowsiness, mental sluggishness, inability to concentrate, bodily aches, poor memory, irritability, fever, chills and night sweats, nightmares, restlessness, insomnia, and emotional instability. Mental depression is another common symptom, ranging from mild to severe episodes of despondency and melancholia. Generalized muscle aches and pains, especially in the back of the neck or in the back and thigh muscles may also be present, as well as edema (fluid retention), particularly around the eye, and tachycardia (rapid heart beat). Gastrointestinal symptoms often associated with this syndrome are bloating, abdominal cramps or pain, constipation, diarrhea, and a coated tongue. Chills and perspiration are also frequently experienced in association with fatigue during food testing of symptomatic patients.

The disorder can begin at any age. It can last from several months to several decades. In some adults the extreme fatigue, bodily aches, depression, and mental aberrations that come from this continuing allergic state can be so severe that they interfere with work and domestic life.

As headache attacks or gastrointestinal upset caused by allergy increase in frequency, the fatigue is more likely to remain even between episodes. Fatigue soon becomes the allergic individual's major complaint. The allergic origin of the fatigue and weakness commonly remains a mystery.

It's not unusual for allergic individuals to sleep up to 15 or more hours for several successive nights to try to overcome their fatigue. Unfortunately, in most cases, these efforts prove futile. The fatigue experienced in allergic fatigue is quite different from the fatigue that naturally follows physical exertion. It cannot be relieved by normal or even excessive amounts of rest. It can only be relieved by eliminating its cause—the allergen.

Instead, the majority of these allergic individuals, many of whom have often sought a variety of medical avenues for relief, are eventually labeled neurotics.

DIFFERENTIAL DIAGNOSIS

Before the diagnosis of allergic fatigue can be defined, a complete medical workup should be done to exclude both organic and functional origins. This should include a comprehensive case history, complete physical examination, and diagnostic laboratory blood testing. Other causes for nervous fatigue include chronic infections and metabolic disorders, including diabetes, hypoglycemia, hypothyroidism, neurological disorders, heart disease, anemia, malignancy, and various nutrient deficiencies. Even if another disease is found, allergic fatigue can still be a causal factor. In some cases, fatigue is caused both by an allergic reaction and an underlying chronic disease state.

THE MONDAY MORNING BLAHS

It is common for people to binge over the weekend on foods to which they are sensitive. This destructive habit is all too often responsible for the Monday morning blahs. If you are feeling blue by coffee break on Monday, sit down and examine what you've eaten during the previous days. Clinical ecologists suggest that rotary diets may help pinpoint food allergies in patients complaining of fatigue when no other cause is obvious. Very often, patterns of stomach upset will disappear following a careful dietary change, and once the new diet has been maintained over a period of several weeks, fatigue and muscle weakness will be replaced by increased amounts of high energy.

FOOD ALLERGIES AND OBESITY

Many obese men and women believe that they are overweight due to heredity, or because they have a thyroid or metabolic problem, or because they simply eat too much. They may blame their lack of self-control or become convinced that they have psychological problems. And yet, some experts believe that roughly two out of three obese individuals suffer from some form of allergy.

Of course, allergy may be only one of several factors affecting an obese person's weight. The presence of a thyroid condition or psychological problems can cause or aggravate a weight problem. Obesity is also related to many diseases including high blood pressure, heart disease, kidney problems, and diabetes. For obese individuals with allergies, the problems of each condition may adversely affect the other. Typically, someone who is obese will have allergic responses more often than his or her nonobese counterpart. The extra weight is a burden on the immune system, and the weaker the immune system, the more one may be affected by one's allergies. Obese individuals also may have increased difficulty breathing, with particularly severe implications for allergic persons with asthma. In many cases, problems will occur due to allergies in combination with other factors.

We store chemicals in the body in fat. Very often, allergies are triggered by a response to chemicals stored in this way. Because the obese person may naturally hold more chemicals in the body, he or she may tend to experience more frequent allergic responses. This also may explain why he or she feels worse, or has strong food cravings, at the beginning of a diet. Chemicals are stored in fat, and as the fat is burned, a large quantity of chemicals is passed into the bloodstream, often causing such cravings.

The mechanism by which an allergy can trigger obesity may be that of the hidden addictive allergy, whereby a person is addicted to the very foods to which he or she is allergic. Often, these are high calorie foods, such as chocolate, cheese, or sugar. So, the person may gain weight because he or she eats these high calorie foods too frequently.

Hunger itself can be an allergic response, and compulsive eating and intense cravings for particular foods may also result from hidden allergies. In some cases, compulsive eating of the food one is allergic to may really be an attempt to stave off withdrawal-like symptoms induced by going without the food for too long. Such withdrawal symptoms might include headaches, drowsiness, irritability, or depression.

Dr. Marshall Mandell, a physician who has written extensively on dietary problems, also notes that some individuals may experience specific food cravings because they know that particular foods have a short-term positive effect on their mood, or provide them with a quick boost of energy. Such positive changes are only short-lived and are usually followed by a drop of energy, a feeling of fatigue, or some other negative mood change such as depression.

Allergies can cause weight problems if they interfere with the body's natural ability to regulate itself. As noted by Dr. Arthur Kaslow, physician and author, both humans and animals naturally attempt to maintain their bodies in a state of biochemical equilibrium known as homeostasis. Unless there is a flaw in their regulatory system, human beings will maintain their proper weight by eating the amounts and types of foods their bodies need to function properly. When the body needs food, it will send out a hunger signal. When it needs water, it sends out a thirst signal. If this mechanism breaks down, an individual may feel hungry when he or she does not really need food. It is possible that allergies can temporarily impair the cells responsible for sending out these signals.

ALLERGIC EDEMA

As noted by several experts, another way that allergies can affect an individual's weight is by causing edema (fluid retention). The edema may be localized to specific parts of the body, such as the ankles, hands, abdomen, or face, or it can spread throughout the body. When it is evenly distributed throughout the body, the individual often doesn't realize it, and therefore, doesn't think that fluid retention has anything to do with the weight problem. Eating food to which one is allergic can cause water retention equal to 4 percent of total body weight.

Edema occurs when an allergen in a food to which the individual is allergic causes some of the body's capillary (small blood vessel) pores to enlarge. The fluid from the blood plasma may then seep into neighboring tissues. These tissues swell with this excess fluid. When the allergen leaves the body, the capillaries return to their proper size. But if the individual continually ingests the allergen, he or she will always have this excess fluid in the tissues, significantly affecting the weight problem.

A way to determine the possible role of edema in a person's weight problem is to try to have that person recall whether he or she ever lost more than 3½ pounds on a reducing diet for a week. That is the largest amount you can burn up even if you were only drinking water. If a larger weight loss ever occurred, edema may have been the cause.

Any initial weight loss on typical reducing diets occurs largely because the diet may eliminate food to which the individual is allergic. For example, if the individual is sensitive to sugar, and the diet restricts the intake of dessert foods, the individual will lose weight beyond that lost from calorie reductions. He or she would lose the extra water retained due to the sugar allergy as part of the edema. Allergic edema would also explain how some individuals can diet and still not lose much weight. This may happen because some food allergen is still in the diet, causing excessive fluid retention and leading to edema.

The orthodox treatment for weight loss is to go on a calorie restricted diet. But be forewarned! This diet may not work if allergic edema is playing a part in contributing to the weight problem. Even the depression many people experience on a standard reducing diet may be allergy related.

An alternative dieting approach is to suggest that the individual initially follow a diet that is well balanced. Then a clinical ecologist can determine which foods or chemicals, if any, are causing any continued weight problems, and have them avoid those substances. A rotation diet may then be introduced to ensure that new sensitivities do not develop.

To help handle food craving in the short term, exercise is highly recommended. It can increase blood flow, bringing needed nutrients to the cells. It can also calm one's mood. Vitamin C as well as vitamin B_6 can also be useful in blocking allergic reactions.

FOOD ALLERGIES AND ARTHRITIS

Some clinical ecologists estimate that from 80 to 90 percent of all cases of arthritis are either allergy induced or are allergylike reactions to some food the patient has eaten. The arthritis may also be related to an environmental factor to which the patient is sensitive, such as gas inhaled from constant proximity to a gas stove. Examining arthritics for both food and environmental allergies may help reduce current symptoms, prevent recurrences of symptoms and minimize the permanent damage that eventually results from joint inflammations.

Studies have shown that, in some cases, arthritic symptoms will lessen if a patient fasts. (Most food allergy symptoms will clear up during a four-day fast.) Studies also report that after arthritis patients fast, the symptoms may reappear if certain foods are eaten. The most frequent foods that caused the reactions were corn, wheat, and meat.

As is true with other food allergy problems, no one specific food causes arthritic symptoms in all patients. Some patients may be allergic to tomatoes while others are allergic to strawberries, wine, or grapefruits. Elimination of the food source from the diet can become an integral part of any treatment program.

For osteoarthritis, there are other factors to be considered. Usually, osteoarthritis is related to a calcium imbalance. Therefore, the imbalance must also be examined and taken into account. Because calcium is deposited in the joints in osteoarthritis, many people assume that the body has too much calcium, while actually the reverse is usually true. While the lack of calcium may be due to a dietary deficiency, it is also often due to a digestive problem. In such cases, the body is not properly handling the calcium it takes in. Therefore, the calcium is deposited in places where it does not belong. Such patients may need supplemental calcium. Vitamin D and vitamin C may also be suggested, since they can aid in calcium absorption by the body.

Dr. Marshall Mandell has successfully treated hundreds of arthritis patients by putting them on a five-day distilled water fast and then allowing their usual foods, one at a time, back into their diet. If a food causes the arthritis symptoms, the symptoms will return when it is reintroduced into the diet and should be permanently eliminated.

This five-day elimination diet can be adapted to allow individuals a way of self-testing specific foods: Keep a food out of your diet for five days, then reintroduce it. If it causes your problems to recur, eliminate it. (For more information on arthritis, see chapter 27.)

Diagnosing Food Allergies

Given the fact that approximately 30 million Americans are estimated to have food and chemical sensitivities, proper testing and treatment of these individuals could have an enormous impact on our individual well-being and on society overall. Some techniques for such testing have been around for some time. Other tests are just evolving.

Patient experience is most important in diagnosing allergies. Environmental medicine specialists now are highlighting the role the allergic individual can and must play in diagnosing and treating his or her own ailment. Articles written in the 1930s reporting the lack of attention paid to patients regarding their conditions could very well be republished today. Unfortunately, very few physicians acknowledged this advice in the past, and few acknowledge it today.

TRADITIONAL TESTING The most common test performed by the traditional allergist is one that really has very little use when seeking food allergies. Still, it is often used. Working well for dust, pollen, mold, animal hair, and insect stings, this is the classic scratch test. The doctor makes 10 to 20 scratches on a patient's arm, using a needle imbedded with the problematical substance being tested. If there is a reaction on the skin, it indicates a sensitivity. But this test picks up reactions only to allergens that stimulate a specific immune response in the body and detects only certain types of antibodies produced by the body with that defensive response.

Another test, developed in the 1960s, relies on screening blood samples. Called the radio-allergo sorbent test, RAST for short, this test is much more expensive to perform than the scratch test and can have more false positives and false negatives.

ALTERNATIVE METHODS A comprehensive medical history might provide significant clues about your allergic profile. A trained clinical ecologist or environmental medicine specialist may find the needed information from such a medical history alone.

Clinical ecologists also use a skin test, evaluating different-sized doses of a questionable substance. The diluted substance is injected into the skin. After 20 minutes, the physician checks for redness and swelling, measuring the size of the skin raised by the suspected allergen. Progressively larger doses of the same suspected substance are administered in this way until the size of the skin reaction no longer increases. All the while, the patient writes down any other symptoms he or she may be experiencing, like headache, stuffy nose, or nausea.

Physicians can use this approach to determine the size of a particular dose of an allergen that might trigger a reaction, or counteract it. It is therefore useful in testing and in treatment.

While this approach has its advantages, it is time-consuming, expensive, somewhat painful, and can test only the part of the food that can be diluted in water. Other parts of the food (that are fat soluble, for instance) may be at cause but will not respond to the test.

A similar test takes another approach, putting extracts of food mixed with glycerin under the tongue, instead of into the skin by injection. While this test is not painful, it also can be time-consuming and expensive.

Another test, employing a technique called applied kinesiology, is based on the principle that there is a reflex response between a suspected allergen and the patient's body, in the patient's muscles. In this test, a doctor offers food to the patient and then measures or evaluates the energy or muscle function after the food is ingested. Here many foods can be tested in each session. However, the results may not be highly accurate, depending on the nature and experience of both the person administering the test and the person being tested.

Newer tests are being developed all the time. Some, like the cytotoxic test, mix blood samples with food extracts and measure how many white blood cells (cells involved in the body's natural defensive system) burst. In allergy smears, samples of different body fluids or secretions are evaluated in the laboratory to look for a specific type of white blood cell. The various immune system cells may also be evaluated. And in the Arest program, radioactive atoms are used to determine how antibodies respond to particular antigens.

HOME TESTS

There are also less technical tests, some of which can even be done at home. A fasting test, which should be done under medical supervision, begins by cleansing your system. Symptoms may still be present or, if your allergy is an addiction of some sort, may have worsened by the second or third day of the fast. Then foods are reintroduced one at a time to check for symptoms. This test should not be done for certain already ill patients, the elderly, the hypoglycemic, or young children.

Another test that can be performed at home is the Coca Pulse test. First find your normal pulse range, by taking it every two hours. Then take it again at specific, regular intervals after eating the suspected allergen. If your pulse rises more than 10 points, the food eaten last becomes suspect. The pulse is rising as a reaction to increased adrenaline in your system. The adrenaline, it is believed, usually is being released in reaction to an allergy.

Another home test involves keeping a food diary, and recording everything you eat for a week. Record symptoms and when they occur as well. After the week, look for a relationship between symptoms and food eaten.

Elimination testing is yet another approach. Eliminate the suspected allergen until symptoms clear up over a 12-day period. Reintroduce the food on an empty stomach. Usually symptoms, if they are to develop, will do so within an hour of testing.

A variation on that is the elimination of all common allergens—wheat, corn, dairy foods, citrus fruits, food colorings, sugar, and foods you may crave, over the course of a week. Then reintroduce the foods, one per day. If symptoms develop, the food may be an allergen. Don't eat it for five more days and then reintroduce it to double-check the result.

A final home test—perhaps among the most effective and sensible of all tests—also doubles as a treatment for food allergies. It is called the rotary diversified diet.

Plan a diet in which you eat no individual food more often than once in four days. After five days, start a food and symptom diary. After reviewing correlations that may crop up through your record keeping, eat any suspected food the next time it comes up in the four-day rotation alone as one full meal. Note symptoms. Eliminate foods that stimulate adverse symptoms from your diet—permanently.

The theory here is that food sensitivities become even more pronounced when a food is eliminated and then reintroduced into the diet. With this diet, your symptoms—and with them the responsible food—are clearly highlighted.

This approach is also useful as a maintenance diet, enabling people who are prone to food allergies to prevent the emergence of new allergies, since they never eat any food too frequently. And even then, if a new food allergy does develop, it is spotted and quickly eliminated.

Treating Food Allergies the Natural Way

Our understanding of allergies has been greatly expanded by the clinical ecologist. Because the traditional allergist only recognizes those allergies that are mediated by the immune system, he therefore can only treat a small portion of illnesses the clinical ecologist would classify as allergies. In addition, the traditional allergist has a limited number of alternatives to offer his patients. Other than avoidance of an allergic substance, the traditional allergist has only immunotherapy—"the allergy shot"—to rely on. With this, the physician administers gradually increasing increments of the substance to which the patient is allergic. It will usually take six months until the optimal dose, that is the dosage at which symptoms are blocked, is achieved. The theory is that the patient uses up his antigens on the allergy shot, and therefore has a higher threshold of response before he will respond badly to an allergen again.

The effectiveness of traditional immunotherapy may be limited only to those allergies directly related to the immune system response. Some experts believe this represents only 5 percent of all allergies. And even within this small group, there are some immune system-related allergies that do not respond to the treatment.

Traditional immunotherapy is not useful, for example, with food allergies or animal dander allergies. Nor is it always effective for dust allergies, for while the physician can desensitize the individual to specific particles that are components of dust, the patient may be allergic to other particles that were not in the allergy shot. And the treatment is a time-consuming process, with no results noticeable until the optimal dose is finally discovered.

THE ELIMINATION DIET

A technique that is used by many allergists that does seem to work on food allergies is the elimination diet. Employed for over 60 years, this plan removes the most commonly occurring food allergens from the diet along with any other foods suspected on the basis of case history or positive test results. In the process of eliminating foods, symptoms usually improve. After avoiding all suspected foods for five to seven days, one food at a time is reintroduced back into the diet. At this point, the patient and doctor observe any recurrence or worsening of symptoms. Some doctors introduce a new food at each meal, while others add only one food frequently for seven days before adding another. If an item causes a symptom, it is then avoided and once again introduced at a later date.

THE ROTARY DIVERSIFIED DIET

Clinical ecologists have improved upon the elimination diet by devising a combined diagnostic and preventive regimen called a rotary diversified diet. In it, certain foods may have to be totally avoided (if one has a fixed allergy), while some may be eaten every four to seven days without ill effects (if one suffers from a cyclic allergy). Rotation diets can be designed to deal with individual food sensitivities. But no food is eaten more frequently than every four days. Rotation diets also help to minimize the stress that pre-existing allergens cause, at the same time preventing future sensitivities from developing. They are also valuable in diagnosing masked food allergies, since our bodies react acutely to allergens reintroduced after four to seven days of abstinence.

Since most food allergies are cyclical rather than fixed, that is, they come and go in varying degrees of severity, a rotation diet is part of the treatment for many allergic patients. Foods to which the patient is sensitive are eliminated and the remaining foods are eaten no more frequently than once every 4 days. Foods you ate on Monday might be repeated on Friday or over the weekend, but not before. For some individuals who are highly sensitive, a 5-, 7-, or even 12-day cycle may be necessary.

The rotation diet ensures against the development of new food sensitivities in a way that simply substituting one food for another does not. For example, if an individual was allergic to wheat, and eliminated it from his diet, but began to eat rice every day, he might develop a sensitivity to rice. Periodic retesting may be recommended several months after you've made the change to a rotation diet. By retesting your sensitivity to some of the eliminated foods, it may sometimes be possible to reintroduce them on a rotational basis.

A rotary diversified diet often is recommended to check for obesity and edema (fluid retention) related allergies. Salt, sugar, and tap water is avoided. Then, for each week over a five-week period, the individual tests a common

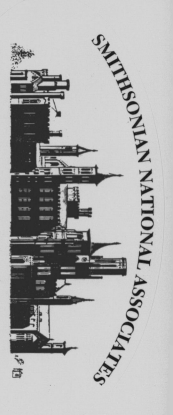

SMITHSONIAN NATIONAL ASSOCIATES

SMITHSONIAN INSTITUTION • WASHINGTON, D.C.

SMT BSTKR

allergen such as dairy foods, wheat, corn, eggs, yeast, pork, soy products, chocolate, or apples. One would avoid each of these foods for four days. If, after five days, the individual has lost five or more pounds, which is then regained when the food is eaten, the test food should be considered an allergen and avoided for at least two months. Then, the food can be reintroduced on a rotational basis, checking to see that it is no longer causing problems. One can continue to test different foods throughout the five-week process.

When following a rotational diet, one should continue to weigh oneself daily, in order to check for edema. Once one has passed the withdrawal period, the avoidance of allergens and a rotation diet can help break food cravings and compulsive eating patterns.

NEUTRALIZING DOSE THERAPY Another technique to treat allergies used by clinical ecologists is the neutralizing dose therapy. This method is especially useful in cases when multiple food allergies are present, and where avoidance of chemicals and medicinal inhalants is difficult, as during the pollen season. A neutralizing dose is determined for each allergen, and when it is injected or administered under the tongue, this dilution can bring about relief from the allergic symptoms.

These treatments are administered in a series during which the dose of the allergen is progressively increased, causing a desensitization to this substance. (They work on the same theory as allergy shots or vaccines. The only differences are in the dilution of the substance and the wide variety of the substances that can be tested in this way.) Eventually, the person can tolerate contact or ingestion of the allergen with only a mild reaction or no reaction at all.

With the neutralizing dose treatment, the allergist is first determining the amount of a particular allergen that causes an allergic reaction. The physician can work with many substances that the traditional allergist would be unable to treat, including foods, chemicals, perfumes, and cigarette smoke. The neutralizing dose approach seems to be effective in 8 out of 10 patients.

Like the traditional allergy shot, the neutralizing dose can be administered by injection. However, it can also be given as drops under the tongue. Instead of taking approximately six months to find the optimal dose, the physician can usually determine the correct dosage in one or two sessions using this technique. Another advantage of the neutralizing dose is that the patient can be given the drops to take at home. It not only works as a preventive measure, but also can block a reaction that has already started.

If a parent discovers that a child who is sensitive to wheat is acting hyperactively, and the parent finds out the child was given cookies at school, the parent can terminate the allergic response—the hyperactivity—by administering the drops. On the other hand, if a parent knows the child will be going to a birthday party and knows the child will most likely encounter an allergic food, the parent can administer the drops in advance to forestall an allergic reaction.

TOTAL ENVIRONMENTAL CONTROL Elimination, rotation diets, and neutralization dose therapy help in the diagnosis and treatment of many allergic disorders. However, for more serious problems that still resist such treatment, total environmental control in a hospital setting may be required.

This may be the case where the allergy is masked or the patient history reveals too little. A person's system can be cleared of all allergens in four to seven days. This is accomplished in the controlled hospital setting, by having patients fast on distilled water only for at least three days, then traditional tests are administered. The controlled environment also assures that the patients are not exposed to any environmental contaminants.

BOOSTING THE IMMUNE RESPONSE Since allergies most often represent an immune system that has gone awry, another important aspect of treatment is finding ways to boost the patient's immune system.

Allergies occur when the immune system has been weakened. Therefore, any strengthening of the immune system should improve resistance to current allergies and reduce susceptibility to new ones. There are several ways in which the immune system may be strengthened. Making sure you are getting sufficient amounts of rest is essential, as is regular exercise. Keeping stress levels to a minimum will also help. You must also be receiving the right nutrients in the right amounts.

Many nutrients have been found to enhance the effectiveness of the immune system. These include vitamin C, beta carotene, vitamin E, selenium, and glutathione. These are all antioxidants, which help to eliminate free radicals from the body.

Free radicals are highly reactive molecules created as a byproduct during the process by which the body converts food into energy. They can easily latch on to cell membranes and DNA, causing cell damage. Free radicals also can develop from many sources, including X-rays, heated vegetable oils and through exposure to ultraviolet light.

Garlic has been found to be an immune stimulant, having both antifungal and antibacterial qualities. Garlic is most effective when eaten raw. It may be either added to one's food or taken as a supplement in tablet or capsule form.

The essential fatty acids are also important to a proper immune response. Many researchers recognize the importance of omega-3 fatty acids, which are found in such oils as linseed and walnut, and in many fatty fishes, like salmon, in warding off both diseases and allergies.

In addition to acting as immune stimulants, there may be other reasons why nutritional supplements may be useful for those with allergies. It has been noted that 200 to 500 mg of pantothenic acid plus 50 mg of B complex vitamins can be useful for allergic individuals. Vitamin C, in addition to its importance as an antioxidant, also has an antihistamine effect, which may benefit those with allergies by reducing the swelling of tissue and cell membranes. One study found that asthmatics taking 1,000 mg of vitamin C daily had 25 percent fewer asthmatic attacks than those receiving a placebo. Another study found that asthmatic children benefited from magnesium supplementation.

STRESS MANAGEMENT Since stress lowers the immune response, reducing stress should help in food allergy elimination. Stress management techniques are available, including progressive relaxation and biofeedback, to recondition the body to learn a new, more healthful way to respond to and deal with stress.

Many other techniques, from self-hypnosis and affirmations ("I have a healthy strong immune system") to visualizations (imaging immune system cells gobbling up invader allergens), meditation, yoga, and tai chi, may prove useful to promote physical and mental relaxation and reduce the stress in our lives.

Stress management techniques can serve to improve the digestion of allergy sufferers. Exercise, in particular, can be an excellent stress reducer. It can lower the levels of anxiety and boost the immune system by helping to eliminate water and toxins from the body and to speed the transfer of nutrients to the cells. It also normalizes blood sugar levels.

Aside from its many other negative affects on the body, sugar is an immune system weakener. One study found that it interferes with the white blood cells' ability to break down many harmful substances. A lack of dietary protein also can damage the immune system. Adequate protein is needed to provide the body with amino acids so that it can produce white blood cells.

PROPER DIGESTION In addition to a weak immune system, some types of digestive imbalances usually have a role in the development of allergies. Since proper digestion requires the secretion of sufficient hydrochloric acid and pancreatic enzymes for easy absorption and utilization of the nutrients in the food we eat, when there is too little of this secretion this process can be altered. One result may be that some portion of the nutrition in the food we eat is not made available to us. The large molecules of protein that should have been broken down by the digestive juices or enzymes go directly into the bloodstream. The immune system reacts to these large molecules as if they were foreign invaders, causing an allergic response to the particular food. To alleviate such allergies, it is vital to restore the digestive system to optimum functioning. Balancing the digestive enzymes may be a way to do this.

Thoroughly chewing one's food is essential to proper digestion since there are digestive enzymes in the saliva that break down starches. If food is bolted down, these enzymes do not have enough of a chance to work, and more will have to be done by the intestinal enzymes. The enzymes may then go out of balance.

A lack of stomach acid also may contribute to digestive disorders. Often, this is the case in allergic children. Also, with age, many adults suffer from a decrease in stomach acid. This can be corrected by taking hydrochloric acid tablets with meals. However, individuals should not attempt to self-medicate in this area. The problem may be either too much or too little stomach acid. Hence, if the individual takes antacid tablets when he or she has low stomach acid or takes hydrochloric acid when he or she is overly acidic, the result may be a worsening of the problem.

37

Allergies in Children

When people think of childhood allergies, they often think of hay fever, asthma, eczema, and hives. But there are many other areas of the body that can be affected by allergies. As Dr. Doris Rapp, a board-certified pediatric allergist and specialist in environmental medicine, informs us, "Allergies can cause headaches or stomachaches; they can affect the bladder, causing your child to wet the bed or to have to run to get to the toilet in time. Allergies can cause leg aches, muscle aches, joint aches, sleep problems, behavior problems, and learning problems. Some children will become tense, nervous, and irritable. Others will become withdrawn and unreachable, hiding in corners and pulling away when you go to touch them. Still others will become very hyperactive and aggressive. Often they will bite, hit, scream, and do all kinds of nasty things.

"Most allergists—including myself for my first 18 years in practice—would not recognize this host of physical and emotional symptoms as having been caused by allergies. But I now recognize that dust, molds, pollens, foods, and chemicals can affect almost any area of the body and can cause all of the problems mentioned above in some individuals.

"Now it would be going too far to suspect that every time a child has a headache it is an allergic reaction, or that every time an adult has a bellyache it is due to food sensitivity. But currently, with conventional medical practitioners, this diagnosis is never even considered and is therefore missed too many times. People will have headaches for years and never once consider whether there might some underlying reason for the headache.

"Environmental medicine wants patients to start to take more control of their health. We want you to pay attention to how you feel. If you don't feel well, or you suddenly can't think correctly; if you're confused, or unusually irritable, or emotionally volatile; if you cry or become upset or angry for no reason; you have to start to ask, 'Why am I having this reaction now? What did I eat, touch, or smell?' Our whole society is geared to go to the medicine cabinet for a painkiller or an antihistamine when we should be geared to get a pencil and paper to record what could be causing this problem at this time.

"After we have educated the parents, they often come in to see us knowing exactly what is causing their child's problems. They can tell if it's something inside or outside the house, if it's a food or a chemical. They can pinpoint the cause."

The Role of the Immune System

According to Dr. Rapp, one of the primary reasons for allergies in children, as in adults, is a poorly functioning immune system. "If the immune system is inadequate, we can develop allergies and environmental illness. One way to strengthen the immune system so that your child is less prone to environmental illness or allergy is by using various nutrients. A helpful resource is the book, *Super Immunity in Kids*, which says, basically: If you take the correct nutrients in the correct amounts, you can strengthen the immune system so that you are less apt to become ill from natural things such as pollen, dust, and mold exposures. You will also be less apt to become ill from exposure to infections."

Are Allergies Affecting Your Child?

Dr. Rapp offers many tips for helping parents to determine whether a child's behavior is related to allergies or environmental factors. "Think back," she says. "Does your child say, 'When I go to school in the morning I feel great!'? Or does the child say, 'I feel great when I leave the house and by the time I get to school I don't feel right'? Or does he say, 'I feel nervous'? Or tired, or irritable, or, 'I have a headache'? If that happens, you have to think, it might be the fumes on the school bus, or what he ate for breakfast, or what he uses to brush his teeth, or the soap that he uses. You've got to think of everything that he came in contact with before he got on the bus, and then what happened when he was on the bus.

"One way for parents to figure out what's causing the problem is to drive the child to school. If you find he can eat, bathe, wash, and do everything else in the usual manner in the morning and you drive him to school and he's fine, then it's probably the bus that is causing problems. And you can check back and forth a couple of times and try to confirm or negate your suspicions.

"Now, children who are sensitive to things in the school will frequently notice that their headache starts within an hour. And the headaches frequently become more intense during the day. By Friday afternoon, the headache will be much worse than it was on Monday morning or on Sunday night. At first the headaches may disappear one to four hours after your child leaves school, but later on, if there are too many exposures during the week, you may notice that they don't get better at night and that it might take the whole weekend for the headache to go away."

It's also a good idea to pay attention to your child's sense of smell.

"Another clue that certain exposures are making your child feel worse is when your child can smell everything before anybody else," Dr. Rapp explains. "She smells natural gas, or smells that perfume across the room, or she can smell food cooking before anybody else. She can smell disinfectants. If these odors bother your child and she can perceive them faster than anybody else, it means that she is probably becoming sensitized to the abundance of chemicals that we have now managed to put in our food, air, water, clothing, homes, schools, and workplaces."

You child's academic performance may yield clues about a possible allergy to something in school. "The child may get an A one day, and an F the next day in the same subject," Dr. Rapp says. "It isn't that your child lost brain cells within 24 hours, but it does indicate to me that you should investigate that school to try to find out what could be causing the problem. Is the school dusty or moldy? Are the ventilation ducts open and clean? Was the basement of the school ever flooded? Does it smell worse on damp days? There is nothing worse in present-day schools than some of the synthetic carpets. They are made of chemicals that cause problems. In addition, they use adhesives that are full of other chemicals that cause even more problems. Many of these chemicals are neurotoxic, which means they damage the nervous system, or carcinogenic, which means they can cause cancer.

"Here is a list of symptoms you may recognize from your child's behavior: The ability to hear, talk, or speak clearly is impaired. Your child suddenly speaks too fast—is hyperactive—or doesn't make sense when he talks. An environmental sensitivity can alter children's ability to write, read, or see clearly. Some children develop blurred vision or double vision by the end of the day because of chemical exposures at school. Some develop red earlobes or cheeks, wriggly legs or dark circles under their eyes. All of these signs and symptoms can be caused by an environmental illness."

Testing for Allergies

"If you suspect that your child may have been exposed to neurotoxic substances—those that actually damage the nervous system—ask your doctor to send you to specialists who can tell you whether the nerve conduction time in your child's body is normal or not," Dr. Rapp continues. "They can do a variety of blood tests to find out if the chemicals that are in the carpets and the adhesives are in the blood."

"The doctor may even make an allergy extract of the air in a room that smells of chemicals. Sometimes the child is exposed to just one drop of the allergy extract of the air of a room—a particular room in the home or school—we can actually reproduce a headache, a stomachache, or problems thinking. The doctor makes the allergy extract the same way one would bubble air through a fish tank: Using a pump to bubble the room air through a salt solution in a tiny test tube. The air bubbles for about eight hours and at the end of this period a solution remains that contains some of the chemicals that were in the air. Then an allergy extract is prepared from this solution which can be injected in the skin, or placed under the tongue. If it causes numbness in the arms, tingling in the fingers, a headache, stomachache, problems with remembering, or a change in activity or behavior within 10 minutes, we have probably collected the problem chemical from the air within the solution.

"Using the new and more precise method of allergy testing called provocation/neutralization, the doctor can then make dilutions of that chemical solution and probably eliminate those same symptoms with one drop of the right dilution of that solution. In other words, if the child develops a headache in a certain room, you can put a drop of the air allergy extract under the tongue and provoke the headache in 3 to 8 minutes. Then you can give the child a five-fold weaker dilution of that same solution and often you can eliminate or neutralize the headache in less than 10 minutes."

Eliminating the Problems

"After you have done a skin test with the allergy extracts, and shown that there is a cause-and-effect relationship between the child's behavior or physical symptoms and a chemical in the school, the next thing is to determine what the school can do to eliminate the problem," Dr. Rapp says. "One of the things they can do is not put carpets in schools. If they do have carpets and they're causing problems, they can take the carpets up and put in hard vinyl tile. In such cases, it is important to insist that they use adhesives that are safe when installing the tile.

"Another big problem in schools is poor ventilation, especially in the winter. Due to the energy crunch we had in the 70s, many schools closed down their ventilation systems to save money and to cut down on the cost of heating. Dust, molds, and chemicals have accumulated at very high levels in these schools. The windows don't always open, and the result is that there has been a gradual buildup, so that more and more children and teachers seem to be adversely affected when they go to school.

"One of the things that you can insist on is that school officials check the ventilation system. There are fast and easy ways to measure the amount of carbon dioxide in a classroom, which can tell you whether the ventilation is good or not. The level should be 800 ppm or less. Relatively simple tests can also be done to measure for certain chemicals, such as chlorine and formaldehyde.

Sometimes, because of poor cleaning of the ventilation systems in schools, the problem is dust and molds, not chemicals. Other times, they put chemicals in the ductwork while cleaning, which really causes trouble because the chemicals then circulate throughout the school, causing illness. Sometimes the intake for the ventilation system is too close to the area where all the school buses line up. The bus drivers let the engines idle for long periods, resulting in all the gasoline fumes and hydrocarbons entering the ductwork intake and circulating throughout the school.

"In one case I encountered, a school had a printing press, and the exhaust pipe from the printing press was at exactly the same level as the ventilation intake on the roof, with the result that all the chemicals from the printing press were going right back in and circulating throughout the school. Some printing press chemicals are toxic to the nervous system and cancer-causing.

"A patient I saw last week has three sons who came home smelling of mop oil, which is used to clean the school. The mother said that the children's clothes smelled so badly that she had to use very hot water to eliminate the smell. One of the boys developed a headache and a burning sensation in his throat. So I asked her to bring some of the mop oil and I just put it underneath his nose and let him take one whiff of the odor. Within seconds, he was complaining of a headache around his forehead on both sides of his temples and he said it was throbbing and that his throat was burning. I gave him oxygen for about 10 minutes and the headache, throbbing, and burning in his throat gradually subsided. We videotaped this reaction.

"There was another child who had trouble only on the two afternoons a week when he went to school. He would be weak and tired, hardly able to stand; he couldn't hold a pencil, clung to his mother, but only on those two days. I sent the mother to the school and asked her to try to figure out what's different in the schoolroom that might be causing your son problems. It turned out that they used a very common disinfectant aerosol in the room, six times a day on the tabletops, to reduce infections. Then they used the same solution on the cot that he napped on. All she had to do was ask the school to stop using that disinfectant and install an air purifier, and the child improved remarkably.

"Then the mother noticed that he had similar problems when he went into the gym, and it turned out that they were using a certain kind of floor wax in the gym. We suggested that they use something that had fewer petrochemicals in it and the result was that he can now be in the gym for 20 minutes. That child had tics and twitches, which is another thing that you see in some children with these allergies. The symptoms disappeared after environmental allergy care.

"I have seen children from all over the country who have problems at school. Some of these children who come to see me don't come in complaining of allergies. But the affected teachers and the children almost uniformly have a history of hay fever, asthma, or eczema. And they have relatives that have these same conditions. Their immune systems are not up to par, or they wouldn't have allergies to start with. But they are the canaries—the first ones to become ill when a school is chemically contaminated, or is too dusty or too moldy. Many children who have these allergies also find that their problems grow worse after their school has been remodeled, repainted, newly carpeted, or refurnished with furniture made of materials that release formaldehyde or other chemicals into the air.

"Children who wheezed a little before, now wheeze a lot. Youngsters who were stuffy once in a while are now congested all the time. Not only do they get nose problems, but they start having infections in the sinuses and their ears. Many of them feel tired and weak when the schools are chemically contaminated. One parent said that her child was too tired to turn the pages of his book. Another said that her child was crying because he couldn't play football anymore because he was just too weak. These are some of the things that are happening in some schools throughout the country, mainly because of dust, molds, and chemicals."

It has been reported that actions taken during infancy can reduce the chance of allergies occurring later in life ("Treating allergies early can reduce later toll," *Family Practice News*, November 15–30, 1990). For example, breast-feeding seems to reduce the risk of allergies later in life. Moreover, if the mother is able to avoid foods to which she is allergic during pregnancy, this further enhances the chances of the child to be free of the allergies. On the other hand, infant exposure to inhalant allergens, smoke, infections, and baby formula in place of its mother's milk, may increase the risk of allergies.

Food Allergies

Medical literature is filled with case studies in which children experience irritability, hyperactivity, insomnia, lack of concentration, poor memory, fatigue, and lethargy. After isolating and omitting all of the allergens from their diets, these sensitive children often improve. Not only do their physical symptoms clear up, but their behavioral imbalances also return to normal. With the control of the allergy, a normal personality is gradually established and maintained.

Among children, the most common sources of food allergies include chocolate, milk, wheat, eggs, and pork. "Ideally," Dr. Rapp says, "your child should eat only organically grown food because it is less contaminated with pesticides, food coloring, or other chemical additives that may be causing your child's adverse reactions. However, in some places, it remains difficult—and expensive—to buy foods uncontaminated by chemicals. Organic foods may be readily available in New York City, but they certainly aren't in many other cities. I encourage people to grow their own vegetables so that they will have their own source in the winter and one which they know does not contain any chemicals."

Dr. Rapp describes several simple ways to determine whether a food allergy exists. Ask your children to talk about how they feel, write their names, and draw pictures before and after eating a meal. Using a peak flow meter or other device, check their breathing patterns both before and after eating. Pulse rate can be monitored as well. "If the pulse is 80 and suddenly after eating it is 120, a food has set off a silent alarm in the child's body, which has caused her pulse to increase," Dr. Rapp says. "So check the writing, the drawing, the pulse rate, the breathing, and how your child feels and looks before a meal and then a half hour or so later. If any of these variables indicates a change for the worse after a meal, one of the foods your child ate may be the cause of the problem.

"Wait for five days before the attempt to find the problem food. It is critical that you wait for five days to get all that particular food out of the body. So for five days, if you have noticed your child had a reaction after eating corn, don't feed your child corn (and tell her not to eat any at school either). Then at 8:00 a.m. on a Saturday, give her the first of the foods she may have been reacting to, and at 10:00 a.m. give her the second possibility one, at noon the next one, and at 1:00 p.m. the next. In this way, you check each food all by itself. Again, check the breathing, the pulse, the writing and drawing, and how your child feels and looks before and a half hour or so after each food.

"Ask your children to write down or tell you their five favorite foods and beverages. The five foods and beverages that they write are probably the foods that are most likely to cause them difficulty. If they wrote down chocolate, cocoa, and cola—which are all different forms of chocolate—it means that chocolate could be the cause of their problems. If they wrote down bread, cake, cookies, pasta, and macaroni, chances are the problem is wheat. If they wrote down ice cream, yogurt, milk, cheese, and pizza, they are probably sensitive to dairy products."

A Final Note

"You can apply the same principles of food isolation to every room in your house and at school or every room at work. Check your breathing (or your child's breathing) before you enter a room, do all the things that I suggested above, and then do them again several hours later. If you find that a particular room is a problem, then you have got to ask, 'Why? What do I smell in this room, what am I touching in this room, what is in this room that could be bothering me? Is it the heating system, the covering on the furniture, the carpet, the floor wax, the furniture polish? Are there items that have been dry-cleaned in this room? Is there an odor?' You'll be surprised at how much you can figure out on your own.

"Also check out the car. Notice how you and your children feel before you get in the car, then check again half an hour later. Compare indoors with outdoors and you'll be able to tell whether it's the outdoor pollution, the lawn spray next door, the mold, pollen, or pollution in the air that is causing problems outside versus inside. You can easily figure out many, many answers by checking your child's pulse, his breathing, and how he writes, draws, feels, and looks. Check these same parameters on yourself as well. If you have high blood pressure, you can even use a blood pressure cuff and check your pressure before and after each of these exposures and you'll turn up answers. By keeping detailed records, you can often figure out the reasons why your children are ill, and many times you can then get rid of the cause and make them feel much better.

"Don't forget to check lavatories. Many children go into the lavatories at school feeling fine, and when they come out they can't think at all because of the chemicals in the disinfectants and deodorants that are used in the lavatories. Don't forget the garage, which has many chemicals in it. Don't forget the attic, which is dusty, and don't forget the basement, which is dusty and moldy.

"Keep in mind: The indoor and outdoor factor that causes more problems than any other is molds. If you live in a moldy house and you are always wheezing, on cortisone, always sick and in and out of the hospital, it could be the moldy house that you are living in that is causing the problem. Sometimes if you live in too much mold, it doesn't matter what kind of treatment you're on. You have to move or get away from the thing that is causing the problems.

"There are some new ways of doing brain imaging that can actually show changes in the brains of some of the people that are exposed to neurotoxic substances. For example, if a child sniffs glue or hair spray or aerosols, you can actually show a characteristic pattern of change in the brain imaging-pattern on the particular individual, which will look different from somebody who has epilepsy or someone who has schizophrenia or depression. They actually produce different brain pictures. I'm sure in a few years, many people who say they are always depressed, or tired, or nervous will be able to have a brain-image pattern taken that will show that specific areas of the brain have been affected by certain exposures or foods."

Patient Story

As Alison's mother, I can honestly say that Alison was born crying. She cried for the first two years of her life. I took her to a clinic at the time and found out she was allergic to corn, wheat, and bananas, which caused her to cry every day, all day long. I took her off those foods, and she became a normal, happy two-year-old. She did well for quite a while until she got a problem with a vitamin deficiency, which caused her to be uncontrollable. I couldn't do anything with her. If I wanted her to get dressed she would scream, rant, and rave. It would take me three hours just to get her dressed.

After reading an article on vitamins, I put her on vitamin supplements. That's when we realized that she hadn't smiled in six months. Then she was fine again, until two years ago, when she started to scream at me all the time, day in and day out, no matter what I wanted her to do, over absolutely nothing. She would scream at me that her shoes were wrong, her hair was wrong.

It would take me all day long just to get her into the shower. At this point she was 10 years old. She should have been bathing on her own. I would go pick her up at school and when she was 70 feet away from me, she would scream, 'Mom, you are early!' And she would go on and on about why I was early. The next day she'd look at me and she'd scream, 'Mom, you are late!' And she would scream the whole way home, until she went up to her room and I would go off somewhere else to get away from her....

Dr. Buttram diagnosed my daughter as having food allergies: to corn, potatoes, chicken, egg yolks, rice, and chocolate. They put her on these sublingual drops and now I have my normal, happy daughter back again. It was a dramatic change. She had become extremely difficult to live with. She would just scream at me about the most ridiculous things. Nothing was ever right. If she got out of bed—Why didn't I wake her up?—Why didn't I let her sleep?—And she would shriek at the top of her lungs. Some days were worse than others.

Now I know that on the days she had a combination of foods or a lot of the foods she was allergic to that she was at her worst. The way that I figured out it was food again was because every once in awhile we would have a great day or two and every once in awhile her diet just happened to not include these things. Then she would be fine. But the next day she'd be right back again with the behavior—totally out of control for long periods of time.

When my mother found out about Alison's behavior, she told me that I myself had been an absolutely horrendous child. Now that Alison had been diagnosed, she understood that I had had food allergies too. Now I understand that children's behavior problems are not always due to what the parent is doing with the child, as far as discipline is concerned. I've had a lot of children; I've been a foster parent for years. When Alison first started this behavior I tried everything in the book and nothing worked. And the thing that told me that something was controlling her, instead of her doing this, was the fact that we would have good days. And it didn't matter what we were doing on a bad day. If I would sit and play with her all day long, and it was a bad day, we would have a bad day. And discipline meant absolutely nothing, because something was controlling Alison.

It was a chemical imbalance in her brain that was controlling her because she had absolutely no control over what she did. It was like the food was controlling her. I related it to the behavior of a manic-depressive or a paranoid schizophrenic who has no control over what they are doing.

Now, when I go to the shopping mall, I see kids who I know have food allergies by the way they are crying. My husband used to say I was crazy, but when Alison was two years old and she would cry, I could tell if it was a food-allergy cry or a two-year-old cry by the sound of her voice. It was a different kind of crying. I have friends who complain about their kids constantly and one child in particular I know has food allergies. And the mother will not take him in to be tested. She'd rather complain about it. The biggest obstacle I see to helping children with behavior problems caused by allergies is making parents understand that there is an alternative. You don't have to live like this. You have to ask yourself, 'Do I really want my child to live like this?'

I feel bad that Alison was so miserable for so long. There are so many kids out there that are this miserable. There are kids in learning disability classes and the parents just don't look any further than their nose. Some parents do make an effort and take their kids to standard allergists who test them, but those doctors may not be able to locate the problem. A friend of mine took her child to a regular allergist who tested him for all the standard things and said he was fine. But he never tested him for half the things to which Alison is allergic and the doctor never questioned the mother about the child's diet.

PART EIGHT

Cancer Treatment and Prevention: Overview and Historical Perspective

In today's society, cancer is epidemic and the single most important medical issue—an issue inseparable from politics and economics. Tens of billions of dollars and an entire industry in which over 800,000 people work full time are involved. The "war on cancer" has led to the formation of an enormous army consisting of the National Cancer Institute (NCI), the American Cancer Society (ACS), and other major cancer research centers throughout the United States.

Each year, just before the ACS's annual fund-raising drive, we are bombarded with news stories of an imminent breakthrough that could change the lives of millions of sufferers. Months after the collection pots have been passed, there is still no breakthrough and the human toll in suffering continues. According to the ACS, more than 1.2 million Americans will be diagnosed with cancer in 1999, and 563,000 will die of it. While we are told that improvement in the treatment of various cancers is just around the corner, and while there have been gains in treating a few forms of cancer, overall we are losing the war.

Part of the reason lies in the strategy of the people who are leading the fight. Their view of the disease is determinedly myopic. To them, cancer is a localized disease represented by the tumor. By excising, poisoning, or irradiating the tumor, the traditional oncologist attempts to kill it in order to save the patient. The allocation of research funds depends on who controls this battle. When the head of the NCI is a chemotherapist, money goes into chemotherapy; if he or she is a radiologist, the money goes to radiology. Unfortunately, the same small group of people have continued for nearly 30 years to dictate where the money goes. At no time has this cartel been receptive to physicians who experiment with more progressive, nontoxic, noninvasive, and most important, unpatentable and hence nonproprietary treatments.

This is not to suggest that established cancer researchers are not interested in finding a cure for cancer. They are dedicated and sincere but are equally eager, I believe, to have their cancer cure be the one that is ultimately accepted. And every company is pushing for its drugs to be the ones of choice.

Forgotten, overlooked, even maligned and denigrated in this pell-mell rush for dollars, power, and control of the golden goose is the fact that a small number of highly qualified physicians and scientists have been able, through a lifetime of work, to succeed in curing and otherwise improving the prognosis of cancer in a certain percentage of their patients. They do not use the word "cure," and I use it only on the basis of the establishment's definition of a cancer cure: alive and well 5 years after being diagnosed with the original tumor. In fact, I have tracked down and interviewed hundreds of alternative practitioners' patients and have found them alive and well 5 years, 10 years, and even 20 years after diagnosis and treatment, even for terminal cancer.

It is true that money and self-interest stand in the way of research on innovative cancer therapies. It is also true that a basic misunderstanding of the nature of cancer prevents the acceptance of innovative therapies. The cancer community is only now beginning to recognize that a person's attitudes, beliefs, and especially diet can affect the outcome or causation of cancer. Only recently have some scientists acknowledged that environment can be a determining factor or that cancer represents a breakdown in the body's overall immune system. Traditional physicians are more reluctant still to acknowledge that treatment that consists solely in removing the tumor with surgery or killing the cells in the tumor with radiation or chemotherapy may end up killing the patient by releasing extra toxins while doing little or nothing to stop the progress of the disease.

The following chapters present an overview and historical perspective on the alternative view that a tumor is merely a symptom and that therapy should focus not on the symptom but on the underlying causes. This view has led to treatment aimed at rebuilding the body's natural immunity and strengthening its ability to destroy or control cancer cells.

The cancer puzzle has not been completely solved. There are still failures in the treatment results of each of the therapists described herein. However, in total, these therapies represent the most logical and advanced perspectives and the best chances for success in the treatment of cancer.

For information on alternative therapies for specific types of cancer, see the following chapters: chapter 55, Breast Cancer and Other Breast Diseases; chapter 56, Cervical Dysplasia, Fibroids, and Female Reproductive System Cancers; and chapter 60, Prostate Conditions.

38

The Cancer Microbe

The lump in Dr. Owen Wheeler's neck was not large, but it was a lot more than a swollen gland. Closer examination confirmed the physician's worst fears. He had a cancer of the lymph glands that had wrapped itself around the major arteries nearby. An attempt at surgery would be the equivalent of slitting the doctor's throat.

As a physician, Dr. Wheeler had seen a great deal of cancer in books, in laboratories, and in his own and other doctors' patients. Now he had to choose a treatment for himself. For him, since surgery was out, it had to be either radiation or chemotherapy. As a medical doctor, he would be in danger of losing his license if he ordered any treatment other than surgery, radiation, or chemotherapy for a similarly afflicted patient. However, from his own experience he knew that the improvement rate for these treatments is 15 percent at best.

Radiation, the doctor soon discovered, would be almost as damaging as surgery to the major blood vessels near his cancer. However, he did not feel ready to subject himself to chemotherapy. Just a few years previously he had watched his father die of the same type of cancer, suffering horribly from the side effects of the drugs used to combat the disease.

Like many other physicians, Dr. Wheeler refused chemotherapy when his own health was involved and began looking into alternative therapies. Ultimately, he decided to go to Dr. Virginia Livingston's clinic in San Diego, California, which featured an innovative treatment based on an unorthodox theory of the nature and cause of cancer, a theory with far-reaching implications for public health. At Dr. Livingston's clinic, Dr. Wheeler's cancerous tumor gradually disappeared.

The Discovery: Dr. Virginia Livingston

Dr. Wheeler did not make the decision to go to San Diego lightly. He knew his life was at stake, but he also knew he was not going to undergo a Johnny-come-lately treatment of uncertain background and unpredictable outcome. He knew that Virginia Livingston was a remarkable physician whose interest in and work on cancer went back two generations. One of only four women to graduate from New York University–Bellevue Medical College in 1936, she was one of the first women residents appointed to a New York City hospital. Her interests then were tuberculosis and leprosy.

Her path to cancer research began indirectly in 1947, when she was asked for a second opinion on a case diagnosed as Raynaud's phenomenon, a circulatory condition that causes ulcerations on different parts of the body. While many of the patient's symptoms resembled those of leprosy, Dr. Livingston thought a more likely diagnosis was scleroderma, a skin disease characterized by hard, knotty patches, which can be fatal if it spreads to the internal organs.

Curious about the apparent similarity of scleroderma to leprosy, Dr. Livingston tested some smears with a special dye designed to detect the presence of tuberculosis and leprosy microbes. The tests were positive, suggesting that these scleroderma microbes were closely related to the tuberculosis and leprosy bacteria.

Dr. Livingston went on to test these organisms on chickens and guinea pigs. To her amazement, almost all the chickens died while the guinea pigs developed hardened patches of skin, some of which looked cancerous. Since cancer in guinea pigs is nearly unheard of, these results raised unsettling questions: Could this microbe from a human being cause disease in chickens and guinea pigs? Could this same microbe transmit disease from animals to humans? Was cancer perhaps infectious? Was it caused by bacteria?

From various hospitals, Dr. Livingston gathered samples of human cancers removed during surgery and put the pathological tissues under the microscope. The microbe was indeed present in every one of the samples. When she isolated and cultured the microbe from the cancer tissues and injected it into mice, the mice developed cancer in about 20 percent of cases. Dr. Livingston decided to call this microbe progenitor cryptocides.

After several years of careful research at Newark Presbyterian Hospital, Dr. Livingston published her findings in the *American Journal of Medical Sciences* in 1950, much to the verbally expressed dismay of many members of the cancer establishment. After all, they had long accepted as an article of faith that cancer is caused by a virus. Medical technology has long been able to develop antibiotics to deal with bacteria but has yet to find any consistently effective protection against viruses. The fact that cancer might actually be caused by a bacteria thus should have come as good news, but the medical establishment refused to give creditability to Livingston's findings by setting up testing procedures to verify or disprove her findings. Instead, the traditional researchers simply continued to voice denial of the credibility of the microbe theory.

Both Dr. Livingston and her opponents—including the ACS—cited as evidence in their favor experiments performed by Dr. Peyton Rous in 1910 which demonstrated that roughly 90 percent of the chickens sold in New York City contained cancers caused by a microbial agent small enough to pass through a filter designed to catch bacteria while allowing viruses, which are much smaller, to pass through. Although Dr. Rous did not conclude this "filterable microbial agent" was a virus, scientists who came after him assumed this to be the case. Dr. Livingston, however, believed her progenitor cryptocides (PC) was in fact the cancer-causing agent discovered by Dr. Rous.

PROGENITOR CRYPTOCIDES (PC) BACTERIA Since PC bacteria are highly pleomorphic (i.e., often assume forms that do not resemble bacteria at all) and have different growth requirements depending on the stage they are in, Dr. Livingston proceeded with extra tests to make certain that she was not dealing with a virus. She discovered that PC would indeed pass through Dr. Rous' filter just as viruses were supposed to do. But then she took samples of the filtered microbes and regrew them in cultures, something impossible to do with viruses, since they are unable to survive outside of living organisms. Dr. Livingston also discovered that unlike viruses, both PC and Dr. Rous' cancer agent could be dried, stored indefinitely, and then reactivated to produce new tumors. For Dr. Livingston, the PC cancer-causing agent was not a virus but was only viruslike. The PC bacteria had to be reincubated and made larger in order to be kept from passing through very fine filters that usually hold back bacteria.

In the course of her research, Dr. Livingston reached another conclusion that put her at odds with the cancer establishment, especially the part of it which believes implicitly in surgery as a first recourse. PC, as Dr. Livingston found out, was present not merely in the cancer but throughout the patient's entire body. In her view, cancer is not a localized disease. Rather, it is a generalized or systemic illness affecting the entire body, not just the particular area manifesting symptoms. Thus, while surgery can be helpful in that by removing cancerous tissue it helps the immune system fight the disease, it is a serious error to think of the tumor or lesions as constituting the disease and of surgery as being the cure. Indeed, from Dr. Livingston's viewpoint, it was no surprise that a patient could develop cancer in a totally different site after a "successful" operation, despite the surgeon's having "gotten it all." Since surgery does nothing by itself to enhance the body's immune system, it may even make another onset of cancer more likely—and more serious.

Dr. Livingston might have concluded that once a drug to combat or at least control PC bacteria was developed, a cure for cancer would be on its way. Careful research on the microbe in laboratory animals, however, convinced her that the solution was far more complex than finding a "magic bullet" to strike down PC. The PC bacteria, she discovered, are a normal constituent of every cell in the human body.

"The microbe is present in people from the time of conception," she stated in a WBAI radio interview in 1987. "It is not always harmful. It is useful, for example, in the knitting of wounds. But when it begins rampant proliferation, it produces a hormone called chorigonadotropin, which promotes tumor growth and is present in abnormally large amounts in cancer tissues."

Dr. Livingston went on to explain that PC normally remains dormant in the cell and emerges only to help in healing after injury to the body. Ordinarily the immune system monitors the production of PC, keeping it at the amount needed to cope with the damage. But when immunity is weakened by stress, poor diet, old age, surgery, and/or other debilitating factors, the body may no longer be able to regulate PC production and PC bacteria may begin to proliferate, releasing chorigonadotropin as it multiplies.

TRANSMISSIBILITY THEORIES Theories about the transmissibility of cancer have alarming implications for public health. Dr. Livingston's experiments convinced her that cancer can be transmitted from human beings to chickens and guinea pigs. This conclusion raises the disquieting implication that the transfer mechanism may work in the other direction as well, allowing cancer to pass from animals to humans.

For obvious reasons, the poultry industry finds such an idea unthinkable. However, Dr. Livingston's chicken vaccine was licensed in California in 1985.

"Cancer is a very serious disease in chickens," Dr. Livingston noted in her radio interview. "Each year many thousands of chickens are lost to cancer. The organism is carried from chicken to chicken, even in the unhatched egg."

If all of these birds were simply "lost," the problem would be confined to the poultry industry, but there is considerable evidence, Dr. Livingston stated, that many infected fowls are finding their way into supermarkets. She believes that the chickens we consume today are just as cancer-ridden as the ones Dr. Rous examined in 1910 when he determined that 90 percent were so afflicted. A March 1987 report on *60 Minutes*, while not concerned specifically with cancer, certainly supported her contention that FAA enforcement is both lax and ineffective in keeping questionable poultry off the market.

The question of whether cancer can pass from animals to humans takes on even wider dimensions when one considers that livestock, often living in cramped and unhealthy conditions, are frequently fed chicken manure because of its high protein content, and are thus exposed to the infectious cancers so prevalent on the poultry farm. But avoiding eating beef and pork, while desirable, is not sufficient, according to Dr. Livingston. Even drinking milk is risky, she asserted, since "about 80 to 90 percent of cattle are carrying leukemia," according to the cattle industry's own literature.

The doctor's views on milk are met with as much skepticism in the dairy industry as her views on meat and poultry are in the meat and poultry industries. But Dr. Livingston's legacy is not without support. Her views are accepted in Europe. In Switzerland and Sweden, where dairy is a major industry, milk from leukemic cows is not permitted to reach the market because the authorities consider it a serious risk to the public health. Such strictures have not been imposed in the United States in part because the U.S. dairy industry simply doesn't believe, and no government authorities will test, Dr. Livingston's theories. The doctor never denied that the expense of enforcing strict quality control and rejecting milk or meat from diseased animals would be tremendous. However, it would also alleviate a great amount of human suffering.

The Treatment: Diet, Vaccine, and Antibiotics

Dr. Livingston pondered this evidence for many years beginning in the 1940s and 1950s and continued gathering data and doing research until she developed a program of cancer treatment diet, antibiotics, and a therapy she called autogenous vaccines. Eighty percent of her cancer patients improved. In 1992, while on a vacation in Europe, Dr. Livingston died. We all mourn her loss. But the challenge her work presents to the medical establishment lives on.

THE ANTICANCER DIET: STRENGTHENING THE IMMUNE SYSTEM The Anticancer Diet is not in itself a cure for cancer, nor is it intended as such; however, it works with the other aspects of Dr. Livingston's therapy to strengthen the immune system. A healthy immune system not only keeps normally present PC under control but combats any disease-causing PC taken in with food. Meats, especially chicken, beef, and pork, are the most likely sources of dietary PC.

Since the immune system of a cancer patient is already seriously depleted, it is necessary to avoid these kinds of foods in order to minimize the influx of pathogenic, cancer-causing PC. For this reason, Dr. Livingston's diet goes beyond the usual tenets of sound nutrition. It emphasizes raw or very lightly cooked fresh food full of vitamins, minerals, and enzymes for rebuilding the body. Refined or processed foods are dispensed with as far as possible. Most animal products are excluded, both because of their suspected ability to transmit pathogenic PC and because they are often full of toxins, hormones, antibiotics, chemicals, and pesticides that deplete the immune system and may interfere with treatment. In fact, the diet Dr. Livingston developed is basically the one which the ACS is now only beginning to promote: primarily vegetarian, low in fats and cholesterol, low in animal products and protein, and high in fresh fruits, vegetables, whole grains, and legumes.

Dr. Livingston stipulated that her patients do the following:
- Avoid the obvious carcinogens and immune system depleters, such as cigarettes, alcohol, caffeine, and drugs, both recreational and prescription.

❤ Avoid the empty calories of foods that are high in white flour and sugar or that have been deep fried.

❤ Cut down on salt and on food high in sodium while increasing consumption of potassium-rich fresh fruits and vegetables.

As patients began to recover, Dr. Livingston allowed them to eat some fish, but chicken, eggs, beef, and milk products remain prohibited, since her research has led her to believe that these foods have a high potential for transmitting cancer to humans. The PC microbes in their pathogenic state are in the animals, and when the animals are eaten, the microbes are transmitted and proliferate in humans.

The most unusual aspect of Dr. Livingston's diet, however, is its focus on abscisic acid, an essential immune nutrient forming part of the vitamin A molecule. As Dr. Livingston stated in her 1984 book, *The Conquest of Cancer: Vaccines and Diet* (Franklin Watts, New York, 1984), "Abscisic acid is the keystone upon which all cancer immunity is built in your body. If you already have cancer, abscisic acid is absolutely critical to your defense, because it actually stops cancer cells from multiplying. If you don't have cancer (or if it is latent in you system), it is imperative that your diet contain high amounts of vitamin A and abscisic acid if you are to immunize yourself against it."

Of course, raw juices, especially carrot juice, and fruits and vegetables high in vitamin A have a prominent role in the Anticancer Diet. However, because many cancer patients have extensive liver damage and therefore are unable to break down vitamin A to obtain abscisic acid, Dr. Livingston's diet also includes a number of foods such as mangos, avocados, tomatoes, and green leafy vegetables that are naturally rich in abscisins. To break down the vitamin A in carrot juice, Dr. Livingston recommended adding a tablespoon of dried liver powder (from organically fed cattle, of course), which contains enzymes that predigest the carrot juice and thus make the abscisic acid available.

AUTOGENOUS VACCINE Besides the diet, Dr. Livingston developed an autogenous vaccine made from the PC in the individual patient. "We make the vaccine," she reported in the 1987 interview, "and as the body builds immune bodies to the organisms, the deleterious effects of the progenitor cryptocides are nullified. But each time we make it, we make it for the individual. It cannot be made for your neighbor, and it cannot be sold."

ANTIBIOTICS Since PC microbes are bacteria, they are vulnerable to antibiotics, and Dr. Livingston found that the administration of safe, nontoxic antibiotics such as ampicillin and penicillin G can reduce the excessive amount of PC in the bloodstream and thereby cause cancerous tumors to shrink. The term "excessive" is used here because, as has been noted, normal amounts of PC do not cause a problem in the healthy body and in fact contribute to one's well-being. It is only when they become excessive that they contribute to cancerous growth in the body.

OTHER PARTS OF THE PROGRAM Other elements of this completely safe, nontoxic program include the following:

- Transfusions of fresh whole blood, preferably from a healthy family member, to reduce the risk of contamination, increase oxygenation, and replenish the body's enzymes.
- Injections of gamma globulin to provide fresh antibodies.
- Injection of spleen extract derived from immunized animals to increase the patient's white blood cell count. White blood cells play a critical role in arresting foreign substances and toxic intruders into the blood.
- Injections of nonspecific vaccines, such as one containing numerous mixed bacteria, for use in respiratory infections and to increase general resistance.
- Supplements and/or injections of vitamins C and B_{12}, plus tablets of vitamins such as A, C, E, B_6, and B_{12}, and minerals to stimulate the immune system.
- Oral supplementation of hydrochloric acid where needed to correct overly alkaline blood caused by digestive difficulties.

Dr. Wheeler's visit to the clinic had a special fringe benefit in that he found a new wife as well as renewed health. But while only one patient could marry the director of the clinic, thousands of others have regained their health and have come home with a regimen that has kept them cancer-free over the ensuing years.

The Patients

Dr. Livingston's ideas about the treatment and prevention of cancer are not purely academic. They have been put to the test in her clinical practice as well as in her laboratory. In The Conquest of Cancer (Franklin Watts, New York, 1984), she listed over 60 cases of patients she treated; these were pulled at random from her files. Of course, not every story is a success story, but the sample does show an improvement rate of 82 percent, a statistic that conventional therapists can only dream of.

EXAMPLE 1: A 66-year old man came to the clinic in 1978, diagnosed with inoperable cancer of the liver. By 1980 the patient reported feeling much better, and tests showed that his tumor had shrunk 50 percent. When Dr. Livingston contacted him in 1983 while writing her book, he said that he was still following the program and was in general good health.

EXAMPLE 2: A 12-year-old boy was diagnosed with Hodgkin's disease. His mother, however, refused to subject him to chemotherapy and brought him to

Dr. Livingston's clinic instead. A year later, his lymphoma was in remission. Follow-up testing revealed that he was totally clear and that a lesion on his liver had disappeared. He went back to school, gained weight, and was soon participating in sports.

EXAMPLE 3: A 51-year-old woman could no longer endure the side effects of radiation and chemotherapy for cancer of the ovaries which had spread to her colon, causing a tumor about the size of a baseball. Her prognosis was terminal when she started treatment at the clinic. A computed axial tomography (CAT) scan and an ultrasound test taken the following year showed no abnormalities. She went back to work, and two years later she was still free of cancer.

None of these case histories, of course, constitutes experimental proof that Dr. Livingston's therapy is effective. Such proof is not likely to be forthcoming, since it is not morally feasible to establish a control group of cancer patients, give them a placebo, and see how many of them die. However, Dr. Livingston always stood ready to put researchers who wished to verify these stories in touch with these patients or any others in her files.

The doctor's work is continued by others in San Diego. Whether her theories will ever find acceptance and be applied in the wider arena of public health in the United States remains to be seen.

39

Peptides and Antineoplastons

Thirty years ago a medical student in Poland took a new and different approach to cancer research. He decided to find out why all people don't have cancer. Everyone is exposed to the same known and unknown causative agents of this disease. What is different about the people who never contract it? Is this difference the key to developing a cure?

The Discovery: Dr. Stanislaw Burzynski

Dr. Stanislaw Burzynski believes so. Now working out of a research facility he founded in 1970 in Houston, Texas, Dr. Burzynski has treated about 2,000 patients with advanced cancer with impressive success since 1977. Most of these people turned to him as a last resort when conventional treatment with radiation, chemotherapy, and surgery had failed. What they found was a therapy based not on the abuse of the body's built-in defense systems but rather on the transformation of cancerous cells into healthy, normal tissue.

Dr. Burzynski's solution lies in a group of chemical substances, part of a larger group of chemical compounds called peptides, that exist in every human body. His research points to a severe shortage of these substances—called antineoplastons—in cancer patients. Simply stated, antineoplastons are a special class of peptides, found in the body, that combat neoplastons—abnormal cells or cancer cells. Antineoplastons could be the vehicle needed by the body to ward off and even reverse the development of these cancerous cells.

Dr. Burzynski has put this theory into action, treating patients by reintroducing antineoplastons into the bloodstream either intravenously or orally with capsules. In many cases, tumors shrank in size or actually disappeared. Some patients even experienced complete remission of their cancers, and years of follow-up study have revealed no sign of any return.

Such results are almost unbelievable. Dr. Burzynski appears to have tapped the power of antineoplastons to naturally "reprogram" cancer cells. His approach could virtually eliminate the need to destroy these cells or remove the tumors they create.

This therapy was not developed overnight. It has taken Dr. Burzynski nearly three decades of research, first in Poland, then at the Baylor College of Medicine in Houston, Texas, and ultimately at the Burzynski Research Institute in Houston. During this time, Dr. Burzynski has zeroed in on the substance he named antineoplaston. But to get back to Dr. Burzynski's original concern, why do tumors develop in the first place?

WHY TUMORS DEVELOP According to his theory, cancer is due primarily to an information-processing error. Good information produces healthy cells; bad information results in cancerous cells. Antineoplastons are important because they carry "good" information to the cells. They can "tell" the cells to develop normally.

All cells start out with specific goals. Some turn into skin, some into blood vessels, some into bone or other body tissues. However, they will never go on to perform these highly specialized functions in the body unless they go through a process called differentiation. Cancer cells, or neoplastons, which everybody produces regularly, never differentiate. They are abnormal cells that the healthy body rejects and destroys because they have not received good information and so have no constructive role to play. When the body is in a weakened state, these neoplastons are not destroyed but rather are left at the mercy of cancer-causing agents that invade the system and "turn them on." They begin to multiply, forming large, constantly growing lumps. They are victims of bad information and assume a destructive role in the body.

This is where antineoplastons come in—as a means of relaying positive messages. Forming various combinations of the substance, Dr. Burzynski sends instructions to the cells that can allow them to differentiate or specialize. He seeks to correct the information-processing error and restore the body's normal defense mechanisms. The beauty of the treatment is that harmful drugs, radiation, and surgery are not required. The body virtually heals itself.

A BIOCHEMICAL DEFENSE SYSTEM According to the research done by Dr. Burzynski and others in this country as well as abroad, antineoplastons are components of a biochemical defense system which parallels our immune system. Unlike the immune system, which protects us by destroying invading agents or defective cells, the biochemical defense system protects us by reprogramming, or normalizing, defective cells. Errors in cell programming may lead to such diverse disorders as cancer, benign tumors, certain skin diseases, AIDS, and Parkinson's disease.

EVOLUTION OF A THERAPY How did Stanislaw Burzynski evolve this amazing therapy? The doctor's progress in medical research is characterized by a rare ability to look further, to take that extra step onto an untried path and go beyond the status quo. Considering that the doctor was born into a family with a passion for learning, these traits aren't altogether surprising. His parents had university degrees, his father a total of five before retiring as a university professor. Stanislaw followed suit, becoming at age 25 one of Poland's youngest men ever to earn both an M.D. and a Ph.D. He began his research at one of Poland's finest medical schools, the Lublin Medical Academy. Its prestigious faculty provided the mentors he needed to shape his embryonic theories on anticancer defense mechanisms.

The Polish government eventually granted him leave to emigrate to the United States, and by 1970 Dr. Burzynski had become a staff member at Baylor College of Medicine. Since his research had been interrupted by obligatory military service, nearly a decade had passed since he had fixed on the notion that the human body must possess a built-in system to resist cancer and similar diseases. He believed that without this system, no one could hope to ward off the cancer-creating "sea of carcinogens" that surround us. Of course, believing that a natural defense system exists does not explain what it is made up of and how it works, but mentors from his university days offered some clues.

From a former chemistry professor Dr. Burzynski had learned about the information-carrying peptides, which are related to the antineoplastons he had yet to uncover. Other clues had come from Dr. Marian Mazur, professor at the Polish Academy of Science and a widely acclaimed authority in the cybernetic field of science. Cybernetics looks at how systems work; one of its key elements is feedback, which provides a way to control and communicate within a system. If cancer cells become destructive because they have received only bad information, the task is not to kill them but to get the right information to them to make them normal and healthy. Cybernetics provides insight into the nature of improving communications within a system so that the desired information or feedback is properly transmitted. A household thermostat is an example of a feedback device: a tool used to close the gap between an actual result—say, room temperature of 90 degrees—and a desired result—a more comfortable 70 degrees.

Dr. Burzynski concluded that active ingredient of the body's cancer defense system might be found in the family of peptides—small blood proteins—which were known to communicate with and affect the growth of cells. Within that system, these substances could operate as a feedback device to correct the difference between actual cancer cells and the desired healthy cells or to reprogram cancer cells with good information so that they could become constructive and vital instead of pathogenic.

Peptides are a popular subject of modern medical research. Nearly 50 different types have been found that can stimulate cell growth. One, known as peptide T, is attracting attention for its potential in treating AIDS. Dr. Burzynski is thus by no means the only scientist exploring the potency of peptides, but he has been at it longer than most and has achieved findings unique to cancer therapy.

An early discovery involved the level of peptides in advanced cancer patients. Their blood samples revealed only 2 to 3 percent of the amount typically found in healthy bodies—a drastic difference. If peptides, as Dr. Burzynski assumed, played a role in the body's natural defense system, these cancer patients had at some point been disarmed. They were victims of misinformation, since there were not enough peptides to carry good information to the cancer cells.

The next task was to determine exactly what kind of peptides cancerous bodies lack. Burzynski put his doctorate in biochemistry to good use, studying the makeup and structure of the deficient substances and uncovering an interesting effect. When applied to tissue cultures, the peptides missing from cancer patients actually suppressed the growth of human cancer cells.

But while progress was evident, the puzzle was far from solved. It was not enough to know that antineoplastons could carry appropriate information to cancerous cells; it had to be determined how to get them to do it in order to ameliorate tumor growths. Dr. Burzynski turned to his knowledge of systems, cybernetic science, and information theory. The idea of using feedback to adjust and correct an obvious imbalance seemed appropriate to the possible role of antineoplastons in treating cancer.

The Treatment: "Reprogramming" Cancer Cells

Dr. Burzynski's concept constituted a scientific leap, yet it appears amazingly simple in light of the most basic function peptides perform: they transmit information to the cells. Some aim to spur on, others to inhibit, cellular growth—but they all do it by sending messages the body can obey.

Dr. Burzynski likens the process to the use of the alphabet: "It's like having 26 alphabet letters—you can create an infinite variety of words." Using the right "code" becomes the key to reprogramming cancerous cells. Theoretically, it is possible to stop a peptide messenger carrying dangerous, damaging goods and hand over a more beneficent, favorable package for it to deliver instead.

The best time to change the peptide code is when cells are new and immature. Guided by good information, the cells can successfully pass through all the normal stages of development. They can gradually take on the special traits they need to serve different parts of the body, in other words, differentiate. When cells differentiate, they have reached maturity.

Imagine being stuck in childhood or puberty, never given the means to change and grow into a finally functioning adult. This is the state of a cancer cell. It doesn't know how to differentiate and mature, because its genetic code is garbled. In a healthy body with a sufficient level of peptides and antineoplastons, good information is quickly communicated to the cancer cell, and the cell is rendered harmless. But when these levels are low, the cancer cell continues to be victimized by the wrong information. Dr. Burzynski's treatment is aimed at ending the cancer cell's confusion. He puts antineoplastons into the bloodstream to carry the proper genetic code, halt the growth of useless tumors, and encourage cancer cells to differentiate.

Antineoplastons are not foreign substances. Because they appear naturally in the body—and evidently are found at a much higher level in healthy bodies—they don't pose a toxic threat. This fact alone sets Dr. Burzynski's approach miles apart from traditional cancer therapies. Radiation treatments and chemotherapy destroy cancer cells but also destroy any other cells in their path.

Other scientists are testing newer methods which have the same objective as antineoplaston therapy, that is, to encourage cancer cells to differentiate. Researchers at Johns Hopkins University, for example, are examining the substance HBMA (hexamethylene bisacetamide). But HBMA is an artificial chemical. The body can be expected to react with greater resistance to a substance it does not produce naturally.

Two significant observations have been made about the side effects of antineoplaston treatment. First, most patients experience virtually no side effects. The few that have appeared have been minor, short-lived, and easily controlled, such as skin rashes, chills, and fever. The second and more remarkable observation is that the treatment can actually create positive side effects in decided contrast to traditional medical treatments. Patients have shown increases in white and red blood cell counts, decreases in blood cholesterol, and stimulated skin growth; these and other effects are known to aid the body's natural healing powers. Antineoplaston therapy has tremendous promise not just in theory but in practice.

However, a new medicine or medical treatment is not accepted overnight. The medical and scientific communities as well as certain governmental bodies set rigid testing standards to ensure the safety and effectiveness of every supposed curative. Antineoplastons are no exception.

Tests and Results

For over 20 years Dr. Burzynski has been subjecting his theory to the testing procedure required to "prove" its worth, and it is holding up well under pressure. More than 60 percent of the patients treated during the Burzynski Research Institute's phase I testing showed considerable improvement, whereas the norm is only 3 percent at best.

PHASES OF TESTING Each phase of testing has different goals. Phase I of Dr. Burzynski's therapy is designed to examine any side effects that may occur and to determine proper dosages of the antineoplaston "medicine." Phase II entails a more specific study of whether and how the medicine acts to reduce or eliminate cancerous growth, and phase III would take an even closer look at these issues, among larger groups of people with the same types of cancer.

When phase I clinical trials began, Dr. Burzynski didn't expect much in the way of an anticancer effect. His aim was to find out how much medicine patients should be given, starting with very small doses that could be increased over time. He had no way of knowing but could only suspect which kinds of cancer would respond best to his treatment. What he expected and what he got were two different things.

The results in the best cases of 20 different phase I trials showed significant anticancer activity. In the most successful trial, not only did more than 60 percent of the patients respond to treatment, more than 20 percent remained cancer-free for over five years. These patients suffered from some of the most serious and difficult to treat forms of cancer, including advanced lung and bladder cancer, and malignant mesothelioma, a type of cancer that results from asbestos exposure and is especially resistant to traditional medicine.

To conduct these phase I trials, Dr. Burzynski had to have some of his medicine on hand. Since antineoplastons are a specific kind of peptide, he and a research team first concentrated on isolating peptides. The substances then were separated into testable fractions to find the traits unique to antineoplastons, specifically, the ability to inhibit the growth of cancer cells.

Once the antineoplastons were located, knowing the coded information in these substances became important. One group seemed effective against specific types of tumors. A second group had a broader effect. One group was labeled antineoplaston A, and was strained and purified until five new coded combinations were found: A1, A2, A3, etc.

These numbered As proved to have the greatest effect on tumors and the least toxic or potentially harmful properties, but one seemed especially powerful. Patients given the antineoplaston A2 in phase I tests had the highest number of complete remissions from cancer. Based on these results, the team decided to purify this A2 substance even further, and A10 was born.

These efforts to isolate the right antineoplaston for certain types of cancer took place while phase I tests were under way. The generalized goals at this stage—to study side effects and proper doses—had yielded some very specific findings. Antineoplaston A3, for example, produced complete remissions of advanced prostate cancer and encouraging results in cancer of the pancreas. Some A combinations were more effective with lung, bladder, and breast cancers; others with malignant brain tumors, for which surgery is usually the only and often futile alternative.

Dr. Burzynski and his team were clearly on firm ground as they entered the next phase of testing. Phase II trials began in 1985 and continue today. Here patients are grouped according to their basic type of cancer. However, depending on how and where those basic types develop in the body, different phase II treatments are tried. For example, in current trials with breast cancer, treatment varies depending on whether the disease has spread to the lungs or to the liver or bones.

By 1992, 24 patients with malignant lymphoma (cancer of the lymphatic system) had already been treated in phase II trials. Chemotherapy had failed to help nearly 70 percent of these patients. Only certain forms of this cancer, such as Hodgkin's disease, have ever shown real success from conventional treatment. But with antineoplaston care, 85 percent showed vast improvement.

The most impressive results have been in brain cancers (astrocytoma stages III and IV and glioblastoma) and metastatic cancer of the prostate.

In a small phase II trial of astrocytoma conducted by Dr. Burzynski, 20 patients were enrolled—13 with astrocytoma stage IV, five with stage III, and two with stage IIB. All diagnoses were biopsy confirmed. All but one patient had received (and failed) one or more prior standard therapies.

Four patients achieved complete remission and two others partial remission. The responses of 10 patients were classified as objective stabilization (less than 50 percent decrease of tumor size). Since the end of this study in May 1990, some of these patients have achieved partial and even complete remission. Even if they are only preliminary findings, such results are impressive in this type and stage of cancer.

In another phase II study of stage IV prostate cancer refractory to hormonal treatment begun in 1988, two complete and three partial remissions were reported in a group of 14 patients. Seven patients obtained objective stabilization.

RECENT SUCCESSES From a 1997 interview, Dr. Burzynski offers us some of the clinic's more current success stories:

"When we started our program, we concentrated on the type of cancers which are uniformly deadly, such terrible types of malignant tumors as primary malignant brain tumors that are known in medical terminology as astrocytoma, glioblastoma, medulla blastoma. These tumors are uniformly deadly. Practically everybody who develops high grade astrocytoma or glioblastoma dies from the disease. There's no cure available, and the death comes quickly, usually within a year.

"We concentrated on the treatment of such highly malignant tumors to prove a point that antineoplastons work. Otherwise, if there are some other treatments available, we could be accused of perhaps using these additional treatments which could make the tumors disappear. But those treatments do not exist. If we are able to eliminate highly malignant brain tumors by the use of antineoplastons, these are the first cases in medical history of this happening. Since we concentrate our efforts on the treatment of such bad malignant brain tumors, of course, most of our statistics concentrate on these tumors. We already finished three clinical trials, phase II trials, in such malignant brain tumors. And we found that the success rate of the patients who are responding to the treatment is between 67 to 80 percent among these trials, which means that only 20 per cent to 33 percent of the patients do not have any proper response to the treatment.

"We already have long-term follow-up for some of these patients, including eight-year follow-up when the tumors disappeared and did not come back. We can say that we were able to not only decrease and eliminate these tumors, but also cure a number of patients from these tumors. We continue to have clinical trials in different types of malignant brain tumors. Currently, we have over 20 different clinical trials in the area of malignant brain tumors, and we are accepting the patients through such trials. If somebody is interested we can, of course, offer him the treatment, and then he can go back home and continue the treatment back home under the care of his doctor.

"The other areas where we have success is the treatment of non-Hodgkin's lymphoma. Certain kinds of non-Hodgkin's lymphoma respond well to chemotherapy and radiation. But we usually see the types which do not respond to these other treatment modalities, such as low grade lymphoma or cases of intermediate or high grade lymphoma, which already fail to respond to chemotherapy and radiation, including bone marrow transplantation. We already have a number of successful treatments in this area, and we are conducting a number of different clinical trials. We can accept patients who would like to be treated. We don't yet have statistics because we did not finish any of these clinical trials yet. We hope to have statistics in various lymphomas perhaps within the next six months.

"We see encouraging results in the treatment of cancers of gastrointestinal tract. Again, we see optimistic results in the treatment of pancreatic cancer, colon cancer, stomach cancer, and cancer of the esophagus. However, the number of cases is still too small to jump to a conclusion. We have clinical trials in each of these areas. Some of these patients are treated by simply taking capsules of antineoplastons. Some other patients are required to take intravenous infusions.

"Another exciting area is the treatment of kidney cancer and cancer of the bladder [although] the success rate is rather small. We have success in certain types of lung cancers, such as large cell type. The other type is non-small types, especially a large cell undifferentiated carcinoma of the lung. But in the other types of lung cancer, it still is hard to tell if you can successfully help these patients.

"In breast cancer, we have few clinical trials, and in certain cases we see successes. In other cases, we see failure. We still have problems when we have extensive liver involvement or lung involvement.

"In other types of cancers, we don't know whether we can have any success or not because the number of patients is too small. There are certain types of malignancies such as sarcomas, for instance, malignant melanoma, where we don't yet have sufficient numbers to come to a conclusion. And there are certain types of cancer where we know that we are not getting good results and we don't accept such patients. For instance, in acute leukemia in children, in Hodgkin's disease, in cancer of the testicles, we usually don't have good results, and we do not accept such patients to our program.

"Of course, there's still a lot to learn, and we hope that as time goes by we accumulate a lot of scientific data which we will prove in which types of cancer antineoplastons work best, and will also prove which types of cancers they don't work at all. It will take some time, but we are committed to continuing our research to have the best results possible."

The Clinic

Most of Dr. Burzynski's patients, during all phases of testing, are treated without being hospitalized. Checkups are conducted every day or every other day for the first two weeks and then less frequently depending on the improvement of the individual patient. The Burzynski Clinic in southwest Houston operates on an outpatient basis, with the average period of care ranging from six months to three years.

There are certain insurance companies that evaluated Dr. Burzynski's program and decided to cover practically every patient who is coming for the treatment. Conversely, there are certain insurance companies that do not pay for the Burzynski treatment. In most cases it depends on the patient's policy. Most of the patients who are coming to the Burzynski Research Institute are in very advanced stages of cancer; they've tried everything possible. Many of them are devastated by chemotherapy or radiation therapy. They may easily catch pneumonia or have bleeding or some other medical complications which require hospital admission. But according to Dr. Burzynski, the great majority of his patients can take treatment at home and can lead normal lives and go back to work and start it soon after they start treatment.

TYPES OF ANTINEOPLASTONS The antineoplastons which have been responsible for the dramatic results mentioned above are manufactured in Dr. Burzynski's plant in Stafford, Texas. According to Dr. Burzynski they are considered a form of chemotherapy since a chemotherapeutic agent is technically any "organized mixture of chemicals that fight a malignancy." However, they do not have the devastating side effects of the traditional class of chemotherapeutic drugs because they are formulations that are identical to proteins that are present in the body. Natural antineoplastons are small proteins isolated from human urine or blood. Synthetic antineoplastons are chemically identical to the natural proteins but are synthetically derived. Synthetics are easier and cheaper to manufacture and are even more efficacious in treating specific cancers such as brain and prostate cancer. Other cancers, though, respond better to the natural substances.

Dr. Burzynski uses a deliberately coordinated assortment of antineoplastons, both synthetic and natural, as the case requires. When he thinks it is appropriate, he refers patients for other types of treatment (chemotherapy, radiation, or surgery) to augment the antineoplaston injection or capsule therapy. While he has had little success with cancer of the testicles and childhood leukemia, he has had astounding results with brain tumors, malignant lymphomas, and cancer of the bladder and prostate.

Other groups have reproduced and are expanding Dr. Burzynski's preclinical work, including researchers at the Medical College of Georgia, the Imperial College of Science and Technology of London, the University of Kurume Medical School in Japan, the University of Turin Medical School in Italy, the Shandong Medical Academy in the People's Republic of China, and the Uniformed Services University of the Health Sciences in the U.S.

The front page of the July–August 1990 issue of *Oncology News* featured an article on antineoplastons, "a completely new type of anticancer agent that is nontoxic and seems to make malignant cancer cells revert to normal." The report was from Geneva, Switzerland, where the prestigious 9th International Symposium on Future Trends in Chemotherapy was held in March 1990. A special session was devoted to antineoplastons where seven papers were presented, including pre-clinical and clinical results by researchers from Japan, Poland, China, and the U.S.

Some of the most exciting preclinical research was reported by Dr. Dvorit Samid from the Uniformed Services University of Health Sciences in Bethesda. She reported that "Antineoplaston AS2-1 profoundly inhibits oncogene expression and the proliferation of malignant cells without exhibiting any toxicity toward normal cells." Dr. Samid explained that AS2-1 does not kill cancer cells, rather it reprograms them to behave like normal cells.

Clinical results of antineoplastons in patients with cancer refractory to other forms of therapy included reports of complete remissions from Japan and the U.S. in inoperable metastatic ovarian carcinoma and advanced stage prostate cancer, respectively.

ATTACKS FROM THE MEDICAL ESTABLISHMENT During the past several years, there have been efforts made by various medical agencies skeptical of the Burzynski treatment to get Dr. Burzynski's license revoked. In response to these efforts, Dr. Burzynski says, "The efforts against us are tremendous. And I did not expect, when I started this program, that I would be harassed mercilessly by the FDA and by some other agencies. Currently, we enjoy peace at the state level. Whatever battles we fought seem to be over. Our main problem now is with the FDA despite the fact that I am approved by the FDA to conduct so many clinical trials. Every patient seen by us is approved by the FDA. The FDA would like to put us out of business without any concern about what would happen to the patients. They are not really worried that the patients who are receiving treatment now will die if they put me out of business. I don't think that effort will succeed because we think and strongly believe that we are doing the right thing; we are saving the lives of many American people, and we will continue."

The Patients

EXAMPLE 1: Mavis once earned her living installing asbestos tiles. In 1970 she learned she had developed malignant mesothelioma—cancer resulting from exposure to asbestos. She was 27 years old.

Surgery was first performed at New York's Memorial Sloan-Kettering Hospital. Some of the tumors pervading her abdomen were removed, along with part of her colon. The operation brought relief but no guarantees and the cancer returned. In May 1979 Mavis underwent less than successful surgery at Methodist Hospital in Lubbock, Texas. More tumors were found, and the disease continued to spread. No conventional cancer treatments could help.

Six months later Mavis came to the Burzynski Institute. She was 36, weak and in intolerable pain. Treatment began with antineoplaston A. Within weeks she had no need for her steady diet of morphine and other drugs. The pain was gone.

Something was obviously going well, though her abdominal tumors were surprisingly unchanged. New treatment was tried with antineoplaston A2. This time more than the pain went away. By April 1980 Mavis was in partial remission from the cancer, with only a few tumors left, and those less than half their former size. By year's end no signs or symptoms of the cancer remained.

Mavis continued to take low-dose antineoplastons for a while, mostly as a precautionary tactic. Treatment stopped in March 1981. Close to a decade of "fatal" disease and pain had ended. Ten years later, she remained in complete remission.

EXAMPLE 2: Rebecca was a heavy smoker; in fact she still is. She is not therefore an ideal patient. Her case is not uncommon, though, and is instructive in that whatever success she has had could be amplified if she would stop smoking. Nonetheless, the lung, liver, and breast cancer she once suffered from is gone.

Rebecca became a patient at the Burzynski Institute in June 1980. She was then 56 years old. Radiation and chemotherapy had failed to arrest the malignant tumor in her lungs and the cancer spread into her lymph nodes and liver. Her Antineoplaston treatment began with intravenous injections of a synthetic preparation called AS2-5.

The results were quick and nearly miraculous. No signs of lung or liver cancer remained after only two months of treatment. Most doctors would expect a rapid return of Rebecca's type of lung cancer, especially because of its spread to the liver, but Rebecca was not a typical case. Her antineoplaston preparation was not typical either, just effective. She's been completely free from this cancer since the end of 1981.

A completely separate breast cancer was first detected in August 1981. A week later she underwent excision of a nodule in the left breast, and on September 11, 1981, she had a modified radical mastectomy for her breast cancer, which was still in its early stages. She was treated with antineoplaston A10 capsules from September 1982 until June 1983 to prevent recurrence of the breast cancer. As of March 1991, her breast, lung, and liver cancers still appeared to be clear.

EXAMPLE 3: Reuben was told by his doctor in March 1978 that his severe bladder tumor could probably be helped only with radiation treatment followed by surgery. He got an affirmative second opinion and underwent treatment.

Surgeons removed as much of the tumor as they could, but Reuben's symptoms became worse. By April he had arrived at the Burzynski Institute—age 47, weak, losing weight, and experiencing painful urination along with blood in the urine. He was given antineoplaston A by intramuscular injection.

Harmful symptoms went away in two weeks; the tumor was reduced to half its size within a month. Over the next year seven cystoscopies—screening procedures for the bladder or tumorous growths—revealed no return of the cancer. Examinations by two consulting specialists in urology supported this evidence, and the antineoplaston treatment was ended in September 1979.

Unfortunately, Reuben's nightmare was not over. Other less severe tumors appeared. Treatment began again in February of 1980, this time with antineoplaston A3. He was given injections daily, over a year's time they were gradually reduced to one a week.

In the end Reuben did triumph over his disease. His last treatment was in 1982.

EXAMPLE 4: Nick could have predicted he would develop cancer if family history was the predicting factor. He had lost two grandparents to the disease, his mother to stomach cancer, and his father to prostate cancer. His son, only 8 years old, had died of malignant cancer that started in the skeletal muscles.

In this case the tragic loss of a child may have helped save the life of the father. At age 39 Nick developed lymphoma, cancer that affects the body's tissue-cleansing fluids, white blood cells, and general circulatory system. His symptoms were widespread: extreme swelling in the legs and stomach; enlarged lymph nodes, liver, and spleen; and a damaging buildup of body fluids. Remembering the agony of his son's chemotherapy and radiation treatments, Nick turned instead to Dr. Burzynski.

Improvement was rapid after treatment began with A2 injections. The swelling was reduced, and fluids decreased in his abdomen. However, the most amazing result showed up a few months later: Nick's liver and spleen were almost back to normal just weeks after his liver had been so enlarged that two x-ray films had been necessary for a complete "photograph."

Nick felt good and returned to work part-time. Only one cancer remained: His lymph nodes still had signs of disease. When he examined the pathological reports on this body tissue, Dr. Burzynski found poor cell differentiation that had not been corrected by treatment. A combination of antineoplastons AS2-1 and A2 was tried on Nick with success. Lack of cancer and any related symptoms pointed to a full remission.

However, the struggle resumed the following year when cancer reappeared in the lymph nodes. Nick came to the Burzynski Institute in May and was responding well to antineoplastons when he fell into a behavior pattern that blocked his progress. He kept making decisions to start and then stop treatments; in addition, an addiction to the drug Dilaudid (hydromorphone) got in the way.

Nick had been on Dilaudid, a painkiller, before coming to the Burzynski Institute, and Dr. Burzynski kept him on it for a while afterward. Later, Nick obtained it illegally and abused it. This addiction led to his failure to maintain the recommended maintenance treatments and resulted in the development of pneumonia after Nick slept in the rain under the influence of drugs.

Despite these complications, treatment continued and a complete remission was finally achieved. Nick died six years later of pneumonia. According to his wife, medical reports showed no signs of recurrent malignant lymphoma.

Looking to the Future

Prevention is the focus of several studies Dr. Burzynski has undertaken. In one study, two groups of mice were exposed to the main cancer-causing agent from cigarette smoke. One group was given food containing an antineoplaston preparation; 80 percent of these mice avoided lung cancer. Among the group that was not given antineoplastons, 100 percent got the disease.

The next step in this research is to use antineoplastons as part of a preventive treatment among humans. Dr. Burzynski believes that this would best be done with apparently healthy individuals who have low levels of antineoplastons. Smokers may well benefit in this respect since they fit this requirement and are therefore prime candidates for cancer and so are in dire need of a preventive program.

The possibilities of Dr. Burzynski's "new medicine" appear endless. Antineoplastons correct (i.e., stop) cancer development in a way the body understands and easily tolerates. Even with phase I treatments, which aren't intended to produce maximum benefits, some patients have emerged cancer-free.

Of course, successful outcomes result from traditional approaches as well. Careful surgery can aid recovery, and chemotherapy has had particular success with rarer types of cancer such as Hodgkin's disease and childhood leukemia. The regrettable part is that these "answers" to cancer can also cause more harm.

Typical and devastating side effects accompany methods to which many patients never respond. Surgery and radiation can lead to serious damage to organs and tissues, and radiation and chemotherapy may drastically undermine the ability of the immune system to fight off even the simplest bacteria and toxins.

What Dr. Burzynski offers is an opportunity to use and strengthen the body's natural defense system. The need to explore and develop antineoplastons and other safe remedies will continue as long as people are exposed to air pollution, radiation, chemicals, ultraviolet rays, and the like.

40

Immuno-Augmentative Therapy (IAT)

The majority of patients arriving at the Immunology Research Center (IRC) in Freeport in the Grand Bahama Islands have been pronounced terminal by orthodox medicine. Many are crippled and unable to walk, others bloated beyond recognition with ascites, an abdominal fluid buildup that is a common symptom of malignant carcinomas. Some have been bedridden for long periods, others are mentally disoriented, and many are in such constant pain that the simplest outing is unthinkable. They come to receive the Immuno-Augmentative Therapy (IAT) developed by Dr. Lawrence Burton, a Ph.D. in zoology who also had a strong background in cancer research. The IRC in Freeport was opened by Dr. Burton in 1977, where he acted as director until his death in March of 1996. Since then, the center has been headed by Dr. John Clement, a British physician who is an internationally respected cancer specialist and who studied with Dr. Burton.

In 1983, Curry Hutchinson was one of Dr. Burton's patients. He recalls that after he had suffered four years from a malignant melanoma that had been partially "removed" from the middle of his back, his doctors and practically everyone else had given up on him. Mr. Hutchinson did not want to continue with traditional medical treatment after the surgery because he knew of too many people who had suffered miserably from chemotherapy and radiation. He investigated the possibility of several unorthodox therapies before deciding to try the Immuno-Augmentative Therapy of Dr. Burton.

His mother took him to the Bahamas as he stood at death's door. She "took me down there in a wheelchair," Hutchinson recalls. "I had about 90 pounds of body weight. I looked like the most pitiful survivor of Buchenwald you can imagine."

At first Dr. Burton was hesitant to treat someone so deteriorated, but finally he relented.

Hutchinson remained bedridden for the first two months there, but then he became strong enough to get up and around and even went to the grocery store. "It is hard to imagine," he remarked, "what a thrill it is to walk into a grocery store when you have not been out of bed for a year. It's like going to Disney World. My mother went home. I started taking care of myself, preparing my meals, and went on with it, slowly but surely." He is still up and around and reports feeling well to this day.

What is going on at the IRC that makes it a fortress of hope for so many cancer "immigrants," most of them outcasts deemed hopeless by established medicine? On Grand Bahama Island, the IRC has taken in people considered doomed. Many are still alive, long after the terminal prognoses given by their traditional physicians and oncologists have come and gone. Others have died but were enabled to survive longer than anyone had imagined possible. Many now lead happy, fruitful lives with much less pain than they had come to accept as an inevitable accompaniment of illness.

Not everyone can be accepted for treatment, unfortunately. Dr. Clement and his staff must first be reasonably sure the treatment they offer is the right thing for the prospective patient's condition. For those patients who are accepted, however, something new appears: a restoration of hope. Many of these patients were told previously that they were dead, and all had life-threatening cancer. The center holds out a small but significant promise to them.

In an interview given prior to his death in early 1993, Dr. Burton was quick to note that IAT "is not by any means a cure for cancer." However, he also relates how "cancer patients who have been treated with IAT... often respond with cessation of tumor growth and, in some instances, with no tumor growth. In many there is actual reversal as well as necrosis [complete stoppage] of the cancer growth."

The Discovery: Dr. Lawrence Burton

The man who made such startling progress in the treatment of cancer had a long career in research. Dr. Lawrence Burton decided to go into cancer research after seeing "firsthand the many horrors of cancer" while assigned as a pharmacist's mate to the U.S. Navy's Cancer Center at Brooklyn Naval Hospital in 1944. In those days, he recalled "the accepted procedure for cancer treatment was radical surgery. If you had a cancer of the foot, the leg was removed at the hip."

After World War II, Burton studied genetics, cancer etiology (the cause of cancer), oncolysis (destruction of cancer cells), and immunology. This culminated in his receiving a Ph.D. in experimental zoology from New York

University in 1955. "My training and experience are classically those of a medical researcher," he said.

After graduation in 1955, Dr. Burton became a research associate at the California Institute of Technology and began to publish the results of his work in leading scientific journals such as *Cancer Research*. Back in New York, he became a research associate at New York University in 1957, moving up to become an associate in oncology in 1966 at St. Vincent's Hospital, a noted teaching hospital. In 1966 he became a senior investigator and oncologist at the cancer research unit while still at St. Vincent's.

Immuno-Augmentative Therapy has its roots in this period of Burton's career. In 1959, Burton and a team of cancer researchers accidentally discovered a tumor-inhibiting factor that reduced or eliminated cancer in a special breed of leukemic mice. Their research progressed well enough so that in the November 1962 issue of *Transactions of the New York Academy of Sciences* they reported on certain natural substances that were capable of causing remission in over 50 percent of the leukemic mice treated.

In the fall of 1965, Patrick McGrady, Sr., science editor for the American Cancer Society (ACS), observed Dr. Burton's experiments and was amazed. In a radio interview, McGrady told my audience, "they injected the mice and the lumps went down before your eyes—something I never believed possible."

McGrady had Dr. Burton and his associate, Dr. Friedman, also with a Ph.D. in zoology, repeat the experiment at the ACS's 1966 Science Writers Seminar. The two doctors, in the presence of 70 scientists and 200 science writers, injected mice having mammary cancer with the serum they had isolated during their research. An hour and a half later, the tumors had disappeared almost completely.

The next day, the results of these experiments received front-page coverage throughout the world. *The Los Angeles Herald Examiner*'s headline read "Fifteen Minute Cancer Cure for Mice: Humans Next?"

Unfortunately, this enthusiastic publicity backfired. As Dr. Burton recalled, "This caused a misleading specter of 'cure' to which no researcher would ever dare lay claim..." Furthermore, when word about the experiments spread throughout the medical community, many traditionally trained physicians questioned their validity, suggesting that the results had been accomplished by trickery.

In September of the same year, Drs. Burton and Friedman were invited to repeat the experiment before the New York Academy of Medicine. This time, in order to avoid accusations of fraud, they had the mice selected by independent oncologists and pathologists. Again, an hour or so after injections with the newly isolated tumor-inhibiting factors, the tumors started to disintegrate. However, there was still little interest in the efficacy of the tumor-inhibiting factors.

During 1970 and 1971, Drs. Burton and Friedman were assisting Dr. Antonio Rottino, a medical doctor on the cancer research team, in treating his cancer patients at St. Vincent's with their antitumor serums. In 1972, however, Dr. Rottino announced that the treatment had to cease. The IAT treatments were considered experimental and therefore unproven and so were not appropriate to use in providing regular medical care.

Also in the early 1970s, Long Island psychologist Martin Goldstone's wife was being treated with the Burton-Friedman technique. She had enjoyed such promising results that when they learned that the treatments had been stopped at St. Vincent's she and her husband and other prominent people in their Great Neck, Long Island, community raised enough funds to establish the Immunology Research Foundation to continue the work of the two doctors.

In 1975 *New York* magazine published an article on the work of Burton and Friedman entitled "The Politics of Cancer—Why Won't the Medical Establishment Pay Attention to These Two Men?" The article drew considerable public attention and inquiry. Senator Howard Metzenbaum of Ohio, whose wife had just died of cancer, wrote a letter to the NCI demanding to know why the public was being kept in the dark about this treatment. He was informed that the NCI was of the opinion that the Burton-Friedman work was nothing new, couldn't possibly be effective, and was therefore not worthy of further investigation or testing.

Perhaps the most important result of the article was that after extensively investigating Drs. Burton and Friedman, Champion International, a philanthropic organization interested in alternative medical therapies, decided to fund the two men's work. Champion International's patronage became all-important three years later, when Dr. Burton decided to relocate his clinic.

The Therapy

The Immunology Research Center moved from Great Neck, New York, to Freeport on Grand Bahama Island in 1977. Since then, over 2,500 terminally ill cancer patients have undergone treatment there. According to Dr. Burton, 50 to 60 percent of these patients experience tumor reduction. Many are able to resume normal lives; frequently they survive five years and more beyond the initial diagnosis (usually made by a traditional attending physician prior to Burton's involvement in the case) of cancer. The five-year survival period is sufficient for the American Cancer Society and the National Cancer Institute to consider a patient cured.

I have visited the IRC on a number of occasions and have analyzed the records of many of Dr. Burton's and Dr. Clement's patients. This investigation has confirmed the remarkable success that IAT continues to have on a regular basis. In sharp contrast to the depressing environment of most cancer hospitals in this country, the attitude of patients at the IRC is one of optimism and hope. Most patients are off drugs and free of pain and report that they feel well. Perhaps the most telling endorsement comes from the family members of non-surviving patients who have continued to support the clinic with financial contributions and moral backing.

Dr. Burton did not believe that we should use the word "cure" in relation to cancer. "Immuno-Augmentative Therapy," he explained, "augments the immune system and enables it to control and combat cancer." But it does not totally eradicate cancer. No therapy does that. Cancer patients, no matter how long the cancer is under control, must always be watchful of their condition to be sure that the cancer does not begin growing again or growing somewhere else. Cancer is not a localized condition but a systemic disease. While it may clear up in one organ, it may flare up in another.

INJECTING BLOOD PROTEINS Immuno-Augmentative Therapy consists of injections of four blood proteins that Dr. Burton discovered and was able to isolate. These proteins are essentially responsible for the control and even shrinkage of tumors. When injected in the proper amounts and at proper intervals, they can help the weakened body do what it would do normally: control the growth and proliferation of cancerous cells.

Dr. Lawrence Burton believed that cancer is primarily a matter of immune impairments. When the immune system is working properly, the cancer cells that occur are quickly arrested and disposed of.

Two questions arise from this explanation. *What exactly are cancer cells? And what causes an immune system to be impaired to the extent that the body can no longer defend itself against them?*

The body's cells are constantly dividing as a normal part of the living and growing process. Each cell has two sets of chromosomes and a single nucleus. For a healthy cell to reproduce, the sets of chromosomes bearing the unique genetic information that makes the cell what it is split and form four sets of chromosomes, while the nucleus splits into two. The single cell then divides into two—a process called mitosis—so that there are two cells instead of one, each with a single nucleus bearing two sets of chromosomes with the same genetic code. This is an endless life process that occurs thousands of times every moment. Dr. Burton's theory posits that approximately 1 out of every 10,000 such cell divisions is endomitotic, or abnormal. In these instances, the cell begins as usual by separating into four sets of chromosomes and forming two nuclei. The problem begins when these nuclei become encased in a single cytoplasmic mold, thereby forming a single cell with a double nucleus and four sets of chromosomes each. This single cell is called a supercell, or neoplaston. It is a cancer cell, usually recognized as being abnormal by the healthy body, which proceeds to destroy it.

This leads to the second question. In cases of cancer, what causes the lapse in the body's immune system that allows the proliferation of these supercells? What allows or causes a person to become vulnerable to the ravages of cancer? Dr. Burton believed that the immune system is overtaxed by the presence of intruders such as viruses, bacteria, and toxins, but he also believes that the greatest damage is done by a person's inability to cope adequately with stress. Although he had not done scientific studies to verify this belief, he was convinced from observation of cancer patients in his care that the damaging effects of stress and negativity are the chief cause of dysfunction within the immune mechanism. According to Dr. Burton, the overly stressed body "stops making antibodies, stops making alpha-macroglobulin, the deblocking protein. Without enough antibodies to attack cancer cells and without enough deblocking protein to restart the process once the waste products of tumor cell destruction are cleared, the cancer grows unchecked. That, I think, is the 'cause' of cancer."

If cancer is indeed caused by stress and other suppressants to the immune system in general and if its occurrence is in the form of abnormal cells that may grow rapidly throughout the body or within specific locales, one is brought back to the matter of how to control this abnormal growth and proliferation. Endomitotic cell division can occur at any time, producing a primary tumor or metastasis. A primary tumor is one where the cancer develops at a particular site; metastases are abnormal cells that have migrated away from the primary tumor and resettled elsewhere in the body. "But," Dr. Burton explained, "it does not matter what the primary [tumor] is: cancer is an affliction of the immune mechanism. When the four proteins of the immune mechanism are operating properly, they can shrink the tumor whether it is primary or metastatic."

Of the four proteins discovered and isolated by Dr. Burton, one is a tumor antibody that can destroy tumors; another is an antibody complement that stimulates the tumor antibody. Without the stimulation from the complement, the antibody will remain inactive. The other two proteins have a direct effect on the destruction of tumors: The "blocking" protein inhibits the antibody to give the body a chance to clear away the toxic waste of tumor destruction; otherwise the body would go into toxic shock. The blocking protein is itself then inhibited by an antiblocking protein. When the blocking protein is prevalent, the antibody and tumor complement are prevented from attacking tumors, which therefore may grow; when the antiblocking protein is prevalent, the blocking protein is held in check, enabling the tumor antibody and complement to actively seek and destroy cancerous cells.

AUGMENTING THE IMMUNE MECHANISM Dr. Burton applied his discovery of blood fractions to create a harmonious balance in the patient's internal chemistry. Once this balance has been established, the patient's body is able to defend itself naturally against the continued proliferation of cancer cells and frequently is able to attack and begin to reduce existing tumors. Dr. Burton's therapy does not attempt to shrink a tumor directly or intervene in the growth of a cancer. It is designed only to "augment an immune mechanism in the patient." The stimulated immune mechanism itself is then responsible for attacking the tumor.

IAT therapy involves two separate stages. The antibody, antibody complement, and antiblocking proteins help the body fight cancer. Every time a tumor cell is destroyed by these three proteins, the fourth one—the blocking protein—is released to inhibit further destruction of the tumor. The role of the protein, as noted above, is not to protect the tumor but to give "the liver a chance to eliminate the waste by-products of cell destruction." The blocking protein actually helps the body recover from the toxic shock caused by killed cancer cells. It plays a vital role not in the actual destruction of cancer but in the body's ability to recover afterward.

IAT involves a careful consideration of the alternating roles of tumor destruction, on the one hand, and the body's recovery from toxic breakdown, on the other hand. The timing of these two processes is all-important. While the blocking protein is eventually deblocked by the antiblocking protein, this process may take too long. During therapy a decision must be made as to when and how aggressively to intervene in this process. The body—especially the liver—must be protected from the toxic waste of the destroyed cancer cells, but it must at the same time be protected from the ravages of the tumor. The attending physician has to decide when the blocking process has given the body enough recovery time. The system is then deblocked by the intravenous introduction of specific amounts of the antiblocking protein, and the cancer destruction continues. The immune mechanism may be bolstered further by the injection of the tumor antibody and tumor complement.

The timing and the quantities of protein introduced are the critical issues. As Dr. Burton explained, "In time, the patient's own body deblocks the system [enabling cancer destruction to be resumed]. But if there is a large amount of tumor, we cannot wait indefinitely while the process is repeated. The patient has a limit. He or she can produce only so much antibody and so much deblocking protein. Thus we have to augment these proteins—once a day, twice a day, as many as six to eight times a day. If the augmentation is done properly, we can produce, to quote the National Cancer Institute, many, many 'spontaneous remissions.'"

However, in a recent interview, Dr. John Clement noted that despite the progress that has been made with numerous cancer patients at the center, success rates are still relative at IRC. He says, "The majority of the patients coming here are already pronounced as terminally ill. We can produce almost invariably some slowing down or even stopping of the cancerous process. And we have been lucky, of course, in a number of patients, we've been able to prevent the cancer, cause a regression. We do not like to use the word cure because even though we may stop the process going on you have to realize that if you've got cancer once you're still the same person and you're likely to get cancer again. You still have the same immune system. You still have the same genetic background. And you are likely to get a recurrence.

"I think it's interesting to note that in the general treatment of cancer if you survive for six years and have no symptoms you're declared cured. You may get a recurrence a year later, but that's called a new cancer."

The Clinic

Ms. Elaine Boise, whose husband, Jack, died in 1985 after more than half a year of treatment at the IRC, talks about pictures she has that remind her of Jack's final months in the Bahamas: "pictures that have surprised doctors... pictures that showed him outdoors, singing, playing the guitar, sailing on a yacht, playing a slot machine at a casino." She recalls "Jack driving a car, going Christmas shopping with me, having dinner out several times in Freeport restaurants."

This is not what most people think of when they are told someone is dying of cancer. They expect instead the kind of person Jack was when he first arrived in Freeport, when none of those activities was possible for him, since he was heavily drugged, sedated, and in a wheelchair. Ms. Boise and her children were amazed by Jack's rapid physical improvement. "It was enough," she recounts, "for us to know that Burton's approach to killing tumors by augmenting the immune system is a valid one clinically, and it is one that should be pursued further."

Perhaps the most remarkable thing about the treatment program of the IRC is that it is essentially nontoxic and noninvasive, unlike chemotherapy, radiation, and surgery, which are either toxic or invasive or both. Chemotherapy, for instance, essentially poisons the body in order to kill the tumor. It is toxic because it introduces a poison into the body, and it is invasive because the poison aggressively invades the cells and tissues of the body. The problem is that the poison is indiscriminate. It kills not only cancerous cells but healthy ones as well. In fact, its invasion of the body is systemic (total), not local, and therefore seriously damages the immune system. It is because of such invasive and/or toxic therapies that cancer is associated with horrible pain and sickness, hair and memory loss, and a generally miserable life.

IRC patients frequently avoided these side effects because IAT uses substances (blood fractions) that occur naturally in the body to bolster the immune system. One patient, Dr. Phil Kunderman, discussing his experience with cancer, explains: "I was so impressed [with IAT], since it seemed such a logical approach. I also was particularly impressed because it had no deleterious side effects, in contrast to radiation therapy and chemotherapy, both of which modalities I had turned down because my own experience as a surgeon proved that these measures were, in an advanced disease at least, [not] all that great."

Dr. Kunderman's story is particularly interesting because he was a leading cancer specialist at the time his cancer was diagnosed. In 1979 he discovered that he had prostate cancer and that it had spread to his bones, particularly the sternum and shoulder, rendering the cancer essentially inoperable. Surgery could do no more than relieve his obstructive symptoms. He had the surgery, but he was told that his prognosis was only one to three years survival.

Dr. Kunderman began therapy at the IRC in 1980. Six years later he reported that he was doing very well and admitted being, "just amazed" by the success Dr. Burton achieved with cancers usually considered hopeless. "For instance," he says, "I know of carcinoma of the pancreas, which in my experience was such a lethal, terrible carcinoma, with remission for as long as 8 or 9 years [as a result of IAT therapy]. In carcinoma of the larynx, the young woman [treated by Dr. Burton] is at least 10 years postlaryngeal. These were such horrible cancers that we never seemed to be able to control; the prognosis was so very bad, and the life span was so short thereafter."

Dr. Kunderman recalls Dr. Burton's associate showing "an x-ray one day of a chest and asking, 'What do you think of that film?'"

"I said, 'Well, it's certainly a big cancer of the left lower lobe, and there is nothing you can offer this patient surgically or by any means.'"

"Then he showed me another film. It was completely clear. He had been on therapy for seven or eight months...."

"I said, 'Well, is this before or after therapy?'"

"He said, 'This is after therapy.'"

"It was an amazing thing. I had never encountered anything like it."

ENTRY GUIDELINES FOR PROSPECTIVE PATIENTS Many people would like to be treated at IRC, but unfortunately, not everyone falls within the entry guidelines set up for prospective patients. During a congressional hearing in 1986, Dr. Clement, now head of the IRC, outlined the criteria for accepting patients at the center:

1. Does the patient have a confirmed diagnosis of cancer?

2. Is the type of cancer one that the clinic has treated successfully in the past?

3. Is the type of cancer one that cannot successfully be treated by other methods?

4. Is the condition one which has failed to be helped with other treatments?

If a patient's condition can be successfully treated by surgery alone, we strongly advise that the surgery be performed. If it is something which can be treated successfully by orthodox therapy, we would not accept the patient. However, if the patient has personally refused orthodox therapy but has a confirmed diagnosis of cancer, he or she may be accepted.

Patients who are accepted are attended by a staff of four medical doctors, two registered nurses, and about 10 laboratory assistants. The nurses collect the medical records the patients have brought with them, try to appraise their general attitudes toward their situation, and then draw blood for the initial immunocompetency test. The clinic's procedures are then explained carefully and in detail to the patients before they are released to meet the attending physician.

STAGES OF TREAMENT Dr. Burton explained the initial stages of treatment from this point on: "When patients get here, we take their blood to test for AIDS and hepatitis, and we use our own tests to see whether their immune systems are functioning. Then they have an interview with one of the four M.D.s. Part of the reason for this is to make sure they are not phony. So far, the ACS has sent three fakes, which the doctors picked up. The ACS and NCI always say that we just want to take the money and run.

"After that, I talk with one of the M.D.s to decide whether to take each patient. Does the patient have a chance [to get better with IAT] or not? If there is no chance, they go home. We don't win any prizes for just taking patients.

"The first three days, they are treated with subefficacious doses [amounts designed only to test a reaction to the substance]. The first day, we give one-fifth of the effective dose. On the next day, if the immune system is working and the patient is killing the tumor, that means the immune mechanism has recognized the proteins in the serum and used them as a signal to begin functioning.

"On day two, one of the proteins is elevated to the effective dose. We do this in stages to determine whether the patient is allergic to any of the individual proteins. Although we have never had a case of this, if there were an allergy we would want to know which protein was the allergen."

If the patient responds well to the increased dosage of one protein, his or her immune system should be elevating one of the two proteins to the effective dose by itself. The next day, two of the proteins are increased to the effective dose and, "if that patient then supplies the amount of the third protein, this is a patient who will probably be able to stop the shots fairly soon, because his or her immune mechanism is good enough that he or she shouldn't have gotten cancer to begin with," said Dr. Burton.

"After the third day," he continued, "the patient gets into another program using the computer, which determines the appropriate doses the patient should receive of each of the three proteins. If the patient has a very high tumor kill, he or she will get only one augmentation. Then, as the tumor goes down, the patient will get two, three, or four augmentations depending on which protein is elevated in the blood and how much of the tumor is being killed. If the patient's immune mechanism is not responding to the augmentations within a couple of days, we will take more a.m. and p.m. blood samples to see if we can spot something wrong.

"The doctors meanwhile test the tumors by x-ray and by palpation. If the tumor begins to soften and shrink, the case is put back in my lap. When the immune mechanism is stable enough that I think the patient can make it, the patient goes home."

At home, the, patient is self-treated. This does not present a problem since these patients are taught early on to inject themselves, using disposable diabetes syringes. Every six months or so, such patients return to the clinic for a week's follow-up to determine whether alterations in the serum are required. Does the patient need more tumor complement and less blocking protein, for instance? If the tumor is breaking down too fast and creating high levels of toxicity, the blocking protein may be increased instead.

The Results

Dr. Burton had particular success with mesothelioma and metastatic colon cancer, two supposedly "incurable" cancers.

MESOTHELIOMA Mesothelioma, or "asbestos cancer," typically attacks the lungs (the pleural cavity), sometimes the stomach (peritoneal cavity), and occasionally the heart (pericardial cavity). It is characterized by a number of tiny tumors initially resembling shotgun pellets that spread and grow rapidly. There is no treatment for mesothelioma according to an NCI treatise on the subject, only pain management. The survival rate is 0. The prognosis is only 2 to 10 months' survival.

The use of asbestos in building has decreased sharply because of the associated health risks. Nonetheless, the treatment of mesothelioma will continue to be a major health priority for many years because of the unusually long latency period of asbestos cancer.

There are no known survivors of mesothelioma in the traditional medical health care system. Dr. Kunderman, a board-certified surgeon, has had considerable experience with this disease since his office was located near Johns Mansville, the asbestos producer. He was eventually afflicted with the cancer himself and chose to place himself under Dr. Burton's care. As mentioned earlier, Dr. Kunderman recovered after being diagnosed as terminal.

It is no wonder that Dr. Kunderman left the United States to seek a nontraditional therapy in the Caribbean. Even though he is a traditional physician, he admits that "our experience with mesothelioma was so horrendously poor. We just threw up our hands toward the end of my years of practice with mesothelioma; we had tried everything, including such radical surgery as removing a whole lung and removing all of the pleura, but still these tumors recurred."

Dr. Burton reported that the average survival rate of his mesothelioma patients was already 47 to 48 months, and a number of survivors are currently residing at the clinic. Some have been released and now live normal lives since, "in contrast to other types of cancer, once you get rid of all tumor cells containing asbestos, the patient is safe," said Dr. Burton. This is due partly to the fact the mesothelioma is strictly an environmental disease and is in no way genetic.

Eleven IRC peritoneal mesothelioma patients were the subjects of a report published in the early 1990s by Drs. Burton and Clement. They had suffered such physical defects as abdominal distension, obstruction, and ascites. The four women and seven men had an immune profile typical of advanced cancer populations: elevated levels of blocking proteins and suppressed levels of deblocking protein and tumor complement. All were "augmented" with injections of immunoglobulin serum antibodies and deblocking protein. The results of the study were as follows:

"Four males and one female are alive, with survival among the five ranging from 22 to 80 months. The mean survival for those living is 43 months, and the median is 52 months. Of the other six cases, mean survival was 23 months and the median was 16 months, with a range of 7 to 50 months. The total subject population represented mean (or average) survival of 35 months and a median survival of 30 months, with a range for all cases from 7 to 80 months."

Dr. Burton's mean survival and survival range results can be compared with those obtained by other researchers working with peritoneal mesothelioma patients who had undergone traditional medical therapies. In 1957 four patients studied had an average survival of 12 months, with a range from 1 to 26 months. A 1960 study showed 12 patients with an average survival of 18 months; survival among these patients ranged from 1 to 60 months. Twenty-one patients surveyed in 1965 had an average survival of 15 months, 45 patients studied in 1972 had an average survival of 6 months, and 68 patients studied in 1974 had an average survival of 9.5 months. Finally, a 1979 study conducted by the University of Missouri dealt with eight patients who had an average survival of 7 months and a survival range from 9 days to 16 months. Clearly, IAT achieves survival rates two to three times those of traditional therapies.

Dr. Kunderman has become convinced "that this approach to the control of cancer in far advanced disease is the right approach in terms of what we know about cancer right now." He spoke of IAT "to a number of my colleagues back home, and they know nothing about it." His surprise is clearly justified: "It just shows how little we out in the field know about this particular type of therapy." He himself was a leading practitioner in the cancer field and had never heard of Dr. Burton until he became a patient himself.

METASTATIC COLON CANCER Dr. Burton had equal success in treating metastatic colon cancer. He noted that "Dr. DeVita, director of the NCI, announced on television around December 1984 that the five-year survival rate for metastatic cancer of the colon is zero. This means that nobody under traditional treatment survived five years. But we have over 10 patients [who have metastatic cancer of the liver] who have lived past the five-year mark and are still alive today."

One of those surviving patients is Robert Beasley, who was diagnosed with colon-to-liver cancer (meaning that the cancer metastasized—traveled—from the site of the primary tumor, the colon, to a remote site, the liver). Beasley says that his doctor "not only could tell I had liver trouble, he could hold the tumors in his hand. That's how bad it was. So he sewed me up and he said, "Take him home. I will not offer him chemo. He has three months to live." Eleven years later, after being treated for this condition by Dr. Burton, Beasley reported that he was in perfect health.

Dorothy Strait is another survivor of colon-to-liver cancer. When she was diagnosed, her surgeon told her that her case was hopeless. Having seen and biopsied her liver metastases and having viewed her liver scans, he gave her a prognosis of three months of survival or less. After being treated by Dr. Burton for a few months, she returned to her surgeon, who was surprised to find no trace of the tumor in her body. Twelve years after the original diagnosis, she was still alive and healthy.

There are many other cases of metastatic carcinoma survivors among IRC patients, with some patients living 7 to 10 years after having received prognoses of less than 12 months' survival. But the traditional physicians who are informed of these drastic turnarounds in their former patients frequently write them off as "spontaneous remissions" rather than giving credit to the "unproven" therapy of immune augmentation. Still, neither the NCI nor the ACS has been able to explain why their "spontaneous remission" rate is zero while that of the IRC is about 1 out of every 10 patients. Dr. Kunderman observes: "That is always the point that is brought up. But in all my years of practice and hundreds of cases of cancer, those remissions in advanced cases have been [so rare that] it's with difficulty that I can recall any.

"So when somebody speaks about spontaneous remission, it's almost like saying, 'Well, it's a miracle.'…I am sure that it happens but I think the cases are few and far between."

OTHER TYPES OF CANCER Commenting on the IRC's success rate in a recent interview, Dr. Clement puts forth the idea that success rates with cancer patients are all relative and vary from one type of cancer to another. He explains, "We have had a lot of luck with colorectal cancers, particularly Duke's grade C. General doctors don't know whether to treat them with chemotherapy or not. We have had good results with that. We have had good results with early prostate cancers, preventing the rather unpleasant use of testosterone depressants or suppressants. Breast cancers, in general, we have varying luck with.

"And the ones we don't have luck with are the ones which grow very, very fast. These are the small cell cancer of the lung, which is typically the smoker's cancer, which has a doubling rate of 30 days, and we just don't have enough time to catch up with that. And the glioblastoma multiformi, which is the worst of the astrocytomas or brain tumors. We don't have much luck with those."

IAT Under Attack

Despite its successful pioneering work in cancer treatment, the Immunology Research Center came under attack from the traditional medical establishment in 1985. The ACS and NCI regard cancer "cure" as their exclusive province, heavily supported by public funding. Many outside efforts were regarded as intrusions and trespasses, and when they departed significantly from traditional treatment approaches, they were suspected of being quackery.

The American cancer establishment finally convinced the Bahamian government that Dr. Burton's Immuno-Augmentative Therapy (IAT) might have involved the use of contaminated blood. The clinic was forced to close on July 17, 1985, but was reopened the following spring after investigation proved that these allegations could not be substantiated. While the clinic was closed, a group of Dr. Burton's patients formed an association dedicated to reopening the IRC. Since most of these patients were Americans, they sought the assistance of the U.S. Congress. A congressional hearing on the matter was conducted in January 1986 by Representative Guy Molinari for the purpose of fact-finding and to make these complaints public. During the hearing, many members of the patient association had a chance to tell the public about their personal experiences at the IRC.

PATIENTS TELL THEIR STORIES TO CONGRESS One of the witnesses was Sherry Costaldo, who was diagnosed as having breast cancer in 1978 at the age of 28 after many doctors had dismissed her, insisting that she wasn't sick. She underwent a radical mastectomy at Memorial Sloan-Kettering and then five weeks of daily radiation and 19 months of chemotherapy, which she was told at the time was only experimental. She recalls that "I was not told that beforehand." Subsequent radiation treatments continued on a regular basis before she suffered a massive seizure on May 31, 1983, resulting from the spreading of her cancer into the brain.

Displeased with what she had come to learn was experimental treatment at Sloan-Kettering, she went to Nassau Medical Center. There she underwent surgery to remove a brain tumor and then endured five more weeks of radiation treatment while she was on Dilantin (phenytoin) and prednisone. She remembers being "extremely ill from the treatment and medication, and seizures occurred periodically." She was "almost always dizzy, disoriented and nauseous, and very ill." She was told she might go on to chemotherapy administered through a shunt in her skull or through the spine, but she would have to suffer even greater pain, and the results were not guaranteed. She returned to Sloan-Kettering, where her ovaries were surgically removed (oophorectomy) in the hope that once estrogen production was stopped, tumor growth might be halted. But on February 10, 1984, a brain scan confirmed that four tumors were lodged in her brain. Her oncologist told her that nothing more could be done. On April 28, 1984, she headed for Freeport and Dr. Burton's IRC, which she had heard was helping many cancer patients.

Although her husband was vehemently opposed to her being treated by Dr. Burton, she underwent IAT therapy for 14 weeks. During that time she was able to get off prednisone completely and eventually found herself "swimming, walking with confidence, and able to take care of my family and myself." She noted her progress from that point on during the congressional hearings: "The improvement has been almost unbelievable, and I am now living a fairly normal life.

"I have taken aerobic dancing, organized and directed a children's choir, and seldom need to rest. I run circles around my husband.

"On May 17, 1985, I repeated the neuromagnetic resonance [brain] scan. My neurologist and I compared the 1984 scan and the 1985 scan; there was no trace of the four lesions, and much of the scar tissue from the massive tumor had depleted."

Ms. Costaldo's neurologist was skeptical about IAT but was both "thrilled and amazed" to see how her health had turned completely around. And Sherry is equally thrilled that IAT not only "saved or extended my life" but accomplished this "without destroying the quality of my life." When the oncologist from Sloan-Kettering contacted her to ask if he could use her recovery as one of his success stories, he was surprised to learn that she had been on IAT. "Oh, my, you mean I am going to have to give Dr. Burton credit for this?" he quipped.

Mary Yevchak began treatment at the IRC in the spring of 1984, only months after being diagnosed as having a large-cell lymphoma of the right lung. Ms. Yevchak had found her traditional medical treatment psychologically distressing as well as ineffective and painful.

"When they started intravenous chemotherapy, my family was told to leave the room," she states. "This was against my wishes because it was such a difficult time for me. The nurses who administered the chemotherapy proceeded to tell me about all the side effects. It would cause hair loss, and I would become sterile. This was especially traumatic to me since I had just been married two years and was looking forward to starting a family. This procedure continued for eight full days around the clock."

She was released in February, but further complications set in the next day. She was put on a combined chemotherapy-radiation program to reduce severe swelling in her head and neck. She soon found it painful to swallow, developed bacterial pneumonia, and was bloated beyond recognition by the large does of steroids that were introduced to offset the radiation damage. During her treatment, Ms. Yevchak was told by her doctor that the "chemotherapy had very little effect, if any, on the cancer," and the radiation, while it did reduce the tumor somewhat, was extremely damaging. During her hospital treatment she was taking 14 oral medications a day, was bloated to nearly 200 pounds, and was completely bedridden. She had already given up when she learned of Dr. Burton's treatment center in the Bahamas. She says, "I was apprehensive at first, but my fears left as I could see a gradual improvement in my appearance and general condition.

"I was immediately taken off steroids, and the bloating started to subside. I became stronger and enjoyed walking short distances for the first time in months, since I was bed- and wheelchair-bound at the time.

"As time went on, I enjoyed more activities, and my outlook on life improved. I was there a total of two months and returned home to continue my daily injections at home. Two weeks later I returned to my job as a schoolteacher and secretary on a full-time basis.

"I visited my oncologist... who gave me a thorough examination, and he could find no trace of the disease, even though he had told me previously that without chemotherapy the disease would spread and tumors would grow throughout my body. It would then be too late for any treatment at all. He also advised me at the time that I had less than a 2 percent chance of living x months....

"At the last visit he could find no evidence of the cancerous condition and stated that it may have been a misdiagnosis; that it could have been a thymoma instead of lymphoma, which is a much less serious condition."

According to Ms. Yevchak, when she told her oncologist that she was going to see Dr. Burton, he stated, "The guy is a quack. He is not going to hurt you, it's only blood fractions, but the rest will do you good. Go down there and have a good time." Says Ms. Yevchak, "He thought I was going to have a nice vacation and come back and die." When she returned and walked into the oncologist's office, Ms. Yevchak quotes him as saying, "Oh, I am in trouble."

Kate Banner was diagnosed with malignant cancer in 1977, with a third of the lymph glands in the lower portion of her colon affected. "So they [the doctors] just did not think that I had too much time," she recalls. Unwilling to suffer through chemotherapy, she insisted, "Keep me comfortable and I will take it from there." She opted for IAT treatment and reported feeling fine at the congressional hearing in 1986. In fact, when she returned home for adhesion surgery, her doctors could not find any sign of the cancer that had threatened her life in 1977. The way Kate Banner sees it, "They have been in my belly, and they can't find any cancer. I think I will stick with Burton."

Living with Cancer, Not Dying of It

Besides IAT's effectiveness against cancer, "Dr. Burton's clinic also provided an ambiance" to Elaine Boise and her family, including her husband, Jack, who did not survive his bout with cancer. She recalls that the clinic "encouraged the most intimate, emotional, psychological, philosophical, and spiritual exchanges between us and among us and our four children, with the result that we are newly bonded now.

"Does it matter, then, that the seven months we spent fighting for our lives in the Bahamas are now counted among the best experiences of my life? It matters. It matters very much....

"The strength and wisdom—that—we could never have obtained through conventional medical treatment. Essentially, at the Immunology Research Center we were not dying of cancer, as we had been at home. We were living it, with many other people. And we savored life with an intensity and a passion that we had not known before, which would have been impossible in an orthodox hospital setting.

"This was the gift, the gift of life that Dr. Burton gave us. Our children and I will be forever grateful."

41

The Whole-Body ("Ganzheit") Approach

The operation to be done that morning at the Maria Hilf Hospital in Mönchengladbach, Germany, in 1931, was routine. The head surgeon, Dr. Sickmann, would perform a mastectomy in the hope of saving a young woman from breast cancer. The operation was nothing out of the ordinary in those days, yet two lives would be changed forever.

The Discovery: Dr. Joseph Issels

Dr. Josef Issels, who had just begun an internship in surgery at the hospital, assisted, first with professional interest and then with growing horror. "The breast was truly a thing of beauty," he was to write in a letter cited in Gordon Thomas' book, *Dr. Issels and His Revolutionary Cancer Treatment* (Peter H. Wyden, New York, 1973), "perfectly formed with the nipple glistening from swabbing with antiseptic.

"Satisfied that everything was positioned properly, Sickmann started to cut. A line of spurting blood marked the progress of his knife. He kept on staring intently at the incision area. I wiped the area clean with surgical sponges and pinched shut the main bleeding points with blood-vessel clamps. Then Sickmann went on cutting.

"Nobody spoke. The only sounds were the rustling of a nurse's gown as she passed over instrument and the click of one instrument following another into the discard tray.

"In 10 minutes, it was all over. Ten minutes to destroy what had taken 20 years or so to form. With a last snip, the breast was cut away like a piece of meat and thrown in the waste bucket."

Dr. Issels was appalled. A few minutes before the patient had been a complete woman. Now she was disfigured forever, not by some ghastly accident but by a skilled surgeon working in a modern hospital. Was the operation necessary?, the doctor asked himself. Had anyone thought of its aftereffects on the woman, now marred for the rest of her days?

The psychological results of the operation were every bit as severe as Dr. Issels had feared. The woman suffered a nervous breakdown, and her husband, not understanding her suffering, divorced her within a year.

Dr. Issels did not waver in his commitment to become a surgeon, but he resolved that he would never assist at or perform another radical mastectomy. Along with this resolve came an implacable hatred for the disease that caused such suffering, a hatred that would lead the doctor to develop and refine his *"Ganzheit"* therapy, to open the Ringberg Clinic in Germany, and to tirelessly devote himself to fighting even the most "incurable" of cancers. Sadly, Dr. Issels died in February 1998. There is no question that his ever-lasting contribution to the lives of thousands of people with cancer lives on.

EVOLUTION OF THE THERAPY Trained as a traditional surgeon, Dr. Issels became aware of the limitations of orthodox therapy when he began treating cancer patients. He became convinced that the successful treatment of cancer required a return to the whole-body approach to the disease. As he once said, "cancer is not just a local disease confined to the particular place in the body where the tumor manifests itself but is a general disease of the whole body."

Based on this approach to cancer, Dr. Issels developed a broad-spectrum therapy to restore and regenerate the body's natural defense mechanisms that complement the specific measures of traditional medicine directed at the elimination of the localized tumor. With this approach, Dr. Issels achieved a degree of success in treating his cancer patients which is unparalleled in traditional medicine.

How did it all begin? In his early years of medicine, Dr. Issels put some of his theories into practice in what he would later call a *"Ganzheit"* or "whole-body" approach to healing. He required that all his patients have infected teeth or tonsils removed, since he strongly believed that they release poisons into the body which lower natural resistance and trigger disease. Proper diet was also considered critical. The usual foodstuffs had to be replaced by biologically adequate ones adjusted to fit the actual organic conditions of individual patients. Chronically ill patients usually had to receive lactobacillus acidophilus, a cultured milk product which served as a ferment substitute to compensate for a loss of efficiency in their digestive systems. Tobacco, alcohol, coffee, tea, and other substances the doctor considered harmful were banned. Whenever possible, long-standing emotional stress was relieved or eliminated. In the meantime, the doctor went ahead with treatment of the particular diseased organ, confident that he was also addressing the root cause of the patient's sickness.

Dr. Issels was soon getting remarkable results with this combination of *Ganzheit* therapy, homeopathy, dietary control, and other therapeutic techniques. His practice became the largest in town, although it did not make him a rich man, since his fees were low and he treated for free those who were unable to pay.

Yet these successes contrasted grimly with his inability to help cancer patients. He knew that his colleagues were equally baffled by the disease, but that knowledge did not ease his frustration. Surgery and radiation seemed to bring temporary improvement, but it was clear that they did not get at the cause of the cancer and could not protect the patient from further occurrences. Surely, Dr. Issels thought, there had to be a way of applying the principles of *Ganzheit* therapy to the treatment of cancer to produce not just remissions but genuine cures. There had to be an alternative to disfiguring surgery, toxic chemicals, and poisonous radiation.

USING HISTORY AS A GUIDE The antipathy Dr. Issels had felt toward cancer in his early years became almost an obsession with the disease. He read everything he could find on cancer and in the process became an expert in medical history. He discovered that cancer, contrary to popular opinion, was not a modern affliction but had been observed by Chinese and Sumerian physicians and described in manuscripts dating back 3,000 years before Christ as resulting from a malfunction in the body's regulatory mechanisms that was to be treated with acupuncture and drugs.

Hippocrates (460–377 B.C.), the founder of Western medicine, was the first to use the word "carcinoma" in referring to malignant tumors, which he believed arose from a "separation of the humors" (blood, bile, and phlegm) and was to be treated with surgery and drugs. But what Dr. Issels found especially noteworthy was Hippocrates' recommendation that the entire body be detoxified and that cancer patients be put on a special diet. Further research showed that for the ancient Greeks, diata, or "diet," referred to far more than what a patient was to eat or drink. The term was closer in meaning to "way of life" or "lifestyle" and strongly suggested abstinence from anything that might be spiritually as well as physically harmful.

The Roman physician Claudius Galen (131– 200 A.D.), the founder of scientific physiology, whose authority had gone unchallenged in Western medicine for over 1,000 years, had also turned his attention to cancer, as Dr. Issels soon discovered. The doctor's interest became more than academic when he read Galen's opinion that cancer is a disease of the entire body, not confined to the site of the tumor.

Moving forward in time, Dr. Issels encountered the world-famous doctor of the Renaissance, Philippus Aureolus Theophrastus Bombast von Hohenheim, better known as Paracelsus, who also felt that the physician's role in treating cancer and other diseases was not to interfere with the body but rather to stimulate the healing processes nature had provided to correct the imbalances in the body that result in illness. Dr. Issels also encountered the pioneer surgeon Ambroise Pare, who shared Paracelsus' view of cancer as a disease of the entire body, and the French thinker Rene Descartes, who thought cancer was caused by abnormalities in the lymph glands. He pored over the work of Percival Potts, the 18th century British physician who was among the first to describe cancer as an "occupational" malignancy when he noticed an abnormally high rate of cancer of the scrotum in young chimney sweeps. In short, no one who might have something useful to say about cancer escaped Issels' scrutiny.

The work of Dr. Edward Jenner, the English physician who had developed a vaccination and checked the scourge of smallpox, seemed to offer special promise in regard to both theory and practice. Although Dr. Jenner had not been successful in treating cancer, he had produced vaccines which had shown promising results against other disorders. Equally important for Dr. Issels, his British predecessor believed that cancer stemmed from inadequacies in the immune mechanisms and that it could have a fatal effect only when the body's natural immunity had broken down completely.

SEARCHING FOR A VACCINE Following this line of thought, Dr. Issels searched for a vaccine that would bolster the body's immune system to the point where it could fight back successfully against cancer. Neoblastine, a vaccine he developed by culturing cancer tissues in a controlled medium many times over a long period to insure safety, seemed to offer some promise. After testing the vaccine on laboratory animals, he tried it on a terminally ill lung cancer patient, together with his *Ganzheit* therapy involving extraction of infected teeth and tonsils, and strict dietary control. Although the patient lived three months longer than expected, the results were ambiguous, since there had been no cure and it was impossible to attribute the patient's improvement to any single factor in the treatment.

Another case, on the surface equally disappointing, occurred when Dr. Issels agreed to treat a woman with an enormous uterine tumor who had already been given up on by her doctors. Heeding her husband's pleas, Dr. Issels agreed to see her but he could do nothing beyond prescribing painkillers and ordering a change in her diet. Nonetheless, the fact that Dr. Issels had undertaken to treat her gave the woman a much better outlook. Until her death two months later, she maintained steadfastly that Dr. Issels' treatments had freed her of pain that drugs had been unable to eliminate.

These patients and others all succumbed to disease and left Dr. Issels little cause for optimism. Yet these cases did serve to convince him that *Ganzheit* therapy had been helpful and to confirm his long-standing belief that cancer is not a mysterious ailment but a chronic systemic illness, to be treated like other diseases of this kind. The tumor, he became convinced, was merely a late-stage symptom, accidentally triggered off but able to grow only in what he described as a "tumor milieu," the result of prior damage to organs and organ systems, especially those involved in maintaining the body's resistance to disease. The disease would never gain a foothold unless the body's defenses were depleted.

Once it had gained a foothold, conventional treatments, Dr. Issels decided, could usually provide only temporary relief. While surgery, by removing large masses of tumor, might stimulate the immune system to regenerate, it was not likely to provide a cure by itself, since the operation could not get at the underlying cause of the cancer. Radiation and chemotherapy, while initially successful, frequently provided only temporary relief. Nonetheless, Dr. Issels did not offer *Ganzheit* therapy as a substitute for the usual treatments but as a supplement which he believed would make the conventional therapies more effective by rehabilitating the entire patient, not just attacking the tumor.

COMBINING TRADITIONAL AND UNCONVENTIONAL METHODS As the number of his cancer patients continued to grow, Dr. Issels began specializing in that disease. In 1950, he took charge of a 30-bed cancer unit at a small suburban clinic, where he put in 17-hour days, treating patients with a combination of traditional and unconventional methods. Surgery was used to remove large tumors. Drugs were administered to improve the functioning of various organs, especially the liver and kidneys, which usually are severely damaged in advanced cancer patients. The body was detoxified through the use of purifying drugs; mild purgatives; a diet high in fruit, vegetables, and grains; and the consumption of large amounts of water, juice, and herbal teas. Homeopathic remedies were used along with vaccines to stimulate antibody production.

Dr. Issels' cure statistics were not numerically impressive, but there was no lack of patients for treatment. Those who came to him were not in the early stages of the disease but were, for the most part, patients whom the medical establishment had been unable to help. For them, Dr. Issels offered the proverbial "last, best, hope" of staying alive, a hope he was sometimes able to fulfill in ways that bordered on the miraculous.

When he was asked to treat Kathe Gerlach in October 1950, Dr. Issels hesitated, since she lived an hour's drive from the hospital and he was reluctant to take the time from his other patients. When he finally acceded to requests from the 41-year-old patient, her husband, and her physician, Dr. Issels was dismayed at her condition. She had an enormous tumor in her uterus which a biopsy had shown to be malignant and inoperable. Edema in her legs had left her unable to walk and she was expected to live only a few days.

Even though the case seemed hopeless, Dr. Issels agreed to treat her at home, since she was far too weak to be moved to the hospital. By mid-October she began to show definite signs of improvement, and by November her pain had subsided. The edema in her legs diminished, although the tumor remained very large.

Dr. Issels drove Mrs. Gerlach to the hospital as soon as she was well enough to be moved. There she began to improve rapidly. Pieces of the tumor were being eliminated, the edema decreased continually, and her circulation improved markedly. By November 25 it was clear that the tumor was regressing. In February of the following year she left the hospital with no detectable signs of cancer.

Mrs. Gerlach, however, was not the only one impressed by this remarkable turn of events. Her surgeon, Dr. Lothar Ley, examined her in March 1951, confirmed Dr. Issels' findings, and offered to refer more cancer patients to him for this unorthodox but clearly successful treatment.

Nearly a quarter of a century later, when Dr. Issels contacted Mrs. Gerlach in connection with his own book, *Cancer: A Second Opinion* (Hodder and Stoughton, London, 1975), he found her leading a normal life with no indications that her cancer might return.

In the spring of 1951, Dr. Issels went to Holland to consult with the Dutch shipping magnate Karl Gishler, who was suffering from prostate cancer that had metastasized to his spine and left him bedridden. His prognosis was terminal.

After much deliberation, Mr. Gishler decided to undergo *Ganzheit* therapy under Dr. Issels' supervision, and the treatment began in mid-May. Over the weeks that followed, Mr. Gishler, despite the progress of the disease that ultimately took his life, remained attentive and alert, interested in every aspect of the treatment. His friendship with and respect for Dr. Issels also grew steadily as he came to know his physician better and understand his deep-seated desire to alleviate human suffering.

These feelings, however, were not shared by the conservative hospital administration, which expressly forbade Dr. Issels to treat any other patients according to his methods. This rebuff led indirectly to another incident that changed the direction of Dr. Issels' career.

THE RINGBERG CLINIC On a visit to Mr. Gishler's bedside, Dr. Issels found the patient in tears not just from the pain of his tumor but from the humiliation of being slapped by a nurse who felt he was being troublesome. Dr. Issels was aghast, but all Mr. Gishler said, as reported in Gordon Thomas' book about Dr. Issels, was that Dr. Issels had to find his own place where he could hand-pick his staff.

In answer to Mr. Gishler's questions about the cost of such an institution, Dr. Issels answered without thinking that 150,000 marks would be about right.

In postwar Germany, 150,000 marks was a considerable sum, close to $500,000 in today's purchasing power, but the tycoon was undaunted.

"Then you will have the money," Mr. Gishler assured him.

On September 21, 1951, the Ringberg Clinic opened in a former hotel in the Bavarian town of Rottach-Egern. Here Dr. Issels finally had a free hand in treating cancer, and here he was able to spend nearly four decades treating patients whom other doctors had not been able to help.

The first patient, Mrs. Lydia Bacher, arrived in an ambulance, bald from radiation therapy and so debilitated by the effects of an inoperable brain tumor that she could no longer speak, hear or see. She was paralyzed in both legs and in the right arm, and her bladder and rectum no longer functioned. Her physicians had discharged her with painkillers, saying that no further treatment was possible. *Ganzheit* therapy, supplemented with daily injections of Toxinal (oxytetracycline), an immunotherapy agent, was started at once.

Within a month Mrs. Bacher's speech had returned, she was able to read a newspaper, her hearing was improving, and her bodily functions were almost normal. By mid-December she was walking, and on March 17, 1952, she left the clinic, completely recovered. Her amazed doctors explained this recovery as a "spontaneous remission," but Mrs. Bacher was only the first of many terminally ill patients to have such a remission at the Ringberg Clinic. She was also the first clinic patient to survive symptom-free past the critical five-year mark which conventional medicine accepts as proof of a cure.

The treatment which practically brought Mrs. Bacher back from the grave and has saved many others from death is not a magic pill or simple potion that produces overnight wonders. Rather, it is a complex and carefully thought out regimen that takes into account every aspect of the patient and the patient's illness and seeks relentlessly to find and correct the imbalance in the patient's being that made it possible for the cancer to arise in the first place.

In 1981, the old hotel was abandoned in favor of a sophisticated medical facility, staffed by four doctors and 25 nurses, and outfitted with the latest equipment for diagnosis and treatment. The documents the patients brought with them pertaining to their illnesses were checked, and the patients were carefully examined to verify the diagnosis. An exact case history was taken, stretching back not only over the course of the disease but over each patient's whole life and, if possible, the lives of the patient's ancestors as well, since Dr. Issels believed that it was necessary to construct a complete nutritional health profile before an effective treatment could begin.

In a memorial tribute to Dr. Issels (*Explore for the Professional*, vol. 8, no. 4), Dr. Karl Windstosser writes that Dr. Issels, "exhausted by the struggle against orthodox medicine's lack of understanding and the windmills of dogma," left Germany in the mid-1980s, first for Florida and then California. "His orphaned clinic," Dr. Windstosser continues, "fell into hands of speculators who thought they might be able to turn a handsome profit by trading on the Issels name, but succeeded instead only in driving the clinic to an inglorious end." The Ringberg Clinic had a good long run before it closed its doors, however. And Dr. Issels continued his impassioned work until just before he died, managing a foundation dedicated to immunological cancer therapy, teaching his philosophy to a new generation, and collaborating with medical colleagues from around the globe, including those carrying on the work of Dr. Max Gerson, described later in this chapter.

The Treatment

Although about 90 percent of the patients he saw had already been designated as incurable and beyond the help of orthodox medicine, Dr. Issels continued conventional treatment if it was possible and appropriate, since he viewed Ganzheit therapy as a supplement to make these treatments more effective rather than as a substitute for them.

In *Ganzheit* therapy as practiced at the Ringberg clinic, once the examination is complete, the doctor tailors the treatment to the patient's individual needs. The patient gets a chart that is filled in every morning and evening, listing the patient's symptoms, whether there is pain, changes in the tumor, the amount excreted, and whether there is vomiting, sweating, etc. When the patient comes in for an appointment, he or she shows the chart to the nurse, who then enters the data on a four-week chart so that the doctor can judge whether the treatment should be stronger or weaker.

TONSILLECTOMY AND TOOTH EXTRACTION As mentioned, all the patients part with infected teeth and tonsils, since Dr. Issels viewed these as sites of infection that place an unnecessary burden on the immune system and act to lower the body's general defenses against disease. Scars and the sites of old injuries are treated with Dr. Huneke's Neural Therapy to eliminate them as sources of infection. Both patients and doctors find tonsillectomy and tooth extraction a strange treatment for cancer and the injection of Novocain (procaine hydrochloride) into parts of the body far distant from the tumor even stranger. But Dr. Issels, although not a devotee of Dr. Huneke's abstruse theories, had seen many cases in which these procedures, often undertaken just to relieve pain, cleared the way for other treatments to attack the tumor.

DIET AND NUTRITION A healthy diet is also a critical element in *Ganzheit* therapy. Most meats are avoided, since meat is difficult for advanced cancer patients to digest and is usually filled with hormones, antibiotics, and pesticides that place further strain on the body. The recommended diet is primarily vegetarian, focusing on organically grown whole grains, fruits, and vegetables, supplemented by enzymes, minerals, and vitamins, with emphasis on A, B-complex, C, and E. Yogurt and acidophilus supplements are used to eliminate abnormal intestinal flora.

Serum activator is administered to bring the metabolism of red blood cells up to normal levels, allowing the release of additional hemoglobin and thus increasing the supply of oxygen to the body's cells.

Organ extracts are supplied to help repair secondary damage to organs and improve their functioning, while a high fluid intake backed up with herbal extracts, DNA, and RNA is used to detoxify the body; improve kidney, lymph, and liver functions; and bolster the excretory systems.

PSYCHOTHERAPY Since *Ganzheit* therapy entails the treatment of the entire patient, individual and group psychotherapy is an important element. Through this treatment, Dr. Issels hoped not only to help the patient come to terms with the disease, but also to remove, or at least alleviate, the psychic stress which he felt could help bring on cancer and hinder its cure.

IMMUNOTHERAPY A major component of the treatment is a highly sophisticated form of immunotherapy, geared specifically to fighting cancer and supported, where necessary, by surgery, radiation, and chemotherapy. This immunotherapy involves a twofold approach: specific immunization against the particular type of cancer to be fought and a general effort to augment the body's natural immune responses.

"Specific immunization works on a well-tried principle," Dr. Issels wrote in his 1975 book, *Cancer: A Second Opinion*. "Once a particular cancer antigen has been identified, it is administered under conditions most favorable for the induction of an immune response that will destroy cancer cells bearing that antigen. This is really no more than an extension of the standard vaccination technique against any infectious disease."

For specific immunization against the tumor, Dr. Issels often administered a vaccine shown to cause regression of malignant tumors which was developed by Dr. Franz Gerlach, a Viennese scientist. Other tumor-specific immunization was effected with standard non-toxic vaccines such as Centanit for carcinoma, Sarkogen for sarcoma, and Lymphogran for Hodgkin's disease.

General immunotherapy is used to bolster the patient's overall immunity and to destroy the "tumor milieu" that makes it possible for the cancer to sustain itself and grow. Here the primary means of attack consists of autovaccines prepared from extracts from the patient's own teeth and tonsils as well as other nontoxic vaccines designed to boost general resistance to disease.

OZONE THERAPY Ozone therapy, although not a direct aid to the immune system, is also used as a means of increasing the oxygen supply to the cells and destroying viruses and bacteria in the bloodstream. This method of systematically exposing portions of the patient's blood supply to medically pure ozone is almost unknown in the United States but has been used against blood-borne infectious diseases in Germany for more than 25 years. Dr. Issels has also found the therapy to be effective in purging the blood of oxidation-resistant pesticides and other toxins.

HYPERPYREXIA (FEVER INDUCTION) Hyperpyrexia, homeopathy's long-sanctioned induction of fever, is also used in much the same way as ozone therapy to make life uncomfortable for the tumor. Once a month patients get a "fever shot," which can raise the body temperature as high as 105 degrees Fahrenheit, where it stays for two hours or so while the patient is under constant medical supervision. In the evening the body's temperature is lowered again.

While Dr. Issels may not have shared the enthusiasm of the ancient Greek physician who remarked, "Give me a chance to produce fever, and I can cure all illness," he knew that fever was a natural reaction of the body to foreign invaders and that it made these invaders more vulnerable to attack. He also discovered that the number of disease-destroying leukocytes in the patient's bloodstream rose enormously after each fever shot and that the patients uniformly reported feeling much better afterward, as their bodies were detoxified. Even localized heating of the tumor area, Dr. Issels discovered, can have effects which, while not as spectacular, were clearly beneficial.

The Patients

To medical practitioners who firmly believe that cancer is largely an incurable disease, Dr. Issels' theories and methods are simply bizarre. To them, the notion that cancer is not a localized illness but a chronic disease that manifests itself as a tumor only in its advanced stages is simply unthinkable, as is the idea that the body, once restored to its normal physiology, is capable of destroying the malignancy. This low opinion of *Ganzheit* therapy, however, is not shared by the patients who have seen it work over the years, some of whom were among the first to be seen at the Ringberg Clinic.

EXAMPLE 1: Nineteen-year-old Thea arrived at the Ringberg Clinic on October 29, 1952. Surgery and radiation had been ineffective against a malignant fibroblastic sarcoma (skin and muscle cancer) that encircled her spine like a snake. Her physicians had sent her home to die and advised her parents to call a priest to administer the last rites. She was not even expected to survive the 600-mile trip to the Ringberg Clinic. But 16 days after beginning therapy, she began to show strong signs of recovery. Three months later, her x-rays showed considerable reduction in the tumor, and one month later she was released from the clinic to return home, where her family doctor had agreed to administer maintenance therapy.

Thea's story seemed well on its way to a happy ending, when she was returned to the hospital in Mönchengladbach, suffering from a secondary fibrosarcoma. Since Dr. Issels happened to be in his hometown visiting his brother, he went to see Thea in the hospital and found her completely resigned to dying.

After some questioning, he learned that Thea had been engaged to be married, when her fiancé canceled the engagement, leaving her desolate. The cancer recurred almost immediately afterward, convincing Dr. Issels that it had been psychologically triggered.

Since radiation had been ineffective in treating the tumor, Dr. Issels suggested that Thea return to the Ringberg Clinic, and her parents agreed. Dr. Issels began treating her in November with Novacarcin, a newly developed immunotherapeutic agent, and by January there was considerable reduction in the size of the tumor. But Thea still lacked the will to live, and Dr. Issels now knew that without a change in her attitude, long-term remission would be impossible.

After carefully considering the options, Dr. Issels decided to visit Thea's former fiancé and tell him about her condition. The man went at once to the clinic to see her, and there was a reconciliation. Thea began to improve rapidly, her tumor shrank, and she was able to return home. Five years after the original diagnosis of cancer Thea got married, and as Dr. Issels notes in his case files, "There has been a complete disappearance of the secondary tumor. The original one remains dormant. Patient is entirely free of any active cancer."

More than a decade later her family doctor found Thea's lung free of malignancy and the original spinal tumor still dormant. His opinion, as given in Gordon Thomas' book, *Dr. Issels and His Revolutionary Cancer Treatment* (Peter H. Wyden, Inc., New York, 1973), was simple and straightforward: "She leads the usual busy life of a mother of three children, and has every reason to expect a full life span."

EXAMPLE 2: Mrs. K. G. was 40 years old when she was first diagnosed as having inoperable stage III uterocervical cancer. At first she responded to radiation treatment, but then an egg-sized recurrence appeared and was unresponsive to radiation. The tumor grew, filling her pelvic area with a solid cancerous mass and blocking her rectal passage so that a palliative colostomy was required. She was admitted to the Ringberg Clinic barely alive.

Ganzheit therapy and immunotherapy were started at once, and within five months all tumor symptoms had disappeared. When Dr. Issels contacted Mrs. K. G. again 20 years later while researching his book, he learned that she was still symptom-free and without any signs of cancer.

EXAMPLE 3: A right-sided mastectomy was done on S. G. to remove a breast tumor. Since biopsies of the cancer tissue revealed that she had a penetrating adenocarcinoma, she was given follow-up radiation treatments that failed to halt the spread of the disease. In six months the cancer had metastasized to both lungs, and the prognosis was hopeless. Three months later, she was admitted to the Ringberg Clinic and was started on *Ganzheit* therapy and immunotherapy. Within two years all the lung metastases had disappeared. When she died at 69 of a heart attack, 15 years after completing the treatment, she was still cancer-free.

Understanding the Distinction Between "Survival" and "Cure"

While skeptics may mutter about "spontaneous remissions," it remains true that three independent studies of Dr. Issels' medical records conducted by highly reputed experts have confirmed a 16.6 percent cure rate among all the terminal patients treated with *Ganzheit* therapy, a figure that no doctor or hospital anywhere in the world comes close to matching. The other alternative therapies mentioned in this section have success rates (five-year complete remissions) ranging from 5 to 15 percent.

To understand the significance of this figure, it is necessary to recall that all these patients were terminal, already given up on by conventional medicine. In the United States, for example, such a patient has virtually no chance of survival, let alone of cure.

This distinction between survival and cure is also crucial. For conventional medicine, "cure" simply means that the cancer patient has survived five years after the initial diagnosis. It says nothing about the state of the patient during that time or at its end. Dr. Issels used a different standard. For him and for the doctors who have studied his work, a cure indicated that the patient in question was free of any detectable sign of cancer: A man or woman who fully expected to die of cancer was alive, healthy, and free of the disease five years or more after beginning treatment.

While even Dr. Issels did not think of *Ganzheit* therapy as the be-all and end-all, his indisputable successes bring one face-to-face with some uncomfortable facts. The tremendous advances in the development of symptom-oriented treatments, which include surgery, radiation, and chemotherapy, have been of benefit to some cancer patients, but these benefits appear to have peaked in the mid-1950s. Notwithstanding the stunning array of new high-tech surgical procedures and chemotherapeutic drugs, traditional medicine has not been able to obtain more than a slight increase in the survival rates of patients. Despite the expenditure of billions of dollars in the war on cancer, there is growing evidence of the limitations of conventional therapies and evidence that statistical manipulations have inflated the amount of actual progress.

Of course, the shortcomings of conventional therapies do not by themselves constitute proof of the accuracy and efficacy of Dr. Issels' theories and methods. But at the very least these limitations should indicate that it is time to take a long, hard look at conventional therapies and the theories behind them. Before the medical establishment is allowed to brand *Ganzheit* therapy as "weird," it should explain why it works in so many cases in which orthodox treatments have failed. Until then, Dr. Issels' explanations are the best one is likely to find.

The Future of Ganzheit Therapy

As mentioned, Dr. Issels continued his fight against cancer throughout his life. In the years before he died, when he was well into his 90s, Dr. Issels and colleagues at the Centro Hospitalario Internacional Pacifico, S.A. (CHIPSA) Center for Integrative Medicine refined a program that combined his comprehensive immunotherapy with the similarly holistic approach developed by the late Dr. Max Gerson, another leader in the alternative medicine field. (See the next chapter for a full discussion of Dr. Gerson's approach to cancer.) The Issels-Gerson Combination Therapy is now being offered at CHIPSA, a modern, full-service 70-bed hospital in Tijuana. Several program plans are available, including supportive therapy, full intensive therapy, advanced therapy, and therapy with hyperbaric oxygen.

42

"Environmental" Approach to Cancer Therapy: Rebuilding the Body's Natural Healing System

W ith the advance of technology, an ever-increasing number of new substances are introduced into the environment each year. These substances range from chemicals, pesticides, and drugs to the byproducts of nuclear weapons and energy. There are also new agricultural and manufacturing techniques such as genetically engineered microorganisms and food irradiation. Until relatively recently the human body, which has evolved over thousands of years, seemed to do a fairly good job of adapting to the changes within the environment. Within the past century, however, the rate at which people have been exposed to new and toxic substances has accelerated so rapidly that the result has been a breakdown in the body's natural adaptation and defensive processes. Certain physicians view this breakdown as one of the major contributing factors to many of today's most dreaded diseases, especially cancer.

The Discovery: Dr. Max Gerson

The theory that cancer is triggered by environmental factors which deplete the body's natural immunity and defensive capabilities is not a new one. In fact, Dr. Max Gerson took an "environmental" approach to cancer therapy over 60 years ago. The cornerstone of Dr. Gerson's therapy is the detoxification of the body through diet designed to rehabilitate the body's natural immunity and healing process.

Although Dr. Gerson died in 1959, his work is being carried on by his daughter, Charlotte Gerson, in the Gerson clinic located on the western coast of Mexico about 30 minutes south of San Diego. Dr. Gerson was eulogized by Dr. Albert Schweitzer, whose wife Gerson cured of lung tuberculosis in the 1930s. Schweitzer wrote in a letter to Ms. Gerson, "I see in him one of the most eminent geniuses in the history of medicine. Many of his basic ideas have been adopted without having his name connected with them. Yet he has achieved more than seemed possible under adverse conditions. He leaves a legacy which commands attention and which will assure him his due place. Those whom he cured will now attest to the truth of his ideas."

FROM MIGRAINES... Dr. Gerson was born in Wongrowitz, Germany, in 1881. The roots of his work date to his early days as a young intern and resident before World War I. At that time he was suffering from severe migraine headaches, which were considered incurable. But Dr. Gerson, after a fruitless search through the medical literature, turned to nutrition to change his body chemistry and gain relief. He was already convinced that contamination of foods by artificial fertilizers and processing has a deleterious effect on body chemistry. He felt that by restoring normal metabolism through a healthy diet, he might be able to improve his migraine condition, and so he started to experiment on himself with certain foods. His first experiment was with milk. He thought that milk, being the first food, was something that even a baby could handle, so that his body should have been able to utilize it properly. But when he drank nothing but milk, his headaches became worse. Then it occurred to him that milk is not normally consumed by adult animals other than humans anywhere in nature and that maybe milk is a foreign substance rather than a natural nutrient in the adult human diet.

Dr. Gerson decided to conduct his next experiments using foods that were more suited for the human type of build and body chemistry, namely, fruits and vegetables. (Contrary to popular belief, human physiology is basically vegetarian and not carnivorous. The human intestinal tract measures 30 feet in length and as such is unsuited to the proper digestion and elimination of meat.) When Dr. Gerson found that he did not experience migraines when he ate nothing but grains, fresh fruits, and vegetables, he began experimenting with single foods to discern their particular effect on his physiology. He found, for instance, that when he ate cooked foods, they often did not agree with him. But it turned out that it wasn't the cooking but the added salt that made the difference. When he ate the same cooked foods without salt, he was able to handle them very well.

Little by little Dr. Gerson began to piece together a menu of foods that he could safely consume, together with a list of foods that would almost invariably give him migraines within a few minutes of his eating them. In the end he arrived at a diet very high in fresh fruits and vegetables and freshly prepared vegetable and fruit juices and very low in fats. Later, in his treatment of tuberculosis patients, Gerson would use a small amount of raw, fresh unsalted butter because it is a good source of the phospholipids which form an important part of the body's defense mechanism, but otherwise the diet was largely free of animals fats, especially cooked fats, and totally free of meats and cooked animal proteins of any sort.

By the early 1920s, Dr. Gerson had succeeded in completely curing himself of migraines with his special diet. He then started extending his findings to patients who came to him suffering from migraines. They too benefited.

...TO TUBERCULOSIS Eventually, although by accident, Dr. Gerson began to use his "Migraine Diet" in the treatment of tuberculosis as well. His daughter, Charlotte, relates how this occurred:

"One time, a patient came to him suffering from migraines and was given what he called his 'Migraine Diet.' When the patient came back after three or four weeks, he told Dr. Gerson that along with his migraines, he also had been suffering from lupus vulgaris, a form of skin tuberculosis, and that with the diet, not only had his migraines disappeared but the lupus had also begun to heal. Dr. Gerson found this almost impossible to believe, because he had learned that lupus was really an incurable condition. But there was the proof before his eyes. He saw that the lesion was healing, and he verified that it had been properly diagnosed and that there had been bacteriological studies showing that, in fact, the man had skin tuberculosis.

"After that, he was able to cure many other patients with skin tuberculosis. This therapy was later verified in large experiments in Munich, involving 450 terminal or incurable cases of skin tuberculosis treated with his Gerson dietary therapy. The treatment was shown to cure 447. From there Dr. Gerson felt that if tuberculosis could be influenced by nutrition, then why only skin tuberculosis—why shouldn't other forms of tuberculosis respond? He applied this same dietary treatment to people with lung tuberculosis, bone tuberculosis, kidney tuberculosis, etc. One of the most famous patients he had at that time was the wife of Albert Schweitzer, who had contracted TB in the tropics. She had been given up because her TB had spread to both lung fields and was quite extensive. Well, among others, she too recovered and lived many, many years, until age 80 or so."

...AND MORE As a result of this healing, Drs. Gerson and Schweitzer became friends and remained so throughout their lives. Dr. Schweitzer followed the progress of the Gerson therapy as it was later applied to a wide variety of diseases, and when he developed adult diabetes, he found relief through Dr. Gerson's treatment. Unfortunately, the American medical establishment has never shared Dr. Schweitzer's high opinion of Dr. Gerson. Instead of being praised, he was persecuted and harassed by his colleagues. Today, forty years after Dr. Gerson's death in 1959, his therapy still remains on the American Cancer Society's "Unproven Methods" list.

The Treatment

THEORETICAL BASIS Before discussing Dr. Gerson's therapy, it is important to look at its theoretical basis. Like the other alternative cancer approaches discussed in this chapter, it differs fundamentally from the traditional medical treatment in that it deals with cancer as a generalized rather than a localized disease. More specifically, it is related to the balance or imbalance in the body's internal chemistry and physiology. According to Dr. Gerson (in *A Cancer Therapy: Results of Fifty Cases*, 4th ed., Gerson Institute, Bonita, California, 1986):

"A normal body has the capacity to keep all cells functioning properly. It prevents any abnormal transformation and growth. Therefore, the natural task of a cancer therapy is to bring the body back to that normal physiology, or as near to it as possible. The next task is to keep the physiology of the metabolism in that normal equilibrium.

"A normal body also has reserves to suppress and destroy malignancies. It does not act in that manner in cancer patients, where the cancer grew from the smallest cellular unit freely, without encountering any resistance....

"In short," says Dr. Gerson, "what is essential is not the growth itself or the visible symptoms; it is the damage of the whole metabolism, including the loss of defense, immunity, and healing power. It cannot be explained or recognized by one or another cause alone."

Dr. Gerson's therapy aims at rebalancing and revitalizing the cancer patient's entire physiology in order to rectify this systemic disorder. It looks for the cause of the illness, works to correct it, and thus not only causes the cancer to regress but prevents it from recurring. Traditional cancer therapy, as has been seen, is not very successful at eradicating symptoms and fails abysmally in preventing recurrences. Furthermore, while the traditional therapies of chemotherapy and radiation may be effective in treating the symptoms of certain relatively rare forms of cancer, they not only do nothing to revitalize the body's immune system, they actually work to suppress it. Gerson therapy attempts to detoxify and rebuild the body's natural immunity and healing power, while traditional medicine administers highly toxic substances which destroy the immune system and often cause secondary cancers. In fact, Dr. Gerson was often forced to turn away cancer patients who had received traditional medical treatments and whose bodies had been damaged beyond hope by these very treatments, not by the cancer.

According to Dr. Curtis Hesse, former director of the Gerson Therapy Center (personal correspondence to Charlotte Gerson), "Ironically, the main problem we actually have in this treatment is not always cancer or disease but the other medications and treatments that the patients have already undergone. In cancer therapy, we do not as a general rule accept any patient who has undergone chemotherapy. From past experience, we know that liver damage and damage to other organs, as well as the immune system, have been such that they do well for a two- to three-week period but then go downhill."

The core of Gerson therapy is a regimen consisting primarily of a saltless and fatless diet of organically grown fresh fruits and vegetables which are usually served raw or as juices. The primary objective of the diet is to detoxify the entire body and rebalance the whole metabolism, not simply to eliminate the symptoms of the disease. "The treatment has to penetrate deeply to correct all vital processes," says Dr. Gerson. "When general metabolism is restored, we can again influence the functioning of all organs, tissues, and cells though it."

FOCUS ON THE LIVER Since detoxification and normalizing the metabolism are major factors in Gerson therapy, Dr. Gerson placed particular importance on the condition of the liver, which is a primary regulator of metabolism. According to Dr. Gerson: "The problem of the liver was and still is partly misunderstood and partly neglected. The metabolism and its concentration in the liver should be put in the foreground, not the cancer as a symptom. There, the outcome of cancer is determined as the clinically favorable results, failures, and autopsies clearly demonstrate. There the sentence will be passed—whether the tumors can be killed, dissolved, absorbed, or eliminated, and finally, whether the body can be restored. "The progress of the disease depends on whether and to what extent the liver can be restored."

The liver's many functions, coupled with its constant interaction with all the other organs of the body, give it a crucial role to play in the maintenance of health. Dr. Gerson and many other scientists have noted that in all degenerative diseases, including cancer, there are varying degrees of liver dysfunction and deterioration. Fortunately, however, while the liver is not easily destroyed and liver damage may not even be detected until liver function has been greatly impaired, the liver is also one of the organs that has the greatest capacity for regeneration. Consequently, the restoration of the liver is a significant objective of Dr. Gerson's diet.

Dr. Gerson's liver therapy is multifaceted. First, animal proteins are eliminated or greatly reduced in the diet because they have been found to interfere with liver medication and impede the body's detoxification.

The ideal diet for patients on liver therapy is the same as that described above for the cancer therapy: low in salt and fat and high in potassium and fresh fruits and vegetables, mostly in juice form.

The juice is also rich in iron and potassium as well as hormones and vitamins which aid in regenerating the liver. The juice is always prepared freshly and is not mixed with other medications which could alter the pH and thereby decrease its efficacy. The restoration of the liver, which may take from 6 to 18 months, depending on the severity of the illness, allows it to detoxify the body and produce its own oxidative enzymes.

Other aspects of liver therapy include liver injections and lubile and pancreatin tablets. The liver injections are composed of liver extract and are given daily for four to six months. They too provide important vitamins, minerals, and enzymes which aid in restoring the liver to its proper functioning. These liver injections are usually combined with vitamin B_{12} injections, which Dr. Gerson believed are important for proper protein synthesis. Cancer patients are often unable to combine amino acids properly in order to form proteins within their bodies.

Lubile (defatted bile powder from young calves) was used more frequently in the earlier stages of the therapy; it is not used for most patients today. However, it is beneficial in cases where the liver is extremely damaged and the whole bile duct system is impaired.

Pancreatin tablets are given during and after the detoxification program is completed as a backup source of digestive enzymes, since those are also deficient in most cancer patients.

According to Dr. Gerson, patients on the therapy actually begin to break down, assimilate, and eliminate cancer tumors. This is accomplished when the repaired liver is adequately producing oxidative enzymes, the general detoxification process (of which the liver is a critical part) is active, and potassium levels throughout the body are adequate.

COFFEE ENEMAS During the period when the body is killing, absorbing, and eliminating the tumor, detoxification is of the utmost importance. Dr. Gerson admitted that in the early stages of development, the therapy did not contain adequate detoxification techniques. "After a tumor was killed," he says, "the patient did not die of cancer but of a serious intoxification with 'coma hepaticum' (liver shock) caused by absorption of necrotic cancer tissue."

Thus, in addition to the other cleansing aspects of the therapy, Dr. Gerson began to prescribe frequent coffee enemas which at the outset of treatment can be given as often as every four hours. This prescription derives from the work of two German researchers who found that caffeine administered rectally causes an opening of the bile ducts, releasing accumulated toxins and causing an increased production of bile, which flushes out these toxins. After these enemas, Dr. Gerson noticed that patients were often relieved of pain such as headaches, fevers, and nausea and could easily discontinue sedation. On the other hand, Dr. Gerson noted that coffee taken orally seemed to have exactly the opposite effect: It caused the stomach to go into spasm and produce a "soaping" over or contraction of the bile ducts. Hence, while regular coffee enemas are an indispensable part of Gerson therapy, drinking coffee is discouraged.

RE-ESTABLISHING POTASSIUM LEVELS Muscles, the brain, and the liver normally have much higher levels of potassium than of sodium. Early in his research, however, Dr. Gerson noted that in cancer patients this ratio is reversed; that is, he found that sodium is elevated in cancer cells and that in the ailing body, potassium is often inactive and/or improperly utilized. He felt that at the beginning chronic disease is caused by the loss of potassium from the cell system; accordingly, another primary objective of Gerson therapy is to reestablish proper levels of potassium in the body.

Because of the specific relationship between sodium and potassium, in which an increase in one mineral causes a decrease in the other and vice versa, one of the first things Gerson advocated is the elimination of salt and sodium-rich foods from the diet.

Additionally, all patients on Gerson therapy immediately begin receiving large amounts of a potassium solution which Dr. Gerson developed after 300 experiments. The potassium compound he used, which is still used, at the clinic, is a combination of potassium gluconate, potassium acetate, and potassium phosphate monobasic. This is administered in the form of a 10 percent potassium solution, which is added to juices 10 times daily in 4-teaspoon doses. The potassium solution is never added to the liver juice because Dr. Gerson believed that it can alter the juice's pH, thereby decreasing its efficacy. After a month, the amount is decreased by about half. The fluid retention and edema (caused by a sodium overabundance) is usually the first thing to disappear when patients are given high amounts of potassium in juices.

Dr. Gerson noted that even in a healthy person it is very difficult to restore potassium deficiencies. In seriously ill people, it may take as long as a year or two before normal levels in major organs are reestablished.

In patients suffering from dehydration, potassium is added to the fluids therapeutically administered in the form of a GKI (glucose, potassium, insulin) solution. According to Ms. Gerson, this solution is not specific to Gerson therapy but is recognized and utilized by the American medical establishment in general. "Dr. Demetrio Sodi-Pallares, a world-renowned cardiologist from Mexico City," says Ms. Gerson, "very much recommends this solution." He agreed with Dr. Gerson that disease is systemic or metabolic. His own research in heart disease has shown that it is not a disease of the heart but a metabolic disease that must be treated with a high-potassium, low-sodium diet.

Dr. Sodi-Pallares found that giving GKI to heart patients with fluid retention is also very helpful. Ms Gerson noted that "This solution helps restore potassium to the cell system. Energy is required in order for potassium to go back into the cell system, and this energy is supplied by the glucose and insulin. We use this solution quite successfully in two ways: first to replenish the patient with fluids, but also to restore potassium to the cells and reduce edema."

DIET All aspects of Gerson therapy revolve around the diet, which is designed to support all the other efforts to rebalance the internal body chemistry. At the clinic, all meals are prepared with fresh, organically grown produce. Nothing is canned, jarred, pickled, frozen, or preserved in any way. Between the juices and the three meals, the total average intake of food for each patient is approximately 20 pounds of fresh raw food a day, mostly via juices.

All refined, processed, and empty-calorie foods are avoided. This includes obviously treated foods such as white sugars and flours and smoked, sulfured, packaged, or mass-prepared products. Other obvious taboos include cigarettes, alcohol, drugs, and caffeine, which are known to deplete the immune system and act as carcinogens. All animal proteins such as meat, poultry, and dairy products are avoided, since they are difficult to digest and hinder, rather than promote, the restoration of the liver.

Both animal and vegetable fats are also avoided as they too can be difficult to digest and can impede detoxification. Additionally, Dr. Gerson found that dietary fats actually have the effect of promoting tumor growth. This accords with cancer research indicating that the higher the level of cholesterol and fats in the blood of cancer patients, the less chance of their surviving. Dr. Gerson slowly eliminated all fats from the diets of his cancer patients and found that the results improved substantially. On the other hand, whenever he added fats (even oils which are low in cholesterol) to the patients' diets, he observed regrowth of tumor tissue. Essentially trial and error, Dr. Gerson found that he was able to control the growth of cancer tissue. With an external tumor, say, a lesion of the breast or skin, when the tumor was practically healed, if the patient was suddenly given a little butter, the lesion would often break open again or a new cancer would begin to grow. When the butter was eliminated, the tumor would begin to regress and heal again.

Consequently, for cancer patients receiving Gerson therapy, fats of animal or vegetable origin are eliminated as much as possible. The only exception is linseed oil, which Dr. Gerson found is particularly well tolerated. For patients suffering from other illnesses, while the diet is essentially low in fat, some raw fresh butter, egg yolks, and low-cholesterol vegetable oils such as safflower oil and sunflower oil may be eaten in small quantities.

Dr. Gerson was a strong believer in the importance of organically grown produce, and as mentioned above, all food used at his clinic must be grown in this manner. Chemical pesticides and fertilizers, he said, essentially poison and denature fruits and vegetables by altering their chemical composition. For instance, he found that many chemical fertilizers cause the sodium content in the affected foods to rise while decreasing potassium levels, which is precisely contrary to what the body requires to restore its healthy metabolic function.

Consequently the benefits of eliminating salt and sodium from the diet while supplementing potassium could be counteracted by consuming foods which had an altered chemical composition because of the manner in which they were produced. Furthermore, chemical pesticides and fertilizers are not washed off most foods by water but actually penetrate the food and thereby poison it. Eating these treated foods brings toxins into the body, where they accumulate, weaken the immune system, and interfere with detoxification.

Part of Gerson therapy for many people is learning how empty refined calories can be replaced with nutritious foods and condiments. For instance, different types of whole-grain breads are used instead of refined white breads; maple syrup, molasses, date sugar, or honey may be substituted for white processed sugars; and certain spices, such as garlic, and foods can be combined so as to enhance their flavor without salt.

The Clinic

Dr. Gerson's clinic occupies facilities on the western coast of Mexico. The clinic is about a block from the beach and has several rooms with an unobstructed ocean view. The other rooms face onto a courtyard garden filled with tropical flowers and trees, benches, and walkways.

Most patients come from the United States by air. They are picked up at the airport by a member of the staff, driven back to the clinic, and assigned a room (all rooms are private). Starting immediately and continuing throughout their stay, all patients receive a glass of freshly prepared juice every hour on the hour, except for one glass which is given on the half hour in order for 13 glasses to be served in a 12-hour period. Within the next hour or so, a staff doctor arrives, examines the patient, looks at his or her records, makes an appraisal, and orders the appropriate course of therapy. Patients who are not in condition to go into the dining room have meals delivered to their rooms. During the day patients are given cod liver oil and vitamin B_{12} shots, and any other prescribed treatment, such as ozone therapy.

Besides the therapeutic techniques, the clinic has excellent facilities and staff to go along with a carefully designed, individually tailored dietary regimen. While the clinic has space for 30 patients, generally the population stays below 25 because of the tremendous amount of work involved in the care of each patient. There is a staff of about 40 people, which includes the kitchen personnel, groundskeepers, doctors, nurses, and cleaning persons. Each patient has a personal doctor assigned upon arrival. There is also a staff doctor on 24-hour call for emergencies.

In addition to medical records and basic personal items, patients are asked to bring a tape recorder for the lectures that are given to help them learn and understand the therapy and to continue it when they return home. The lectures are on food preparation, juicing, the specific medications, the typical healing crises that occur on the program, and restoration of the body's normal healing functions.

THE MEALS Three full vegetarian meals are served each day. Usually, breakfast is served at 8:00 a.m. and consists of freshly squeezed orange juice, oatmeal with fresh stewed fruit, and a special whole-grain rye bread. This bread is made mostly of rye flour with a small amount of wheat or another whole grain. It is unsalted, made with very little yeast, and served toasted without butter.

At breakfast patients also receive the first of their special juices. Along with the potassium supplement, in six of the 13 daily juices there are three drops of half-strength Lugol solution (an iodine/potassium compound). A small amount of thyroid extract is also added. Dr. Gerson felt that the iodine and thyroid supplementation is extremely important in helping to reactivate the immune system. He found that this iodine-thyroid combination is especially important in the first couple of weeks. The patients receive five grains of thyroid, the full regular thyroid extract with Lugol's solution, not thyroxin or eytomel or any of the fractionated materials.

Four times a day starting at breakfast, patients also receive three tablets of pancreatic enzyme (pancreatin), which helps restore the stomach acid, as most patients with chronic degenerative disease have low stomach acid and need to have supplementation of these materials in order to be able to digest properly. In addition, they receive a 50 mg tablet of niacin six times a day.

After breakfast and from then on during the course of the day, a glass of juice is served every hour on the hour (except for the one served on the half hour). There are five glasses of apple and carrot juices in a 2:5 and 3:5 proportion, and four glasses of various green leaves juiced with a little apple to make them more palatable. All the juices are supplemented with the potassium solution.

Lunch, served at 1:00 p.m., begins with a large plate of fresh mixed raw salad which contains a wide variety of green and other vegetables. It is spiced with a little bit of apple cider vinegar and mixed with a few herbs and a little water so that it is not too strong.

In the very last year of his practice Dr. Gerson found that cold-pressed, good-grade linseed oil was very helpful to his patients, and that it was the only oil or fat they were able to handle and digest. This was important because during all the years he had been treating cancer he had looked for an oil that would help the body transport vitamin A, which is an oil-soluble vitamin. Since the carrot juice and the liver and green juices all contain very high levels of vitamin A, which cancer patients need to reactivate the immune system, Dr. Gerson felt that he also needed some form of fatty substance to transport the vitamin. He finally found that linseed oil filled the bill since his patients could handle it without any new tumor growth. Gerson therapy thus includes a few tablespoons of linseed oil in the diet. Usually patients are started on two tablespoons daily (it can be used as an oil dressing for salads at lunch and dinner). After about a month the oil is cut down from two tablespoons to two teaspoons daily.

The second item at lunch is a soup that Dr. Gerson called Hippocrates soup. Dr. Gerson found that certain combinations of foods and herbs have a very beneficial and detoxifying effect on the body. This soup is a combination of celery, onion, leek, potato, and tomato; it is cooked and mashed and is quite tasty. Garlic can be used for extra flavor.

The soup is followed by a cooked vegetable plate, usually two vegetables and either a baked potato or potato salad that is made without eggs or mayonnaise but may consist of diced potatoes in a vinegar and flax oil sauce. Neither salt nor butter, cheese, nor any fatty substance are added to the foods, but most patients report that after a while they lose the need for these condiments and enjoy the natural flavors.

In the course of the day, patients also receive a shot of crude liver extract with B_{12}, which is important for helping to restore the damaged liver.

THE "HEALING CRISIS" The next phase in the therapeutic process is what Dr. Gerson described as a healing crisis. This is an activation of the body's defenses, and often takes the form of fever as the immune system begins to be functional again. Ms. Gerson says that "almost invariably, once the patient begins to produce a fever, this is followed by a tumor reduction. It seems as though the fever helps the body break down and dissolve the tumor tissue. Along with the fever comes flulike symptoms such as aches and pains all over the body. If, for instance, the patient has had symptoms of arthritis, the arthritis often flares up during this period. Usually within 24 hours or so, the healing crisis abates, the arthritis, for instance, is gone, and the tumor tissue is reduced.

"This healing crisis can be quite severe in cases where the body is getting rid of accumulated heavy toxic materials. These toxins are removed through the coffee enemas, but sometimes the patient will have a very irritated colon because these materials literally burn as they are being released. In those cases, we alter from the coffee to chamomile tea enemas, which are soothing and help the body release toxic materials which have built up. We see that type of problem with patients who have been medicated a lot with tranquilizers and antidepressants. The latter are especially toxic. When they have been used a fair amount, the patients suffer a lot as they are released from the body. We have to give these patients chamomile tea enemas, peppermint tea and chamomile tea by mouth, and oatmeal gruel—all are soothing."

Usually these reactions last no longer than three to four days, and when they are over, the patients claim to be much relieved and improved, with a better appetite. Sometimes, if patients have experienced a good deal of weight loss, they become ravenously hungry. This is part of the body's normal healing process. Ms. Gerson tells of a 38-year-old patient with liver and pancreatic cancer who had been told in October 1986 that she would not survive past Christmas. She was on 12 morphine tablets a day and had lost 25 pounds. In two days she was free of pain and off the morphine, went through a healing crisis with fever, came out of it after about six or seven days, and started to be very hungry. Every time she went to dinner, she took food back to her room so that she could have an extra meal or two in the middle of the night. This patient not only survived past Christmas but told Ms. Gerson in mid-1987 that she was feeling wonderful and had resumed most of her normal activities.

OZONE THERAPY Ozone therapy, used in Europe for decades but still considered an unproven method in the United States, is one of the most effective new techniques added to Gerson therapy. In an interview Ms. Gerson explained what is used: "Ozone actually, in chemical formula, O_3. Plain oxygen that we breathe all day in our air is O_2. Now, that little extra oxygen atom that's loosely attached… comes off easily and is highly active…. It circulates very quickly through the bloodstream and attaches very quickly to the red blood corpuscles and is released, among other places, at the tumor site. The ozone molecule [is] extremely active and can directly attack and destroy malignant tissue….

"The ozone can be used in many ways. We have used it, for instance, as an insufflation into the rectum. The patients can easily hold it, and it is then absorbed directly into the bloodstream. It is also extremely effective in colon cancers…. It can be put into the vagina for tumors in the cervix or uterus. It can also be given intravenously; ozone gas can be injected into the veins without any adverse effect. This is something that makes people worry a bit, because they still remember the horrible exterminations done on prisoners in concentration camps. By simply injecting air into the vein, you can cause spasms of the heart and death. But this isn't air; it's oxygen and ozone. This has to be done properly, with very, very thin needles so that the bubbles that go into the vein are very, very tiny. And they disperse very quickly in the blood and are picked up very rapidly by the red blood cells. If it's done slowly, there is absolutely no adverse effect. To be quite sure of that, I'm usually the first one to get any of these new techniques done on me. I've had it done a couple of times; I've had as much as 20 cc of ozone gas put into my veins and I'm here to talk to you about it. We also use room ozone generators, so you can breathe air augmented with ozone; it goes through the lungs very quickly and into the bloodstream.

"Ozone has been proven to be very effective at killing viral and bacterial infections. The ozone can be used, and has been used, by pediatricians, for instance, in cerebral infections. They have removed a little bit of cerebral fluid and put it into the spine, and it works very well. So ozone happens to be one of the best and totally nontoxic antibiotics. In some patients infections and even certain anaerobic parasites can be quite easily eliminated with these ozone injections. Besides that, there is a feeling of well-being in the patients who are given ozone because it increases oxygenation and energy. Ozone is also, with its extra single oxygen atom, an excellent scavenger of free radicals, in other words, a very good detoxifying agent. It's altogether a wonderful material, and we feel that since we started using it quite extensively within the last three or four years, we have vastly improved our results."

The Patients

Cancer patients have been treated with Gerson therapy for over fifty years, and the results have been amazing, especially in contrast to those reported by conventional cancer specialists and agencies. The therapy was administered at treatment centers in New York and then California before the establishment of the new Gerson Therapy Center in Mexico in 1977. It was at this time that statistical analyses began to be recorded. A 40 to 50 percent improvement rate was recorded in terminal patients, and an 80 percent improvement in early to moderate cancer cases.

The following are examples of the types of improvements patients have experienced using Dr. Gerson's therapy. In 1946 Dr. Gerson appeared before a Senate subcommittee considering appropriations on cancer research. The first two cases described here are those presented by Dr. Gerson at the hearings. He was then treating cancer patients at Gotham Hospital in New York City.

EXAMPLE 1: A 15-year-old girl had been treated for a tumor in the spinal cord. She had been paralyzed and her father had been told that she would die. When she came to Dr. Gerson, she couldn't walk or feed herself. In front of the Senate, approximately eight months after beginning Dr. Gerson's treatment, she could move her arms and hands, and her tumor had vanished. Now, over 40 years after her appearance before the Senate, this woman, who in 1945 was given approximately six months to live, is still alive. "I have been tested throughout the years," she writes, "and there is no sign of any tumors." She concludes by saying, "I truly hope that our government will soon open its eyes to the truth, even if it does hurt the canned food business."

EXAMPLE 2: In this dramatic case, the patient had had a malignant lymphatic sarcoma that resulted in very large tumors of the abdomen, neck, groin, and other areas. After going to two hospitals, she was informed that nothing more could be done. A year on Dr. Gerson's diet changed her life completely. When she was presented to the Senate, there was no sign that she had ever had cancer.

Additional cases, 59 of which are discussed in detail in Dr. Gerson's book, are no less dramatic.

EXAMPLE 3: A 17-year-old girl was admitted to the hospital with a tumor on her upper lip, which had grown progressively larger since age two years. She had undergone two operations to remove the tumor, but it continued to undergo "rapid growth and possible development sarcoma." She also had a lung tumor, and she said that "12 tumor specialists told Mother that I would never get well and that there was nothing they could do!" A few years later 12 smaller tumors were discovered all over her body (on her jaw, eyelid, arms, etc.). Within one month on Gerson therapy the tumors were no longer palpable, and a month later they disappeared.

She went off the diet for two years when she got married, and three years later she developed a brain tumor which caused dizziness and impaired vision. She decided against the operations recommended by her doctors and began intensive treatment with Dr. Gerson. One month after she had begun the therapy her eye specialist noted "a phenomenal improvement." The last report received by the patient's mother noted further improvement of the overall well-being of the patient.

EXAMPLE 4: A 30-year-old man was diagnosed with melanosarcoma (a skin cancer) which was spreading over his body. He had undergone surgery once for removal of tumors. New nodules appeared two months later, and doctors recommended radical surgery of both axillae and removal of the left half of the neck and neck muscles as well as removal of glands in the groin. Refusing surgery, the patient started Gerson therapy, and within a few weeks all glandular nodes had disappeared. Three years later the patient wrote the following to Dr. Gerson:

"I am now more vigorous and stronger than ever. The long 18 months to two years which we spent in following your orders have paid off with the very best of health. At present I weigh 187 pounds and am full of pep and health. I have worked harder this year than in any year of my life and I eat a well-balanced diet of all normal, healthy food." He remains well today.

Dr. Gerson's daughter, Charlotte, relates some of the cases which have been treated with success at the new clinic. She notes that all these patients arrived at the clinic with independently confirmed cases of cancer and with complete medical records from their physicians (x-rays, tests, and surgical and full diagnoses). She stresses that the primary reason that the clinic does not do its own medical reports is that the results are often so striking that when the clinic did records in the past, doctors did not believe them and tended to accuse the clinic of falsifying the records.

EXAMPLE 5: An eight-year-old boy, Teddy, arrived at the clinic blind and completely paralyzed. He had undergone surgery in March 1985 and had been diagnosed as having a malignant brain tumor, the same type of tumor which recently took the lives of baseball's Dick Howser and ex-CIA director William Casey. By the middle of summer of that year his condition had deteriorated substantially. When he arrived at the clinic, although he had had surgery, an external tumor had started to grow from the back of his head and he had lost speech, sight, control of his bladder and bowel, and the use of his limbs. He had been given up as hopeless by his attending physicians and was not expected to live more than a month or so.

He was put on Gerson therapy at the clinic and remained on it upon his return home. A year and a half later his mother wrote to Ms. Gerson that Teddy had regained all functions with the exception of his eyesight. Two years later she reported that there was a slight improvement in the acuity of his vision; he still could not see, but otherwise he was doing very well. Notwithstanding his handicap, Teddy was not enrolled in a school for the blind but was put in a regular school, in which he was doing exceptionally well. At the end of the school year in 1987 Teddy received a letter from the principal of the school congratulating him on his academic performance and announcing that he had made the honor roll. Teddy remains alive.

EXAMPLE 6: A woman arrived at the clinic with a confirmed diagnosis of breast cancer with bone metastases. She had had a mastectomy but subsequently the cancer had spread. When she arrived at the clinic she had six "hot spots" in the spine and one in the shoulder. Her outlook was extremely poor and she was in considerable pain. She started on Gerson therapy around October 1985. In September 1987 she reported to Ms. Gerson that not only did she have a clear scan, she was horseback riding three times a week, was in excellent shape, and had plenty of energy. These results should be compared with those of orthodox treatment, in which a breast cancer with bone metastases does not have any chance of recovery no matter what type of therapy is used (surgery, chemotherapy, or radiation).

PART NINE

Chronic Conditions

43

Digestive Disorders

I n examining digestive disorders, one must realize that there are no special clinics where research and treatment focus exclusively on these disorders and that there are no particular pioneers in the field of digestion. One reason for this is that digestive disorders are not often clearly diagnosed as such. Usually a determination is made that a patient has cancer, arthritis, or renal failure, but these conditions may be directly related to chronic digestive disorders that have gone undetected for a long time. While you may be undergoing extensive, costly, and toxic treatment for a diagnosed disease, it is possible that only the symptoms of your disease are being treated, not the underlying cause.

HOW DIGESTION AFFECTS YOUR TOTAL HEALTH It is up to you to be aware of the great effect that digestion has on your total health. If you suffer from a disease you must—with the help of a physician who is knowledgeable in this area—determine how maladies related to digestion can cause a variety of disorders ranging from constipation to colon cancer. In fact, virtually every disease can be ameliorated to some extent by taking appropriate steps to correct digestive problems.

However, since few specialists truly understand the complexities of digestive disorders, you should use the information in this chapter to find the sort of health care you need if you suffer from a disease that may be related to poor digestion and nutrient absorption. Even if you do not suffer from any ailment, read this chapter carefully to make yourself aware of what causes and what alleviates digestive disorders.

Many people go through life with chronic digestive problems—fatigue, nausea, and flatulence, for instance—and assume that this is a normal state of affairs. Any complications that result are rarely understood as being connected to the underlying problem with the digestive mechanism. Disturbances that obviously do have something to do with digestion—diarrhea, constipation, and the like are usually dealt with by taking over-the-counter drugs such as laxatives and antacids. You may think that you have a "weak" stomach or that these problems are just "a part of getting older," and so you may end up taking these drugs habitually, unaware that they can exacerbate the problem.

After reading this chapter, you will be in a position to take positive steps toward rectifying any slight imbalances you may have detected on your own or toward preventing these disorders from occurring in the first place. Proper digestion is primarily a lifestyle choice: You can use your understanding of this physiological process to take control of your own health and well-being.

Traditional vs. Alternative Approaches

The differences between traditional and alternative medicine are particularly evident in the treatment of digestive disorders.

THE TRADITIONAL VIEW Under the traditional medical paradigm, a person is generally deemed healthy unless he or she has a major breakdown in the digestive apparatus or a major disease. In essence, the paradigm says that health is the absence of disease.

Traditional physicians are more used to treating symptoms than correcting the causes of disease. For this reason, one of the most common problems in digestion—because it is a cause rather than a symptom—is one that is rarely considered in traditional medical practice. This is the *malabsorption syndrome*, or the failure of the body to absorb the nutrients that have been ingested, a failure often related to a digestive lapse. The problem here is that even though a food is eaten and goes through the whole digestive system, the nutrients, minerals, and vitamins frequently do not get into the blood and hence do not penetrate the body at the cellular level. Instead, the undigestible elements are eliminated as waste byproducts.

Traditionally trained physicians are very skilled at identifying and treating conditions when they have reached a severe disease state. Their approach to diagnosis and treatment is anatomical in nature; they use sophisticated technologies to evaluate the anatomy of the digestive tract—the stomach, pancreas, small intestine, colon, and liver—and look for evidence of tumors, polyps, ulcers, and other problems. These technologies include endoscopy, the upper GI series, barium enemas, colonoscopy, and liver scans. However, orthodox physicians are less likely to search out or treat an underactivity, sluggishness, or suboptimal function. Even when such conditions are detected, they are often not considered significant.

The standard therapies for digestive problems include medications such as Tagamet, Zantac or Pepcid for stomach problems or Azulfidine or prednisone for inflammations of the colon. Although these medications may give relief, they tend to suppress the symptoms without getting to the root of the problem and repairing the faulty digestive mechanisms.

Additional problems may arise from the fact that many traditional physicians are also specialists and tend to be compartmentalized, focusing only on their own area of specialization. For example, they may not make a connection between various diseases and improper digestion. Specialists will tend not to integrate the fact that a joint problem may be related to a digestive problem, because they are looking only for the condition in which they specialize. The typical patient suffering from these two connected problems will end up going to a joint specialist for the first disorder and to a gastroenterologist for the other, and it is likely that the two specialists will remain separate. A connection between the two disorders may never be made.

Finally, traditional medicine generally gives limited attention to the role of the diet in digestive ailments. For instance, a gastroenterologist will usually consider the role of food only when it is obviously connected to a disease, such as with lactose intolerance; or when patients report a direct connection between eating a specific food and a symptom (e.g., when they eat a tomato they get diarrhea).

THE ALTERNATIVE VIEW The digestive process, like all body systems, produces a wide spectrum of symptoms when it is not functioning properly. Complementary physicians consider mild or moderate symptoms to be signs of suboptimal functioning in the digestive system. These symptoms include burping, a feeling of indigestion, and constipation. Traditional physicians, by contrast, generally overlook these symptoms and focus their attention on the severe end of the spectrum, where symptoms such as vomiting or bleeding often call for immediate and aggressive orthodox treatments.

Complementary physicians may also use special machines that are not in wide use by traditional physicians, even though these machines are of the highest scientific standards. For example, a complementary physician may use a Heidelberg gastrogram to analyze the level of stomach acid. Although this machine was scientifically devised at the University of Heidelberg and is widely used in Germany, it has relatively few followers in the American medical community.

Complementary physicians often analyze the body biochemistry via sophisticated blood laboratory testing that goes beyond traditional medicine's use of the standard SMA-24 profile to identify major digestive disorders.

Complementary physicians tend to treat via natural substances such as foods, herbs, or homeopathic preparations. Also, supplements which contain concentrated forms of vitamins and minerals are fundamental elements of body rebalancing.

Complementary physicians tend to be attuned to the concept of mild malabsorption since they frequently see the end product of this condition, namely, deficiencies of nutrients. Thus, they are more likely to focus upon this possibility.

Complementary physicians tend to view body functions in a holistic manner so that they are attuned to the relationship between digestion and vitamin and/or mineral deficiencies related to malfunction of such conditions as arthritis, anemia, and disturbances of the glucose mechanism.

Finally, complementary physicians are very interested in the foods eaten, the frequency, the quantity, and whether any specific foods seem to cause irritation or other reactions. Thus they tend to test for food sensitivity as part of a complete analysis of body function.

Why Digestive Problems Occur

The digestive process consists of four main steps, which involve: (1) hydrochloric acid in the stomach; (2) pancreatic enzymes, as food is entering the first part of the small intestine, known as the duodenum; (3) bile, from the liver and gallbladder; and (4) the absorptive processes in the small intestine. If any of the organs involved in digestion are faulty in any way, the efficiency of the absorptive process can diminish and the body will not be receiving the nutrients it needs.

INSUFFICIENT PRODUCTION OF STOMACH ACID Insufficient or suboptimal production of stomach acid, which is not an illness but a sluggish stomach, is the single most common digestive problem, especially in those over the age of 40. In the presence of low stomach acid, food digestion in the stomach is impaired and thus protein and minerals are not digested efficiently. Many persons with this condition of insufficient acid suffer with burping and belching after meals.

As people age, their physical energy tends to weaken, which can affect basic body functions. Because it takes a great deal of energy to make stomach acid, a very strong chemical substance, suboptimal stomach acid production tends to be a common problem as we grow older.

PROBLEMS WITH THE PANCREAS AND ITS DIGESTIVE ENZYME PRODUCTION The pancreas is a gland which produces pancreatic enzymes for digesting protein, carbohydrates, and fats. After the stomach does its part, it empties its contents into the duodenum. This partially digested food, called chyme, is a thick, acidic liquid and the pancreas must first neutralize this acidity and make it alkaline before digestion can proceed further.

Therefore, the first juices from the pancreas are alkalinizing juices to offset the stomach acid. If these pancreatic enzymes are suboptimal or insufficient, or if the interplay between the release of chyme from the stomach (about one teaspoon at a time) and the production of pancreatic enzymes is off balance, difficulties will result. Very often, when a patient complains of digestive problems from two to three hours after eating, the pancreas is the culprit. Many of these problems, which involve carbohydrate and/or protein and/or fat digestion, are a result of faulty pancreatic function.

PROBLEMS WITH BILE The liver produces bile, which is stored in the gallbladder and sent into the small intestine through the bile duct. This alkaline fluid is partly responsible for fat absorption by emulsifying or breaking down fats into smaller particles.

The liver is a major workhorse of both digestion and the detoxification of the body, and it can be overtaxed by a poor diet or by any inefficiencies in the digestive process. If the production of stomach acid or pancreatic enzymes is sluggish, this sub-par functioning can be a major stressor on the liver.

PROBLEMS WITH THE SMALL INTESTINE When the chyme is released from the stomach into the small intestine, the pancreas produces and releases large quantities of alkaline pancreatic enzymes, which are the next phase of digestion and which also protect the duodenum from the acidic chyme. The digested food then moves further down the small intestine into the jejunum, where food absorption takes place. The nutrients are then carried through the bloodstream to various parts of the body to provide energy and maintain general health.

MALFUNCTIONS OF THE ILEOCECAL VALVE One of the main problems that can take place in this region involves the ileocecal valve, which is located between the small and large intestines. Diarrhea and constipation are often associated with malfunctions of this valve. It is the valve's job to open when the contents of the small intestines are ready to pass through, to let a certain amount through and then to close. However, if the valve stays open too long, or is too tight or closed, problems can occur.

Mainstream medicine does not appreciate the importance of the ileocecal valve in the digestive process, largely because the valve's location makes it difficult to visualize. Faulty heart valves, by contrast, are well appreciated and well studied by traditional medicine, which uses highly technical anatomical equipment to take pictures of the heart valves.

If the ileocecal valve remains in the open position, it can enhance diarrhea, because everything is flushing through too quickly. Food passes through the digestive apparatus so rapidly that the absorptive process is impaired. In addition to the rapid transit due to the open valve, the movement of food progressing in the normal forward direction may reverse, as the contents of the colon backflush, or move retrograde.

The colon is the "garbage disposal" area, whereas the small intestine is the "kitchen" area. Therefore, a backflush of waste material puts a biochemical stress on the small intestine and irritates the liver as well. In short, the waste material makes a mess in the kitchen. The material may be absorbed into the bloodstream, causing various toxic reactions.

If the ileocecal valve is too tight or too closed, this can cause constipation. The tight valve, by not facilitating the passage of the small intestine contents into the colon, retards the entire digestive flow, which leads to infrequent bowel movements, or constipation.

Unfortunately, most people are unaware of this valve and its importance in the regulation of proper digestion.

IRRITATION OF THE COLON When the stomach acid mechanism and pancreatic enzyme system do not work properly, undigested particles of food or actual pieces of food may reach the colon, also called the large intestine. This not only irritates the colon, but also leads to flatulence because the undigested food will be fermented by the friendly and not-so-friendly bacteria residing in the colon.

The colon may be irritated throughout its entire length or in any of its anatomical parts: the ascending colon, the traverse colon, or the descending colon. Often, the most common pattern is that all three parts are out of balance. In this case, the patient should consider how he or she handles stress because the colon may be the organ in which various stress elements are manifesting themselves. In addition, caffeine often leads to a general colon irritability.

When the irritation occurs in the descending colon only, there has been found to be a high correlation with food intolerances or allergies in his testing of hundreds of patients. Therefore, the person needs to keep a careful food diary to identify frequently eaten foods and those he or she suspects are culprits in allergic reactions. Foods that commonly prompt allergic responses must be identified in the diet as well. These include gluten foods (wheat, barley, oats, and rye), sugar, peanuts, citrus fruits, dairy products, soybeans, corn, and caffeine.

An irritation of the ascending colon alone means that its ecology is off balance. For example, there may be an overgrowth of yeast because the ascending colon becomes a fermentation factory of sorts when undigested food particles reach it. The unfriendly bacteria that live in the small and large intestines may be especially likely to overgrow if the production of stomach acid is so low that the digestive system becomes under-acidified, or excessively alkaline. A highly alkaline environment favors the growth of yeast, which may then exceed the usual niche it maintains within the ecological population of the colon.

Symptoms of Digestive Disorders and Related Health Problems

Digestive system disorders can be placed in two main categories: those that are clearly and directly related to digestion, and those that are ultimately digestion-related in origin, but are a step or two removed from the digestive process, and therefore more difficult to connect with digestion.

Symptoms of digestive system disorders in the first category are more easily recognized. The most common include burping, belching, flatulence (intestinal gas), a feeling of indigestion, undigested food in the stool, or a feeling of food "just sitting there." When such symptoms are present, it is relatively easy to connect the problem to some malfunction in the digestive process.

But other symptoms are not so quickly connected to digestion. These are problems that occur over time and are related to the long-term inefficiency of absorption of nutrients and/or an insufficiency of nutrients in the food to begin with, both of which can lead to deficiencies. Because such problems are not directly connected to digestive difficulties, hardly anyone realizes that they have anything to do with digestion. Such disorders include:

GUM PROBLEMS: Many problems with receding gums, bleeding gums, and periodontal gum disease have a lot to do with a deficiency of calcium and other nutrients, including vitamin E, GLA (gamma-linolenic acid), bioflavonoids, and vitamin C. Suboptimal production of stomach acid can lead to malabsorption of minerals, especially calcium and iron.

ANEMIAS: Many cases of anemia can be linked to low stomach acid levels, because iron is not absorbed efficiently. Other factors can include blood loss, heavy menstrual cycles, and low iron in the diet.

OSTEOPOROSIS: This disease, so common in elderly women, results from a deficiency of calcium and many other minerals, which can be accentuated by digestive malfunctions resulting in malabsorption of calcium.

OSTEOARTHRITIS: Insufficient stomach acid production can lead to lack to proper absorption of dietary calcium. Eventually, this results in a deficiency of calcium, where osteoarthritis is a major component of a long-term deficiency of calcium in the body due to malabsorption, leading to breakdown of the joints.

SKIN DISORDERS: Poorly nourished skin is another common result of malabsorption due to digestive problems. The skin may show minor symptoms, such as blemishes, dryness, scaling or a tendency toward irritation. These are often due to dietary deficiencies and/or poor absorption of calcium, zinc, vitamins A and E, and essential fatty acids.

HYPOGLYCEMIA: Also called "low blood sugar," this condition is related to nutritional deficiencies, including low zinc, chromium, and manganese, which are associated with uneven levels of glucose in the blood.

In addition to the ailments related to long-term malabsorption, there may also be illnesses of the digestive apparatus. These include:

GASTRITIS: This condition is an irritation of the stomach, very much like an "internal sunburn," which can cause some of the discomfort of indigestion in the stomach. Some people with gastritis (type B) harbor a bacteria called helicobacter pylori. This bacteria is unique in its ability to live in the acid environment of the stomach, where it is able to create a protective coating. Many people with gastritis also have problems with absorption of vitamin B_{12} and may develop macrocytic anemia as a result.

GASTRIC ULCERS: Up to 80 percent of those with gastric ulcers (of the stomach) have helicobacter pylori in their systems. While stress may impair the immune system and allow the bacteria to take hold, it is not the main culprit in most stomach ulcers.

DUODENAL ULCERS: These are severe irritations of the small intestine. Some studies show that up to 80 percent of people with duodenal ulcers also have helicobacter pylori present.

Dr. Martin Feldman's Approach to Digestive Wellness

Dr. Martin Feldman, a traditionally trained physician who practices complementary medicine by emphasizing his own concept of soothing, replacing, and repairing faulty digestive mechanisms, is a true innovator among alternative physicians. A former assistant clinical professor of neurology at Mt. Sinai Medical School, Dr. Feldman now practices general medicine treating a wide variety of conditions including allergy, low immunity, skin problems, arthritis, diabetes, hormonal imbalances, headaches, and other brain-related symptoms such as poor memory, poor circulation, irritability, and sleep disturbances.

Over many years of practice, Dr. Feldman has found that a surprisingly large number of health disorders are related to a suboptimal digestive process, which lessens the body's ability to absorb the vital nutrients needed for proper functioning. Rather than taking the traditional approach of waiting for symptoms to develop into full-blown disease states, Dr. Feldman strongly believes in treating sluggish conditions before they develop any further. By identifying and treating digestive system disorders when they first begin, he believes that a large number of degenerative diseases may be avoided.

Many of Dr. Feldman's patients have been dissatisfied with standard methods of treatment. They often report that side effects of standard drugs were bothersome and did not correct their condition.

"Through years of observation, I have learned from my patients," explains Dr. Feldman, "and I have found that when more sophisticated methods of testing are used, it turns out that inefficient digestion or malabsorption is frequently present and leads to a variety of other problems." He estimates that at least one-third of the patients seeking his help have digestive difficulties. He has found this to be particularly so in regard to people with osteoarthritis, gum disease, skin problems, anemia, and hypoglycemia. In response to his patients' needs, Dr. Feldman has worked out various nutritionally oriented therapies which have proven successful in the treatment of many of these disorders.

In his approach to diagnosis, Dr. Feldman makes full use of standard medical procedures and tests, including a complete medical history and comprehensive blood laboratory analyses. In addition, he also uses a noninvasive technique, based on acupuncture pressure points, to test the strength of various internal organs and mechanisms.

ACUPUNCTURE AS A DIAGNOSTIC TOOL One of the most interesting and innovative aspects of Dr. Feldman's approach is his use of acupuncture meridians for diagnosis. With this technique, he can determine which components of a patient's digestion are sluggish by testing the level of electrical activity in their specific meridians, including those for the stomach, pancreas, small intestine, ileocecal valve, colon, and liver. If the flow of energy in a given meridian field is deficient, that aspect of digestion is often suboptimal.

As Dr. Feldman explains it, "Acupuncture theory has taught us that there are many energy flows throughout the body. The energy flow is quite specific along anatomical pathways. These pathways were very well worked out for centuries in China. Traditional acupuncture intervenes by inserting needles into specific acupuncture points to either improve the flow of electrical energy through that flow channel or meridian, or to reduce the flow. Whereas acupuncture electrical information and its electrical pathways are mainly used as a therapy to rebalance either over- or under-energy flow, the under or deficient electrical flow often reflects an organ weakness. Thus, the liver with an entire acupuncture meridian can be tested by measuring the over or under electrical activity in its meridian. Although acupuncture is thought of almost exclusively as a therapeutic modality, it has equal value as a diagnostic tool."

Because he uses acupuncture theory only for diagnosis and not for treatment, Dr. Feldman has no need for needles. Instead, he has developed his own method of using these meridians to profile the component parts of the digestive apparatus and pinpoint areas that are underactive or suboptimal in strength. In this way, he can determine the energy flow or lack of flow and thus assess the body's function.

As he describes it, "Without needles, without any invasion of the body, we can profile the liver's energy, the stomach's energy, the pancreas's energy, the small intestine's energy and the colon's energy. We can see which areas are the weakest, where imbalances are occurring and where the problems are most severe." And all this can be accomplished in minutes.

GASTROENTEROLOGY STUDIES Once these areas of weakness are identified, Dr. Feldman can then focus on them using other modalities, if needed. At times, the diagnostic input of a gastroenterologist might be required when a specific anatomical or physical determination is needed. The gastroenterologist would decide upon the technical study or studies required, which might include the use of x-rays or visualization with tubes, such as a gastroscope or a colonoscope, allowing the specialist to look directly at the stomach or the colon.

A NEW VIEW OF BLOOD TESTS Dr. Feldman considers the results of standard laboratory tests in his diagnostic analysis of a patient. These tests can also yield important data if viewed in a complementary fashion. The tests that are readily available and inexpensive are the SMA-24 blood tests, the complete blood count with differential, the sedimentation rate, an analysis of the urine, and measures of long-term glucose levels and thyroid levels.

Once Dr. Feldman has laboratory results, he can then look for indicators of suboptimal functioning in the digestive system, such as a slight elevation of SGOT enzymes on an SMA-24 blood test. The SGOT, an enzyme found in liver cells, can double or triple in the presence of hepatitis. Traditional physicians will generally look for such extremely elevated levels and tend to disregard slightly elevated levels. Dr. Feldman, however, considers that even a small increase in the level of this enzyme can indicate that the liver, while not diseased, is off balance and in need of attention. As he explains, "I'm looking for the early evaluation of an imbalanced or a suboptimal liver, not a very diseased liver."

Lab tests can also disclose blood indicators of malabsorption, such as:

(1) the presence of macrocytic anemia, an enlarged red blood cell anemia that is associated with vitamin B_{12} deficiency;

(2) the level of ferritin, one of the forms of iron stored in the body, which if relatively low is an early indicator of a low metabolism of iron;

(3) the level of total protein in the blood, which when relatively low (especially if there is adequate dietary protein) can indicate malabsorption of protein; and

(4) low body levels of minerals such as calcium, magnesium, zinc, manganese, chromium, and selenium, which are very common with malabsorption. Deficiencies of fat soluble vitamins such as vitamins A, D, and E are also common. The water soluble vitamins, including B complex and C, are generally less affected because they are more easily absorbed.

INFECTIONS OF THE DIGESTIVE SYSTEM As another diagnostic tool, Dr. Feldman considers the results of laboratory tests for bacteria and parasites. For example, helicobacter pylori antibody levels in the blood, which may reflect the presence of these bacteria, provide an important clue to duodenal or gastric ulcers. Tests for these bacteria are performed by specialty laboratories.

Similarly, a test may reveal the presence of parasites in the digestive tract. These parasites, Dr. Feldman notes, "are becoming more and more widespread in the population," and are another cause of digestive problems. Traditional testing methods involve taking random stools and looking at them under a microscope to try to find cysts or other parts of the parasites.

Now, however, there are more sophisticated methods of finding parasites. The newer tests look for special stains or, more importantly, monoclonal antibodies that will attach even to small fragments of the parasite or its cysts. The attached antibodies are visualized under the microscope. Thus, these sensitive tests identify the biochemical markers of parasites, so that it is no longer necessary to literally find the parasites themselves. For example, this type of test can detect the marker of giardia, parasites that primarily inhabit the duodenum and upper small intestine, which previously were very difficult to diagnose via their visualization. Also, sophisticated analysis of the stool with culture of bacteria and other organisms yields important information regarding the ecology of the flora of the colon.

TREATMENT Once he has identified the areas of weakness of the digestive apparatus, Dr. Feldman can begin to formulate a plan to soothe, replace, repair, and rebuild faulty mechanisms. The treatment chosen depends on diagnostic findings, including the areas of dysfunction—stomach acid, pancreas enzymes, bile, small intestine; whether and where irritation is present; and whether any pathogens are present, such as parasites or unfriendly, harmful bacteria. To correct any of these problems, Dr. Feldman's treatment relies heavily on natural substances, including vitamins, minerals, herbs, and occasional homeopathic preparations.

The first step in this process is to soothe any parts of the digestive system that are irritated, whether the stomach, the small intestine, or the colon. Various herbal-type preparations, such as marshmallow, slippery elm, and aloe vera may be used for this purpose. Aloe vera, in particular, can help soothe the ileocecal valve, the ascending or descending colon, or the entire digestive tract when it is irritated.

Next, it is important to replace whatever is insufficient or suboptimal. When deficiencies of stomach acid are determined, oral acid tablets (such as betaine hydrochloride or glutamic acid) may be prescribed in order to optimize the stomach acid phase of digestion. However, Dr. Feldman warns that this therapy must be supervised by a knowledgeable practitioner so that the patient does not take the wrong type of acid. Other natural substances, including zinc, folic acid, intrinsic factor, and duodenal substance, can help get the stomach back on track to produce its own acid.

For problems with low production of pancreatic enzymes, oral analogues of pancreas enzymes may be swallowed after the meal to augment this phase of digestion. There are many varieties of vegetarian enzyme products on the market, and Dr. Feldman matches up the type of product used with his analysis of the pancreatic energy field.

EMPHASIS ON REPAIR

The most crucial step in Dr. Feldman's treatment is repair. The concept of repair of suboptimal function is not a high priority of the American model of medical treatment.

Traditional physicians might consider the use of oral medicine to replace pancreatic enzymes. The main therapies related to the stomach are Tagamet, Zantac, and similar pharmaceuticals which suppress the production of stomach acid. The focus of concern is heavily weighted toward ulcers or other anatomical maladies.

Although the pharmaceuticals that control stomach acid have their place, the mainstream paradigm does not go beyond that to address the issue of cause: What is the root cause of the faulty mechanism and how can it be repaired?

Often, Dr. Feldman's approach to repair includes two phases: (1) eliminating negative influences on the organ in question, including foods that provoke allergic reactions, irritants such as caffeine, and poor food choices (such as fatty and denatured foods) that stress the digestive system; and (2) using natural therapies to rebuild the suboptimal or sluggish component(s) of digestion.

Obviously, the vitamins, minerals, and herbs used in the repair process will vary with the needs of each patient. However, Dr. Feldman's treatment formulas often make use of the following substances:

STOMACH: Cabbage juice, licorice, zinc, vitamin A, n-acetyl-glucosamine, marshmallow, ginger, and cayenne. Natural therapies such as goldenseal and a citrate bismuth can help to combat an infection of helicobacter pylori, although an antibiotic may be needed as well to eliminate the bacteria.

ILEOCECAL VALVE: Lipid soluble chlorophyll, aloe vera, slippery elm bark, and whole echinacea. An increased consumption of water can also help to repair a closed valve.

COLON: For an imbalance of the ascending colon: bifido bacteria (which can help rebalance the ecology of the colon), fructooligosaccharides (FOS), insoluble fiber, and calendula. For a parasitic infection of the lower digestion: grapefruit seed extract, black walnut herb, artemesia, and homeopathic antiparasite remedies. For a general irritation of the colon: aloe vera, lipid soluble chlorophyll, butyric acid, Jerusalem artichoke flour, inulin, 1-glutamine, a mix of soluble and insoluble fiber, calcium, and magnesium.

LIVER: Lipo factors, including choline, methionine, and inositol, milk thistle, herbal formulas that combine a number of herbs, and homeopathic solutions.

Food Allergy and Digestion

Foods to which a person is allergic or sensitive are considered as invaders or chemicals by the body's immune system. Thus, they irritate and weaken the digestive apparatus. Because of this, it is vital that the patient be educated in terms of diet and food allergies. This is a rather complicated procedure, given our present-day American diets.

For instance, it is quite common to find that persons consume large amounts of foods to which they are, in fact, allergic. Many of our food products contain hidden ingredients that must be recognized and avoided. For example, many products contain corn syrup for sweetening and persons sensitive to corn should avoid them. Wheat is another common allergen that is often hidden in our foods. Thus, learning how to read food labels in this way and choosing food correctly is a critical part of treatment.

Food allergies and sensitivities are a major source of digestive trouble. They may be hereditary but may also result from cerebral or gastrointestinal reactions or sensitivities to ingested substances. Wheat, for instance, very commonly incites a cerebral allergy, and a large proportion of the population suffers from gastrointestinal allergies to milk. These kinds of food allergies are responsible for such symptoms as headaches, fatigue, rapid mood swings, heart palpitation, diarrhea, constipation, and shortness of breath. Besides milk and wheat, other common food allergens are corn, eggs, beef, citrus fruits, potatoes, and tomatoes.

Digestive malfunctioning can be the cause of complications when allergens are present. If there is a deficiency of the gastric juices or pancreatic enzymes, for instance, a food will be in the system for a much longer time than it would if there were adequate amounts of acids and enzymes to break it down readily and on schedule. If the food sitting in the system is one to which the body is sensitive, that sensitivity will be heightened by the delayed action of the digestive mechanism. Furthermore, if protein molecules are not broken down into small enough particles because of faulty digestive processes, the larger units entering the bloodstream will be treated like foreign invaders by the body's immune system, and an allergic reaction will ensue.

Children possess less developed gastrointestinal systems than adults, and so they often suffer from obvious food allergies. Later in life, though, as the digestive system becomes more sophisticated, these allergies are manifested in less obvious ways. Even if the symptoms are not the same, the underlying allergy may be. A child who has suffered milk-associated asthma, for instance, may have severe acne as a teenager. The milk allergy is still there, but its symptoms have moved to a different organ system, often misleading the patient and physician into thinking that the original allergy has been outgrown.

Allergies often manifest as disease forms. If a person responds negatively to a food substance so that heart palpitations or gastric distress reactions result, that person may seek and receive treatment from a cardiologist or gastroenterologist. The patient may ultimately be subjected to invasive and taxing drug and/or surgical treatments that have side effects far more debilitating than the original food allergy.

HIGH-PROTEIN DIETS High-protein diets pose a special problem with respect to food allergies. People who consume a lot of protein usually tend to have it in their systems around the clock. This is because it takes at least four to seven hours for proteins to be digested, and if the protein is fried, deep-fried, or charcoal-broiled, it can take even longer. If a person starts the day with bacon and eggs and then has a sandwich of cold cuts and cheese at lunch, more meat and maybe milk at dinner, and even a late night snack of milk or ice cream or pizza, that person will have protein in his or her system all the time.

If any substance—in this case, protein—sits in a person's system virtually all the time, two things will occur. First, the person will almost certainly develop an allergy to it because of overexposure. Second, the person will probably not be aware of the allergy because his or her system will never be without the substance long enough for him or her to notice its ill effects when he or she ingests it versus the clearing of those symptoms while he or she is without it. The negative symptoms then become cumulative and chronic and begin to be manifested as disease states. Digestion is usually strained, and the different disorders that appear are generally regarded as signs of poor health, which becomes tolerated as unavoidable or is attributed to genetics or age.

FOOD ROTATION Food rotation is one way to help alleviate this problem or to treat it at home as an adjunct to whatever medical care you are receiving. Don't eat the same foods day after day, because no matter how healthy and nutritious they are, you will not benefit from them if you body rejects or reacts negatively to them. Wheat, for example, is an excellent food, but because it is found in practically every processed food, it is also a very common allergen. Therefore, it must be rotated in the diet with other grains. Eat it no more frequently than every fourth day and in no more than a 4-ounce portion at each meal. Then there is a good chance it can be eaten without causing an allergic reaction.

All foods should be rotated in this manner. Even if your body is not responding negatively in an overt way, you may be having hidden reactions to many different foods. Even if you are not, by overusing a food—eating it too frequently and in oversized portions—you may eventually develop an allergy to it. Try to make a routine of rotating all foods and avoid eating processed foods as much as possible because certain foods, such as corn and wheat, are ingredients in many of them. (See chapters 11 and 13 for further discussion of rotation diets).

Lactose Intolerance

Lactose intolerance is an almost universal digestive disorder. Probably two-thirds of the world's adults cannot tolerate lactose, which is found in milk and all milk products. This substance is very poorly absorbed in the digestive systems of most adults, with the notable exception of Scandinavians and other northern Europeans. When lactose-sensitive people continue to eat dairy products, they begin to suffer from a wide range of symptoms, which include abdominal cramping and bloating, chronic nasal discharge or postnasal drip, puffiness under the eyes, gas, and diarrhea.

Lactose intolerance is a malabsorption of lactose caused by a deficiency of lactase, the enzyme responsible for milk digestion. Lactase breaks down lactose into the readily digestible forms glucose and galactose. If it is absent or deficient, lactose remains undigested in the system. Some passes through the blood and is excreted in the urine, but most ends up in the large intestine. The lactose molecules draw water out of the tissues and into the intestinal cavity, while the undigested glucose is fermented by intestinal bacteria. Carbon dioxide is given off during this process, and diarrhea, bloating flatulence (gas), and belching may result.

The lactase deficiency can be caused by damage to the intestinal mucosa; this damage may be brought on by acute infectious diarrhea in infants. Malnutrition, cystic fibrosis, and colitis also have been known to cause lactase deficiency. Even in the absence of these traumas, lactose deficiency is very common.

The most obvious remedy for lactose intolerance is to stay away from milk and all milk products. Also, keep in mind that lactose is found in many vitamins and most processed foods, and so it is best to avoid processed foods and request from vitamin manufacturers a full disclosure of their exact ingredients. It is important to eliminate lactose from the system completely in order to recover from its ravages. Another option may be to purchase a commercially prepared lactase supplement which boosts your supply of lactase and enables you to better digest the lactose. Some lactase-deficient people, however, can still eat a few fermented milk and dairy products without negative consequences. These items—primarily yogurt, buttermilk, and cottage cheese—must be tested on an individual basis to determine one's reaction to them.

Gastritis

Gastritis, another very common digestive disorder, involves an inflammation of the mucosa lining the inner wall of the stomach. The inflammation is accompanied by such symptoms as nausea, vomiting, and loss of appetite. In the acute form, gastritis can be caused by infections and/or the ingestion of corrosive agents such as alcohol and aspirin. In the chronic form, gastritis is a serious condition which may be the cornerstone of degenerative diseases such as ulcers.

The treatment of gastritis should include the elimination of any substance (an allergen or anything else that is difficult to digest—fried foods, etc.) known to be causing or aggravating the condition. The diet should include lots of liquids and small amounts of soft foods such as soft-boiled eggs and oatmeal. Vegetables should be steamed to maximize their digestibility and reduce their acidity. A blood chemistry test should be performed to determine what (if any) vitamin deficiencies exist, since they often play an important role in this disorder. Vitamin deficiency related to gastritis is responsible for many complications, among which are a prickly sensation in the skin, loss of memory, depression and general weakness.

Pressure Diseases

Another group of disorders associated with the digestive system have been termed pressure diseases, because they are caused by a pressure buildup that results from failure to eliminate waste efficiently. They include diverticulitis, hemorrhoids, hiatus hernia, and appendicitis, among others.

DIVERTICULITIS Diverticular disease is the most troublesome and widespread of these conditions. It occurs when the muscle rings encircling the colon, which move along bulk matter, become clogged. Try clenching your fist and then imagine that mud is stuck in the creases of your hand. The crease can be thought of as diverticula, and the mud in them is the result of food being trapped in the creases of the digestive organs. When bulk and fiber are lacking in the diet, the colon must deal with a mass of food too dry to be pushed along with ease, and so it becomes overworked, overstressed, and overstrained. Its membranes eventually herniate, or rupture, and it is these ruptures that are called diverticula. When there are many diverticula—and there can be hundreds—they tend to become inflamed and cause more acute symptoms. This condition is known as diverticulitis. Approximately one in four people with diverticular disease develop these acute symptoms.

Diverticulitis barely existed before the 20th century, but now is said to affect one-third of all adults middle-aged or older, half the population over 50, and two-thirds of the population over 80. It is the most common digestive disorder of senior citizens.

Research on the genesis and development of diverticular disease has shown that it results from a gross lack of fiber in the diet. The refining of carbohydrates seems to be the main culprit here, since this condition is almost wholly absent in cultures where whole grains, legumes, vegetables, and such are the mainstays of the diet and where processed foods are not used. Diverticular disease is also limited mostly to the wealthy nations of the west and is rarely seen in underdeveloped areas. In India and Iran, the disease is seen only in the upper classes, whose dietary regimens are not unlike those of the industrial working classes in the west.

The traditional treatment for diverticular disease has been to give the patient stool softeners to help the stool pass through the system and expanders to force it out. Given for about two weeks, these agents are typically administered along with antibiotics. Until recently, doctors also put these patients on low-residue, soft food diets. Since it has been shown that this sort of diet exacerbates the condition, the diet has been replaced with a fibrous diet that helps the colon begin processing waste more efficiently and with less strain. Bran is usually prescribed, and patients are often told to avoid milk products and spicy foods since these tend to produce abdominal pain, pressure, and gas.

Alternative treatments for diverticular disease may include the above suggestions, but will add to the patient's diet other abdominal and intestinal cleansers taken orally. These include cellulose, hemicellulose, pectin, and noncarbohydrate lignin. Celery, brussels sprouts, broccoli, and especially beet juice will also help the condition. Bran should be unprocessed because this type has a shorter intestinal transit time and helps increase stool weight. The diverticula pockets may be cleansed with dietary supplements of chlorophyll, chamomile, garlic, vitamin C, zinc, nondairy acidophilus, pectin, and psyllium. Instead of medicinal antibiotics, good amounts of garlic may be used since garlic is a natural antibiotic.

HEMORRHOIDS Hemorrhoids, closely associated with constipation, are another pressure disease. Constantly straining to push dry, compacted stools out of the system causes the veins in the rectal and anal passages to become distended and engorged with blood. The veins become weakened, lose their elasticity, and can no longer carry blood properly; they allow the blood to pool instead, creating a ballooning effect.

When the hemorrhoids are internal, they can become obstructive to stool passage. With constant pressure being exerted against them, they may rupture and bleed and, in severe cases, hemorrhage. External hemorrhoids, also called piles, are very sensitive and may grow to the size of golf balls.

It is estimated that half of all Americans over 50 years of age have hemorrhoids and that hemorrhoidal treatment is a $50 million a year industry. Most of the profit comes from sales of suppositories. Suppositories are given to shrink and lubricate hemorrhoids to prevent them from rupturing. Alternative treatments for hemorrhoids center on hygiene, diet, and exercise. If you increase your intake of water, vitamin C, and fiber and exercise regularly, the blood trapped in the hemorrhoidal veins will be reabsorbed into the body and the problem will be cleared up. However, it will recur unless you integrate these changes into a new, more healthful lifestyle.

HIATUS HERNIA Hiatus hernia is another condition related to constipation and low-fiber dietary regimens. Like the other pressure diseases, it is essentially a modern-day Western disorder affecting primarily middle-aged and older people. There are no warning symptoms until it causes a sharp pain just below the breastbone. Caused by the body's straining to evacuate stool, it is a condition in which part of the stomach wall becomes extended and pushes up against the diaphragm and the skeletal system. Obesity may contribute to the condition, which also sometimes develops during pregnancy.

The traditional treatment of hiatus hernia usually includes antacids, a bland diet, and sometimes surgery. These steps are adequate to relieve the pain, and you certainly should follow the suggestions of your physician. The alternative (or even complementary) approach is aimed at going beyond alleviation of the painful symptoms by establishing a dietary regimen that can reverse the condition while ameliorating the source of discomfort. Since constipation due to a low-fiber diet is frequently the cause of this condition, make sure to get plenty of high-fiber bulk foods. In the case of the obese, losing weight may also help. Before resorting to surgery, you may want to explore other alternatives, such as the treatment developed by Dr. Nathaniel Boyd in New Hope, Pennsylvania, in which a saline agent is injected into the stomach-lining tissue, causing it to tighten and retract from the diaphragm.

APPENDICITIS Another pressure disease, appendicitis, is caused mainly by troublesome elimination. The most common abdominal emergency in the Western world, it is brought on by continuous constipation, straining during stool elimination, and anal retention—failing to evacuate solid waste when the body tells you to. By delaying your bowel movements, perhaps because you are too busy to be inconvenienced, you confuse your body. The water from fecal matter begins to be reabsorbed, and the dry, hard stool that is left will pass only with great pain and difficulty. In the meantime, you strain the muscles that must retain this mass and eventually train them to delay normal elimination.

Some people learn to have a bowel movement only once a day or even once every two or three days. You should have two or three bowel movements a day, depending, of course, on what and how often you eat. When there is not enough dietary fiber to move food and waste readily through the digestive system, pressure builds up and blocks the passage of stool. Bacteria accumulates and backs up into the three to six inch long appendix which is attached to the large intestine. The appendix becomes inflamed and infected, and an appendectomy must be performed.

To see how critical the issue of fiber is here, consider the 6,000 appendectomies performed in the United States each week compared with only a handful per year in rural Africa, where processed fiber-depleted food is virtually nonexistent. This again is a pressure disease that can be avoided or even treated with a high-fiber diet consisting of complex carbohydrates.

Ulcers

Ulcers are a disorder of the digestive tract that afflicts between 10 million and 14 million Americans, including 2 million children. About 1 in 10 men and 1 in 20 women suffer from ulcers. Ulcers are sores, or lesions, that can be found anywhere in the body.

Ulcers occur most often in the duodenum, which is the upper portion of the small intestine. The duodenal ulcer is usually found in the first few inches of the duodenum. The second most common type is the peptic or gastric ulcer, which affects the stomach.

Some ulcers are slight abrasions of the internal mucosal lining; others advance to the stage where they totally perforate the stomach or intestinal wall. Their three stages of development are known as perforation, penetration, and obstruction. In acute perforation, the ulcer eats through the wall of the abdomen. This is the most serious state and causes the greatest number of deaths. Surgery to close the perforation is virtually unavoidable.

Penetration is the stage where the patient usually awakens at night with severe pain in adjacent areas of the body—the back, liver, and so forth—not just to the stomach. This transfer of effect to other organs makes the ulcer diagnostically elusive. Obstruction is the stage in which swelling caused by inflammation affects the stomach and the opening to the small intestine.

The vast majority of ulcers are caused by the helicobacter pylori bacteria, a fact discovered just two decades ago by Dr. Barry Marshall, an Australian physician. Today, it is known that this bacteria accounts for 80 percent to 85 percent of all digestive ulcers. These bacteria take up residence in the lining of the digestive tract and then contribute to the breakdown of that lining, resulting in a lesion or crater.

This discovery overrides the prior concept that ulcers generally are caused by the production of too much hydrochloric acid or stress. A number of government panels have begun to reach a consensus opinion that most ulcers are indeed caused by helicobacter pylori and that the medical community should routinely test for the bacteria to diagnose and treat ulcers.

TRADITIONAL TREATMENT In recent years traditional physicians have in fact moved in the direction of testing for the bacteria. However, they generally limit their treatment to the use of antibiotics to combat the bacteria and acid-production blockers such as Tagamet and Zantac to prevent the stomach acid from irritating the broken-down tissues in the mucosal lining.

The mainstream use of antibiotics is commendable because it addresses the cause of ulcers, a bacterial infection. However, the heavy reliance on acid-production blockers is troublesome for two reasons: the drugs do not address the real issue, which is why the bacteria have proliferated in the digestive wall; and since the natural stomach acid opposes the bacteria, the acid-production blockers may reduce the body's ammunition against the infection.

In the process, these drugs also may lessen the effectiveness of the overall digestive process. The stomach's role in digestion is to produce acids that help to digest foods. When that mechanism is suppressed by acid-production blockers, the body may not digest foods efficiently and absorb nutrients. Thus, a patient may suffer from malabsorption.

ALTERNATIVE APPROACH As a complementary physician, Dr. Feldman advocates a much more comprehensive approach to the treatment of ulcers. In addition to removing the bacteria, he says, the treatment should accomplish three goals:

(1) helping the stomach to heal the erosion; (2) rebalancing the stomach acid production so that it works properly; and (3) optimizing the immune system so that the body can protect against a reinfection.

Dr. Feldman's approach to diagnosing and treating ulcers generally includes these steps:

DIAGNOSING THE CONDITION

The mainstream medical community uses endoscopes and upper GI x-rays to determine if an ulcer actually exists. Dr. Feldman may call on these diagnostic techniques as well to obtain as much scientific data as possible on the status of an ulcer.

Like a growing number of physicians, he also uses tests performed by specialty laboratories to identify the presence of helicobacter pylori. However, these tests have not yet progressed to the point that they can reliably detect the antibodies for the bacteria in every patient. The reason is that the bacteria are located in the inner wall of the stomach or duodenum, which is an open space. That means the body's blood antibody circulation may not reach them and the test may produce a false negative result.

Given this imperfection in the blood antibody testing, Dr. Feldman also draws on his clinical judgment in the diagnostic process. If the blood laboratory test is negative but his clinical experience suggests the presence of helicobacter pylori, he may conduct a therapeutic trial by having the patient take some natural substances that combat the bacteria. He can use this technique because the substances are safe and well tolerated, producing very few side effects. Dr. Feldman then monitors the patient to determine if the therapy reduces his or her symptoms.

OPPOSING THE BACTERIA

Both antibiotics and natural substances can be used to fight the helicobacter pylori infection. For antibiotic treatments, Dr. Feldman favors the use of amoxicillin because it is usually effective and well tolerated by most patients.

In addition, he may combat the bacteria at a second level with natural therapies. These include goldenseal, an herb that has antibacterial properties, the mineral bismuth in a citrate form, and various combinations of homeopathic solutions. Because homeopathic solutions function primarily as transmitters of energy, Dr. Feldman can test the effect of specific homeopathic products on the body's acupuncture-meridian energy fields.

HEALING THE ULCER

In addition to removing the bacteria, it's important to help the body heal the ulcer irritation or erosion. Dr. Feldman uses a variety of natural treatments to heal the digestive lining. These include cabbage juice, aloe vera, licorice herb, and n-acetyl-glucosamine, a nutrient complex. Other substances that soothe the irritation and thus promote the healing process are marshmallow, ginger, cayenne, and an herbal combination called Robert's Formula.

TESTING FOR FOOD ALLERGIES

Food allergens tend to irritate the stomach, making it harder to heal an ulcer or any other irritation of the stomach or intestines. Therefore, any foods to which a patient is allergic should be eliminated from the diet. To identify such offenders, Dr. Feldman will test a patient's reaction to various food substances by placing them upon the taste portion of the tongue. The brain-taste mechanism, which is very highly developed, has the ability to ascertain if a given food substance is a danger to the body.

REBALANCING THE ACID-PRODUCTION MECHANISM

Paradoxically, many patients with ulcers have a low production of stomach acid. As Dr. Feldman notes, the low-acid environment allows the helicobacter pylori bacteria to get a foothold in the mucosal lining, while a normal acid level would tend to provide some antibacterial protection.

In addition to allowing the bacteria to grow, a low acid production can cause other problems. One is that food will sit in the stomach for a long period of time and ferment abnormally due to the lack of sufficient stomach acid. This fermentation then produces abnormal acids that irritate the stomach and the ulcer. The result: you end up with the paradox in which people with low stomach acid experience the symptoms of a high acid production. They may take antacids to suppress the symptoms, but that remedy doesn't correct the true problem. The stomach must work efficiently so that food does not ferment abnormally.

Dr. Feldman has found that many patients suffer from this problem, so he puts a strong emphasis on reoptimizing the stomach's acid mechanism. Again, he uses a variety of natural therapies to get the acid-production system back on track. These remedies include zinc, folic acid, intrinsic factor, and duodenal substance. In some cases, he also prescribes oral acid supplements, which may assist the acid mechanism in strengthening itself. This latter treatment requires careful supervision to ensure that a patient takes the proper form of acid in the proper doses.

REPAIRING THE IMMUNE SYSTEM

As a final phase in his treatment of ulcers, Dr. Feldman focuses on rebuilding the immune system. The logic here, of course, is that the immune system must be working at its maximum level to fight the bacteria that causes most ulcers to begin with. This part of the treatment consists of nutrients that serve as the building blocks of the immune system. They include vitamins A, E and C, bioflavonoids, gamma linolenic acid (GLA), essential fatty acids, zinc, and selenium.

WHAT TO AVOID As a final note, people who suffer from ulcers should avoid ingesting items that exacerbate the condition. These include alcohol, nicotine, aspirin, coffee, soft drinks, salt, high-oil nuts, and even raw fruit (except bananas). Foods that are excessively spicy and difficult to digest should be avoided as well, since more pepsin will be secreted to deal with these foods.

Thus, you don't want to eat a lot of high-protein foods, especially those accompanied with high levels of fat. Animal foods require more gastric involvement and should be avoided if possible. If you do eat meat, at least trim the fat; also, avoid overcooking, deep frying, and charcoal broiling since these processes make the molecules bond more tightly so that more digestive effort is required to break them down.

Carbohydrate foods have their own protective buffer in the natural state (brown rice and whole grain and vegetables), but once they are refined (white flour and white rice, cakes and pastries) the buffer is stripped away. Therefore, avoid denatured, processed carbohydrates. Vegetables are usually quite acidic, so avoid those causing gas (turnips, cucumbers, brussels sprouts, broccoli, radishes, and cauliflower), especially in the raw state. Vegetables will be less acidic if you cook them, preferably by steaming since it does not destroy their fibrous structure. Raw cabbage juice has been found to be quite beneficial.

While ulcers require special diets, there are general guidelines for good health. No chapter on digestive disorders could be considered complete without suggesting the sort of dietary modifications that you should undertake to both avoid and overcome these conditions.

44

Chronic Fatigue Syndrome

C hronic fatigue syndrome poses a major problem for traditional medicine, which has fumbled in its treatment to the point of sometimes claiming the illness does not exist.

But chronic fatigue is a major problem in the United States. Millions do not have the energy they once had. This goes from those having just a little bit of energy to those with a maximum depletion, who are in bed, unable to function. This chapter will look at different courses and natural therapies, nutritional and psychological, to help people, especially as many traditional healers have abandoned the field. We ask: What is the natural approach?

Definition

Our readers may recall Charlotte Perkins Gilman's classic short story, "The Yellow Wallpaper," written at the turn of the century. It focuses on a woman who feels lethargic and constantly worn out. However, since her husband, a doctor, cannot find any organic cause, he refuses to believe she is really sick. He keeps telling her to lie down, although this "rest cure" is not working and even making her sicker. This common female complaint in the 19th century provides a striking parallel to the reception of chronic fatigue syndrome, which many practitioners, not finding its cause, have tried to ignore.

Dr. Neenyah Ostrom, author of *America's Biggest Cover-Up*, underlines that chronic fatigue syndrome is very difficult for the average doctor to diagnose especially because the government agency charged with creating a definition of the illness has come up with one so misleading that nobody can figure out what the illness is supposed to be. In late November 1995, there was a meeting at the

Centers for Disease Control and Prevention in order to discuss changing the definition of the disease. It turned out researchers wanted to define it out of existence, so that anyone who is tired can be said to have chronic fatigue syndrome. Ostrom argues, "If you speak to any clinicians who see people with this condition, they will tell you it is very easy to diagnose. They can tell within moments of talking to a patient whether the patient has it, since the symptom complex is so unique."

Why is it that for 10 years Americans with a debilitating illness were not recognized as having a disease? They were simply told that chronic fatigue syndrome does not exist. Dr. Dean Black says, "You have to go back to the last century and you will read about women suffering from nervous disorders—so many of them that clinics had to be set up to care for them. There was always the search for a cause, but one couldn't be found and so, without a cause, doctors wouldn't say it was a disease. It had to be in the patient's mind. This is not a new way of sweeping things under the carpet."

Dr. Ostrom mentions, "Since there are debates in the government on whether chronic fatigue syndrome exists or not, very few therapies have been tested for chronic fatigue patients."

Dr. Black brings up another historical example to explain the current difficulties traditional medicine has in coming to grips with chronic fatigue syndrome. He says that we need to go back to the origin of the current paradigm, in the 17th century, when Rene Descartes promulgated his doctrine of universal doubt, which held that one could know nothing without scientific method. "People would say things to Descartes, but he would explain them away, saying, 'I can see this, this, or this equally plausible alternative.' He felt we could only know things for certain if we have a scientific method whereby we can define truth in a rational, cause and effect manner. Now that method had a certain amount of rules, one of which was there had to be a straight line between a single cause and a single effect. Deviate from that and you introduce so much complexity that the idea of certainty is lost.

"Medicine's power base is the idea of its basis in certainty, which hinges upon the concept of a single, linear, cause-effect relationship. That's why medicine is always looking for a single causal factor. This is called the theory of specific etiology."

In reference to chronic fatigue syndrome, Dr. Black alludes to the situation of Epstein-Barr, which was initially thought to cause chronic fatigue syndrome, although later this theory was challenged. "That is why they were so happy to discover this EB virus," he explains. "It seemed marvelous to them because it served to justify the single cause idea. Yet, as has been frequently pointed out, everyone may have Epstein-Barr [it is so widely distributed]. Chronic fatigue syndrome is caused by many factors operating together. But this idea has been excluded by traditional medicine, which refuses to come to grips with multifactorially generated disease. So medicine's reluctance to accept this multifactorial explanation is because it holds to this idea of absolute truth, which requires simplicity and must have one cause and one effect."

Dr. Andrew Gentile stresses that we need to be able to differentiate between chronic fatigue syndrome and other health problems. Since chronic fatigue syndrome has no known cause, we need to rule out other disorders that we know the cause of. The working definition provided by the government for this disease says there is no other illness at the root of it. Distinguishing it calls for great care, since feeling fatigue is ubiquitous as a symptom of many diseases, such as anemia, low thyroid, hypoglycemia and a variety of other illnesses. These other illnesses must be clearly ruled out.

Dr. Gentile calls chronic fatigue syndrome a degenerative disorder that causes fatigue and has flulike symptoms. The fatigue is not a simple tiredness, it is an exhaustion accompanied by feelings of unwellness. Often patients are bedridden for months. The chronic fatigue syndrome—a syndrome is a disorder that contains a collection of symptoms, but is not necessarily a disease entity—includes sleep disturbance as one of its manifestations. The patient is not able to fall asleep or stay asleep and does not feel refreshed or restored after much sleep. The other symptoms have to do with cognitive and intellectual functioning. As Dr. Gentile describes, "Patients will go from one room to another and when they get to the new space, they can't remember why they are there. They can't remember the name of a colleague they worked with for years. There are difficulties in concentration and an inability to read complex texts. So there are cognitive symptoms, sleep disorder, flulike symptoms, frequent sore throats, tender lymph nodes and often fevers and chills."

Diagnosis

Dr. Martin Feldman says the first step in the analysis of any patient who comes to him with fatigue, whether mild, moderate, or severe, is to profile the patient to see how he fits with the five major categories or possibilities of the syndrome. It is not, by any means, that every patient with the syndrome has these problems, but they are a good place to begin tests in case of weaknesses in the areas. These five indicators, with Dr. Feldman's comments, are (1) An immune viral breakdown, leading to low adrenal function. "You'll find that almost all chronic fatigue syndrome people have low adrenal function once you test the adrenals properly"; (2) Thyroid imbalance. "A large proportion, though a little less than half, have these issues"; (3) Vitamin B deficiency; (4) Hypoglycemia; and (5) Cerebral allergies. Within those five indicators are found almost all people with chronic fatigue syndrome.

For Dr. Feldman, after these tests, the next phase is testing thymus, spleen, and the lymphatic system. He states, "It's very easy yet very hard to test the thymus because you have to use electrical energy. You could test the T and B cell counts. That's easy to do but it's very expensive; so, in daily practice, it's easier to test thymus electrical energy. You can also do this for the spleen. When we have a circuit, like a weak thymus circuit, we can try any aspect of therapy within the weakened circuit to obtain a resonance in a way that will help that circuit be strengthened and come up."

Dr. Gentile is more concerned with self diagnosis. "If you feel you have chronic fatigue syndrome, ask yourself these questions: (1) Am I not just tired but have had debilitating fatigue for six months? (2) Do I have flulike symptoms? (3) Can I not find any physiological cause? (4) Do I have pronounced sleeplessness? (5) Do I have low stress tolerance so that if I take a short walk or try any sport, I feel vaguely ill and tired? If you answer yes, you may want to consider a fuller assessment of yourself by a physician."

Dr. Majid Ali states that most physicians have a tendency to focus narrowly on one or two aspects of a problem. But, he says, "I don't think trying to find a diagnosis for one or two symptoms is terribly important. What is important is how the patient describes his suffering. We need to think of what things we can do at a molecular and energetic level to relieve his suffering and restore his health.

"I've seen patients whose lives have been devastated by chronic fatigue syndrome. They've gone through all these drugs, antivirals, steroids. With each drug, they get better initially and then nose-dive. What do we do?

"Think of chess. In chess, the queen is the most powerful and the pawn is the weakest piece. But as a good chess player knows, there are many games in which the lowliest piece, the pawn, can take that all-powerful queen. This can be done by a player who is able to 'read the board.' And I think what a good holistic physician has to be able to do is read the board. What I mean is look at the patient's whole situation and then, as a doctor, ask yourself: 'Should I first work on the kitchen, what the patient eats, or should I first work on self regulation, control of breathing and so on, or must I first create some hope, make them talk to other recovering patients and take a workshop?'" Making the correct choice of initial therapies should take precedence over minutely analyzing the symptoms.

Causes

VIRAL POSSIBILITIES Although many resist the multicausal explanation for chronic fatigue, as Dr. Gentile notes, some healers have been able to develop such an explanation. "There is now the feeling that a single cause is not sufficient, and, moreover, in the world of treatment, it is now much more productive to work on caring for the symptoms than on continuing on a quixotic search for a single cause. Healing is really the charge of medical research."

Dr. Feldman tells us that chronic fatigue syndrome is an entity of severe fatigue with a 50 percent reduction in capacity. There is a continuum of fatigue problems, and chronic fatigue is on the low end. "One will find two factors involved," he states, "first, a flulike infection, either a new or renewed one, and often, though not necessarily, a history of such infections, whereby the viral mix—for there may well be more than one virus involved—weakens the immune system. The second point is that this immune system difficulty somehow pulls down hormonal function. Almost all patients with this syndrome have low adrenal function and many have low thyroid function. So we have a hormonal mix-up causing fatigue, but behind this is the viral disease pulling down the immune system."

According to Ostrom, "What is probably behind the chronic fatigue disorder is a virus that was first found in AIDS patients. It is called human herpes virus 6 (HHV-6). What is interesting is that there are two types of this virus, one form is found very widely in the general population and the other is found in people with cancer, AIDS, chronic fatigue syndrome, and other immunological problems. That virus can attack the immune system very effectively and I believe it will eventually be found as instrumental in causing chronic fatigue syndrome, AIDS, and some forms of cancer."

Dr. Gentile adds that a plethora of studies look at viruses in connection with this syndrome. One theory has it that there is a single viral agent. In fact, he states, "I have heard chronic fatigue syndrome being called a number of things: from Epstein-Barr to mononucleosis.

"Epstein-Barr was brought into the discussion by way of a lab in Philadelphia, which exclusively studies this virus. One of the lab assistants was negative for current and acute Epstein-Barr virus, but during the course of the study the assistant developed the symptoms of chronic fatigue syndrome. He was treated and found to be positive for Epstein-Barr virus. So we had the first studied case in which a person went from Epstein-Barr negative to Epstein-Barr positive at the same time as he had all the symptomatology for chronic fatigue syndrome. That began a flurry of studies investigating the Epstein-Barr connection. We now know there is not a high degree of correlation between the symptoms of chronic fatigue syndrome and Epstein-Barr serological titers. So Epstein-Barr is probably not the cause of chronic fatigue syndrome."

Dr. Gentile goes on to note that the Epstein-Barr virus is widely distributed in the populace. Most people have it by age eight. So there is not a clear discrimination between those who have it and those who do not. We would expect many more people to be ill with chronic fatigue if it was indeed Epstein-Barr that was causing it. As a result, this candidate for being the cause of chronic fatigue syndrome has fallen into disfavor.

"However," he persists, "several other candidates have presented themselves, including HHV-6 (formerly called HBLT), which is a B lymphocyte virus and was being studied by the National Institutes of Health. But again, studies showed that this virus is very widely distributed and thus could not be the distinguishing agent that was responsible for the syndrome. There are other studies proceeding. Wistar, a renowned laboratory in Philadelphia, is looking at a retro virus, HTLV-2, as a possible cause."

Dr. Neil Block reminds us that quite a list of viruses have been implicated in some forms of fatigue syndrome. These viruses include, along with Epstein-Barr, herpes, coxsackie, adeno, and entero viruses as well as a number of lesser known ones. He echoes Dr. Gentile in saying, "The one that has received the most attention, Epstein-Barr, has not panned out as an answer and, indeed, in some sufferers, it plays either a very minor role or no role at all. But it can't be dismissed. And most cases deserve to be tested with an Epstein-Barr viral titer to determine the antibody status, whether there is or has been current or past infection with the Epstein-Barr virus."

Other viruses that have been implicated are the long-lasting sequelae or aftermath from the hepatitis virus, the mononucleosis virus or influenza virus, all of which have been known to cause a fatigue two or three months after the original virus has disappeared.

Dr. Majid Ali says, "It's very enlightening to look at Epstein-Barr. I come from Pakistan and for us Epstein-Barr was not a kissing disease. Because of poor sanitation, all of us were exposed to the virus as children. But we came through the exposure with intact immune systems. Our immune systems fought off the Epstein-Barr and we acquired a certain resistance. In this country, people will get infectious mono or Epstein-Barr (those are the same thing) later. They get it in college or high school. It's the so-called kissing disease. They will be sick for four or five weeks and lose some weight. They'll be tired for some months and then snap back."

However, he states, there is a different possible scenario. Think of people in their 30s and 40s, with good jobs. They are not fit and are under tremendous stress. Their nutrition is awful, and now comes Epstein-Barr and it floors them. "The problem," Dr. Ali states, "is not that Epstein-Barr is more virulent; the problem is their molecular defenses are shattered. Their bodily ecosystems are destroyed and so they have no ability to fight back. So whether Epstein-Barr is a devastating terminal attack on their immune system or a garden variety illness they can easily get over depends on the state of their previous health. You give Epstein-Barr to little children and they generally survive very well. In fact, they generally don't even know they have this disease. So the issue is not the power of the virus but of our defenses."

Dr. Gentile states, "The consensus among practitioners is that a single virus probably does not cause this illness. We have to carefully distinguish between cause and trigger. Clearly, a virus may trigger a cascading set of events in various body systems: neural, endocrine, cognitive, hormonal. A variety of abnormalities may be found in these systems, but if viruses do trigger these imbalances, then they quickly hide within the normal cells—which does usually happen with viral behavior—while their effects wreak havoc in the body system."

It is as if the virus triggers something in the immune system wherein the system cannot find its way back to homeostasis, failing to self regulate. There is a breakdown each time the immune system is stressed by toxic load from the environment or food allergies or when infections are reactivated. The flare-ups and relapses occur and reoccur frequently, reproducing all the symptoms. These relapses then compound themselves. If a patient is not sleeping every night, then symptoms like exhaustion and a deranged immune system crop up.

"We know, by the way," Dr. Gentile adds, "that the rhythms of this illness dovetail nicely with 90 minute circadians. In sleep, we have a REM cycle that occurs every 90 minutes, and this is the cycle by which our immune system is synthesizing proteins. The immune system works lock and key with this cycle. But if one has a sleep disturbance caused by a virus or a set of viruses from this disorder, one's sleep will be off and so the immune system will be off."

ENVIRONMENTAL FACTORS AND ALLERGIES Dr. Ali looks to the surrounding environment and lifestyle as playing causal roles. He relates that the immune system gets injured by environmental pollutants, such as mold, formaldehyde, and pesticides, as well as by allergic foods or by nutritional aspects, by stress and by lack of physical fitness. He gives equal emphasis to all four areas.

Dr. Michele Galante also sees the importance of allergies. "The patients I have seen have been very allergic, not only to pollens and airborne agents (as from grasses and trees) but especially to foods and to chemical sensitivities. These are people that are so sensitive that they cannot be exposed to perfume, nail polish, gas fumes, carbon monoxide, or even just paint, as from a freshly painted room. They are so debilitated that a short exposure will give them headaches, a weakened condition, even emotional states. Chronic fatigue syndrome is closely connected to allergy."

Ostrom seconds this notion. People who have chronic fatigue syndrome will often develop allergies they have never had before. For instance, they will exhibit violent allergic reactions to medicines and show new food sensitivities. In patients with chronic fatigue syndrome as well as AIDS, a portion of the immune system shuts down, another portion, which causes immune reactions, is revved up, almost 100 percent. These people respond immunologically to things that, before they got sick, their immune system would not have recognized.

Some of these allergy causing substances are unavoidable. Chemicals in our environment, aside from those in our foods (the coloring, preservatives and so on), are everywhere. There is chlorine in our water, the air is filled with pollutants; things that were not in our ecological system 50 or 60 years ago. Recent phenomena that accompany technological advances, such as the mercury in silver amalgam dental work, is weakening our systems. These chemicals in and of themselves do not necessarily have so strong an impact, but all together, day after day, for many years, overloads the liver and immune system. Electromagnetic influences, previously ignored, are now under discussion. Many believe the cathode rays from computers influence the electromagnetic fields of the body, for instance, as well as the electromagnetism of cellular phones, radio waves, TV waves, things relatively new to our environment."

FOODS AND YEAST INFECTIONS Dr. Ali says we should take children as our models since they learn quickly and change eating patterns to ensure health. He sees children with fatigue and attention deficit disorders. After tests you find the child is allergic to wheat, dairy, peanuts, sugar. You tell the mom she has to change everything she feeds him and she is ready to collapse. But talk to her six or nine months later, once she knows all the other wonderful food options she has, and she is happy. The child resisted at first, but then his problems began to clear up. Halloween came, he nose-dived. He began to clear up again. Thanksgiving, he nose-dived. Christmas, he nose-dived. Children learn more quickly than stubborn adults. Knowledge allows us to change in accordance with what we learn.

Dr. Galante also focuses on food, pointing to processed foods, white sugar, white flour, hydrogenated products, and chemicalized foods, all lacking vitality. People are eating these foods in far too great a quantity. Through food therapies which remove these foods, at least in the less severe cases, he has seen relief from hypoglycemic reactionssuch as mood swings and manic depressive symptoms.

Another problem in chronic fatigue syndrome is candida, both external and internal.

Dr. Ali reminds us, however, not to go looking for a doctor to cure us of yeast since it is in our bodies. "You do not want to get rid of it, but rather achieve 'gut balance,' and restore the gut ecosystem." Candida is just one possible problem; he tests for the nine different kinds of yeast. Of the yeasts, candida is not number one in terms of the body making antibodies against it, though candida is number one in terms of total population.

METABOLIC REGULATION What about the relation of chronic fatigue to metabolic regulation? We can understand metabolic immune depression in relation to chronic fatigue syndrome. When glucose production is up it brings on a level of hypoglycemia, with a high degree of glucose in the blood causing an increased level of insulin in the blood. Because of poor utilization of glucose, fatty acids come to the surface, increasing in the blood in order to provide a sufficient level of energy. A high level of triglycerides will occur and the immune system will be depressed because it needs a new army of T-lymphocytes, which are not being produced because of derangement in lipid metabolism.

VITAMIN AND HORMONAL DEFICIENCY Dr. Neil Block relates these problems to lifestyle. Those who do not have the best lifestyle, such as the smokers, drinkers, and those who do not breathe the best air, often lack B nutrients, which affects the immune system. Even if you are taking a number of vitamin B pills, make sure you are on a multi B regimen, so none of the B vitamins begin to get scarce in the body.

Lack of C, E, and beta carotene can also affect your immune system, as well as a lack of minerals, particularly, calcium, vanadium, copper, magnesium, potassium, molybdenum, boron, iodine, selenium, and chromium. The trace minerals are especially important for organ function.

Dr. Block also points to hormonal imbalances, particularly thyroid imbalance (especially hypothyroidism) found in females in a prevalence of six to one over males. It tends to develop spontaneously between the ages of 20 and 50, although it can come at any time, often from unknown causes. The rare causes, which are the ones known for this disease, are because of a superabundance of iodine in the body or a deficiency of iodine, the latter being unlikely in our society, where we have iodized salt and other sources. Another rare cause is that of a person consuming too many of certain vegetables, such as cauliflower, broccoli, or brussels sprouts, which tend to bind the active ingredient and inhibit thyroxin production.

Other hormones frequently out of the normal range are the adrenals. "There are a number of tests we can run for this, none of which is perfect," Dr. Block continues, "for, we have to remember, the adrenal gland is really two organs in one. On the inside, the adrenal medulla is making adrenaline and its brother noradrenaline. And then there's the outer coating, the adrenal cortex, making cortisonelike substances, related to our immune system and blood sugar control, and corticoid steroids. The last thing the adrenal cortex is important for is modulating the male and female hormones that are in conversation with the pituitary gland and primary sexual organs.

"And, lastly, some chronic fatigue syndrome patients have imbalances in gender hormones. It is not unusual to have imbalances in the estrogen that governs the ovary function or to have imbalances in other governors such as LH from the pituitary gland or in progesterone."

People will come to him with complaints, such as lack of menstruation or milky discharge from the breast, breast tenderness or more menstrual cramps than usual. Meanwhile, every month he has one or two men come who are low on testosterone blood scores, though with this one must test the degree of free testosterone to validly interpret the blood test. This last group makes great strides when given carefully measured dosages of male androgens.

Dr. Galante remarks, "The allopathic drugs, conventional drugs, antibiotics, and steroid usage are major influences. The use and abuse of these drugs, in childhood, for example, sets up chronically weakened conditions that will extend into adulthood and contribute to a predisposition for chronic fatigue. These drugs are suppressive in nature, not curative. They themselves impose an illness upon the system. This may be one of the largest of the causal factors."

Dr. Ali heard of a young person suffering from chronic fatigue syndrome who went to a medical clinic and was given a prescription for steroids. We know steroids suppress the immune system, so why would anyone give someone with this disorder these drugs? Steroids can create a sense of euphoria for a couple of days, of well being which is false. An unenlightened patient will take the steroids; an enlightened one will reject them.

PSYCHOLOGICAL FACTORS Dr. Gentile tells us that the disorder seems to reduce stress tolerance. Sufferers cannot exert themselves or will relapse into a fatigue, whether they try to walk or swim. He has had patients who had been marathoners before contracting the illness. They report the same onset. They had been working hard then got sick with fever and chills. The illness waxed and waned. They would feel better at times and go back into running but then quickly relapse. For these patients, stress cannot be tolerated, either in physical or psychological form, and will exacerbate the illness again and again.

Dr. Block adds that the stresses that affect and elevate the chronic fatigue syndrome patient are the same ones that affect us in everyday life. These cause faltering in many bodily systems, such as in the neurotransmitters, which are missed in examinations by many doctors who are not aware of GABA, dopamine, serotonin, and other neurotransmitter chemical levels.

Dr. Paul Epstein says a key tenet of naturopathic medicine is to do no harm and treat the underlying cause. If a person has chronic fatigue syndrome, that is a diagnosis—they have a suppressed immune system (another diagnosis) documented by blood tests and other measures. What caused this? It may be improper diet, then the patient will need to eat properly. But we need to ask why he adopted that diet in the first place. It may be stress, but we can ask what caused the person to follow certain patterns of reaction to stress. As we treat the patient, going through all the different problems layered one on top of the other, we eventually get in contact with the person's core self.

One way to get into this is through the inner child. A lot people have been influenced by John Bradshaw's work on recovering and healing the inner child and on seeing the connection between the wounds and scars of childhood which may have led us to create lifestyles that are addictive. So, even as I help the person medically, by advising on diet, stress reduction and so on, I remember this. If we do not touch deeper problems, healing may not occur.

Natural Remedies

Dr. Dean Black states that we were born to interact with the environment in a particular way. So we ask what is right for the body as it exists in the natural world. If we interact out of line with the body, we become sick. If we act properly, we become better. It is as simple as that. Natural health does nothing more than sustain the body's operations as they ought to be sustained.

"If you look at the body from an overall point of view," according to Dr. Galante, "from an environmental point of view, focusing on the bug is not going to be productive. As sophisticated as modern medicine is (so advanced we can tell all the amino acids and proteins in the body and get pictures of them), we cannot help the person who's got the difficulty. That seems to be a problem."

Dr. Ali thinks this is because so many doctors proceed from a flawed paradigm, the prevailing model of disease medicine. "A physician read one of my monographs and said, 'Ali, I know what you're talking about. We are disease doctors, while you are a health physician. I have difficulty relating to you because unless you give me the name of a disease, I don't know how to behave.' That's a paradox. I believe there'll come a time when people will not even go to doctors. They'll be coming to me, not so they can get drugs, but so they can get off drugs."

Dr. Galante summarizes his ideas in this way: "Why is medicine having so much trouble today? Because it doesn't have the answers. That's why we're in a crisis. That's why people are turning to natural therapies as they see the conventional approach is not curative but suppressive. That's why I exist."

FINDING THE RIGHT TREATMENT Dr. Gentile brings forward some related ideas. "Several key points about finding treatment for chronic fatigue syndrome involve the choice of an empathetic expert who believes the disease exists. It has reached the level of scientific respectability and most practitioners and medical examiners believe it exists. It is important to have someone up to date on in the literature and who has seen, minimum, 50–100 patients—someone who understands the ups and downs of the disease and is aware of the number of different treatments that have developed."

He points out a number of ways to locate a credible expert. For one, there are chronic fatigue syndrome support groups in every major town in our country and now worldwide that have lists of physicians who have tended to specialize in the disorder. There are national groups such as the Chronic Fatigue Syndrome Association. They maintain a list of doctors who understand the disease and have treated it and are sympathetic and believing.

"This last trait is so important," Dr. Galante explains, "because many sufferers have gone through scores of doctors. We're treating a woman now who has already seen 75 physicians all over the world. She was ready to give up because she feels people do not believe her. So, a critical part of treating this illness is belief. A second thing to bear in mind is, this being a chronic illness with a wide range of symptoms, it will tend to fall between the cracks of all the medical sub-specializations. With this disease, it will not be adequate to go to a single physician. It would be worth considering putting together a team, which would include a GP/internist, one who works both with traditional and alternative therapies; an allergist/infectious disease specialist; and a psychologist/psychiatrist. This team could coordinate so as to work out a treatment plan. They could collaborate and work so the client understands what is coming next. And if these treatments don't work, they could determine why that might be, and what would be worth trying next."

THE SPIRITUAL ELEMENT Dr. Ali tells us that when dealing with a chronic, devastating illness like this, hope and the spiritual element are two elements essential for long-term success. She has had case histories that truly stretch the bounds of credulity. "Creating hope is a very easy thing to do; sustaining hope is diffi-cult but it is central to healing. Before I see a patient, he or she has seen at least seven specialists. They've had biopsies, CAT scans. When they come to me, it's not that easy to simply reassure them that they'll get better, after they've seen the previous failures. But, fortunately, by the time they get to me, they've lis-tened to some of our tapes, read our books, and, most importantly, have talked to some of the other patients who have gotten better. So when they come in, and they've seen our nursing staff, our ancillary staff, they see we are all seri-ous. If they ask how my program differs, we say this: they do not have the option to remain sick."

VITAMIN THERAPIES A nurse is making up an intravenous (IV) chronic fatigue syndrome protocol with vitamin C, magnesium sulfate, pantetheine, calcium, pyridoxine, and a multivitamin formula. She says patients who come in are very tired, have joint pains, headaches, and memory loss. These IVs help repair cell membranes and boost the immune system, which will then hopefully function better. About 90 percent of her patients have responded well. Dr. Ali will usu-ally order a set of five to begin with, she says, and after that he can measure their response, see how deep their problem is and whether they require further drugs.

"I see these drips as jump-starting the cellular enzymes," Ali says. "The enzymes, which are detoxification enzymes, are dependent on minerals and vit-amins. If I feel there is enough time, when the patient is not acutely ill or has been chronically ill for a number of years, I will try to use a more conservative approach. But when I see people with severe, incapacitating fatigue, I use the IV. In fact, in one of our studies where we compared one group who had the IV and one group who didn't, we saw the IV speeds up the recovery process."

Dr. Ali continues, "We have 14 different formulations or protocols to man-age different clinical problems in our IV drips. For chronic fatigue syndrome, we use C, magnesium, calcium, pyridoxine, pantetheine, zinc, B vitamins, molybdenum, potassium, copper, and selenium. Most of our protocols have 15 to 18 items, and we change their quantities depending on the individual's state."

Ostrom notes that the antioxidants, with C, E and A, will be efficacious in treating chronic fatigue syndrome, as they are with AIDS, since in both cases they are entering the same immunological battle. In these cases, the systems are under fierce attack from free radicals, viruses, and, in some cases, bacteria. The supplements help to re-equilibrate and repair damage done by the molecules and help boost the immune system.

"First, we have to get the vitamins really right," Dr. Feldman urges, "since they are the building blocks of the immune system. People suffering from chronic fatigue syndrome are deficient in such things as A, B_5, B_{12}, E, bioflavonoids, the essential fatty acids, zinc, selenium, and GLA (gamma linole-ic acid). All those must be put into order before we can proceed further."

For immune strength or immune power the following supplements are recommended:

A (as pure A)	10,000 to 20,000 IU
Beta carotene	15,000–25,000 IU
B$_6$	100–200 mg (be tested for reaction first)
C (buffered)	To bowel tolerance. Try a sago palm not a corn source. Buffering neutralizes acid.
E	300–600 IU
Quercetin	250–1,000 mg
Pycnogenol	150–300 mg
Essential fatty acids	100–350 mg (obtainable from sunflower, sesame, safflower, evening primrose or soybean oils, and black currant, a tablespoon a day)
Zinc picolinate	20–50 mg
Selenium	100–300 micrograms (oceanic)
Coenzyme Q10	100–300 mg

Dr. Neil Block discusses his treatment: "If proteins or amino acids come out low, we can try to individually supplement the amino acids. If minerals are lacking, they can be given individually or in tandem, trying to operate by an economy of scale, so a patient doesn't have to take from more than 10 to 15 bottles at a time. As for hormonal imbalance, I have 20–25 percent of my chronic fatigue syndrome patients on thyroid. I prefer to use the more natural brands of thyroid. Again, I believe in giving both the male and female hormones. We also have to try to adjust the pancreas and adrenals. For the pancreas use chromium or chromium picolinate. For adrenals, the glandulars or homeopathics and sometimes things like licorice tend to help multiple hormones. If we are working on the pituitary, use glandulars, the homeopathics, and on rare occasions, I use a lot of the amino acids to try and build neurotransmitter activity. The amino acids to be used are arginine, tyrosine, and phenylalanine. Tryptophan was also once useful to me until they took it off the market. I'm also not afraid to use, correctly and in small doses, items obtained from the pharmacy. What I tend to shy away from are the tranquilizers, such as Valium or Librium. I do make use of antidepressants on occasion."

Often his patients have seen other physicians and holistic healers and they may need only one or two things to turn the body around on multiple levels. With neurotransmitters being easily adjusted nowadays, with items like the less toxic antidepressants such as neurotrytamine, neuroiptamine, and the newer Paxil and Zoloft, which lack drastic side effects and have a response beginning in two to four weeks, they're worthwhile. It's nice for a patient who has suffered two, four, six years, to take these new agents and, within two to four weeks, get at least some indication of the direction in which they are going."

Ostrom mentions another new drug which may yet be helpful: Amplygin, currently in FDA trials, appears to fix a very important immune system antiviral pathway. Found to work on AIDS, it has yet to be proved against chronic fatigue syndrome.

Dr. Galante opines antibiotics can certainly be called for when all else fails, where the system has been debilitated, perhaps by too much drug use before. However, the state we are aiming for is where the energy in the body will overcome all problems.

HERBAL THERAPIES Herbologist Letha Hadady says that the tradition of herbology is very rich in China with many herbs to choose from for healing the immune system. One is a form of ginseng called Dang Shen. Another herb is astragalus. In her view, when used together, the first lifts our energy up and the second sends our defenses to the surface.

After using these herbs, we should act to kill germs and viral infection with such herbs as honeysuckle flower, andrographis, and dandelion. When we have built strength and killed germs, we must build blood using Chinese blood tonics, such as Han Yin Sow, called eclipta alba in Latin and growing wild in the American Southwest. It builds blood without any side effects, such as inflammation. You can take this every day in powdered form. Other immune strengthening agents are Chinese ginseng, dandelion, false ginseng, astragalus, andrographis, eclipta alba and honeysuckle.

She also mentions, Fo Ti, which builds blood while it keeps us cool.

When you fight viral infection with herbs, she reminds us, you have to do a number of things. One part of herbal treatments is taking antibiotic and anti-inflammatory herbs, like dandelion, a cleansing agent that keeps us cool. It can be put in salads, soups and found in the health food stores as capsules.

Honeysuckle flower grows outside in the garden. Boiled as tea, it will eliminate a sore throat and fever as well as kill pneumonia, staph, and strep germs.

There are three types of ginseng: American, Chinese, and false. The American type provides more moisture, more saliva and is good after a fever. Chinese ginseng, called Ren Shen, gives us energy. Dang Shen, or false ginseng, makes us feel stronger, without feeling hotter. All can be used in soups.

Cayenne pepper plays a role in health, increasing circulation and making us feel stronger. It can be used by those who do not find it irritating.

There are also herbs for relaxing the nervous system. One is Siberian ginseng, which can be taken as an extract or in capsule form. Valerian, taken in capsules, can quiet the nervous system. "For people who are depressed," Hadady says, "we need to bring them to their center as a way to be grounded and to feel more whole. Use ginger and mint. Mint helps to bring the worries out of the head and ginger helps to burn them away, because it is digestive and heating so it brings us warmly to our centers. They make a good combination."

High Energy preparation is the name of an herb mixture that uses Western and Oriental ingredients. It has guttacola, American ginseng, demianna, red clover, peppermint and cloves, which strengthens the adrenals and lungs.

Hadady adds that cloves and hot water will pick up your energy, and make you breath deeper.

DIETARY CHANGES Dr. Majid Ali sees eating right as a measure to prevent or combat chronic fatigue syndrome. Carbohydrates, like corn and wheat, are big culprits. One should eat healthy substances, such as wild and brown rice or unusual grains such as fatigue and spelt. Soy products are also very good, as is teff. The other good sources of carbohydrates are lentils and different types of beans. Tomatoes, potatoes, and yams are okay, but in moderation. Foods which have white flour are a no-no, as is white rice. The best sources among the grains are brown rice, amaranth, quinoa, soy, teff, and spelt.

Lentils, beans, eggs, and protein drinks are good sources of protein. Egg is excellent, but many people are allergic to it. Dr. Ali also recommends protein drinks in the morning—their amino acids give sustained energy. Sugar and carbohydrates, by contrast, provide a roller coaster effect—they are useful only when doing an endurance type of physical activity, in which case you need carbohydrates. But most people do much better without sugar and carbohydrates.

Dr. Ali does not insist his patients follow a vegetarian diet, but recommends little beef. Unusual meats, like venison or pheasant are better, he states. "We provide a list to patients of places where they can order such meat. Cornish hen and turkey are fine. Hunted fish (deep sea fish) are good. Cultured fish are not recommended. They're beginning to put fungicides into fish raised in fisheries. If you are going for fish, do the deep seas ones. (Unless you have serious mercury sensitivity, then you should avoid fish.)"

He feels eating certain fats is essential, but one should avoid oxidized, processed, denatured fats or animal shortening, corn oil, palm oil, and coconut oil. If you do not have milk sensitivity, butter is possible. You can make ghee by taking butter, warming it and taking the white part off. It is delicious and those who cannot tolerate butter can still tolerate ghee. Use virgin olive oil, the type you find in Italian stores. Avocado oil is an excellent source of monounsaturates, but if it is processed stay away. For supplemental oils, flaxseed is excellent. People should make a habit of using flaxseed on their salad dressing.

Dr. Galante prescribes using a lot of live foods that can be taken right from nature without cooking, like raw fruits, vegetables, and sprouts. They can provide tremendous energy, with a lot of enzymes and nutrition. They take little energy to digest and give much energy back.

Think of all the varieties of vegetables: red leaf and green leaf lettuce, mustard greens, red and green chard, arugula, broccoli, beets, carrots. Turnips and parsnips, both root vegetables, are very high in calcium. Green leafy vegetables give needed chlorophyll and oxygenate your blood. Radishes, red and green peppers, eggplants are excellent and ginger can be used to flavor any juice. Celery is a good diuretic and cabbage is high in beta carotene, as are all the green leafy vegetables. Sprouts are the best source of protein, put into a salad it will add to anything you are eating. An ounce of wheat grass, which is high in chlorophyll, is equal to 22 ounces of the choicest vegetable you can imagine.

HOMEOPATHY Homeopathy is Dr. Galante's specialty; it has been very effective against chronic fatigue syndrome, and is probably quite different from what people are experiencing with other treatments. Homeopathic remedies are given in microdosages, all made from natural substances, effective in treating and curing many conditions.

To talk about one particular therapy, though, is not appropriate, Dr. Galante explains, since the essence of homeopathy is that each individual will have selected for him or her a remedy based on his or her unique physical constitution and manifestation of symptoms. He points out that the homeopathic healer will select a remedy that is uniquely fitted, mentally and physically, for a particular sufferer's makeup.

ACUPUNCTURE Registered nurse and acupuncturist Abigail Rist-Podrecca points out that the *chi*, or bioelectrical energy, flows through pathways in the body. When there is a disease process occurring, she says there is a blockage. Acupuncture needles—there are actually 365 points that can be used—open the blockages and let the energy flow smoothly through meridians. The other thing that occurs is that the needles dilate the blood vessels, so you get more blood flowing through the area, more oxygen and more nutrients into the area, and this aids all forms of health.

Needles are presterilized in ethylene gas. After they are used, they are thrown away in an infectious waste container so there is no cross-contamination question in the process. "If you do go to an acupuncturist," Rist-Podrecca cautions, "one of the first things I would ask as a patient-consumer, is whether they are using presterilized needles."

TAI CHI One of the benefits of *tai chi* is that it increases one's awareness both internally and environmentally. "Then you can choose which to work on, whether there is something physically wrong or something in the environment that needs to be corrected," says Eric Schneider of the Northeastern Tai Chi Chuan Association.

He tells us the practitioners can use the energy in their bodies to go toward the conflict and resolve it rather than spend time worrying. We are born with a certain amount of energy, called pre-birth *chi*. You may know a person who can go out and party all night and wake up the next morning at 6 a.m. fine. Another person will do the same partying but the next morning be unable to get out of bed. This is due to differences in the natural reservoir. The practice of *tai chi* can increase the natural storehouse.

According to Schneider, the environment has energy, brought into the bodily system through the simple breathing apparatus. You have to cultivate a part of your body that can observe phenomena dispassionately, without having to grab onto every experience and run with it, to get yourself in stressful situations and say quietly, 'Oh, so this is what is happening now. What can I do about it? What are my options and how am I feeling?' In this way, you can soberly assess your experience.

Tai chi is a 10 year practice. Practitioners say, '10 years great gain, 3 years small gain.' It takes 10 years to get what is called the *gung chi*, the task framework so the body has a certain way to contain energy. Gradually, as the mind starts to cultivate and stay with the body, the whole system starts to grow. This is not a quick fix. "In fact," says Schneider, "in my opinion, any practice that is to have profound value cannot be done quickly. Everything that has lasting effect takes time."

IMAGERY AND HEALING Dr. Paul Epstein uses a type of visualization in his practice. He says imagery is a therapeutic technique that assists people to explore through words and symbols so they can understand the language of the subconscious.

"In exploring this," according to Dr. Epstein, "usually what comes up is the issue that is at the core of what will be the healing. When we are dealing with people, they may get in touch with childhood wounds or abuse from the past that needs healing. Perhaps they'll get in touch with the fact that the work which they are doing is not real work.

"In one such case, with a person suffering from chronic fatigue syndrome, we found the illness was a case of a person trying to get love. She had not let go of trying to get love from mom and dad. She was still stuck at that place. And the pain and the grief of not having that love were not only weakening her immune system, but keeping her stuck in the unhealthy way she was living her life."

Dr. Majid Ali reiterates some of Dr. Epstein's message: "What I demonstrate to my patients is that the way you look at the world around you determines the biology under your skin. If you can be in a self-regulatory, healing mode, your brain activity, heart activity, muscle energy, skin energy, will all be functioning positively. Or you can be trying to figure things out, think everything through in an overly intellectual way, and your biology will be as up and down as the New York skyline. This is the stress mode and it causes disease. Another mode is an even, steady state mode and that is a resting mode.

"Our goal is to perceive this energy in these modes and understand how the energy profoundly affects the electrophysiological profile. Can we allow this energy to guide us into the healing mode? We want a transition from an ordinary, thinking, nervous stressful mode that causes disease to a nonthinking, meditative, deep respiring mode that makes us well. That is our goal."

A Holistic Health Model

REALIGNMENT OF THE VITAL FORCE Dr. Michele Galante ties it all together: "A homeopath will tell you that a person cannot be well if he or she is feeling ill at ease in mind or heart. Just having a physically healthy body is not enough.

People want more. We are not saying the doctor and homeopath has the key to make people happy, but we can say that homeopaths do work to make people feel emotionally better. There is a realignment of what's called the vital force, which causes the person to get well. We all have this capacity. The body is a living, tremendously powerful organism and it can heal itself. It healed itself before there were antibiotics and it will heal itself long after antibiotics fall out of favor."

THE SELF-HEALING PROCESS Dr. Epstein elaborates on his earlier position: "What's needed in treating chronic fatigue syndrome or AIDS or such problems is a new approach. Not looking for the quick fix or what will work for everybody, but for an approach that is individualized, holistic and one that empowers the patient to get involved in the cure and gives that patient belief and hope that healing is possible.

"There are two points in my treatment that I've been told by patients have helped them most. That I have given them hope and belief that healing is possible, and I have shown them that there are things they could do to help themselves. I don't heal anybody. Doctors don't heal anybody. They support people as they heal themselves."

A physician's work, in his opinion, is to support the self healing of each individual and to help them through the process.

Dr. Epstein wants to help patients listen, explore and understand the message of their disease, which is the key to unlock the door to recovery. After the diagnosis, medications, natural or other, there still has to be an exploration healing for this person. We might have conditioned immune-suppressant responses built into our attitudes, beliefs, the way we live our life, the way we think and the way we eat. An illness cannot be fixed from the outside; there is no magic bullet for chronic fatigue syndrome. People heal themselves by engaging in a self-healing process, by looking at their life and its meaning.

It may seem rather complicated, but it is not. It is based on the knowledge that we do not get sick over night. The condition may manifest suddenly in certain symptoms, but it took years and years to arrive. And it was not from one virus; not just Epstein-Barr or herpes or parasites, low blood sugar, or electro-magnetic pulsations. It was a combination of all of them.

In order to detoxify, it takes time. It might take you a year to really cleanse. You need a rational diet so you can get rid of the food polluting your system. Bring in the healthy foods, exercise, meditation, acupuncture.

If you are what you eat, eat what you appreciate becoming. Remember, the mind is a powerful healer and also a powerful slayer. Surround yourself with positive thoughts and people who will support your endeavor to live a natural lifestyle. Chronic fatigue syndrome can be cured. Everyday you can be processing health and overcoming disease.

45

Diabetes

Diabetes is a serious condition that in the late 1990s affects nearly 16 million Americans a year. Today diabetes is the third leading cause of death in the United States and a primary cause of new cases of blindness, renal disease, and nontraumatic amputations. In 1997, the total annual estimated cost of diabetes was $98 billion.

Causes

Diabetes is closely associated with heart disease, and the incidence of both conditions increased when Americans began to change their diet patterns.

Under normal circumstances, insulin is released by the pancreas in response to elevated levels of sugar in the blood. It promotes transport and entry of glucose to muscle cells and various tissues, thus lowering blood sugar levels. In the diabetic, part of the process is interrupted due to either a deficiency, resistance, or insensitivity to insulin.

INSULIN DEFICIENCY For many years, it was thought that diabetes was purely and simply a deficiency syndrome, in which the body did not produce sufficient quantities of insulin for proper glucose metabolism and assimilation. More recently, it has been learned that many diabetics do produce enough insulin, but their cells do not take it in. The problem is then due to insulin insensitivity or resistance.

INSULIN INSENSITIVITY Insulin enters cells at points known as receptor sites. When these receptor sites become plugged up by fat, cholesterol, inactivity, and obesity, insulin cannot enter. As a result, glucose stays in the blood and creates hyperglycemia or high blood sugar. This excess sugar is diagnosed as diabetes. In these cases, there is not a need to increase insulin production but a need to enhance insulin sensitivity. The person needs to work at making their own insulin more efficient, and simply increasing the amount of insulin will not do that.

INSULIN RESISTANCE This is a closely related phenomenon, in which there is also a sufficient or even overabundant supply of insulin. Here, allergic responses prevent insulin from doing its job. Usually, allergies to specific foods suppress the activity and efficiency of insulin. Different factors may be responsible for a disordered carbohydrate metabolism in different people. Wheat, for instance, may create symptoms of high blood sugar in one woman and corn may affect another. Offending substances can be determined on an individual basis with food allergy tests.

Types of Diabetes

Juvenile or type I diabetes is the most serious form of the disease; it usually manifests itself in childhood or teenage years. This form of diabetes is characterized by a true insulin deficiency. It apparently results when the pancreas is damaged from some exotic viral infection or even a highly toxic state. The disease may also be a genetic condition. Since juvenile diabetics have an insulin deficiency, they have to receive insulin regularly, and generally for life.

Maturity-onset or type II diabetes is more of an acquired disease. It is often precipitated by chronic excess weight from poor diet and/or lack of exercise. It may also be brought on by overconsumption of stressor foods or other allergens that are insulin resistors. This form of the disease is characterized by complications of insulin resistance and insulin sensitivity rather than, in most cases, a true deficiency of insulin. For this reason, maturity onset diabetes can frequently be non-insulin-dependent.

Symptoms

Often there are no symptoms present, especially in the beginning stages of type II diabetes. The prediabetic state can be accompanied by obesity, especially when it is centered at the waistline and just above the waistline. Classical diabetic symptoms are more often experienced by type I diabetics and include frequent urination, especially at night, great thirst and hunger, fatigue, weight loss, irritability, and restlessness. Progressively, the eyes, kidneys, nervous system, and skin become affected. Infections and hardening of the arteries commonly develop. In type I diabetes, coma from a lack of insulin is an ongoing danger.

The Shortcomings of the Traditional Medical Approaches

INSULIN Before the development of insulin in the 1920s, diabetic patients had a bleak prognosis. Sufferers saw the condition rapidly go from bad to worse as complications such as blindness, gout, and gangrene developed. Overall life span was drastically shortened.

In the beginning, insulin appeared to be a miraculous drug, and in fact it probably was. The life span of diabetic children was extended from months to decades. Today, many of these children live normal, productive lives.

The problem with insulin is that it is prescribed to all diabetics, not just those with true insulin deficiencies. While insulin addresses the immediate crisis by lowering blood sugar levels, it does little to correct long-range problems. In fact, many adverse effects can be heightened by aggressive insulin therapy. Insulin stimulates the development of antagonists in the body that counteract its blood-sugar-lowering effects. When a diabetic receives insulin, the person's blood sugar begins to fall. The body immediately responds to the falling levels of blood sugar by stimulating growth hormones and epinephrine. These hormones keep blood sugar levels elevated because the brain needs sugar.

The result of aggressive insulin therapy is a rebounding effect. Blood sugar is high, so insulin is injected. This makes the level plummet as the blood sugar is forced down by the insulin. But that drop cues the insulin antagonists to quickly raise blood sugar again to meet what the body perceives as a life-threatening situation.

This constant fluctuation of blood sugar levels leads to a wide range of long-term disorders. In fact, clinical experience shows that diabetics treated aggressively with insulin have a 40 percent greater incidence of eye problems than those treated moderately. Despite this finding, it is still common for diabetics with worsening eye problems to be treated more and more aggressively.

Insulin may also contribute significantly to inner arterial wall damage, which is a major problem among diabetics. The incidence of heart attacks and strokes is five to eight times greater among diabetics. About 75 percent of all diabetic mortality is due to heart disease brought on by hardening of the major arteries.

Other complications that may involve insulin use are related to the damage done to the microvascular vessels, particularly those leading to the eyes, kidneys, and peripheral nerves. As these arteries become thickened and brittle, they become less and less functional, and it becomes increasingly difficult for blood to pass through. In the eyes, sudden surges of blood sugar put extra stress on the retinal blood vessels. If the stress is repeated, as it frequently is in diabetics, the vessels will hemorrhage and break. Over time, many hemorrhages will occur and blindness will result. After glaucoma, this is the most common cause of blindness in older people.

In the kidneys a similar succession of events frequently results in a renal insufficiency and in an inability to eliminate nitrogen waste from the body efficiently.

Insulin's interference with proper blood circulation, involving both large and small vessels, is also responsible for a high incidence of neuritis and gangrene, which frequently lends itself to peripheral tingling in the fingers and toes, a loss of feeling, and amputation. Sexual dysfunction is also related to this. Most of these complications occur after repeated exposure to fluctuating blood sugar levels.

Many of the secondary problems associated with diabetes, then, result from the indiscriminate overuse of insulin and the failure of the medical profession to employ natural, noninvasive, and efficacious methods of holding diabetic symptoms in check. Although 90 percent of diabetics are type II, they have been lumped together with type I as being able to benefit from insulin treatment in cases where blood sugar remains consistently and dangerously high. Type II, maturity-onset diabetics can be non-insulin-dependent in most instances, and should not be treated with aggressive insulin programs prescribed for type I juvenile diabetics, who are, generally, insulin dependent. A great many people who need insulin can drastically reduce the amount needed by incorporating a wider spectrum of treatment approaches beyond just maintaining blood sugar levels.

ORAL HYPOGLYCEMIC MEDICATIONS Insulin is not the only culprit in traditional diabetes treatment; there is also a group of oral hypoglycemic medications that stimulate the secretion of more insulin and thus lower the blood sugar level. Some even act peripherally; that is, they awaken and increase the number of sensitive receptor sites so that there are more locations for glucose to enter the cell. This peripheral action, in effect, makes insulin go further. It extends its potential efficacy more than it could by merely increasing its presence in the bloodstream.

These oral agents—which include Orinase, Diabinase, Tolinase, and other pharmaceuticals—are a cause for concern because of their potential adverse side effects. They have been shown to greatly increase heart disease and death due to heart attack. What we are looking at is a disease in which heart disease is a risk factor being treated with drugs that drastically increase the likelihood of premature heart attacks.

DIETARY RECOMMENDATIONS Although insulin has been at the center of traditional diabetes treatment, some attention has also been given to dietary modification. Unfortunately, the greatest part of the dietary advice given is not well founded and may contribute to a worsening condition.

There are several shortcomings associated with the standard diabetic diet. First, the diabetic is told to avoid all carbohydrates, since these foods eventually break down into glucose. But no distinction is made between simple sugars and complex carbohydrates. Fiber is also denigrated because it is considered a carbo-hydrate, which it is not. In addition, there is no attempt to relate allergic respons-es to specific foods. The dietary advice commonly given only worsens the diabet-ic's condition and is responsible for many side effects and complications.

Unlike simple sugars, complex carbohydrates are beneficial. Although both are broken down into glucose, the latter do not go directly into the blood-stream. While simple sugars immediately enter the blood, complex carbohy-drates go through a long process of digestion and only very gradually release sugar into the blood. Therefore, they do not then contribute to the high blood sugar levels, as do simple carbohydrates. Instead, they stabilize and improve health.

While diabetics are told to stay away from potatoes and rice, they are advised to eat more protein. They are, in effect, being told to jump from the frying pan into the fire. First, protein is high in fat and cholesterol, especially when it is derived from animal sources. Fat accumulates in the blood and sets the patient up for cardiovascular disease. In addition, it clogs receptor sites, which thus become more desensitized or resistant to insulin. Blood sugar inevitably rises, causing the doctor to prescribe more insulin or oral medication in an attempt to stabilize the blood sugar.

Large amounts of protein are also related to accelerated kidney damage. This is because protein must be immediately processed by the body; it cannot be stored. This puts a great stress on the nephron cells, which filter the body's toxins. Many diabetics suffer from kidney deterioration as a result and must receive dialysis or a kidney transplant. Studies show that the elimination of meat from the diet is often enough to reverse kidney damage.

The Benefits of the Natural Approach

Despite its severity, diabetes need not be as debilitating as it usually is. While there is currently no cure, there are ways of enhancing the body's natural defens-es through nutrition, avoidance of allergy-producing substances, and exercise. A healthy lifestyle and alternative approaches to treatment can decrease the amount of insulin or oral medications needed by some persons; others may be completely weaned off these substances. The goal of treatment can and should be to build up the body's ability to function as independently as possible.

When changing to a more holistic approach to treatment, it is important not to immediately discontinue any medication, including insulin. Instead, a preventive medicine physician should assist in the gradual transition. With a doctor's guidance, an insulin dependency may be reduced or completely elimi-nated with time. Complete elimination, however, is not always possible.

Physicians who practice alternative approaches to treating diabetes for the most part employ a program combining exercise and dietary modification aimed both at better nutrition and at weight loss, where indicated. Insulin and medications are used only as second- and third-line approaches. This sort of program usually controls the disease and its ancillary complications in a less invasive, more efficacious manner, in a short period of time.

While maturity-onset diabetics respond most dramatically, even juvenile diabetics may be able to reduce their insulin dependency. More importantly, they are able to alleviate many of the insidious complications that have come to be thought of as intrinsic to diabetes.

DIET Since diabetes and heart disease are so closely related, Dr. Atkins recommends that some people with diabetes follow a Dean Ornish program, in which they drastically cut down on dietary fats. The best diet consists of organic vegetarian foods, eaten raw, sprouted, steamed, baked, or stir-fried with little or no oil. Those who have a true insulin disorder will not fare well on a high-carbohydrate diet, since diabetes is a carbohydrate metabolism disorder.

"It is important to know who needs carbohydrate restriction versus who needs fat restriction," Dr. Atkins says. "To determine that, there are a variety of tests, including a cholesterol profile in which we look at the ratio between the triglycerides and the HDL. When a person has a blood sugar disorder leading to a lipid disorder, the ratio is extremely high. To be really safe, the number should be approximately the same, or the HDL should be higher than the triglycerides. It is perfectly appropriate to spend five or six weeks on one diet and then get all of your parameters checked again, and then five or six weeks on the other diet, and get them checked again. In that way, you can make an intelligent decision."

EXERCISE An exercise regimen is crucial for burning calories and normalizing metabolism, and is especially important for overweight adults who tend to be inactive.

Exercise also heightens the body's sensitivity to insulin. By lowering cholesterol, it lowers triglyceride levels in the blood, making cells more available for glucose assimilation. This is why the insulin requirements of diabetic athletes always drop while they're engaged in swimming, soccer, and other sports. Athletes also notice an increase in their insulin requirements when they cease their physical activities for any extended period of time.

Athletes are not the only ones to benefit from exercise. Ten to 20 minutes of light exercise after each meal helps to reduce the amount of insulin necessary to keep blood sugar levels under control. A brisk walk gets the body's metabolism working a little bit faster so that the absorption of food is more easily distributed. That prevents blood sugar from rising too high.

An exception to the rule is for diabetics with heart disease. In these patients, exercising after eating may precipitate an angina attack because of the transfer of blood from the intestines to the legs and other parts of the body.

FOOD ALLERGIES Testing for food allergies can determine which foods are responsible for insulin resistance. Clinical experience has shown that this approach to treatment is the most useful way to get to the root of adult-onset diabetes and to reverse the condition. Patients can usually be weaned off insulin, since an insulin deficiency is not the cause of the problem. Eliminating allergy-producing foods may also foster weight loss. This occurs because people crave foods when they are allergic to them. When these foods are taken out of the diet, the desire for them eventually stops.

To determine whether a specific food is causing hyperglycemia, a doctor can monitor a patient's blood sugar before and after a specific food is eaten. Foods that raise the blood sugar cause allergic reactions and should be eliminated.

SUPPLEMENTS In addition to diet and exercise, the following supplements are important to know about:

CHROMIUM PICOLINATE. Chromium helps normalize glucose levels in insulin-dependent diabetics.

MAGNESIUM AND POTASSIUM help to maintain a glucose tolerance level.

ZINC is essential for normal insulin production.

ENZYMES. Digestive protylase, amylase, and lipase.

VANADYL SULFATE may be the most important mineral for diabetes. It was discovered in France in the late 1800s and used to control diabetes before insulin appeared. It works at the cellular level and is most effective when taken three times a day.

HERBS Plants containing phytochemicals with antidiabetic properties, in order of potency:

Cichorium intybus (chicory)
Rauvalfia serpentina (Indian snakeroot)
Thymus vulgaris (common thyme)
Arctium lappa (gobo)
Carthamus tinctorius (safflower)
Passiflora edulis (maracuya)
Opuntia ficus-indica (Indian fig)
Taraxacum officinale (dandelion)
Tetrapanax papyriferus (rice-paper)
Canavalia ensiformis (jack bean)
Linum usitatissimum (flax)
Pueraria lobata (kudzu)
Hordeum vulgare (barley)
Inula helenium (elecampane)
Althaea officinalis (marshmallow)
Oenothera biennis (evening primrose)
Avena sativa (oats)

Triticum aestivum (wheat)
Medicago sativa (alfalfa)
Panicum maximum (guinea grass)

Plants containing phytochemicals with insulin-sparing properties, in order of potency:
Cocos nucifera (coconut)
Plantago major (common plantain)

TOPICAL TREATMENT FOR DIABETIC ULCERS Diabetic ulcers plague many patients with this disease and cause a condition that is often serious enough to warrant amputation. This tragedy can be averted with a simple solution. According to clinical studies, raw, unprocessed honey is an ideal dressing agent for almost every type of wound or ulcer. It sterilizes the area, and often works even after antibiotics fail.

HOMEOPATHY The remedy Mucokehl, from Germany, may actually reverse diabetic neuropathy. People using this remedy get feeling back in their extremities, and their eyesight improves.

CHELATION THERAPY Chelation therapy is known to reduce diabetic retinopathy and foot ulcers. (See chapter 33 for an in-depth discussion of chelation therapy.)

Monitoring and Preventing Diabetes

Diabetics and those who wish to prevent diabetes can do a great deal to monitor themselves. It's important to look for the presence of antibodies that attack some part of the body to defend against an ingested allergen. This is easy to see if the symptoms are blatant, but not if they are subtle. The thing to look for is a general lowering of the body's immune response. The best way to see this is to go five days without eating the food (or any of its relatives) you wish to test. If you want to test milk, abstain from cheese, ice cream, and all other dairy items or processed foods that may contain milk as an ingredient. After five days, eat a meal consisting of just milk and eat generous amounts of it. Then tune in to your body's response. If you experience headaches, stomachaches, pulse rate changes, increased heartbeat or blood sugar, depression, lethargy, dizziness, or even delusions, you can see that your body has reacted negatively to this substance. In other words, you have an allergic response to it. You will have to back off from it. Leave it alone for 12 weeks initially. When it is reintroduced into the diet, it must be rotated with other foods. Eat it in modest amount no more often than once every four days.

"Of course, there are a lot of good things about that four-day basis," says Dr. William Philpott, a prominent diabetes researcher and clinician. "You will eat... 30 or 40 kinds of foods instead of the half dozen you've been eating. This is a very wholesome thing. To have the necessary nutrition you will have a wide range of foods." It is a good idea to try introducing new foods into your diet, ones that you have never thought to have. Try to eat no foods more frequently than twice a week.

Dr. Philpott recommends that you invest in some diabetic equipment so that you can quantitatively monitor your blood sugar an hour after each meal. "At least 110 is optimum," he says, "and 160 or beyond is high blood sugar. Before the next meal, test your blood sugar again to make sure it is at least 120 before starting your next meal. If not, wait and exercise. Get it down before your next meal. Monitor your pH from saliva— it should be 6.4. If it is below 6.4, you are having a reaction to the food. Measure your pulse; if it varies drastically, you are reacting to the food. Blood pressure is more significant. Physical symptoms, mental symptoms, and blood sugar are the most important. They are absolutely essential. It will take about 30 days to do this."

Patient Stories

Dr. Julian Whitaker, who has worked with many diabetic patients, had considerable success with a program that emphasizes diet, vitamin and mineral supplements, exercise, and practical education. He describes a 27-year-old patient who was taught to use these essential tools:

> *He was on insulin for about six months and was also having hypoglycemic reactions. When we saw him, he was taking only 10 to 12 units of insulin per day and his blood sugar levels were very low. Whenever you have a situation like this, you can cut down on the insulin and then eventually get off it completely. We measured in his blood a protein called C-peptide which measures the body's production of insulin. If his pancreas was not producing insulin, his C-peptide would be about zero. This patient had a close to normal C-peptide, meaning that his pancreas was producing insulin. We put him on a program to sensitize his body to the lower levels of insulin his pancreas was producing. This included exercise, a low-fat diet, and vitamin and mineral supplements.... It has now been about nine months, and he has been without insulin. His blood sugar level would go to about 140 or so after breakfast, but then he was told to exercise, and when he keeps up his program, his blood sugar level stays under control. I think this indicates that you have a very powerful tool in diet, exercise, and minerals which is patently ignored by most physicians treating diabetes as they systematically utilize insulin and the oral drugs in their diabetic patients.*

Another case of Dr. Whitaker's illustrates the shortcomings and even abuses of traditional diabetic treatment and at the same time provides an idea of how an alternative approach may be more appropriate and efficacious.

Five years before I first saw this patient, he had had mild high blood pressure for which he was started on diuretics. He used hydrochlorothiazide, a thiazide diuretic. This drug has a tendency to lower potassium and elevate blood sugar, findings that are well known and listed in The Physicians' Desk Reference, but it is still the most commonly used prescription medication worldwide. The patient's potassium level dropped, he developed some cardiac arrhythmias, his blood sugar level began to go up, and his problem was diagnosed as high blood pressure plus diabetes. He was placed on oral medications that failed to lower his blood sugar, so he was placed on insulin. When a patient like this gentleman, who did not have any diabetes to speak of but had a drug-induced form of diabetes, is placed on insulin, his blood sugar drops to a very low level. The body responds to this low level by generating glucose from the liver and shooting the blood glucose up very high so that when the highs and lows are checked, the physician feels the patient is out of control and increases his insulin level; this, of course, only increases the rebound, or the up and down characteristics, of the blood sugar. This is what happened. He not only was having much higher and much lower blood sugar levels, he was having one or two hypoglycemic attacks a day. He kept going back to the hospital with this problem, and when he arrived there, his blood sugar would be high so they increased his insulin. He was taking 130 units of insulin daily and was also taking additional medication for cardiac arrhythmias and high blood pressure, which he didn't have, and 17 prescription pills daily.

When we saw him, we realized that he had not had any dietary advice at all. This, I think, is in some way systematic malpractice. We very rapidly took him off of all of his medications. When we instituted a low-fat, high-carbohydrate diet plus an exercise program under close monitoring, we were able to test his blood sugars two to three times a day. We cut his insulin in half in two days and then eliminated it after another two days. For nine days he went without insulin, and his blood sugar never went back up again. We stopped the diuretics and gave him additional potassium. His blood sugar never went back up again, and he was able to lose some weight in the short time he was with us. When he went home and continued the low-fat, high-carbohydrate diet plus exercise, his weight continued to drop; he lost, I think, an additional 20 pounds. Over this period of time, he never required medications again. Here he had been treated by two board-certified, highly specialized, highly respected physicians in his community, who had been doing—and I went over his chart very carefully—everything appropriately, according to standard methods of practice. In other words, it is currently acceptable that some kind of drug is given for mild elevations of blood sugar. The practice isn't even frowned upon. It's also currently acceptable to prescribe a diuretic for mild blood pressure elevations, even though the diuretic may cause problems down the line.

Following these currently acceptable methods of therapy, the patient was rapidly deteriorating not from any diseases he had but from the treatments he

*was given. We were able to use diet and exercise to cut through the require-
ment for medications, and he is still, a year and a half later, not taking any
medications. Now he's quite a bit healthier. I think the diabetic patient is
prone to excessive drug use not only in the treatment of his initial condition
but also in the treatment of conditions associated with diabetes. But when you
use a diet-exercise program to cut through that, you can eliminate a tremendous amount of prescription medication, as was done in this patient.*

Dr. William Philpott's treatment is based on the detection of insulin resistance
factors in specific food and chemical allergies as they affect the individual
patient's ability to utilize available insulin supplies efficiently. He describes what
happened in his treatment of a 60-year-old man who was a diagnosed type II
maturity-onset diabetic:

*He was placed on an oral medication which he took twice a day. However, I
saw him 11 years after that diagnosis at his present age. His fasting blood
sugar was usually around 300. The doctors said, 'We are going to have to go
to insulin.' He was very weak—just terribly fatigued and depressed, too. He
had read my book Victory over Diabetes (Keats, New Canaan, Connecticut,
1983), and wanted to give it a try before he went on insulin. When he came
to me he was not on insulin yet, he was just ready to be put on insulin. I simply put him on foods that he just never would be addicted or allergic to and put
him on intravenous vitamin C, B6, calcium, and magnesium for about four
days in a row....*

"*By the time we reached the fourth day his fasting blood sugar was normal. On the sixth day, we started feeding him foods that he more commonly
used. One of those foods was wheat, and within 1 hour his blood sugar was
270. At about three or four hours it had normalized and we were able to give
him another meal. With rye, it was 275. On garbanzo beans it was 206, millet was 189, and even milk was 176. Oatmeal was 206. So we had at least a
dozen foods that gave him high blood sugar. Actually the most important was
the wheat which he ate religiously every day.*

*We find the cereal grains containing gluten wheat and rye, oats, barley,
buckwheat to be the most serious reactors. Through the years, only sugar and
glucose have been used as the criteria for response, but we found much higher
reaction to wheat....*

*As we studied him we grew a fungus from his mouth and from his stool
and rectal area called Candida albicans. He also had rather high antibodies.
A lot of diabetics are made toxic by this organism.*

*We spotted that and found that he was deficient in magnesium and folic
acid. We found that he was using 400 mg of caffeine, by coffee, a day. This
was an important factor that was helping to disorder his functions. Now
knowing the foods he reacted to, leaving them out of the diet for at least 12*

weeks while treating his infection and making his nutrition optimum, we were able to very quickly leave him with good energy, good control, and no high blood sugars at all anymore.

Instead of going on insulin... here we have him strong with no high blood sugars at all and absent of infections. If we had just given him insulin and paid no attention to this fungus infection, he'd still be toxic. If you monitor him from any standpoint you wish, this man doesn't have diabetes. That's the difference between the types of symptom management: just giving insulin to cover this insulin resistance that he had. We measured his insulin, and actually he had a normal amount of insulin.

It was the same problem of insulin resistance that we see in these cases. Now... he knows that the disease process is not deteriorating him any more. The consequences of this deterioration are rapid spreading, depression, weakness, infection by fungi and viruses, and soon the whole degenerating disease process. Now we have him on a high-fiber diet... which will feed the right kind of bacteria. There will be good bowel function, moving the toxins out of the body, which is necessary.

But this is a very small part of what you need to do. People should lose weight and should use this kind of diet, but there is something much more central to this disease process, which is the insulin resistance to the food and your ability to isolate which foods prevent your body from using insulin properly.

46

Acquired Immune Deficiency Syndrome (AIDS)

Probably the most popular new musical on Broadway in the 90s was Rent. Although it suffered from a saccharine quality, it was a crowd pleaser because it mirrored something in the times. The central characters were a pair of couples—one straight, one gay—and all four members of the group were HIV positive. One dies of AIDS in the course of the drama; but even more important for the theme of this chapter is the fate of the straight male's former girlfriend. When she found out she was positive, she committed suicide.

This death is, if anything, more tragic than the AIDS death, insofar as it's partly driven by an establishment-induced myopia. The plain fact is: It has not yet been proven that HIV (human immunodeficiency virus) causes AIDS, though there is an association between the two. Moreover, if the woman killed herself, it's probably partly because she only knew about AZT and the other drastic treatments touted by conventional doctors. She was probably unaware of the less toxic, more natural treatments we will explore in this chapter.

In 1984 at a conference in Maryland, Dr. Robert Gallo claimed to have isolated the HIV retrovirus, which he conjectured was the active agent causing AIDS. The press front-paged the story, not only lauding Gallo and his fellow researchers, but predicting a cure was just a short distance down the road.

Well, 15 years have passed and we find that in relation to AIDS, we are not on the high road of hope but slogging through a quagmire of failed studies that provide little sense or information about how the disease proceeds, unworkable treatments, and toxic drugs that kill as fast as they cure. That's the bad news coming from the medical establishment. The good news is where the establishment failed, that is, in the accuracy of their doomsday predictions about the inevitable, plaguelike spread of AIDS. AIDS has not spread with either the speed or decimating broadness that was foreseen. On the other hand, if there is to be any good news on the treatment front, it will have to come from the alternative doctors who eschew AZT and toxic "cocktails" to concentrate on such healing remedies as the use of nutritional and lifestyle changes as well as oxygen and ozone therapies.

In this chapter, we will comment briefly on some of the problems with the conventional understanding and treatment of AIDS, and remark on the fact that AIDS has not spread as widely as it was one time feared it would. We will devote the bulk of the chapter to the alternative treatments for AIDS that do seem to be working.

Does HIV = AIDS?

In 1984, Dr. Gallo found the presence of HIV in the majority of the AIDS sufferers whose blood he tested. From this he concluded that HIV causes AIDS. So far this is still the best evidence that HIV = AIDS, but it relies on a peculiarly strained logic.

Even if the HIV virus were found in every AIDS patient, this alone does not settle the question of what causes the syndrome. HIV could simply be a cofactor, an agent which is necessary but not sufficient to create AIDS. Prominent AIDS researcher Dr. Root-Bernstein writes in *The Scientist*, "We also thought we knew that HIV alone is sufficient to cause AIDS. But such researchers as Luc Montagnier... and many others... now believe that cofactors are necessary and, therefore, that HIV by itself cannot cause AIDS."

The case for labeling HIV as partially, not wholly, the cause of AIDS is summed up well by Dr. Root-Bernstein. He notes, "All AIDS patients do have multiple, well established causes of immunosuppression prior to, concomitant with, subsequent to, and sometimes in the absence of, HIV infection." If HIV infection in AIDS patients is always found with other debilitating conditions— he lists the seven conditions: "chronic or repeated infectious diseases caused by immunosuppressive microorganisms; recreational and addictive drugs; anesthetics; antibiotics; semen components; blood; and malnutrition"—then it seems reasonable to conclude that these factors are as necessary as the presence of HIV to bring on the disease.

THE NATURE OF THE RETROVIRUS HIV is a retrovirus and part of the controversy swirling around it is whether a retrovirus could be powerful enough to play a determinative role in creating the AIDS disease.

First, we need to describe a virus. A virus is an extremely simple organism that contains genes (strands of DNA or RNA holding the information needed by the virus to copy itself) within a shell with, possibly, an outer membrane around that. The virus is so absolutely simple it cannot reproduce, feed itself, or carry out any other functions on its own. To survive, it has to get into a living cell and use that cell's machinery. It can only survive as a parasite, though; perhaps surprisingly, these viruses are not always detrimental to their host. A virus may move from cell to cell, leaving its own genetic material behind as it travels. In the best of cases, this new material may be valuable, and, if nothing else, will account for increased genetic diversity.

A retrovirus is a particular, only recently discovered, subtype of virus. To understand its action we need to step back a minute and look at how genes operate. Until 1970, it was believed the DNA in a cell's nucleus was the sole possessor of the genetic code. When it was necessary to direct cell operation, RNA (a messenger version of the code, created on the DNA template) would be manufactured and sent out to carry the DNA's orders. This seemed to be an adequate explanation, except for viruses. They were so simple they could only contain either RNA or DNA, not both. However, while a DNA-carrying virus could be easily understood—it entered a host cell and used its DNA to form RNA out of materials from the host cell—the operation of RNA-carrying viruses seemed inexplicable. In 1970, biochemists Howard Temin and David Baltimore overthrew accepted thinking by showing that certain types of RNA could themselves manufacture DNA. They deservedly won a Nobel Prize for their findings. This is relevant to our study because it led to an explanation of how RNA-carrying virus operated successfully. Once it entered a likely host, it used the host's machinery to manufacture its own DNA, which then took over operation of the host cell. A virus that functions in this manner, as does HIV, is called a retrovirus.

Where this causes a problem for AIDS researchers is that it adds yet another puzzling element to the disease, since the retrovirus, in general, is not actually threatening and tends to leave its host unaffected by its presence.

Harvey Bialy, editor of the science journal *Bio/Technology*, rounds out this point by mentioning, "HIV is an ordinary retrovirus. There is nothing about this virus that is unique. It does not differ substantially from all the benign retroviruses.... It contains no gene different enough from the genes of other retroviruses to be a possible AIDS gene."

He also remarks that HIV uses all of its genetic information when it first infects a cell. "It doesn't hoard any for later use, so there is no conceivable reason HIV should cause AIDS 10 years after infection, rather than early on when it is unchecked by the immune system."

Why AIDS Hasn't Spread as Predicted

For the moment we can leave these problems to be sorted out by the scientists, since we want to turn to the less speculative question of what inroads AIDS has made into the world's populations.

Predictions based on the HIV theory have failed spectacularly. Here are the bare facts. AIDS in the United States and Europe has not spread through the general population. Rather, it remains almost entirely confined to the original risk groups, mainly sexually promiscuous gay men and drug abusers. The number of HIV-infected Americans has remained constant for years instead of increasing rapidly as predicted.

These statements may seem bold to the point of being outrageous to anyone who keeps up with the AIDS story by following it in the mass media. However, there is one thing that escalating predictions of the ravages of AIDS conveniently tend to leave out of their reports. That, in many cases, when a report of a sudden increase of AIDS patients is made, it is accompanied by a redefinition of what the disease is

Recall that people only die indirectly of AIDS. AIDS weakens the immune system and then they die of another disease, such as tuberculosis. Now suppose—and this is not a theoretical case—a fatal disease that was not classified as AIDS-related is reclassified as AIDS-related. Obviously, you would be adding the people who had died of that disease previously to the AIDS death list and driving up the figures.

As I said, this is not hypothetical. In January 1993, the Centers for Disease Control (CDC) changed the definition of AIDS so that anyone who had a low CD4 blood cell count was defined as an AIDS statistic. According to the previous definition, a person did not have AIDS until he or she came down with an AIDS-related disease. Is it any surprise then, after this redefinition, that the CDC's 1993 report said the disease was exploding? The reported cases had doubled from about 48,000 to about 107,000. However, a task force for the Society of Actuaries didn't fall for this explosion. Robert Maver, speaking for the task force, said the increase was artificially produced, created by widening the net of people who were considered to be suffering from the disease. He commented, "Under this new category [low CD4 level] alone, more than 50,000 cases were added to the 1993 total."

Nor is this some kind of anomaly in the reporting of AIDS victims. The definition was also altered and expanded in 1985 and again in 1987.

Although there is not the time in this chapter to deal with the similar numbers game being played with the statistics of African AIDS victims, similar hanky-panky is going on with AIDS predictions there as I will show at length in a book forthcoming from Seven Stories Press.

The statistics bandied about in the area of AIDS are subject to much distortion so let's have the real figures.

According to author Neville Hodgkinson:

Predictions of HIV's spread… have turned out to be not just inaccurate, but completely ill-conceived. In countries such as the UK where relatively careful testing and screening programs have been established, estimates of the numbers of people testing HIV-positive are lower than they were seven to eight years ago. An anonymous screening survey published in 1993 came up with an estimated total of 23,000, hardly an epidemic in a nation of 55 million people... AIDS cases outside the original 'risk groups'... are almost nonexistent in such countries: a cumulative total of sixty-three in the UK.

Similar low numbers for AIDS cases outside of the risk categories are found in New York City, 66 out of 37,600. In the U.S. as a whole, Hodgkinson points out, "estimates as of November 1995 put the total number of people testing HIV positive at between 630,000 and 897,000, lower than a previous, long-standing Public Health Service estimate of around 1 million people."

C. Geshekter noted in 1995 that new AIDS cases in San Francisco had declined 90 percent since March 1992.

The book *Sex in America: A Definitive Survey* (University of Chicago Press, 1994) concluded that "AIDS is, and is likely to remain, confined to exactly the risk groups where it began: gay men and intravenous drug users and their sexual partners."

Geshekter notes further, "If we examine the numbers involved, we see why AIDS is not spreading among the general population." Since 1981, there have been 476,899 cases of AIDS have been reported in the United States. "But over 90 percent of the victims suffered from hepatitis, malnutrition, drug abuse, previous infections that required antibiotics, or had a sexually transmitted disease before any exposure to HIV."

At this point, the reader might wonder why projections have been and continue to be so flawed. In the book *Rethinking AIDS*, P. Plumley lists three reasons why public health officials tend to vastly exaggerate the number of people that will get AIDS in the future. "(1) no one wants to appear complacent; (2) the worse the epidemic is projected to be, the more money will be available for public health work; and (3) when the numbers turn out to be lower, the officials can take credit for having done a good job of AIDS education."

Of course the downside of this is that the money the public health officials have accrued by pumping up the number is largely wasted, because it is not properly targeted. David Mertz points out, "Only 5 percent of all U.S. AIDS educational materials are directed at gay men. Instead, a sizable majority of safe-sex material is targeted to young, white heterosexuals. Injecting drug use receives similar short shift in these materials." This results in a dangerous squandering of resources.

Problems With Conventional Treatments

RESTRICTED OPTIONS The first difficulty is that conventional programs are restricted in purview almost exclusively to drugs. If one brings up measures to help the AIDS patient that go beyond ingesting pharmaceuticals, according to

Dr. Dean Black, "This opens up the door to all the lifestyle measures that medicine has so long discounted, the idea that it could be in the behavior of the AIDS victim, in the diet, in the lifestyle in some fashion."

Researcher Bill McCreary points to the absurdity of doctors who ignore their own intuitions about the people they are treating to await orders from on high:

> Doctors say it's not approved by the FDA so we can't touch it.... Doctors usually do a better job because they're there, they know the patient.... Today, the doctor works from a cookbook that is issued out of federal government. They have to abide by that cookbook or they may be found guilty of malpractice.

AZT: A SUSPICIOUS PAST The major recipe in that cookbook now is AZT, widely prescribed as the "approved" AIDS treatment. AZT was developed as a chemotherapy agent in the late 1960s for the treatment of leukemia, but was never patented by its creator, Dr. Richard Beltz, after he established that his chemotherapy compound was "too toxic for even short term use" and "caused cancer at any dose." Because of this, AZT was never used for its intended purpose as a cancer chemotherapy. Laboratory studies revealed some of its side effects to be hair loss, weight loss, muscle loss, anemia, and the very same pneumonia associated with AIDS. The drug was then shelved.

The drug's antileukemic mechanism of action is to kill growing lymphocytes by termination of DNA synthesis. The rationale of AZT therapy is simple, if not naive: the retrovirus HIV depends on DNA synthesis for multiplication, and AZT terminates DNA synthesis. Thus AZT should stop AIDS.

It should—but there's one catch. As Huw Christie explains, "Cancer cells, which AZT was designed to kill, grow faster than normal tissue cells, the idea therefore being that, when incorporating AZT, they die more quickly than normally replicating cells too. When the treatment is finished and the chemotherapy stopped, the normal tissue cells can set about making up for their own lower rate of loss." Studies show, on the other hand, that no more than 1 in 1,000 lymphocytes are ever infected by HIV—even in people dying from AIDS. Since AZT cannot distinguish between an infected and an uninfected cell, 999 uninfected cells must be killed to kill just one HIV-infected cell.

In 1984, the U.S. Department of Health granted a contract for AZT to Burroughs-Wellcome which remarketed AZT to AIDS doctors as an "antiviral." AZT was first given to human beings in the initial AIDS treatment trials.

A campaign was then waged to get every HIV-positive person on AZT. Researcher John Lauritsen explains, HIV-positive patients "were told that they should go for what was called early medical intervention. There were slogans put out, 'Put time on your side.' The early intervention meant purely and simply AZT. And rather than putting time on the side of these people, what the drug did and is doing is to terminate their lives."

Here's another difference from cancer treatment. In cancer, you begin to take chemotherapy after you contract the disease. AZT, as we saw, originally developed for chemotherapy, would be the first "chemotherapy" prescribed as a preventative before a person shows any symptoms.

Activist G. Hazlehurst put it like this: AIDS "is the only disease I know of where treatment with powerful drugs is begun several to many years prior to the actual onset of any illness, when there is still the possibility it may not even develop."

HOW AZT AFFECTS THE IMMUNE SYSTEM The public is kept in the dark about these facts. As a result, when people are diagnosed as HIV-positive and prescribed AZT, they believe their sudden decline and impending death is attributable to AIDS and not the drug.

Dr. Martin Feldman told me, "The current drugs on the market, primarily AZT, tend to severely weaken the immunity and make the body have to work harder to have immune strength. The body uses up its basic nutrients in the process. Really, the body is fighting against the AZT."

Another commentator notes that if you give AZT indefinitely, so that every six hours the patients take 250 mg of AZT, they are going to "lose weight, they become anemic, they lose their white cells, they have nausea, they lose their muscles.... That is what you call AIDS by prescription."

AZT challengers agree that it can only weaken the immune system further. Dr. Dean Black castigates the developers of the drug for the whole rationale of the treatment. "By virtue of determining to substitute for the immune system, by attacking this alien agent with a drug, medicine has literally replaced the body's immune system. What can it do but become weak?"

A number of advocates of alternative treatment tell us that we need to change the focus of treatment toward "stimulating, activating, and increasing" the body's antibody system. "Since it is the evolutionary responsibility of the cytotoxic T-lymphocytes to destroy infected and abnormal self-cells, increasing their numbers would be beneficial." The best direction of treatment, according to this perspective, would be to help the body to use the immune system it already has instead of forcing it to tolerate an artificial one.

Since we've brought up the subject of better treatments, let's move on to three doctors who have already developed alternative treatments.

Alternative Treatments

A number of alternative treatments are having some success with AIDS. In this chapter we will highlight three of the newer approaches, pairing each description with a brief mention of a doctor who has pioneered the approach as well as the histories of some of the patients he has worked with. The three approaches are (1) supporting the body's own methods of healing and defense by bringing nutrient levels up to optimal levels; (2) working on improving the body's metabolism using a special fatty acid preparation; and (3) elevating the level of oxygen in the blood to boost the immune system and cell activity.

Optimizing Nutrient Levels: Dr. Christopher Calapai

In an article published in a scientific journal, Cohen and Kutler note that in evaluating the health conditions of HIV-infected persons, before they showed any disease symptoms, most had poor nutrition. They had decreased body mass, fat, and protein, resulting from malabsorption. They would be eating but their bodies were not adequately breaking down the food and assimilating its nutrients. A further study, "Influence of HIV Infection on Vitamin Status and Requirement," points out that a vicious circle will result from this malabsorption. "Once occurring, malnutrition leads to immunosuppression, infection, and mucosal damage... resulting in further malnutrition."

Poor absorption of nutrients will weaken the immune system, then, but Dr. Christopher Calapai sees the body's inability to profit from food nutrients as stemming not only from absorption problems, but from anorexia and high resting energy expenditure (REE). REE means that the body is overstimulated. While it should have slowed during rest, the metabolism is still using up nutrients at an accelerated pace. In any case, the HIV-infected patient is either not getting or using too quickly the nutrients he or she needs to support bodily functions.

It is no question that certain vitamins are needed to maintain immune response. These include E, B_6, C, and beta carotene. Studies of the elderly, who generally have impaired immune systems, have long shown that these vitamins, taken as supplements, will improve immune response.

In fact, there is evidence that certain vitamins as well as herbs can counter the progress of AIDS as they bolster the immune system. Let's pause to highlight some of the more notable successes that have been seen with these types of therapies, many of which are used by Dr. Calapi.

VITAMINS AND OTHER NUTRIENTS In a forthcoming work, I will have a 100 pages to detail the vitamin and herbal supplements that have been used for treating AIDS patients with positive results. In this briefer space, I can only touch on some of the substances that have recorded good results.

GLUTATHIONE

Glutathione is an antioxidant that protects against cellular damage. It stimulates lymphocytes that help defend the body against viral illnesses, such as AIDS. When N-acetyl-cysteine (NAC) is given to a patient, the body will convert it to glutathione.

A study in *Nutrition Review* indicates that HIV-positive individuals are deficient in glutathione. On the other hand, results have been reported from a number of studies that indicate HIV activity is reduced by glutathione's presence.

Dr. Joan Priestley gives her HIV-infected and AIDS patients intravenous glutathione, because, she says, "Glutathione specifically attacks the AIDS virus in about four different steps."

Speaking at a 1991 AIDS symposium, Dr. Calapi stated:

When we add glutathione intravenously with vitamin C, we see a significant turnaround in the patient's comfort, attitude, and well being... NAC taken intravenously can inhibit reverse transcriptase [HIV replication] activity better than 90 percent. There is no drug available for any treatment or disease that can do better than 90 percent with minimal or no side effects.

VITAMIN A (BETA CAROTENE)

Beta carotene is a safe form of vitamin A, which stops damage from bodily pollution, bolsters the immune system, inhibits viruses, and prevents premature aging.

A study done by Dr. Semba of Johns Hopkins showed that a vitamin A deficiency was associated with HIV-positive and AIDS patients. It concluded that this deficiency was a serious risk factor in the disease. In a different study, Dr. Semba's team found that a lack of vitamin A was positively correlated with death from AIDS.

On the other hand, a number of studies chart improvements when beta carotene is administered. In one, 11 HIV-positive patients received 60 mg of the vitamin per day for four months. They recorded an increase in natural killer cells and other vital parts of the immune system, which HIV infection tends to diminish. Another study was done on 10 patients who had just gotten off AZT and began taking 120 mg a day of beta carotene. Although one died a few months into the treatment, the other nine experienced an HIV burden diminution, clinically measured improvements in health, and evaluated themselves as having a better quality of life.

VITAMIN C (ASCORBIC ACID)

Vitamin C is one of the stars among the vitamins in treating AIDS. Basing his opinion on numerous clinical studies, Dr. Robert Cathcart confidently states, "Vitamin C can double the life expectancy of AIDS patients." He says that his treatment, which involves using massive doses of buffered ascorbate of 50 to 200 grams every 24 hours (in combination with other treatments for secondary infections), will produce a clinical remission of the disease that shows every evidence of being prolonged if the treatment goes on.

Other doctors report similar results. Dr. Raxit Jariwalla, a virologist from the Linus Pauling Institute, says, "In laboratory cultures of HIV-infected cells... vitamin C can significantly suppress both the activity and replication of the AIDS virus."

Joy DeVincenxo, who is HIV positive and has used massive doses of vitamin C, explains, "A lot of doctors... do not believe in giving me vitamin C... [but] without it, I know I wouldn't have stayed stable for so long."

These statements are supported by a host of studies, such as the one that appeared in the volume *Nutrition and AIDS*, which summarized the results of various examinations of C's value. The authors point out, "A striking property of ascorbic acid is its ability to inactivate viruses and inhibit viral growth in their host cells." Experimental studies reported in the same volume show that vitamin C will directly interfere with HIV replication, carrying the assault on the disease into the enemy's camp.

VITAMIN E

Vitamin E is an antioxidant that seems to prevent many diseases caused by environmental stressors. It is found in fish and vegetable oil, nuts, and whole grains. However, the majority of Americans do not get enough of this vitamin in their foods and need supplementation.

Studies are piling up showing that vitamin E is a warrior against AIDS. One study showed that the administration of 50 mg/kg per day over five days already began to inhibit the replication of HIV. Another study showed that if the dosage of E was increased 15-fold (to 160 IU/liter), immune system functions that had been suppressed by HIV presence were restored.

HERBAL TREATMENTS

Again, we can only skim the surface in mentioning some herbal treatments that have shown themselves as powerful agents in working against AIDS.

Vital work has been done in the area of herbal therapies by The Institute for Traditional Medicine in Portland, Oregon, in looking at how Chinese herbs can be used in treating AIDS. The founder of the institute has developed a specific herbal combination, which combines strong tonic herbs with those that fight inflammation and infection. Of 150 patients who have undergone therapy with this herbal formula over three months, 76 percent experienced an increase of energy, and 62 percent of the patients who suffered from diarrhea saw a cessation of the problem. Other symptoms were similarly improved.

Dr. Chang of the Sun Yat Sen Medical Center also found a mix of Chinese herbs to work strenuously against AIDS. He found that extracts from 11 different herbs inhibit the activity of HIV. Dr. Quingcai Zhang notes these Chinese herb treatments are effective because they work with the body to fight infection, rather than, as do such drugs as AZT, by trying to override the body's own creative functioning.

Let's look at some of the herbs that have a good reputation for working against HIV.

ASTRAGALUS

Astragalus root has been used for centuries in China because it was thought to strengthen the immune system. Current research shows the truth of this belief since astragalus is now known to correct T cell (part of the immune system) deficiency and promote antiviral action.

A study at the University of Texas showed that taking astragalus extract stimulates T cell production in healthy animals and restores it in cancer patients who have seen their T cell production impaired. In another study, involving 19 cancer patients with weakened immune systems, an extract of astragalus induced such a complete recovery that it was noted, "People whose immune systems were devastated by cancer experienced full restoration of immune function."

Of course, studies need to be conducted on AIDS sufferers, but astragalus's aid to the immune system is evident.

GARLIC

Garlic has a number of antitumor and antiviral mechanisms. It stimulates the immune system's productions of phagocytosis, which eliminates abnormal cells from the body. It is toxic to some abnormal cells and inhibits the implantation of others. It has even proven effective against some bacteria that do not respond to antibiotics.

In fighting AIDS, it is especially good in eliminating the opportunistic infections that plague AIDS patients once their immune systems have been weakened.

A German study of seven AIDS patients who were given five grams of garlic daily found that five showed significant improvements in their T cells, along with other improvements in health and fewer outbreaks of opportunistic infections.

GINSENG

Numerous studies of ginseng's benefits were conducted in Russia in the 1960s and 1970s. Norman Farnsworth collected and translated many of these studies, which indicated that various types of ginseng acted to normalize body temperature, enhance the body's ability to resist infection, improve cells' ability to dispose of the byproducts of metabolism, and counter the effects of environmental pollution.

Its effects in treating AIDS patients have also been shown. In a study by Y. K. Cho and others, Korean red ginseng improved weakened immune response in subjects infected with HIV.

LICORICE ROOT

Licorice root has also been effective in stopping the HIV virus from replicating, according to a scientific study. The study, done at the World Life Research Institute, recorded no toxicity to normal cells.

The plant is known to strengthen the immune system by increasing macrophage activity and that of interferon-gamma, both vital actors in combating infections and viruses. Licorice is a detoxifying agent and has anti-inflammatory, antiallergic, and antispasmodic properties.

ST. JOHN'S WORT

Studies at New York University have shown that St. John's wort contains two potent chemicals that are highly effective in preventing the spread of retroviruses, like HIV, both in laboratory samples and in patients.

One of the researchers, Meruelo, found that one of these chemicals would stop the spread of AIDS, even crossing the barrier into the brain, which serves as a reservoir of HIV cells, to combat the disease there. Meruelo comments that St. John's wort's "antiviral activity is remarkable both in its mechanism... and the potency of one administration of a relatively small dose of the compounds."

PHYTOCHEMICALS Before moving on to the lifestyle components that form part of Dr. Calapi's program, I want to call your attention to a new area of research in supplementation that I believe will have a lot to offer toward helping AIDS patients in years to come. This is the area of phytochemicals.

Phytochemicals are disease-preventing or healing substances found in edible plants, such as those found in licorice root, which are believed to account for the plant's valuable immune-system strengthening qualities that have already been outlined.

These chemicals are found in frequently consumed foods such as fruits, vegetables, grains, legumes, and seeds as well as in less common foods such as soy and green tea. They have already been associated with the prevention and treatment of four of the leading causes of death in this country: cancer, diabetes, cardiovascular disease, and hypertension. Although not enough studies have been done on these substances, those that have been done hint that quite large benefits are to be expected from these substances.

One example of such studies is the research on limonene, found in citrus fruits, which shows that it increases the body's production of enzymes that help it dispose of potentially carcinogenic substances. It is well known that people whose diets are heavy in fruits have lower rates of most cancers than those who don't have such diets. Many are attributing this low cancer rate to the effect of the phytochemicals.

I believe as the new millennium opens, these phytochemicals will begin to play an important role as healers of ravaged immune systems and in counteracting and inhibiting the growth and existence of AIDS.

LIFESTYLE CHANGES

DIETARY MODIFICATION

Dr. Calapai's treatment program involves both building up the body with proper nutrients and calling on his patients to make lifestyle changes. Before actually laying out his program and profiling some of the patients who have maximally benefited from it, let us investigate the type of lifestyle changes that have proven effective in both his therapy and in that of other doctors.

Research supports the long-term efficacy of dietary counseling and use of nutritional supplementation for AIDS patient to increase or maintain weight, restore lean tissues, and lessen the effects of the disease. These factor could help decrease mortality as well as improve bowel function.

Patrick Donnelly, program coordinator for the Whole Foods Project, says AIDS patients must be made aware of the need to eat nutritious foods. He advises working with what are being called "the new four food groups, which are grains, legumes, fruits, and vegetables." These foods are high in antioxidants. and have nutrients like beta carotene, vitamin C, zinc, and selenium. Such nutrients are not found in the high-fat, high-protein standard American diet. Donnelly says, "We're trying to get people to look at a new way of eating that is not about providing calories so much as supporting the immune system."

Another member of the project staff, Richard Pierce, comments, "You only have to look at this food [we provide] to see that it's full of life…. The vitality of the food is what nurtures us. "

Along with eating healthy food, one must learn to avoid the foods that contribute to the growth or virulence of the disease, counterproductive foods, particularly yeast and sugar. Yeast is a natural part of our makeup but it can wreak havoc on the body when it gets out of control. Sugar is an immune suppressant. If one takes 100 grams of sugar, it will cut antibody production by 50 percent for 24 hours.

EXERCISE

Studies have shown that regular exercise has long-term benefits on the biological condition of HIV and AIDS patients as well as on the course of the illness. Researchers have found that exercise will improve a patient's health at all stages of the disease. Moreover, it seems that complications of the disease will be delayed by exercise.

ACUPUNCTURE

Acupuncture has proven to be one of the most popular treatments that HIV-positive people have turned to since 1982. One study followed the development of acupuncture for AIDS treatment in the United States and found that people with HIV who use the treatment have extended survival rates. In addition they regularly report a substantial reduction in symptoms and side effects from HIV-related drugs. Acupuncture frequently provides relief from AIDS-related diseases, and most patients report a reduction in fatigue, abnormal sweating, diarrhea, and acute skin reactions after four to five treatments. Some patients have a 15- to 20-pound weight gain and return to long hours of work.

Abigail Rist-Podrecca, a registered nurse, notes that acupuncture works by "dilating the blood vessels, so that the vessels can open. You get more circulation, more of the nutrients, more oxygen flowing through those meridians [the places where the acupuncture needles are stuck]."

She believes one of the reasons AIDS patients weaken is because they lose ability to take up nutrition through the intestines. Acupuncture acts to reverse this digestive problem as well as working on the lungs and other bodily centers.

Studies conducted at the Lincoln Hospital Acupuncture Clinic in the Bronx, the AIDS Alternative Health Project in Chicago, and with the Quan Yin Herbal support program in San Francisco have reported symptomatic relief and overall physical improvement in patients with AIDS they have treated with acupuncture needles.

REFLEXOLOGY AND AROMATHERAPY

A couple of unusual techniques that have shown positive results so far with AIDS are reflexology and aromatherapy.

Reflexology is a form of relaxation treatment. It was used in a program with AIDS patients run in Uganda in 1993. Four months after the program began, 85 percent of those treated noted pain relief, better relaxation, and better sleep after the reflexology sessions.

Aromatherapy is the use of plant essences in healing. Pure oils are used, some of which have already proven to have antifungal and antiviral effects.

Teopista studied the effect of aromatherapy when it was used in conjunction with other therapies to see if it would lessen the need for toxic drugs. Using 80 randomly selected AIDS patients, the study concluded that the group that utilized aromatherapy, in contrast to the control group, reported fewer aches and pains, faster healing of wounds, greater physical strength, and a better ability to cope.

HOW DR. CALAPAI'S PROGRAM WORKS As mentioned, Dr. Calapai's program centers on nutrition and lifestyle changes. When he first sees a patient, he asks him or her to bring in a week's worth of diet history, which he goes over very carefully. He immediately tells the patient how important it is to institute lifestyles changes that will provide strong benefits. These changes include immediately stopping smoking and alcohol usage.

He orders a detailed diagnostic protocol that includes blood evaluations of cellular, mineral, vitamin, hormone, and viral and antigen levels. He also does aggressive testing for common infections, such as herpes and tuberculosis (TB), which can contribute to the progression of the disease. He is flexible and allows a patient to take the antiretroviral drugs if that patient so desires. He also lets the patient consult other doctors.

Once he has the test results, he uses them along with the patient's history to devise dietary recommendations. Here we have it in his own words:

In review of the blood testing… I sit down with my patients, give them a five-page handout as to what they should eat, what hey shouldn't eat. I like to try to get them away from red meat, get them more towards a vegetarian diet.

DR. CALAPAI'S PROGRAM: RESULTS Let's hear what Dr. Calapai says about his results and then describe a few of his patients. "Many of the patients that I have put on the protocol after two weeks or so say they're feeling very good." He continues, "They have a lot of energy; they're sleeping better…. The overwhelming majority say they feel better in a number of ways."

He has had patients who have followed his nutritional and lifestyle alteration program and, though they have very low T cell counts, have been free of coughs, colds, and any other opportunistic infection for a year.

He feels confidence in his protocol and comments, "AIDS is a syndrome where people are dying relatively rapidly, so I don't know how appropriate it is to wait until there's firm and hard data before recommending some of these safe, nontoxic treatments." His general position is that, given that many people are not finding that the conventional treatments do not work, "We have to try and use the safe things—the herbs and nutrients—and see how much help they can offer the patient."

Now we can review a couple of his patients.

A 32-year-old Caucasian female, when she came to the doctor in January 1992, was HIV positive and having headaches, sinus congestion, and fatigue. Testing showed her T cell count was 616. (The T cells, parts of the immune system, are taken out of action by HIV retroviruses. A lower count indicates the inroads of the disease.) The patient was put on the protocol and by September her T cell count was up to 1,000. She feels good and has not had any opportunistic or other infections.

A 32-year-old Caucasian male came to Dr. Calapai in February 1993 with a three-year history of being HIV positive. He had hepatitis B in the past. He was deficient in magnesium, vitamins A, B$_6$, and D. After going on the nutritional and lifestyle alteration program, his vitamin and mineral deficiencies were corrected. He exercises regularly, his weight is stable, and he is energetic.

These and other of Dr. Calapai's patients whose cases I studied showed a substantial improvement in health status in a short time. This is testimony to the efficacy and intelligence of his program.

Improving Metabolism: Dr. Emmanuel Revici

Dr. Emmanuel Revici's program is similar to Dr. Calapai's insofar as it also affirms that AIDS must be dealt with by supplying nutritional deficiencies. However, it is much narrower in locating the deficiency only in certain fats. At the same time, it is broader in that it is based on a well worked out philosophy.

This philosophy, though not based on Chinese medicine, does resemble the Oriental system in seeing the body as driven by two crosscurrents. Elsewhere in this book, I make mention of Chinese thought on ying and yang. Traditional Chinese medicine sees these two energies as creating the body's vitality. The body's health depends on their balance. Similarly, Dr. Revici sees two basic processes in the body: the anabolic, which builds up, and the catabolic, which breaks down. He writes, "The two antagonistic intervening factors... act alternately, each being predominant for a period of time. The result is... an oscillatory movement with successive passages from one side to the other of the average value." When an organism is working normally, it maintains its characteristic rhythms and intensities by means of this oscillation. However, when there is a breakdown, it will be because the alternations are lopsided and either catabolic or anabolic influences are unduly dominating. It is as if a pendulum's swing were being artificially pulled to one side.

In the case of AIDS, as he sees it, there is a deficiency in certain of the body's phospholipids (a type of fat), which normally play a role in disease prevention. He traces the course of the disease: A primary viral infection occurs, which brings about the weakening of the body's line of lipidic defense. This is followed by secondary, opportunistic infections which are allowed to run wild due to the body's lowered defense threshold. Then comes an exaggerated catabolic imbalance whereby the body's breakdown of substances is outrunning its construction of others.

The treatment called for in such a case is a four-pronged one. To deal with the viral infections, antiviral agents should be introduced into the system. To deal with the lipid deficiency, these lipids have to be reintroduced by injection. For the secondary opportunistic infections, proper antibiotics are applied. And for the catabolic imbalance, balancing agents are prescribed.

PATIENT STORIES Let's look at a few of Dr. Revici's patients to see what results he has been getting.

> *A 27-year-old man was diagnosed HIV positive in 1986. He complained of tiredness, headaches, and night sweats. He was treated from April 1987, continuing through the present. Around the time of his initial HIV-positive diagnosis, his CD4 count was 625; subsequently, it stayed around 650 until February 1992, when it was reported to have doubled to 1,310. In March 1993, he reported "feeling very well," with "no complaints except mild weakness."*
>
> *A 30-year-old man was diagnosed HIV positive in 1990. He came for treatment in 1992 with memory difficulties and cervical, axillary, and inguinal adenopathy. At the time of his initial HIV-positive diagnosis, his*

absolute CD4 was 243. After three months of treatment, it had risen to 636. In April 1993, the adenopathy remained and there was a mild oral thrush.

A woman was diagnosed HIV positive in 1985, at the age of 24. She came for treatment in 1989. At that time, she came she had carcinoma in situ of the cervix, fatigue, nausea, and complained of constipation. Over the course of her treatment, her T4 counts nearly doubled from 600 to 1016. As of May 1993, she was well, working, and continuing treatment.

All in all, I examined ten of Dr. Revici's cases and about them I can make these generalizations. Of these patients, only three seem not to have improved during therapy. Yet, of these three, one, though worsening in immunologic markers, nevertheless felt "well" at the end of ten years of treatment. Another, though his T4 count also declined considerably over four years of treatment, was still "feeling fine" at the end of that period.

Thus, of the ten patients, eight currently (or recently) report feeling well after an average period of 5.2 years of therapy. Five of the eight also report no remaining symptomatic complaints; and two of those have had a marked improvement in immune markers. All are currently continuing in therapy.

This treatment, which I would emphasize uses nontoxic substances, has had results decidedly better than those averaged by treatments based on AZT consumption.

Oxygen and Ozone: Dr. John Pittman

Dr. John PIttman's treatment is based on the use of ozone and oxygen. Before describing his treatment in more detail, it will be helpful to give some background on medical applications of ozone with viral infections.

Certainly, oxygen is an essential nutrient. It is, in fact, the most essential, as it is the only one which must be continuously available, at pain of quick death. As we all know, life ceases if the supply of oxygen is cut off for more than a few minutes.

Those observations are so taken for granted that we hardly think about them further. Specifically, have we thought in any depth about how ubiquitous "hidden" hypoxias (health-problem-causing lack of oxygen) may be? This might be one approach to explaining the sometimes surprising therapeutic effectiveness of oxygenation therapies, of which the application of ozone to HIV infection is one of the newest.

A number of studies, such as ones by M. Carpendale and colleagues and another by Wagner and other scientists, indicate

that ozone inactivates the HIV virus at low and safe concentrations.

Carpendale reports, "Ozone... has been shown to inactivate human immunodeficiency virus (HIV) in serum at noncytotoxic concentrations."

It has been conjectured that ozone kills HIV cells. Ozone is also able to strengthen immune responses.

TREATMENT PROTOCOL Ozone therapy is a prime component in Dr. John Pittman's Carolina Center for Bio-oxidative Medicine where he and his staff treat and study patients with AIDS, HIV, and other immune-compromising conditions. Dr. Pittman believes that ozone can arrest the progression of AIDS' diseases and turn the syndrome into a manageable condition. He values ozone's ability to help alleviate chronic problems that plague patients, including dermatological conditions and low level infections. He also notes a relationship between ozone and improved T cell and CD4 counts. Best results occur when an intensive series of treatments are taken every four to six months.

Dr. Pittman uses ozone as an integral part of a wider treatment protocol, which he carefully described to me: "The first 10 days of their program entails a modified juice fast. Everyone drinks fresh pressed vegetable juices and no solid food." Patients are then put on an intensive detoxification program. Nutritional supplements are given. The patient begins autohemotherapy. This involves the removal of blood from the body, so it can be filled with ozone, then reinfused.

After five days of autohemotherapy, Dr. Pittman says, "if the patient has tolerated that... we begin with the direct intravenous infusion of ozone gas... on a daily basis, gradually increasing concentrations and volume until we observe a healing crisis in the patient." The patient will experience fevers, chills, and sometimes flu symptoms. When the healing crisis passes, the doctor tapers off dosage and concentration, and goes into lower doses, "which have a more immune stimulating effect."

Concurrent with ozone therapy are other intravenous therapies, which include intravenous vitamin C and mineral infusions as well as EDTA chelation therapy. The doctor also employs acupuncture and other dietary therapies throughout the program.

Although I was not able to obtain the same detailed case histories from Dr. Pittman that I had from the other two practitioners we have discussed, I did gather very positive anecdotal evidence, including the story of a man who came to the clinic with a CD4 count of 42. In two weeks of intensive therapy, his count soared to 285.

As you can see, Dr. Pittman believes in a nontoxic multifactorial approach in the treatment of AIDS. He says, "I think the approach for AIDS has got to be one from a multimodality standpoint. There is no one single approach. It is only through the combination of appropriate antiviral therapy, immune stimulating therapy, diet, and detoxification programs that a patient is really going to be maintained and have any hope of improvement."

Alternative Health Therapy Concepts

Theories and methods that seem very different can have broadly similar results. All three of the treatment approaches we mentioned have, at the very least, reversed some of the symptoms of HIV infection in some patients, and have improved the quality of life, according to the patients themselves, in many.

The three approaches are not mutually exclusive. Is there any reason why they should not be used together, complementing each other? For example, it was noteworthy that some of the reported actions of the vitamin C infusions used by Dr. Calipai were very similar to those of the ozone infusions used by Dr. Pittman. Both were found to be highly effective in inactivating many viruses, and HIV in particular; and both seemed to augment the effectiveness of the immune system. Perhaps if they were used together, the effects of each would potentiate each other, with results better than either alone.

One of the very important advantages of many of these "nonconventional" methods is that, whether or not they are effective (and there is evidence that some are), they are generally safe. Most nutritional and herbal methods cause far fewer side effects than the pharmaceutical and surgical methods now in favor. This is a major argument for permitting them to be used at the discretion of the individual.

That is a reason for not bringing these modalities under the regulatory authority of the state or organized medicine. It is a matter of constitutional freedoms. But there are also strong economic arguments. The costs of these "alternative" techniques are almost always far lower than the treatments now approved by organized medicine for the same disorders. Thus, encouraging the use of these other approaches can save the American public, both as taxpayer and as health-care consumer, vast amounts of money.

Yes, the physicians whose work with HIV infection we have examined approach health and illness from different perspectives. But they do share a basic world view that separates them from the practitioners of conventional medicine.

According to the conventional view, my body consists of congeries of mechanisms, with subsystems that can be adequately understood separately, with little regard to the status of all the myriad other subsystems. The view of the body found in alternative healthcare is one which sees its level of interconnectedness as far higher. In a healthy organism all the subsystems are supporting each other in myriad ways (most of which are not yet observable or understood). In the first (allopathic) world view, most disease originates through the breakdown of some one mechanism, or a few discrete mechanisms; disease then is to be treated by fixing (or bypassing) the defective mechanism(s). In the second (holistic) world view, however, disease has to do not only with individual mechanisms, but with weakenings of many kinds of couplings between mechanisms, and with overstressing supporting systems through excessive demands for support. In this view, the total system can be strengthened by adding inputs that may rouse relatively quiescent supporting subsystems to become more active, as well as by giving additional resources to many different supporting systems—therapeutic strategies that are emphasized in the work of the three doctors we have used as examples.

Thus, depending upon whether you share the view of the first or second group of health workers, your attitude toward your own health will vary. If you have the traditional view, you will tend toward passivity ("comply with doctor's orders: take your prescribed medicine"); while with an attitude like that of the alternative therapist, you will tend to be active ("take responsibility for your own health, learn all you can, make your own choices"). Perhaps, by this time, you won't be surprised to find that, according to their view of health, long-term AIDS survivors fall into the second camp. Let's close by looking at some of their portraits.

Survivor Portraits

Literature on long-term survivors with AIDS is replete with anecdotal evidence linking survival to such things as holding a positive attitude toward the illness, taking control of one's health, participating in health-promoting behaviors, engaging in spiritual activities, and taking part in AIDS-related events.

Survivors are very pragmatic problem-solvers who educate themselves about alternative treatments, nutrition, and exercise. If something isn't working for them, they change it. Fred Bingham shows how he actively participated in his own healing process.

> *I was given a diagnosis of full blown AIDS in October 1989. I went into the hospital where I was given AZT.... By the time I left the hospital, I could hardly walk.... I was a wreck and I was scared to death.*
>
> *Then I started an incredible journey of researching journals and other anecdotal sources. I was trying to find out how to deal with HIV in a very scientific way...*
>
> *The protocol that I've been on to maintain my health is multifaceted. It compasses a broad array of nutrients, including herbs, vitamins, minerals, trace elements, amino acids and live cell glandulars. Today, I have a completely normal immune system.*

Long-term survivors have another feature in common; they avoid AZT and other toxic antivirals. Rather than take toxic antivirals, more and more patients turn to unconventional therapies, such as those we have been describing.

While AIDS survivors generally do not follow mainstream treatments, they are not loners. They maintain good relationships with their friends, families and doctors, and often belong to support groups. Bill Thompson, an AIDS survivor and activist says, "It was through… the help of my friends, I learned about carrot and beet juice and I went out and got a Champion juicing machine. That's how I've been maintaining good health."

Another feature of long-term survivors is they reject the view that HIV-positivity means early death. They are passionately committed to life, believe in the possibility of survival, and surround themselves with people who will love and support them. They make major lifestyle changes, including in their sex lives, and in most cases, they have given up drugs and alcohol. They have also dabbled with dietary changes.

A writer who studied the lives of survivors says:

> They all talked about what they called "emotional house cleaning." Usually after they had survived their first major opportunistic infection, it represented a crisis to them and they did some soul-searching. They either repaired relationships, or ended them. And all but two talked about a rebirth of spirituality. Half had returned to the religions of their childhood— although none in a fundamentalist, judgmental way—and half spoke more generally of the sense that there was a meaning to suffering…. This gave them a sense of purpose in the here and now. The were not done with life yet. They had a reason to stick around.

This is part of the prescription then, if you are HIV positive or have AIDS. Check out the alternatives, change the negative features of your lifestyle, stay aware of the spiritual aspects of reality, be committed to your friends, and become aware that your life has meaning. Then you'll be there for the long haul.

47

Migraines

Twenty-three million Americans suffer from migraines. One in five women are affected, as compared to only one in twenty men, making women four times more susceptible to this widespread health problem. Children also experience migraines.

Causes

It is now believed that these headaches occur when sudden dilation of blood vessels create pressure on the brain. There are numerous triggers for migraines. Below, Dr. Mary Olsen, a chiropractor from Huntington, New York, who specializes in craniosacral adjustments and applied kinesiology, describes the eight most common reasons for their occurrence.

ALLERGIC REACTIONS "Allergies can be dietary or environmental," Dr. Olsen says. "Dietary triggers can be to foods, food combinations, or additives in foods. Alcoholic beverages, particularly red wine and beer, are among the most common causes of migraines. Tyramine, a chemical found in cheese, smoked fish, yogurt, and yeast extracts, may be involved. MSG, which we find in Chinese cuisine and most processed foods, is often implicated, as is sodium nitrate, found in cold cuts and hot dogs. Aspartame, a commonly used artificial sweetener, may lower serotonin levels in the body. Some researchers believe that this contributes to severe headaches. Chocolate and other foods containing caffeine can also be dietary triggers. In addition, people can have allergies to such common foods as wheat, dairy, corn, and eggs. A person can have environmental allergies to toxic fumes emitted from modern products found in the home."

Today, the theory favored by environmental medicine specialists to explain how allergy-related migraines may occur describes an antigen-antibody reaction, initiated by an allergen, and started as an immune reaction in the tissues where antibodies are localized. The allergen reaction induces the release of chemical mediators like histamine and noradrenalin. The excruciating pain associated with migraines occurs as a direct result of the allergic response: The antigen-antibody reaction affects the temporal arteries in the skull, causing the vessels to expand, with resultant thinning of the vessel walls and subsequent fluid leakage. As a result of the edema (fluid retention), the brain begins to swell, pressing against the inflexible skull structure. The intense pain is mainly due to the stretching of surrounding sensitive tissues in the area of the swelling.

HORMONAL FLUCTUATIONS "Women suffer from migraines to a much greater extent than do men," Dr. Olsen continues. "Of these women, approximately 60 percent correlate headaches to their menstrual cycle. The major contributing factor is the hormone estrogen. We know that women who take oral contraceptives are more susceptible to severe migraines, and that women experience less frequency and severity of headaches after menopause, when there is a sharp reduction of estrogen. Unfortunately, the widespread use of estrogen replacement therapy has resulted in many women having a return of these headaches. Although the exact relationship between migraines and estrogen is unknown at this time, we do know that estrogen affects the central nervous system, including the systems involving serotonin, which can be involved in the development of migraines."

CRANIAL FAULTS "Malposition in cranial bones or cranial faults is another factor contributing to migraines. Trauma to the head, such as striking the head on a car door, or birth trauma, may be enough to lock a bone into a particular position. A whiplash injury may also result in cranial faults."

MERIDIAN IMBALANCE "The applied kinesiologist or acupuncturist checks for a meridian imbalance. Meridians are twelve bilateral electromagnetic channels of energy in the body, identified within the Chinese science of acupuncture. Blocked energy or chi (or qi) within a meridian causes dysfunction, including migraine headaches."

UPPER CERVICAL SUBLUXATION "Another common cause of migraine is the cervical subluxation in the upper part of the neck. This is especially prevalent among people who use the telephone as a regular part of their work. The tendency to hold the phone between the neck and the shoulder forces the vertebrae in the opposite direction. You also see this with people who tend to read in bed. Propping the head up in one direction causes the vertebrae to shift, which puts stress on the nerves and contributes to the migraine."

LOW MAGNESIUM LEVELS "A number of studies have noted that many people suffering from migraines have low levels of magnesium in their blood. This is true too of people who suffer from fibromyalgia, a myofascial condition that can cause severe pain to the head, mimicking a migraine."

OVER-THE-COUNTER AND PRESCRIPTION MEDICATIONS "If you use aspirin, acetaminophen, mixed analgesics, or other acute care medications to get rid of your headaches, you actually may be causing them. The use of these painkillers is the single most common reason for migraines. They are called rebound headaches, and this is why they occur. When you take a painkiller often, the body gets used to having a certain amount of that drug in the bloodstream. When the level falls below that threshold, the body begins to experience withdrawal symptoms. One of these symptoms is headaches. If this situation exists, any preventive treatment for migraine will be undermined."

STRESS "Although stress is not a cause in itself, it can exacerbate the effects of the headache or cause an increase in frequency."

Symptoms

Migraines differ from regular headaches in that they usually occur on one side of the head. They can be accompanied by nausea, vomiting, sensitivity to light and sound, fatigue, weakness, irritability, and vision problems. An aura sometimes precedes a migraine. Usually, this is a visual phenomenon that may appear as a flash of light. However, other sensory systems can be disturbed, causing the aura to appear as numbness, tingling, odor hallucinations, language difficulties, confusion, or disorientation.

General Guidelines for Alternative Treatment

Although exact treatment depends on a patient's individual needs, Dr. Mary Olsen suggests general guidelines for treating migraines brought on by different factors. Of course, combination approaches are often indicated as well.

MIGRAINES CAUSED BY FOOD ALLERGIES. "Since migraines don't necessarily follow immediately after ingesting a food, it may be difficult to make a connection between a particular food and the resultant headache. We often have patients keep a food diary to record what is eaten and physical reactions. That makes it easier to correlate foods with delayed reactions. If we suspect that a particular food is troublesome, the patient is asked to place a sample of that food under the tongue. If there is a sensitivity, a muscle that tested strong previously will weaken. Pulse is also evaluated for such changes as increases in intensity or frequency. Treatment can be as simple as removing the offending food from the diet."

MIGRAINES CAUSED BY ENVIRONMENTAL ALLERGIES. "If the migraines appear to be caused by environmental allergies, the British Migraine Association recommends keeping houseplants. Different plants have the ability to absorb different toxins. For example, spider plants absorb the formaldehyde released from particle board, plywood, synthetic carpeting and new upholstery, while chrysanthemums protects against the toxic effects of lacquers, varnishes and glues. If you don't feel like keeping a lot of chrysanthemums around the house, the same effect comes from drinking an herbal tea made with this flower."

MIGRAINES CAUSED BY HORMONAL IMBALANCE. "To keep hormones in balance, supplementing the diet with vitamin B_6 and evening primrose oil around the time of the menstrual period may help restore hormonal balance enough to forestall migraine attacks."

MIGRAINES CAUSED BY CRANIAL FAULTS. "Since migraines involve the cranial nerves, patients suffering from migraines should always be examined for cranial faults. These faults are extremely difficult to evaluate, due to the subtle movement of bones, but correcting them can be key to healing.

"One of my patients only partially responded to treatment after we corrected other findings that contributed to her headaches. Although the frequency decreased, she still reported migraines. At first, she had a general examination for cranial faults with no positive findings. Finally, after examining every single sutral point (or area of articulation) along the frontal bone in the forehead, we found the problem and corrected it. Her headaches stopped. In this case, the patient had an internally rotated frontal bone. Applied kinesiologists find this to be the most common cause of migraines from a cranial fault. This is particularly true if the patient reports eye pain with the migraine.

"The correction for this is done in three steps. First, pressure is applied to the posterior aspect of the palate on the side of internal rotation. Then a light pressure is applied on the lateral pterygoid muscle, located behind the upper molar in the mouth. Next pressure is applied to the medial pterygoid on the opposite side. That completes the treatment."

MIGRAINES CAUSED BY MERIDIAN IMBALANCE. "The task of the practitioner is to balance the energy by stimulating the meridians. There are various ways of accomplishing this. Acupuncturists use needles, while applied kinesiologists prefer to stimulate the meridians with a finger.

"There are three acupressure or acupuncture points helpful in treating migraines. Lung 7 is located about two finger-widths from the crease in the wrist, on the thumb side of the anterior part of the arm. Bladder 67 is found at the nail point of the little toe, and gall bladder 20 is located between the mastoid and the occipital protuberance in the skull. These are stimulated in a circular or tapping motion until there is an effective change."

MIGRAINES CAUSED BY UPPER CERVICAL SUBLUXATION. "The chiropractor can remove the subluxation with an adjustment to the proper area."

Migraines caused by low magnesium. "I have found a combination of magnesium and malic acid helpful. A health care practitioner should be consulted because the dosage varies with each patient."

MIGRAINES CAUSED BY MEDICATION. "These individuals must gradually wean themselves away from drugs, with the help of their doctor. When they are no longer dependent on these medications, treatment can begin."

MIGRAINES CAUSED BY STRESS. "Studies in England suggest that the herbal remedy feverfew can reduce the frequency of migraines. Feverfew has sedative qualities and can be taken as a tea. One cup per day is usually effective. In addition, relaxation techniques, such as meditation, progressive muscle relaxation, and yoga can help to reduce stress. Regular moderate exercise, such as swimming or walking, also lowers tension and creates a psychological sense of well-being."

Dr. Jennifer Brett, a naturopathic physician from Stratford, Connecticut, also comments on the benefits of feverfew: "An important study reported by the *British Medical Journal* back in 1983 found that one to two capsules of a freeze-dried extract of feverfew would prevent most migraines from occurring."

Specific Alternative Therapies

SUPPLEMENTS In addition to feverfew, Dr. Brett makes the following recommendations: "When feverfew is taken with magnesium, in doses of 250 to 500 mg daily, and Ginkgo biloba, most people notice a significant reduction in the number of migraines, even to the point of disappearance. This includes people who suffered daily. Many people come to me who have had no success with more conventional treatments. After starting them on feverfew and magnesium, they get a significant reduction in the number of headaches and the severity of pain. Even when they have headaches, they tend to be less frequent and less painful. In my experience, this combination will work for more than 70 percent of migraine sufferers.

"Some people find that they need to add the nutrient niacin. Niacin causes flushing in many people, and it is exactly this flushing that stops the migraine headache. By taking the blood out of the head and into the skin in the form of a flush, the migraine can be aborted before it even starts."

HERBS Plants containing phytochemicals with antimigraine properties, in order of potency:

Myciaria dubia (camu-camu)
Malpighia glabra (acerola)
Momordica charantia (bitter melon)
Portulaca oleracea (purslane)
Phyllanthus emblica (emblic)
Rosa canina (rose)

Capsicum annuum (bell pepper)
Capsicum frutescens (cayenne)
Carya glabra (pignut hickory)
Nasturtium officinale (berro)
Spinacia oleracea (spinach)
Phaseolus vulgaris (black bean)
Carya ovata (shagbark hickory)
Oenothera biennis (evening primrose)
Helianthus annuus (sunflower)
Allium schoenoprasum (chives)
Chondrus crispus (Irish moss)
Basella alba (vinespinach)
Brassica chinensis (Chinese cabbage)

REFLEXOLOGY Applying pressure to the feet can alleviate migraines because specific reflex points correspond to the head area. Reflexologist Gerri Brill says the most benefit comes from a routine that encompasses all body systems. Here she gives a detailed description of her program:

CREATING A COMFORTABLE ENVIRONMENT. "I start off by getting you to feel relaxed. Sometimes I use a foot basin to soften and warm up the feet. Then I have you lie down on my massage table while I explain the anatomy of the foot and the idea that each part corresponds to an area of the body. The big toe relates to the head and the little toes relate to the head and sinus. Under the toes is a ridge that corresponds to the neck and shoulders. The chest/lung area corresponds to the ball of the foot. The narrow part is the waist area, and at the heel you have the small and large intestines, the sciatic nerves, and the lower back."

RELAXING BREATHING. "There is a special place on the foot that corresponds to the solar plexus. This is a little notch just below the ball of the foot. The solar plexus is the seat of the emotions. By placing my thumb in this little notch, as you inhale, and releasing as you exhale, I help you to let go of a lot of stuck feelings held inside. It helps promote relaxation and is good to do at the end of the session as well."

WRINGING THE FOOT. "As you lie down, I wring out your foot three times or so, as if I were wringing out a washcloth. That helps the foot relax."

LUNG PRESS. "This is where I press the fist of my right hand into your chest/lung reflex, while holding your foot with my left hand. This area is on the pad of your foot, directly beneath the ridge of the toes. As I press, I slowly bring the flat of my fist down to the heel. I repeat this action three times. It is another relaxation technique."

FOOT-AND-TOE BOOGIE. "Next I do what is called the foot boogie. That means rocking your foot back and forth to loosen it up. Then I do the same with your toes. I place my hands around each toe as I shake your toes back and forth. It sounds silly but it feels great."

ZONE WALKING. "Zone walking is performed with the outer aspect of the thumb. If you place your thumb on your lap, it is the area that rests on your lap. It's important to keep fingernails short so as not to dig into anyone. Using the outer aspect of my thumb, I start way down at the heel. I mentally divide the foot into five zones, with each zone leading to a different toe. Starting at the outside portion of the foot, the fleshier part, I bend the working thumb at a 45 degree angle, and apply pressure as I creep up the foot ever so slightly. Each move is no more than a sixteenth of an inch. There are a lot of nerve endings in the feet, and I want to hit all of them. Applying a steady pressure, I work my thumb upward, all the way to the tip of the toe. When I reach the top of the toes, I go back down to the heel again to repeat the process. These steps are repeated for all five zones. By covering the whole body in this way, I help to create an equilibrium."

SPINE REFLEX. "Now I am at the inside aspect of the foot. That's the spine reflex, and it is very important because the spine supports you and holds you erect. I start at the bottom by your heel with my thumb. Again, I work with the outside corner of my thumb held at a 45 degree angle, and walk up your spine. I go all the way up to the big toe. Then, I turn around and thumb-walk down, using little steps and steady pressure. I don't want to hurt you, but I do want to exert a good amount of pressure since this is pressure therapy."

SHOULDER AND NECK REFLEX. "Now I move to the ridge underneath the toes. This corresponds to the neck and shoulder line, and it is important for headache relief because when people have tension and headaches, their neck and shoulders are usually tense. Again, I use the thumb-walk. I start at the outside of the big toe and thumb-walk to the ridge. I bend the toes back slightly to get inside. This is repeated until I get to the little toe. Then I turn around and thumb-walk back."

HEAD AREA. "The big toe relates to the head, so of course I want to work this area. I place the fingers of my right hand over my left hand, and thumb-walk down the fleshy part of your big toe. I divide the big toe into five zones and work down each area using very, very tiny bites or steps. My aim is for twenty-five bites on that big toe. That covers the whole area. I do that five times. This is very important."

BRAIN REFLEX. "Rolling my index finger over the top of the big toe stimulates the brain and relieves aches caused by migraines. Often this area feels sensitive because of crystal deposits that accumulate. These deposits need to be broken up."

HEAD AND SINUSES. "After finishing the big toe, I move to your little toes. Again, using my thumb, I divide each toe into three zones and thumb-walk, using little bites. This is repeated three times on each toe. This is another place that I feel tiny grains of sand. Breaking these up is the main way to relieve migraines."

CLOSING THE SESSION. "Just to make the session complete, I go back to the top of the foot while supporting the heel with the fist. I finger-walk with the right hand between the little bones on the top of the feet. This area helps the lymphatics, chest, breast, and also part of the back. Massaging here helps you to achieve a state of balance. Then I work around the ankle areas. The ankles relate to the reproductive organs and alleviate headaches caused by PMS. That's just one foot. Now I wrap up the foot that was worked on and start over on the other side. Afterward, I massage both feet at the same time, which is very soothing.

At this point, you know that the session is coming to an end. Once again, I massage your solar plexus area and have you take a deep breath. Finally, I do a nerve stroke to soothe the feet. This is where I ask you to imagine taking in peace and balance with each breath. This promotes a profound sense of relaxation. At this point your session is over, but you should rest a few moments instead of getting up quickly. Just relax and acknowledge how great you feel. Be sure to drink some water after your session to flush out the deposits."

Migraines in Children

Children suffering from migraine tend to be sensitive, nervous, and temperamental, with various behavior disturbances as common predisposing factors. Preceding the actual attack, the child may be noticeably lethargic and may refuse to eat, possibly complaining of abdominal discomfort as well. Often, the child's temperature is elevated and may gradually rise to as high as 104 degrees F. during an attack. This fever may draw attention away from the diagnosis of migraine in favor of a diagnosis acute infection, especially when other symptoms are present, such as abdominal pain, nausea, and vomiting. Acute appendicitis may be erroneously suspected. The array of symptoms typical of migraines in children are often misdiagnosed, particularly as these differ substantially from adult symptoms.

Migraine headaches, unfortunately, are not uncommon in childhood or even infancy. And while migraine sufferers most can most often trace the onset of the headaches to the period of early adulthood, early symptoms occur during childhood in nearly one-third of cases.

Children five years of age and under often suffer from what are called "allergic syndromes," sometimes involving bronchial asthma with migraine symptoms as a secondary condition.

In the vast majority of childhood cases of migraine, hereditary factors seem to be present—with a close relative also having migraines.

Among the factor that may precipitate a migraine attack during childhood are food allergies, sleeplessness, irregular meals, fatigue, extended exposure to bright sunlight, and visual stimulation (e.g., movies or television).

Patient Story

Dr. Olsen on one patient's treatment:

A patient of mine complained of headaches once a month, two days prior to her period. They occurred on the left side of her head and were debilitating, resulting in extreme fatigue and irritability. During this time, she felt that she was of no use to herself or her family, and she would go into a depression.

We made several recommendations. The first was a regular program of exercise, which for her meant walking daily. Exercise helps raise the level of endorphins in the body. Endorphins are the body's natural pain reliever and tend to elevate mood.

Our diet recommendations included the restriction of salt, caffeine, alcohol, and sugar. We added 200 mg of magnesium glyconate and a gram of fish oils each day. Many patients respond well to this.

It is also important to allot extra sleep at this time, particularly for women who have hormonally related migraines.

Her treatment was completed with a balancing of the cranial bones, which allowed the pituitary, the master gland that influences the menstrual cycle, to function properly.

On the Research Front

A hot treatment—literally—for cluster headaches is capsaicin, the substance that makes chili peppers hot, which has shown great promise in trials. Other natural treatments that have been the focus of research include a combination of vitamin D and calcium; magnesium supplementation; riboflavin; pyridoxine, used to combat medication-induced migraines; lithium, which raises choline levels (low in cluster-headache sufferers); omega-3 fatty acids; and feverfew.

Research has borne out many patients' claims that red wine, coffee, cow's milk, and chocolate are indeed migraine triggers. The effectiveness of an elimination diet, commonly avoiding preserved foods, dairy foods, and citrus, among others, has been shown in several studies.

Biofeedback is another effective treatment for migraines, along with chiropractics, relaxation techniques, and exercise. Most startling in its simplicity is the use of an elastic band around the head to ease migraine symptoms, which showed remarkable effectiveness in one recent study.

48

Thyroid Disorders

The thyroid gland is an important component of the immune system. As Dr. Stephen Langer, who practices preventive medicine in Berkeley, California, explains, "The thyroid gland is a little butterfly-shaped organ at the base of the neck that puts out a teaspoon of hormone a year which affects the metabolism and acts as a cellular carburetor for every cell in the body—from our hair follicles down to our toenails. As such, the thyroid can be implicated in just about any kind of condition you can think of.

"If a person's metabolism is hypo-functioning, everything is going to be slow. In a book I wrote called *Solve the Riddle of Illness*, I explain why upwards of 40 percent of the population may have subclinical hypothyroidism and not detect it by the traditional blood chemistry work that's done at their general practitioner's office. The symptoms of low thyroid include weakness, dry coarse skin, slow speech, coarse hair, hair loss, weight gain, difficulty breathing, problems with menstruation, nervousness, heart palpitations, brittle nails, and severe chronic fatigue and depression.

"Now if you get somebody with a constellation of symptoms like that they're going to be sick and tired of feeling sick and tired. Plus they're going to feel depressed all the time because they're going from one doctor to another, sometimes with two or three or four pages worth of complaints, and the doctors tell them it's all in their head, or that they should go home and learn to live with it."

Dr. Hyla Cass, a holistic psychiatrist, emphasizes the importance of thyroid inflammation, or thyroiditis, as a root cause of a variety of emotional and physical problems. She also describes difficulties today in establishing the diagnosis of thyroid disorder in the face of continuing skepticism from conventional physicians. According to Dr. Cass, "When the thyroid isn't working properly, the immune system is impaired, and this sets up a vicious cycle. You have a person whose immune system is depleted and who is anxious; they're told by regular doctors that the problem is all in their head, that there's nothing physically wrong with them. So then they feel worse."

Hypothyroidism

Hypothyroidism is a condition marked by deficient activity of the thyroid gland. "To treat someone with hypothyroidism," Dr. Langer says, "I put them on as little as a quarter of a grain of thyroid, which is a newborn-infant dose, and this produces a radical change in the way the person functions. Of course, for someone who has low thyroid function, I also use orthomolecular nutrition and a lot of clinical ecology techniques along with treating the thyroid gland.

"Recently I treated a patient who was the wife of a doctor and the mother of two young children. She basically came in and told me that she didn't want to go on living. She was so tired all the time, and so depressed, that she couldn't keep her head off the pillow after two o'clock in the afternoon. If she didn't go to bed, she would just fall apart. I did a history and physical on her and we made some dietary changes, but basically this woman was profoundly hypothyroid. We put her on a quarter of a grain of thyroid, which is what I start my patients with before building them up very gradually. A quarter of a grain is the smallest dose available. It's such a small quantity that most pharmacies don't even carry it, because when doctors order thyroid they don't even think to order so small a dose. But a quarter of a grain of thyroid was enough. Within a three-week period, this woman not only regained her mental health, but she was out taking tennis lessons, which was shocking even to me because although the treatment usually works it usually takes a longer period of time. So, just that amount of metabolic support was enough to turn this person's life around.

"Another person I treated was a 62-year-old woman who was a member of the Catholic clergy. She had been a nun for at least 30 years when I met her and I will never forget this woman. She came in bloated, profoundly depressed, and fatigued. The only thing that kept her going was basically overworking her adrenal glands. She came in and told me that when she was 12 years old, she went under a dark cloud. When I saw her it was 50 years later, and by that time she had been through 30 or 40 different doctors, including internists, endocrinologists, psychiatrists, and psychologists of various sorts. One of the first things that showed up in her—which I thought was a very positive sign—was that she was freezing all the time. When we did a basal body temperature on her, it never went above 95 degrees. Basal body temperature is a person's resting temperature when she wakes up in the morning. However, when I did a blood workup on her, all her thyroid hormone levels were within normal limits. I empirically placed her on a dose of thyroid that we gradually built up to about four grains a day, which is quite a high dosage. She's one of the few people I've treated who has needed that high an amount. Within three months, her depression of 50 years' duration was totally gone.

"Now, obviously she was bitter and angry that she had been suffering for all that time. But the organic feeling that she had of overwhelming fatigue totally disappeared within a three-month period of time, and I've seen that response in thousands of patients over the years. A small dose of thyroid, combined with things like nutritional support and eliminating food allergies, can really turn a person's life around."

Thyroiditis

Over the past 15 years or so, it has become apparent that some people with thyroid conditions have normal thyroid hormone levels and are suffering from another condition known as Hashimoto's disease, or autoimmune thyroiditis.

What triggers an autoimmune response? Dr. Langer explains: "Imagine autoimmune thyroiditis to be like rheumatoid arthritis of the thyroid gland. A person can have rheumatoid arthritis, which is an autoimmune condition where the body puts out antibodies to the joints. Frequently people with rheumatoid arthritis stay in long periods of remission. When they are under a great deal of stress, the body puts out antibodies to the joints and all their joints swell up. Similarly with the thyroid, if a person gets stressed out for any reason whatsoever, the body can start pumping out antibodies to the thyroid gland. The thyroid becomes acutely inflamed and the hormone which should not be in the system starts escaping. The clinical term for the gland is an 'escaping gland.' The hormone escapes from the gland and it's almost like pumping speed into your system."

Dr. Langer notes that "There is a very precise blood test that any doctor can order called the autoimmune thyroid antibody test, and most of the people who I suspect have thyroid conditions and have normal thyroid hormone levels will have an elevation in their antithyroid antibodies. If they have an elevated antithyroid antibody level, they have the symptoms that go along with low thyroid, which can be any one of 125 symptoms that we enumerate in *Solve the Riddle of Illness*."

Like hypothyroidism, thyroiditis can cause a number of psychological symptoms. Dr. Langer explains: "With thyroiditis people get anxiety attacks and panic attacks for no apparent reason. They could be sitting and reading a book. All of a sudden they will develop a cascade of heart palpitations and fearfulness. I've had a number of patients who have been rushed, almost on a monthly basis, to the emergency room to be worked up by cardiologists because their heart was pounding over 200 beats a minute. Cardiologists would do EKGs and echocardiograms and tell them to go see a psychiatrist who would work them up, not find anything, and then put them on an antidepressant or a

tranquilizer, and actually make the condition worse. When you have an undis-
covered organic basis for a psychological problem, being put on psychotropic
medication is like sitting on a thumbtack and being put on pain pills for the rest
of your life. It has about the same effect. It wears the system down, and as a
result the patient's condition not only does not improve but will in fact deteriorate, because the underlying cause is not being treated.

"To treat patients with thyroiditis, I put them on a trial dose of thyroid and
continue to monitor their thyroid hormone levels. Most of these people wind
up taking between one and two grains of thyroid a day and their thyroid hormone levels still stay normal despite the fact that their levels were supposedly
normal to begin with. More importantly, they get a complete remission of
symptoms, many of which manifest themselves as psychological symptoms."

A large number of Dr. Cass's patients also have thyroiditis. "I really can't
emphasize the importance of this problem enough," she says, "because thyroiditis often accompanies the mixed infection syndrome, which can consist of
any combination of the following: parasites, candida, and the viral syndromes—
including the Epstein-Barr virus and the cytomegalovirus. Psychological components include depression, anxiety, and even panic attacks.

"To treat thyroiditis, I've done nutritional consults on people that were
under the care of other physicians. When I suggested that they had thyroiditis
and that it was to be treated with low doses of thyroid hormones, I was met with
skepticism from the other doctors.

"When people have these long-standing chronic conditions, they can
become extremely depressed. They feel like they can't go on anymore, particularly when their body has been so wracked by the continuing illness. Also, some
of the mixed infection of thyroiditis and the parasites or other viruses can actually affect the brain directly. Thyroiditis and its accompanying infections affect
the central nervous system along with every other organ of the body. So people
come in extremely depressed, both as a reaction to their prolonged illness and
as a primary symptom of the illness—and this is usually totally overlooked.
That's why it's crucial to do a good medical workup on a patient whose disorder may at first appear purely psychological in origin."

"There is one more connection to be drawn between depression and the
thyroid dysfunction," Dr. Langer adds: "poor libido. One of the classic symptoms of depression is a loss of interest in sex. Those people who in the past were
sexually active, but who all of a sudden or gradually started to lose interest in
sex, will be diagnosed as being depressed right away. Men come into my office
by the score—many of them young—who have potency problems, and they
can't figure it out because they have no apparent organic illness. As a result,
they get performance anxiety, and if that continues long enough, they wind up
getting severely depressed. But I have found that if you go to the root cause of
their depression, very often it's the thyroid that's malfunctioning.

"If a person develops an acute depression that leads to a sexual dysfunction—which it frequently does—a doctor would be remiss if he or she didn't look for an imbalance in the thyroid. Patients have got to start taking their health destinies into their own hands and demanding that doctors do thyroid testing and look for auto-immune thyroid disorders and nutritional imbalances, which are frequently the underlying causes of sexual dysfunction and depression."

Who is Affected?

"The constellation of problems associated with thyroid disorders occurs not only in middle-aged people but also in young people, and not only in women, but also in men," Dr. Langer says. "While thyroid disease, particularly autoimmune thyroiditis, is classically considered to be primarily a disease of women, this is just not true. I have seen as many men as women who are suffering from autoimmune thyroiditis and, I might add, from hypothyroidism. Men are really given short shrift and aren't even given the requisite diagnostic tests in many instances to rule out thyroid disease because the medical profession thinks that this is strictly a woman's disorder.

"Moreover, I have seen teenagers and children who are acting out, who are written off as hyperactive, when they may be suffering from a thyroid disorder. Very young children or teenagers express their emotions differently from adults. Sometimes they get written off as being mentally retarded or having minimal brain dysfunction. Then they're given any one of a number of different drugs and placed in special classes. Many times, these young people have thyroid disorders that can be easily treated. But because thyroid dysfunction often leads to frequent infections, these kids are placed on antibiotics. Then they wind up with an overgrowth of yeast in their gut that in turn causes a low-grade inflammation in their gastrointestinal system. As a result, they don't adequately digest their food, so the body starts regarding the food as a foreign invader and puts out antibodies to the food. The child starts exhibiting the classic symptoms of food allergies, which are psychiatric complaints: anxiety attacks, depression, forgetfulness, inability to concentrate, even full-blown panic attacks.

"In a lot of these cases, you can actually isolate and eliminate the foods that cause an anxiety attack, but merely removing the food is not enough to get to the underlying cause of the disorder. Frequently patients have food allergies because of a pre-existing condition in their digestive systems which has to be addressed. The presence of such a pre-existing condition can cause immune system alterations which result in autoimmune dysfunction. So this is a vicious circle. One of the chief target organs of autoimmune dysfunction is the thyroid gland. You get autoimmune thyroiditis."

Alternative Therapies

"The question for holistic clinicians to ask themselves, regarding each individual patient, is where they're going to intervene," Dr. Langer says. "Different physicians will intervene at different places, depending upon their background and interests. I try, to the best of my ability, to get to the root cause of what's going on. If I am having difficulty figuring out the cause, then I try to intervene at a point in a person's imbalance that will cause the least disruption to their lifestyle and give them the best results for the least amount of money in the quickest period of time. Frequently, that turns out to be treating with small doses of thyroid and altering eating habits. In my clinical experience, I have found that with the thyroid and nutritional support, very often a person will get better. The thyroid is not a lifetime treatment and can be removed after the person's condition has been stabilized. Thyroid treatment is inexpensive, works rapidly, and when done properly it is absolutely nontoxic.

Dr. Allan Spreen, a general practitioner who specializes in nutrition-based medicine, reminds us that while thyroid supplementation is an important modality, it is not fail-safe. "I'd love to say that correcting thyroid function is a panacea. While it doesn't work 100 percent of the time, if a patient comes in complaining of fatigue and depression that is linked with the physical findings of foods not digesting well, and cold extremities, then an underactive thyroid may be the root cause. People come and say, 'Oh, my husband says, Don't touch me with your feet at night because they're just ice cold.' These are the same people who are comfortable in a room when everybody else is boiling and they're freezing in a room when everybody else is comfortable. Their thinking seems to have slowed down, they just don't seem to be able to concentrate like they used to, and they don't remember lists the way they used to.

"In this kind of a situation, once I find that their blood levels of thyroid are normal, I go back to the old school of Broda Barnes, who, 40 or 50 years ago, did axillary temperature testing. I ask my patients to keep a record of their early morning basal body temperature. If their basal metabolic rate based on early-morning body temperatures is really low, then I consider them to be candidates for thyroid supplementation. In axillary testing, Broda Barnes talked about temperature ranges between 97.8 and 98.2 degrees Fahrenheit, which is lower than the 98.6 people think of as normal. But the axillary temperature is taken in the armpit first thing in the morning, using a mercury thermometer that stays there for 10 minutes before they get up. If their temperature is, much of the time, down in the 96.8, 96.7, 96.5 range, I at least consider the possibility that the person needs low doses of natural thyroid, which is still available.

"Thyroid is a prescription drug, but it can be broken down into very low doses. Some doctors who use this type of testing use synthetic thyroid. I prefer to prescribe natural thyroid in very low doses. If a person responds—either their temperature rises or their symptoms lift—then I retest them to see if their blood levels of thyroid have changed. Many times a person with this profile of symptoms who takes thyroid will feel better, and their blood tests will have remained unchanged, including their thyroid stimulating hormone and their actual thyroid hormone levels. So the blood testing has missed the diagnosis, and yet the person feels well with the increased, but undetectable dose of thyroid hormone."

Patient Stories

I came to be treated by Dr. Spreen only after first following the conventional route in medical treatment. In 1988, I was in my fifth year of infertility treatments, had taken multiple infertility drugs, and wound up severely depressed, which caused me to lose 35 pounds in two months. I couldn't sleep, I had panic attacks, the whole horrible group of symptoms associated with depression. The doctors put me on the conventional Xanax treatment for three years before I met Dr. Spreen, who was helping me with some other related medical problems. I had hair loss, skin problems, nail-biting problems. I had aches all over my body, especially in my legs. Dr. Spreen got me on a vitamin regimen, which made me feel somewhat better.

Then… Dr. Spreen put me on very low doses of thyroid and immediately—within two to three weeks—all the problems I just mentioned were gone. Now I had had thyroid checks three times during the whole time when I was being treated for infertility, and the blood tests had always come up negative. But I knew that in my family there were thyroid problems. There are at least six members of my family that I can think of who have thyroid disorders, but mine just never showed up on my tests. After taking these very low doses of thyroid, my skin problem cleared up, I stopped biting my nails, and my legs stopped aching. The mild depression I was still suffering from all of a sudden in August vanished. I felt great. I slept like a normal person again. I had energy. People started commenting on how I seemed to be like my old self again. It was like getting a new lease on life!

I feel rather fed up with the original doctors I went to see. They treated me like I was an hysterical woman who needed to get a grip on things. I have never told them about my recovery using alternative methods because I don't think they'd be receptive to it.—Jenny

I had hives, some kind of an allergic response, about five years ago and it progressed to the point where I had hives on my vocal cords. It was a pretty serious allergic reaction, for which I was first treated with antihistamines. Later, I was treated with prednisone. When small doses of prednisone given every other day didn't help, my doctor began increasing the dosage until I was taking 70 mg every day. After about six weeks I started declining physically from taking this tremendous dose. I gained about 50 pounds. I had conjunctivitis in both of my eyes. I had open sores. I was so weak I was almost bedridden. I did find another doctor who slowly weaned me off of the prednisone. But when it was all over, my immune system had been damaged. I had a lot of viral illnesses that are usually associated with chronic fatigue syndrome. I could scarcely get out of bed, and I couldn't lose all the weight I had gained. So I went from doctor to doctor. I was living in the Midwest at the time and many of these doctors said, 'Your metabolic system has been altered by prednisone. Too bad, but you will never lose that weight. And prednisone can damage the immune system. Too bad, but your immune system has been damaged.' No one could offer me any help at all.

I first went to Dr. Atkins in New York and he was a lot of help to me. It was through Dr. Atkins and his association with Dr. Huggins that I learned about dental amalgams, because when your immune system is depleted you are much more susceptible to any kind of toxins, including mercury leaching from mercury amalgam fillings. It was causing me a great deal of trouble and I did have those removed.

Then I moved to California and I had heard, previous to my moving, about Dr. Slagle and her work with depression. In fact, I referred friends to her, friends I had made in California, and they had these miraculous cures from depression after two weeks of taking B-complex and amino acids. But I didn't think of going to her myself for quite awhile because I thought of her as someone who only treated depression. In fact, like many alternative physicians, she treats the whole person. She had worked with fatigue a lot, and she first tested me thoroughly and found that my thyroid and, in fact, my whole endocrine system, was not functioning properly—most likely as a result of prednisone. She picked up subtleties in the test that other doctors ignored. She has the philosophy that a body should be healthy and whole. She doesn't need gross parameters of unusual test results to say something is wrong here. So she was able to discover that I had a rather unusual problem in my thyroid and she was able to treat it.

When I began seeing her I still had very limited energy. Even though Dr. Atkins had helped me lose weight so I looked normal, I still didn't feel normal. In one day, I could either go to the grocery store or go to a doctor's appointment. That was all I could do. The remainder of the day I had to rest. I went to Dr. Slagle and after she began treating my thyroid I had a leap of improvement. I regained my energy. She also gave me amino acids, which heightened my mood. Even though I hadn't thought I was depressed—and I still don't think I was—generally the amino acids made me feel healthier. And while I don't have the energy of a lot of people around me, I can pretty much function normally, which is a miracle. It has been a five-year struggle and I'm finally living practically a normal life.

*Here's what I have learned from my experience. You simply cannot go to a traditional physician and carelessly allow that doctor to treat your symptoms with drugs. Traditional physicians tend not to look at the whole person, but to give drugs to ameliorate the symptoms, or to treat individual problems without regard to what that treatment does to the rest of the body. I learned to use tremendous caution when entrusting my body to someone. If you're going to trust your body to someone, you should know a lot about the physician. You should know whether the physician treats the whole person and sees you as more than an allergy or a gallbladder.—*Helen

Dr. Hyla Cass describes her experience with one patient:

I recently saw a young woman who came in depressed, tired, unable to get up on the morning, and feeling overwhelmed by her work responsibilities. Her history revealed that she was often cold, especially in her hands and feet (she even wore socks to bed), had thinning hair, dry skin, constipation, and was losing the outer part of her eyebrows. I suspected an imbalance in her thyroid. When I asked about thyroid disease, she said that it had been suspected before, but her tests had been normal. I checked her thyroid hormones, including thyroid antibody levels.

Often despite 'normal' blood tests, there is an underactive thyroid. Dr. Broda Barnes' technique of monitoring thyroid function through body temperature is used by many alternative practitioners. Although this patient's thyroid hormone blood levels were normal, she did, in fact, have antithyroid antibodies, confirming a diagnosis of Hashimoto's thyroiditis. This is an autoimmune disease, treatable with thyroid hormone, antioxidants, and adrenal support. Her signs were those of hypothyroidism, indicating that the circulating hormone was being rendered ineffective. With Hashimoto's thyroiditis, there are often also intermittent signs of hyperthyroidism, or overactive thyroid, such as irritability or heart palpitations.

I prescribed thyroid hormone from natural (animal) sources, and asked her to monitor her body temperature, so I could adjust the dosage. She asked whether this supplementation would suppress her own thyroid function, and whether she would be taking it for the rest of her life. The answer was 'no' on both counts. The treatment actually supported her own gland, allowing it to heal. Within 10 days of starting the program she was feeling alive again.

PART TEN

Women's Health Throughout the Life Span

Although this is beginning to change, there has in the past been little research on women's health issues. And in many cases the research done on health issues affecting men and women equally has emphasized the men's side and understated differences pertaining to women.

The natural healing tradition, however, has always emphasized women's problems, since at many points in modern history, the natural healer was the only person women could go to have their problems taken seriously and taken care of. And natural healing techniques were often nearly exclusively a woman's domain. Just as doctors have traditionally been men, and midwifes and nurses traditionally women, women are still mostly excluded from the highest levels of the medical establishment—where the decisions are made as to which types of treatments to favor (typically those that rely on expensive drugs or even more expensive machines and procedures) and which to ignore (typically those involving substances that are not patent-protected, like vitamin C, or techniques that could be practiced by unlicensed, and hence uncontrollable, practitioners, including massage and herbal treatments).

We are at a moment in history when alternative approaches have, in theory, finally been accorded a newfound legitimacy in the eyes of the medical establishment. It is only right that now more and more people, and especially women, will turn to the long, strong, and wonderful natural healing tradition. International in scope, it spans many cultures and synthesizes ancient folkloric remedies together with cutting-edge technologies.

If doctors practicing Western medicine in the conventional way are going to ignore women's issues, let's see if the alternative medicine community can take up the slack. Let's see if we can help women keep themselves healthy by emphasizing good nutrition and all the individual alternative therapies that address the specific health concerns of women.

49

Menstruation and Pre-Menstrual Syndrome (PMS)

Painful and difficult periods are so commonplace in our society that some women have come to think of them as normal, but they are not normal at all. Many experts feel that the symptoms of dysmenorrhea are related to our dietary practices, as well as to unresolved emotional difficulties.

Menstrual Cramps

"What causes menstrual cramps?" asks Dr. Pat Gorman, an acupuncturist and educator from New York City. "In addition to toxins found in foods with preservatives, additives, and caffeine, they are due to putrid proteins found in dairy and red meat. These foods contain a lot of hormones that upset the system. In addition, foods fried in heavy oils cause problems and should be cut out immediately by any woman interested in getting rid of dysmenorrhea."

Dr. Gorman adds that the Chinese attribute this condition in part to pent-up anger and frustration. "If you are not happy with your life, if you are angry with people, you must work this out. The liver, which stores blood and prepares it for the period, is also responsible for anger. That's not a Western concept, but with my patients I find that working out anger helps the liver to relax. As a result, there is far less of a problem with dysmenorrhea."

Dr. Marjorie Ordene, a gynecologist in Brooklyn, New York, agrees that hormonal and psychological factors cause painful periods and explains the underlying factors: "What causes dysmenorrhea is exaggerated uterine contractions. These contractions are mediated by receptors in the uterine lining that are stimulated by hormonal and psychological factors. Hormonal factors that stimulate the uterine receptors have actually been isolated. They are chemical messengers called prostaglandins. Two things are clear. People with menstrual cramps have an excess of prostaglandins, and there is an imbalance in the type of prostaglandin they produce."

She adds that eating foods one is allergic to can increase prostaglandin production: "For example, many women are sensitive to yeast, and eating baked foods, breads, pastries, and processed fruit juices, can cause an increase in prostaglandin production."

SYMPTOMS There are different types of menstrual pain. Usually it is experienced as a spasmodic cramp, but there can also be an achiness, a feeling of heaviness in the lower abdomen, or discomfort in the lower back or thighs. Other symptoms may include nausea, vomiting, loss of appetite, diarrhea, headache, dizziness, tiredness, anxiety, and depression.

Dysmenorrhea usually begins at the onset of menstruation, lasting a few hours, but it can begin pre-menstrually and remain several days. According to traditional Asian medicine, if the tongue has a thick white coating, the problem is the result of too many of the wrong type of proteins, while a thick yellow covering signals toxicity from protein.

CONVENTIONAL TREATMENT Medical doctors often prescribe medications, such as ibuprofen, to inhibit prostaglandins. While these work to relieve menstrual cramps and accompanying symptoms, problems occur when drugs are taken month after month. Side effects can include gastrointestinal bleeding, decreased blood flow to the kidneys, and leaky gut syndrome, a condition that allows undigested food particles to enter the blood.

ALTERNATIVE TREATMENT

DIET

Changes in diet can decrease overproduction of prostaglandins and restore normal balance. Cool, green foods help reduce hot stabbing pains and inflammation. It is good to eat foods such as organic grains, legumes, oatmeal, and steamed green vegetables. Deep sea fish such as salmon, tuna, or mackerel can be included, as well as flaxseed oil. Hot spices should be avoided, as well as fried, greasy foods, sugar, salt, alcohol, and stimulating foods such as garlic and onions. Foods that produce allergies should be eliminated as well.

Women who have nerve-related menstrual pain can benefit from tofu, but should stay away from too many cold raw salads, hot spicy foods, and even white potatoes. Herbalist Letha Hadady suggests this soothing recipe: warm tofu cooked with sweet spices, like pumpkin pie spices or nutmeg. This quiets the nerves and helps a woman feel nurtured and relaxed.

Dr. Anthony Penepent, a physician who practices natural hygiene, helps patients with painful menses by placing them on a strict hygienic regimen. "I put them on a fast one day before the onset of their period. In serious conditions, I might have them fast one day and then prescribe juices or juice blended with salad and fruit for the following days until they complete their menses."

SUPPLEMENTS

Evening primrose oil and magnesium citrate are two supplements that may be taken. Taken throughout the month as a daily supplement, evening primrose oil prevents headaches and blemishes that occur just before the period. Magnesium deficiencies are common and result in the release of prostaglandins that cause spasm and pain. Magnesium is antispasmodic and helps relieve the problem. Take 300–500 mg daily and work up to bowel tolerance.

HERBS

The following herbs help to alleviate menstrual problems:

Gardenia and philodendron. These are popular in Chinese medicine, and can be obtained by prescription from an herbalist.

Corn silk tea. This helps to get rid of the bloating that comes from too many hormones stored in the blood. Women's Rhythm also eliminates bloating. This formula can be found in certain health food stores or ordered from Kahn Herbs.

Xiao Yao Wan. This wonderful remedy, which can be purchased at pharmacies in Chinatowns in major cities, helps digestive processes. Not only does this formula relieve painful periods, it also alleviates anger.

Green tea. Green tea is cooling and satisfying, with very little caffeine. A pinch of tea can be added to a pot of boiled water, steeped for five minutes, and sipped throughout the day. People experience an energy pickup from digestion being activated, not from nerves being stimulated. Helps soothe sharp, stabbing pains.

Aloe vera juice or gel. Either can be used to eliminate headache, irritability, fever, stabbing pain, blemishes, and bad breath associated with menstrual cramps. Aloe also reduces acid from the stomach and liver, and is slightly laxative. Just add to juice, tea, or water.

Dandelion. This helps to break apart impurities in the system. Can be bought as capsules or tea.

Sarsaparilla. Sarsaparilla helps hot, stabbing pains brought on by inflammation. Sarsaparilla is anti-inflammatory, antiseptic, diuretic, and soothing.

Valerian. This is a sedative herb that makes a woman feel quieter, more relaxed and grounded. It is especially good for nervous women who experience insomnia, anxiety, crying jags and emotional upsets, and other nervous problems. Valerian quiets the nerves that go to the uterus.

Yunnan Pai Yao. This combination of herbs helps reduce heavy bleeding and stabbing pain. By increasing the circulation, internal bleeding is healed, and swelling and pain are reduced.

HOMEOPATHY

Homeopathy was developed in Germany over 200 years ago by Dr. Samuel Hahnemann, and means "like cures like." The same substances that cause a disease in a healthy individual can heal an ailment in a sick person, when diluted and given in minute proportions.

Homeopathic physician Dr. Ken Korins explains that the dilution process is what makes homeopathic remedies so safe: "Homeopathy is a vibrational medicine. We are dealing with very subtle energies. Substances are given in extremely small dilutions that cannot possibly have any toxic effects. In fact, if you were to analyze these substances, you would not find a trace of the original material in the final dilution."

The correct homeopathic remedy is the one that most closely matches the symptoms that manifest themselves. Dr. Korins recommends that dysmenorrhea sufferers choose among the following:

Colocynthis. This frequently indicated remedy is useful when you have a severe onset of sudden cramps, particularly on the first day of menstruation. Emotionally, there is an intense irritability and anger associated with the menstrual cramps. A key indication is that you feel better when your knees are pulled up toward the stomach, and held with firm pressure.

Magnesia phosphorica. This helps spasmodic cramps with bloating. The key indication for this remedy is that you feel better from warmth. Magnesia phosphorica and colocynthis will help alleviate the symptoms in 85 percent of the cases.

Pulsatilla. A key indication for pulsatilla is variation; the cramps and the flow of bleeding are changeable. The pains themselves are typically cutting and tearing, and may be felt in the lower back or kidney region. Generally, you feel worse in warm stuffy rooms and better in the open fresh air. Emotionally, you tend to be mild, gentle, and weepy when entering the menstrual state and prefer the company of other people to being alone.

Viburnum. This is indicated when the menses are very scant and often late. In fact, they may only last a few hours. When you get cramps, the flow of the blood stops. Cramps tend to radiate to the sacrum and the thighs. You may feel faint or like passing out.

Cimicifuga. This is indicated for spasmodic, cramping pains. The pains radiate across the pelvis from one thigh to the other. It is often associated with a premenstrual headache. Increased flow results in more pain. Emotionally, you may feel nervous to the point of being scattered, and often somewhat depressed.

Chamomilla. This is helpful if you are either hypersensitive and insensitive to any pain. Emotionally, you tend to be irritable and contrary. Someone brings you something that you ask for, then you don't want it. During intense periods, you may become dependent on coffee and other stimulants and sedatives. Another symptom is anger. When you become angry, your symptoms become worse.

AROMATHERAPY

Aromatherapy also may help. Marjoram, clary sage, and lavender are wonderful analgesics. Eighteen to 20 drops of oil added to a lotion or oil and massaged into the abdomen and lower back helps to relieve menstrual pain. Breathing in the cooling fragrances of rose, lavender, or sandalwood can alleviate sharp, stabbing pain.

Last but not least, there is stress management. Deep abdominal breathing, meditation, tai chi, and other mind/body disciplines eliminate frustrations and anger that bring on pain. Additionally, it is helpful to slow down the pace of life from the time of ovulation to the period.

Abnormal Blood Flow: Amenorrhea and Menorrhagia

Amenorrhea and menorrhagia are medical terms for abnormal blood flow. Amenorrhea refers to the cessation of bleeding, or very light and infrequent periods, most often caused by an abnormally functioning hypothalamus, pituitary gland, ovary, or uterus as a result of drugs or surgery that removes the ovaries or uterus. "Bulimics and anorexics also exhibit this pattern," notes Dr. Pat Gorman. "Sometimes this is caused by excessive dieting and overexercise driven by self-hatred. Not accepting who she is, a woman thinks, 'I've got to make myself thin, beautiful, and perfect.' If this is going on at the end of the cycle, when toxins are being released into the system, the woman is aggravating her body to the point of saying, We're not going to give up this blood. We desperately need it. Forget ovulation, forget periods."

With menorrhagia the opposite scenario occurs, and there is profuse bleeding. The condition can be debilitating, sometimes bad enough to warrant immediate attention at a hospital's emergency ward. "The Chinese say menorrhagia is caused by excess toxins and heat in the blood from foods containing preservatives, additives, and caffeine, especially coffee. It's like water in your car radiator becoming low," Dr. Gorman says. "The engine will overheat and explode. Alcohol adds more toxicity because it constantly removes water from the blood. As water diminishes, it heats up the blood. When the blood is what we call 'hot,' or fast-moving, it's very hard for the body to hold it in. It can't stop the bleeding."

The emotional profile of the menorrhagic individual is someone who sees herself as a victim. Dr. Gorman explains, "This person feels the need to serve everybody. She does not know how to set boundaries. Whatever anybody wants, they get. She keeps pouring out her energy and pouring out her blood."

Dr. Vicki Hufnagel, a gynecological surgeon and activist for women's health rights, adds that heavy bleeding is often a sign of an underlying problem in the female system, especially when it is accompanied by pain. The problem is frequently due to a hormonal imbalance. "Anything can throw off a cycle," says Dr. Hufnagel. "Emotional stress, insomnia, too much estrogen in the system, or too little light, as in the winter. Other physical problems that can cause menorrhagia are fibroids, polyps, and a malfunctioning thyroid gland."

Oriental medicine can diagnose amenorrhea and menorrhagia by examining the skin. Amenorrhea manifests as pale, sallow, slightly yellowish skin from a deep lack of blood and nutrients. Often this is accompanied by a great deal of emotional anxiety. With menorrhagia, the tongue has a red tip and tiny red dots. When the condition is long-term, a woman can become anemic.

Before you can restore the blood flow in patients with amenorrhea or menorrhagia, you must discover the reason for the problem. Once the cause is addressed, periods should return to normal.

HORMONAL BALANCING Dr. Hufnagel says that hormonal dysfunctions in women with menorrhagia can be corrected with oral doses of natural progesterone. "Often, the creams women are using are not adequate because they don't cause a rise in the blood level. We often have to give what we call oral physiological levels of progesterone. I give women natural hormones, in a cyclic manner, the way her body should be getting them."

Hormone balancing is also accomplished through diet. Fatty diets cause higher levels of estrogen in the system, which, in turn, can cause menorrhagia. Lean diets, and exercising with weights, produce more testosterone, which, in turn, helps to balance hormones and put an end to menorrhagia.

NATURAL HYGIENE APPROACH Dr. Anthony Penepent says that amenorrhea is one of the easiest conditions to correct. Mostly it stems from undernourishment and can be corrected with a diet that includes two green salads daily, using romaine lettuce, fresh lemon juice, olive oil, and some brewer's yeast. You should also include two pieces of fresh fruit and two soft boiled eggs in the daily menu. Where amenorrhea is caused by a thyroid condition, a thyroid supplement is needed. Additionally, if stress is in the picture, the stressful situation must be remedied. For more serious cases, additional dietary intervention is necessary. Usually, small changes in diet are all that are needed.

Dr. Penepent says, "Even if the woman doesn't follow a completely natural hygienic regimen and is not vegetarian, she still can get tremendous results simply by increasing the amount of green leafy vegetables in the diet and providing concentrated nutritional sources, such as eggs and unsalted raw milk cheese."

HERBS The following Chinese herbs have specific effects on the blood and are needed at different times of the monthly cycle. Dr. Pat Gorman recommends working with a health practitioner to create an individual protocol and to monitor progress, but offers these general guidelines:

At the beginning of the cycle:

Dong quai. High in vitamins A, E, and B$_{12}$, this blood-builder can be taken most days of the month, up to the point of menstruation, or just before it begins if there are strong pre-menstrual symptoms. "You don't want to be building blood if you are having trouble moving that blood," Dr. Gorman warns.

Women's Precious. This formula is a tremendous blood builder, taken after the period ends for about three weeks. Women's Rhythm is then used the following week.

At the end of the cycle:

Gardenia. This is taken when PMS symptoms arise. By moving blood that is stuck, gardenia helps to relieve that heavy, bloated feeling.

Women's Rhythm. This helps release a woman's blood. It is usually taken a week before the period to help move toxins out of the organs. (Women's Precious and Women's Rhythm are formulas that can be found in some health food stores and ordered directly from Kahn Herbs.) Can be taken every day:

Floradix with iron. This wonderful product is available in most health care stores. Liquid Floradix is superior over the dry form because it contains more live nutrients.

Toxic Shock Syndrome (TSS)

Toxic shock syndrome is a rare, but serious—and sometimes fatal—disease. The victims tend to be tampon users under the age of 30—and especially those between 15 and 19. This sudden and serious disease affects persons with severely compromised immune systems, who are poisoned by a strain of bacteria, called *Staphylococcus aureus*, phage group I. This type of staph produces a substance called enterotoxin F, which can overpower and destroy a weak body.

Toxic shock syndrome is linked to the introduction of tampons with four new ingredients, in the early 1980s. Before then, tampons were made primarily of cotton. In the 1980s, though, highly absorbent polyester cellulose, carboxymethyl cellulose, polyacrylate rayon, and viscose rayon came into use. Three of these new ingredients were soon taken off the market; today, only one of the new ingredients, viscose rayon, is in use. Today's tampons are either entirely viscose rayon or a blend of cotton and viscose rayon. In addition, the tampons on the market today may contain an assortment of chemicals, including pesticides used in growing cotton, chemicals used in the manufacture of viscose rayon (lye, sodium sulfate, and sodium hydroxide), and dyes (some of which have been considered carcinogenic since the 1950s).

One theory of the reason for TSS is that the vagina is normally an oxygen-free environment, which limits growth of dangerous bacteria. However, air is trapped between the fibers that make up tampons. When that air is inserted in the vagina along with the tampon, the possibility of toxin production increases. Even after the tampon is removed, some of its fibers may remain.

TSS was originally thought only to affect women who wore high-absorbency tampons. But now it is known to affect newborns, children, and men as well. Initial indications can include a high fever, headache, sore throat, diarrhea, nausea and red skin blotches. These signs can be followed by confusion, low blood pressure, acute kidney failure, abnormal liver function, and even death.

A severe case of TSS is a medical emergency that may necessitate hospitalization. However, there are many natural ways to support the system once a crisis is over for quick recovery and prevention of recurrence.

ALTERNATIVE REMEDIES FOR TOXIC SHOCK SYNDROME Dr. Linda Rector-Page, author of *Healthy Healing: An Alternative Healing Reference*, developed a protocol for healing from TSS out of necessity: "I actually came close to death on an operating table from TSS. I had to bring my body back, and I did it herbally. It took a couple of years, and now I can speak from experience."

HERBS

Dr. Rector-Page's personal ordeal gave her a great deal of confidence in the power of natural remedies. The following herbs helped her to overcome toxicity, restore immunity, and return to health:

Ginseng. Both Panax and American varieties are general tonics that balance and tone all body systems, as well as improve circulation. Ginseng should not be used when there is a high fever.

Cayenne and ginger. These nervous system stimulants can help the body recover from shock. They can either be taken internally or applied to the skin in compresses.

Hawthorn extract. Hawthorn speeds up and normalizes the circulation, and restores a sense of well-being.

DIET

In addition to herbs, Dr. Rector-Page ate super-nutritious foods that could be easily digested and quickly utilized by her failing system. These foods included high-potency royal jelly, bee pollen, wheat germ, brewer's yeast, and unsulfured molasses. The addition of green drinks, including chlorella, barley grass, spirulina, and wheat grass, supplied her with high potencies of vital minerals. "All these go into the body very quickly and help it to recover, even from a death situation," explains Dr. Rector-Page. "By going on a program of concentrated nutrients, I was eventually able to create a state of health that was better than before."

PREVENTION OF TOXIC SHOCK SYNDROME Alternatives to tampons have included sea sponges. However, sea sponges are no longer sold as menstrual products. A 1981 report alleged risks from embedded sand, chemical pollutants, bacteria, and fungi. No additional studies were done, but the Food and Drug Administration (FDA) halted menstrual sponge sales. Another alternative is called the Keeper, a rubber cup that sits in the lower vagina. The Keeper may hold an ounce of menstrual blood, and should be emptied several times a day.

This device does not promote the growth of bacteria in the vagina. However, the Keeper is not widely available. Tampons that are 100 percent cotton, and thus present less risk than modern superabsorbent tampons that may also contain added chemicals, are available in many health food and natural goods stores.

Pre-Menstrual Syndrome (PMS)

PMS is more widespread in Western societies than in primitive cultures, because of diet and lifestyle. Dr. Michael Janson, an orthomolecular physician from Cambridge, Massachusetts, and author of *The Vitamin Revolution*, says, "Sugar, caffeine, and alcohol precipitate or worsen symptoms and should be avoided. This is because a lot of patients with PMS have frank hypoglycemia. Their sugar levels fluctuate up and down. Eating sugar sends blood sugar levels way up, and the body responds by dropping sugar levels way down. Additionally, caffeine, even when taken in small amounts in the morning, can aggravate symptoms, such as breast tenderness, and sleep disturbances."

The effects of PMS can range from mild to severe and vary from person to person. They may include bloating, cramps, headaches, swelling, fluid retention, low back pain, depression, abdominal pressure, insomnia, sugar cravings, anxiety, irritability, breast tenderness, mood swings, and acne.

ALTERNATIVE THERAPIES FOR PRE-MENSTRUAL SYNDROME

DIET AND NUTRITION

According to Dr. Janson, the best diet to lessen the symptoms of PMS is high in fiber and complex carbohydrates, with small meals and snacks in between. This helps to regulate blood sugar, and in many cases is enough to reduce or eliminate PMS symptoms. Herbalist Letha Hadady recommends cool green foods such as salads and the avoidance of hot, spicy, and acidic foods as well as the elimination of coffee. Some people, however, need more help and can benefit from vitamin therapy, exercise, and a stress management program.

When symptoms are severe, diet alone may not be enough. These nutrients may prove useful:

Vitamin B_6 (pyridoxine). This has a number of helpful properties for alleviating PMS. As a smooth muscle relaxant, it can decrease cramps. As a diuretic, it reduces fluid retention, swelling, and breast tenderness. Between 200 and 400 mg should be taken daily. Vitamin B_6 can be taken throughout the month, rather than just pre-menstrually. One hundred mg in a B-complex vitamin can be taken the first two weeks of the period, and an additional 250 the last two weeks of the cycle. More B_6 increases the need for magnesium.

Magnesium. Magnesium calms the nervous system and relieves anxiety, depression, irritability, nervousness, and insomnia. As an antispasmodic, it alleviates cramps and back pain. Magnesium also helps reduce cravings for sweets. Between 500 and 1,000 mg may be needed.

Gammalinolenic acid (GLA). GLA is a precursor to prostaglandin-E1, a hormonelike substance that helps to regulate neurological and hormonal functions. Prostaglandin-E1 helps reduce muscle spasms, cramping, sugar cravings, mood swings, depression, anxiety, irritability, acne, and to some extent breast tenderness. It also reduces inflammation and decreases the stickiness of the platelets, which prevents blood clotting. GLA is found in evening primrose oil, borage oil, and black currant oil. Borage oil is the most concentrated source of GLA, containing 24 percent GLA, the equivalent of six capsules of evening primrose oil. One 1,000 mg capsule of borage oil provides a daily dose of 240 mg GLA.

Eicosapentaenoic acid (EPA). This oil found in fish and flaxseed oil produces prostaglandin-E3, which helps to alleviate breast tenderness. Flaxseed oil is fragile and should not be used in cooking. It can be used in salad dressings or over cooked foods.

Vitamin E. 400–800 IU can reduce cramps, breast tenderness, and fibrocystic breasts, which often swell up before the period.

Multiple vitamin/mineral supplement. A balanced multivitamin/mineral supplement can help to balance the system.

EXERCISE

Exercise helps to improve mood, reduce cramps, eliminate excess fluid, and control sugar cravings. Aerobic exercises should be performed three to four times per week.

HERBS

Herbalist Letha Hadady finds these Chinese herbs useful for alleviating symptoms of PMS:

Lungtanxieganwan. A Chinese remedy that alleviates anger associated with PMS.

Xiao Yao Wan. Helps relieve PMS symptoms of depression, poor circulation, indigestion, and bloating.

Women's Harmony. Increases circulation.

HOMEOPATHY

The homeopathic remedy chosen should correspond to the symptoms described; only one should be used for best results. Sometimes it's a matter of trial and error; if one does not work, try another. Dr. Ken Korins, a classically trained homeopathic physician in New York City, recommends these remedies for PMS.

Lachasis. This helps most physical and emotional symptoms that accompany PMS, such as headaches, right ovarian pain, breast tenderness. It may be indicated if PMS symptoms stop once menstrual flow stops. Also, symptoms get worse with heat and with constricted clothing around the abdomen. Emotional indications are restlessness, paranoia, and a tendency to be talkative.

Laccaninum. Think of this remedy when the only symptom is a painful, swollen breast. Pain leaves once the menstrual flow begins. There is a tendency to be irritable.

Bovista. Gastrointestinal symptoms occur before the period, such as diarrhea. There may also be traces of blood before the actual flow begins. Subjective and objective feelings of swelling occur throughout the body, even through the hands, causing a tendency to feel clumsy.

Pulsatilla. Emotional symptoms of PMS, such as a weepy, mild disposition. There is a need for consolation from others. Strong craving for sweets.

Natmur. Emotional state is melancholy and sad, and worsens with attempts to console by others. Headaches occur before, during, or after period. Craving for salty foods and an aversion toward sex at the time of the period.

Sepia. For sadness, depression, indifference, and feelings of discontent and discouragement about life. Often a colicky pain is felt before the menses. There may also be a sensation of the uterus dropping, as if it would fall through the vagina due to congestion in that area.

Folliculinum. This is a new French remedy that can be given on the seventh day of the cycle in a 30 to 200c potency.

PROGESTERONE

Progesterone promotes youthfulness, and is beneficial against cancer and fibrocystic breast disease. Dr. Michael Janson says additional progesterone is especially important for women exposed to exogenous estrogens, found in pesticides, food additives, drugs and other chemicals in the environment. These lead to an overload of estrogen and a deficiency of progesterone. Progesterone is extremely helpful for treating PMS symptoms in such cases.

REFLEXOLOGY

Reflexology is a science and an art based on the principle that we have reflex areas in our feet that correspond to every part of the body. Massaging specific reflex areas in the feet help to improve the functioning of specific organs and glands.

Laura Norman, a certified reflexologist from New York City, describes three reflexology techniques:

Thumb walking. "This technique can be used on the bottom, tops and sides of the feet, although it is most used on the bottom. The procedure entails bending the thumb at the first joint and inching along the bottom of the foot like a caterpillar, pressing from the heel up to the toe. The right hand is used on the right foot. Taking little tiny bites, press, press, press the whole bottom of the foot."

Finger walking. "This is done in the same way, but bending the finger at the first joint, using the tip of the finger on the outside edge."

Finger rotation. "This is where you rotate the finger into the foot."

Massaging the feet with the above techniques, using a nongreasy, absorbent cream, warms them up and helps promote overall relaxation. For addressing specific problems, reflexology must be applied to specific areas.

Knowing where to massage is fairly simple, as reflex points on the foot correspond to the way the organs and glands are distributed within the body. Laura Norman explains, "If you were to imagine your body reduced, and superimposed onto your feet, the points would be laid out just as they are in your body, from top to bottom. The top of the body is the head, and the toes reflect everything in the head area—the eyes, nose, ears, mouth, teeth, gums, jaw, brain. The ball of the toes represent the chest area, the heart, lungs, bronchial tubes. Then the center of the foot is the internal organs. Working down to the heel and ankle area, you find the pelvic area and reproductive organs. For PMS, these are the points that need to be massaged.

"The pelvic and reproductive organs are located in the heel and ankle area. The uterus point is midway between the ankle bone and the heel, on a diagonal. Thumb walking should be performed around the ankle on the big toe side of the foot. The thumbs should be pressed down, like a caterpillar, all over that inside ankle. Then a circular rotation performed with the thumb can be done on that midpoint. Finger walking can also be used over that area.

"Next, work should be done on the reflex areas that correspond to the ovaries. That is located on the outside of the ankle. With the right foot cradled on the left leg, find the high spot on the ankle bone. Square off the back of the heel and draw an imaginary diagonal line. Divide this line in half and that is where the ovary point is. This outside point of the foot is not visible and must be measured by feel or by using the index or middle finger of the left hand as it wraps around the bottom of the heel. This reflex point is almost always more sensitive than the uterus point, so care should be taken not to use too much pressure. It should help to get the blood circulating.

"Following this, the reflex to the fallopian tubes should be addressed. That goes across the top of the ankle, from ankle bone to ankle bone, on the top of the foot. This connects the ovaries to the uterus. What you need to do is finger walk from one ankle bone to the other across the top of the foot. Two fingers can be used here, one from each hand.

"Although the focus is on the reproductive organs and glands, all systems should be massaged, as the entire organism is interrelated. It is important, therefore, to massage and press on the entire foot to help all-over relaxation. Sliding the thumbs across the bottom of the feet serves this purpose and feels wonderful."

Reflexology for PMS helps most when performed three or four days before, and during, menstruation. First the right foot is worked on, while resting on the left leg. Then the same actions are repeated on the left side.

Patient Stories

There are two basic areas of concerns that I had. Number one, I had a very troublesome menstrual cycle. Number two, I have certain characteristics that place me at a slightly higher risk for breast cancer than other women. Because of these two factors, I wanted to go beyond the traditional Western medical approach. Certainly, I wanted to use what Western medicine had to offer, like getting regular examinations, but I also wanted to take an additional step. That's why I sought herbal remedies and holistic health care.

Back in November 1993, I went to a health care seminar given by Letha Hadady on breast health. I was very impressed by the information that was given. I made an appointment with Letha after that, and the remedies she gave me were very helpful.

Before I had the herbal remedies, my menstrual cycles were extremely heavy, I had mood swings, and I was very prone to exhaustion. I was extreme-ly irregular. When I started taking the herbal remedies, the menstrual cycle became very regular again, approximately every thirty days. The flow was more regular, the cramping was easier to deal with. The mood swings disap-peared, and I became balanced. My own body told me that this was certainly working for me. The herbs have made a fundamental difference in my life.

The Chinese herbs are different from American herbs because they are given in combination. They address a number of symptoms at one time, and they are also cost-effective, which I think is important for many people today.

This is something that a woman can choose to use in conjunction with reg-ular health care approaches: self-exams, medical care, proper nutrition, and addressing emotional health.—Claudia

I had a job I loved, but it was very stressful. I wound up with amenorrhea for a few weeks. Since I am not yet premenopausal or even perimenopausal, I was upset by that.

I heard of a product from a friend called Eternal, an herbal tincture that contains damiana leaf, saw palmetto, and a lot of other wonder substances that help with hormonal rejuvenation. My friend had been on Premarin for almost 20 years because of hot flashes after a hysterectomy, and found great relief from Eternal. I tried it, and to my relief, it counteracted the effect the stress was having, and brought my periods back. Everything is back to normal, and I no longer have a problem.—Susan

Twenty-five years ago, I had my first reflexology experience. My friend Judy came to visit me from California. At the time, I was suffering from terrible menstrual problems. I was pre-menstrual, bloated, headachy, achy, and feel-ing awful all over.

She said to me, "Laura, I've been studying something called reflexology, that is such a powerful tool to help you feel better all over, and especially with the menstrual condition." Judy had me take off my shoes and socks, lie down on my bed, and prop my feet up on some pillows. She pulled up a chair to the end of my bed, dimmed the lights, put on some music, and applied some hot, wet washcloths to my feet. She started to rub and press and squeeze my feet with the washcloths. It felt incredible to start with. Then she began massaging my feet with some cream, and this was heavenly. Next, she started to apply pressure to very specific parts of my feet, which she said corresponded to various parts of my body.

I felt fantastic. I was floating. I had never felt so deeply relaxed in my entire life. My symptoms completely disappeared. Afterward I was energized. I was so clear-thinking and productive. At that time I was in college studying for exams, and under a lot of pressure.

Judy continued to work on me, and I continued to find out more about reflexology myself to help myself. I saw a tremendous difference, and it totally changed the course of my life. As a result of pursuing this for my own healing, I ended up doing this professionally, and started a whole career in reflexology.

Now I have been practicing reflexology for 25 years and have seen incredible results with all kinds of conditions in all walks of life. I've seen it work on little infants and children and seniors.—Laura

50

Sexual Dysfunction in Women

Psychologist Dr. Janice Stefanacci says that sexual dysfunction stems largely from a society that offers people no models of normal healthy sexuality. "If we look to the media," she says, "we see things that are totally aberrant in terms of frequency and potency. We see relationships portrayed between males and females where there is power and domination, or submission and seduction. Role models of healthy sexual communication and actualization are virtually nonexistent. People need a sense of what is normal.

"They also need time to think about sexuality as an integrated part of their personality. Our culture is very fragmented in this regard. Many, many people, men and women, never spend time thinking about their sexuality. In fact, if you were to take an informal survey and ask people, 'What is sexuality?' a good proportion of them would say, 'It's sex. It's something you do, maybe in the bedroom, maybe at night.' Nobody is really sure how often you are supposed to have it or how long it is supposed to last. Most people don't realize that sexuality is a completely integrated part of their personality as much as actualizing in education or interpersonal relationships. Sexuality is very much a part of who we are, how we present ourselves in the world, what we do, and how we think of ourselves. Our adequacy and our self-esteem is tied up in our sexuality."

How Society Defines Sexuality

Our society defines sexuality entirely according to male standards in which sex is a performance, and orgasm is the primary, and perhaps only, yardstick for gauging satisfaction, and hence sexual "function." Some sex researchers are beginning to question the whole concept of sexual dysfunction, promoting broader and less rigid definitions of sexual response and pleasure. "The Masters & Johnson model of sexual response—excitement, plateau, orgasm, and resolution—is very performance-oriented," says Rebecca Chalker, a women's health activist whose forthcoming book, *Secrets of Women's Sexuality*, explores ways in which feminists are redefining male standards. "After desire and willingness, the only other compulsory element is pleasure," Chalker points out. "Pleasure and intimacy are the real goals of sexual activity, and if you look at it that way, the concept of sexual dysfunction simply collapses."

Nevertheless, women may worry when they have difficulties achieving orgasms, especially with a partner, and men become concerned if they have difficulties in controlling ejaculations and in getting erections. Both women and men are also distressed when they don't feel sexual attraction. In fact, most people who seek out counseling do so for difficulties with sexual communication and the lack of sexual desire. (For a discussion on sexual dysfunction in men, see chapter 58.)

Early on, through regular masturbation, boys learn what feels good and how to reliably get orgasms. Girls often wait to begin sexual exploration until they initiate sexual activity and miss out on the benefits of self-exploration. "Learning about sex from boys or men isn't the best thing for women," Chalker says. "Their efficient, orgasm-oriented model doesn't necessarily encompass women's needs and preferences. For example, the repetitive thrusting of intercourse is a pretty efficient way for men to get orgasms, but many women don't easily get orgasms this way. Many need very specific manual stimulation. Another problem is that men get their orgasms relatively quickly, and are then ready for a nap. On average, it takes women much longer to become fully aroused and able to have really strong orgasms." Chalker points out that the biggest difference between women's sexuality and men's is that women have an innate ability to have multiple orgasms. "But under the male standard, many women simply don't have the opportunity to discover this phenomenal facet of their sexuality."

Many sex therapists recommend that women explore their sexual response through masturbation, using a vibrator, sex toys, and sexy videos to stimulate sexual fantasies. You may also want to experiment with things like aromatherapy, oils, and herbs. After sufficient homework, you can try integrating these changes into sex with your partner. Another important change heterosexual couples can make is to try rewriting the "intercourse script." That is, plan to have sexual sessions where intercourse will not take place. Try giving each other maximum pleasure just with your hands. Men can also learn the time-honored technique of postponing intercourse, and hence ejaculation. This ensures that women have time to become fully aroused and can get the maximum pleasure from a sexual session.

Chalker points out that there are two powerful aspects of our sexuality—the physiological and the psychological—and that "neither can live without the other." Unfortunately, psychological problems are the more difficult to deal with and manifest themselves variously. Single people suffer when they cannot find a suitable sexual partner, while people in long-term relationships may find that they are no longer attracted by their partner. In this regard, counseling, as well as exploring a variety of books that are available, can be very helpful. Many people search for aphrodisiacs to stimulate sexual desire, but some research suggests that sexual images—in literature, photographs, or videos—are also quite helpful in stimulating the release of sexual hormones. The booming market in erotica would seem to affirm this idea.

"Today, we have enormous resources available to help with sexual problems that we didn't have a few years ago," Chalker notes. "I've reviewed some of the herbal aids and remedies here, and I encourage the reader to explore the wide range of resources available in book stores or by mail order."

Alternative Therapies

NUTRIENTS Studies show that a heightened libido and orgasmic intensity are related to blood levels of histamine. Women who have low histamine levels tend to experience low sexual excitement, while those with a high level are more able to sustain orgasms. Nutrients that increase histamine levels include vitamin B$_5$ and the bioflavonoid rutin. Broccoli, parsley, cherries, grapes, peppers, melons and citrus fruits are good food sources.

AROMATHERAPY "Aromatherapy is fantastic for helping women regain their sense of sensuality," declares aromatherapist Ann Berwick. These are some of the oils she recommends:

Rose is wonderful for enhancing feminine qualities. It bring out the loving, tender side of us that wants to surrender. Men who have trouble showing their emotions or opening up to their partner can benefit from rose as well.

Clary sage heightens sensation. It takes you out of your body and into a different realm, allowing you to relax and enjoy the romance.

Sandalwood is a wonderful oil for people not in touch with their physical side. It is very earthy and very deep.

Jasmine restores self-confidence in people who have been through traumatic sexual experiences. It can help women who have been abused or who are emotionally closed off from damaging relationships.

"By blending different oils, you can create a formula that enhances the sensual side of your nature," says Berwick. She suggests adding them to the bath or using them while massaging a partner or in self-massage. A personal perfume can be made and used daily. "Surrounding yourself with these glorious scents is a wonderful help."

NOURISHING THE KIDNEYS Registered nurse and acupuncturist Abigail Rist-Podrecca explains sexual dysfunction from an Eastern point of view: "Chinese medicine looks to the root of the cause, rather than just the symptoms, and the root seems to be the kidney. The kidneys are called the roots of life. Everything stems from the kidney, they say."

Weak kidney function can be diagnosed in Oriental medicine in multiple ways, including facial diagnosis: "Under the eye is the thinnest tissue in the entire body," explains Rist-Podrecca. "You can see through the skin there. If the blood is not being cleared by the kidneys, and detoxified, then you will see a darkness under the eyes. People will say, 'I haven't had enough sleep,' but it goes beyond that. In Chinese medicine, it says that the kidneys are not functioning optimally, so the blood isn't being cleansed."

She goes on describe various factors that can drain the kidneys. "Cold can deplete the kidneys. Many people can't tolerate cold. This is so because in the winter time, the kidney's function becomes suppressed, much the same way as the sap in a tree runs to the core and into the roots. When people have a compromised kidney situation, where it isn't functioning optimally, they can't stand the cold weather.

"Overwork and tension can also weaken kidney function because the kidneys and the adrenal glands (the adrenal sits on top of the kidney) are considered one and the same in Chinese medicine. So too much stress, and too many chemical toxins, deplete kidney functioning." Hundreds of Chinese herbs nourish kidney function. Here Rist-Podrecca names a few:

Har shar woo. This is an essential herbal formula for nourishing kidney function. It is also said to darken the hair. Hair, bone, teeth, joints, and sexual functions are tied up with the kidney energies. When you energize the kidneys, you affect all these different areas. When combined with dong quai, har shar woo helps the type of kidney dysfunction that causes low back pain.

Romania is a dark black herb that is high in iron and helps to nourish the blood and improve kidney function.

Dong quai resembles a cross section of the uterus, and has an affinity for this area of the body.

HERBS Plants containing phytochemicals with aphrodisiac properties, in order of potency:

Vicia faba (broad bean)
Catharanthus lanceus (lanceleaf periwinkle)
Euphorbia lathyris (caper spurge)
Passiflora incarnata (passionflower)
Panax ginseng (Chinese ginseng)
Punica granatum (pomegranate)
Malus domestica (apple)
Zea mays (corn)

Sexual Abuse

Abuse against women is a problem of staggering magnitude, and it occurs in every socioeconomic and ethnic group. In the United States, it is estimated that 1.8 million women are beaten every year by current or former partners. About 15 percent of women using primary care clinics have been assaulted by partners.

Sexual abuse, even more than physical abuse and battering, is a profoundly invasive violation. It takes what is most pleasurable to us, our sexuality, and turns it into a nightmare of powerlessness and revulsion. Sexual abuse happens to girls and boys, women and men, of all ages. If you have been sexually abused, the most important thing you can do is seek out a counselor, program, or support group that can guide you to recovery and help you become aware of the many resources now available. In addition, there are soothing, empowering products and therapies that may also aid the healing process.

No one deserves to be abused. If you have been abused, you are not the one who has done something wrong. Seek out local support groups, shelter, and legal help. Your state may have a hotline for abused women. The National Coalition Against Domestic Violence may have a local branch near you. Check the Yellow Pages under the following headings: Social Services, Battered Spouses, and Abuse. If danger is imminent, dial 911.

Traditional Chinese Perspective on Sexual Abuse

Traditional Chinese medicine sees sexual abuse as an attack on one's energy field. Left uncorrected, this results in physical as well as psychic disturbances. Phyllis Bloom, from the Center for Acupuncture and Healing Arts in lower Manhattan, describes imbalances which commonly occur, and tells how acupuncture, Chinese herbs, and essential oils can help to restore equilibrium and health:

"There are three levels of energy in the body: the protective level, the nutritive level, and the constitutional level. With sexual abuse, any and all of these can be affected. It depends on the situation, for example, whether it is an acute situation or a chronic one that has gone on for a very long time. If the attack is severe, that can cut through all layers.

"The protective level is the surface. It is what we use to defend ourselves. When this level is affected, it can manifest in several ways. A person I treat, who was sexually abused, continually gets flus, sinus problems, and illnesses. This is because her protective layer is overworked and has fallen down. Sometimes people have back pains because they were attacked from the back.

"When the protective layer is overworked, the body delves deeper and undermines the nutritive level. At this level, blood is created and energy flows through all of the organs. People who have problems at this level commonly have problems with various systems. They have digestive or respiratory problems, for example. They often have blood problems too. Women can experience tremendous pain during their periods or stabbing pains in the pelvic area. Other possibilities are masses, fibroids, and cysts. Disturbances in blood also affect a person's ability to express herself in the world. Women suffer from this a great deal."

YUNNAN BAIYAO "One of the most common formulas for correcting psychic and physical trauma is called Yunnan baiyao, meaning the white medicine from Yunnan province. This herbal combination helps the body redirect the blood flow from traumatized areas where the blood becomes stuck. It creates new channels. Once this flow is established, we can work on healing deeper layers of trauma."

ACUPUNCTURE "Chinese medicine has a five-element system that includes fire, water, metal, earth, and wood. When the nutritive level is affected, the fire element is disturbed. This element is responsible for relationships, intimacy, and boundaries. The organs associated with it are the heart, the heart protector or pericardium, and the small intestine.

"The heart is the center of who we are. Sexual abuse is a shock to the system, and shock is absorbed by the heart. When the heart is affected, we may see memory blocks, insomnia, palpitations and arrhythmia. Acupuncture can help. Sometimes Yunnan baiyao can help as well. The acupuncture meridians primarily emanate from the chest out to the inner side of the arm. One in particular that we use is called the Spirit Gate."

AROMATHERAPY "The essential oil sandalwood can help with palpitations, nervousness, insomnia. Just one drop is needed on the center of the chest."

51

Pregnancy

A woman undergoes numerous internal changes during each stage of pregnancy. These physiological changes are described by nurse practitioner and massage therapist Susan Lacina.

FIRST TRIMESTER. "The fetus grows rapidly, and the mother's body changes to support this swift development. Hormonal balance changes. Human chorionic gonadotropin hormone (HCG) is needed for development. As it is released, it causes many discomforts, such as breast tenderness, digestive problems, nausea, and vomiting. Progesterone levels increase and may cause mild hyperventilation, heartburn, indigestion, and constipation. Increased blood flow and its change in composition contribute to fatigue, overheating, and sinus congestion."

SECOND TRIMESTER. "The placenta takes over the hormone production, and the levels of HCG drop. Along with that, the discomforts of nausea and vomiting ease up. Physical growth of the fetus crowds the abdomen, and a woman's body expands to accommodate the growth. Fetal production of thyroid stimulating hormone (TSH) begins in the 14th week and causes the mother's thyroid level to increase. This can lead to irritability, mood swings, mild depression, increased pulse rate, and hot flashes. Adrenal hormones become elevated and remain that way until delivery. This may cause impaired glucose tolerance and swelling. Skeletal structure becomes softer and more flexible to allow for expansion. If a woman doesn't have enough muscle flexibility in her joints, she will have some pain, as tight muscles do not allow for these adjustments. She may experience sciatic nerve pain down the lower back to the back of her legs due to the extension of the pelvis, especially at the joint of the sacrum and the pelvic bone. The growing baby puts pressure on the inferior vena cava and can cause light-headedness, nausea, drowsiness, and clamminess. Prolonged reduction of blood flow can cause backaches and hemorrhoids. Lying on the side decreases this problem.

"From the 20th week on, the uterus expands by stretching muscle fibers. Abdominal muscles and ligaments stretch to support the uterus, and there may be abdominal pain. There is an increase in melanin production, causing darkening of the nipples and a line called linea nigra down the abdomen. If the lymph drainage system is not functioning well, an excess of melanin in the skin can cause brown spots. A well-functioning lymph drainage system is believed to keep melanin levels down so that brown spots do not occur. Increased progesterone causes sinus congestion, postnasal drip, and bleeding gums. Increased capillary permeability may cause the hands and feet to swell."

THIRD TRIMESTER. "As the baby continues to grow, the expectant mother changes her posture to shift her center of gravity. Heavier breasts can cause shoulders to slump forward. The spine is pulled out of alignment, and commonly causes backaches. The growing fetus also compresses the veins and the lymphatic system. That can cause ankle edema and varicose veins. There is increased pressure on the intestines and bladder, causing frequent urination and constipation. Pressure on the sciatic nerve can cause more lower back and leg pain. As the diaphragm starts to rise, breathing becomes more difficult. Insomnia is common."

The Benefits of Massage and Other Types of Bodywork

Lacina tells why a pregnant woman and her unborn child benefit greatly from massage. "We tend to think of a baby in utero as being cut off from the world," she says. "In reality, the child within is a conscious being that responds to sounds, emotions, and the inner environment that its mother creates, either through her sense of well-being or lack of it."

Here Lacina describes how maternity massage promotes a comfortable and healthy pregnancy:

RELAXATION AND STRESS REDUCTION. "This is the most important reason for a massage, and there are significant medical reasons why this is so. Research shows that prolonged stress builds up abnormal levels of toxins and chemicals in the bloodstream. These are passed through the placenta to the baby. Minimizing the buildup of toxins can be achieved by periodic deep relaxation. Relaxation increases the absorption of oxygen and nutrients by the cells of the muscles. When oxygen and nutrition increase, the woman has more energy. Some doctors also believe morning sickness and nausea are eliminated by lowering stress levels."

IMPROVED LYMPHATIC DRAINAGE. "Massage assists the lymphatic system in eliminating excessive toxins and hormones. Unlike the heart, the lymphatic system has no pump. It moves freely until muscles tighten up, but when muscles become too tense, either from the fetus or from stress, lymph movement decreases and the concentration of toxins rises. In the lower extremities, the growing uterus can inhibit lymph drainage, leading to swelling, varicose veins, hemorrhoids, and fluid retention. By relaxing the muscles, massage helps stimulate lymphatic drainage of toxins. It decreases the development of varicose veins by its draining effect and helps reduce swelling in the legs."

BETTER OVERALL MUSCLE TONE AND ELASTICITY. "A woman's body must expand to accommodate the growing fetus. Hips widen, and abdominal, lower back, and shoulder muscles stretch. Legs must accommodate increase in weight. Massage promotes flexible muscles, joints, ligaments, and tendons. It also helps decrease muscle spasms and leg cramps by getting rid of lactic acid buildup, and can alleviate the pain caused by sciatic nerve pressure. Added flexibility helps the muscles that are needed for labor."

HORMONAL BALANCE. "Massage balances the entire glandular system. An overactive thyroid gland becomes less active, thereby decreasing irritability, mood swings, and hot flashes. An underactive thymus gland is stimulated, which increases its ability to fight infection. The alternating relaxation and stimulation that massage provides helps a woman's body function in a more balanced manner."

Maternity massage lessens symptoms associated with each stage of pregnancy. Additionally, it eases and quickens labor, and helps afterward, In the first trimester, Lacina says, "Massage must be gentle so as not to interfere with hormonal balance. Gentle pressure with the fingers on the bridge of the nose, under the eyebrows, under the cheekbones, and under the forehead can relieve sinus congestion."

In the second trimester, Lacina continues, "Concentration is on stimulating lymph circulation, decreasing edema in the hands and feet, and working on breathing problems by massaging the chest. Massage at this time also helps increase flexibility in the muscles, joints, ligaments and tendons. Additionally, it can reduce sciatic pain and muscle spasms. To alleviate hemorrhoids, pressure can be applied to the crown of the head, for 15 seconds three times a day."

And in the third trimester, "Massaging the lower hips and the area near the sacrum helps reduce back pain. Stimulation of the lymph system and blood circulation continue, especially from the thigh to the abdomen. As delivery time approaches, the massage therapist can teach the mother and her partner shiatsu and acupressure points that stimulate and speed up delivery. At about 34 weeks, peroneal massage can be learned and applied."

Lacina also discusses peroneal massage: "This is a gentle stretch of tissues in the area between the vagina and rectum. Learning peroneal massage increases the mother's awareness of the muscles she needs to relax during the actual delivery and decreases her chances of having an episiotomy, an incision made to enlarge the vaginal opening at the time of birth. The actual procedure is as follows: Using warm vitamin E or vegetable oil, the mother places clean, oiled thumbs or index fingers an inch to an inch-and-a-half inside the vagina, and firm, gentle pressure is applied downward and outward. Stretching continues until a burning sensation is felt. This is held for a few minutes. Performing this once or twice a day, up until the time of delivery, can result in an easier birth."

"Massage during labor helps to reduce pain and anxiety by offering relief from muscle contractions. The stimulation of certain acupressure points can speed up labor."

POSTPARTUM MASSAGE "Postpartum is the name given to the six-week recovery period after birth," Lacina explains. "During this time, hormones readjust and the uterus involutes (returns to its pre-pregnancy size). Massaging the abdomen in a circular motion helps the uterus to contract and helps to expel blood.

Massage also helps to stimulate milk flow. The following techniques can be applied for this purpose: (1) The pressure point at the base of the sacrum can be held for about 15 seconds, and then released. (2) Breast massage is another technique that can be used. Using some light oil, a woman circles her breasts with her fingertips. She places the hands flat on the breasts, starting at the nipple, and moves outward and up. That helps the glands to release milk. (3) Additionally, there is an acupressure point at the top and middle of the shoulder. If that is held for 15 seconds, milk production is helped. (4) Pressing the point between the sixth and seventh ribs (at the nipple level on the breast bone) helps to release milk."

Lacina points out that there are instances when massage should not be used. Contraindications include vaginal bleeding or bloody discharge, fever, abdominal pain, systemic edema (excessive swelling), sudden gush of water, severe headaches, blurry vision, excess protein in urine, diabetes, high blood pressure, heart disease, and phlebitis.

ACUPRESSURE POINTS The following acupressure points may be helpful:

Thumbs can be applied to the sacrum, at the bottom of the spine, and walked up the spine to the waist. Each point is held for about five seconds.

The point in the center of the buttocks is pressed in as the mother exhales and released as she inhales.

Thumbs can be pressed along the shoulder blades between the spine and the scapula.

On the legs, pressure can be applied to spleen 6, an acupressure point located approximately three inches above the ankle, on the inside of the leg right below the tibia bone. Holding this spot for 10 seconds and then releasing it helps to stimulate uterine contractions and speeds up labor.

The uterus point is on the inside of the foot, just under the ankle bone. The ovary point is on the outside of the foot, under the ankles, near the heel.

Squeezing these points at the same time for about 10 seconds and then releasing them, helps to speed up labor.

Breast and nipple stimulation helps to create oxytocin, the hormone that helps the uterus to contract.

ALEXANDER TECHNIQUE The Alexander technique differs from massage in that the pregnant woman is actively engaged. Kim Jessor, of the American Center for Alexander Technique in New York, makes an analogy to a piano lesson: "We talk about being Alexander teachers, the people who come to us are students, and the context is a lesson. So while the results are very therapeutic, I don't think of the work as a therapy but rather as a learning process. This is significant in that it empowers students to take charge in the changing of their movement habits."

The Alexander technique is based on the concept that all of us know how to move comfortably as children, but lose that natural flexibility over time. The method teaches people how to move freely again, which is especially valuable for women undergoing the stresses of pregnancy. Jessor explains this concept with a story: "I was watching my 15-month-old son in the playground as he squatted down to pick something up. There was something extraordinary in watching that particular movement. It was so easy, so organic, so direct. It's the kind of movement that most of us have lost contact with.

"That made me think of a film that I saw of women in Brazil giving birth while squatting. They were working in harmony with gravity to push their baby out. While squatting is not a preferred method of delivering babies for Western doctors, it actually is one of the most efficient positions for a woman to be in to birth her baby and it is used in many cultures around the world.

"In an Alexander lesson with a woman who is pregnant, I actually work quite a bit on guiding her in and out of a squat. It's one of her movement options. Whether or not she, in fact, gives birth squatting, I think that it is a really useful way to begin to open up the pelvis.

"Young children have a certain freedom of movement that most of us lose contact with. One of the objectives of the Alexander technique is to restore that freedom of movement, which is important and wonderful for all of us, but particularly important for a pregnant woman dealing with the demands of pregnancy."

The Alexander technique is an experiential process. Real changes occur in the presence of a teacher who guides the student with hands-on training. "This is one of the special aspects of the Alexander technique," Jessor says. "You can learn a new way of moving because a teacher's hands gives a new stimulus to your nervous system. After a lesson, people tell me, 'Wow, I feel so much lighter,' or 'I can't believe how easily I am moving.' This is because they are actively participating in the lesson. But it is also a function of the Alexander teacher's hands giving that experience."

Jessor describes some of the ways the Alexander technique helps women during and after pregnancy:

LOWER BACK PRESSURE IS RELIEVED. "In pregnancy, women are contending with additional weight in the front of the body, which creates more pressure on the lower back. I find that most people bend over from the waist, keeping the knees straight, and pulling the head back into the spine. This creates a lot of pressure in the back. If you do that over and over, day in and day out, it starts to wear on the body. Imagine trying to do that and being pregnant at the same time; there is even more stress. I might work with a pregnant woman on a movement like bending over. I actually put my hands on her, guiding her through the movement of bending, so that she gets an experience of moving in a new way. I have had two women come to me during their second pregnancy who had a lot of back pain the first time around. Both reported little or no back pain because they learned to move in new ways that no longer put pressure on the lower back. I really feel that back pain in pregnancy is not inevitable."

BREATHING IMPROVES. "Lots of pregnant women have breathing difficulties. There is a good reason for this; with the uterus growing and expanding, there is less space for the internal organs. The diaphragm has less room, so it is more difficult to breathe. The Alexander technique teaches students how to move with less downward pressure on the organs. This minimizes breathing constriction. A study on the Alexander technique and respiration, performed by a Dr. Austin at Columbia Presbyterian Hospital, here in New York, found significant improvement in breathing capacity after a course of lessons."

REST IS ENHANCED. "Fatigue and exhaustion is another issue in pregnancy, especially in the first and third trimesters. Women need to rest a lot, and there is an effective way to learn that in an Alexander lesson. This is not a movement component of the work, but involves lying down on the table. I have a woman lie down on her back in the beginning stages, and on her side as the pregnancy gets further along. I help her learn how to release unnecessary tension. It is easier to do this in the lying-down position because the student is not contending with gravity. The table lesson teaches the pregnant woman how to consciously release excess tension, which enables her to really rest and recuperate."

LABOR IS EASED. "Labor is an intense situation where a woman must learn to deal with pain and fear. The Alexander technique teaches the skill of releasing muscles between contractions. By fully letting go, the woman does not remain tense in response to the pain. Rather, she is able to conserve energy. When I gave birth, I worked with another Alexander teacher for labor support. She put her hands on me and gave me verbal direction. As a result, I was able to release more effectively between contractions. Husbands of pregnant students come to me for labor support lessons where they learn to be more available to women as they give birth."

STAMINA INCREASES AFTER DELIVERY. "There is a lot of very challenging physical labor in being a mother. Again, there is much bending. There is also a lot of lifting. It is very important to pay attention to how you are doing this. I work with a new mother on ways of bending efficiently to pick up her baby. Recently, I taught someone how to bend over and pick up a stroller while it had a 35-pound child in it. Also, the way that the baby is handled is very much affected by the way the mother is using her body. The better the use, the greater the sense of support and security for the child."

BREAST-FEEDING IS EASIER. "Breast-feeding also includes the component of bending. You tend to move toward the child as you are nursing, and there is the possibility of compressing your body. The Alexander technique teaches you how to maintain a sense of ease and balance while breast-feeding the baby throughout the day."

Jessor concludes by saying that there are less tangible, but equally valuable, benefits from working with the Alexander technique during pregnancy. As a woman becomes aware of different options in movement, she simultaneously opens up to greater options in her thinking: "Women begin to realize that they can make different kinds of choices about the kind of birth they want to have, where they want to have it, and who they want to use for labor support. In the same way that they begin to find freedom in movement, they find greater options in terms of the choices they make about their pregnancy."

Nutritional and Lifestyle Considerations

The best insurance for a well baby is to follow a highly nutritious whole-foods diet. What you eat now will impact the health of your child later. According to nutritionist Gracia Perlstein, "When a woman is considering pregnancy, it is important that she address her diet to see how healthful it is, as many difficulties have their root in prenatal deficiencies. Scientific studies reveal that birth defects, and even problems that develop much later in life, can be prevented when the mother has excellent nutrition. I would like to include the father there too, because the quality of the sperm is also very important." Since the most crucial stage of embryonic development occurs in the first few weeks, before a women realizes that she is pregnant, good quality foods should be eaten all the time.

Eating properly means selecting unprocessed or minimally processed foods. A wide assortment of whole grains, legumes, vegetables, fruits, nuts, and seeds supplies multiple nutrients. "So many people eat the same 10 or 20 foods over and over again," Perlstein says. "In traditional cultures, people have much more variety. I would like to emphasize that supplements should only enhance an excellent diet. Make the effort to eat high-quality, nutrient-dense foods. That means whole foods, the way nature produced them."

The body intuitively knows what it needs to support new life, and paying attention to its messages can be a helpful guide. "A woman's body is very wise when she is pregnant. Many women can't stand the look or smell of coffee or cigarettes, even when they used to smoke or drink coffee several times a day," states Perlstein. She adds that worrying about eating the right foods all the time is stressful and can produce more harm than good. But nutrition education can benefit women with highly processed diets, who need to learn about better food choices. "Vegetarian women may crave animal foods or be drawn to dairy when they are pregnant. Usually it is good to pay attention to these cravings, but to respond in the most wholesome way possible."

Wholesome means organically grown. Pesticide-free fare is better for everyone, of course, but vitally important for young children and developing fetuses, according to recent research. Dairy and animal products should be from creatures naturally raised. One reason for this is that pesticides and other contaminants tend to concentrate in an animal's tissues. The higher up the food chain, the higher the concentration of toxins. Fortunately, many health food stores, and more and more supermarkets sell the healthful varieties.

Animal products, when a part of the diet, should be eaten in moderation. Although protein needs increase, they can be abundantly obtained from vegetarian sources, which are less toxic than their animal counterparts. Excellent vegetarian protein sources include fortified soy milk, tofu, tempeh, beans, nuts, and seeds, for example.

The increased need for calcium is similarly fulfilled in such a diet: "Many women do not realize that there are excellent sources of calcium other than milk and dairy. There are green leafy vegetables, fortified soy milk, tofu, almonds, and many other calcium-containing foods. If you eat a diet rich in fresh vegetables and fruits, you tend to get quite a bit of calcium. If you want a supplement, calcium citrate is easiest on the stomach. Other forms sometimes cause digestive upsets or constipation. Definitely avoid calcium-depleting foods—coffee, chocolate, and sodium."

Perlstein adds that eating several small meals throughout the day offsets common complications: "Hunger, not calorie counting, is the most reliable guide to eating during pregnancy. Five to six small, nutrient-dense meals per day is a sensible ideal. This is a good habit to develop in the last trimester of pregnancy, when the organs in your stomach are somewhat constricted, and good in the early stages to prevent nausea. It keeps the blood sugar from falling, and nausea has a lot to do with low blood sugar."

Water should be pure and taken in adequate amounts. Eight to 12 glasses are recommended to help flush out toxins from the liver and kidneys: "Many people do not drink enough fluids," notes Perlstein. "This is especially important during pregnancy because the woman is filtering the waste for two bodies."

Beyond an excellent diet, Perlstein recommends the following daily nutrients for pregnant women:

Multiple vitamin/mineral supplement

Vitamin C

B_{12}

Zinc
Vitamin E–400 units
Folic acid

Folic acid, which is also contained in green leafy vegetable and whole grains, is especially important in pregnancy because science has shown it to prevent neural tube defects. Even when included in the diet, extra folic acid should be taken in supplement form as it is fragile and easily damaged by heat. Additionally, acidophilus helps prevent constipation and other types of colon problems.

Extra iron may be needed, but a woman should have her hemoglobin tested first, just to be sure. Research shows that excess iron in the system can have damaging effects.

Raspberry tea throughout the pregnancy strengthens uterine muscle. It contains fragine, a smooth-muscle relaxer. In the final stages of pregnancy, it can be combined with black cohosh, squaw vine, and peppermint to relax the pelvis, speed up delivery, and make delivery less bloody.

Ginger is one of the best natural remedies for nausea, especially when accompanied by small, frequent, meals, fresh air, and plenty of rest. Ginger can be taken as a capsule or tea.

(Other herbal tips: A washcloth soaked in ginger or comfrey tea and applied to the area promotes healing of an episiotomy. Rosemary added to bath water relieves tension and back pain. Adding jasmine and clary sage to a bath has an uplifting effect, and prevents postpartum depression.)

WHAT TO AVOID DURING PREGNANCY Equally important is knowing what not to take in. Nutritionist Gracia Perlstein lists substances that can harm a growing fetus:

HARMFUL HOUSEHOLD CHEMICALS. "First on the list of what to avoid is chemical exposure to toxic household cleansers. Natural food stores are a good source for environmentally harmless cleansers of various kinds. You want to avoid fumes from paints, thinners, solvents, wood preservatives, varnishes, glues, spray adhesives, benzene, dry cleaning fluid, anything chemically based and questionable. Stay away from household pesticides. I want to emphasize again that you don't want to go spraying for fleas, roaches, or ants with commercially available pesticides when you are pregnant or looking to become pregnant."

RADIATION. "Avoid radiation and x-rays, especially during the first three months. If a doctor feels an x-ray is required, be sure to mention that you may be pregnant. Ask if it can be put off until after the first trimester, if possible."

CERTAIN HERBS. "Basic rule of thumb is not to have bitter herbs, such as goldenseal and pennyroyal. Many books list these herbs specifically."

ANTIHISTAMINES. "You want to avoid antihistamines. That includes some from the natural food stores such as ma huang and osha root."

LAXATIVES. "If you are having problem with constipation, adequate fluids, whole grains, and fresh vegetables should correct that problem quite easily. You want to avoid senna, castor oil, and cascara sagrada as well as diuretics, including the herbs buchu, horsetail, and juniper berries. If you drink adequate fluids and don't consume excess sodium or animal protein, your kidneys should be able to filter without water retention."

HAIR DYES. "Avoid dying your hair with chemicals. Nonchemical hair dyes are available, which usually do the trick."

HORMONES. "Hormones are another reason to stay away from commercial meats."

SUBSTANCE ABUSE. "Of course, you need to stay away from intoxicants and strong substances, including cigarettes, alcohol and recreational drugs."

HIGH TEMPERATURES. "Avoid very high temperatures for a prolonged period—for example, hot tubs or saunas."

TOXIC SURROUNDINGS. "As much as possible, avoid stress, negative people, and aggravating situations. Instead, try to spend quality time alone and with loved ones, people who are supportive. Spend time in nature. Read inspiring literature. Listen to beautiful music. This has a beneficial effect on your mental and emotional state. That, in turn, affects your baby's biochemistry."

Exercise During Pregnancy

The American College of Gynecologists and Obstetricians (ACOG) endorses physical activity during pregnancy and has created specific guidelines for the dos and don'ts of exercise:

Pregnant women derive health benefits from a mild to moderate exercise routine. Exercising 60 minutes, three times per week, is preferable to intermittent activity, but some benefit can be derived from shorter durations as well. Sometimes little oxygen is available for aerobic exercise due to the body's increased oxygen demands. Therefore, a woman should begin an aerobic activity slowly, and gradually build to capacity. She should not push too hard, and certainly not to the point of breathlessness. Pregnant women should not exercise in the face-up position after the first trimester. This position limits blood supply to the baby.

Standing for prolonged periods of time, doing heavy work in the standing position, and exercising at high intensities are to be avoided. These activities are associated with diminished birth weight in newborns. It's better for women to engage in non-weight-bearing activities such as cycling and swimming, rather than exercises like running. Non-weight-bearing exercise minimizes risk of injury and allows activity levels to remain closer to prepregnancy levels, right up to delivery. A woman should be aware that her center of gravity is different, and that she might lose her balance when exercising. Anything that could involve falling over, or even mild abdominal trauma, should be avoided.

Pregnant women require an extra 300 calories per day in order to maintain their normal metabolic rate. Exercise increases the need for more calories.

A pregnant woman must be careful not to raise body temperature with vigorous workouts, especially in the first trimester. Excessive body heat in the mother can adversely affect the development of brain tissue in the baby. The threshold for this is a body temperature of about 39.2 degrees C, which is 100 or 101 degrees F. The conclusion here is to exercise, but never to the point of raising body temperature. Pool exercises help to dissipate heat.

Chiropractor Richard Statler answers some commonly asked questions on the subject of pregnancy and exercise:

WHEN SHOULD A PREGNANT WOMAN NOT EXERCISE?

"Basically, every pregnant woman can benefit from starting an exercise program at any point in pregnancy. However, there are certain exceptions to this rule. In these situations, an expectant woman should avoid or limit exercise:
   Pregnancy-induced hypertension
   Premature rupture of membranes
   Incompetent cervix
   Persistent second or third trimester bleeding
   Premature labor during the prior or current pregnancy
   Intrauterine growth retardation
Other medical contraindications include thyroid, heart, vascular or pulmonary conditions. Women with medical problems need a physician's evaluation to determine whether an exercise program is appropriate."

HOW MUCH EXERCISE SHOULD A PREGNANT WOMAN GET?

"How much exercise a woman is capable of largely depends on her fitness level before pregnancy. Someone who has never exercised should not begin a heavy program. Nor should someone who was an avid exerciser completely give it up. For a marathon runner to suddenly stop because she is pregnant can be as problematic as a nonrunner deciding to run marathons during her pregnancy."

WHAT ARE THE BENEFITS OF EXERCISING DURING PREGNANCY?

"Statistics show that women who exercise during pregnancy usually have an easier, shorter labor and safer delivery. There are fewer premature births. During pregnancy the woman feels more energetic and vital, and less stressed. Exercise alleviates a good portion of discomfort from back pain or sciatica. By stabilizing the blood sugar, exercise can even help women who are diabetic. Mothers who exercise see quicker recovery times after delivery.

"One benefit to exercising in a group program is the social aspect. An exercise group can provide informal support. First-timers speak to women who have been there, and get real-life input and suggestions. That's important in this day and age, when people no longer live with extended families who traditionally passed down such wisdom."

HOW DOES EXERCISING AFFECT THE BABY?

"When a mother exercises, she gets more oxygen and is able to pass that to her baby. Better nutritional delivery, better oxygen, and better blood flow can only be helpful. There is also less complication with labor and birth, and that can mean a healthier baby."

Dr. Statler says that exercises geared toward opening up the pelvis are particularly important in preparing women for delivery: "The pelvic area is where the baby sits. It must expand so that the baby can pass through. The pelvis has three contact points. In the front is the pubic bone area; in the back are two sacroiliac joints, one to the left and one to the right. Those joints can stretch and open up to allow the pelvis to expand. Although hormones secreted during this time allow the pelvis to open up tremendously, placing the woman in the typical birth position of lying on her back compresses the sacroiliac joints. We can potentially lock up two-thirds of her ability to stretch."

Stretching exercises are key for opening up this area. Here are three that Dr. Statler recommends:

HIP STRETCH. Stand with feet shoulder-width apart. Rotate on the balls of the feet until the heels are turned out. In this position, do a half squat, keeping the back straight. It may help to do this while leaning against a wall. It can also be done on a supermarket line, while holding onto a shopping cart. An alternate way of doing the exercise is seated. Once again, feet are shoulder-width apart, and feet are flat on the floor. Shimmy forward slightly to keep from sitting back in the chair. Lean back a little bit to take the weight of the body off the hip joint. That allows for better movement. Place a child's volleyball or play ball between the knees and hold it there. Pivot on the balls of the feet to turn the heels out, keeping the heels flat on the floor. Now gently squeeze the ball while pushing the legs together and internally rotating the thighs toward the midline. Hold for 10 seconds and relax.

Either of these exercises is great for opening up the hip and sacroiliac joints. They prepare the mother for delivery by developing more stable joints throughout pregnancy.

PUBIC STRETCH. This exercise helps the front of the pelvis by using motions that are opposite to those used in the previous exercise. Standing, with feet one shoulder-width apart, turn toes and thighs out. Bend knees slightly. As before, this can be done in a supermarket while holding on to a shopping cart. In the seated position, sit on the floor with soles of the feet together and knees apart. Use the back against the wall for support. Pull the feet as close to the body as is comfortable. Place the hands on the knees, and gently press the knees down and apart from each other toward the floor. Hold that for thirty seconds while breathing deeply. Repeat two or more times. Never do any bouncing or jerky motions. These are slow stretches.

CAT ARCH. Lie on all fours so that hands and knees are touching the floor. Arch the back like a cat, while slowly inhaling. Allow the back to return to the flat back position while exhaling. Do not curve the back in. Hold for a few seconds and relax. Repeat 10 to 15 times.

Aromatherapy

Aromatherapist Ann Berwick reports that in Europe, where aromatherapy is scientifically studied and widely prescribed, hospital maternity wings utilize essential oils for their soothing and uplifting mind/body effects: "There is a report of one woman who had severe anxiety throughout her pregnancy. They gave her neroli oil, which helped to keep her blood pressure down and allowed her to go into delivery in a more relaxed state. During delivery, she was given lavender and clary sage to relax her uterus. Clary sage is also slightly euphoric, so it helped her to cope mentally with the birth." Here are some formulas to try before, during, and after birth:

As an antidote for nausea and vomiting, peppermint is effective when a very dilute amount is rubbed into the stomach or inhaled.

For relaxation, 8 ounces vegetable oil, 13 drops lavender, 2 drops geranium, and 10 drops sandalwood can be massaged into the skin or used as a compress.

To clear nasal congestion, a teaspoon of eucalyptus oil can be added to a cold air humidifier or pan of hot water. The steam inhaled lessens congestion.

To help heartburn, place 2 to 3 drops of diluted peppermint oil on the back of the tongue.

Five drops rose oil, 12 drops clary sage, and 5 drops ylang-ylang in 2 to 3 ounces vegetable oil can be used as a massage oil during labor.

To prevent stretch marks, massage 2 ounces wheat germ oil, 20 drops lavender, and 5 drops neroli oil into thighs.

To soothe sore nipples, mix one pint cold water, one drop geranium oil, one drop lavender oil, and one drop rose oil.

After an episiotomy a sitz (shallow) bath is helpful, especially when 2 drops of cyprus oil and 4 drops of lavender oil are added. Soak for 15-20 minutes.

To promote milk production, take two drops fennel oil with some honey water, every two hours.

Hemorrhoids will be helped by 5 drops of cyprus oil, added to the bath.

The astringent action of cyprus and lemon oil constricts varicose veins. A few drops can be added to a body lotion and applied to the veins morning and evening.

Homeopathy

Homeopathic physician Stephanie Odinov Pukit lists a variety of remedies for all stages of pregnancy. She begins with treatments for morning sickness, noting, "Along with the dry biscuit in bed with a hot beverage, homeopathic remedies can be extremely important at this time."

SEPIA. Ambivalence is the key word here. There is a conflict between self-preservation and the urge to procreate, which makes wanting a child questionable. The woman becomes angry and irritable and feels as if a black cloud hovers over her. Although her appetite is insatiable, heavy pains worsen with smells or thoughts of food.

PULSATILLA. This is the opposite scenario. Pulsatilla is an excellent remedy for the woman who is cheerful, sweet, somewhat helpless. The person is warm and may throw the covers off at night. She becomes worse with emotional excitement. Nausea comes and goes and is characteristically worse in early evening.

NUX VOMICA. This is a wonderful remedy for soothing the nerves after a woman has abused her body with alcohol, drugs or coffee. She tends to be constipated. She tends to wake up at night to think about business because she is ambitious and driven.

ARSENICUM. The picture here is a person constantly anxious about her state of health. She always runs to the doctor fearing that something is wrong. The woman tends to have burning pains. She has great thirst and takes little sips. Symptoms are usually exacerbated at midnight.

COCCULUS INDICUS. This remedy specifically helps motion sickness. The woman tends to lose sleep and to be constantly exhausted. She may be nursing children, or caring for someone. The woman feels dizzy standing and better when lying down. She is worse in fresh air.

Petroleum may be needed if there is a voracious appetite followed by persistent vomiting.

BRYONIA. The person has strong sensitivity to smells and may have connective tissue and arthritic problems. Nausea becomes worse with motion.

Dr. Odinov Pukit suggests these remedies for problems that occur in the latter stages of pregnancy:

SEPIA OR PULSATILLA. In the third to sixth month, the fetus presses high up in the abdomen, causing heartburn, shortness of breath, and indigestion.

These remedies also help hemorrhoid problems. The one chosen depends on the other symptoms manifested. Sepia is for a gloomy disposition, while pulsatilla is for a sweet nature.

CARBO VEGETABILIS. The woman is slightly heavy and tends to have indigestion and shortness of breath due to poor oxygenation. Although she tends to be chilly, she prefers open windows with the air directly on her.

BELLIS PERENNIS. As the baby drops into the pelvis, pressure is felt on the organs in the lower part of the bladder. Pain and arthritis may occur as a result. Bellis perennis is specific for pain in the uterine area or groin. The woman might be walking when all of a sudden her legs weaken from a sharp nerve pain. After childbirth, when arnica has done its job and there are still some lumps remaining in the tissues, bellis perennis is also excellent.

KALI CARB. This is for women with back pain, especially those who tend to wake up between 2:00 and 4:00 in the morning. This individual's personality is somewhat crabby and closed. She is vague and evasive about answering questions. Pains are better with pressure and rubbing. The person tends to be anxious and chilly.

ACONITE. High-potency aconite is wonderful to use when there has been shock or fright. Arnica and calendula may be useful for this purpose as well.

In addition, Dr. Odinov Pukit works with abnormal presentation. She finds that homeopathic remedies can help turn the baby over when used between 32 and 36 weeks: "Pulsatilla works in 40 percent of the cases, and other remedies are used when they match the woman's constitution. A wonderful remedy for that woman in general may help in that specific area as well."

Midwife Jeannette Breen finds homeopathy useful during labor, and after birth. "I seem to be using more and more homeopathic remedies since I've been seeing the advantages." These are a few she recommends:

ARNICA. Starting a month before delivery, regular application of arnica directly to the nipples prevents their later tearing and cracking with breastfeeding. After birth, arnica quickens recuperation. Calendula can be used in the same way.

CALIFILUM. May help a stalled labor. This is specific for a weak uterus or a uterus running out of steam. The woman often experiences weakness, exhaustion, trembling, and shivering. Sharp, brief, unstable, and painful lower uterine contractions fail to completely dilate the cervix and push the baby.

GELSEMIUM. May be indicated as a follow-up to califilum. Also good for neuralgia, rheumatic discomfort, and pains in the bladder and vaginal area. The person tends to be thirsty and chilly.

CIMICIFUGA. Also good for stalled labor, especially when woman is becoming fearful, hysterical, and exhausted, and the pains are becoming erratic. This tones the uterus, calms it down, and helps it to become more coordinated.

Breen cautions that homeopathic remedies should not be used as a quick fix. "There is not always a pill to take care of every problem in labor and birth. Sometimes you have to be patient. That's what midwives are good at. They try to be as patient and supportive as possible during this time."

Dr. Odinov Pukit adds that after birth homeopathic remedies can help newborns as well: "If the baby is distressed, we might need arnica rescue remedy. Carbo veg is wonderful if there is cyanosis with some respiratory effect. And arsenicum if the baby is born lifeless."

Water Birth

Jeannette Breen is a great enthusiast for using water during labor: "It has a wonderful analgesic quality, which is much better than an epidural. Being immersed in water provides tremendous relaxation. It does not take the pain away, but women do report feeling less pain in the water. They feel less effect from the pull of gravity. Their movements are very easy, and there is much better tissue relaxation, which means there is almost no tearing in a water birth. It is also easier for the baby because the mother is more relaxed and moving freely. She is not stuck in one position. It is easier for the baby to negotiate the pelvis and to slip out in a warm, moist environment that is quite familiar."

Social Support

"Two keys to a normal healthy pregnancy and birth are a healthy diet and good social support," says Breen. "Those seem to be overlooked, especially in traditional maternity care in this country. The focus is on diagnostic testing, but not a lot of emphasis is placed on healthy diets, other than prescribing women prenatal vitamins and iron. There is no question that a high quality diet rich in all the nutrients can make a woman's whole body work more efficiently and effectively.

"Social support creates an environment of love that is all-important but too often overlooked in hospitalized birthing environments that focus solely on technology. No one can have the baby for the pregnant woman; she has to do it herself. But if she is surrounded by love and support, rather than fear and technology, she is able to give birth in a very intuitive, instinctual way which is satisfying and safe."

Corrective Vaginal Surgery Following Episiotomy

In the United States, about 80 percent of women give birth by episiotomy. Of those operations, approximately 90 percent are improperly performed. "Doctors are just not instructed in how to do this surgery," says Dr. Vicki Hufnagel. "All you have to do is go to your local medical school, get out the textbook on obstetrics, and look at what an episiotomy is. It will have a drawing, and a discussion that says to put one or two sutures here, and one or two there. They are teaching physicians to close an entire organ system in just one or two layers. If you were to close a laceration on your face in one or two layers, your muscles wouldn't work, your face wouldn't work. You'd be a real mess. We are teaching students how to close the vaginal vault area in a manner that is not allowable in other places. That is the standard of care that we have, and it is completely unacceptable."

Incorrectly performed episiotomies result in problems down the road. Without support of the vaginal muscles, the cervix pushes through the vagina. It appears that the uterus is being forced out, when really it is not. Doctors mistakenly diagnose a prolapsed uterus and commonly recommend a hysterectomy. Tragically, 100,000 to 200,000 women with this misdiagnosis receive this operation each year.

Corrective surgery easily ameliorates the problem. Repairing the vagina is a simple procedure that can be performed in a doctor's office. It takes all of 45 minutes, and patients can go home the same day.

Postpartum Depression

Depression after childbirth affects thousands of women each year. Although the exact cause is unknown, hormonal shifts after birth, particularly drops in progesterone, may play a large role. Research also links the condition to low levels of the neurotransmitter serotonin. Emotionally, it is often connected to difficult labor and disappointments after birth.

Symptoms range in degree, but are generally worse than a temporary feeling of the blues immediately following childbirth, according to Dr. Marjorie Ordene, a complementary gynecologist from Brooklyn, New York: "Postpartum depression is defined as a gradually increasing sullen mood and a loss of interest and enthusiasm starting around the third postpartum week. This is different from the baby blues, which is a frequent and common occurrence in the normal population. The blues happens the first week postpartum, and basically goes away by itself. We are talking about something much more severe." In the worst-case scenario, women can become sick for years, and lose touch with reality.

ALTERNATIVE THERAPIES FOR POSTPARTUM DEPRESSION

HOMEOPATHY

Homeopathic physician Dr. Jane Cicchetti recommends that women try the 30c potency of the remedy that best addresses their symptoms. If this does not help, a visit to a homeopathic physician can provide more individual support:

Sepia. Sepia may be needed after an exhausting delivery, after giving birth to two or more children at once, or after having several children. The woman feels completely worn out and depressed. Physically, she feels as if her uterus might fall out, and finds herself crossing her legs a lot. Often there is an actual prolapse of the uterus. Emotionally, a woman who loved her husband and children suddenly has an aversion to them. In fact, she has an aversion to everyone and wants to be alone. She becomes irritable and angry if anyone bothers her, and has an aversion to sex. The woman cries often but cannot understand what is wrong; in fact this problem is caused by a hormonal disturbance rather than an emotional one.

Natmur. Natmur is for chronic grief. The woman is introverted and dwells on past, unpleasant memories but keeps them to herself. She tries to put on the appearance that everything is fine, and becomes aggravated if someone tries to comfort her.

Ignatia. Ignatia is for postpartum depression brought on by emotions. It is needed when disappointment follows childbirth. A woman imagines an ideal pregnancy and birthing situation. When that does not work out, she feels extremely let down and depressed. These feelings may occur after a stillbirth or a miscarriage. There is uncontrollable sobbing and sighing, and a rapid change of emotions, which are often contradictory. Depression is acute, while natmur depression is chronic.

Arnica. This commonly needed remedy is useful for depression, upset, and malaise brought on by bruising, soreness, and pain that lasts a long time. Arnica helps heal the physical trauma, and improves the mother's energy and emotional state.

Pulsatilla. Pulsatilla is given when a woman cries a lot and wants to be taken care of. She needs to attend to her newborn baby, but feels as if someone should be attending to her. This individual will eat sweets and other goodies to alleviate overwhelming feelings of sadness and loneliness. The woman often is warm-blooded and enjoys the fresh air. She is happier walking around outside, and much happier if she can be with people.

Cimicifuga. This remedy is used less often, but is very important for those who need it. Cimicifuga is derived from black cohosh, a powerful herb for treating hysteria and female complaints. It is needed when a woman feels as if a dark cloud of gloom has settled over her. She fears losing her mind. Often this stems from a very difficult delivery where the woman had a mini nervous breakdown, feeling at one point as if she was going insane. This leaves her with a great fear of ever having a baby again. Often she has alternating states. When she is not under this dark cloud of gloom, she becomes excitable and talkative, jumping from one subject to another in an almost hysterical fashion. Cimicifuga heals the nervous system.

Kali carbonicum. This deep mineral remedy is indicated for women who become anxious and irritable after a delivery that leaves them feeling weak.

Easily startled, they want to be left alone and have an aversion to being touched. They tend to be chilly and to have insomnia from 2:00 to 4:00 a.m. Further, they are regimented and have trouble going with the flow of caring for a new baby. Often these symptoms follow a delivery that primarily consists of back labor. Sciatica develops to some degree, which then leads to this emotional state.

Phosphoric acid. Here a woman is extremely disappointed from physical or emotional shock. She may have lost the baby, or something might be wrong with it. A loved one may have died at the time of birth, or she may be affected from the loss of much bodily fluid during delivery. Indifferent to everything, the woman lies in bed with her face to the wall. It is as if her emotions have completely disappeared. She doesn't want to talk, think, or answer questions.

Cocculus. This is a remedy for fatigue and emotional depression brought on by loss of sleep. The woman feels drunk and may go through the day feeling dizzy and staggering. These feelings are brought on by sleep deprivation.

Aurum metallicum. For profound depression characterized by total hopelessness, self-destructive behavior, and a longing for death.

These remedies can make a difference because they get to the root of the problem. Regarding conventional treatment methods that use antidepressants, Dr. Cicchetti says, "Women just suppress their symptoms, and their health does not really get any better."

NATURAL PROGESTERONE

"Studies show that postpartum depression can be prevented by treating women with progesterone," reports Dr. Marjorie Ordene, a gynecologist from Brooklyn, New York. "Companies that make natural progesterone recommend taking a half teaspoon twice daily, starting a month after delivery. Since postpartum depression is supposed to start three weeks after giving birth, it makes sense to begin using the natural progesterone cream at that time."

VITAMIN B$_6$

According to research, vitamin B$_6$ raises serotonin levels. Patients given B$_6$ for 28 days after delivery did not have a recurrence of postpartum depression.

MISCARRIAGE

Surprisingly, two-thirds of all pregnancies end up as miscarriages. One reason for this phenomenon is that many women miscarry before they even know that they are pregnant. Most commonly, genetic abnormalities precipitate the problem. Embryos develop wrongly, and a woman's body naturally aborts the fetus. Endocrine system imbalances are also associated with miscarriages. Women in their late forties have an especially difficult time carrying full-term, due to hormonal changes that accompany aging. Poor thyroid gland functioning can also interfere with pregnancy, as can intercourse during pregnancy. Another cause of miscarriages is low-grade infections, which are often the result of sexually transmitted diseases. Women do not consciously realize a problem exists, but the body knows, and rejects the fetus. Bladder infections are also common; as the uterus enlarges, it places great pressure on this organ. Miscarriages may also occur when women are hard on their bodies. These women push themselves to the limit by overexercising and undereating to the point of anorexia. Their unhealthy state doesn't provide enough nutrition for themselves or their fetus.

PREVENTING MISCARRIAGES When a miscarriage occurs more than once, a woman needs to have a thorough medical workup. Once the problem is understood, it is often correctable. If a woman is having intercourse during pregnancy, for example, she may simply need to take precautions. Using a condom during intercourse can prevent a miscarriage because it keeps male prostaglandins out of the female system, which, in turn, prevents premature uterine contractions. Low-grade infections must be cleared up, and increasing the intake of liquids and vitamin C can sometimes do the trick. Mixing four ounces of strawberry juice with four ounces of water is an especially good source of vitamin C, which acidifies the urine and helps prevent bladder infections. More serious infections should be cultured, and treated appropriately. Sometimes, this means antibiotics. Older women, who are having a difficult time holding on to a pregnancy due to hormonal changes, may need low doses of progesterone, about 25 mg, in suppository form.

BREAST-FEEDING FALLACIES

Following are corrections to common fallacies related to lactation and breast-feeding:

Nipple soreness is not related to skin color.

The lactating breast is never empty.

All women do not experience pain during each breast-feeding.

Nipples do not get tougher with nursing.

Creams and oils on the breast are not encouraged for nipple soreness; vitamin E toxicity could be a concern because of liberal applications, and pesticide residues are a concern in sheep-fat-derived lanolin.

Engorgement may be experienced by newly breast-feeding mothers but is almost always indicative of inappropriate or infrequent suckling.

The let-down process is not a singular event, but occurs continually during suckling.

The human nipple is different from artificial nipples: it can stretch two to three times its nonsuckled length. It contains 15 to 20 pores, which spurt a fine stream of milk. The milk ejection occurs in a rhythmic fashion. The nipple remains elongated only with active suckling. It does not drip continuously.

Noninfectious mastitis rarely requires antibiotic therapy; infectious mastitis includes temperature elevation and flulike systems as well.

Extra fluid intake is not needed for breast-feeding; drinking to quench one's thirst is sufficient.

The lactating mother's breasts become full usually between one to three days after the infant starts suckling.

Colostrum, which is a highly concentrated source of protein and antibodies, is produced as early as the third month of pregnancy.

Women with inverted nipples can breast-feed.

Healthy babies do not need supplemental feedings before the mother's milk comes in.

Breast milk helps reduce bilirubin concentrations by coating the small intestines, reducing bilirubin recirculation.

Additional water or glucose given to the infant reduces total caloric intake and reduces the coating action of milk feedings.

Human milk is far superior in all aspects to artificial formula.

Source: K. G. Auerbach, "Breast-Feeding Fallacies: Their Relationship to Understanding Lactation," *Birth* 17, no. 1 (March 1990): 44–49.

On the Research Front

Morning sickness has been the subject of much recent research; among treatments found effective by studies are acupressure on the pericardium 6 point, or the use of a wristband that puts pressure on this point; vitamin B_6 supplementation; and powdered ginger capsules. One study concludes, however, that morning sickness may not be an unmitigated evil; it is connected with a lower miscarriage rate and may serve to protect the fetus from food poisoning.

Research has indicated that cesarean sections, as well as being associated with greater risks to mother and infant, are often unnecessary. Women who have had one cesarean section may later give birth vaginally, however; in the United States, the number of women giving birth vaginally after an earlier C-section has risen in recent years. Another encouraging statistic is that, according to one study, women over 35 years old generally have no more complications and bear children with less infant mortality and fewer congenital anomalies than younger women, although they do more often require surgical intervention to give birth.

Another subject of studies has been birthing positions; several studies have concluded that use of upright posture in a birthing chair is as safe as the traditional semirecumbent posture, and may allow less pain during labor. Water birth is another method that has received recent attention. Other strategies that reduce labor pain include biofeedback during labor, acupuncture, transcutaneous electrical nerve stimulation (TENS), Lamaze training, and hypnosis. Many studies have pointed to the advantages of birthing centers or midwife-attended home births over hospitals, and demonstrated their equal safety.

52

Female Infertility

Approximately 2.5 million American couples are unable to conceive. The question of what can and should be done to conquer infertility is not only a complex medical issue. With the advent of more and more advanced techniques for getting around nature's roadblocks to conception, it can also be a thorny ethical dilemma as well, with high emotional stakes.

Causes

Among the reasons for infertility in women are endometriosis (see chapter 54); poor diet; deficiencies in folic acid, vitamin B_6, vitamin B_{12}, and iron; heavy metal toxicity; obesity; immature sex organs; abnormalities of the reproductive system; hormonal imbalances; and genetic damage from electromagnetic radiation. (Issues related to male infertility are discussed in Chapter 59.)

It may be surprising to learn that the birth control pill, and other sources of estrogen, can add to the problem. Barbara Seaman, an advocate for women's health issues and author of *The Doctors' Case Against the Pill*, the publication of which led to detailed product warnings being included in birth control pill prescriptions, concludes that the chemicals in the pill may increase infertility in three ways: by suppressing the natural productions of hormones; by increasing the risk of sexually transmitted diseases (STDs), especially chlamydia; and by upsetting the assimilation of nutrients.

"Fertility experts confirm that many women who have been on the pill for a long time have problems re-establishing their monthly cycles. In Switzerland, Fabio Bertarelli, the billionaire owner of the largest company to manufacture fertility drugs, publicly states that he owes his fortune to the birth control pill. In

1993, Bertarelli told the *Wall Street Journal* that his typical customer is a women over 30, who has been taking birth control pills since she was a teenager or in her early twenties. When she got off the pill, her normal cycles did not come back."

Seaman adds: "Fact is, there are a lot of nutritional issues involved. If a woman has been on the pill for a long time, she may be very low in folic acid; vitamins B_1, B_2, B_6, B_{12}, C, and E; and trace minerals zinc and magnesium, all essential to normal fertility. Sometimes just getting on a really good diet with really good supplements can get her back into a fertile cycle without needing heavy-duty drugs. It should be noted, however, that any dietary supplements used should be low in vitamin A, niacin, copper, and iron, the levels of which tend to be elevated in pill users."

Another reason the pill affects female fertility is that it promotes the growth of chlamydia, Seaman says. "This condition has reached epidemic proportions in the United States, with over half a million new cases yearly. Chlamydia causes pelvic inflammatory disease, which can then cause sterility. Usually, the first time it strikes, chlamydia does not render a woman sterile. Woman who get the condition once should give up the pill at once."

Symptoms

After 10 years of fertility tests and treatments, Carla Harkness, frustrated by the lack of consumer-oriented literature on the subject, consulted over 100 medical specialists and put together *The Fertility Book*. Harkness sees infertility as an emotional life crisis that is largely unacknowledged by society: "Reactions include grief and mourning, loss of self-esteem, and impaired self-image. Couples often have difficulties communicating with one another. Their sexual relationship is tested and damaged. All in all, it is a traumatic experience."

She adds that an early end to pregnancy, due to miscarriage, produces the same frustrations: "The failure of a fertilized egg to implant is amazingly common. Often up to 50 percent of fertilized eggs do not make it past the initial two-week period to implantation. Up to 20 percent of confirmed pregnancies are miscarried in the first trimester in women under 35 years old. As a woman approaches 40, that number can exceed 25 percent, and by the age of 45, the miscarriage rate is almost 50 percent. The emotional impact of miscarriage is similar to infertility. There is often grief and mourning that are not accepted as genuine mourning in our society. Couples often hear things like, 'I guess it was meant to be,' 'Something was wrong,' or 'You'll have another.' That is often of little solace to someone feeling this kind of loss."

Assisted Reproductive Technology

"The laboratory options have just exploded in the past decade for infertile couples," Harkness reports. "In 1978, the first 'test-tube' baby was born in England through a process called in vitro fertilization. Since then, the process has been instituted worldwide. There are now over 260 clinics practicing some form of that kind of laboratory fertilization, which is now called assisted reproductive technology or ART.

"Now the boundaries have even exceeded menopause. Before you had the practice of donor sperm for artificial insemination. Now there is the ability to fertilize donor eggs from younger women with the husband's sperm, and to implant those eggs in an infertile woman who is over 45 or 50. She is able to carry a child to term that is not genetically related to her. These kinds of options have all become available, and they offer a great deal of hope to many couples."

ETHICAL ISSUES While modern advances in fertility treatments offer a wealth of new possibilities, the other side of the coin is that they raise ethical concerns. "A number of religious groups have raised questions about the intervention of technology in the natural process of reproduction," Harkness explains. "There is also a theme of pronatalism at any cost here, emphasizing that to be complete as couples or as women, people absolutely must birth a biological child. Another big issue revolves around extending maternal age past nature's deadline of menopause. Before, women in their mid-40s probably weren't able to get pregnant because their bodies would stop that function. Now, it is possible for women in their 50s and 60s to become pregnant. This raises such questions as, Is that putting too much demand on their bodies? What about the age difference between them and their children? What about obligations to aging parents while having little ones in midlife? Additionally, there is a legal and moral question revolving around the status of unused, frozen embryos in the event of death and divorce.

"There are further questions surrounding the availability of this expensive technology to those without the means or the medical insurance. Unfortunately, these treatments are quite expensive. From the moment you walk into a specialist's office asking for an evaluation, you start incurring costs in the hundreds of dollars for examinations and tests, all the way to thousands of dollars for the in vitro techniques. It's about $10,000 per cycle for a straight in vitro lab procedure, all the way up to $15,000 if egg donor in vitro fertilization is utilized."

Many women distrust scientific intervention. Problems with IUDs have caused pelvic inflammatory disease resulting in infertility. DES (diethylstilbestrol, an estrogen replacement often used as a "morningafter" pill in the United States, even after it was linked to cancer and anomalies of the vagina and cervix) has been another big problem, as has thalidomide. Now there is a concern about using female hormones to stimulate ovulation. With most infertility treatments, whether the problem is due to the man or woman, it is mainly the women who undergo the drug treatments, the surgeries, and so forth. What are the long-term effects of exposing women to these drugs?

NATURAL OPTIONS Dr. Marjorie Ordene believes that while there is a place for technology in fertility, women are too quick to seek out these methods, and suggests trying these natural options first:

LEARNING TO RECOGNIZE OVULATION

Women should learn to recognize their time of ovulation by taking their temperature first thing in the morning, before getting out of bed: "Usually, temperature rises in the second half of the cycle, two weeks before menstruation. The mucus that is produced around the time of ovulation has a clear and slippery quality. This is the kind of mucus that is needed for the sperm to penetrate the cervix."

HEALTHY LIFESTYLE

Women should follow a healthy diet and a basic exercise program.

EMOTIONAL AND SPIRITUAL WORK

Often, a woman has apprehensions about becoming pregnant that need to be addressed. It may be reassuring to talk to the inner child and let her know that even though there will be another child, the little girl in her will still get the attention she needs. This kind of spiritual work is often important in achieving pregnancy.

Eastern Naturopathic Approach to Fertility

The traditional Eastern approach to fertility depends less on modern technology, and more on time-tested knowledge. Dr. Roger Hirsch, a naturopathic physician from Santa Monica, California, explains Chinese philosophy and infertility treatments based on this point of view: "We look at making the abdomen happy. This is an aphorism for correcting the digestion, menstruation, and hormones, so that women can conceive. Of course, raising the man's sperm count and sperm motility is important as well, because it is not just the woman who is infertile in an infertility situation. A key to this is the way the blood flows in the pelvic cavity."

INCREASING PELVIC BLOOD FLOW A study of endometriosis-induced infertility was performed in China and published in the *Shanghai Journal of Traditional Chinese Medicine and Medicinals* in 1994. Forty patients were treated with neon laser acupuncture, retention enemas, and injection into the endometrial nodes with common sage root, which is a blood-vitalizing or blood-moving herb. In the 40 patients treated, the size of lumps diminished and symptoms disappeared in 17. Thirteen women conceived. Among these, six had suffered from fallopian tube blockage and seven from ovulatory dysfunction. There was a total amelioration rate of 97.5 percent.

SEXUAL HYGIENE Another important consideration in reversing endometriosis and infertility is good sexual hygiene. There was a study done with Israeli women several years ago that showed them to have a low percentage of endometriosis as a cultural group. This was related to sexual hygienic laws in the orthodox Jewish religion which says that you can't be with a man during menstruation. Chinese medicine says the same thing. Having intercourse during menstruation causes an imbalance of energy and results in the migration of endometrial tissue into the pelvic cavity.

HERBS In Chinese medicine, herbs are used to tone renal/adrenal function because reproductive function is related to the kidney and its related complex. The actual viability of the eggs for a woman over 40 is related to kidney yang function.

One of the herbs very good for kidney yang is called herba epimeti, which translates in English to "horny goat weed." This is an aphrodisiac that the Chinese discovered by watching goats become sexually active after eating this particular plant. They put the plant into the herbal formula for women who are kidney yang deficient, and they noted that it increased sexual desire.

Deer antler is a renewable resource from the deer, which grows every year. Lutaigou is the gelatin that comes from boiling the deer antler. This is wonderful for helping women over 40 who are trying to extend their egg-producing years. It helps slow down the biological clock.

In the European system, we have wormwood, which creates more circulation in the pelvic cavity. The Chinese use this along with daughter seed and fructose litchi, a little red berry.

A lot of people know about dong quai. This helps the circulation in the pelvic cavity. Also used is cortex cinnamomi, which is not the cinnamon you put in your mulled cider, but a thick bark cinnamon.

ACUPUNCTURE In China, acupuncture has been used in the treatment of infertility for centuries. The first published account of this is seen in medical literature dating back to 11 A.D. The Chinese look at five principal organs—the liver, spleen, heart, lung, and kidney—and use acupuncture to release blockages from these systems so that energy or *chi* can move freely. This helps the body return to good health. Promoting fertility is one benefit that can be obtained.

Acupuncture to kidney points releases psychological blocks that interfere with reproduction. Dr. Roger Hirsch uses the treatment to help patients overcome deep-rooted fears connected to sexual abuse: "If there has been early abuse, rape, or incest, there sometimes is a problem with hormone maturation. In other words, fear causes the hormones to become dormant. This is related to the kidney, as this organ controls reproductive function, endocrine function, and hormonal function. I needle points along the kidney meridian to help establish a connection between the heart and the uterus. I also use the Bach flower remedies walnut and crab apple. Walnut breaks links, and crab apple cleanses."

Dr. Hirsch connects another psychological issue—low self-esteem—to endometriosis and infertility: "In treating self-esteem issues, I work on the heart and kidney points. The acupuncture points that seem extremely valuable for this are pericardium 5 and 6. If a practitioner is having a problem with understanding whether or not a psychological issue is involved in the infertility, and the patient does not know what the issue is, pericardium 5 can be needled. If something is holding the person back, that will bring an event or dream to memory, and the patient will understand why she is stuck. In treating self-esteem issues, we may also release stress by needling the heart 7 point, heart 9, and sometimes heart 7 to heart 5.

"We also address conception vessel 17, which is between the breasts. This is a very important place for women because it opens their energy. It also helps relieve liver *chi* congestion or stuckness. Remember, the liver and the liver hormones, both in Chinese and Western medicine, govern the flow of blood in the pelvic cavity."

Additional Naturopathic Approaches

Dr. Joseph Pizzorno says that as a naturopath and midwife he saw numerous infertile couples and discovered two causes of the condition that were not generally recognized by the orthodox medical profession. "The first was pituitary insufficiency. The pituitary gland was not secreting enough of the hormones needed to stimulate the ovaries to mature, ripen and produce a viable ovum. Most of these women had been on birth control pills for long periods of time. Even though they had been off it for several years, their pituitary never functioned fully again."

"With these women I did two things. I gave them an herbal concoction using herbs that are commonly used for women's health problems, which are supposed to stimulate proper pituitary functioning. I also gave them raw pituitary gland from an animal. There were surprisingly good results with this treatment. A urine test beforehand measured the level of hormones from the pituitary. If a patient had low hormone levels, I would then use this protocol with them. A surprising number became pregnant once their urinary hormone levels returned to normal.

"The second major cause was pelvic inflammatory disease, where there were infections in the fallopian tubes, the little tubes that go from the uterus to the ovaries. Infections leave scars. Then the ovum cannot penetrate the tube and get into the uterus for fertilization.

"An age-old hydrotherapy procedure, called sitz bath, helps end this problem. A woman gets two big pots of water. (We use washtubs that are about three feet in diameter.) One tub gets filled with hot water (as hot as she can stand it).

When a woman sits in it with her arms and legs out of the tub, the water level reaches her umbilicus. The other tub gets filled with ice cold water. That tub is filled to the point just below the umbilicus. In other words, there is more hot water than cold water. The woman sits in the hot water for five minutes, and then in the cold water for one minute. She alternates back and forth three times.

"The first time a woman does this, she will find it startling. But after a while she will actually start to like it. She does this every day. After a few treatments, she starts getting a discharge. As near as we can make out, this discharge is the body throwing off scar tissue and toxic material in the ovaries. This is a particularly dangerous time for a woman to have intercourse. The ovaries are starting to open up, and there is a high probability of an ectopic pregnancy. The egg will only be able to go partway down the tube since the tube is not yet open enough for it to get all the way into the uterus. We therefore tell women no unprotected intercourse for at least three months while doing these treatments every day. Again, a surprising number of them become pregnant."

RESTORING THYROID BALANCE Even as far back as the 1930s, alleviating low thyroid conditions was found effective against infertility. Dr. Ray Peat, author of *Nutrition for Women*, says, "Over the last five years, I have worked with quite a few women, some who have tried for as long as 10 years to get pregnant. Several had spent as much as $100,000 on other treatments. Consistently, within a few weeks of correcting their thyroid, they get pregnant."

To keep thyroid levels up, women should snack frequently and eliminate unsaturated fats. Although touted as beneficial, recent studies show them to inhibit thyroid secretion. More high-quality protein may be needed, especially by women following a weight loss program or vegetarian diet. A daily minimum of 40 grams is recommended. Taking a thyroid supplement for a short period of time can greatly help. "People whose thyroid function is suppressed can benefit from a week or two of thyroid supplementation," Dr. Peat advises. "They don't need to take this indefinitely."

NATURAL HYGIENE Dr. Anthony Penepent practices natural hygiene which he has known about his whole life. In fact, he says that it made his own birth possible: "Members of my family were natural hygienists before I was born. Back in the 40s, my mother fasted for 30 days at Dr. Christopher John Cursio's hospital in Rochester, New York, the Castle of Health, so that she could conceive and retain pregnancy."

Dr. Penepent follows the principles of natural hygiene when treating any medical condition: "Over the years, I have seen many wonderful things happen with natural hygiene which would not have been possible with allopathic medicine." Explaining infertility, Dr. Penepent says there are many causes, but that all of them can be treated similarly: "There are many mechanisms that can come into play. You can have basic amenorrhea or failure to ovulate. You can have any variety of hormonal imbalances, or fallopian tube obstruction. In 40 percent of the cases it is not the woman's fault, although she may take the blame to save her husband's ego. The man may have a low sperm count, depressed sperm motility, or abnormal sperm morphology. These are all possibilities. Then again, conception may occur but the egg or ovum may not have sufficient nutrients for the embryo to develop. What happens then is you have unrecognized spontaneous abortions that make it appear as if the woman is infertile, when in actuality she just has a nutritional deficiency.

"In many cases, an infertile woman can conceive and go on to have a successful pregnancy with a minor amount of dietary change. In the case of the fallopian tube obstruction, it may be necessary for her to fast for several days. I remember one patient, a rabbi's wife, who was childless. Because of their religious beliefs, it was absolutely essential for her to bear children. In her particular case, I put her on a fast for several days and followed that up with a nutritional regimen. She was able to conceive within six months."

SUPPLEMENTS The right nutrients can make a difference in whether or not pregnancy is possible:

Colloidal silver. When chlamydia is causing infertility, colloidal silver helps to clean up the system.

Vitamin E. High doses of vitamin E balance hormone production. Under the guidance of a health care professional, an individual should start slowly and gradually increase dosage.

On the Research Front

Promising substances for the treatment of fertility are sarsaparilla root; kelp, which is used for this purpose in Asia; 6-methoxybenzoxazolinone (6-MBOA), a nonestrogenic component of young rapidly growing plants. Chinese drugs in combination with clomiphene citrate and progesterone have proved more effective than treatment with either Chinese or Western drugs alone, and a Chinese technique combining moxibustion and acupuncture has had some success in treating infertility. Factors shown to contribute to difficulty conceiving are smoking, even moderately; exposure to nitrous oxide; and environmental hazards like pesticides, methyl mercury, and lead in tap water.

53

Infections

Vaginal Yeast Syndrome (Candidiasis)

Dr. William Crook, author of *The Yeast Connection and Women*, says that yeast overgrowth is the result of antibiotics, and that women are especially susceptible: "The yeast we're talking about normally live in the body of every man, woman, and child. It's called Candida albicans. When you are healthy, there are no problems, but when you take a lot of antibiotic drugs you begin to get complications. Antibiotics knock out the normal, friendly bacteria while they are fighting off enemies. As a result the yeast overgrows, and a woman may get a vaginal yeast infection, a child may develop thrush or diaper rash, and a man or woman may get bloating, constipation, and digestive symptoms.

"But that's not the major problem. This yeast puts out toxins that weaken the immune system. It so disturbs the interior membrane of the intestinal tract that you absorb food allergens that would normally be excreted. People truly become sick all over."

CAUSES "There are several reasons why a woman is more susceptible to yeast infections than a man," says Dr. Crook. "Since her genitalia is internal, yeast is able to grow on the warm anterior membranes of the body. The little tube going from the urinary bladder to the outside is only a fraction of an inch in a woman, whereas in a man it is many inches long. This allows the bacteria to get up into the woman's bladder much more easily. Women have 50 times more urinary tract infections than men, and they are given antibiotic drugs as treatment.

Birth control pills further promote yeast growth. So does pregnancy. And teenage girls with a few pimples on their face are much more likely to run to the dermatologist and get tetracycline, an antibiotic that makes yeast grow."

Nutritionist Gracia Perlstein adds these causes to the list: "Some women are susceptible at the end of each month's menstrual flow. Low estrogen levels present at menopause, and also pregnancy, where the rate of infection can be as high as 20 percent toward the end. Also women who have diabetes have an increased risk.

"Stress is another factor. Many people have two or three jobs. They are running around, eating on the run, not really paying attention to their diet. When people do that, they tend also to overdo sweets and processed foods that weaken the immunity and set up a perfect environment for the candida overgrowth."

Complementary physician Dr. Robert Sorge says candida is the result of drug pollution. In addition to antibiotic overuse mentioned earlier, he adds the following: "The most likely candidate for candida overgrowth is a person who has been on steroids, hormone medication, cortisone, the entire gamut of prescriptions and over-the-counter drugs, especially ulcer medications like Tagamet and Zantac, and oral contraceptives. As far as I'm concerned, the sugar and junk food diet that most people have is also a drug."

SYMPTOMS Classical symptoms of a yeast infection are itching, redness, irritation, and a cottage-cheese-like curdly white discharge. Symptoms are not always obvious, but a gynecologist can often confirm whether or not a yeast infection exists by looking at a smear under the microscope or creating a culture to see if yeast colonies form.

Clearing up immediate symptoms is relatively simple. Many over-the-counter preparations, including homeopathic remedies, exist for that purpose. The trick, according to Dr. Marjorie Ordene, a holistic gynecologist from Brooklyn, New York, is to treat the overall yeast syndrome, not just the local infection. "Often the vaginal itching will be the impetus for the person to come to the doctor, but it is not the only problem they have. Unless the whole person is treated, the yeast is bound to recur." Dr. Ordene breaks down symptoms of a yeast syndrome into five categories:

General symptoms: low energy and fatigue, brain fog, depression, headaches, muscle and joint paints, memory loss, extreme sensitivity to chemicals, recurrent urinary infections, light-headedness.

Digestive symptoms: gas, bloating, intermittent constipation and diarrhea, indigestion, intestinal cramps.

Respiratory symptoms: chronic post nasal drip, frequent coughs, sore throats, colds, asthma, allergies.

Skin problems: eczema, itching, rashes, fungal infections.

Hormonal problems: menstrual irregularities, menstrual cramps, premenstrual syndrome, mood swings, problems with the endocrine glands, hypothyroidism, hypoglycemia or diabetes.

DIAGNOSIS Since the intestines serve as a reservoir for much of the yeast, a stool study may reveal an overgrowth. Excess yeast here indicates that yeast is present in other parts of the body, including the vagina, and causing recurrent yeast infections.

A simple skin test may reveal a yeast allergy as well. Red or itchy skin indicates a problem. Often the results are seen quickly, within 10 to 15 minutes, although sometimes there is a delayed reaction or none at all.

These tests are not always reliable, according to Dr. William Crook: "Although we physicians generally like to have a test that can say you do or do not have a particular condition, such as a chest x-ray to see whether your heart is enlarged, there is not presently a single, simple laboratory test that can say whether you do or do not have a yeast-related problem. If a woman has a vaginal infection, a lab study of the secretion may help identify the yeast. Sometimes a culture may. But they are not 100 percent accurate. They may not be more than 50 percent accurate. There are studies done on stools because yeast grows there, but those are not reliable either. The best we can do is to suspect it, and then to note the response of a person to a sugar-free special diet, and oral antiyeast medication, both prescription and nonprescription."

ALTERNATIVE THERAPIES FOR YEAST INFECTIONS

A YEAST-FREE DIET

A yeast-free diet is both diagnostic and therapeutic. If a woman feels better when following the diet, this indicates a yeast sensitivity. The diet should be observed for several weeks at a minimum, and may be followed indefinitely. Some people feel much better and choose to eat this way permanently. Foods can be added back gradually, however, to see their effect. If symptoms recur, the reintroduced food should be avoided.

Avoid sweets. The relationship between sugar and yeast was seen in a study performed at St. Jude Hospital in Memphis, Tennessee, where mice who were fed sugar had 200 times greater yeast concentration than mice who were not. Yeast feeds on sugar, causing many symptoms, especially digestive problems such as gas and bloating. Avoiding sugar entails more than just not adding granulated sugar to cereal or tea; it means checking labels and staying away from corn syrup, maltose, artificial sweeteners, fructose, corn starch, sodas, and lactose, a milk sugar found in dairy products.

Avoid foods containing yeasts and molds. These include baked foods such as breads, muffins, cakes, cookies, and other refined carbohydrates, commercial fruit juices, tomato sauce (unless homemade with fresh tomatoes), foods containing vinegar, pickled foods, smoked foods, alcohol, fermented foods, smoked meats, dried fruits, mushrooms (except for shiitake), pistachio nuts, and peanuts. Leftovers may be moldy as well.

What you can eat are healthful foods that do not contain yeasts and molds. Included are whole grains, such as brown rice, millet, amaranth, quinoa, and barley, as well as fresh vegetables. Lots of steamed green vegetables are particularly beneficial because they are abundant in purifying chlorophyll. Also allowed are sea vegetables, whole wheat matzo, sourdough rye bread, popcorn, tortillas, tofu, miso, plain yogurt, lean meats, fresh fish, organically fed, free-range poultry and eggs from free-range chickens. Organic extra virgin olive oil, when used sparingly, can inhibit yeast overgrowth, according to recent studies. Raw garlic or lightly cooked garlic helps get rid of candida in the intestines.

SUPPLEMENTS

Sometimes diet alone is not enough. After all, yeast has been in the body for years. These supplements provide additional needed help:

Flora. The flora found in lactobacillus acidophilus and bifida bacteria can be taken in powder form or as sugar-free yogurt. The effectiveness of flora was noted in a New York Medical School study of women with recurrent vaginal yeast infections. Those eating sugar-free yogurt had fewer infections than those who did not. Flora repopulate the intestinal tract with good bacteria, which in turn crowd out the yeast. The effects of flora are temporary, so the powder or yogurt should be consumed on a daily basis.

Antifungal, antiyeast agents. Over-the-counter preparations, such as citrus seed extract, kyolic garlic, caprylic acid, pau d'arco, and berberine, may be helpful. Sometimes prescription agents such as nystatin are needed. These remedies get rid of excess yeast only. Since they are not absorbed into the blood, they are safe to take, even during pregnancy and while nursing.

Homeopathic candida. Helps desensitize the body to yeast.

Garlic suppositories. Simple insertion of a clove of garlic into the vagina has a powerful healing effect. *The New Our Bodies, Ourselves* suggests that the clove should be peeled but not nicked, and then wrapped in gauze before inserting.

A strong body is better able to rebalance its health. In addition to supplements that target yeast infections specifically, these nutrients provide overall nutritional support:

Multivitamin/mineral supplement. Formulas containing zinc, magnesium, yeast-free vitamins, trace minerals, and essential fatty acids boost immune function and help prevent recurrent yeast infections.

Chlorophyll cleanses the intestines and purifies the blood.

Essential fatty acids. 3,000 mg of evening primrose, borage, or black currant seed oil daily in three divided doses, or one tablespoon of organic flaxseed oil. (Never cook flaxseed oil, and keep refrigerated.)

Vitamin C. 3,000–5,000 mg daily in three divided doses helps fight infections.
B complex. 50–100 mg with each meal combats stress.

HERBS

The following Oriental and Western formulas can help alleviate yeast problems:

Digestive Harmony and Herbastatin. Digestive Harmony is a combination of bitter herbs that work together to cleanse the digestive tract and other internal organs of yeast infections. Herbastatin gets rid of yeast caused by phlegm.

Yudaiwan. This Chinese remedy helps to eliminate creamy discharges.

Ku shen. Used as a wash to clean the vagina.

Garlic. Excellent for fighting infections. Can be eaten raw, lightly cooked, or taken in capsule form. Odorless brands are sold in health food stores.

Black walnut tincture. Thirty drops three times daily, added to water before meals.

Pau d'arco. This has wonderful immune-enhancing and antifungal properties. As a tea, three to four cups can be taken daily.

Summa. This is another good herbal tea for helping the immune system.

Also helpful are goldenseal, bearberry, Oregon grape, German chamomile, aloe vera, rosemary, ginger, alfalfa, red clover, and fennel.

COLON THERAPY

"My battle with candida lasted a long time," says colon therapist Tovah Finman-Nahman. "I tried everything, including a strict diet, antifungals, and vitamin C drips. But I never got it under control until I started doing colonics. Then I saw quick results. The gas and the bloating went away, and my chronic fatigue amazingly disappeared. I have seen similar results with a lot of people who come to see me. I can't stress how good colonics are."

What makes colon therapy such an effective treatment? First, it creates a clean internal environment. "We want a good environment so that flora can grow and flourish. That is paramount when we have candida overgrowth," says Finman-Nahman. Second, colonics calm an irritated colon: "Herbs can be added to the water, such as pau d'arco, which has antifungal properties. Yellow dock can also be added to soothe any inflammation. Fennel can be used to dissipate gas and eliminate the bloating that a lot of people with candida tend to get. Aloe vera gel is absolutely wonderful. It is very soothing to an inflamed colon. And of course, it can be taken orally in the form of aloe vera juice.

"In conjunction with colonics, psyllium can be taken orally. This moisturizes impacted fecal material in the congested colon, which further aids cleaning.

"People ask, 'How many colonics should I get?' That depends on the individual. The more the merrier. For a healthy person I recommend at least 10 in a series, and then a maintenance program. Sometimes, it can take as long as six months to get candida under control because it is a very hearty bacteria. When yeast is at the point of being candidiasis, it can grow through the colon walls and run rampant. The more we cleanse, the better our chance of getting it under control and regaining health."

AROMATHERAPY

Tea tree oil is scientifically shown to be antifungal, antiyeast, and antiviral. One tablespoon of the oil added to a pint of water, and used in a douche, helps to eliminate yeast infections. This can be followed with the placement of acidophilus tablets or capsules into the vagina to reestablish proper vaginal bacteria.

LIFESTYLE FACTORS

Nutritionist Gracia Perlstein notes these important habits for minimizing the incidence of vaginal infections:

Wear underpants with a cotton crotch so that air can circulate. Avoid pantyhose or any tight-fitting clothing for the same reason.

Develop good toilet habits of always wiping from front to back. This keeps anal bacteria from entering the vagina. Avoid feminine hygiene sprays and powders, which can cause irritation. Douching is not necessary; a healthy vagina is naturally clean.

Keep stress under control. Take a few deep breaths. Go for a brisk walk in the open air. Do something to alleviate the stress that builds up.

HOMEOPATHY

Since homeopathy treatments are chosen according to symptoms, deciding on a remedy depends on the quality of the discharge and the sensations, according to Dr. Ken Korins. Here he offers some of the major remedies for vaginal yeast infections:

Pulsatilla. This remedy is often indicated in vaginitis. The woman has a thick, yellowish-to-green discharge. Sometimes the consistency is milky or creamy. Mentally, she is often moody, gentle, and weepy, and craves sympathy.

Silica. The main symptom is an itching of the vulva and vagina. It is sensitive to touch. The discharge tends to be thin, and sometimes curdly.

Kreosotum. The person has violent symptoms. Discharges are excoriating, burning is profuse, and there is a foul odor, as well as violent itching and a burning and swelling of the labia. Discharge tends to be yellow and may actually be a watery, bloody type of consistency.

Hephera sulph. Symptoms are similar to silica, but more chronic. There is itching of the vagina, particularly after sexual intercourse, and it often has an odor similar to that of old cheese. Both hephera sulph and silica can be used to treat sores or cysts, particularly Bartholin cysts.

Kali bichromium. Here discharges tend to be thick, green, and sometimes jellylike.

Alumina. Discharge is thick and transparent.

Nitric acid. Helps when there are sores or ulcers on the vaginal mucosa. The sensation tends to be a sharp, sticking pain. Discharges are brown. Often, there is a stain on underwear that leaves a yellow perimeter.

Mercurius. The discharges are excoriating but greenish and bloody. There is a sensation of rawness.

Medorrhinum. Discharge is thick and acrid, with a sensation way up in the uterus.

Herpes

In the 1970s herpes was a cause for widespread concern, but it took a back seat to AIDS in the 1980s and 1990s. While not as deadly, herpes is more prevalent, causing pain to most of those afflicted. Over half the population gets cold sores from time to time, the result of herpes simplex virus 1 (HSV1). Others become afflicted with shingles, a herpes zoster infection, years after they get chicken pox. Additionally, people get Epstein-Barr, the form of herpes that causes mononucleosis. Still others break out in genital herpes, an infection caused by herpes simplex virus 2 (HSV2). All in all, the number of men and women with herpes is greater than 80 percent.

CAUSES Herpes is a contagious virus that lives at the base of the spine in the nerve cells. Periodic attacks occur whenever the immune system is below par. Any kind of emotional, mental, or physical stress can lower the body's defense system and create the perfect climate for an outbreak. Common physical stressors include illness, menstrual periods, vaginal yeast infections, too much sunlight or friction (which breaks down skin cells), allergies, and certain foods. Genital herpes can be sexually transmitted. Pregnant mothers can transmit the virus to their unborn children via blood or through direct contact with infected tissue during delivery. Prescription drugs that lower immunity can set off an attack: such medications include antibiotics, steroids, and antidepressants.

SYMPTOMS Genital herpes causes surface sores on the skin and lining of the genital area. In women, sores can appear on the cervix, vagina, or perineum, which may be accompanied by a discharge or vaginal blisters. There is often a burning sensation, especially at the onset of an outbreak. Other symptoms may include urinary problems, fever, and lymphatic swelling. Intercourse is painful and should be avoided during an outbreak to prevent sexual transmission. HSV2 occurs intermittently and usually lasts from five to seven days.

As the name implies, oral herpes tends to attack the skin and mucous membranes on the face, particularly around the mouth and nose. These cold sores tend to appear as pearl-like blisters. Although they are short-term, they can be irritating and painful. Herpes zoster, the result of the varicella zoster virus, causes agonizing blisters on one side of the body, usually on the chest or abdomen. Pain is usually felt before effects are seen, the result of overly sensitive skin covering the affected nerve. Symptoms may last from a few days to several weeks.

CONVENTIONAL TREATMENT FOR HERPES There is no conventional medical cure for herpes, although drugs are commonly given to lessen symptoms. The most famous of these is acyclovir, also known as Zovirax, which supposedly reduces the rate of growth of the herpes virus. Herpes medications have many potential side effects, including dizziness, headaches, diarrhea, nausea, vomiting, general weakness, fatigue, ill health, sore throat, fever, insomnia, swelling, tenderness, and bleeding of the gums. In addition, acyclovir ointment can cause allergic skin reactions.

NATURAL REMEDIES Herpes sufferers will be glad to learn that natural remedies are often highly effective in shortening the length of outbreaks and in diminishing their frequency. Following are some of the important ones to know about.

NUTRITION AND LIFESTYLE CHANGES

When herpes strikes, it is always a good idea to rest and eat lightly. Short fruit fasts, with plenty of pure water and cleansing herbal teas, can be very helpful. Good herbs to include are sage, rosemary, cayenne, echinacea, goldenseal, red clover, astragalus, and burdock root. Beneficial bacteria, such as those found in non-dairy yogurt, or supplements of lactobacillus and acidophilus, support the digestive processes necessary for the maintenance of the immune system. Other nutrients that directly enhance the immune system include garlic, quercetin, zinc gluconate, buffered vitamin C, and beta carotene or vitamin A. In addition, 500 mg of the amino acid L-lysine, taken two to four times a day, can produce excellent results. Bee propolis is anti-inflammatory, while B vitamins combat stress. Also good are bee pollen, blue-green algae, and pycnogenol.

Nervous system stressors, such as caffeine, alcohol, and hard-to-digest foods like meat, should be avoided, especially at the onset of an attack. Foods high in the amino acid arginine, such as chocolate, peanut butter, nuts, and onions, are also associated with higher incidences of outbreaks.

Since stress promotes outbreaks, it is important to make time for activities that alleviate tension. Many possibilities include biofeedback, yoga, meditation, deep breathing, and exercise.

Toothbrushes should be changed frequently, and completely dried before reuse to prevent reinfection. Soaking them in baking soda also fights germs.

HOMEOPATHY

According to Dr. Erika Price, a practitioner of classical homeopathy and holistic healing, classical homeopathy is the most effective form of treatment for people with the herpes virus: "The properly chosen remedy will motivate and empower the individual's own defense systems to fight back against anything harmful to it," she claims. Unlike orthodox medicine, homeopathy does not suppress ailments. This is very important because when you suppress a disease, it doesn't go away but goes somewhere else deeper inside of you. Deeper means it goes to a more important organ than the skin. Homeopathy has no adverse effects and can only be of benefit. When the patient's physical, mental, and spiritual nature are taken into account, a cure can be found. The following remedies may prove extremely helpful:

For cold sores:

Natrum muriaticum. When sores are on the lips, especially in the middle of the lips, the 30c potency should be taken twice a day.

Phosphorus. Cold sores that manifest above the lips, accompanied by itching, cutting, and sharp pain, need the 30c potency twice a day.

Petroleum. For cold sores that erupt in patches and become crusty and loose around the lips and mouth, petroleum is indicated. A 9c potency is needed three times a day.

Apis. Apis helps cold sores around the mouth and lips that are accompanied by stinging, and painful blisters that itch and burn. A 6c potency is needed three to four times daily.

For female genital herpes:

Natrum muriaticum. This is indicated when the herpetic lesions are pearllike blisters and the genital area feels puffy, hot, and very dry. A 6c potency may be beneficial when taken four times a day.

Dulcamara. Women who tend to get a herpes outbreak in clusters on the vulva or on the hair follicles around the labia and vulva every time they catch a cold or get their period probably need dulcamara in a 12c potency two to three times a day.

Petroleum. This may help if herpes eruptions form in patches and the sores become deep red and feel tender and moist. Outbreaks usually occur during menstrual periods, and most often affect the perineum, anus, labia, or vulva. A 9c potency should be taken three times a day.

For shingles:

Arsenicum album. This benefits most cases of shingles, especially when the individual feels worse in the cold, worse after midnight, and better with warmth. If taken at the onset of an attack, it is best taken in a 30c potency twice a day for two to three days. After the first three days, arsenicum album is indicated if there is a burning sensation in the areas that were affected by the zoster eruptions (typically the chest and abdomen). At this point 12c, taken two to three times a day, is best. This remedy is excellent for the getting rid of the burning sensation that is often present.

Hypericum perforatum. This is a wonderful remedy for any kind of nerve pain. It is indicated whenever there is intense neuritis and neuralgia, with burning, tin-

gling and numbness along the course of the affected nerves. Hypericum perforatum should be taken in a 30c potency, two to three times a day, as needed.

When taking homeopathic remedies, Dr. Price reminds patients to not
touch them directly, as that may disturb the vibration of the medicine. Rather,
they should be placed under the tongue until dissolved. Coffee, mint, camphor,
and chamomile must be avoided, as they work against the remedies. It is also
important to note symptoms; as they change, so must the remedy.

AROMATHERAPY

The use of essential oils has recently gained popularity in the United States,
where it is used widely in skin and body care products. But its medicinal value
has long been accepted in other countries, particularly France, where, in many
instances, its antimicrobial properties make it an acceptable replacement for
drug therapy. Aromatherapist Valerie Cooksley, author of *Aromatherapy: A
Lifetime Guide to Healing with Essential Oils*, says that pure essential oils, properly used, can heal cold and canker sores. One mouthwash she recommends
combines five drops each of peppermint, bergamot, or tea tree oil to raw honey,
which is used as a carrier. This is important, as oils do not mix with water alone.
The mixture is then added to a strong sage or rosemary tea. Rinsing with the
formula several times a day balances the pH of the mouth and helps to heal
infections. Using this daily may even prevent outbreaks.

Additional spot treatments alleviate pain and restore health. One that
Cooksley recommends involves dabbing a cotton swab with myrrh oil and
applying directly onto cold and canker sores. Another aromatherapist, Sharon
Olson, dabs a cotton swab with diluted tea tree oil and places that on the cold
sore to kill the virus. She follows this up later with lavender, which soothes the
sore and stimulates the growth of new skin. The addition of fresh aloe vera gel
further promotes healing. A side benefit of the therapy is its ability to lift the
spirits. "When I get a cold sore, I get depressed," reveals Olson, "so I usually
inhale some rosemary or basil to lift my spirits and clear my mind."

HERBS

Plants containing phytochemicals with antiherpes properties, in order of
potency:

> *Myrciaria dubia* (camu-camu)
> *Glycyrrhiza glabra* (licorice), plant
> *Viola tricolor hortensis* (pansy)
> *Sophora japonica* (Japanese pagoda tree), bud
> *Oenothera biennis* (evening primrose)
> *Malpighia glabra* (acerola)
> *Glycyrrhiza glabra* (licorice), root
> *Sophora japonica* (Japanese pagoda tree), flower
> *Coffea arabica* (coffee)

Aesculus hippocastanum (horse chestnut)
Rhizophora mangle (red mangrove)
Citrus limon (lemon)
Camellia sinensis (tea)
Abrus precatorius (crab's eyes)
Podophyllum hexandrum (Himalayan mayapple)
Mangifera indica (mango)
Origanum vulgare (wild oregano)
Phyllanthus emblica (emblic)
Allium cepa (onion)

Urinary Tract Infections and Inflammations

Urinary tract infections (also known as cystitis and bladder infections) are quite common, accounting for approximately six million office visits per year in the United States. E. coli and other bacteria that inhabit the large intestine are most often responsible, due to the closeness of the urethra and vagina to the rectum.

Dr. Jennifer Brett, a naturopathic physician from Stratford, Connecticut, says only 60 percent of people with symptoms of urinary tract infections (UTI) have true infections; the other 40 percent have inflammations. Three types of infections and inflammations that Dr. Brett commonly sees are true urinary tract infections, urinary tract inflammations, and interstitial cystitis, a more distressing form of inflammation that can last for months or even years.

CAUSES The cause of urinary tract inflammations is unknown, but some doctors believe it may be due to viruses, food allergies, candida in the colon, hormonal changes, new sexual partners, or vigorous sexual activity. Similarly, some believe that interstitial cystitis may be from candida or allergic reactions to foods and additives. "These irritants inflame the pelvis and bladder, and the body responds by increasing blood flow to the area," Dr. Brett explains. "Pelvic congestion causes further irritation and pressure on the bladder. Again, the body responds by sending more blood. This becomes a vicious cycle."

HIGH-RISK GROUPS

Dr. David Kauffman, a specialist in women's urological problems, says that there are basically four types of women at high risk: "The most common patients are young, sexually active females. Another large group at risk are post-menopausal women. In fact, 8 to 10 percent of all women over 60 will get a bladder infection at some point. We also see a lot of patients who are hospitalized. The risk of bladder infection increases about 5 percent per day for every day that a catheter is in place. For this reason, medical doctors try to get catheters out as quickly as possible. The last high-risk group are patients with neurological problems. An example would be multiple sclerosis, where patients do not completely empty their bladder.

"Many sexually active women get cystitis as a result of intercourse because the bacteria that normally live in the vaginal vault area get pushed up into the urethra. A woman's urethra is only about an inch and a half long, while in men it is much longer. In females, it doesn't take too much for bacteria to migrate from the outside of the urethra to the inside of the bladder. That's why we see so many more young women with bladder infections.

"It is very important for women to know that their partners are not giving them infections. The bacteria starts in their vaginal area and simply gets pushed into the bladder during intercourse."

HORMONAL IMBALANCE

"You might be asking yourself, why don't all sexually active women get bladder infections? There are many reasons for this. One of the more interesting ones has to do with the woman's hormonal environment. We know that there are estrogen and progesterone receptors on the lining cells of the urethra. In some women bacteria sticks to these receptors due to hormone levels. Imagine bacteria as little organisms with Velcro hooks. Picture the lining cells of the urethra with the opposite kind of hooks. Bacteria just hooks on to the Velcro on the receptor sites. In most women, the urinary stream washes away most bacteria. But in these women, the hormonal environment will not allow for it to be expelled that easily. These are the women we see in our office with recurrent bladder infections."

Dr. Kauffman adds that postmenopausal women tend to get urinary tract infections for this reason as well. Their low estrogen levels cause their urethral linings to be "stickier" for bacteria. "One way to treat that is simply to administer low-dosage estrogen cream into the vaginal vault, about once a week," he advises. "Many women are on estrogen pills, but that does not have the same protective influence on the urinary tract as does estrogen cream."

WEAKENED IMMUNITY

Dr. Linda Wharton, a naturopathic physician and acupuncturist from New Zealand and author of *Natural Woman Health: A Guide to Healthy Living for Women of All Ages*, says that recurrent bladder infections reflect a state of lowered immunity and weakened vitality: "Remember that cystitis is an infection, and as in the case with all infections, individuals with lowered nutritional status, poor cellular health, and lowered immunity are much more susceptible to its threat. Women don't always develop acute cystitis each time a stray bacteria finds its way into the bladder. As is often the case with many other genitourinary infections, it is common to play host to these potentially problem-causing bacteria for weeks or months or even a lifetime without them actually resulting in acute symptoms. It is only when the health of the whole body is reduced that an explosion of this bacterial population takes place. This may occur, for example, when a woman goes through a period of great stress, such as a divorce or the death of a loved one."

STRUCTURAL PROBLEMS

Dr. Wharton adds that other causes of cystitis are often overlooked: "Pelvic floor muscles can weaken as a result of pregnancy and childbirth. When these muscles are weakened, the bladder may prolapse and bulge forward into the wall of the vagina. If the back part of the bladder droops below the neck of the bladder, it becomes virtually impossible to empty the bladder properly. This leaves an almost permanent reservoir of urine in the bladder. In time, the stagnant urine becomes a haven for bacteria to multiply, should they be present."

Dr. Wharton further states that a prolapsed transverse colon, brought on by childbirth, age, abdominal fat, poor posture, and spinal problems, can result in bladder compression. In time this can cause the transverse colon, which lies across the abdomen, to sag, compressing the organs beneath it, including the bladder. Blood flow is impeded, and the oxygen-starved bladder becomes ripe for infection. She adds, "This same downgrading of tissue health can occur as a direct result of a chronic back problem. All the pelvic organs receive nervous impulses from the spine, and a chronic lower back problem can interfere with these nervous impulses from the spinal cord." Wharton advises women with these concerns to see an osteopath or chiropractor.

CONSTIPATION

According to Dr. Wharton, "Waste materials are excreted from our bodies through several different channels. The bowels excrete in the form of feces; the lungs gets rid of toxins in the form of carbon dioxide; the skin eliminates toxins as perspiration; and the kidney and bladder pass toxins out in the form of urine. If any one of these waste disposal systems is functioning inadequately, it places an excessive load on the others. If you only manage a half-hearted bowel movement every two or three days, you are placing undue stress on your kidneys and bladder, as accumulated toxins are passed out this way instead. In a sense, then, there is actually a direct link between chronic constipation and repeated urinary tract infections."

SYMPTOMS Typical symptoms of urinary tract infections and inflammations are frequent urination, a sensation that the bladder is never quite empty, and a burning sensation upon urination. Often women get up at night to urinate. There may be cramps, and the urine may be dark and foul-smelling. In severe cases, there may be blood in the urine as well.

DIAGNOSIS A diagnosis of cystitis is usually made by collecting a midstream urine sample, and testing for the presence of bacteria. If the problem stems from an inflammation, no pathogenic bacteria will be found in the urine. Further, a vaginal culture will not reveal vaginal secretions.

CONVENTIONAL TREATMENTS FOR URINARY TRACT INFECTIONS The usual treatment for cystitis is a course of antibiotics, and standard therapy for chronic cystitis generally consists of repeated rounds of the same therapy.

In the long term, this practice may actually exacerbate the condition rather than cure it. It is well known that broad-spectrum antibiotics are indiscriminate killers that destroy colonies of friendly gut bacteria along with problem-causing organisms. Once the delicate gastrointestinal microflora is upset, less desirable strains of bacteria proliferate, virtually unchecked. This includes E. coli, the prime cause of cystitis, and candida overgrowth, a suspected cause of inflammations.

Dr. David Kauffman says that antibiotics should be a last-ditch effort, used only when various holistic protocols fail to achieve results. Even then, mild medicines should be used: "What of women who do all the right things, and still come back with bladder infections? In these cases, we need to turn to more traditional medical approaches. The gold standard for treating patients who do everything right and still get infections is a very gentle, bacteriostatic antibiotic. A bacteriostatic antibiotic does not kill the bacteria, but limits bacterial growth. It is gentler on the system, and generally does not cause yeast infections or GI disturbances. I am not big on taking antibiotics, but this is a better alternative than constant infections."

Dr. Jennifer Brett reports that radical therapies are sometimes used for persistent cases: "Treatments I have read about in recent medical journals include surgery to cut nerves to reduce irritation to the bladder, hormonal therapy, and even antidepressive medications to help women sleep better, even though this doesn't get at the root cause of the problem."

NATURAL TREATMENTS

FOR CYSTITIS

For cystitis sufferers, it is important to drink plenty of pure water, about one 8-ounce glass each hour. "If you are in agony and you don't know what to do, start drinking water, and don't stop," advises Dr. Linda Wharton. "Stay away from tea, coffee, soft drinks, and alcohol, but drink plenty of water."

Unsweetened cranberry juice or cranberry capsules also may help. Cranberries change the pH of the urine, making it more acidic and less hospitable to bacteria. It also contains powerful antibacterial substances. In fact, studies reveal that as little as 15 ounces of cranberry juice cause an 80 percent inhibition of bacterial growth. Bacteria loses its ability to cling to the bladder wall, and must exit the system along with urine. Other research indicates that cranberry juice combined with vitamin C acidifies the urine further. The effect is therefore much greater when both are taken together.

Other drinks useful for temporarily acidifying the urine include lemon juice and water, buttermilk, or simply mixing two teaspoons of apple cider vinegar into a glass of water. Drink any of these substances three or four times a day.

During an acute attack of cystitis, the diet can be temporarily changed to further acidify the urine. Dr. Wharton warns that this is recommended only for short periods of time, during an acute infection: "Eat plenty of acidic foods, such as grains, nuts, seeds, fish, dairy products, meat and bread, and cut back on fruit and vegetables."

An ascorbic acid form of vitamin C acidifies the urine, and should be taken to bowel tolerance with cystitis or any infection. Bowel tolerance is where the stool becomes quite loose, almost to the point of diarrhea. Any time the body is fighting an infection, it tolerates large amounts of C, sometimes as much as 10,000 to 15,000 mg orally each day (and even more intravenously). Ascorbic acid should be taken every two to three hours since it is water-soluble, which means that it is rapidly excreted from the body.

Dr. Wharton says that ascorbic acid fights infections in several ways: "Vitamin C concentrates in very high levels in the urine and exerts a direct bactericidal effect. It also supports systemic immune system function by helping to activate neutrophils, the white blood cells most involved in the front line defense against infection. It also works to stimulate the production of lymphocytes, which are important for coordinating immune function at the cellular level."

In addition to vitamin C, think about vitamin A. An easy way of supplementing with this vitamin is to use halibut or cod liver oil capsules, up to 25,000 IU a day, during acute phases of infection. Vitamin A helps protect the mucous membrane lining of the bladder and urethra from irritation during infection. It also improves antibody response and white blood cell function. Just a word of warning here: if you are pregnant, do not supplement with these high doses of vitamin A, as it has been associated with birth defects. Beta carotene, with which the body can make vitamin A as it is needed, is a safer alternative.

Zinc is essential for increasing white blood activity in response to infection. When cystitis is acute, approximately 50 mg elemental zinc is needed daily.

The classes of herbs used to treat cystitis include antiseptic herbs, demulcents, and diuretics. Antiseptic herbs for bladder infections include uva-ursi, buchu, goldenseal, juniper berries, and garlic. "Think garlic whenever you have any type of infection, including cystitis," says Dr. Wharton. Demulcents soothe inflamed mucous membranes inside the bladder and urethra, and include marshmallow root, juniper berry, and corn silk. Diuretic herbs stimulate the production and excretion of urine, which helps to wash out bacteria. Common diuretics are parsley and goldenrod.

Dr. Wharton recommends these old naturopathic herbal remedies for treating burning urine: "Mix together equal parts of fennel, burdock, and slippery elm. Steep a teaspoon of this mixture in a cup of boiled water for about 20 minutes. Have one cup before each meal, and one before bed."

She also recommends flaxseed tea or a combination of uva-ursi and buchu: "For either tea, use one teaspoon of the dried herb(s) to a cup of boiling water. Again, let it steep for 15 to 20 minutes. Then drink one cup, three or four times a day. The results more than compensate for the awful taste."

Dr. Joseph Pizzorno adds this bit of advice: "After sexual intercourse, women should wipe the opening to the urethra with a dilute solution of Betadine or a strong solution of goldenseal tea to wash away any bacteria that may have been forced up into the urethra."

Hydrotherapy is another traditional naturopathic method for helping people overcome the discomforts of cystitis. Sitz baths or hot compresses stimulate blood circulation and remove toxins from the pelvic area. Dr. Wharton explains how this is done: "You can use a hot compress by dipping a small hand towel into a basin of water, as hot as you can possibly tolerate it. Ring out the water and quickly apply the cloth to the area just above the pubic bone. As the cloth cools, repeat the process. In total, apply the compress eight or nine times. Repeat this process two to three times throughout the day. It actually feels wonderful and gives quite a bit of local relief to the symptoms.

"Alternatively, you can try making a sitz bath. Fill a small tub with water, once again, as hot as you can bear it. Add six drops of bergamot oil, and sit in the bath so that water actually covers your pelvis and lower abdomen. Stay there for around half an hour. As the water cools, keep replenishing with fresh, hot water to keep the water up to a hot, even temperature. Just a word of warning: If you have a problem with a weak heart or high blood pressure, hot sitz baths aren't really for you. You are better off just using a local compress."

Dr. Wharton reports impressive results in the treatment of chronic cystitis with acupuncture, when it is accompanied by lifestyle and dietary changes: "Usually an acute attack of cystitis responds to two to four acupuncture sessions, spaced two or three days apart. Chronic cystitis sufferers often benefit from an extended course of acupuncture treatment to prevent the reoccurrence of their problem."

Essential oils can enhance any treatment program, according to aromatherapist Ann Berwick. To help clear up a urinary tract infection, 18 to 20 drops of juniper and cedarwood can be added to one ounce of lotion and massaged into the lower abdomen. Also, six to eight drops of juniper, bergamot, or sandalwood can be added to a sitz bath or full bath.

FOR INTERSTITIAL CYSTITIS

When the diagnosis is interstitial cystitis, Dr. Jennifer Brett says the best idea is to "remove congestion from the pelvis." To remove the source of irritation, it is a good idea to be tested for food allergies to see if a food is causing an antibody-antigen reaction and irritating the bladder. It is also important to test for candida in the colon because candida can cause irritations and antibody reactions that irritate the bladder. Next, check to see that the hormones are in balance. If they are not, they can be treated with vitamin B_6, evening primrose oil, and herbs.

Doing aerobic exercise every day helps to remove blood congestion from the pelvis. This means walking, jogging, swimming, bicycling, anything that moves the blood. Specific exercises to remove the blood involve turning upside down. In yoga, this is accomplished with the headstand or shoulderstand. It can also be achieved by raising the legs up and bicycling. But if there is a back or neck problem, a simple solution is the slant board. This can be made simply by taking an old door or a couple of one-by-four boards. One end can be placed on the couch, and the other end on the floor. Once it is stable, the person lies upside down, that is, with the head near the floor and the feet near the couch. The blood is automatically pulled out of the pelvis by gravity, and moved into the chest and head. Remaining too long can cause dizziness; 5 or 10 minutes works for most people.

A low-acid diet decreases irritations. High-acid foods to omit are red meat, dairy, shellfish, and citrus fruits. The diet should include whole grains, beans, and vegetables. Essential fatty acids, such as those found in flaxseed oil, evening primrose oil, and fish oils, can help reduce inflammation. In interstitial cystitis, they are key for reversing the cycle of irritation and blood congestion. Useful herbs are marshmallow, corn silk, slippery elm, and goldenrod.

"If you follow these basic points," says Dr. Brett, "within three to four weeks, you are likely to notice that your ability to sleep through the night is improved, and that your cramping and pain during the day is significantly lessened."

FOR NONBACTERIAL URINARY INFLAMMATION

For urinary inflammation not caused by bacteria, Dr. Brett suggests avoiding foods that encourage candida growth, such as wheat, simple sugars, white flour, pastries, candies, alcohol, aged cheeses, vinegar, and even fruit. She also says to avoid known food allergens. It is a good idea to get a test to determine if there are any other foods in the diet that are acting as irritants.

Again, one 8-ounce glass of water every hour is needed. It is also a good idea to drink a glass of water and to urinate immediately after sexual intercourse. This tends to reduce bladder irritation that sexual intercourse may cause.

It is also important to avoid tight-fitting pants, nylon underwear, and pantyhose. They encourage candida growth in the vaginal tract, which irritates the bladder and urethra.

In addition, take vitamin C (2,000–6,000 mg buffered), vitamin B_6 (100–200 mg), and four to six capsules of evening primrose oil. Herbs that soothe the bladder include althea or marshmallow, corn silk, slippery elm, and goldenrod.

The homeopathic remedy cantharis is often effective in reducing bladder and urethra irritations.

ORIENTAL PERSPECTIVE ON URINARY TRACT INFECTION Dr. Jennifer Brett explains that traditional Chinese medicine views cystitis as the end result of an accumulation of damp and heat in the bladder: "Often there is a weak flow of *chi* (energy) in the kidney and the spleen meridians. Weakness of spleen energy leads to the formation of damp in the body, which, in turn causes a stagnation of energy. As in nature, whenever anything builds up, there is friction. A stagnation of chi eventually leads to the development of heat, what we in the West interpret as cystitis.

"Spleen *chi* is easily injured through dietary indiscretion. Overeating can damage the spleen *chi*, as well as drinking with meals, or an overconsumption of damp-forming foods, such as dairy products, chilled foods or drinks, and raw fruits and vegetables. Greasy foods, such as take-out foods, also damage spleen *chi*.

"What you do with your mind actually affects spleen energy as well. An overuse of the mind, particularly through chronic anxiety and worry, or through many years of overstudying, also tends to deplete spleen energy.

"When the cooling yin energy of the kidneys is weakened, cystitis becomes much more likely as well. Kidney yin is consumed with age, but it can also prematurely diminish through lifestyle. The long-term overwork, stress, and exhaustion that form a part of many American lives these days, along with an overconsumption of alcohol and too much sex, all deplete the vital kidney energy." Acupuncture, combined with lifestyle changes, can help to balance energy and eliminate cystitis.

Preventing Infection

Long-term preventive changes obviously make a lot more sense than simply dealing with each acute infection as it arises. Here are some simple personal hygiene measures to reduce the likelihood of reinfection:

After a bowel movement, wipe from front to back, away from the vagina.

Encourage your partner to wash thoroughly before any sexual contact.

Avoid the transfer of bacteria from the anus to the vagina during lovemaking.

During a period, change pads and tampons frequently.

Do not wear tight-fitting jeans or nylon pantyhose or pants. Cotton pants and stockings with garters allow more air flow and ventilation.

Make a habit of drinking lots of water. Aim for seven to eight glasses each day. This keeps the urine dilute so that bacterial proliferation is less likely. It also prompts frequent urination, which washes out problematic bacteria. Reduce intake of coffee and tea.

Make a habit of emptying your bladder frequently. Research shows that women who ignore their urge to urinate for long periods of time are much more likely to develop cystitis. The motto here is when you need to go, go right away. Urinate after sexual intercourse. This will help to wash out any of the bacteria that may have been pushed up into the urethra.

Try not to urinate before sex so that more bacteria is pushed out after sex. A glass of water right before intercourse will further increase the volume of liquid in the bladder for the washout of bacteria later on.

If infections are an ongoing problem, try this. Take a detachable shower and direct a stream of water into the vaginal area before sex. This will dilute the bacteria and decrease their numbers so that less bacteria gets pushed up into the bladder during intercourse.

Avoid chemical irritation to the urethra by staying away from perfumed or colored personal hygiene products. Diaphragms and birth control pills, as a means of contraception, often promote urinary tract infections and should not be used by women who tend to get the condition. Condoms or a properly fitted cervical cap are better.

See a registered osteopath or chiropractor if you think you may have a spinal problem that can be contributing to your recurring cystitis.

"Remember that your bladder health reflects your overall health," says Dr. Linda Wharton, "so take a good look at your lifestyle. Ask yourself, "Do I eat a nutritious, balanced diet? Do I get enough relaxation and sleep? Am I under stress?" Maybe you drink too much coffee or alcohol or smoke or use recreational drugs. If your lifestyle is unhealthy, your body will be too."

54

Endometriosis

E ndometriosis is a condition in which the glands and tissues that line the inside of the uterus (the endometrium) grow outside the uterine cavity. Normally, cells build up in the uterus each month in preparation for pregnancy. They serve as a nest for an incoming embryo. When pregnancy does not occur, the lining sheds and appears as menstrual flow. With endometriosis, cells may attach themselves to the fallopian tubes, ovaries, urinary bladder, intestinal surfaces, rectum, part of the colon, and other structures in the area.

Causes

The exact cause of the condition remains a mystery, though several theories exist as to why it happens. These are some possible explanations:

Retrograde menstruation. Blood flows backward, instead of outwardly. It is thought to go out the fallopian tubes and into the pelvic and abdominal cavity. Once there, cells from the exiting blood implant themselves outside the uterus onto other tissues.

Lymphatic channels. Cells of the endometrium lining go through lymphatic channels, or migrate via blood, and then implant themselves outside the uterine cavity.

Genetic predisposition. Certain families are predisposed to the condition.

Immunologic failure. The immune system is deficient in some way, causing tissue to proliferate in abnormal areas. The thought is that through some type of immune deficiency, endometrial tissue gets activated at different times in the cycle through hormonal and chemical influences.

Childbearing. Childbearing in combination with methods of contraception may be responsible.

Symptoms

Endometriosis can produce slight or severe pain, ranging from mild cramps to agony and dysfunction. Pain results from swelling, inflammation, and scarring of affected tissues. It is usually cyclical, and most commonly occurs just before menstruation. Some women have pain during sexual intercourse any time in the month.

Where and to what degree pain is felt depends on the location of the endometrial tissue and the degree it has spread outside the uterus. Some women have pain during urination due to implants on the bladder. Some have pain during bowel movements due to colon and rectal implants. There can be ovarian pain or pain radiating to the back, buttocks, or down the legs. Upon a manual gynecological examination, there may be pelvic pain due to inflammation and scarring.

Internal bleeding may occur as well as nose bleeding or bleeding from another orifice, at certain times of the month. Any cyclic bleeding is suspect for endometriosis. Other symptoms that sometimes appear include bladder infections, fatigue, and lower back pain. Endometriosis may result in infertility when it interferes with ovarian function.

Diagnosis

Endometriosis can be suspected in the presence of one or more of the symptoms listed above, but the only real way to confirm a diagnosis is with a surgical procedure, known as a laparoscopy, which allows the doctor to actually see and biopsy tissue. Sonograms and MRI scans may be helpful, but they are not definitive in making the diagnosis.

Proper diagnosis is important, because while endometriosis is considered benign, it can become malignant.

Conventional Therapy

Treatment usually consists of medical prescriptions for pain control and reduction of endometrial growth. Antiprostaglandin medicines, such as indomethacin, ibuprofen, and Naprosyn, are often given to reduce pain.

Another popular pharmaceutical, danazol, is also used for this purpose, but in some women it does not provide total or lasting relief. Studies show danazol to have a good effect after surgery to remove adhesions. After some of the adhesions have been removed, it may help an infertile woman become pregnant. A side effect of the drug is that it may increase cholesterol, especially the LDL variety, which is implicated in accelerated arteriosclerosis. Adverse effects of all the above drugs can include weight gain, edema, decreased or increased breast size, acne, excess hair growth on the face and perhaps even in the developing fetus, and deepening of the voice.

Hormones are sometimes given to fool the body into believing it is pregnant, since pregnancy seems to retard or prevent the development of endometriosis. This method appears to have some benefit, but side effects include depression, painful breasts, nausea, weight gain, bloating, swelling, and migraine headaches. Since side effects can be fairly severe, this is not a popular method. Newer compounds, called gonadotropin-releasing hormone compounds, are sometimes given by injection. These suppress the pituitary gland from releasing the female hormones FSH and LH, causing what is called a clinical pseudomenopause. They help to reduce pain in many women, and to decrease the size and volume of endometrial tissue after surgery.

Through the advanced surgical technique of Female Reconstructive Surgery (FRS), developed by Dr. Vicki Hufnagel, the uterus and ovaries can be repositioned, thus reducing the deep pelvic pain that is associated with endometriosis.

Alternative Approaches

IMPROVING IMMUNE FUNCTION Dr. Tori Hudson, a naturopathic physician from Portland, Oregon, believes there is most support for the immunological weakness theory of endometriosis because women with the condition have altered immune cells, and fewer T-lymphocytes. By improving immune function with supplements, diet, and botanicals, she claims to help many patients: "I've seen women with severe pelvic pain, who were scheduled for surgery one month from the date that I saw them. My treatment helped them to recover completely without the surgery." She adds that most, but not all, women respond to her protocol, which is designed to stimulate a maximal immune response.

The basic program consists of the following antioxidants: vitamin C, to bowel tolerance, up to 10,000 mg; beta carotene, 150,000–200,000 IU; selenium, 400 mcg; and vitamin E, 800–1,200 IU. Changes in the diet are made to further stimulate the immune system. This is accomplished by lowering fat, adding whole grains, vegetables and fruits, and eliminating immune system inhibitors such as coffee, sugar, alcohol, and high-fat foods. Foods such as cheese and meat have high amounts of estrogen and are omitted, as estrogen aggravates the disease. A mostly vegetarian diet is best for lowering estrogen and stimulating the immune system.

Two botanical formulas are included. One contains chaste tree berry, dandelion root, motherwort, and prickly ash in equal amounts. One-half teaspoon is taken three times daily. The other formula contains small doses of toxic herbs that must be carefully prescribed by a naturopathic physician.

In addition, Dr. Hudson sometimes prescribes natural progesterone made from wild yam. The wild yam extract is converted in the laboratory to natural progesterone.

THE CHINESE HOLISTIC APPROACH Dr. Roger Hirsch, a naturopathic doctor in Santa Monica, California, who specializes in Asian medicine, says that the Chinese approach to gynecological imbalance is a holistic one: "What do I mean by holistic? It treats the mind and body as an integral unit like a gloved hand. If you move the hand, what is moving, the glove or the hand? The body or the mind? They move in concert. If there is a psychological, emotional, or spiritual imbalance, it may show up on the physical plane, and cause a 'stuckness' or endometrial situation."

The Chinese diagnose endometriosis by looking at the way the blood flows in the body, specifically in the pelvic cavity. This is determined by the appearance of the root of the tongue, which represents the pelvic cavity. "If a woman has endometriosis, there will be raised bumps and papillae in the back of the tongue and perhaps a greasy yellow coating," he says. "If you look at the back of your tongue in the mirror and see raised bumps that are red and fiery, especially during the time of menstruation, you may well have endometriosis."

HELLERWORK: A FORM OF BODYWORK Hellerwork is a bodywork technique derived from rolfing. Both modalities are similar in that they work to improve body structure with deep tissue work, but Hellerwork is different in that it is not painful. Certified Hellerwork practitioner Sarah Suatoni gives an overview of the process: "There are three components to Hellerwork. There is a hands-on part, which feels much like a massage, a movement educational aspect, and a mind/body dialogue aspect. I will talk about each of these.

"In the hands-on process, we analyze the body much as a chiropractor would, looking at the posture, or the structure as we call it, to determine which parts of the body are out of balance. We look to see which myofascial tissue connections are creating this misalignment. Then we work with our hands to release it. That, in a sense, is also the beginning of movement education, because this isn't done to the client but with the client. In other words, I put my hands on a spot, and we work closely together with visual images or deep breathing to help the person identify the misalignment, feel it, and then release it.

"The second part of the work is movement education, in which we do very simple everyday movements. We look at how a person sits or stands. In the case of a computer programmer, we look at how they sit at their computer and use their arms. We look at whatever it is that may be contributing to the dysfunction in the body, and then we begin to look at how we can have the person move in a way that will not create the same problem.

"Last, but certainly not least, is mind/body dialogue. We work under the belief that our emotional patterns, memories, and attitudes are reflected in our bodies. In the same way one needs to look at a movement pattern in order to shift some sort of physical dysfunction, one needs to look at emotional patterns or beliefs in order to shift those as well. We dialogue with clients in order to identify underlying emotions or memories. Then we look at how clients might better facilitate emotions or memories, so that they are not manifesting them through physical dysfunctions.

"This work is a process where people come in for 11 sessions. Once a week for an hour-and-a-half is ideal although other time frames are possible. Each session touches upon a different part of the body and different aspects of the being."

HOMEOPATHY Homeopathy is another holistic therapy that addresses underlying emotional causes. Dr. Anthony Aurigemma has been treating his patients homeopathically for 10 years and claims that the therapy is completely safe and highly effective. "There is no doubt in my mind that something actually happens and that it helps people," he says. "I utilize the remedies because I see them work. What spurs me on is the continuous improvements of most of the patients I see."

Patient Stories

Dr. Aurigemma outlines one patient's progress with homeopathy:

A 35-year-old woman, who was diagnosed with endometriosis via laparoscopy in 1991, came to my office in February 1993. She had a history of migraine headaches, vaginal yeast infections, pain beginning in her hips and going down to her knees, as well as mid-month pain in the uterine area, shooting, throbbing ovarian pain, pain while running, and pain after overeating. Premenstrually, she experienced headaches, anger, bloating, crankiness, and sensitivity. She had headaches the last day of her menstrual cycle, and the day after the menstrual cycle ended.

In homeopathy, part of the diagnostic process includes an assessment of how people appear. These were some of her personality characteristics. She was bright, lively, and pleasant. Even though she seemed to be in pain, she was not irritable. She said she alternated between being warm and chilly and that she easily got overheated. In addition, she claimed to be spontaneous and very quick to act. Also, she was an animal rights activist who took in strays. She said that she did not harbor anger. Instead, she tried to get things out in the open. In terms of her eating habits, she was not a very thirsty person. She liked to drink cold water and herb teas, and she would occasionally have a glass of wine with a steak dinner. She said that she liked salads, spicy foods, and borscht, but that creamy foods were too rich. She smoked one to two cigarettes per day, two or three times per week.

Her fears included claustrophobia, not liking to be in tunnels, elevators, or crowds. Thunderstorms bothered her. She was somewhat weepy at sentimental movies.

I studied her symptoms, personality characteristics, foods, likes and dislikes, and fears. Based on this information, I came up with a particular homeopathic remedy which I asked her to take twice a day, four or five days a week.

Approximately three months later, she reported feeling 70–80 percent better. Her uterine pain and headaches had decreased, pre-menstrual symptoms were less severe, and there was an almost total disappearance of her yeast infection. At that point, she was given one single dose of the same remedy, but in a higher potency. I gave this to her in the office and it was not repeated.

A month later, she returned, and said that she was improving further. There were no headaches at all with her period and very little pain. The yeast flared up, but then got better. On that visit, I gave her no remedy at all and told her to come back in three months, or if symptoms started to return.

Three months later, in September, she came back with some return of headaches when the period was stopping. Even so, headaches were still about 50 percent better than they had been in the first place. The yeast infection was 90 percent improved, and the monthly pain was about 75 percent better overall. This is without any further remedy.

At this point, I gave her another dose of the same remedy to take daily, five days per week. That was three months ago. Since that time, I have not seen her. She reports being between 75 and 80 percent better overall, and 90 percent better with her yeast infection. These subjective estimates of health are given to me by the patient, since there is no physical way to measure improvement. She is more functional, better able to do things, happier, and pleased with the treatment. She plans to continue.

Her symptoms are fewer, and certainly less intense. In seven months, her periods became easier, and between periods she feels more comfortable. There were no side effects from the remedy other than an aggravation of her yeast infection for a few days which then subsided. That was due to a higher potency of the remedy. Homeopathic remedies can aggravate symptoms. Very often that aggravation is a sign that the remedy is correct and is bringing things to a head, getting the body to focus on the problem, and then getting rid of it.

She is functioning better, she is less uncomfortable, but we do not know whether or not the endometrial tissue has shrunken or gone away. The only way to really know that is by doing another laparoscopy, but a person is unlikely to undergo surgery when feeling better.

Linda describes her experience with endometriosis:

I had constant abdominal pain from the endometriosis for 21 days out of every month. For many years, I took 8 to 10 aspirin a day and sometimes stronger painkillers. In four years, I had been to three gynecologists, two internists, and a gastroenterologist. I had laparoscopic surgery and then was given Lupron injections. Lupron is a drug that blocks estrogen and causes the endometrial tissue to shrink. After three months on Lupron, the pain from the endometriosis was gone, but there were some terrific side effects. Hot flashes interfered with my sleeping. I also had a lot of trouble with joint pain. But by far the worst side effect was loss of bone density. This is the reason why you are not supposed to take drugs like Lupron for more than six months in your lifetime. After I stopped taking Lupron, the endometriosis came back within a month or two. At that point, my gynecologist said my best options were another drug that could also affect bone density or a complete hysterectomy. It seemed as if I didn't have any acceptable options left.

At that point, I found Dr. Lonsdorf, an Ayurvedic doctor, who recommended certain herbal mixtures for me. She also suggested other simple measures that are simple to follow and of benefit to everyone: sipping hot water throughout the day to aid digestion, eating the main meal in the middle of the day and eating less toward the end, cutting down on meat and working toward a more vegetarian diet, getting to bed by ten and up by six—that is, trying to get more in touch with the circadian rhythms—using massage to stimulate circulation, and practicing meditation to calm the mind.

I incorporated as many of these suggestions into my life as I comfortably could. Within a few weeks, the pain from the endometriosis was almost completely gone. I have been under Dr. Lonsdorf's care for almost a year and a half and almost never have any discomfort anymore. I have much more energy and am much calmer. Some other problems I had, like low blood sugar, have also cleared up. In fact, the Ayurvedic medicine helped me so much that my husband and both our daughters see Dr. Lonsdorf now.

Dr. Anthony Penepent describes one patient's success treating her endometriosis with natural hygiene:

One woman came to see me who was on prescription narcotic medication for the pain. The medicine gave her no relief, and she was at the point of wanting a hysterectomy to get relief from the pain. I put this woman on a natural hygienic regimen for a couple of weeks. First, she fasted for five days. Then she followed up with a nutritional plan.

Let me briefly describe a typical hygienic regimen. The patient has a breakfast consisting of a vegetable juice or a vegetable/fruit juice combination, a blended salad, a piece of fruit, perhaps some hot cereal and a couple of soft boiled egg yolks. For lunch the patient has a vegetable juice or vegetable/fruit juice combination, a blended salad, a cup or a little more than that, a piece of fruit, and then some raw nuts or unsalted raw milk cheese. For the evening meal, the patient starts with juice again, blended salad, tossed salad, steamed vegetables such as string beans, broccoli, or escarole. Then she goes on with the main course, which includes a steamed potato or yam, natural brown rice or other whole grain, and a legume. I also might supplement the meal with egg or cheese, depending on the protein needs of the woman. Of course, there are variations for individual patients.

Following this general plan, this patient was pain-free at the end of one month. That was 10 years ago. Right now she is pregnant with her second child, whereas before she was infertile. Natural hygiene has tremendous implications for endometriosis. There is absolutely no reason why a woman should have pain or be infertile because of such a simple condition.

What I can see from my perusal of the literature is that endometriosis is plainly a condition of liver toxicity, where the liver is failing to completely break down the estrogen hormones that the body is manufacturing. These breakdown products wreak havoc in the form of endometrial tissue in the pelvic cavity.

55

Breast Cancer and Other Breast Diseases

B reast cancer is the most frequently occurring cancer in women. There were 180,000 new cases in 1998 and 43,500 fatalities. In 1950, 1 in 20 females were diagnosed with the disease; today, the number has risen to 1 in 8.

Causes of Breast Cancer

Dr. Michael Schachter, a complementary physician from Rockland County, New York, describes some of the key factors in the development of the disease:

ESTROGEN "Women whose menstrual periods start when they are relatively young have an increased risk for developing breast cancer, as do women who have a late menopause," explains Dr. Schachter. "This suggests that a woman who has a longer exposure to female sex hormones during her lifetime is at greater risk for developing breast cancer, and that estrogen, the female sex hormone that stimulates cell growth, may play a role in its formation. Women who have no children, and also women who have children but do not breast-feed, also have an increased risk. This suggests that the other female sex hormone, progesterone, may have a protective effect.

"Other known and accepted risk factors include an increased alcohol intake, a diet high in fat, being overweight, and a family history of breast cancer. Some of the reasons for this is that fat tissue can make estrogen, and alcohol tends to stimulate its production. In summary, most risk factors seem to be associated with increased lifetime exposure to estrogen, decreased lifetime exposure to progesterone, or a combination of the two.

"Estrogen and progesterone tend to balance each other in the body. Excessive estrogen or reduced progesterone may lead to a condition known as estrogen dominance. The symptoms of estrogen dominance include water retention, breast swelling, fibrocystic breasts, pre-menstrual mood swings and depression, loss of sex drive, heavy or irregular periods, uterine fibroids, craving for sweets, and fat deposition in the hips and thighs.

"Estrogen tends to be transformed into two major metabolites in the body. They can be called the good and the bad estrogen, just as there is the so-called good and bad cholesterol. The bad estrogen, known as 16alphahydroxyestrone, favors the development of breast cancer, whereas 2-hydroxyestrone seems to protect against it. Certain chemicals stimulate the formation of one or the other."

XENOESTROGENS "Now that we've seen that the role of estrogen is very important," Dr. Schachter continues, "this leads to a discussion of something called xenoestrogens. *Xeno* means foreign, and xenoestrogens are chemical substances that are foreign to the body, but behave like estrogens. These substances mimic estrogen's actions. Some xenoestrogens can reduce estrogen's effects. These varieties, which are rapidly degraded in the body, usually occur in plant foods such as soy, cauliflower, and broccoli. They protect against the development of breast cancer. Other xenoestrogens, typically synthetic ones, appear to stimulate cancer growth.

"We are living in the petrochemical era. This period began in the 1940s as a result of technological advances in the procurement of oil, and the manufacture of its products. In 1940 one billion pounds of synthetic chemicals were manufactured; by 1950 the amount had increased to fifty billion pounds; and by the late 1980s, 500 billion pounds of synthetic chemicals were being produced annually. Many of these compounds are toxic, mutagenic, and carcinogenic. The majority have not been adequately tested for toxicity, let alone for their environmental and ecological effects.

"Approximately 600 chemicals have been shown to be carcinogenic in well-designed, controlled, and validated animal experiments. And within the scientific community, the overwhelming consensus is that chemicals carcinogenic to animals are also carcinogenic to humans. In large-scale epidemiological human studies, approximately 25 chemicals have been proven carcinogenic. For each of these 25 chemicals, animal research established carcinogenicity one to three decades earlier, making the animal studies all the more significant.

"Many synthetic chemicals behave as these bad xenoestrogens, particularly pesticides, fuels, and plastics. They do so in various ways. Some enhance the production of the so-called bad estrogens that I mentioned earlier, and others bind to estrogen receptors, inducing them to issue unneeded signals to increase cellular growth. Xenoestrogens may enter the body through animal fat, as they tend to accumulate in fatty tissue and tend to concentrate as you go up in the food chain.

"Xenoestrogens tend to be synergistic so that a mixture of tiny amounts of many chemicals may have dire effects. As an example, at Mount Sinai, in New York City, Dr. Mary Wolf found that levels of DDE, a relative of DDT, were higher in 58 women who developed breast cancer compared to those who had not. At Laval University, 41 women who had estrogen-responsive breast cancers had higher concentrations of DDE. And in a 1990 study of breast cancer and pesticides in Israel, a strong relationship between the two was shown. In the 1970s Israeli women had one of the highest breast cancer mortality rates in the world, but in the 10 years that followed a 1976 ban on several organochlorine-type pesticides, the incidence of breast cancer declined 20 percent, while it increased in all other industrial nations, strongly suggesting that the pesticides had a major causal effect on the development of breast cancer. Prior to the ban in Israel, some dairy products there had pesticide residues as high as 500 percent above U.S. levels, and residues in human milk were 800 times that level."

POOR LYMPHATIC DRAINAGE Dr. Schachter describes the relationship between xenoestrogens and poor lymphatic drainage: "When xenoestrogens cause breast cancer, they do so by accumulating in the fatty tissues of the breast. It is the job of the lymphatic system to drain toxic substances from the tissues. Poor lymphatic drainage may therefore play a role in breast cancer formation.

"The lymphatic system is a specialized part of the circulatory system that functions as a central component of the immune system. It consists of fluid called lymph, derived from blood and tissue fluid. The lymph moves through the lymph vessels, called lymphatics, back into the bloodstream. Lymph contains cell debris, nutrients, waste products from the cells, hormones, toxins, and many other substances. It is the microenvironment of the cells. Lymph flow does not move along like the blood through the contraction of the heart, but is dependent upon other factors, such as muscle contraction that massages the outside of the lymphatic vessels, breathing, which pulls lymph along with each inhalation, pressure from the pulsation of the arteries, changes in posture, and passive compression of soft tissues. Therefore, it is very sensitive to constricting external pressure that can impede its flow.

"This leads to practical implications. It may be somewhat surprising to learn that bras may play some role in lymphatic blockage and in the development of breast cancer. Over 85 percent of lymph fluid flowing from the breast drains to the armpit lymph nodes. Most of the rest drains to the nodes around the breast bone. Bras and other tight clothing can impede this lymphatic flow, thereby trapping toxic chemicals in the breast. The nature of the bra, its tightness, and the amount of time it is worn influences the degree of blockage.

"This was popularized recently by Sydney Ross Singer, Ph.D., a medical anthropologist, with the publication of his book, *Dressed to Kill: The Link Between Bras and Breast Cancer*. In this book Singer describes an epidemiological study that he carried out, which shows a very strong link. This study is similar to the early studies that showed a relationship between smoking and lung cancer. In fact, its results were even stronger. Women who wore bras more than 12 hours daily had a 19 times greater chance of developing breast cancer than those who wore bras less than12 hours a day. And women who never wore bras seemed to have an even greater protection against breast cancer.

"The message to women is to wear bras as little as possible, and when wearing them to choose one that is least constricting. When a woman does not wear a bra, lymph flow through the lymphatics in the breast will be less impeded, thus promoting removal of toxic chemicals from the tissues of the breast," Dr. Schachter concludes.

X-RAYS Dr. John Gofman, M.D., Ph.D., and professor emeritus of molecular and cell biology at the University of California, Berkeley, sounds the alarm on the harmful effects of x-rays in his book, *Preventing Breast Cancer*.

The effects of x-rays take years, even decades, to manifest, which is why orthodox medicine does not pay attention to this danger. Indeed, x-rays are standard practice for medical diagnosis and treatment. "The incubation time is what has led organized medicine exactly in the wrong direction," says Dr. Gofman. "In the first half of the 20th century, medicine looked at treatments in this way. If you gave someone poison, the effects would be seen in weeks or months. They did not think in terms of years or decades. What we have learned about x-ray-induced cancer is that a very small proportion occur in the first few years after the x-rays are administered. But most of them take 10, 20, even 50 years. Women with breast cancer, who are 45, 50, or 60, are thinking, 'Why me? I haven't done anything wrong.' What these women are not thinking about is what they were exposed to early in life. In the early 1940s, for example, pediatricians in New York City, Rochester, and the Pacific Northwest were giving children fluoroscopic examinations 12 times a year for the first two years of life as part of their well-baby examination. Fluoroscopy is far worse than x-rays because the beam is left on for a long time. This laid the foundation for the development of breast cancer, and other forms of cancer, later in life. If you really want to know the story about breast cancer today, you have to ask yourself, What happened 30, 40, and 50 years ago?"

It is not the radiation itself that persists but chromosomal damage, Dr. Gofman says: "Inside the nucleus of every one of our cells is a string of DNA organized into 46 chromosomes. That's a treasure. Damage to your chromosomes is going to be there for the rest of your life."

Dr. Gofman bases his claims on well-documented research published in the 1960s and 1970s, as well as his own work. "Ian Mackenzie, a great Nova Scotia physician, discovered the relationship between breast cancer and medical x-rays when he studied women who had been in tuberculosis sanitoria, and who had received a treatment known as pneumothorax. This was a wonderful treatment that injected air into the chest cavity to rest the lung. It saved many lives.

Unfortunately, during the course of treatment, these women were given 100, 200, or even more fluoroscopic exams to check whether the air had been placed in the lungs. Twenty to 30 years later, Mackenzie's work showed a 20-fold increase in breast cancer in these women. His results were published in 1965 in the *British Journal of Cancer.*

"Many people doubted his findings, saying that if he was correct we would have seen breast cancer in Nagasaki and Hiroshima. Turns out nobody looked to see if this was the case. So one of the members of the Radiation Research Foundation looked, and found exactly what Mackenzie had found.

"Arthur Tamplin and I raised a flag in the *Lancet* by saying that the Wanabo and Mackenzie studies suggest that breast cancer is one of the easiest cancers to induce by radiation. Today, everybody who is anybody in medical science knows that breast cancer is related to ionizing radiation, such as medical x-rays.

"A couple of years ago, I tried to answer this question—not whether x-rays cause breast cancer, but what part of all breast cancers are being caused by x-rays? My estimate was about 75 percent. Everybody said, 'Oh, that's too high. It must be much lower.' Since that time, I've done much more extensive work, and I have changed my numbers from 75 percent to better than 90 percent. Moreover, I now have enough data on a variety of other cancers to say that most cancers, not just breast cancer, are caused by medical x-rays."

Whether Dr. Gofman is 100 percent right or just partly right, whether medical x-rays are a primary cause of breast cancer and other types of cancer, or merely an important secondary factor that until now has been ignored by our government and the medical establishment—in either case, women need to recognize the seriousness of the problem and to insist that radiation exposures be as minimal as possible.

"If you have a serious problem and you are told you need an x-ray, I don't want to stand in the way of your getting that x-ray," says Dr. Gofman. "But I want to be very sure that you are not getting a dose that is 2, 4, 8, or 20 times higher than is needed. I think there is room for at least a 3- to 4-fold reduction in dose, possibly even a 10-fold reduction. Every community should insist that their radiological facilities produce evidence that their dose is low. Mammography is a lesson in what you can do when you are pushed to the wall to do it. In the 1970s, radiologists were giving 2, 5, and 10 rads per mammogram. When they were told that this would cause more cancers than it helped cure, they went to work and got the dose down to 3/10 of a rad or less. That is a 20- to 50-fold reduction in dose. Getting the dose down further should be a major national priority. If we do that, we are going to bring about the single most significant reduction in cancer incidence in this country. That's real prevention."

HIGH-FAT DIET Earlier, Dr. Michael Schachter gave one explanation why fat can cause breast cancer. Here, Dr. Charles Simone gives another reason why fats generate disease: "We know that fatty foods actually convert normal cells into problematic cells. Consuming high-fat foods, particularly unsaturated fats, increases free radical production, damaging the cell membrane. At this point, the damaged cell has two choices. It can die. That's fine, because if it dies you make another one. Or it can repair itself. In the repair process, a cell can go awry and metamorphosize into a cancer cell. So fats cause free radicals which damage cells, which in turn try to repair themselves, and transform themselves into cancer cells."

Additionally, Dr. Simone cites these other two factors as leading contributors: "We know that tobacco is the number two cause of cancer in our country, and the number two cause of breast cancer as well. Regarding alcohol, we know that two to three drinks per week is enough to confer a two- to three-fold risk of getting cancer of the breast independently of everything else. So the number one, two, and three causes of breast cancer—high-fat diet, smoking, and alcohol consumption—are totally within our control."

Diagnosis and Prognosis

Initial symptoms of breast cancer include thickening, a lump in the breast, or dimpled skin. Later on there may be nipple discharge, pain, ulcers, and swollen lymph glands under the arms.

Once breast cancer is diagnosed, the prognosis depends on the course of the disease. Dr. Michael Schachter explains: "The staging of the breast cancer involves the size of the cancer in the breast, whether or not it has spread or metastasized to regional lymph nodes, and whether or not it has metastasized to distant organs. The more lymph nodes involved and the greater the size of the tumor, the worse the prognosis. Stage zero is limited to the topmost layer, and the five-year survival rate is about 90 percent. In stage four, in which cancer has metastasized to lymph nodes above the collar bone or has distant metastases to organs such as the liver, lungs or brain, the five-year survival rate drops to 10 percent."

While the possibility of a positive diagnosis for breast cancer is terrifying, it is empowering to know that there are steps to take to prevent the condition, that minimally invasive treatments are often beneficial, and that it is possible to avoid a recurrence.

Natural Approaches to Prevention

Naturopathic physician Dr. Tori Hudson says, "I believe that breast cancer is a preventable disease. Just look around the world. Women in our culture have one of the highest—if not the highest—incidences of breast cancer, while women in Japan have the lowest.

"The reason is diet. To make a big story simple to understand, cultures that have a vegetarian diet, or are closest to a vegetarian diet, have the least breast cancer. That's how it all pans out no matter how you look at it. This implies that cultures that eat less fat, and less animal fat, have the least amount of breast cancer. So the big picture is really clear. Eat a lot of vegetables, fruits, and whole grains and beans. Those foods provide protection."

Letha Hadady, an herbalist and educator, visited China to learn why Chinese women had such a low incidence of breast cancer as compared to American women and those in other Western nations. While diet was a big part of the picture, she learned that other factors came into play. In order to prevent breast cancer, Asians build immunity through diet, cleansing herbs, and the avoidance of pollution, stress, negative emotions, smoking, alcohol, and radiation: "They have much cleaner habits than we do." In addition, Hadady made this important discovery: "I found it quite interesting that breast cancer is considered a disease of melancholy in China. That feeling of heaviness in the chest leads to poor circulation and excess phlegm. This leads to two conclusions. Increase circulation and you have a better chance of prevention. And reduce phlegm. The easiest way to reduce phlegm is to stay away from foods like cheese, chocolate, fried foods, and milk. You will not find dairy in the diet in China. Their diet tends to be grains and greens."

In his book, *Breast Health: A Ten Point Prevention Program*, Dr. Charles Simone outlines the following plan for optimal breast health:

Optimize nutrition

Take antioxidant supplements

Avoid tobacco

Avoid alcohol

Avoid estrogens

Exercise

Minimize stress

Become spiritually involved

Increase awareness of sexuality

Get a good regular physical examination, starting at age 35

Re-examining Conventional Assumptions

When a diagnosis of breast cancer is made, minimally invasive therapy may be just as effective as more intrusive standard medical approaches, according to Dr. Robert Atkins, a well-known advocate of holistic medicine: "Women develop a lump in their breast and appropriately have a mammogram or biopsy which leads to the diagnosis. At this point the trouble begins. The doctor gives the patient two choices: a mastectomy or a lumpectomy with radiation. A paper... on this reported a third option that was every bit as good regarding survival rate and life expectancy. That was simply to do a lumpectomy without the radiation."

Dr. Atkins goes on to say that unbeknownst to women, after diagnosis and treatment, there is much a woman can do to regain total health: "The biggest fallacy of all is when doctors tell patients after therapy that they've done all they can do and there is nothing left to do. This ignores the whole concept that people can get healthier by enhancing all their internal systems to make sure that the neoplasia, the process of forming cancer, no longer takes place. In other words, cancer is not the tumor itself; cancer is a process.

"Once you know that, you can ask, 'What can nutrition do?' You learn that it can help in multiple ways. First and foremost, free radicals trigger the formation of cancer, and the recurrence of cancer. Nutritional antioxidants can help to slow down the formation of free radicals. Additionally, plant foods have antioxidant and immune-enhancing properties."

Alternative Approaches to Treatment

DIET AND NUTRITION To prevent and reverse free radical damage to breast tissue, Dr. Steven Rachlin, an internist in Syosset, Long Island, has his cancer patients follow this daily protocol:

Emulsified vitamin A (up to 50,000 IU)
Beta carotene (up to 100 mg)
B_1 (400 mg)
B_6 (500 mg)
Folic acid (3,200 mcg)
Vitamin C (up to 5 g)
Coenzyme Q10 (270 mg)
Flaxseed oil (1 tbsp)
Cat's claw (1800 mg)
Melatonin (up to 10 mg)
Shark cartilage (1 mg per kg of patient's weight)
Pycnogenol (150 mg)
Essiac (several ounces)
Pancreatic digestive enzymes (up to 40 g)
Aloe vera juice (9–12 ounces)

Dr. Michael Schachter adds that trace minerals play a vital role in the prevention of free radical damage: "The body contains certain antioxidant proteins, such as SOD (super oxide dismutase), which helps neutralize oxidatively induced free radicals. SOD requires three minerals, zinc, copper, and manganese, to function properly. Deficiencies of any one of these minerals may predispose to oxidation damage, with a resulting increase of susceptibility to breast cancer.

"Adequate amounts of calcium and magnesium are also important. Considerable evidence exists supporting the role of selenium in preventing and treating cancer. A dosage of 200 mcg daily is safe, and large amounts may be given with monitoring. Chromium and molybdenum may be supplemented as well, and these are also important.

"Recently I have begun to use the whole range of trace minerals in colloidal form as a supplement. That's a liquid form where the minerals are bound to organic chemicals. We use about 70 different minerals. Many of these minerals are in trace amounts, and have already been shown to be essential, and are probably lacking in our synthetically fertilized soil. I believe these colloidal trace minerals will play an important role in bolstering the immune system."

As mentioned earlier, a diet that is largely vegetarian and low in fat, mainly consisting of whole fresh foods, such as vegetables, fruits, whole grains, nuts, and seeds, protects against breast cancer. In addition, certain foods are medicinal in their ability to protect against breast cancer. They include:

Soybeans, soy products, and lima beans. Isoflavones and phytoestrogens found in soybeans, soy products, and lima beans protect against cancer. The low incidence of breast cancer among Japanese women is largely attributed to the widespread use of soybeans.

Flax. The omega-3 fatty acids in flax seeds and oil protects against breast cancer.

Fish. Fish high in omega-3 include salmon, tuna, sardines, mackerel, and herring.

Cruciferous vegetables. Vegetables such as broccoli, cauliflower, and brussels sprouts contain cancer-fighting substances.

Mushrooms. Reiki, shiitake, and maitake mushrooms have strong anticancer properties.

Hot, spicy foods, oily foods, and stimulants such as coffee, black tea, drugs, and alcohol should be avoided. Water should be pure, free from fluoride, chlorine, pesticides, and other synthetic chemicals. Many urban and suburban water supplies cannot be trusted and need filtering. As some filters remove chemicals and chlorine but not fluoride, a reverse-osmosis type of water purifier is recommended.

Natural herbal substances are a veritable gold mine for protecting women against breast cancer. Some herbs to know about are listed below:

Carnivora (Venus fly trap). This powerful herb is popular in Europe but less known in the United States. In Germany, it is even used to wipe out cancer that already exists.

Essiac. This is a Native American herbal combination that has a synergistic effect in putting an end to cancer and in its prevention.

Cat's claw. This formula is used by the Peruvian Indians for the prevention and treatment of cancer.

Evening primrose, borage, and black currant seed oils. All these supply gamma linolenic acid, known for its strong anticancer activity.

Xiao Yao Wan. This combination of digestive herbs increases circulation, builds blood, and breaks apart fibroids. The Chinese say it prevents breast cancer caused by phlegm and feelings of melancholy, which impede circulation to the chest. Xiao Yao Wan is available in Chinatowns throughout America.

Dandelion. Helps prevents cancer by breaking up phlegm and eliminating it from the system. Excess phlegm can turn into tumors.

Astragalus. A wonderful immune-strengthening herb that can be used in cancer prevention or as an adjunct to cancer treatments. Letha Hadady says, "It has worked wonders for my friends on chemotherapy who take this between sessions for strength." Add one teaspoon of astragalus powder to some pure water, and drink once or twice a day. Or try Astra-8, a combination of astragalus and other immune-strengthening remedies in capsule form, found in health food stores.

EXERCISE Dr. Michael Schachter notes, "Any activity that removes accumulated toxins in the breast reduces the chance of women developing breast cancer. Studies show that aerobic exercise is associated with decreased cancer risk, as exercise promotes lymphatic drainage and sweating helps remove toxins from the tissues."

"Although I am not aware of any direct studies showing reduction of breast cancer with a detoxification program using saunas and certain nutrients as done with the Hubbard method of detoxification," says Dr. Schachter, "I do know that this procedure has been clearly shown to reduce pesticides and other toxic chemicals in the bloodstream and in fat tissues. Since high levels of these substances increase the risk of breast cancer in women, reducing them with this detoxification method should help to reduce the risk of breast cancer to women."

MASSAGE Lymphatic detoxification is aided by manual lymphatic drainage (MLD), a simple method of massage, using light, slow, rhythmic movements to stimulate the flow of lymph in the body. Massage therapist James Kresse notes that this is especially important for women suffering from lymphedema, a condition that often occurs after a mastectomy: "When our lymph nodes are not functioning properly, or have been irradiated or removed, an excessive accumulation of stagnant waste occurs. The lymph system becomes overloaded, thus forming lymphedema.

"MLD should be applied directly after surgery, rather than when a massive edema has formed. This will guard against any possibility of a blockage in the system or alleviate any that exists. Studies in Europe show that severed lymph vessels regenerate with constant MLD therapy. The therapy makes the scars from the mastectomy more subtle, which increases the mobility of the arm. It also lessens pain from surgery and the uncomfortable sensitivity that occurs."

IMMUNO-AUGMENTATIVE THERAPY (IAT) In the 1950s, Dr. Lawrence Burton and a team of researchers discovered IAT, a nontoxic, noninvasive method of controlling cancer by restoring the patient's own immune system. Although the therapy demonstrated success, Dr. Burton left the United States after medical politics prohibited him from practicing here. In 1977 he opened the Immunology Research Center in Freeport in the Grand Bahama Islands, where thousands receive treatment for the disease. (See chapter 40 for more information on IAT.)

Since Dr. Burton's death, Dr. John Clement, an internationally respected cancer specialist who studied with Dr. Burton, heads the center. Dr. Clement gives an overview of how the treatment works: "The intellectual basis of the treatment is that many cancers can be controlled by restoring the competence of the patient's immune system, as the body's complex immune-fighting system may well be the first, best, as well as last line of defense against many cancers.

"The method we use is similar in any type of cancer we treat, although each patient has her treatment tailored to the results of her own blood test. We do not deal with toxic chemicals in any way. We assay the blood for the factors we believe are aiding the patient's own cancer. By identifying these factors, we are able to control them, put them back into balance, and hopefully destroy the patient's cancer."

Regarding breast cancer, Dr. Clement says: "We have had patients with breast cancer who have had no other treatment other than IAT for upward of 20 years who have no recurrence of disease. While we are still claiming only to control their cancer, you will see that to all intents and purposes, by any kind of medical description, they have been cured."

Dr. Clement reports less success with patients who come to him after extremely arduous chemotherapy and those with advanced cancer where there is a loss of bone marrow and fluid collection in the abdomen or pleural effusions in the lungs.

Addressing other forms of cancer that affect women, Dr. Clement states that IAT is often successful with cancer of the cervix if it is caught early, even after surgery. Additionally, lung cancer, which is becoming more widespread among women, and which is generally untreatable by conventional methods, can be more successfully treated with IAT. "We have a good measure of control with adenocarcinoma of the lung and with squamous cell carcinoma. If fluid is present, however, which indicates a more severe type of disease, very often we do not have much control. Nor do we have much luck with the type of cancer that is associated with smoking, the small-cell lung cancer. This is because small-cell lung cancer grows rapidly. Tumors will double in size in just 30 days. Our treatment does not work quickly enough to do these patients much good." As for ovarian cancer, Dr. Clement states, "We have been lucky. We have been able to control this cancer in people even after metastases and recurrences of the cancer following operations and chemotherapy."

MIND-BODY CONNECTIONS Exploration into the effects of outlooks and emotions on health and disease processes has opened up an exciting area of science, known as psychoneuroimmunology. Researchers have discovered that the mind, nervous system, and immune system interact with one another at the cellular level. When we feel joy, we enhance our healing mechanisms. Conversely, when we feel fear or hopelessness, we generate disease.

Dr. Carl Simonton, coauthor of *Getting Well Again* and *The Healing Journey*, is one of the early pioneers in this field. In the late 1960s, as a radiation oncologist, he noticed that emotional factors and patient attitudes influenced the course of treatment. His research led him to an extensive body of literature, where he learned that the three biggest mental influences on cancer are a tendency to respond to stressful situations with hopelessness, bottling up of emotions, and perceived lack of closeness to parents. This understanding prompted Dr. Simonton to look at the influence of counseling on the course of treatment. He discovered that survival times doubled, quality of life improved, and there was a better quality of death in association with counseling efforts.

Dr. Simonton firmly believes that emotions drive healing systems and that the imagination and standard counseling can be used to increase a patient's will to live: "The emphasis of our approach is to focus on what is right with the individual. We ask, What are the person's goals and aspirations? What are their main sources of inspiration and creativity? What is their sense of purpose and destiny? As people become clearer and more connected to these concepts, they rediscover a strong desire to live. That in turn enhances their inherent healing mechanisms.

"As we explore these areas, we begin to address those things that interfere with achieving these very important aims. One primary culprit is unhealthy beliefs. To demonstrate this, I would like to give an example of a patient that I have worked with for over 20 years. This 36-year-old woman came to me in 1976 with metastatic breast cancer that had spread to her ribs and spine. Her father was a physician, and her husband's family had run a retail store for three generations. She was involved in helping her husband run the family business.

"Her religious and spiritual life were important to her. It was a great source of strength. She wanted more time to be involved in religious administration and spiritual counseling. As she began to pursue these areas, her beliefs about how she should be the good daughter, the good wife, the good mother, came into play. These beliefs were all quite rigid, allowing virtually no freedom for her own creativity. Over time, we helped her to make a shift in these beliefs and behaviors, which was central to her recovery.

"She has been free of disease for 15 years. Currently, she is weller than well and runs marathons. The family store burned down about 10 years ago. Now she works primarily in church administration, doing religious and spiritual counseling, which is what she always wanted to do."

Dr. Simonton emphasizes that there is a relationship between all types of cancer and rigid thinking: "Here we tend to be controlled by beliefs about how we should be or have to be. That allows very little room for the expression of the spirit. Becoming aware of the direction that our life force wants to go is essential for renewing vitality and healing power. It becomes important to listen to the voice within and to develop ways of enhancing that. This takes practice."

Dr. Simonton says the way we use our imagination can mean the difference between success and failure in treatment: "In our imagination, we must think about the things we do for ourselves that are helpful. There are three areas that we need to look at: our beliefs about treatment, our beliefs about the body's ability to heal itself, and our beliefs about the disease itself. When a person is first diagnosed with cancer, if she shares the common cultural perspective, she believes that cancer is strong, that the body is weak, and that treatment is harsh. In keeping with these beliefs, a person is going to experience much in the way of undesirable side effects and less benefit. As we look at those beliefs, we find that they are not at all compatible with reality; cancer is a weak disease composed of weak cells. It is important to remind ourselves that our bodies have always been able to recognize and destroy cancer cells since before we were born. Shifting those images helps healing to occur."

Fibrocystic Breast Disease

Fibrocystic breast disease is caused by overcongestion from foods that clog the system, such as wheat, dairy products, refined foods, and fats. Caffeinated products, such as coffee, tea, chocolate, and soft drinks, are hard on the body and add to the problem, as does a sluggish thyroid, which makes metabolism more difficult and leads to constipation, causing a buildup of toxins. Toxic accumulations worsen congestion and can manifest as breast lumps (cysts). Stress further accelerates the condition.

Fibrocystic breast disease shows up as single or multiple breast lumps. Cysts are usually harmless, but are related to a higher-than-normal chance of breast cancer later on. Mammograms determine whether or not breast lumps are benign.

DIET AND NUTRITION A diet high in complex carbohydrates can make a difference; fruits, vegetables, grains, beans, and some fish are recommended. Red hot peppers, cayenne pepper, and regular or daikon radishes cut through mucus and help to eliminate breast lumps.

These nutrients offer extra help when combined with a cleansing diet:

Antioxidants. Selenium, and vitamins A, C and E.

Magnesium. Magnesium cleanses by entering cells and forcing out excesses of calcium and other minerals.

Iodine drops. Iodine speeds up the metabolism of the thyroid gland. As the metabolism perks up, breast lumps tend to disappear. Iodine drops from seaweed can be obtained in the drugstore in a saturated solution of potassium iodide or Lugol solution. There is also an Edgar Cayce remedy called Atomodine. In addition, health food stores sell iodine drops as liquid kelp. Before using iodine, a thyroid blood test should be done to check for thyroid antibodies. This ensures that there is no thyroiditis, an inflammation of the thyroid gland.

Herbalist Letha Hadady recommends the following plant remedies to break up congestion in the chest, and release phlegm and mucus from the system before they lead to more serious problems:

Xiao Yao Wan. This formula is a combination of digestive herbs that increase circulation, build blood, and break apart fibroids. Xiao Yao Wan is available in Chinatowns throughout America.

Dandelion. Dandelion tea or capsules can be taken everyday to break apart fibroids.

EXTERNAL TREATMENTS

Castor oil packs. According to medical psychic Edgar Cayce, stimulating liver circulation ends constipation. Substances that clog the body and form breast lumps are then eliminated. To do this, rub castor oil on the skin over the liver. Cover with a towel, and place a heating pad over it. Do this for 20 minutes each day.

Peppermint oil. Rubbing peppermint oil on breast lumps diminishes them by stimulating circulation.

Phytolaca oil and hydrotherapy. Dr. Joseph Pizzorno has found success with this combination treatment: "We have a woman put a hot compress on her breast so that it gets real warm. She then covers the area with phytolaca oil. Following the application, she covers it with a cold pack. We combine herbal medicine with hydrotherapy to help the cysts drain out of the breasts. I use that treatment with a lot of women, and have had quite a good response."

YOGA Dr. Gary Ross, a family physician and certified yoga instructor, recommends yoga poses, meditation, and breathing exercises for alleviating fibrocystic breast disease brought on by stress and a sluggish thyroid. These three postures increase blood flow to the thyroid and chest area:

Shoulder stand. On a mat or thick blanket, lie flat on your back. You may choose to place a rolled towel under your neck. Raise your legs over your head so that your body is in a U formation. Rest the elbows firmly on the floor and support the back with both hands. Adjust your body so that it is completely vertical. Then press the chin against the chest. Hold still as you breathe slowly, concentrating on the thyroid gland. You may only be able to do this for several seconds at first, but work up to one minute. To come down, lower the legs slowly toward the head. Then lower the back to the floor one vertebra at a time. When the back is on the floor, continue to lower the legs gradually until you are once again flat on your back. Do this once in the morning and once in the evening. For full benefit, follow with the fish pose.

Fish pose. Lie on your back. Legs can be straight or folded. If straight, place hands under buttocks, with palms down. Otherwise, hold onto crossed feet. Resting on the elbow, arch the chest and neck back. The head should be on the floor, but do not apply pressure there. Support should come from your elbows. Do not bend the neck too far back as that can impede circulation. Focusing on the thyroid, breathe deeply in this position, holding for 30 seconds.

Cobra. Lie face down, with elbows and palms down to the floor or mat and palms beneath the shoulders. With a smooth, gradual motion, raise the eyes upward, then the head, neck, and spine, one vertebra at a time. Allow the area below the hips to remain on the blanket. Hold the pose and then come out of it using reverse motions that are equally slow and gradual. Breathe in as you come into the posture, hold the breath while in the cobra, and breathe out when coming down.

In addition to these yoga asanas, Dr. Ross advocates deep breathing exercises for bringing more energy into the chest area. Visualization creates a mindset that helps lumps to disappear. Further, meditation creates spiritual and mental tranquility conducive to healing.

Breast Implants

Are breast implants really a problem? Going by news reports, the woman without medical training is bound to be confused. One report attests to their safety, while the next one says they are terribly damaging. Dr. Vicki Hufnagel, a gynecological surgeon and activist for women's health rights, offers the following view based on cases she has seen and her reading of the literature:

"I have seen plenty of women with breast implants who are dancers, actresses, or models, and I have seen terrible, terrible results. I have seen deformed breasts, and I have seen women who are fatigued, depressed, and in pain. Where their skin was once soft and supple, it is now hard and wrinkled. They look like they have aged 20 years.

"We did blood studies of women with implants and found antigens to the silicone. All their immunological studies were abnormal. To my mind, many of these women are experiencing a silicone reaction. It is real, not a figment of crazy women's imaginations."

Dr. Hufnagel adds that all implants cause damage from silicone, even those using saline: "A lot of women say, 'I'm going to have a saline implant and it is going to be safe.' That's a myth. All implants made are made of silicone. Saline is put in a silicone holding capsule."

Fragments of silicone react with tissue, even when the capsule remains intact. Dr. Hufnagel learned this after operating on a patient to remove saline implants and sending tissue to pathology for an analysis: "This was big news, and I flew to Washington with it. Here a woman with a saline implant, without a rupture, without a leak, with silicone only being used to hold her saline, gets silicone in all of her chest wall tissue."

Removing implants to reverse the problem has never been a simple option. Women who consider this choice are often talked out of it by surgeons who tell them that their breasts are too stretched out and that they will look terrible afterward. "Women are too scared to do anything about it," Dr. Hufnagel says. "They are afraid that they are going to look worse than they did before the implants were put in, which probably was fine to begin with. A lot of this image issue about having breast implants is probably due to social problems that we have in our society."

Indeed, once the implants are removed, women's breasts cave in and become grossly deformed. This sad state of affairs prompted Dr. Hufnagel to devise new surgical methods for restoring breast appearance during breast implant removal.

SURGICAL RESTORATIVE PROCEDURES Dr. Hufnagel's challenge was in figuring out how to take implants out without having breasts cave in. She reports success using an argon beam: "I asked myself, 'How do we shrink the dead space that has been created in a woman's body from tissue being pushed out?' I use the argon gas to send a heat-fiber type of electricity in a spraylike manner. This will not burn the body but it will shrink tissue. We take the whole chest wall, where this envelope is, and we shrink it. That prevents massive deformity.

"We operated on two small, thin women who had large implants in very small chests. Normally, they would have been deformed had we removed their implants. But we have had good outcomes. We really think we've hit on something.

"Also by using the argon beam, we are ablating the reactive tissue and allowing new healthy tissue to grow in its place. This is breakthrough surgery." Dr. Hufnagel adds that ending the need for such operations depends on psychological and sociological factors. "The silicone problem is going to be with us as long as women don't like themselves."

Before surgery, Dr. Hufnagel advises women to learn as much about silicone as they can, to get a complete diagnostic workup, including a silicone antibody test, and to follow a good vitamin program. "Surgery is stressful to go through, so build up your body," she advises. "Not too much vitamin C for the first two weeks, as it will increase scar formation. You want higher amounts of A and E. Avoid C until two weeks after surgery.

"Learn everything. Ask questions. Ask to look at pictures of women who have had their implants removed. If they don't remove the capsule, be sure that they at least biopsy it and submit it for tissue analysis to look for silicone.

"Finally, report your case to the FDA. Every case should be reported. That doesn't mean that the government is going to take action. But if we have enough people, someone someday may stick their nose in the file and find out, 'My goodness, after the FDA retracted their announcement on silicone, they got all of these reports and still did nothing.'"

Lymphedema

Lymphedema, a swelling of the limbs due to collecting lymph fluid, affects 1 percent of the U.S. population. As health practitioner James Kresse explains, "There are two types of lymphedema. The first is primary lymphostatic lymphedema, an inherent condition that predominantly affects women in their mid-30s but which can manifest at birth or during adolescence. The second is more common, and frequently occurs in patients who have had mastectomies or the removal of malignant tumors. The large increase in the incidence of breast cancer and subsequent mastectomy operations is one of the major reasons for the rise in lymphedema today. Secondary lymphostatic lymphedema can occur from six months to three years after the initial surgery."

SYMPTOMS Lymphedema appears as a swelling or skin thickening of a limb. It is important to detect the condition early, and this can be done in several ways. Kresse advises, "Notice any jewelry becoming tighter over a short period of time on the affected limb. Or squeeze the affected limb for 10 seconds. If an indentation is noticed, notify your surgeon immediately. Or measure your arm with a cloth tape measure around your wrist and forearm. If you notice an increase in the circumference of your arm, call your surgeon right away."

MANUAL LYMPHATIC DRAINAGE (MLD) Lymphatic detoxification is aided by manual lymphatic drainage, a simple method of massage, using light, slow, rhythmic movements to stimulate the flow of lymph in the body. "This type of therapy is very, very light," says Kresse. "It's almost featherlike. We're working on the parasympathetic nervous system. A regular massage stimulates the sympathetic nervous system. That is our fight or flight nerve. The parasympathetic nervous system is our night nerve, our rest and relax nerve. This is the nerve that lymph drainage affects in order to calm the patient down."

COMPRESSIONAL BANDAGING In addition to MLD, compression bandaging is used to apply pressure around the affected limb. Exercises performed with the bandage enhance muscular contractions that help with lymph flow.

LIFESTYLE CHANGES Kresse states, "If lymphedema is not brought under control with a combination of MLD, specific exercises, and a low-protein/sodium diet, along with combined decongestive therapy or the use of pneumatic pump, the affected limb can swell to an unsightly size and become life-threatening.

"There are dos and don'ts that a person should be aware of. Just to mention a couple, as far as the dos are concerned, the person needs to practice meticulous skin care with the use of pH-balanced lotions and creams to protect the skin. Following a good nutritional program consisting of lots of fruits and vegetables is helpful. Salt and fatty foods should be eliminated, and protein intake limited. It is important to maintain an optimum weight, as obesity contributes to lymphedema. Exercise such as swimming, walking, and stretching is excellent. Incorporating deep diaphragmatic breathing techniques, along with specific exercises taught by an MLD therapist, is good. While sleeping, the patient can elevate the limb by tilting the mattress or by placing pillows under the arm. Antibiotic solutions should be carried at all times, for incidental cuts, scratches, or bites. Infection should be treated at the first sign.

"Precautions to take include not subjecting oneself to extreme temperature changes, such as hot tubs, saunas, steam baths, or other thermal treatments. Care must be taken when using instruments on the infected limb, such as the instruments used in manicures and pedicures. Pets must be watched to see that they don't scratch or bite. Blood pressure readings, injections, vaccinations, or acupuncture should be avoided on the infected arm. Constrictive clothing and jewelry should not be worn. Heavy prostheses can cause excess pressure on the infected limb. Care must be taken when cooking, gardening, or doing daily chores. Finally, heavy objects must not be lifted. This can cause a lymphedema right away or somewhere down the line."

Other therapies that help lymphatic conditions include rebound exercise, ozone therapy, enzyme therapy, colon hydrotherapy, deep breathing exercises, and a good vitamin and herbal program.

Patient Stories

I have always been interested in holistic medicine, and I was a great fan of Carlton Fredericks. In 1989, when I discovered a lump in my breast, I sought help directly from a holistic doctor, Dr. Robert Atkins. I went to him before any diagnosis because I knew that if I had to have surgery, I wanted to see someone who was open-minded to alternative therapies.

The lump was malignant, and I had a modified radical mastectomy. Fortunately, my lymph nodes were clean, but the tumor was not a hormonal tumor and it was a very aggressive one.

I started therapy with Dr. Atkins, consisting of a low-carbohydrate diet. That meant absolutely no caffeine, and no sugar of any kind. I was also on a program of vitamins and nutrients targeted to my specific problem. Once a week, I was given an intravenous drip of an anticancer formula developed by Dr. Atkins, which was largely vitamin C.

Soon after surgery, I had a problem. The tumor grew back into the incision. Both the surgeon and Dr. Atkins advised radiation, which I was given for five weeks. While I was undergoing radiation, I did the IV weekly, and it alleviated any side effects of the radiation. I wasn't tired, and I was able to work half-days.

A month or so after the radiation, the tumor came back again in the area of the incision, and again it was removed. I continued Dr. Atkins's therapy. That was almost seven years ago, and I haven't had a problem since. I am still on the diet and the vitamin program. The intervals between the IVs have been extended to two months.

There is no question in my mind that Dr. Atkins saved my life.
—Marylou

I got breast cancer 10 years ago, when I was 39. I had conventional surgery but would not undergo chemotherapy or radiation. Since I had no positive node involvement and no metastases after surgery, I was told that I was fine and that there was nothing else to do. But because it was a very large tumor, and an aggressive one, I was concerned about it. Since I had been involved with natural medicine for a long time and pretty well educated in it, I started to search for ways to prevent the return of the cancer.

I discovered a lot of things. I went on a one-year program of injections of a formula that was mostly mistletoe. I had to get the prescription for the vials and send away to Switzerland for the formula. I injected myself with the herbal formula.

I did a lot of reading, and I took courses in Chinese herbology. I learned about several herbalists, and studied with Letha Hadady over the years. I took several workshops with her, where I learned about Chinese herbs and the whole philosophy of Asian medicine as well as the Ayurvedic and the Tibetan systems. Over the years, I have taken formulas of Chinese and Western herbs.

The results are difficult to show concretely. All I can tell you is that I don't have cancer and that 10 years later, after having had a very aggressive kind of tumor, I am still fine.

I believe in natural medicine. I also believe very firmly that it is important to have a practitioner, to not use the local health food store as your medical advisor. Everybody has to be examined individually.—Rita

When I was 46, my doctor found tumors in my breasts and my uterus. He screamed at me to see a surgeon, but I refused. The reason I said no is because of what happened to one of my best girlfriends, Kimberly. Kimberly was 34, beautiful, and very sensitive, with a wonderful husband and three stepchildren. She found a lump on her breast and went to the doctor. Her mammogram was negative but they did a biopsy anyway and found that it was can-

cerous. Three days later, she had her breast lopped off. That was followed up with lots of chemotherapy. Her hair fell out and she vomited 24 hours a day. She couldn't keep any food down. Then they did radiation and her skin burnt up and two of her ribs broke. Most people don't know how dangerous radiation is. I had seen enough. I wouldn't touch any of that medicine with a 10-foot pole.

I decided that I was going to try to heal myself using entirely natural means. By the way, I was already in a stage 4 situation, and my doctor had given me two months to live. So I had this deadline. I had to get well by February 15th.

Norman Cousins, who wrote a bestselling book about healing through laughter, says that a doctor shouldn't tell a patient that he or she is terminally ill. When you tell someone they are going to be dead in 18 months, they die in exactly 18 months. To counter that, I gave my immune system the opposite message. I had to get well in two months. Otherwise, I would lose my breasts, my uterus, and probably my house and my studio too because I don't have health insurance. I believe in giving yourself a deadline in a positive way, rather than in a negative way. Giving your body a positive deadline sets a healing situation in motion because. And of course, the brain is the main master of the immune system, so what you tell yourself will influence what happens to your body.

I got a lot of books out of the library. One said to eat brown rice. Another said to visualize. Still another said to do psychological work on yourself. I decided that I needed a whole program covering every single aspect of my life. I called my program MOTEP, Marathon Olympic Tumor Eradication Program. It's a funny title, but it shows how hard I worked on it.

First of all, I joined a Y and swam one mile per day. While I was swimming, I would incorporate Dr. Carl Simonton's visualization technique. I had used it before to get rid of a lump in my neck that I got from using acrylic paint. So I did have some experience at "self-lumpectomy," and this is what I was attempting to do.

I started to talk to myself in a very positive way, visualizing the tumors as shrinking and going away. This occurred during the Gulf War, so I would visualize a Scud missile actually hitting my breasts, and little white particles of the tumor floating into the water. I would actually see this. Then when I would take a sauna after the swim, I would visualize the tumor as actually melting.

All day I would invent these very aggressive visualizations. When you visualize, you don't want passive imagery, such as snowflakes or Tinkerbell sprinkles. Those are ineffective. You want to use very aggressive imagery: sharks eating your cancer, or Pacman, or Scud missiles hitting your tumor. It helps to believe that you can conquer this disease. So I believed 100 percent in my program.

My program also consisted of special foods based on the macrobiotic diet. I ate whole grains and fresh juices, vegetables and fruits, and some fish. No meat and no dairy products were included. I had lots of carrot juice because the beta carotene is very healing. I also meditated and chanted to get rid of stress.

There are two major points in my program. One is to detoxify the body and the other is to de-stress because your body cannot heal if you are full of heavy-duty anxiety. You want to calm your body down with meditation, chanting, and other spiritual activities, such as white-light meditation, in which you visualize a white light cleaning out your body.

I also got myself into group therapy because this has been shown to extend the lives of cancer patients. Furthermore, I healed my relationships. People in good relationships with social support are the ones who live the longest. So you want to mend your relationships or get out of them. If a relationship is destructive, you don't want to be in it. A woman in my group is going through a terrible divorce and she has breast cancer. She decided to go away to Puerto Rico to Ann Wigmore's healing place for awhile. I think that's the best thing she can do. She needs to get away from her stressful situation so that her body can heal.

I broke up with a boyfriend and turned him into a friend because he was causing me a lot of distress. He was going out with other women and bringing out feelings of jealousy and anger in me. I cleaned out all those negative emotions from my body.

One month later, my body went through a horrible healing reaction, called inflammatory breast cancer. My breasts turned bright red and hard as a rock, and my left arm was totally paralyzed. Unfortunately, inflammatory breast cancer is not recognized as a healing reaction. If a surgeon cuts the body at that time, the patient dies immediately from the trauma. Women need to support their bodies at this time. Then they have a great chance of living through it.

I continued with my program throughout my healing crisis. Three weeks later—this is one week before my appointment—I knew I had won the battle. My yellow-green hue disappeared and natural color came back to my cheeks. Two days later, both tumors were gone. This was five days before my appointment. My body responded to my deadline.

My doctor was shocked not to find any lumps. He examined my breasts three times to be sure. He looked for my uterine tumor, but that was gone too. He finally said that I should make a video about my experience. That's when I decided to write my book, Keep Your Breasts: Preventing Breast Cancer the Natural Way.

Women around the country are using this program to get well without subjecting themselves to surgery or drugs. And we have had outstanding results. One woman changed her mammogram results in only 10 days from the time she told them to clear, and she was high-risk. Another woman dissolved a lump in only two weeks. Once you have the information, it's easier to utilize than if you have to look here and there and try to piece it together like I did.—Susan

A 24-year-old woman came to me with benign breast lumps on one breast. She had had a lifelong history of severe constipation, requiring laxatives and enemas. On top of that, she basically lived on muffins, breads, and coffee.
The first thing we did was take her off all caffeine. That included coffee, tea, chocolate, and soft drinks. To eliminate the congestion, we asked her to stop eating muffins and bread.
This was a start, but it didn't address her constipation problem. I investigated that further and found that she had a mild case of subclinical hypothyroidism. This means that her blood tests for thyroid function were normal, but clinically she felt sluggish and constipated, with slightly dry skin, and a low body temperature. This condition is crucial to correct; when thyroid function is low, the body is unable to metabolize excessive amounts of congesting foods. I put her on a low dose of natural thyroid. That, coupled with dietary changes, antioxidants, magnesium shots, and castor oil packs, absolutely changed her life. The breast cysts and constipation went away. Her energy picked up. It was absolutely amazing.—Dr. Gary Ross

I had been overexposed to the sun and wound up with a severe toxic reaction. It was sun poisoning that went one step further and became lymphedema. Instead of just having blisters on the surface of the skin with lymphatic fluid in them, my lymphatic fluid was backed up. The lymph nodes weren't clearing them up, and it wasn't coming to the surface the way it should. So, I wound up with a severe case of lymphedema. My ankles were the size of my knees, and I couldn't really walk. I let myself get dehydrated because I couldn't even take going to the bathroom. It was the most horrible thing I ever encountered.
I finally dragged myself to the Healing Center after three or four days of agony. That's when I began alternative treatments. I had a vitamin infusion, using 75,000 mg of vitamin C. I had lymphatic massage and was prescribed homeopathic remedies. I was also prescribed huge amounts of bioflavonoids, as well as quercetin, essential fatty acids, and lecithin.
I also used magnets, which were great. Not only did they help the lymphatic drainage, but they freed me from pain. I applied those to my legs—first ceramic magnets, and afterward electromagnets. These really helped with circulation and healing.
I had great relief and was once again able to walk normally instead of dragging my feet.—Susan

56

Cervical Dysplasia, Fibroids, and Reproductive System Cancers

Cervical Dysplasia

Cervical dysplasia is an abnormal growth of cervical tissue caused by the sexually transmitted human papilloma virus (HPV), the same virus that is responsible for cervicitis, genital warts, and possibly cervical cancer. These conditions can be detected with a Pap smear.

The likelihood of a woman contracting cervical dysplasia increases with intercourse at an early age, having unprotected sex with several male partners, smoking, birth control pills, and weak immunity. Naturopathic physician Dr. Tori Hudson explains, "Women who have intercourse at an early age are more vulnerable to getting genital warts and cervical dysplasia because the cells of the cervix at that age are more susceptible to being infected by the virus.

"Smoking is the biggest factor in acquiring cervical dysplasia and cervical cancer. If you smoke, and you are exposed to the virus, you are much more likely to develop dysplasia, and you are much more likely to develop cervical cancer from your dysplasia. We know that the nicotine itself actually lodges in the glands of the cells of the cervix. When exposed to the virus, the DNA can change to take on more abnormal features. If you have genital warts and you smoke, it is much more likely that they will turn cancerous as well.

"Oral contraceptives are known for creating a folic acid deficiency, and folic acid deficiency is associated with acquiring cervical dysplasia, and having the disease progress to cancer."

Dr. Hudson describes cervical dysplasia as a progressive syndrome that develops over time: "After initial exposure to the virus, there is no indication that anything has changed. Later, immune changes may occur. Warty tissue may develop, then mild dysplasia, moderate dysplasia, severe dysplasia, carcinoma in situ, and then invasive cancer." Since these symptoms are not evident upon physical examination, Pap smears are necessary.

PREVENTION AND DIAGNOSIS OF CERVICAL DYSPLASIA Since HPV is sexually transmitted, the conditions associated with it are preventable. Notes Dr. Hudson, "Cervical dysplasia, genital warts, and cervical cancer are all sexually transmitted diseases. That should make an impression on all of us, because it really dictates how we should protect ourselves.

"Obviously, we shouldn't smoke. We should protect ourselves by having safe sex and a healthy immune system. If you take birth control pills, it is advisable to take folic acid. A good maintenance dose would be 800 mcg daily. Those are the main ways to protect against cervical dysplasia and genital warts." Additional preventive daily supplementation may include 1,000 mg vitamin C and 25,000 units of beta carotene.

To catch the condition early, Dr. Hudson stresses yearly Pap smear exams. Statistics show that the longer women wait between Pap smears, the higher the incidence of cervical dysplasia and cervical cancer.

Before treatment, it is essential to get fully diagnosed to determine the stage of the illness. If a woman has an abnormal Pap smear, her partner needs to be examined by a urologist for warty tissue. Otherwise, they will be passing the virus back and forth and reinfecting each other. Diagnosis by a licensed, well-trained, alternative practitioner will determine if a woman is a candidate for natural treatments only or whether she needs to integrate these approaches with conventional methods.

CONVENTIONAL TREATMENT FOR CERVICAL DYSPLASIA Conventional medicine usually does nothing to treat mild dysplasias and genital warts. "Basically, they wait to see if it gets worse," says Dr. Hudson. "Often the body can reverse mildly abnormal states to normal on its own, as the body has an extraordinary ability to heal itself. But when it can't, then the disease progresses, and the downside of waiting becomes apparent."

In the later stages, aggressive measures may be taken. The preferred conventional treatment is known as LEEP (loop excisional electrosurgical procedure), which uses an electrical wire to cut out abnormal tissue. This is less expensive and less traumatic than the method of treatment previously used, called cone biopsy or conization. In advanced disease states, a hysterectomy may be needed to save a woman's life.

NATUROPATHIC TREATMENT Women with cervical dysplasia often have excellent results using naturopathic approaches. Dr. Hudson notes, "In the results of a research study that I conducted at the College of Naturopathic Medicine in Portland, we treated 43 women with varying degrees of cervical dysplasia.

Through my treatment protocol, 38 of the 43 reverted to normal, three partially improved, and two had no change, meaning they didn't get better and they didn't get worse."

Dr. Hudson's protocol consists of three parts: systemic, local, and constitutional treatment. An overview of her therapy is outlined below:

SYSTEMIC TREATMENT

Beta carotene. 150,000 IU daily.
Vitamin C. 3,000–6,000 mg daily.
Folic acid. 2.5–10 mg daily.
(Note: High doses of folic acid must be prescribed by a naturopathic physician. After three months, the amount of folic acid is decreased.)
Immune herbal formulation

LOCAL TREATMENT

Vitamin A suppositories
Herbal suppositories

CONSTITUTIONAL TREATMENT

Dietary changes
Use of condoms
Avoidance of smoking
An optimal immunity diet is low in fat, and high in whole grains, vegetables, and fruits. Immune system inhibitors such as coffee, sugar, alcohol, and fat are omitted.

At the end of three months, it is very important to follow up again with a health practitioner, and to obtain another Pap smear. Sometimes a biopsy is also needed.

Fibroids and Uterine Bleeding

Fibroids are growths, composed of muscle tissue and usually benign, that attach themselves to the inner or outer wall of the uterus. One in five women over 35 has them; the majority of these women are African-American. These tumors grow in response to estrogen levels. Medically, they are also referred to as fibromyoma uteri and leiomyoma uteri.

Complementary physician Dr. Robert Sorge says that fibroids are nature's way of encapsulating toxins that result from an unhealthy diet and lifestyle: "Most of our patients with this condition consume tremendous amounts of coffee. As far as I'm concerned, this is something that every person concerned about their health must stop drinking. Diet sodas, greasy fries, pizza, potato chips, doughnuts and danishes, and other devitalized foods add to the problem."

Registered nurse and licensed acupuncturist Abigail Rist-Podrecca adds that Oriental medicine sees fibroids as the result of blockage to the uterine area: "This can be caused by anger, emotional upsets, or a history of problems with menstruation, where it is either late or prolonged. Sometimes, after an abortion, the endometrial wall will still have some cells from that particular pregnancy. Further down the line, that can develop into fibroids."

SYMPTOMS Small fibroids are symptomless, but when they grow, they may result in painful periods, bladder infections, and infertility. Uterine bleeding is another common symptom, explains Rist-Podrecca: "If the fibroid is located on the inside of the uterus lining, then you will have this uterine bleeding, which usually sends women to the gynecologist, where they opt for hysterectomy. If the fibroid is located on the muscle wall, then there is not so much bleeding, but the fibroid will continue to grow."

Dr. Sorge adds that bleeding is the body's attempt to restore balance, according to naturopathic medicine: "Circulation and oxygenation of the uterine muscles and blood vessels is diminished, and metabolic waste products begin to build up. Bleeding is the sign of a highly toxic condition attempting to correct itself."

CONVENTIONAL APPROACHES TO FIBROIDS

MYOMECTOMY

Small fibroids that do not cause problems are sometimes removed by a procedure known as a myomectomy. This procedure removes the fibroid only and does not interfere with a woman's ability to have children.

HYSTERECTOMY

For larger tumors, or fibroids that cause heavy bleeding, hysterectomies are standard treatment. Dr. Herbert Goldfarb, a gynecologist and assistant clinical professor at New York University's School of Medicine, reports that the majority of these operations are unnecessary, as well as dangerous: "Each year 750,000 hysterectomies are performed, and 2,500 women die during the operation. These are not sick women, but healthy women who go into the hospital and do not come out. Surgical procedures have morbidity, which means complications, and they have mortality, which means death."

In addition, hysterectomy can be psychologically destructive: "Some women want the operation and are all right about it, but most women feel like lambs being led to slaughter. They really don't want to have this procedure done, but their physicians give them no alternative.

"A new laser procedure, called myoma coagulation, has the potential to end the use of hysterectomy for fibroids once and for all, but most people don't know about it. My book, *The No Hysterectomy Option*, was written in response to my frustration at having a technology to help women avoid hysterectomies, but women not knowing about it. Sometimes women need hysterectomies, but often they are told they need them for frivolous reasons. My book is designed to help women understand when it is needed and when other options are available. I always like to say that hysterectomy may be indicated, but it may not be necessary. Our best customer is an informed consumer.

"We could avoid hysterectomies in well over 50 percent of the patients now having them. Breaking it down, somewhere between 10 and 20 percent are done for cancer. At this point, I am not going to say that these can be avoided, although some of the ones done for precancerous conditions of the cervix can. But hysterectomies for conditions like endometriosis are not needed. Endoscopic, laparoscopic procedures, and judicious use of alternative medications will control these conditions. Regarding fibroids and bleeding, we can take care of this with myoma coagulation if the condition is caught early enough."

ALTERNATIVE THERAPIES FOR FIBROIDS

MYOMA COAGULATION AS A MEANS OF AVOIDING HYSTERECTOMY

Dr. Goldfarb has lectured extensively to doctors on myoma coagulation (also called myolysis), which has enabled him to successfully prevent hysterectomies in hundreds of women with fibroids and uterine bleeding.

The typical candidate for the procedure is the woman uninterested in reproduction, since the uterine wall may become too weak to support pregnancy. Also, the size of the tumor must be 10 cm or less (approximately 6 inches). If the fibroid exceeds this size, it can be reduced with the medication Lupron. Dr. Goldfarb explains: "Lupron reduces estrogen levels in the body, and temporarily reduces the size of fibroids. With Lupron, we get a 30 to 50 percent reduction in size."

Once the tumor has become smaller, coagulation can be performed, which shrinks it another 50 to 75 percent and puts an end to the problem: "When we do this procedure, we literally undermine the tumor by destroying its blood supply. As we put needles around the fibroid, it turns blue, showing that the blood supply has been interrupted. Fluid and blood go out, and the tumor shrinks. It becomes stringy tissue and just sits there, becoming very small, which eliminates the need for removal. The patient has no symptoms and can go about her life without the need for further surgery."

The cost of myoma coagulation is equal to other operations, but cost-effective in the long run: "The good news is that patients come into the hospital in the morning, have the procedure done, and go home in the afternoon. That saves the insurance company significant amounts of money. Also, these patients go back to work within a week so that there is very little cost in terms of disability."

DIET AND EXERCISE

Since fibroids grow in response to estrogen, nutritionist Gracia Perlstein advocates the natural lowering of estrogen, through diet and exercise, as a first-line defense against fibroid growth.

"Research shows that an over-fatty diet increases estrogen in the diet, and we know overweight women produce more estrogen. So the first approach would be dietary.

"The best diet for a woman attempting to decrease the size of her fibroids, or at the very least keep them from getting any larger, consists of whole foods, and is semivegetarian or vegetarian. The best protein sources are from vegetables and include whole grains, especially millet, amaranth, quinoa, buckwheat, whole grain oats, and brown rice. A wonderful way for cooking whole grains is to put one part grain to four parts water in a slow cooker. Before going to sleep, turn the cooker on low or automatic shift, which starts high and lowers. When you wake up in the morning, you have a creamy, delicious whole-grain cereal. That's a wonderful way to eat whole grains every day.

"Eat small quantities of legumes daily. Soybeans and foods made from soy, in particular, contain isoflavones that discourage tumor growth. Foods made from soy include tofu, fortified soy milk, miso, and tempeh. A variety of other beans can be used to make wonderful ethnic dishes and include black beans, adzuki, pinto beans, chickpeas, mung beans, lentils, and lima beans. Grains and beans are your best source of proteins.

"If you eat meat, I recommend eating only small quantities of it, no more than 3 ounces per day. Three ounces fits into the palm of your hand. It should be only from animals that are free-range and grass-fed, with no hormones or antibiotics. A good way to get animal protein is to make soup stock with chicken or fish bones. Simply put them in pure water and simmer, with a little organic cider vinegar, for a couple of hours or overnight. Red meat, poultry, and conventional dairy products, which are fed hormones, should be avoided entirely.

"The liver detoxifies excess estrogen, so you want to support liver function by avoiding all recreational drugs, alcohol, fried foods, coffees, and any processed or refined foods. Be sure to drink at least two quarts of pure water a day to help your bowels and kidneys. You are trying to remove excess estrogen from the system, and this is supported when your organs of elimination work properly."

"Regular exercise will reduce excessive estrogen levels. Most people are familiar with the fact that hard-training women athletes sometimes reduce their estrogen levels to the point where they stop menstruating. We are not after that kind of effect, but regular exercise is very beneficial and helps the body remove excess estrogen."

SUPPLEMENTS

For further uterine support, Gracia Perlstein recommends the following supplements and herbs:

Balanced oil supplement. One tablespoon daily. Balanced oil supplements are a mixture of flax, borage, and other unrefined, natural, organic oils.

Multiple vitamin/mineral supplement.

Iron and herb supplement. This should be taken if there is anemia from heavy bleeding. Avoid high doses of iron as they are implicated in cancer and heart disease.

Vitamin E. 400 units, twice daily.

Silica supplement.

Vitamin C with bioflavonoids. 1,000 mg, five times daily divided over the course of the day.

Evening primrose oil. 100 mg, three times daily.

False unicorn root. Fifteen drops of the tincture in a small amount of water can be taken every hour when there are acute uterine problems.

Shepherd's purse. Fifteen drops of the tincture in a small amount of water, three times a day, may stop excessive bleeding.

White ash may reduce size of fibroids.

Perlstein asserts that such a comprehensive program of diet and lifestyle changes, geared toward reducing excess estrogen, gives the body the tools it needs to shrink fibroids or keep them from growing any larger. In addition, the side effects of such a program are wonderful: "You will be slimmer and have more energy than you would using conventional methods, which have harmful effects."

NATURAL HYGIENE

Complementary physician Dr. Anthony Penepent recommends fasting for excessive uterine bleeding, short of life-threatening situations where the woman needs hospitalization: "This condition signals liver poisoning. During the course of the month, a little fasting might be in order, in addition to a very strict hygienic regimen, to straighten out the condition. I have had patients with all forms of dysfunctional uterine bleeding, and to my recollection, I cannot remember any woman who followed my instructions who did not have a good result."

OIL-SOLUBLE LIQUID CHLOROPHYLL

Dr. Joseph Pizzorno says this old natural therapy can quite effectively put an end to abnormal uterine bleeding. Oil-soluble liquid chlorophyll is available in capsules. Two to three are usually taken two to three times a day.

Dr. Pizzorno says that for some unknown reason, the chlorophyll seems to relieve this condition: "Many people think this works because it improves clotting, but it turns out that women with abnormal uterine bleeding do not have clotting abnormalities. So why it works is not clear. But the bottom line is, it works quite well."

HERBS

Abigail Rist-Podrecca says the following herbs are good to stop dysfunctional uterine bleeding when taken under the supervision of a Chinese herbal practitioner:

Poo wha. Made from bee pollen.

Er jow. From the hide of an animal.

Chuan xiong (Ligusticum wallichi). Regulates bleeding by the amount taken. Too much causes uterine bleeding, and too little stops it.

Han lian cao (warrior's grass). Helps tone the spleen and uterine and stops intense uterine bleeding.

ACUPUNCTURE

Acupuncture points that relate to the uterus are found on the ankle. Rist-Podrecca explains how electrical acupuncture to this area helps reduce fibroids: "We use a small electrical current. This makes the uterus contract and expand. It palpates the area slightly to get the body to recognize that the fibroids are there, to increase circulation, and to start vibrating them so that they are released."

HOMEOPATHY

Consider the following remedies for uterine bleeding and fibroids:

Ipecac. Dr. Marjorie Ordene, of Brooklyn, New York, recommends this remedy to stop acute hemorrhaging with bright red blood. "When given in the 200 potency, every 15 minutes, ipecac slows down the bleeding. That's two pellets under the tongue, until the bleeding actually stops. I have had success with a number of patients, and other physicians have reported this as well."

Dr. Ken Korins says the two remedies to think of first for heavy bleeding are shina and sabina.

Shina. This is for heavy, dark, blood that forms clots and leads to debility and exhaustion.

Sabina. Also for clots, but here the blood is bright red. When large clots are being expelled, there is a laborlike pain that radiate from the sacrum to the pubis.

In addition, these are other formulas to consider:

Secale. Women who need secale have dark blood that is almost black. Periods are profuse and prolonged.

Phosphorus is indicated when there is bright red blood with no clots.

Trillium. Bleeding is very heavy and bright red. The person characteristically feels faint and dizzy after bleeding. Periods occur biweekly, and are worse with any slight movement.

The following remedies are specifically for fibroids:

Aurum muriaticum. This remedy is for fibroid, when there are no other symptoms. There is no heavy bleeding and no particular discomfort. It may help reduce their size of the fibroids.

Hydrastinum muriaticum. Has been known to cure large fibroids, especially when they seem to be on the anterior wall of the uterus, pushing on the bladder and causing symptoms of urinary frequency and pain.

Reproductive System Cancers: Ovarian and Cervical

Women are susceptible to ovarian cancer and carcinomas of the uterine cervix, either cervical or endometrial cancer. Of the three, ovarian cancer occurs most often, and is growing in frequency. It usually manifests after menopause, especially in women who have few or no children, who were unable to conceive, or who gave birth later than the average age. Other factors that place women at risk include a past history of spontaneous abortions, endometriosis, type A blood, radiation to the pelvic region, or exposure to cancer-causing chemicals, such as asbestos.

Cervical cancer is associated with promiscuity at an early age, a genital herpes infection, and multiple pregnancies, while endometrial cancer is related to a history of infertility, failure to ovulate, the use of drugs containing estrogen, and uterine growths.

SYMPTOMS OF REPRODUCTIVE SYSTEM CANCERS Uterine cancers are easier to detect in the beginning stages, and tend to be more treatable, whereas ovarian cancers are rarely discovered early on, and are terribly damaging to the individual's quality of life.

Abnormal bleeding in the vaginal area, especially after menopause, is the chief sign of endometrial cancer. Sometimes there is pain in the lower abdomen or back. A Pap smear does not always catch endometrial cancer early on, but it can be detected with a surgical exam of the uterus.

In the early stages of cervical cancer, symptoms are usually absent, although there may be a watery, vaginal discharge or spotty bleeding. Signs of advanced cervical cancer include dark, odorous vaginal discharges, fistulas, weight loss, and back and leg pain. One's chance of survival increases with early discovery through yearly Pap tests.

Women should look for these early indications of ovarian carcinomas: abnormal vaginal bleeding, weight loss, and changes in patterns of urination and bowel movements. While a Pap smear will not detect ovarian cancer in the beginning stages, it may be discovered through annual pelvic exams.

CONVENTIONAL TREATMENTS Contemporary treatments for ovarian cancer are a disappointment in that while they can make cancers disappear for weeks or months at a time, they will, in fact, fail in the end, as the cancer returns with a vengeance to finish the job. In fact, orthodox survival rates for ovarian cancer patients are only between 5 and 10 percent. Cancers of the uterine cervix initially exhibit higher success rates with surgery, which may involve the removal of the uterus (hysterectomy), as well as both ovaries and the fallopian tubes (salpingo-oophorectomy), in addition to x-ray and hormone therapies. But there is no guarantee that the cancer will not return.

Gar Hildebrand says that more patients would triumph over reproductive system cancers if a combination of approaches were employed. He states, "No one should be treated by a single specialty, and then watched in hopes that the cancer will not come back. It's not scientifically justifiable, nor is it acceptable to the patient. Sitting and waiting just causes horrible, immune-suppressing anxiety.

"Let's say a woman with an ovarian cancer has just been admitted to Memorial Sloan-Kettering Cancer Center. The first thing the doctors will do is a laparotomy. She will be opened up, and a surgeon will get the bulk of the tumor out. I have no problem with that.

"But the second step [should] definitely not be to use drugs that kill tumors. Tissue damage always accompanies cancer; unless it is addressed, the cancer is sure to reappear. In other words, throughout the body, tumor toxins cause cells to lose potassium, and to swell with extra salt and water. This state is worse around the tumor itself. Often times a treatment that goes into the bloodstream fails to penetrate to a tumor effectively because the tissue next to the tumor has no immunity. What's really needed, then, is for the patient to be stabilized physiologically. The ideal treatment would be for the person to receive nutritional salt and water management, a diet that nourishes and corrects the water retention in the cells. We're going to feed the whole body to try to get the tissues back to normal functioning."

ALTERNATIVE APPROACHES TO REPRODUCTIVE SYSTEM CANCERS

DIET AND NUTRITION

Hildebrand recommends a diet that detoxifies and stimulates cells back to health. "Doctors have long been aware that most cancer patients have an aversion to meat. They'll smell it and gag; that's a self-defense mechanism. It's absolutely essential for these people to stop taking in heavy proteins—animal proteins and sometimes even heavy vegetable proteins, like legumes—for a while, just to clear up. The tumor's converting that stuff into caustic chemicals, related to the ammonia we use in our laundry machines. It's those chemicals that create damage systemwide.

"We can also detoxify the body by supplying oodles of plant chemicals, called phytochemicals. These foods can be eaten cooked or raw, and should include vegetables of all sorts, fruits, and a few whole grains. Fruit and vegetable juices are especially important. You have to flood the system with nutritious fluids, such as carrot and green leaf juices. Apple juice should always be added because apples contain a material that is very good for cellular energy. If you put those juiced phytochemicals into the body every hour, these cancer patients will have their cellular enzyme systems speeded up so that the individual cells can spit up toxins.

"Eating an excess of empty calories and proteins creates toxicity that causes the immune system to overproduce white blood cells that aren't very adept at what they do. Once you restrict protein and calories and get the nutrient level up, these patients' immune systems become intelligent again. They stop making excess stupid white cells, and create more lymphocytes interested in more types of challenges. In other words, you get a very lean, mean immune system."

COFFEE ENEMA

Hildebrand explains how coffee enemas are used: "These enemas have been used by thousands of cancer patients, outside the realm of traditional medical care, because they work. Boiled coffee in retention enemas stimulates the liver's enzyme system, which in turn causes great relief from pain in cancer patients. The liver has more than a thousand documented medical functions. When we help it to work better and faster, the cancer patient's overall physiological condition changes, sometimes within hours, and certainly within the first several weeks of treatment. You have a whole different person. People come off gurneys and out of beds, excruciating chronic pain is eased, and addiction to morphine is broken.

"Every three minutes, all the blood in our bodies goes through our liver. Our livers and small intestine walls have an enzyme system with a fancy name that we will call GST for short. This enzyme system naturally responds to cancer in the body by going up, and the coffee enema has been shown in laboratory experiments with rats, and in later experiments with humans, to produce increased liver bile flow, and to stimulate the GST enzyme system. In fact, it's raised to 700 percent of normal levels of activity. When the GST system is running that fast, it can effectively remove tumor toxins from the bloodstream. And it doesn't take very long. The effects of these coffee enemas will last for sometimes four, six, or eight hours before a feeling of discomfort and pain around the tumor returns. They're that effective.

"You have to know how much coffee to use: a quart of water with three tablespoons of coffee boiled in it. That's cooled and strained, not filtered, because a filter would remove some of the molecules that stimulate the GST enzyme system. The coffee is safely taken into the colon, while the person is lying on his or her right side, retained for 10 to 15 minutes, and then released. Patients doing this without the supervision of a physician should know that anything cooler than 100 degrees is going to cause cramping in the intestines."

HYPERBARIC OXYGEN

"We're also going to try to increase circulation with full-body-immersion oxygen therapy," Hildebrand continues. "Hyperbaric oxygen treatment is given in a diving chamber that used to be used to treat the bends. There's been a lot of fascination with ozone in cancer treatment in the alternative field. But what we found is that ozone applications only raise tissue oxygen by 25 to 50 percent, whereas hyperbaric oxygen can predictably raise oxygenation by 800 to 1,000 percent. This means that tissue around the tumor, which doesn't have enough oxygen to function, can get sufficient oxygen for energy production. This will also allow the tissue to repair itself by producing a high-potassium, low-sodium environment, so that this edema can come out of the tissue."

COLEY'S TOXINS

Hildebrand states that this treatment has the most glorious record of any treatment in the cancer literature, especially when combined with the Gerson diet program, consisting of hourly glasses of fresh juice and coffee enemas: "I am hopeful that much interest will be sparked in this therapy because, right now, the only reports I've seen of long-term survival for ovarian cancer patients have been from a combination of these approaches.

"The word toxin is a little confusing, because Coley's toxin is not really a poison. It refers to a bacterial endotoxin that is an immune stimulant. I would put that directly into the abdominal cavity once the tissue around the tumor has been stabilized.

"Coley was a physician who searched the literature for cancer treatments after a heartbreaking experience of losing a child patient to the disease. Much to his surprise, he found a skin infection called erysipelas. Erysipelas is caused by a streptococcus that causes a skin fever of 105 to 106 degrees. This fever causes an inflammatory infection which interferes with tumor action.

"Coley constructed a live erysipelas vaccine, which was too toxic at first. Some patients died, but others experienced a tumor regression. He went through a lot of trial and error, and eventually settled on something which we now call Serratia marsecians. He mixed the serratia and the strep in a ratio of 1,500 cells to one, and then crushed the mixture through a microfilter to liberate the internal toxins of the bacteria. This liberated antigens, which would in turn cause the immune system of the patient to think that there was a chronic infection that had to be fought.

"Coley's toxins seem effective due to the fact that the immune system, when turned on, can cause a lot of dust to rise. These patients need to be put into an intensive care unit, and hooked up to monitors, just in case of a problem, although there have never been any heart attacks or kidney failures reported in the 900 cases that have been thoroughly studied. Then a tiny amount of toxins is administered intravenously for four hours through a drip. About two hours into the process, the immune response begins. The patient will develop chills and shaking and that last for about half an hour to 90 minutes, followed by a rise in temperature of about a degree every 10 minutes. Once that temperature hits 105 or 106, the ICU staff lies them down or puts in a suppository of Tylenol to stop it.

"The reaction is the immune system's response. This is not a poison. This is not a toxin. It's not like chemotherapy making your hair fall out or causing bone marrow suppression. The Coley's toxins are much more like what happens when your immune system decides to cure you of an infection. So the symptoms are more flulike, without the nausea and vomiting. After the second or third IV application, patients usually get sleepy and actually nod off. The fever lessens progressively. In other words, there's a honeymoon period.

"Coley himself said that if you don't keep these up for at least three or four months, in booster dosages, you won't get a permanent response. The literature reveals that gains are lost when Coley's toxins are given in lower concentrations or for shorter durations. But when properly used, there is an extraordinary 50 percent cure rate in advanced, inoperable uterine and ovarian cancers."

THE BENEFITS OF AN OVERALL APPROACH Gar Hildebrand re-emphasizes the importance of utilizing any and every cancer protocol that works: "We believe that it's time we stopped living in an either/or world, where orthodoxy is over on one side and the marginalized alternative professions are in the trenches and foxholes, and nobody talks. We believe it's time to get the doors and windows of communication open, so that we can find the context for each of these treatments and the way they fit together.

"Our own experience reveals that using the nutritional approach takes a toxic load off of the immune system and speeds up intracellular enzymes, so that they can repel toxins and pull them from the blood rapidly. Calorie and protein restrictions, and a diet high in nutrients, can lead to sensitization of the tumor. Years of experience shows that diet therapy alone can produce monthly fevers. And tumors may or may not regress through those fevers. But if you stimulate the immune system when those fevers are hitting, you have a much greater chance of tumor reduction. That's why we suggest the marriage of these disciplines, and the respectful recognition of the role of every aspect of anticancer medicine that's ever been developed."

Patient Story

I still have cervical cancer, but I am working on overcoming it through a number of approaches. I watch my diet very carefully. I feel that my condition is in an early enough stage where I can handle it nutritionally. But it's not just nutrition that I have to deal with. I have to deal with all the emotions that help to create disease in the body. It's also a matter of detoxing. I do colonics and a lot of juicing. I take supplements. And I do meditation, and exercise.

The major reason I started to see a nutritionist was, of course the wake-up call, the cervical cancer, which was just diagnosed three months ago. But I had also had ulcerative colitis for almost twenty years.

I feel like I now have energy again. I exercise at least several times a week, which was literally impossible before. I even had trouble getting up a flight of subway steps without feeling exhausted at the top. So I have several different things that I am working with: nutrition, meditation, and detoxification. I'm working on it.

Now I have to find a gynecologist who is holistically oriented because my primary care physician dropped me after I refused to have a hysterectomy. I feel very lucky. I feel that someone else trying to deal with this would have followed the recommended course of action and would have given up their reproductive rights, allowing themselves to be mutilated, and always fearful of having the cancer reappear.

Also, I feel that the cancer is nothing more than a wake-up call. Your body is saying, "Hey, something is wrong here. You're out of balance. You need to address this, this and this." If you don't, disease is the end result. Now I am vegetarian and doing a lot of things differently. If I didn't, I might not be alive now. I might be at a higher risk for the cancer to spread throughout more of the body. This doesn't mean that I am 100 percent there. I still have a lot of work to do. But I feel very hopeful.—Morgan

57

Menopause

Menopause marks the end of the female reproductive cycle, which typically occurs between the ages of 45 and 50 but can happen anywhere from 40 to 60, or earlier as a result of surgery or illness. Perimenopause, the beginning stage, normally occurs over a period of years, and may take as long as a decade. Many women harbor misconceptions about the nature and effects of menopause; in cultures where menopause is less feared, symptoms are virtually nonexistent, and in fact menopause is anticipated as a rite of passage into a stronger, wiser time of life.

Causes and Symptoms

During menopause, the ovaries shut down, and estrogen, a hormone produced by the ovaries, diminishes and eventually stops. The symptoms of menopause are the result of the body's readjustment to the absence of estrogen.

One of the first symptoms perimenopausal women experience is a change in the frequency of their menstrual cycle. The time between cycles may increase or decrease, or it may skip a month. Usually blood flow is reduced, but, occasionally, women experience heavy, irregular bleeding. Another common symptom is hot flashes. Additionally, women may experience dry skin, mood swings, depression, irritability, vaginal dryness, night sweats, bladder infection, fatigue, and sleep disturbances.

Before menopause, estrogen is produced by the ovaries; afterward the adrenal glands take over. Women with healthy adrenal glands at menopause therefore experience less traumatic changes.

Misconceptions about Menopause

MENOPAUSE CAUSES A LOSS OF SEX DRIVE

According to clinical psychologist Dr. Janice Stefanacci, society expects menopausal women to lose their sex drive, but this does not have to be the case. "Many women fear that they are going to lose their passion and sexuality. Really, only a small portion of women who go through menopause have their sex drive adversely affected. For these women who lose their sexual desire or have difficulty becoming and staying aroused, help is available. But most women do not experience sexual arousal problems, and many report feeling more sexual because the risk of pregnancy is gone."

MENOPAUSE CREATES PSYCHOLOGICAL PROBLEMS

Dr. Linda Ojeda, author of *Menopause Without Medicine*, says many women see menopause as the beginning of the end. "They believe that life is going to be downhill from this point on. They no longer think of themselves as youthful, as able to contribute to society. They fear that their behavior will become erratic, hysterical, and out of control. This is not true. When we reach 50, we do not turn into these raging maniacs, and we are not more susceptible to clinical depression. In some women, however, lowered levels of estrogen, endorphins, and serotonin, the hormones that affect mood, can create mood swings. Levels can be raised naturally in these women.

"We know that beliefs and attitudes affect the transition," she continues. "In Asian countries, symptoms are virtually nonexistent. In these countries, menopause is looked at as an important event in a woman's life. She now has more prestige and is viewed as a wise, older woman. Women anticipate this time of life with relish. If you are approaching menopause with fear and trepidation, you need to examine your attitude."

MENOPAUSE IS A DISEASE

The medical community has created this belief by stressing the need for hormone replacement therapy. In reality, menopause is not a disease but a natural transition that should be dealt with naturally. Dr. Ojeda wants women to know that there is a science behind safe, effective, holistic methods for helping women through this transition period easily.

Dangers of Hormone Replacement Therapy

Dr. Bruce Hedendal of Boca Raton, Florida, expresses concern regarding hormone replacement therapy as it is practiced in this country today. "The powers that be would like us to believe that they are using hormones. They are if your own body is making them, or if they are from plant estrogen sources, like soy products and yams. But Premarin, the most commonly given synthetic, is actually from pregnant mares' urine. Ten million women take Premarin in pill or patch form.

"Most people are told that estrogen prevents osteoporosis. This is true to some degree. Around menopause, the benefits of synthetic estrogen replacement therapy is effective for five to seven years only. It slows down the bone loss, but it does not reverse it in any way, shape, or form. The studies have shown that 8 to 10 years after menopause is finished, there are no benefits to estrogen replacement therapy on bone loss.

"The average woman would be surprised to learn that synthetic estrogen has some very serious side effects. I've talked with a lot of holistic doctors. Their opinion is that synthetic estrogen has definitely been shown to increase the risk of cancer of the breast. They have been toying with this concept for years. Of course, the makers of Premarin and other synthetics say no, but the research now confirms this as true."

Dr. Robert Atkins adds that estrogen therapy has one side effect that people don't talk about: insulin resistance. "This syndrome is characterized by low blood sugar, high blood pressure, or high insulin levels. But the most frightening one of all to most women has to do with upper body obesity." The good news is that natural therapies often make the need for synthetic estrogens unnecessary.

Natural Alternatives

DIET Dr. Jane Guiltinan, a naturopathic physician from Seattle, Washington, says, "A lot of women don't know that there may be alternatives to estrogen replacement therapy. There are some very good plant sources of estrogens in some of our foods. In fact, you can get significant amounts of plant estrogens. They have been shown in several research studies to improve menopausal symptoms.

"The food that has the highest content of estrogen is soy. Soybeans, tofu, tempeh—anything made with soy—will contain plant estrogens. Oats, cashews, almonds, alfalfa, apples, and flax seeds contain smaller amounts of estrogen. A woman emphasizing those foods in the diet can experience significant decreases in her hot flashes."

Studies suggest that too little magnesium in the diet causes hot flashes. Magnesium can be found in whole grains and beans and soy products.

Sugar, which can cause hot flashes and other menopausal symptoms, should be avoided. Sugar, coffee, and alcohol adversely affect the blood sugar and can disturb the emotions.

VITAMINS AND MINERALS The following nutrients provide an additional boost to good health in the menopausal years:

Multivitamins. Women need a natural multivitamin/mineral supplement containing higher amounts of magnesium than calcium, and high amounts of B and C vitamins. A good multiple vitamin helps build the adrenal glands, which lessens emotional symptoms.

Vitamin E. This vitamin is known for its ability to rejuvenate the reproductive system and alleviate hot flashes. Low amounts of FSH and LH are related to hot flashes, and Vitamin E helps to increase levels of these brain hormones. It also helps lessen vaginal thinning and dryness. Mixed (beta, delta, and gamma) tocopherols are best as they are found together in nature. D-alpha tocopherol is also preferred over synthetic vitamin E. Generally, 400 IU per day should be taken in the beginning. The dosage can be gradually increased to 600 IU, although some women may need up to 800 IU.

Zinc. This mineral supports ovarian function. A good source is zinc picolinate. It can also be taken as an amino acid chelate or as zinc methionine. Twenty-five to 30 mg per day is generally needed.

B complex. B-complex vitamins are important throughout life, but there is an extra need for these during menopause. They can be obtained from whole grains, and green vegetables. B_5 and B_6 are especially helpful during menopause (300–400 mg B_5, 150 mg B_6 per day). Folic acid, in prescription doses, is a valuable replacement for female hormones, according to Dr. Carlton Fredericks.

Essential fatty acids. EFAs, which are precursors to the natural hormones in the body, are very important for both men and women. People on low-fat diets should pay special attention to this. A diet too low in fats can lead to an increased risk of cancer and aging. Omega-6 fatty acids can be found in flaxseed, sesame, pumpkin, and safflower oils. Omega-3 fatty acids are found in fish oil capsules or fish. Both are needed. EFAs help prevent or treat vaginal dryness.

Vitamin D. The best source of vitamin D is sunlight. It can also be taken in supplementation (400–600 IU per day), although caution should be taken not to get too much of this vitamin. Another source of vitamin D is salmon oil. People living in polluted environments need more vitamin D.

Calcium. Calcium is essential for the prevention of osteoporosis; supplementation should begin before the onset of menopause. There are many forms to choose from. Dairy is a poor source because many people have an intolerance to it. Calcium citrate is easy to digest, as it is already in an acidic medium. Calcium carbonates are alkaline and therefore more difficult to digest. Amino acid chelate is an excellent source of calcium. Calcium lactate is another good source. Calcium gluconate can be made into a powder and mixed into drinks; 1,300 mg per day, from food and supplemental sources, is the recommended dosage. If it is not being absorbed well, more may be required. Each person should be analyzed to see the amount needed.

Gammalinolenic acid (GLA). This is available as evening primrose oil, borage oil, or black currant-seed oil; 200 mg per day is recommended.

Boron. Research shows boron to be a precursor of both female and male hormones.

OTHER SUPPLEMENTS Additional products that help create hormones include:

Pregnelalone. Taking 25–30 mg a day serves helps the body create female hormones.

DHEA. Natural DHEA, found in wild yam extract preparations, rejuvenates the body.

Progesterone cream or serum. Progesterone is a woman's rejuvenating hormone, which protects against cancer and fibrocystic cysts and increases the beneficial effects of thyroid hormone. In addition, it guards against osteoporosis by putting calcium back in the bones. After menopause, progesterone can be taken three or four weeks out of the month. Wild yam cream contains progesterone, and can be purchased over the counter. Oral natural progesterone can also be taken.

Estriol. This is a natural, friendly estrogen that has been shown to inhibit breast tumors in animals. Some gynecologists are beginning to recommend Estriol for menopausal women, as being safer and more effective than synthetics.

Triple Estrogen. This formula is 80 percent estriol. The remaining 20 percent is made from estrone and estradiol. Estriol provides protection from breast tumors. Together, estrone and estradiol help protect against osteoporosis and cardiovascular problems. There are no negative side effects.

HERBS

Chaste berry. Sold under the trade name, Vitex, chaste berry is commonly referred to as the menopausal herb because it alleviates many symptoms, including hot flashes, vaginal dryness, and mood swings. It works by raising the progesterone level.

Ginkgo biloba. Studies demonstrate ginkgo's effectiveness in leveling mood swings.

Ginseng normalizes brain hormones. It balances body temperature and is effective in preventing hot flashes.

Wild yam contains beneficial progesterone, the precursor of estrogen. This gives a woman the building blocks needed to create more hormones.

The following herbs may also prove beneficial: licorice root, black cohosh, dong quai, alfalfa, red clover, sarsaparilla, and blessed thistle.

HOMEOPATHY The homeopathic remedy chosen should correspond to the symptoms described. According to Dr. Ken Korins, a classically trained homeopathic physician in New York City, only one should be used for best results. Sometimes it's a matter of trial and error; if one does not work, another can be tried. These are some of the remedies Dr. Korins recommends for menopause:

REMEDIES FOR HOT FLASHES:

Lachasis. Heat is felt all day long, while cold flashes may be experienced at night. Once the flow begins, all the symptoms disappear. Symptoms are worse with pressure and heat, and better with the onset of discharges or flows. Increased sexual desire is also associated with a need for lachasis.

Belladonna. There are many hot flashes. The face looks red and feels hot, and there is hot perspiration coming from the face and a pounding, throbbing, congested feeling in the head. Often there is dryness. Condition improves with resting quietly in the dark. Symptoms worsen with light, cold air, and sudden jolts. Emotionally, the state can border on hysteria with rages.

Glonine. Hot flashes are focused, with pressure in the head and feelings of congestion. There may be an associated rise in blood pressure at the time of the flashes. Symptoms are worse with heat and better with cold air. Emotionally, there is a fear of death and mental agitation.

Amyl nitrate. Flashes of heat are accompanied by headaches. Often they are associated with anxiety and heart palpitations.

Manganum. Hot flashes are associated with nervous system depression. The body does not want to move. Symptoms improve when patient is lying down. Emotional state is peevish and fretful. There is a loss of pleasure in joyful music, but a profound reaction to sad music.

REMEDIES FOR FLOODING (irregular periods which stop for awhile and return very heavy); these remedies may also help younger women with extremely heavy periods:

China. There is heavy bleeding, with dark, clotted blood. This leads to debilitating fatigue. Symptoms get worse with drafts and light pressure, but better with strong pressure and heat. Emotional symptoms are apathy with a strong disposition toward hurting other people's feelings (not the normal state).

Sabina. Characterized by heavy, bright red, clotted blood. Expelling the clots is painful, and radiates from the sacrum to the pubis. Emotional symptoms are irritability and a dislike for music.

Secale. Periods are profuse and prolonged. Blood is almost black. Symptoms worsen with heat and improve with cold.

Phosphorus. There is easy, frequent bleeding of bright red blood, often with no clots. The emotional state is low-spirited, with multiple fears. Also, memory may decrease. Another symptom is constant chilliness.

REMEDIES FOR VAGINAL DRYNESS AND THINNING:

Sepia. The vaginal area is itchy and dry. There is a sense that the uterus is falling out of the vagina. There is also a loss of libido. Symptoms tend to be worse with standing, cold and rest, anything that causes venous congestion. Symptoms are improved with anything that increases venous flow, such as motion. Emotionally, there is an indifference to loved ones, sadness, and a tendency to weep easily.

Natmur. Vaginal dryness makes sexual intercourse very painful. Discharges tend to be acrid and burning. There is often a loss of pubic hair. Emotional state is one of depression and irritability, which is worse with consolation. Symptoms also tend to worsen around ten o'clock in the morning.

Bryonia. Vaginal dryness is accompanied by severe headaches. Any motion is painful and distressful. Condition gets better with rest.

Nitric acid. Vaginal dryness reaches the point where the mucosa fissures, causing splinterlike sensations in the vaginal area.

EXERCISE Regular exercise can reduce the frequency and severity of hot flashes. This is because follicle stimulating hormones decrease. For best results, it is a good idea to begin exercising before menopause begins. Otherwise, it may trigger hot flashes. Exercise also alleviates mood swings and depression by naturally raising serotonin and endorphin levels in the brain. The best exercises to engage in are dancing, brisk walking, running, swimming, biking, and tai chi. Additional benefit is derived from cross-training, doing different exercises on different days. The advantage is that it prevents any one part of the body from becoming overdeveloped.

AROMATHERAPY "Aromatherapy is truly holistic because it is a mind and body treatment," states Ann Berwick, author of *Holistic Aromatherapy and Women's Health*. "I think this is part of the secret of its power." Berwick uses essential oils to help alleviate a number of conditions, including hormonal imbalance in women going through menopause. "Cyprus, fennel, and clary sage are believed to have estrogen-like effects. For overall balancing, I recommend to my clients that they use these oils in a lotion or body oil, and apply to their body two or three times a day. When women are experiencing hot flashes, I also suggest that they breathe in peppermint or basil on a Kleenex throughout the day. I find that a great help for most of my clients."

AYURVEDIC MEDICINE: "THE SCIENCE OF LIFE" Ayurveda means "the science of life." It is a system of medicine widely used in India for the past 4,000 years. Menopausal women report relief and rejuvenation from Ayurvedic formulas using herbal phytoestrogens and phytoprogesterones. Ayurveda believes that balance is the key to perfect health. It basically determines which body/mind type a person is and, based on that system, helps people choose the type of foods they should eat and the type of exercise best for them. For more information, read *Perfect Health* and *Ageless Body, Timeless Mind* by Deepak Chopra.

REFLEXOLOGY In chapter 49, Laura Norman outlines reproductive system reflex points. Here she gives additional information on specific ways to relieve menopausal symptoms: "For menopause, in addition to working the reproductive organs, I also would encourage you to work your thyroid gland, as this will help take over when the ovaries stop producing estrogen. This is how to find this point: the base of the toes reflects the neck area where the thyroid is located. At the base of your toes, press your thumbs and thumb-walk across that ridge, particularly in the base of the big toe.

"Another area to massage is the adrenal gland reflex point. You are on the big toe side of the foot. Go about a third of the way down your foot. You are under the ball of the foot, in line with the big toe. If you press your thumb into that area, it will provide energy when you feel fatigued.

"Also, the pituitary gland, which helps all the other glands to work, is located in the center of the big toe. Pressure applied there helps stimulate that area. Both feet should be massaged equally."

PART ELEVEN

Of Special Concern to Men

When many people think of the Hong Kong cinema, what immediately comes to mind are gangsters or kung fu fighters. However, the Chinese, whose doctors have given great attention to sexual dysfunctions, such as impotence and infertility, also have created many films that dwell, often in a comic manner, on these matters. I'm not talking about pornography but raunchy ribaldry as in the film *Sex and Zen*. At the beginning of the film, the hapless hero accidentally has his penis cut off. He wanders from magician to quack to alchemist, trying to find a replacement. One offers to take one from an animal, and another fashions a prosthesis out of tin.

The earthy comedy's underlying comment is on the importance of sexual expression to Chinese culture, something we will have reason to be thankful for in these next few chapters as we note, among other remedies, Chinese herbal formulas used for men's health problems.

58

Sexual Dysfunction in Men

Impotence is of concern to men everywhere as has recently been highlighted by the sensation caused by Viagra, a "wonder drug" that has restored potency. It soon turned out that Viagra was not as wonderful as it was cracked up to be. We will begin this chapter with a few remarks about this pharmaceutical in a discussion that will also delve into the psychological causes often behind impotency. We will also make some mention of the natural slowing down in sexual activity that accompanies aging. At a certain stage, we will see, repeatedly using Viagra or other drugs to stimulate an erection may be an unwise act of forcing the body to go beyond its natural bounds. Then we will bring up the subject of male menopause, which is not just a time for a man to look backward at what he has lost in aging, but to look ahead at what positive changes he can make and new plateaus he can reach. Then we will look at herbal remedies for impotence as well as those that come from Chinese medical theory.

Impotence, Aging, and Viagra

Dr. Michael Tierra is a consultant who has 25 years of experience with Chinese medicine. His East West Clinic is located in Santa Cruz, California. He is the founder of the American Herbalists Guild and has written a number of books on herbal medicine, including *Chinese Traditional Herbal Medicine*.

He told me told me about a patient he was seeing. "I had a gentleman about 70 years old, who had tried Viagra with poor results. He would get an erection but he had no desire for his partner. I had him check on the drugs he was taking."

Dr. Tierra explains that the drugs an older man will take often have impotence as a side effect. A doctor imagines a man of 75 or so shouldn't even think about sex, so he won't mention the side effect.

"This particular gentleman was taking Coumadin, a blood thinner to prevent heart attack. I think this particular drug may have been causing the impotency."

This doesn't mean, Dr. Tierra cautions, that once the patient had adjusted his medication, he should return to Viagra. "With Viagra, the body is being forced to do something it is not naturally inclined to do. This is asking for trouble. If you don't find the cause of your impotence, and you just force your organ to perform, you may be exhausting some latent resources in your body." Moreover, Viagra has side effects, such as heart attacks.

"The issue here," according to Dr. Tierra, "is a man needs to recognize that as he ages, he needs to slow down. But there is so much ego involved in sexual performance [that he refuses to acknowledge aging]."

I spoke further about this with Jed Diamond, a licensed psychotherapist and leader in the men's movement, who has published all over, in *The Wall Street Journal*, *The New York Times*, and other places. His latest book is *Male Menopause*.

He points out that to think of Viagra as the only treatment for impotence is stifling the possibilities. "Erective dysfunction is very common," he says. "There are a number of viable treatments. Viagra is only one way." He mentions the many natural alternatives such as L-arginine and ginkgo. These two release the nitrous oxide mechanism, in the same way Viagra does, that allows for a relaxation of the blood vessels in the penis, which allows for erection to occur.

Diamond continues, "Right now the situation around Viagra is bad. It's being prescribed like candy, rather than, as it should be, recognized as a very potent drug."

Diamond shares this anecdote: "I was on a TV show with a woman whose husband had taken this drug. The couple had had a good sex life but they wanted to make it just a little bit better. He was in his 60s. He went home from the doctor's, took the Viagra, and, in the middle of lovemaking, went into convulsions and died. The wife said, 'I don't know if it was the Viagra or something else.' Maybe he would have died anyway. The point was the Viagra had been prescribed by a urologist who didn't know this man very well, hadn't taken a good medical history. So, don't take those drugs without checking into them, seeing how they will affect your particular physiology."

Dr. Michael Tierra notes that the Viagra craze is partially ego-based. Men feel a psychological pressure to perform. "But few men are good lovers because they don't realize that women are slower to get aroused and so these men are not catering to the women's needs."

Such attitudes make them think they should have sex more often than they are really capable of having it. According to Dr. Tierra, a man at age 50 should be having sex once a week. By 60 or 70, he should cut back to once or twice a month. That's sex with ejaculation. He points out, in Chinese erotic thought there is a concept unknown in the West: sex without ejaculation is a gratifying possibility. Women can have sexual fulfillment without ejaculation, and men need to learn more about this path. Men need to become better lovers.

Moreover, there is a physical reason to occasionally practice this type of sex. Chinese doctors argue that ejaculation depletes energy and so should be done with moderation.

As one ages, there is a natural drying process and the vital secretions will lessen. That's why people wrinkle as they get older. There are not enough vital secretions in the body. Women will have dryness of the vagina as they age.

You've heard of young people being referred to as "ripe" or "luscious." These folk idioms contain the observational truth that the body is touched by plentiful secretions when we are young.

As we age, these secretions are at much more of a premium. You don't want to waste these secretions.

Male Menopause

The aging as it first becomes evident in the middle of middle age is now being called "male menopause."

Think about this. Every six seconds another baby boomer turns 50. With these tens of millions of people aging, there is a wake-up call going out. Say you're an average guy, who's just hit the big 50. You worked on your career, your family. You got the best education that's available. But did you pay attention to your health. Did you think somehow that because you were so knowledgeable, so successful, that by proxy your health would do well?

Maybe you misconstrued what it means not to be overweight. You think because you're not overweight, then you're not sick. I've got news for you. There are people who are processing cancer or diabetes or heart disease, and they are not overweight.

Probably back in the 1960s, you were into eating naturally, and living in a clean way, but somehow it all fell by the wayside.

A man's midlife crisis is now called male menopause. The symptoms of the crisis, according to Diamond, are drops in testosterone, and DHEA, among other things. These are measurable changes, but their significance varies as does the rate of drop. As a man reaches this stage, there is also increased fatigue, and a loss of memory, especially short-term memory. There's going to be a weight gain, even for those who exercise and keep fit. There will be emotional changes, often increased indecisiveness, fearfulness, anxiety, and depression. There will be sexual changes, including a lowering of sexual desire, particularly toward a partner a man has been with for a long time. There are difficulties with erections and less of a general feeling of well being.

Dr. Eric Braverman, author of *Male Sexual Fitness*, gives more details on how aging affects sexuality. "Men begin to experience a sexual decline after age

30. The biological reasons for this decline are a falling testosterone level, falling amounts of growth hormones, and lower DHEA levels. These declines are programmed into the body in the same way a woman is programmed to experience menopause around age 50." At that age, women are no longer fertile and their bodily changes reflect this. Men can be fertile till age 80, but their sperm counts start declining by age 40 or even at 35."

Sexual frequency also begins to slow down, although men may not notice this change until age 50 or 60. But a majority will begin to experience a deficiency in the hormones mentioned from about age 40. There is a reduction in the ability of the gastrointestinal (GI) tract to absorb nutrients. The brain slows down, losing 10 milliseconds of speed per decade, and losing alpha waves.

Diamond says there are a number of courses a man can take as he experiences these changes "Some men will react by saying, 'This is old age. We have to accept it.' Other men react by trying to go backwards to return to their youth. Maybe they try to find a younger woman or buy a sports car. Whatever the attitude, there's much more positive ability to move ahead if a man takes care of his health." As he sees it, this is the crucial period that determines if the second half of a man's life will be powerful, productive, and passionate or whether it will be a time of ill health, despair, and depression.

Male menopause comes along from about age 40 to 55, although, in unusual cases it could range from as early as 30 to as late as 65. With men there is more of a bell-shaped curve for its onset than there is for female menopause. For the female, it takes place in a much narrower time period, around age 45.

Now these are not just hormonal and physical changes, but they are accompanied by psychological changes. A man begins to question, asking, "What have I done with my life?" and "What have I done that was significant?" There are also spiritual changes as the man begins to ask bigger questions, such as, "Is there something to life beyond just acquiring things?" Suddenly, a man may feel the need to pursue a calling, not just a career.

Often at this age, a man becomes a mentor, teaching some of the things he has learned to younger men. This is so essential because without that you have younger men growing up without role models, with a feeling that older men don't care about them. And you have older men who are saying, "I've had a career. I've raised a family. But there's something missing." That missing component is the feeling of giving something back.

Society needs this mentoring. This is an opportunity the male menopause can offer. The chance to take on something larger, which will not only be good for the man but for youth and society. Also at this stage, friendship and intimacy grow more important as well as having a partner one can get to know more deeply.

"Now I'm often asked," Diamond told me, 'what can women do to help men who are going through male menopause?' For one, they have to try to understand what is going on. Second, women have to take this seriously, because there can be erection problems, depression problems. This is not just a mild transition.

"And third," Diamond added, "this time can be looked forward to. We don't have to look at this period as if doors were only being closed. They are also being opened. It can be a wonderful time if we will understand it."

Holistic Approaches to Sexual Dysfunction

Having seen the general parameters of this stage in a man's life, let's look some recommended therapies for impotence.

Dr. Braverman recommends a holistic approach, saying, "My practice is holistic toward treating sexual dysfunction. The penis is an organ like any other organ in the body so we follow the key principles of healing we would with any other organ."

When he finds a man is having a problem, he checks a number of physical functions. He checks blood flow. "If it is retarded, we will use niacin, chelation, even Viagra, to increase blood flow to the penis."

He also looks at whether the nerves to the penis are healthy. Here he looks for any influence of diabetes or neuropathy.

Careful measurement must precede treatment. "There is no substitute for measuring," Dr. Braverman says. "No one can manipulate a patient's testicles and say, 'Yep, there's enough testosterone there.' No doctor or healer can look at someone's belly and say, 'The liver is certainly making enough growth hormone.' It just can't be identified without tests. We have to measure it all."

There are markers whereby doctors can measure statistically the level of anxiety or the level of depression that may be associated with sexual dysfunction. They can accurately determine the levels of testosterone, DHEA, and so on. "This is no guessing game," Dr. Braverman says.

Dr. Braverman's practice differs from that of conventional physicians in that he looks at the whole picture. Sexuality is not just related to the penis. Where testosterone is low, of course, the penis is affected, but also the general health levels are going down. The DHEA, which is coming from the pancreas, liver, and brain, is dropping, and these organs are also touched.

Also, when a person is anxious, depressed, has insomnia or emotional upsets, this will have an effect on the brain. Any failure in the bodily system will weaken sexual functioning.

After looking at the circulation and the nerves, Dr. Braverman's major concerns are the adrenal glands, the growth hormone axis (brain, pancreas, and liver), the GI tract, and the brain. If there is weak absorption in the intestine, for instance, this will cause an overall bodily imbalance.

"What's exciting about all this," Dr. Braverman says, "is that if we look at the body as a whole and work with that, we can get better results than from just treating the genitals alone."

According to his experience, growth hormones can yield dramatic results in men in their 50s, 60s, and 70s. And DHEA can also be very impressive. To help sustain an erection, there are various agents that make the erection last longer, so men can have better sexual experiences. He sees these and other new treatments creating "a new age in the treatment of sexual dysfunctions."

Dr. Braverman recounts some of the more dramatic cures he has witnessed. There was a man who hadn't had sex in nine years. He was the victim of a stroke. He went on DHEA growth hormone and testosterone. This restored him sexually.

"I had a 72-year-old man," Dr. Braverman says, "who told me he was interested in having sex once a week. After we got him started on growth hormones and other substances, he found himself having it six times a week."

The funny thing, he mentions, is that usually when you treat men and improve their libido and performance, you end up treating their partners too, because the partners are not ready for this.

Another incredible case. A man in his 60s was having memory problems. Dr. Braverman began treating his hormonal imbalances, which also affected his sex drive. His wife had mentioned that, in 30 years of marriage, he had been a low sex person. The treatment had gone on a while and his wife came in. She couldn't believe the change. "'Wow,' she said, 'I wish we had come to you earlier.' This was a low sex man who seemed to have little need for human warmth. We changed around his whole attitude. Not just his desire for sex, but he was hugging, touching, feeling, experiencing a sensual relation to another person in a way he never had before."

Herbal Treatments

Besides going to a doctor and setting up a well-rounded treatment, there are a number of natural methods that can be used to overcome impotence. One is the herbal approach.

C.J. Puotinen, a noted herbalist, explains that the best herb to choose depends on the cause of the problem. If it can be put down to an arterial blockage, ginkgo biloba, widely regarded as a memory tonic, can help increase circulation, as has been documented in European studies. If you take 240 milligrams (mg) of ginkgo daily, it should relieve impotence due to arterial blockage. Ginkgo biloba is best taken as a standardized extract because the constituents are not readily assimilated by the body. It does not break down well with alcohol either so it's not effective as a tincture or crude extract. Throughout Europe you can get this herb in capsule form, although though this is not so popular in the United States.

More generally, Puotinen's two most common recommendations are yohimbe bark, which is a strong aphrodisiac, and damiana, "which is a gentler, more romantic, milder herb. The latter is suggested as a first choice when dealing with problems of impotence, since it has fewer adverse side effects."

Yohimbe bark, because of its strength and side effects, is often taken in combination with other herbs. It should not be taken by those with high blood pressure, heart or liver disease, diabetes, kidney problems, or by anyone who uses alcohol, tranquilizers, or antihistamines. When you are taking it, you should not be consuming such things as liver, cheese, or red wine. In fact, with all these restrictions, the bark sounds more like a pharmaceutical than some of the other herbal preparations.

Puotinen doesn't recommend a given dosage, since it is best taken in one of the combinations available in health food or herbalist stores. These combinations should be used according to the directions on the label.

The root is often taken with damiana, stinging nettle, and green oats. Incidentally, a few years ago, a Chinese corporation accidentally fed carp it was raising these last two herbs, and the fish's reproduction increased.

Puotinen says that in *The Male Herbal*, by James Green, the following dosages are recommended: "Take two tablespoons of yohimbe bark and add them to two cups of water. Make a tea by simmering for 10 minutes. Add one gram of vitamin C to stop nausea and aid in assimilation. Drink one or two cups. If you feel any side effects, such as gastrointestinal problems, then try smaller dosages or take the bark in blends. This bark should only be used for a short period of time. It's not something you want to repeat more than once in a day. This is not a tonic."

For most of the other herbs, such as green oats, when they are taken in a tincture, one or two droppers full should be taken once or twice each day for nine or ten days. If the effect is not achieved, dosage should be increased. If you take them in capsule form, one or two capsules two or three times a day is usually recommended.

General Facts About Herbal Treatments

Herbalist C.J. Puotinen notes that herbal remedies come in three broad categories: tonics, medicinals, and poisons.

Tonics are very safe and can be taken over a long period.

Medicinals have side effects. They should be taken in small dosages for a brief time under an expert's guidance.

Poisons are only to be used with an expert's advice, in minute quantities in a tightly controlled protocol.

One way these herbs are available is in raw or crude tinctures. A tincture of this sort is an alcohol extract made by putting one of these herbs in combination with vodka or another grain spirit. These extracts are named "crude" because you are not dealing with one chemically manufactured in the laboratory.

(In chapter 60, we detail how you can make these crude extracts on your own.)

Other Nutritional Remedies

Amanda Crawford, an herbalist from California, offers some additional nutritional recommendations. She has a degree in phytotherapy from Britain's College of Herbal Medicine and is a member of the National Institute of Medical Herbalists.

Nutritionally, she says, the first place to start is with fat-soluble vitamins, particularly A and E. These can be taken in supplement form or in foods.

"I recommend eating six pieces of organic fruit every day. Any fruit a man likes: oranges, apples, papayas, blueberries, pears, all through the list. Go out and spend money on the most inviting fruits available in the market."

You might want to work on preventing cardiovascular disease with the supplements that are good in that area. B vitamins can be obtained by n eating whole grains. Garlic can be taken—two to four cloves a day or 1,000 mg as a supplement. Also take magnesium, from 50 to 100 mg a day. This is also rich in many foods.

Chinese Medicine

Another approach, which also uses herbs, but is based on a more systematic analysis of the underlying causes of the problem, is that of Chinese medicine.

Dr. Michael Tierra says Chinese therapy begins by trying to uncover the root causes of the problem.

To grasp the Chinese system, it will be useful to begin by briefly outlining the two basic energy principles that it sees as guiding life. These are yin and yang. Yin is connected to the parasympathetic nervous system and hormones. Yang is the sympathetic nervous system and is responsible for stimulating hormones.

Impotency is said to stem from one of three possible debilities intimately involved with the yin/yang duality. Let's list them and their accompanying treatments.

Blood deficiency and stagnation, arising from poor circulation. The indications of this state are weakness, anemia, and paleness. Dong quai is recommended here. Although it is commonly given to women after menstruation to restore the blood, it can also be useful in this instance.

Yang deficiency is due to an androgenic hormone deficiency. Here the male hormones need to be strengthened. This type of impotency can be recognized by coldness, weakness, and spontaneous perspiration. What would be useful here might be rehmannia and eucommia. They should be taken in combination at 15 grams per day, broken into two doses. Dr. Tierra adds, "They are regularly taken together because the Chinese don't see one herb as totally answering a medical problem. Chinese herbs act to augment systems in the body. Often a preparation will avail itself of a primary herb and a helping herb that reduces possible side effects of the primary herb." Such formulas are especially indicated for complex conditions, which involve more than one system in the body, or when a strong effect is needed, since a combination of herbs will generally be stronger than a single herb.

Deer antler and Chinese ginseng are also helpful in this situation. Take three or four grams of both twice a day.

Yin deficiency. This is the evident cause of impotency when the person is run-down, weakened, often thirsty and suffers from night sweats, dryness, and insomnia. Rehmannia Six is indicated in this case.

Ashwagandha can also come in handy. This is an herb that builds potency. It is not a stimulant but a gradual enhancer. It needs to be taken over a few months. After one or two weeks, there will be increased vitality accompanied by less tension, a good combination. Take three drops in a teaspoon twice a day.

A couple of Chinese herbal formulas have proven generally useful. One is schisandra chinensis, which helps with excessive sweating, excessive urination and discharges of all kinds. It is like a mortar that holds the *chi* energy of the body.

A second useful one is epimedium grandiflorum. The epimedium is a flower that is grown in shady areas and used as an ornamental. Its Chinese name, Yin Yang Huo, translates as the "horny goat herb." It was used to increase the sexual activity of animals. Use 6 to 12 dried leaves, boiled in two or three cups of water for one half hour. Drink one or two cups twice a day.

Gary Null's Protocol for an Alternative to Viagra

yohimbe bark extract	100 mg
anise	20 mg
velvet bean	20 mg
cardamom	20 mg
cinnamon	20 mg
ginkgo	30 mg
ginseng	30 mg
muira puama	400 mg
oat	30 mg
wolf berry	30 mg
ashwagnanda	30 mg
country mallow	30 mg
saw palmetto	30 mg
nettler root	100 mg
ginger root extract	50 mg
zinc L-monomethionine	10 mg
L-arginine	1,000 mg
phoshatidyl choline	500 mg

59

Male Infertility and Related Problems

In chapter 52, we discussed infertility from the female perspective. In this chapter, we look at some of the alternatives now available to address male infertility. This chapter will also include some recommendations for the treatment of infections and other problems of the male genitalia. Many of the herbs and formulas we recommend in this chapter can be taken as teas, so we include a brief discussion of how to brew or decoct teas.

The Chinese Perspective

The Chinese say that male infertility is caused either by a deficiency of sperm creation or by the sperm's lack of motility. Sperm motility does make a difference. Without that capacity to move in the seminal fluid, there will not be a high probability of conception since the sperm is not getting where it has to go.

According to Dr. David Molony, author of The *Complete Guide to Chinese Herbal Medicine*, a licensed acupuncturist and certified herbalist as well as the executive director of the American Association of Oriental Medicine, the Chinese formula tze pao san pien, which increases potency, is one of the best methods to treat infertility. He says, "American ginseng is useful, since it is not overly hot. Infertility may be because a person thinks too much, which produces a too-hot condition in the body." The ginseng should be taken in doses of 500 mg, spread out over the day in two or three capsules. If it is to be used as the root, use two slices to make tea and also chew on any leftover root.

Deer antler also is useful. It can be found not only in Chinese herb stores but even in Chinese grocery stores in ampoules you can drink. However, Dr. Molony cautions, if you have a lot of heat, are irritable, and have high blood pressure, don't take the antler. It is a stimulating preparation. It has to be counterbalanced with a yin element that will cool you down.

(In the previous chapter on sexual dysfunction, we discussed the yin and yang principles of Chinese medicine. Basically, each is a type of energy whose balance in the body is necessary for health.)

If you are yin deficient, on the other hand, you will need a tonic such as Rehmannia Eight, which is safe for everyone and includes warming agents, or Rehmannia Six, which is cooler and damper. Both of these preparations will work to restore your ability to have a normal sex life.

"In general," Dr. Molony says, "the problem of Americans is that they are too hot. They overdo stimulants, even overdo vitamins. People will take so many vitamins that the yin, the cooling element in the physiology, is sucked up. With extreme yin deficiency, you will not be able to ejaculate or even relax enough to get an erection."

With infertility, one of the problems of the patients is an inability to relax. They need to slow down and get to know their partner. One helpful preparation to help relax, not a Chinese one, is kava kava. Take the 30 percent kava in a 200 mg dose, three times a day. It will have no negative side effects.

Also it's good to use general tonics, such as ginseng. You can use astragalus to build up the immune system. If you have a deficiency in any aspect, a tonic will help you rebuild.

When you take herbs, remember they tend to be damp. Taking too many will slow down your metabolism. If you are taking them, be aware of your general state and note if you seem to be slowing down and feel as if you are walking in oil. Carefully monitor your intake.

Dr. Michael Tierra, a consultant with years of experience with Chinese medicine, says that because the balancing of yin and yang is so important, an herb should be taken that addresses both sides of the energy equation.

"Infertility," he explains, "will be caused either by a yin or yang deficiency. In this case, though, there is a planetary, that is, broadly effective, Chinese formula that addresses both sides of the deficiency at once. Called, Wu Zi Wan (The Five Herbs of Creation), it will tonify both kidney yin and kidney yang equally."

Also useful for this problem is ashrwagandha. Avoid the imports of this herb from India, though, because they may have a high bacteria count.

Dr. Tierra notes that ginseng is also valuable for those with an energy deficiency. If you have little energy or a weak digestion, six to nine grams taken in two doses should prove valuable. It can be taken as tea. Try the Chinese or Korean red varieties, not American. "The little bottles you can buy in stores are not serious helps to our health because the amount of ginseng in them is too minute," he warns. "You'd have to drink a case of them to feel any effect."

If you get the ginseng root, you can break off a chunk with a hammer and suck on it all day. You can also brew it up as the Chinese do in a ginseng cooker. A cooker, which can be purchased in Chinatown, is a ceramic cylinder with little feet on the bottom so it will stand up in boiling water. You fill it with water and the root, then place it inside a second pot that is filled with water itself. Place it on the stove and bring the water in the outer pot to a boil. It functions like a double boiler. You leave the little jar inside the pan and leave it to simmer for hours. You don't actually have to buy the Chinese pot. You could put a Mason jar in a pot of water and achieve the same effect. This is also a fine way to make herbal teas since it seems to combine decoction and infusion all in one.

Other Herbal Remedies

There are a number of other herbal remedies that are useful in relation to infertility, according to herbalist C.J. Puotinen. If the problem seems to stem from the circulatory system use gota kola and ginkgo. Also said to enhance fertility are stinging nettles and green oats. Although there have been no clinical studies on these substances, anecdotal evidence certainly supports their value.

The tonic and adaptogen herbs are also quite helpful. Tonics are herbs that act to restore and strengthen the whole system. They produce normal tone, gradually improving overall function.

The oats and nettles as well as dandelion can be taken daily. They boost the whole system, improving everything in the body, which will have an indirect effect on infertility.

The adaptogens are a type of the tonics. They gradually correct imbalances. The most widely known adaptogen is ginseng. These tonics lower or raise blood pressure that is out of whack, and bring blood sugar into the normal range. They will slow a too-rapid pulse or, alternately, speed up and strengthen a sluggish one. In the same manner, they will recalibrate a reproductive system imbalance.

Other helpful adaptogens recommended for men with fertility problems are astragalus, Siberian ginseng and the Chinese herb fo-ti. All of these have followings among herbalists, who believe that over long periods, they correct imbalances that lead to infertility and other health problems.

Regarding ginseng varieties, the two normal types are American and Chinese. (The Siberian one is of a different variety.) Puotinen notes, "The American herbalists don't make fine distinctions between these ginsengs. They feel their effects are all more or less the same. Some people use both Siberian and American ginseng at the same time; others will start with one and then switch to the other if they are not achieving a good effect. According to Chinese medicine, though, each is different in its effects."

Herbalist Amanda Crawford has some additional advice. For one, she thinks it would be better if we were all eating a more Mediterranean diet. "This would be one rich in garlic, rosemary leaves, and olives, taking them not as supplements but as part of eating a wide variety of natural foods." She says we should add to that the herbs that help the liver, such as dandelion root and leaf. Taken as a tea, dandelion will make you feel more grounded and will have untold benefits. Take one cup a day for three weeks. Its effects will start subtly but become clearer after drinking the tea every day for a week. In the second week, the man will feel an increase in power. In the third week, he will feel as invincible as the dandelions that keep coming up on the lawn.

Blue vervain is another herb for the liver. It has a bitter taste. Take one half of a teaspoon, diluted in water before meals, morning and night for six weeks to get the best benefits. It acts to balance hormones, liver, and blood. "In the pre-Christian herbal traditions," Crawford says, "it was said to make you true to your self. When we talk about infertility, it's never far from questions that pertain to both the emotional and spiritual sphere."

Tribulus is an herb used in the body-building and sports community. It increases testosterone and growth hormone in the body as well as sperm count. It was traditionally used in India as a counter to infertility and as an aphrodisiac. It can be taken in a 250 mg capsule twice a day. However, Crawford says, "This is a fairly strong herb. It may not be your best option to increase testosterone without knowing why you have low testosterone in the first place. Doing that may be asking for trouble. I urge men, especially those who may not be as fit as body builders, not to begin with this herb without first consulting your physician."

A safer way to improve infertility is with zinc. Its helps with spermatogenesis and prostate problems. In the following chapter, we talk about necessary dosage and in what form it should be taken.

Arginine is an amino acid. Again, don't take this by the bucketful. Too large a dose can exacerbate dormant infections. Since there are small but appropriate amounts of arginine in organic whole foods, such as oatmeal, sunflower seeds, and even cocoa, avail yourself of those ways of ingesting it.

Herbalist Amanda Crawford makes this suggestion for a good cold-morning breakfast containing the amino acid arginine as well as other nutrients:

Some old-fashioned oatmeal—none of that instant gunk, which is of no value to your body—but that made from rolled oats, organic when possible. On top you can put some flax seeds and some dried fruits, such as blueberries for the bioflavonoids. Eating that morning medicine will help nourish your reproductive health and anchor your sense of health from the inside out.

You need to get the essential fatty acids that can be found in nuts and fish. This can be supplemented with omega-3, about two grams in gel capsules per day.

These are some of the things men can do for infertility. They might also take a moment to relax. Drink a simple cup of dandelion or chamomile tea and reflect on what you would like to bring into the world as you nurture you fertility.

Infections

The herbal approach can also be used for other common problems of the bladder and urethra.

"For urinary tract infection," herbalist C.J. Puotinen says, "cranberry juice is recommended." It is often thought of as a source for women with these infections, but it can also be used with men. It helps maintain a healthy pH balance within the urinary tract, preventing bacteria from adhering to the lining or walls of the tract. So infections can't get a foothold.

One can also used buchu to treat infection as well as small stones and fluid retention. Buchu is both a diuretic and urinary tonic. It can be taken for long periods of time. Puotinen also talks about corn silk, "which is simply that found on the ears of corn," as another tonic. "One can't overdose on corn silk," she says. European goldenrod also can be taken.

Other useful herbs are juniper berries, which can be taken in small quantities, and barberry. Any infection in the bladder area can be cleared up very easily by using barberry, especially when it is taken in combination with cranberry juice, which will cover its offensive taste, or in capsule form. Few would take it as a tea, although that is a possibility. It should be made as a decoction, not brewed, tea.

Other Problems of the Male Genitalia

Dr. Michael Tierra gives the following recommendations for handling inflammation of the testicles and discharge from the penis. "These conditions require herbs that are anti-inflammatory and diuretic at the same time. These would include yellow dock root, chaparral, and goldenseal. Use 30 drops of each. Ideally, they should be taken in combination to get a broader, synergistic effect."

One good combination is:

30 drops of verbaris
30 drops of goldenrod
30 drops of yellow dock root
30 drops of gentiana

Garlic should be taken separately, one or two cloves a day to combat infection.

Premature Ejaculation

This problem often has a psychological basis, but it may have physiological causes also. The Chinese would say it is due to a yang deficiency and its associated coldness. It can be treated with a rehmannia/eucommia combination called you qui wan or with Rehmannia six. Astragalus would also be effective. You qui wan can be brewed as a tea, with four or five cups decocted down to two cups. It can also be taken as a dried extract, where a person swallows a teaspoon with water.

How to Prepare Teas: Brewing and Decocting

While most everyone knows how to brew tea—just put the leaves in a closed sieve and let them steep—not everyone knows how to decoct a tea or realizes which substances should be decocted and which should be brewed. Herbalist C. J. Puotinen explains the distinction:

"Most teas are brewed as infusions. They are steeped as you steep a Lipton teabag. You pour boiling water over the herb then let it sit for 5 or 10 minutes. Afterwards, you strain the herb particles and drink the brew."

A decoction, by contrast, is made by taking a pan of water, putting in the herb, bringing it to a boil, and then immediately turning down the heat and letting it simmer for 5 to 15 minutes. Let it stand off the stove for another 5 or 10 minutes before drinking.

Barberry, for example, having leaves that are thick and leathery, requires decoction rather than infusion.

60

Prostate Conditions

T he prostate is a small, walnut-shaped gland below the bladder. Its job is to provide the seminal fluid that combines with sperm. The prostate is both a gland and a muscle. It creates this fluid and the muscle pumps it out. As a gland, it needs fluids and as a muscle, it needs exercise. This second function is often overlooked.

The prostate gland has to be considered in relation to the whole body. Depending on how toxic the body is, you are going to have diseases related to the prostate and other systems. Among the conditions that can affect the prostate are prostatitis, prostate enlargement (prostatic hypertrophy, benign prostatic hyperplasia), and prostate cancer. (For an in-depth look at the alternative views on and treatments for cancer, see chapters 38 through 42.)

Warning Signs of Prostate Problems

According to Dr. Lawrence Clapp, the author of *Prostate Health in 90 Days*, who has a background in homeopathy and body work, typical warning signs of prostate problems include hesitation in urination, undue urgency in urination, and the feeling that you have to get up at night to urinate. If you want a more scientific measure of whether there are problems on the way, have a hair analysis. If this analysis shows that zinc and copper are not in a balanced state, then you are headed for trouble.

Evidence of an inflamed prostate can also be back pain. A lot of men don't realize that back pain can be produced by prostate difficulties. They simply have pain in the back. If you have pain with fever, pain with stools or with cloudy urine, then that's prostatitis.

Benign prostatic hyperplasia (BPH) refers to the enlargement of the gland. This gland encircles the urethra, and as it enlarges it can put pressure on it, pushing it shut; this is what causes urination problems.

Prostate cancer, one of America's leading malignancies, may or may not be associated with symptoms. This generally slow-growing cancer often goes unrecognized in many older men, who ultimately die of other causes. Some men experience urinary or other problems. A PSA (prostate specific antigen) test—although not always reliable—is often used to diagnose the disease.

Who is Affected and Why?

"Surprisingly," Dr. Clapp says, "prostate problems are occurring in younger and younger men." Prostate problems are endemic in our society. At about age 40, 10 percent of men have a slight enlargement of the gland. By age 50, 50 percent have some enlargement. By age 80, 90 percent show symptoms. "Many traditional doctors are even saying, prostate problems are inevitable," Dr. Clapp continues. "I don't agree."

So what causes a prostate difficulty? "One way this problem begins," Dr. Clapp explains, "is that in our sex lives we pick up bacteria from our partners. These bacteria remain in the prostate." The prostate can't handle them all or handle the variety of them so this causes infection. And this infection languishes until the prostate becomes inflamed or enlarged.

A second reason for prostate problems is diet. In most countries in the world, men do not have these problems. But in the United States, their occurrence is partly conditioned by the use of tobacco, alcohol, rich and spicy foods, fats in red meat, and by overeating. All these things weaken the prostate, so it can't fight back against bacteria so well.

Prostate problems have also been tied to the pesticides we use. These pesticides are loaded with estrogens and chemicals designed to work on the reproductive systems of insects. Unfortunately, they build up in our systems. "I remember," Dr. Clapp recalls, "as a boy growing up, we kids used to run behind the DDT truck that sprayed the neighborhood [to kill mosquitoes]. They still do that spraying in Florida." These pesticides get into all our foods. It's on the grass the animals eat. Even if you wash your vegetables very carefully, which is helpful, you'll still be getting the pesticides that have worked their way into the inner membranes of the plants.

Israel outlawed the use of pesticides more than 10 years ago. Now cancer is down 60 percent. That's highly suggestive.

A swollen prostate also can be caused when pituitary production, stimulated by stress or alcohol consumption, converts testosterone into dehydrotestosterone, which is harmful.

One final reason for some prostate problems, which is almost comic, is tight underwear. Frequently this underwear will cut off circulation.

Conventional Treatments

Dr. Harry Preuss, professor of medicine and pathology at Georgetown University Medical Center, and author of *The Prostate Cure*, tells us about the conventional treatment for prostate problems:

"The standard approaches are through surgery or drugs. There is an operation in which the prostate is reamed down to a good size. There are also laser and microwave approaches in use. There are also drugs that can be taken to relax the prostate and allow the urine to flow out. These will be administered over a matter of months and may have quite adverse side effects."

In the case of prostate cancer, the conventional approach may involve prostatectomy (surgical removal of the prostate gland), radiation, and/or chemotherapy.

Dietary Remedies

According to herbalist Amanda Crawford, good prostate health requires a man to stay away from alcohol, tobacco, sugar, the fats and acids in red meat, and dairy products, which are particularly harmful, not just because of the fats but because of the enzymes. It is also imperative to avoid processed foods. At the same time, increase the amount of fiber you eat. Use organic fruits, vegetables, and whole grains. You'll also want to cut out the cappuccino, cafe mocha, and espresso. Try green tea instead. Crawford explains: "It has a little bit of caffeine. Caffeine in small doses helps our body. This green tea gives us a gentle lift and it has fewer negative side effects than coffee."

Herbal Solutions

Herbalist C.J. Puotinen states that the standard herbal remedy for prostate problems is saw palmetto. It is the easiest herb to find, the easiest to use, and the most likely to bring fast results. It may have gastrointestinal side effects, however. The majority of users experiencing serious prostate symptoms will experience benefits in 5 to 10 days after beginning its use.

Amanda Crawford adds that saw palmetto, the biggest selling herb in America, will decrease symptoms; it is clear from the research it will actually decrease the size of a gland that is already swollen. The way it works is this: As a man ages, his testosterone drops and his estrogen levels begin to rise. The prostate absorbs some of this estrogen but saw palmetto will inhibit the absorption so the gland either reduces in size or ceases to swell. This type of estrogen accumulation also seems to account for breast cancer. When estrogen accumulates in an organ and isn't doing anything there, it causes problems by becoming a site of inflammation.

The saw palmetto is a berry native to Florida and South Carolina. It smells funny and doesn't taste very good but it's rich in oils and beneficial plant compounds. It used to be given to livestock or people after a period of high stress, such as a drought. It has a nourishing effect on men, aiding the essential fatty acids, although its effects are not yet fully understood.

Crawford advises taking two grams of the dried berry per day. "You need to get the extract in a kind of solvent that is natural but good at extracting oils. There are some very good extracts on the market today. If you're using the extract, take 320 mg a day. Take this for a minimum of a month to see if it's working well. It works best at a minimum of three months of consistent use. For many men, they may be taking it a year to see the best benefits. In capsule form, take 160 mg, two or three times a day. It is useful to combine it with pygeum Africanum, which is excellent at 40 mg three times a day. This can be mixed with pumpkin seed oil as the three work together."

Pygeum, though, may have side effects, including vomiting, nausea, indigestion, and other gastrointestinal difficulties. This occurs in 13 percent of users, which is a high percent. This brings up the point that people are used to thinking of medicinal herbs as being completely free of side effect, but this is simply not true. Only tonic herbs are clear of adverse reactions.

There are further costs. Pygeum is taken from areas in Africa where the environment has been weakened by industrial farming. Besides, people who are politically conscious about how they spend their consumer dollars may not want to support some of the things going on where these plants are harvested. It might be better to use plants that are indigenous to North America, ones that are abundant and not endangered.

Saw palmetto also works very well with nettle root. One teaspoon of the root extract two times a day, morning and night, will reduce the nocturnal need to rise and urinate.

Prostatitis, with painful urination, discharge, and other problems, requires an appropriate diagnosis from a doctor. In addition to what the doctor prescribes, one might want to take a tea of mixed herbs. The recipe for that is as follows:

damiana leaf	2 ounces
echinacea root	4 ounces
ginger root	⅓ ounce
hydrangea root	1 ounce
licorice root	⅓ ounce
stinging nettles	⅓ ounce

Take one ounce of this mixture and steep it—don't boil it—for 15 minutes. Then strain that out. It should be taken for eight days. It nourishes the immune cells and decreases inflammation. And it won't get in the body's way of healing itself.

Dr. Preuss calls our attention to another herb-based remedy. "One natural product that I recommend to help with prostate problems is sernatin." This is a water-soluble extract from flower pollen, mainly derived from rye, dried, mixed, and given in a capsule. This extract has been proven, in double-blind, placebo experimental studies, to be as good or better than pharmacological agents. There are 10 good clinical studies done in Europe and Japan that show the benefits of sernatin. It has been as shown that 60 to 80 percent of sufferers get some relief from symptoms that are bothersome to them. Besides, they won't have the serious side effects that would come with medication.

The only downside is a mild upset stomach, which is reversible by stopping the sernatin or reducing the dosage. This adverse reaction affects 3 percent of takers, which is not that high, since it is a reaction that would affect 1 or 2 percent of those taking a placebo.

The dosage is two pills two or three times a day, amounting to about 63 milligrams in total. This extract is commonly used in Europe and Japan, but not so much in the United States.

For the inflamed prostate, also take such substances as hydrangea extract in doses of 20 drops or 30 mg.

How to Make Herbal Extracts

In these chapters on men's health, and other chapters throughout the book, we have repeatedly talked about the vital use of herbs in the healing process. It might be worthwhile to pause briefly and talk a little more about herbs. Since we have dwelt on the value of herbal extracts, we'd like to mention how you would go about making your own extract if you so desired. Herbalist C.J. Puotinen tells us, "One way these herbs are available is in raw or crude tinctures." A tincture of this sort is an alcohol extract made by putting one of these herbs in combination with vodka or another grain spirit. These extracts are named crude because you are not dealing with one chemically manufactured in the laboratory.

You can make these crude extracts on your own in forms that often are more effective than products you can buy over the counter. Let's explain how would you go about doing that, using as an example the preparation of saw palmetto berry, which, as we have seen, is a useful substance to use to work on prostate problems.

You can find the saw palmetto berry in any herbal store. It has a distinctive aroma. Select high quality berries, ones that look like real berries, not shredded wheat. They have a discernible taste and color. These will be dried herbs unless you live in the Southeast or Florida, where they grow.

Take a small amount, say one cup of the dried herb for a four quart jar. Fill the jar one quarter full with the berry, then half or three quarters full with the vodka, rum, brandy or a neutral grain spirit. Many U.S. herbalists prefer 80 proof vodka.

Cover the herbs with the alcohol for a period of several hours to a few days. They will expand as they absorb the alcohol. Keep an eye on the alcohol level so that you always have a margin of a couple of inches above the dried plant material. Then leave the jar sealed in a warm place, but out of direct sunlight for four to six weeks. Some will even prefer eight weeks. Some will go by the lunar cycle, bottling it at the new moon and keeping it in the container for two full moons, which is about six weeks. Shake it every couple of days. By this time the alcohol has absorbed as much of the plant's constituents as it is likely to. Now strain the liquid into a measuring cup and then pour it into amber glass bottles for long-term storage.

You might also choose to pour the liquid into another jar with dried palmetto berries in order to create a double or, eventually, triple strength extract. That would be very effective and can be taken in a smaller dosage. With the double strength extract, you can read the recommended dosage and cut it in half.

It is a time-consuming process, but the extract prepared in this manner will be of better quality than what is bought in stores.

Some people are afraid of using extracts that have been prepared in this way because they anticipate negative effects from the alcohol on their biochemistry. Don't forget, though, that the more concentrated the extract, the less alcohol it has in it. Also remember the dosages are measured in droppers or teaspoons. You will not be taking a large amount.

However, if you want to avoid alcohol, you can use other liquids such as vegetable glycerin or cider vinegar, using the same count you would use for spirits. These substances are not as effective because they don't dissolve all the constituents of the herb as alcohol would, nor do they have the preservative qualities. Alcohol tinctures will last for years.

The Chinese Perspective

Dr. Michael Tierra, author of *Chinese Traditional Herbal Medicine*, also recommends saw palmetto as herbal treatment of the prostate. However, drawing on the wisdom of Chinese medicine, he points out that there are different causes for prostate dysfunction. Thus, to treat the problem intelligently, one must begin with the cause.

If kidney deficiency is to blame, indicating a problem in the endocrine system, it is necessary to strengthen this system. Rehmannia Six or Eight, both Chinese herbal preparations, are called for. Six if for a yin deficiency; eight for a yang deficiency.

The basis of Chinese medicine is not, as in Western medicine, to see the prostate problem as a single disease, but to break the disease down into components and see how it is individually manifesting. Each symptom is addressed by an herb, and the symptom picture in general is handled by an herbal combination.

Kidney deficiency that creates a prostate problem can be further divided into three basic types. First there are problems due to poor circulation in the pelvic region. These can be treated with lovage, Chinese salvia, red sage, or red peony. Second are problems in the urine flow, so that it is slow or incomplete. These problems should be treated with diuretic herbs, such as water plantain, which is grown in the United States, or fu ling. Third, there may be problems with swelling, which should be dealt with by utilizing herbs, such as seaweed, particularly kelp. Another incredibly effective herbal remedy from China is Kit Kat pills, which will treat swelling as well as frequent urination.

In all cases, about nine grams a day of the herbs should be taken. Dr. Tierra prefers if his patients take the herbs in a tea. He gives them a combination that will include several herbs. A patient takes four or five cups of water, cooks them down to two, and then drinks one cup in the morning and one in the evening.

David Molony—herbalist, acupuncturist, and author of *The Complete Guide to Chinese Herbal Medicine*— adds that for an inflamed prostate, gentiana formula is helpful because it includes herbs that cool the inflammation, as would antibiotics, and has a diuretic effect, increasing urination. This formula can be purchased in a Chinese herb store. The usual dose is eight pills, three times a day.

Zinc and Other Minerals

Anne Louise Gittleman, author of *Super Nutrition for Men*, who has a private practice and consults around the country, believes that a lack of trace minerals is connected to prostate problems.

First, let us recall the importance of these minerals. They allow us to use ingested proteins by helping produce the enzymes that break down these proteins into amino acids that are usable by the body. If they are not broken down, these incoming proteins are toxic to the body. These elements are precursors to all hormonal functions and so are especially important to men.

Most people in our society assimilate only 20 percent of the protein they take in because they are deficient in trace minerals. They may lack them because the purifying and processing of food in our current agricultural methods, along with acid rain and other environmental factors, mean that these minerals are being lost from our plants and diet. We are a mineral-deficient society, which compromises our overall health.

Gittleman highly recommends that men include supplemental trace minerals in their health plan. These minerals will help balance pH, detoxify lymph, and build and re-establish enzyme and hydrochloric acid production. They will also aid in carrying oxygen to the cells.

For many men, they may be the missing link to a healthy prostate.

One important trace mineral is zinc, which is especially important because in many states it is deficient in the top soil. It is vital in the production of testosterone and for muscle strength, which declines with age. Zinc can be depleted from the body by the use of sugar, coffee, and alcohol. You need zinc piconalate taken twice a day; B$_6$; and pituitary prolactin.

Herbalist Amanda Crawford also recommends increasing zinc. She says you can get this by eating pumpkin seeds. If you're taking the zinc in tablet form, you might need to take 30–50 mg a day, which is a high dose. So she says it's better to get the mineral through the seeds. Pumpkin seeds, aside from being high in fiber, have the essential fatty acid cucurbitacin. We know this has a beneficial effect on men's health generally and on the prostate in particular. The pumpkin seeds can be taken with almonds, sesame seeds, flax seeds, or milk thistle seeds. The latter are good for the liver and protect the body against some of the compounds that have been associated with prostate cancer. Six hundred to 1,200 mg a day of milk thistle seeds are indicated.

You could take a handful a day of each of these seeds: pumpkin, flax, and milk thistle. Crawford says not to tie yourself to one or the other. "Perhaps you could have them in a protein shake each morning or sprinkled on a salad. So you are eating these foods as your medicine and it becomes interesting. You don't have to swallow yet another pill."

Manganese is another valuable mineral since it acts to stabilize blood sugar. It can be obtained from nuts and seeds. Selenium and chromium are two other necessary minerals. Chromium contributes to keeping muscle mass lean, balancing blood sugar, and helping individuals lose weight. Vanadium is a favorite of weight lifters and also helps with blood sugar metabolism.

Massage

Prostate problems can also be treated with massage. For the massage oil, you'll need a carrier oil to which small amounts of the essential oils will be added. For the carrier oil, use olive oil, almond oil, or any cold-pressed oil. Don't use a vegetable oil. Add to this oil the essential oils; these are aromatherapy oils, derived by steam distillation from herbs. Take a few drops of these herbal oils. One recipe calls for 5 drops of either lavender or thyme oil. Then add 10 drops of cypress or fir to add an evergreen fragrance. To that add 10 drops of eucalyptus and rosemary, for a cleansing fragrance. Put this in one fluid ounce (two tablespoons) of the carrier oil.

Massage this into the prostate area and into the whole lower abdomen and even into the back. Massage the gland, which is four or five inches into the rectum, for 15 or 20 minutes. The swelling frequently goes down immediately as fluids are cleared by finger pressure. You may see a shiny black waste that is liberated and comes out.

Massage the deep muscles around the prostate gland between the testes and the rectum. This will have an uplifting and antidepressant effect.

An even simpler way to pamper the prostate requires little effort. Invert your posture. Get a slant board and lie on it for 20 to 30 minutes a day or use yoga to take some of the pressure off the area. Let gravity give you a massage.

You may also try an enema, using first hot water and then cold water to expel stagnant fluids.

Acupuncture

Dr. Michael Tierra also has found acupuncture to be a good measure to be taken in relation to prostate problems. "It should be done on a weekly basis," he states. "There are points to be touched on the inner legs and abdomen. This will not be as effectively reached by acupressure. Acupuncture must be done."

PART TWELVE

Health, Beauty, and Longevity

In the largely unread, fourth book of *Gulliver's Travels*, the hero comes to an island, near Japan, where a race has realized mankind's dream of living forever. The irony is that these immortals all wish they were dead, because, though they have lived hundreds of years, these have been miserable years, since they have all the infirmities of the aged, such as blindness, deafness, arthritis, and senility. Jonathan Swift's satirical thrust can be applied today, when we consider the following facts. Americans are living longer than ever before, but most are unable to enjoy longevity because its potential pleasures are canceled out by the prematurely early encroachments of aging.

In the following chapters, we look at how aging affects many of the body's systems, including the brain, and the natural techniques now being used to reverse it. In addition, we look specifically at two "health and beauty" areas that are not only affected by the aging process but also are cause for concern at other times of life: teeth and hair.

61

Reversing the Aging Process Naturally

I
n the next 10 ten years, 50 percent of the United States population will be over 40, but unlike their parents these baby boomers are not accepting diabetes, high blood pressure, arthritis, overweight conditions, and high cholesterol as the necessary companions of aging. They are looking for ways to stop premature aging.

When we start to get older, especially when we have not been living the healthiest of lifestyles, we begin asking: Can I detoxify? Can I reverse premature aging? Can I get back more energy, energy I didn't have since I was young? As we will see, if one is willing to take the steps to live in a healthy and natural way, the answer is Yes.

In this chapter, we will look first at what causes premature aging, both physiologically and in our deficient lifestyles, and then look at a program to reverse this aging. The program is all-sided and includes proper eating habits, exercise, the use of muscle and mental relaxation techniques and the adoption of a mental attitude that faces life bravely and honors it in all its forms: human, animal, and vegetable.

Causes of Premature Aging

Why do so many of us look older than our years? What are the forces, inside and out, that seem to pushing so many people to an early grave, or if they don't literally kill them, weaken them so their vitality, strength, and *joie de vivre* are far below what they could be?

In our society, we have accepted the idea of being overweight, of having high blood pressure, high triglycerides, high cholesterol, and arthritis, as inevitable accompaniments of getting older. Since so many people have these problems, we think of them as normal. Even the doctor will say, when you get to be a certain age, these situations are to be expected and, since they are irreversible, accepted.

Of course, many people in the alternative medicine community disagree. We now know that it's possible to live to 100 and beyond, staying healthy longer and thus "rectangularizing" the aging curve.

Dr. Martin Feldman, a traditionally trained physician who practices complementary medicine, supports this stand. "We need to have optimum energy as we grow old, not accept the diminishment many find encroaching as they grow older."

Joint disease, Dr. Feldman points out, is an area where medicine has accepted a reversible condition as inescapable. There is now an epidemic of joint disease in the United States. The majority of people over 60 have either early, moderate, or late osteoarthritis. Conventional doctors call it a wear-and-tear disease of the joints that appears naturally, which sounds nice, as if the joints wear out like the parts of a car, but it is nonsense. The disease is the product of deficiencies and occurs when the joint is not being nourished. A nourished joint will remain healthy.

Dr. Feldman has seen marathon runners in their 70s and 80s who use their joints 10-fold or even 50-fold more than a normal person and yet their joints remain robust. (See chapter 27 for a full discussion of joint disease.)

FREE RADICAL DAMAGE The body may age before its time because it is carrying too much toxic load due to things it is exposed to environmentally and biochemically, coming especially from the dust and chemicals we ingest daily. This assault weakens the repair mechanisms and leads to a vitamin and nutrient deficit.

According to Dr. Ross Pelton, author of *Mind, Food, and Smart Pills*, the primary cause of premature aging is free radicals. Dr. Denum Harman of the University of Nebraska first developed the theory of how these radicals act to accelerate aging. The radicals are electrically imbalanced molecules that do tremendous damage at the cellular level. If we look down into the body, into the cells, we find their individual powerhouses, the mitochondria. In the mitochondrias' folds are super coiled strands of DNA. An invading oxygen free radical can zoom into the mitochondria and hit one of the DNA's paired bases, distorting the whole segment. A repair enzyme will quickly move to the site and return the DNA to its original shape. But this is a process that gradually wears the body down.

OTHER CAUSES Dr. Hal Huggins highlights another cause of premature aging, the mercury in silver amalgam fillings. Mercury does not just sit there—you inhale it and it goes into your lungs. You eat and chew, wearing it away, so it goes into your stomach and digestive system. There it undergoes metastasization, forming methyl mercury, a highly toxic substance. (See chapter 63 for more information on this hazard.)

How to Take Supplements

The first thing to look at as a means of reversing aging is supplements. Most people do not know how to properly take vitamins and minerals. You must follow the law of compensation. If you smoked, used sugar or caffeine, if you have been an angry person who held in your anger, if you have not honored the life force, not exercised, not been fulfilled, you must work to compensate for these deficiencies.

One-a-day supplements are the easy way out. I have met people who say, "I eat meat. I eat sugar. But it's all right because I take my one-a-day vitamin." My friend, that does not work. The body cannot be lied to. After 30 or 40 years of the body's debilitation by an unhealthy lifestyle and environment, a little pill will not do the trick. You need to detoxify and cleanse the body.

Another illusion is the idea of the recommended daily dose, given by drug companies and conventional physicians. This is not the best way to think about health. These recommendations are like the minimum wage. Is that what we are interested in, minimal health? Or do we want optimal health? These dosages of supplements, which are now called recommended daily values, are very substandard if one wants a long-term healthy lifestyle.

You have to know what your bodily state is and plan accordingly. I would suggest one level of usage for healthy people who know they are healthy, while, for those processing diseases, there is a quite different level of use. The person becoming conscious of his or her health will need to consult a nutritionist who can design a personalized supplement program to meet an individual's needs.

WHY SUPPLEMENTS ARE SO CRUCIAL The reason supplements are crucial is that, as a person ages, certain fatty acids, amino acids, and members of the main groups of nutrients are lost. Scientists are looking into this issue and already know that choline, tyrosine, glutathione, cystine, vitamin E, zinc, and chromium are poorly absorbed and deficient in older people. Meanwhile, as these substances grow scarce, there is a buildup of heavy metals, such as aluminum and lead. These can be removed from the cells with chelation. Vitamin C and zinc are also useful in flushing them out. Most importantly, as the body loses necessary nutrients they have to be put back in for optimum physical and mental functioning.

At the same time, free radicals, growing more common in the body as we age, have to be fought. Remember, when you eat meat, drink alcohol, and are around pollutants, then the body creates free radicals. They cause skin to wrinkle in the sun, they foster cancer, arthritis, and heart disease. However, nutrients, called antioxidants, such as beta carotene and vitamin A, are able to neutralize the effect of the radicals, slowing down the aging process.

DHEA: THE MOTHER OF ALL HORMONES Dr. Richard Ash has talked to his large New York City radio audience about the revivifying power of DHEA, called the mother of all hormones, which is a key underlying ingredient for the productions of the adrenal gland. He tells us that when the body is under stress, the adrenal gland requires cortisone and adrenaline, more highly in demand during such times. If these hormones are overused, they will become depleted as will DHEA, the precursor of these substances.

A lack of DHEA, he explains, will cause all sorts of negative consequences for the immune system. Often at age 80, a person will have 1/20th of the DHEA he or she had at age 20. Once the capacity and reserves of DHEA have been eaten up, chronic diseases will be harder to combat due to a weakened immune system. One of the earliest signs of DHEA depletion is an inability to get REM sleep, which will cause insomnia. An uninformed doctor may prescribe sleeping pills, which will not get at the root of the problem. This deficiency will also cause poor sugar regulation, a hyperglycemic symptom, since with low DHEA, a person will not be able to tolerate sugar in the diet, so will have to eat more frequently. Other common symptoms are palpitations, sweating, confusion, poor concentration, and not being able to cope with everyday stress.

Dr. Ash points out that with a low amount of DHEA, there will be less salivary IGA, which is a substance found in the gastrointestinal (GI) tract. When IGA is depleted or absent, there will be more antigen penetration in this area as well as food and chemical sensitivity reactions. There may be inflammation of the tract, a condition called "leaky gut," whereby certain unwanted foods and chemicals get into the body system. Then autoimmune disease may arise when the body attempts to defend itself against these unexpected intruders. Dr. Ash notes that by administering DHEA and building back up salivary IGA, we can diminish food sensitivity, lower toxic load, and restore the GI tract, getting back an intact immune system, and thus treating the cause not the symptoms.

PROGESTERONE, ESTROGEN, AND TESTOSTERONE Dr. Eric Braverman has found that counteracting the aging process has to be undertaken on an individual basis. His treatments look at each patient's individual hormone imbalance, brain mapping, attention span, memory problems and cardiac and exercise capacities. Once this is examined, the patient needs to be nutritionally correct. He recommends natural yam extract which contains PET (progesterone, estrogen, and testosterone), all the hormones that are essential. Progesterone has anticancer properties and helps with the calming of the brain. Estrogen strengthens the bones, has anticancer effects, especially in the colon, aids memory and gives cardiovascular protection. Testosterone reduces the side effects of other hormones, and helps keep the sex drive vigorous through a person's 50s, 60s, and beyond. For a woman, the ovary produces all three of these substances, but as Dr. Braverman puts it, "If the ovary dies, you must resurrect it. If you permit an organ to die, you allow yourself to die. We must stop this if we want abundant life. We replace depleted hormones with PET, and missing adrenal with DHEA."

BIOFLAVONOID COMPLEX Another invaluable supplement is the citrus bioflavonoid complex, which can be obtained from lemons, plums, and oranges among other fruits. With an orange, one can cut open the skin and right below is the nutrient, the bioflavonoid. Another bioflavonoid that is good is rutin, which comes from buckwheat. If one is going to take the bioflavonoid in pill form, I would recommend 300 mg per day for a healthy person, while a person in poor health should take 500 mg. As for the rutin, the proper dosage for a healthy person is 25 mg per day, while the ill person may take up to 50 mg.

BLUEBERRY EXTRACT Blueberry extract is good for the eyes. During World War II, the RAF gave this to its pilots to improve night vision and strengthen the immune system. Red cabbage extract is also important. There are cultures that lack a variety of foodstuffs, but they eat cabbage and obtain its antibacterial, antiulcer properties. Cabbage, eaten juiced or steamed, will prove very healthful.

RED WINE CONCENTRATE Red wine concentrate also has life-enhancing effects. A few years ago a study was made of the people living in a certain area in France. This was a group who had a high cholesterol diet, who ate creams, cheese, and meats to such a degree that one would expect them to show a high level of cholesterol and heart disease, seeing that coronary trouble and high cholesterol go hand in hand. Yet, they did not have many heart problems, and the only thing that seemed to be counteracting the effect of this diet, distinguishing them from other groups with similar diets, was red wine. This is what the study showed.

I looked into it. It could not just be the wine, because alcohol in general is not beneficial, in fact, it destroys nutrients. It had to be something in the wine. It had to be the bioflavonoids, antioxidants, in the red wine. If this is so, you don't need the wine. Why not take just the grape, for from the skin and seeds comes an antioxidant, which can be obtained as a pill. Recommended daily dosage for the healthy is 50 mg, and for those not in good health, up to 200 mg.

GREEN TEA If you lived in China, you would probably be drinking green tea and taking green tea extract. We know it has anticancer properties. It is an immune system stimulator. Decaffeinated green tea is very beneficial.

BETA CAROTENES Beta carotenes are helpful and can be obtained in all the green, red, and orange fruits and vegetables. As I've said previously, six to nine servings a day of fruits and vegetables are ideal.

GLUTATHIONE Glutathione is good for the immune system but it is not easily assimilated by the body so it should be taken with something that produces it in the body, such as intacytelsistine. Recommended dosage is 200 mg a day for the healthy and up to 400 mg for those not in the best of health.

VITAMIN C Of all the nutrients, though, the single most important is vitamin C. Its benefits are multiple. This vitamin is important for the skin, giving it that youthful elasticity. This is because it produces collagen, the connective cell tissue, which holds the muscles and skin together. It helps the body produce interferon and increases leukocyte activity. It aids the thymus gland, the liver and the brain, while acting to prevent arthritis, cataracts and heart disease. It seems it helps with everything. A healthy person should take 2,000 mg a day, spread out over the course of the day. For the unhealthy person, I have seen people take, under medical supervision, up to 150,000 mg in intravenous (IV) drips.

At the Healing Center of New York City, they use IV drips of vitamin C and other nutrients to counteract the aging process. Dr. Howard Robins points out that toxins and free radicals are stressful to both the body and mind. When the body is in pain, fatigued, and under attack from heavy metal and other pollutants, which we come in contact with on a daily basis, this weakens us as well as affecting our minds adversely. With the IV vitamin C, we cleanse the body. The Healing Center also uses drips with other nutrients, such as EDTA, as a way to cleanse the heavy metals from the body and keep viral problems under control, by destroying viruses and keeping them from replicating. These drips will also help boost the energy level.

VITAMIN E Another life-giving supplement is vitamin E. People with herpes, chronic fatigue syndrome, hepatitis, and even AIDS have miraculously improved by taking large doses of the vitamin. Dr. Wilfred Shute, up in Canada, working with his brother, has treated over 30,000 patients in his decades of medical practice. He has helped with intermittent claudication, diabetes, gangrene and so many other conditions. Recommended dosage of this vitamin may be 800 units, sometimes 1,000 or up to 1,600 units.

OTHER IMPORTANT SUPPLEMENTS AND HERBS

Sea algae. High in trace elements, antioxidant cofactors, flavonoids, and carotenoid.

Coenzyme Q10. Every cell in the body needs this coenzyme to create energy and build stamina.

NADH. Also known as coenzyme 1, NADH is a naturally occurring substance in the body that supplies energy to the cells, allowing them to live longer.

Thymus extract. Pure oral thymus extract enhances immune function and helps reverse the aging process.

Tyrosine. Strengthens the thyroid and adrenal glands, protecting against stress.

Fo-ti. Rejuvenates the endocrine system and is an excellent digestive tonic.

Ginkgo biloba. The ginkgo tree has survived for hundreds of thousands of years due to its powerful immune system. An extract of the leaf of the tree improves circulation to the microcapillaries of the brain and heart so that needed nutrients and oxygen can get to all the tissues.

Ginseng is the best-known longevity herb. For centuries, the Chinese have revered ginseng for its rejuvenating effects. Research has shown that ginseng can stop free radical damage associated with aging. It helps people focus better when under stress, and increases overall energy levels.

Gota kola. Elephants, who browse on gota kola, are known to have excellent memories and to be long-lived. Gota kola is useful for increasing vitality and endurance, and may lower blood pressure.

Hawthorn berries support circulation and cardiac function.

Milk thistle protects liver function. The liver releases toxins from the body, promoting health and youthfulness.

Eating Right for Long Life

I was pleased, both by what I saw and what it signified, when I went to the Dallas market, one of the largest in the United States. In it, there are hundreds of fruit and vegetable stands. Most cities in the U.S. have a farmers' market, open at least one or two days a week, but the Dallas one is open 365 days a year. It has six large hangers, each the size of a football field. The success and popularity of this market signifies that people in the area are into buying fresh, healthy, and inexpensive foods. Many Americans who want to get back to what is important are going back to organic. Looking at the vastness of this market, one realizes how much variety one has to choose from. This is where your good nutrition comes from. This is where we should be shopping for our meals if we want to reverse the aging process.

Take the papaya. It enhances digestion, is rich in beta carotenes, rich in calcium, and magnesium.

You can buy an organically grown head of broccoli at the Dallas market and it may have 90 percent more nutrients than a commercially grown head, taken from land where the soil has been denatured. If you do not have the nutrients in the soil, you are not going to get them in the produce grown in that soil. Buying these organic foods and paying a few cents more, is certainly an improvement over the $1,000 or $100,000 you will pay fighting the diseases acquired from a lifetime of bad eating habits.

VEGETARIANISM A number of doctors testify to the benefits of a healthy vegetarian diet. Dr. Martin Feldman, talking about patients in his nutritional program, says his group is doing better on lowering cholesterol than any comparable group. He states, "We did not select people to come in to work on cholesterol problems. We are using a total assault on the lifestyle without focusing on cholesterol. The level of reduction is superior to that found in any prior drug study [where drugs were used to cut down on cholesterol]. It is extremely important that we can achieve this reduction without drugs. Drugs are expensive and have side effects. Also, we do not know what long-term problems may arise with them."

Dean Ornish has shown that a vegetarian diet can help clear the arteries. The findings of my study group supports this claim. We found we could lower cholesterol, lower the triglycerides, lower the percentage of body fat, aid digestion, shorten the transit times of food almost by half, remove constipation, and create better sleep habits, so we could shorten a person's needed sleep (often by two hours a night). That is reversing the aging process.

ENZYMES Nina Anderson, author of *Over 50, Looking 30*, notes that organic foods are also valuable because they contain enzymes. Our present diet depletes our body's enzymes. Anderson says the problem is that we eat too many cooked foods, which are overly processed, causing the pancreas to work overtime. Americans have some of the largest pancreases of any human being.

What happens after you eat a Thanksgiving dinner? Anderson asks. Ninety percent of the food at the dinner is cooked. After we eat, everyone wants to go to sleep. That happens because the pancreas is going crazy trying to put out enough enzymes to digest the meal. (Enzymes are what allow nutrients to be used. For example, you have enzymes in the heart that allow magnesium to be used. Without that enzyme, magnesium will not get to the heart.) It has to call for reinforcements from another source of enzymes, the metabolic enzymes. They are in the organs, killing the viruses and fighting disease. All of a sudden they are called out to help digest food. But what do you think happens when they have left the front lines?

"If you want to avoid degenerative disease, those debilitating diseases," says Anderson, "then you should take enzymes. They'll fight the battle for you. You'll stay young and you'll look young."

Your skin is a reflection of your internal health. With proper diet and the use of enzymes, she tells us, your age spots will disappear, moles will shrink, and the lines on your face will thin. Those are some things you will notice. They are external changes and not as important as internal regeneration. Still, they have value since people are concerned with not looking old. If you keep taking enzymes, your internal organs will stay young and healthy and you will feel good.

Now where do we get these enzymes? Enzymes are the catalysts of life. Raw foods are loaded with enzymes. Fruit and vegetable juices are filled with enzymes. When food is processed, the first things taken out are enzymes. Why? Because the enzymes are what allow the food to ripen, though, if it ripens far enough, it rots. So to stop it from ripening and rotting, so that it can be sold longer, these enzymes must be destroyed. But if you destroy the enzymes, you destroy the food's life force. It will have carbohydrates, vitamins, fats, and minerals, but not its life force.

Enzymes can be used externally as well as internally for youthful effects: "There are amazing enzyme treatments for the skin," Anderson says. "Papaya enzymes are wonderful. Or you can mix a plant enzyme powder and put it on as a mask. Not only does it take the lines out of your face, but it fills them in and builds up collagen. It can also get rid of age spots and shrink moles. When you use enzymes as a mud pack when you come in from the sun, it fights free radicals that otherwise might foster melanoma."

A FINAL NOTE ON DIET All in all, our diet is crucial to our outward and inward appearance and health. Think of Italy and the Mediterranean. You see people with magnificent skin, lovely and supple, and this is because of the oils and other healthy foods in the diet. The Mediterranean diet includes a lot of oils and beans, a lot of white beans, garlic, onions, herbs, fresh food, a lot of organic. They have wines, but ones rich in bioflavonoids and the essential nutrients. They eat food that helps the heart, and deoccludes the arteries.

Diet is crucial. Eat less. Eliminate saturated fats and the excess protein that we take in which creates toxicity in our body, in our liver, while making us feel sluggish. These fats and protein creates edema and dehydration. Go vegetarian and organic. That is a major part of the recipe for maintaining vitality and health.

Detoxification Therapies

CHELATION THERAPY Dr. Martin Dayton from Florida, board-certified in family medicine, chelation therapy, and clinical nutrition, says that chelation therapy has multiple benefits, and long life is one of them: "Dramatic increases in life span are found with chelation. While there are no longevity studies per se, this conclusion is implied indirectly by studies which show a lessening of killer degenerative diseases. In fact, chelation favorably impacts all four major causes of death in the United States [heart disease, cancer, cerebral vascular disease, and lung disease]."

During the chelation process many beneficial changes occur at the cellular level. A manmade amino acid, called EDTA, is administered to the patient via intravenous drip. Once in the bloodstream, EDTA attaches itself to heavy metals such as lead, cadmium, and mercury and holds onto these toxic substances until they exit the body through the urine. Dr. Dayton explains why removal of these substances is vital to good health: "The toxic material prevents normal function and repair. For example, lead prevents normal enzymatic processes so that the body cannot function properly and repair itself. This leads to premature aging and the premature development of disease. Removal of toxic material through chelation keeps the body functioning optimally." (See chapter 33 for more discussion of chelation therapy.)

COLON CLEANSING Colon cleansing is an ancient and time-honored health practice for rejuvenating the system, used in Egypt over 4,000 years ago. Later, Hippocrates taught these procedures in his health care system. The large intestine, or colon, is healed, rebuilt, and finally restored to its natural size, normal shape, and correct function.

Colon therapist Anita Lotson explains the procedure and some of its physical and psychological benefits: "There are several stages of therapy. The first segment involves cleansing, a thorough washing of the large intestine. The colon is irrigated by a technique whereby water is gently infused into the large bowel, flowing in and out at steady intervals. Through this method, water is allowed to travel the entire length of the colon, all the way around to the cecum area. The walls of the colon are washed and old encrustation and fecal material are loosened, dislodged, and swept away. This toxic waste material has often been attached to the bowel walls for many, many years. It is laden with millions of bacterium, which set up the perfect environment for disease to take route and entrench itself in the system, wreaking havoc. As this body pollution is eliminated, many conditions—from severe skin disorders to breathing difficulties, depression, chronic fatigue, nervousness, severe constipation, and arthritis—are reduced in severity, providing great relief, especially when augmented with dietary changes and other treatment modalities.

"The next phases are the healing, rebuilding, and finally restoration of a healthy colon, functioning at maximum efficiency for the final absorption of nutrients, and the total and timely elimination of all remaining waste materials. During the healing phase, we begin to infuse materials into the bowel that will cool inflamed areas and strengthen weak sections of the colon wall. Flaxseed tea, white oak bark, and slippery elm bark all soothe, lubricate, and introduce powerful healing agents directly into the large intestine. These herbal teas may be taken orally as well. Simple dietary changes have been made by now, such as the addition of water. This simple measure spells the difference between success and failure in alleviating many bowel conditions. I ask all my clients to double their intake of water.

"I love to see people's change in attitude from the time they come in to the time that they leave. Sometimes people are very irritable when their bowels are backed up. They're often depressed, and sometimes nasty. By the time they leave, you can see a smile and a bounce in their step. It's a different person altogether."

MAGNETIC HEALING Susan Bucci is a holistically trained nurse who has spearheaded the development of magnetic healing products. "Magnets oxygenate tissues and allow cell walls to absorb more oxygen," she explains. "They promote mental acuity and normalize pH balance by increasing alkalinity. Restorative sleep is enhanced. Therapeutically, they stop pain, fight infection, and reduce inflammation and fluid retention. Over time, fatty and calcium deposits dissolve and the circulatory system opens up. Put that all together and you've got healing from A to Z. Take that a step further: if you achieve optimal well-being, you can actually live a long, productive life."

In addition to promoting overall well-being, magnets can eliminate many specific signs and symptoms of old age. Bucci reports these antiaging benefits from her own use of magnetic healing techniques: "My energy level has increased. I used to have chronic fatigue in the worst way, but now that's gone. My immune system is functioning much better, so my susceptibility to viruses and colds has decreased dramatically. Allergies are basically gone, and there are no more killer sinus headaches. My circulation has improved so that I withstand weather a whole lot easier. Wounds heal quickly, and my spider veins have disappeared. Also, I was headed for an early menopause, but now my menstrual cycle is very much on track, very regular.

"Hair, skin, and nails have definitely improved. My hair grows faster, and has a much better quality to it. Within two weeks of using magnets on a daily basis, I was able to see new, thick, dark, hair growing. My grays started falling out and disappearing. I was going to color my hair about four years ago and I still haven't touched it with an ounce of anything. My skin definitely looks and feels younger. And my nails grow so well that if I break one, it doesn't upset me. I know that it will grow right back."

How is it that magnets can do so much? Simply stated, magnets perform a wide range of benefits because we are magnetic beings who derive energy from the earth's magnetic field. Bucci explains, "One reason we get sick is that the earth has lost a good deal of its magnetism which leaves the body in an unbalanced state. Additionally, we are bombarded by unhealthy energies." Magnets create overall benefit by restoring internal harmony.

It is important to realize that any old magnet will not do. The negative pole restores health and good energy to the system, while exposure to the positive pole is detrimental. This has been repeatedly proven in studies where a variety of creatures, from earthworms, mice, and chickens to larger animals, live twice as long as untested control groups when exposed to negative field magnets, and half as long when exposed to positive fields. Bucci recommends unipolar magnets, marked by the Davis and Rawls system with an N or the word negative and a green label. "That's the healthy side, and that's the one we face toward the body." Negative field ions support biological systems, which help the body to heal itself. "The body is an amazing machine with a remarkable capacity to cure itself," Bucci says. "Give it a boost in the right direction and it does the rest on its own. The negative field is completely safe and risk-free."

Bucci finds that magnets work best when worn on a daily basis. During the day she wears a magnet over her heart to improve circulation and oxygenation.

"It keeps the heart open and flowing and sends all that wonderful oxygen throughout my body," she says. At night, she takes the magnet off and sleeps with her head on a magnetic mattress pad. This is because the most important benefit while sleeping is increased melatonin production from the brain's pineal gland. "People are running out to buy melatonin, but guess what? We can encourage our own melatonin production.

"People ask me how long magnets should be worn. Generally speaking, the longer you wear them, the more healing takes place. You can wear them all night and during the day. Generally, the body will tell you when it has had enough. It also will tell you when a condition has healed, although you should check with a physician just to make sure."

Kinesiology

John Etcheson, an expert in kinesiology, says this discipline is an acupuncture-related science developed by the Chinese. It focuses on learning what foods and herbs are best used and assimilated by an individual. With this knowledge, a proper supplementation and diet can be devised that is finely calibrated to an individual's biology.

Etcheson, also an herbalist, states that in kinesiology, "First we need to test a patient's polarity to find out if it's balanced."

He demonstrates with a female client. She extends her left arm, shoulder level, away from the body. The patient has placed her other hand flat on the top of her head. That's a positive energy position. Etcheson pushes down on her extended limb, asking her to resist the pressure. She can hold her own against his pressure. Now she turns the hand on her head over. That is negative. This time when the hand on the head is reversed, the extended arm can be pushed down more easily. Etcheson explains this is a normal reaction based on the differences in polarity. If the patient were strong either way she placed her atop-head hand, she would probably be dehydrated or need to work with his thymus to balance her body.

Next, again with the left arm extended at shoulder level, the patient holds a nearly empty canister against her solar plexus with her other hand. The extended arm is weak and can be forced down easily. Next the right hand holds a canister filled with honey or another organic substance against the solar plexus. Now the arm is stronger and cannot be forced down. This is because the body knows the honey's nutritional value. In the nearly empty canister was a little table sugar, which is without value to the body. This same experiment might have been done, by the way, by placing alternating substances under the tongue. This is one way we can see the body's reaction to different herbs and foods.

In kinesiology, these food reactions are studied more precisely to determine proper individual diet.

Exercise

What kind of exercise can slow aging?

One valuable type is power walking or racewalking. Franco Pantoni, a U.S. National Champion racewalker and racewalking coach, discusses this exercise. He compares racewalking to running. "The difference from running is the speed at which we travel. This exercise was established in 1908. It's great for both the body and mind. Most people don't know that Harry Truman and Albert Einstein were walkers. I have a picture of Einstein walking—he was a very fast walker—and a journalist is trying to keep up with him."

This exercise will increase the amount of oxygen in the blood. As mentioned, one reason the body ages is that free radicals cause cellular damage. Free radicals are generated by a lack or low level of oxygen in the tissues. A slight decrease in oxygen in the tissues will be accompanied by an increase in the pesky free radicals. Vigorous exercise will combat this problem.

Pantoni describes the exercise by saying that the posture for free walking is to keep oneself very straight and light on the feet as if an invisible wire pulled one up from the top of the head. The hips are kept very loose. The inclination forward is 4 or 5 degrees, bending forward from the ankles, not waist. He tells us to lean forward as if you were about to fall forward. Stride forward, planting the heel first, keeping the leg straight, toes up. The arms is are bent at a 90 degree angle at the elbow and held in front of the chest. The hands are closed but not clenched tightly. The arms are held about six inches in front of the chest. As you move, swing them between the chest and waist, with a pumping motion, an easy, natural motion, working all the muscles in the upper body. The faster you go, the faster you pump, bringing your heart rate above 120.

"But as you go, think about relaxation," Pantoni coaches. "You have to think relaxed. Sometimes, there are so many things you are aware of: arms, feet, hips, but if you can become relaxed, you will profit. You will reach a point where you get that feeling of locomotion, where everything gets fluid. You are gliding, easy."

The *Medical Tribune* recently reported that senior citizens do not exercise enough. By exercising, the article meant going to a gym for a full workout, exercising all the muscle groups. It is hard enough to get the average person to do an aerobic workout or to go swimming or biking. Less than 5 percent of us exercise daily. When you factor in all the diseases due to faulty diet and lack of exercise, you have disaster.

One exercise that is easy to do at home is sit-ups. Doing them properly will tighten your stomach and abdominal muscles. Place a pillow on top of your ankles and anchor the feet under a bed. In doing them, never put your hands behind your neck, because that will pull the neck and spine up and can throw your spine out of place. Instead, cross your arms over your chest. Only come up about nine inches, which will be enough for you to get complete expansion and compression. Exhale coming up and inhale going down.

Another simple exercise can be done with equipment available in most gyms. It is the slow and rhythmic lifting of weights from a seated posture, doing the lift from 10 to 15 times. The general formula to go by is that if you want muscles that are big, bulky and have greater strength, then use a heavier weight and less repetitions. If you want muscles that are lean and fast, use lower weights and more reps. I would suggest 15 reps, 3 sets.

For strengthening the shoulders, upper chest and upper back, lift barbells of a comfortable weight, going from the arms hanging toward the waist till they are at shoulder height. As you move, don't crane your neck, but practice deep breathing, allowing deep releasing of oxygen.

Remember, an average gym will have about 20 pieces of equipment, but that does not mean you have to use all 20. If you tried to use them all, many of the exercises you would do would be redundant. You might be using a slightly different grip, but you would be working the same muscle group as on a different machine. You can work out on the slant board and any of the crunch machines, but the most important thing to keep in mind is to exercise everything: the hamstrings, calves, abdominals, upper chest, shoulders, arms, and neck.

Relaxing and Coordinating the Muscles

FELDENKRAIS: RELIEVING MUSCLE TENSION AND STRESS Where exercise strengthens and adds to muscle suppleness, sometimes, bad patterns of movement or chronic tensions have established problems in the joints or muscles. Feldenkrais is a practice that helps eliminate the problem of poor movement habits.

Sharon Oliensis, a guild-certified practitioner, talks about her discipline. "Dr. Moishe Feldenkrais developed this method to relieve chronic muscle tension and stress. It uses very gentle movements. Either the student does them to him or herself, guided by the instructor, while lying on the floor, or the student lies on something like a massage table and the teacher uses a hands-on approach, taking the student through gentle movements so that he or she lets go of a chronic holding or stress pattern. This helps the student develop a greater sense of ease and flexibility so breathing and coordination improves."

Oliensis runs her hand lightly over the back of a clothed, standing male patient. She senses the curve of the spine and muscle development along the spine. Everyone's spine is different. As her hand moves up and down its length, the student directs his awareness to the point she is touching. Together, they make discoveries about its length and shape, as well as it sensitivities and insensitivities. One of the principles is to bring awareness to those parts of our body of which we were previously unaware, and develop the knowledge to alter old patterns. Then, she tests freedom of hip movement.

The patient lies on his back. "I lift his legs and press down through the soles of his feet to see how movement transfers up through his skeleton, through the pelvis, ribs and up to the top of his head. Then I can see and he can feel what is the pathway a movement most easily takes and where there are resistances to the movement. Based on that, combined with what he has told me, I can judge what to work on in any individual session. Part of the therapy is his body learning beneficial patterns, which comes of his learning to differentiate between parts of his body that are relaxed and parts which are still tense. Normally, the part that has been worked on will feel more in contact with the table, larger, wider, smoother. The side not worked with will feel as if rising off the table. The key for the nervous system is to learn a new way of behaving and recognize, simply enough, that one can feel this way or that way, relaxed or tense."

YOGA Another means of keep the body young and the muscles flexible is to relax and strengthen it with yoga.

Yoga instructor Mary Dunn says yoga is a way to help alleviate the aches and pains and tensions that come from daily living as well as the general malaise and fatigue that may overtake a person.

When you come home from work with legs feeling tired and heavy, Dunn says, do a modified shoulder stand. With the back on the floor and a pillow under it, lift legs up and point them to the sky, bracing them against the wall. This will open up the chest and lungs, make the shoulder and the breath relaxed, so you can leave the tension of the day behind.

One of the methods of yoga is stretching. Most of our experience of stretching comes when we have to do some work, reaching for something on a shelf, for instance. Yet, if we were asked to replicate that reaching motion, we would feel constricted, because we were not stretching properly. We need to train the nervous system so as to bring consciousness into the body so all the joints are open. When we have opened all of them, we have stretched the nerves that accompany those muscles. When we relax, they relax, and since the nerves go back to the brain, it relaxes too.

Energy Practices

CHAKRA PSYCHOLOGY Aside from dealing with muscular tensions produced by our stressful environment, it is necessary to develop methods of channeling our energy, not letting it get dammed up and frozen the way our muscles can be when we do not know how to relax them. Indian and Chinese methods can play an important role.

An Indian practice, chakra psychology, is related to yoga and focuses on the energy we receive through breathing.

Shyam Bhatnagar of Sri Center International of New York City tells us there are seven chakras along the spine that influence our nervous system. It takes years to develop awareness of these nodes—six to seven years for the first.

Each of these chakras can teach a form of awareness:

- body awareness;
- gender;
- social identity;
- consider ourselves lovers of the divine, people who love nature and mankind;
- the arts and creativity;
- androgyny, resolving sexual dualities as well as being the center for meditation; and
- what reality is and what the underlying substratum is on which we superimpose our simplifying projections. At this last chakra can be found divine consciousness.

Bhatnagar tell us a number of practices, both enjoyable and beneficial, lead to a deepening experience of the chakras. First, synchronize breathing with the respiration of the cosmic bodies in heaven. We need to be aware of these bodies. The sun affects us most because it is our father. Without the sun, there would be no life on this planet. Second is the moon. These two heavenly bodies have a relationship and our body is constructed based on this relationship. To get in tune with this relationship, we need to do breathing exercises.

The right nostril is the solar or sun-dominated one, while the left is moon dominated. Conversely, the right brain hemisphere is lunar while the right is solar. When you are predominantly breathing with the left nostril, your right hemisphere will be more dominant. Breathing predominantly with the right nostril, you will find the left hemisphere in control. At any time, one of the nostrils will be dominant.

It may seem from casual observation that you are using both nostrils equally, Bhatnagar states, but there is a slight difference. There is a way to determine dominance. Place the thumb first under one then the other nostril. Breathe in, breathe out. Next time you do this, be aware of the temperature. Whichever side feels cooler is more open. If your digestion is not good, lie on the left side after and before eating, he advises. If you are in a situation in which you feel you cannot express your feelings, lie on the right side. When the right side is open, you will have more courage to express yourself. This is help you can get from the cosmic forces.

MEDITATION A way to keep our senses alert and relaxed is through mindfulness meditation.

Beverly McGregor, Ph.D., a psychologist and founder of The Health Institute in Dallas, points out the value of mindfulness meditation. "It has to do with being aware of what is around us at every moment. In practice, we can learn to be calm and centered. When stressors come up, we can respond in a better way. We can be fully present in what is happening.

"You may be watching a sunset or seeing a lake. Suddenly a thought comes up—'I wish this other person were sharing this with me,' for instance. Suddenly we are thinking of something else, and not fully present with the lake."

Mindfulness meditation helps one to escape distracting and, hence, detracting thoughts that stop one from living in the moment.

Attitudes and Belief Systems

The expression "our health care system" is a misnomer. It has never dealt with being healthy. You have to focus on keeping yourself healthy. Pasteur was only one half right. He recognized that there were germs and they played a role in illness. That's correct. But he was wrong when he said the germ would cause the disease. The milieu your body is in will cause the disease. Germs will alter depending on your body.

A funny thing I have wondered about is why so many people interested in health are sick. Some of the sickest individuals I have ever met are in the health movement. It is not all about a deficiency of nutrients. I have studied the healthiest individuals I could find. And afterwards, along with Dr. Martin Feldman, I developed a protocol for wellness that will optimize a person's over-all life with, among other things, diet, supplements, exercise, and positive life affirmations. Anyone who has followed this regimen has seen substantial, sometimes radical, improvement.

Life is not so simple that you can change one thing and see real improvement. For that, you have to change the whole field.

Number one is attitudinal change. With the wrong attitude, you will become sick. Negative attitude, meaninglessness, bad disposition, these always lead to disease. The disposition is the catalyst.

In poorer foreign countries, I will often meet people without the material wealth we have, but they have meaningfulness and purpose. They have balance. People in their 70s up to their 90s, loving and honoring life, not feeling angry or rejected.

A healthy person looks for a message in a crisis. Before he or she overreacts, he or she assesses the situation. Nothing is so bad it cannot be dealt with. Nothing you cannot survive. Look beyond the crisis toward solutions. You may not be able to change the crisis, but you can shift attitude and remain focused and balanced.

Meaninglessness exacerbates physical and psychological conditions. Stop beating up on yourself. Take the responsibility to love yourself. Most people are lovable if they let their real self show.

Shyam Bhatnagar puts it like this. "Some people seem to say, 'I don't like myself, but I want you to love me.' That's cheating. If a person starts to cheat on you, it's unfair. You have to love yourself first. Otherwise, there is dependency."

Stop making excuses. There is no need for any illness. But to say this, you must be willing to look into those dark places in your psyche that you have avoided or denied. Be willing to be consistently disciplined in your eating, in meditation. The moment that you are helpless—you pig out or you get angry— it is all for nothing. Then, it is gone. And how many games do you have to play before you realize you always lose?

Dr. Stan Huff, a licensed professional counselor, talks about changing yourself: "Visualization and imagery will help a person change some negative messages, escape old roles or the tyranny of negative experiences so as to replace these with a more positive set of roles and messages. A person can replace these counterproductive stories with more affirmative ones that fit better with who you deserve to be."

He explains that visualization is an active form of meditation that allows the patient to see images in the mind's eye that can influence the emotions and reduce stress. It gives the person new options and choices in ways to relate to the world.

Honor the Child Within You

You have to start honoring the little child within you. The child is the healer. I have never seen an adult who did not use this child as a vehicle for healing. A child has wonderment, acceptance, openness. Children do not reject you because you are black or white. They do not care. They love you for being you. I see these deadly serious people hanging out in doctors' offices. They are not using their inner child. No way is healing going to happen.

Quiet that mind. Find out how healthy you want to be. On a scale of 1 to 100, how healthy do you want to be?

Dolores Perri tells us, "Don't believe anyone who says you cannot do it. When I see people in their 80s running marathons, people cutting down their cholesterol without drugs, I know you can do it."

Put all the parts of wellness together. If you leave out one part because it is inconvenient, then you have problems. Put them together and you will reverse the aging process and be able to look forward to productive later years when you will be passionately alive.

62

Brain Aging

O ne of the most disturbing symptoms of aging is diminished brain function, which can cause everything from forgetfulness and loss of concentration to Alzheimer's and other serious diseases. Fortunately, modern research reveals that much can be done to keep the brain in top form your entire life.

Symptoms of Brain Aging

Dr. Eric Braverman says that brain aging affects people differently and brain health is a preventative process. "Even when you feel halfway decent in your 50s, 60s, and 70s, parts of your body may be breaking down," he cautions.

The part of the brain affected determines which symptoms manifest themselves. "Individuals age in all different shapes and forms, just as a face can have wrinkles on the brow or wrinkles under the eye," Dr. Braverman says. "The area of the brain that slows down can affect such things as general memory, concentration, or logic."

Nutrition and Supplements

Another leading researcher in the field of antiaging, Dr. Ross Pelton, author of *Mind, Food, and Smart Pills*, contends that our brains do not have to deteriorate as we age: "It is simply poor nutrition and abuse that allows this condition to develop. Virtually everyone can enhance their memory, learning capabilities, and intelligence." Dr. Pelton helps his patients optimize brain functioning with two goals in mind: to slow down or stop the brain aging process, and to optimize the function that we have.

First and foremost, Dr. Pelton recommends building total body health with a healthy diet. An organic vegetarian diet supplies the body with more protective nutrients and healthful fiber, and at the same time decreases toxins. Additionally, he believes that everyone should take a high potency multivitamin/mineral supplement and extra antioxidants with each meal: "We are no longer looking at the Recommended Daily Allowance (RDA) as the level of nutrients appropriate for people. I say RDA stands for Really Dumb Allowance. It's more like the minimum wage, the minimal amount you can get by on. If we want to get into lifestyles of antiaging and life extension, we need to consider not only healthy diets but a program of optimal nutritional supplementation. Antioxidants are among the most important protectors against the aging process in general and against brain aging in particular. They will stop the onset of senility, Alzheimer's disease, and other brain injuries."

SPECIAL BRAIN NUTRIENTS Then Dr. Pelton utilizes special nutrients to enhance the brain:

Flaxseed oil. This major brain nutrient is the greatest source of the essential fatty acid omega-3 (eicosapentaenoic acid, or EPA). Omega-3 gets converted into another fatty acid, which nourishes the fat cells in the brain. One tablespoon of flaxseed oil is needed daily. It should be refrigerated, not cooked, and taken with the largest meal of the day.

Hydergine increases oxygen to brain cells, and makes a person less susceptible to free radical damage and aging. Dr. Pelton says this is one of the most important substances for preventing brain aging due to its oxygenating capabilities. Hydergine is available in the United States, although as a prescription drug; Lucidril and Piracetam (see below), which have similar properties, must be ordered from overseas. Although classified as drugs by the FDA, Hydergine, Lucidril, and Piracetam do not have any side effects, according to Dr. Pelton— only positive effects on memory and the prevention of brain aging. Overseas mail order sources sell Hydergine in 4.5 mg tablets, while in the United States it is only available in 1 mg tablets. The higher dosage, taken twice a day, is highly effective in helping people with early signs of memory loss.

Piracetam. This prescription drug is not available in the United States; however, it is available in over 85 other countries worldwide, where it is appreciated for its remarkable qualities and its complete lack of toxicity. Like Hydergine, Piracetam is powerful for preventing brain cell destruction caused by a lack of oxygen. Piracetam also can increase the flow of electrical information between the left and right hemispheres of the brain, a process known as superconnecting. It has proven effective in treating the learning disorder dyslexia. When used in conjunction with high-potency lecithin, Piracetam is highly effective in helping some Alzheimer's patients improve cognition, memory, and recall.

Lucidril, as its name suggests, makes you more lucid. This exciting drug can actually reverse brain aging. Dr. Pelton explains: "The primary yardstick in brain aging is the buildup of lipofusion, the result of free radical damage over the years. This buildup is really cellular garbage that collects and coalesces inside the cells into a black, tarlike mass. In elderly people you can see this in the skin as liver spots or age pigment. It is theorized that when 60 to 70 percent of the brain cell is clogged, it breaks down and stops working. That's when the symptoms of senility kick in very quickly. Lucidril actually dissolves and flushes out these garbage deposits from brain cells and restores the brain cell to a much younger state." Lucidril has been shown to extend the life of laboratory animals and to enhance intelligence, learning, and recall.

Depranil. This drug has been shown in animal studies to prevent the destruction of a specific group of neurons in the nigra striata, the area of the brain that goes bad when people develop Parkinson's disease. Moreover, it helps enhance intelligence and cognition when 5 mg are taken, once daily.

Melatonin is one substance from the armamentarium of alternative medicine to get free play in the mainstream media recently; you've probably already heard a lot about melatonin. This is a brain hormone produced by the pineal gland, and it diminishes with age. Three milligrams once daily taken at bedtime can help normalize sleep cycles.

DMAE is a naturally occurring but little-known B vitamin that enhances memory, boosts natural energy, and improves sleep. Additionally, it helps learning problems in children that have short attention spans. DMAE is safe, but if too much is taken, it can produce mild headaches, insomnia, and muscle tension.

Brain Electronic Activity Map (BEAM)

Dr. Eric Braverman has mapped brain aging and how nutrients influence this process. Using a test called the Brain Electronic Activity Map (or BEAM), a technique developed at Harvard Medical School and refined, strengthened, and expanded by Dr. Braverman, the brain's level of electric activity is studied. This is a crucial area of concern because such things as substance abuse, hormonal imbalance, chronic fatigue, anxiety, hypertension, and even Lyme disease, may affect the brain and cause premature aging. Often an electroencephalogram (EEG) or MRI will show nothing wrong, while the BEAM test reveals the brain has been suffering from stress. It gives a window on the brain and how it is aging. So, as Braverman says, he is using "the BEAM that lights the path to wellness."

He relates that one thing this test registers is the speed of brain cycles, since slowing is a key marker of aging. The normal healthy rhythm of the brain is 10 cycles per second of alpha waves. Compare this to the heart's normal rate of one cycle per second. Since the brain is intense and complex, it functions more quickly than the heart. As people age, though, their brain rhythm will decrease to nine, eight or seven beats per second. There will be a drop out of Alpha rhythms and an increase of Theta waves.

This can occur prematurely for many reasons including head trauma, Alzheimer's and abuse of such substances as cocaine, marijuana, and alcohol. When these causes operate, the frontal and temporal lobes will be found to be aging in an accelerated manner. Aging will also be increased by whiplash, metabolic disorders, loss of circulation and the "toxic home syndrome," which refers to the damage that can be done to the body by things such as cleansers that vaporize, pesticides, and herbicides that are found around the house or garden. Add to that possible harm from fluorescent lights and electromagnetic pollution. The latter is caused by the electromagnetic grid we all live in, surrounded by digital clocks, VCRs, CD players, computers, sleeping blankets, cellular phones and beepers, and microwave ovens. These appliances transmit negative electrical resonance—the opposite of what our bodies need, causing damage to our chromosomes and tissues. These stresses hurt us slowly, in small ways, causing cumulative degeneration, creating subtle discrepancies in how the body functions.

Dr. Braverman notes that a computerized spectral analysis will pick up how these factors have affected the brain. A PET scan, which tells about the metabolism of the brain, can be correlated with a BEAM test, which may be recording not only weaker brain electrical activity but a loss of metabolism of the neurotransmitters.

Other Natural Therapies

Dr. Braverman believes that each person must be individually tested to determine weak areas of brain function and to devise a program that addresses specific needs. For overall general improvement, he endorses these important therapies.

AMINO ACIDS AND OTHER BRAIN NUTRIENTS Amino acids build up in particular areas of the brain that need help. The dopamine system responds to the essential amino acids tyrosine and phenylalanine. Melatonin, mentioned above, helps sleep and slows down aging by supporting the pineal gland. Choline builds memory, while gabba, available as gabbapentin, helps anxiety disorders. Choline, phosphatidyl serine, ginkgo, tryptophan, tyrosine, and phenylalanine all boost brain voltage.

CHELATION THERAPY As described in chapter 61, chelation therapy pulls out aluminum and other heavy metals from the bloodstream, resulting in improved memory. It can also reverse or prevent other destructive conditions associated with the aging process, such as arthritis, hardening of the arteries, cataracts, and strokes.

ELECTROSTIMULATION Amino acids and neurotransmitter precursors are more effective when accompanied by electrostimulation of the brain. A TENS unit, worn on the forehead and left wrist, helps drive these substances along a good pathway. A cranioelectrical stimulation (CES) device also helps electrical fields, and additionally enhances the entire neurotransmitter system.

EXERCISE Research shows that the whole neurotransmitter system of the brain can be improved through exercise.

MEDITATION Meditation connects the body and mind electrically, creating harmony between the brain and other body systems.

NATURAL HORMONES Three hormones from natural sources help to slow down the aging process: progesterone, testosterone, and estrogen. Without natural estrogen, the hair thins, the nails break, the bones rot, and the brain weakens. Estrogen improves the absorption of nutrients into the brain, especially improving dopamine levels. Progesterone protects from the side effects of estrogen. Additionally, it is calming to the brain and improves sleep. Testosterone enhances the sex drive, builds stronger bones, and gives greater physical strength.

PHYSICAL TOUCH Neurotransmitters are adversely altered when people are in isolation, when they don't have love in their life.

63

Holistic Dentistry

urn-of-the-century author and editor Frank Harris wrote, "Doctors tell us that men commonly dig their graves with their teeth." Not only is this done by improper diet, but by not taking care of one's teeth or even by putting poisons in one's mouth. In this chapter, we want to look at how eating right can add to the health and capability of your teeth, while eating the wrong substances, such as sugar or chocolate, can damage your teeth by reversing the natural fluid flow in the mouth.

We will also evaluate the way people treat their teeth when they are diseased. We will find that typical treatments for repairing damage, such as silver amalgam fillings and root canals, are much more hazardous than claimed. More shockingly, we will find that many say the fluoridation of water, a public health practice established in most major cities, is not only dangerous to our bodies but has no positive benefits for teeth at all.

Healthy Diet, Healthy Teeth

The first thing to think about when it comes to healthy teeth is whether we are following an appropriate diet, which will be reflected in the condition of the gums and teeth.

Think of the general practitioner of yesteryear. One imagines this doctor making a house call on an ailing patient. His first request on seeing this patient was "Stick out your tongue." He wanted to see the tongue's color.

Dr. Victor Zeines, the author of *The Natural Dentist*, reminds us that this practice, far from being quaint and outdated, can still be used to make a good, first diagnosis of medical problems. In fact, Chinese doctors, who also ask to see the patient's tongue, have a book that discusses 280 diseases that can be detected from the state of the tongue. Today, such problems as the following can be diagnosed by inspecting the tongue. For example, a *white tongue* indicates that toxins are coming out of the body (this will be observed in people with a cold or the flu), *cracks* in the tongue indicates vitamin deficiency, *yellowish gray or yellowish green tongue* indicates gallbladder or liver trouble, and a *brownish or grayish green tongue* indicates intestinal or stomach problems.

The mouth is indicative of the body's general state of health. If you have a cavity, it is the end result of general physical problems of the whole body not just the isolated tooth.

What is decisive for the health of the teeth? It is simply eating a proper diet. Let us look at the research in this area.

HISTORICAL PERSPECTIVE Famed dental researcher Weston Price wrote a book, which he worked on in the 1920s and 1930s, based on studies of the teeth in people in native cultures. People that followed traditional ways, eating simply prepared food, indigenous to the region where they lived had teeth in good condition with no malformation, or crowded placement. As soon as they adopted a Western diet of canned processed food with white sugar and white flour, their dental health deteriorated. Children born to parents on a Western diet had occlusion and malformed teeth. Price even saw that children born before the introduction of Western foods had healthy teeth, while children in the same family born after the new diet was instituted had poor teeth.

He concluded reasonably that the nutrition in Western cultures is the main cause of dental problems.

WHAT TO AVOID When a person is not eating properly the body becomes acidic, so minerals are pulled out of the mouth to travel into other parts of the organism. The teeth weaken in an acid environment while acid-based bacteria begin booming. A cavity arises from a mineral deficiency followed by an invasion of bacteria.

Sugar is a main culprit in this process, though not in the way popularly understood. Many believe sugar gets in the mouth and sits on the tooth, wearing it down. The real problem with sugar is that it reverses the fluid flow. This flow normally goes from the tooth's pulp chamber into the mouth. Sugar alters this, sending materials in the mouth into the tooth's internal environment, irritating the inside of the tooth, creating cavities. Caffeine, found in coffee, tea, chocolate, soft drinks, and pain medication also creates this inversion, based on a change in the hormonal balance; it also encourages diseases such as multiple sclerosis (MS) and arthritis.

WHAT TO EAT We know what you should not eat, but we still have to ask what foods are best suited for our mouths. The way the human jaw is set up and the chewing motions made are geared toward a fruit diet. Such a diet of fruit, along with nuts, seeds, and root vegetables will create an alkaline state in the body as opposed to the acidic state current American diets support. This is another reason to adopt the vegetarian diet we talked of earlier.

In the United States we have a high level of stress, a polluted environment and deficient diet. Food often comes to us shipped over long distances, losing many of its nutritious qualities in the trip. We need to make up for those lost qualities with vitamins and minerals.

The average person should first take a calcium and magnesium vitamin, from 800 to 1,500 mg/day. Men need about 800 mg while women need higher dosages, with the largest dose needed by pregnant women. A calcium supplement is necessary for strong teeth, while a B complex will help people keep up their energy levels.

Folic acid can help the body utilize nutrients, aids the functioning of the nervous system, and is particularly useful for pregnant women since it prevents neural tube damage.

Coenzyme Q10 will oxidize cells, while vitamin C taken in dosages of 6,000 mg/day will keep the gums healthy and strong. Mineral supplements are also helpful.

Drinking juices is a good way to obtain the recommended five vegetables a day in your diet. Carrot juice is an excellent beverage, high in calcium. A 12 oz serving of carrot juice can have as much as 600 mg of calcium.

Green leafy vegetables are also high in calcium. Traditional culture held that chewing on kale was the fastest way to get white teeth. This idea probably is based on recognition of kale's high calcium content. Kale can be juiced and mixed with carrot or apple juice, perhaps with a drop of lemon.

The Truth About Mercury Fillings

Even a person eating a healthy vegetarian diet can have problems with his or her teeth and go to a dentist for help. Yet the shocking fact is, a patient can go to a dentist to solve one problem and leave, apparently cured, but actually in a more imperiled state.

The common treatment for dental caries are fillings. But what are we putting in our mouths? A large percentage of the commonly used filling is mercury. The current silver filling is typically composed of 14 percent silver, 1 percent zinc, 12 percent tin, 26 percent copper, and 52 percent mercury. This amalgam has a higher proportion of mercury than fillings had 20 years ago. Eighty-five percent of the American population has these fillings.

For over 150 years we have been told these fillings are safe, the most durable available. This is not true, argues Lydia Bronte, a health researcher. The amalgam in the filling constantly leaks mercury into the mouth and saliva, where we swallow and inhale the mercury, which then gets into the tissues.

Her claim has been substantiated by a 1996 Toxicological Profile released by the Department of Health and Human Services. In discussing the dangers of mercury it states, "One of the most likely forms of exposure is by absorbing mercury vapor released from dental fillings. Most silver-colored dental fillings are about 50 percent metallic mercury and slowly release small amounts of mercury vapor."

In the early 1970s, Dr. Hal A. Huggins, the director of the Huggins Diagnostic Center, found that mercury could leak from the fillings and damage the body. As he puts it, people with these fillings have "little time bombs in their mouths." Huggins says mercury is coming out in measurable amounts. This opinion is backed up by Dr. Warren Levin, who remarks that studies have shown if you chew gum, then put a probe in your mouth to test the air, the level of mercury vapor registered is enough to exceed what OSHA (the Occupational Safety and Health Administration) classifies as a safe level for industry.

Up until 1985, the American Dental Association (ADA) repeatedly declared that mercury never escapes from fillings. Then they had to acknowledge that it did leak. Still, even with the leakage, ADA Online, the ADA's Website, declares the fillings safe.

SYSTEMIC EFFECTS OF MERCURY What effect does mercury have once it gets in the body? Mercury will act to deactivate enzymes that utilize zinc and other agents. Dr. Alfred V. Zamm points out that this inactivation will affect every cell making them slowly dysfunctional. The enzymes are shut down when mercury substitutes for the minerals necessary for enzyme operation.

Other diseases or health problems will be exacerbated by the presence of mercury, including such illnesses as multiple sclerosis, Lou Gehrig's disease, leukemia, tremors, chronic fatigue syndrome, Parkinson's disease, and Alzheimer's disease. Moreover, memory is affected adversely, and depression and anxiety can occur.

The most common symptoms of mercury toxicity are fatigue, depression, inability to concentrate, memory deficit, gastrointestinal tract problems, kidney problems, and frequent infections.

Further symptoms include brittle nails, lack of energy, sensitivity to cold and heat, dry skin, dry hair, irritability, and mood swings. The neurological symptoms include nervousness, headaches, and hypothyroidism. Everyone who has the fillings is bound to have some problems with the thyroid since mercury interferes with its operation and with the absorption of the thyroid hormone into the body. A person who has a hypothyroid condition due to the presence of mercury will test normal on thyroid blood tests but will have all the symptoms.

Mercury will also affect the presence and functioning of the T cells, which control the human immune system. An important study on this subject is "Effect of dental amalgam and nickel alloys on T-lymphocytes" by Eggleston, D. (1984) *Journal of Prosthetic Dentistry*, Vol. 31, No. 5. The study took patients'

T cell counts. The subjects were then given mercury fillings, the count was taken a second time, and the amount of T cells went down 35 percent. The fillings were then removed, and lo and behold the T cell count climbed back to its previous level. The article's conclusion was that mercury and nickel in these fillings adversely affect the quality and quantity of T cells.

Other important studies drawing attention to the danger of mercury are Palkiewicz, P., Zwiers, H., Lorscheider, F. (1994) *Journal of Neurochemistry*, vol. 62, pp. 2049-2052, and Duhr, E., Pendergrass, C., Kasarskis, E., Slevin, J., and Haley B. (1991) *FASEB Journal*.

When patients have mercury fillings removed from their mouths, they often see improvement, although it may be held back by the mercury already in the body. Dr. Michael Schachter has seen patients both whose blood tests have gone from abnormal to normal once silver fillings were removed and victims of MS and chronic fatigue syndrome whose conditions have markedly improved once fillings were taken out.

Dr. Zeines has seen improved memory, better sleep, and less nervousness. He notes patients suffering from arthritis, cirrhosis, MS, autoimmune diseases, chronic fatigue syndrome, and heart disease have registered marked improvement.

REMOVING FILLINGS THE HOLISTIC WAY Removing these fillings is not an easy task and the process is potentially dangerous since taking out the amalgam could accidentally release mercury.

Dr. Howard Hinton, a holistic dentist, stresses that the removal must be done under the care of both a physician and a dentist. The patient must be on a good diet and should undergo laboratory tests to determine how he or she is eliminating the mercury. Ideally, the removal should be carried out in a sterile, bubble chamber—a round room with a laminar air flow circulating through the space; negative ion generators, to charge particulates in the air; and processed water and air. A rubber dam is used in the mouth to reduce exposure and the filling is removed with extreme care. (The highest absorption in the body is in the mouth.) During the operation, high suction and lots of water is used to reduce the presence of mercury vapor.

Once the fillings are removed, one still has to detoxify the body. A lack of health improvement may be due to the fact that mercury is still in the body.

Dr. Elmira Gadol, another practitioner of holistic dentistry, speaks of a treatment to aid the body after the fillings are out that detoxifies the brain. When a cell is toxic with heavy metal, it can not easily eliminate it since the cell wall has a changed ionic balance, but an anesthetized cell will release the metal.

Garlic supplements will help the body eliminate the existing mercury toxins and selenium can be taken to neutralize the metal. Mercury found in fish from polluted waters is less toxic than that from fillings, since the fish's body will have produced selenium to neutralize the poison. (Note that caffeine will act to retain mercury in the body.)

Once the fillings are removed, hair analysis should be done to see what other heavy metals are in the body. These metals interfere with cell processes, such as the oxygen going in and the carbon dioxide going out. These metals also have to be drawn out or problems will remain.

Some patients can be helped by taking intravenous vitamin C. Also, various chelating agents can be prescribed. These agents will attach to the mercury and take it out of the body in urine or feces.

Hot baths with Epsom salts and baking soda are also recommended as a way to bring out the mercury. In working on detoxification, various methods should be tried alone and in combination. Whichever is doing the best job should be used.

Root Canals

A second common dental procedure, root canal, poses another problem; it may leave hidden bacterial pockets that prove a breeding ground for disease.

In theory, root canal procedures are worthwhile. A root canal is undertaken when the tooth's pulp cavity has been entered by decay and the nerve is infected and dies. The tooth too may die, its insides, cleaned out by decay, may fill with pus. A root canal treatment cleans out the ruined area and, as Dr. Warren Levin, director of Physicians for Complementary Medicine, explains, fills it with gutta percha (a substance derived from tree resins).

Remember that the tooth is filled with dentin tubules, running from the inside of the structure to the outside in which bacteria could sit, producing toxins which transfer into the system. A study some years ago took teeth that had root canals and ground them up. Some of the powder was placed under the skins of rabbits. They found that if a patient had arthritis, the rabbit got it. If the patient from whom the original tooth came had heart disease, the rabbit contracted it, and so on. Clearly, bacteria was still carried in the teeth after the root canal had been performed and it could carry disease into the body.

This research was never publicized until the book *The Root Canal Cover-Up* by Dr. George E. Meinig, recently appeared.

Dr. Huggins, explaining the process of bacterial transfer in detail, says that whenever you put anything in the tooth for the root canal, bacteria will get into the dentin tubules and flow from the pulp chamber to the outside of the tooth. Though in a root canal procedure bacteria is cleaned from inside the tooth, it cannot be cleaned from the tubules. Sometimes on the surface of the tooth dentists are finding toxins extruded from the tubules that are similar to those produced by botulism.

A second problem may arise. The teeth sit in a kind of hammock, called the periodontal ligature. When a root canal is performed, the dentist must take a round drill, or burr, and cut out about 1 mm of the bone of this hammock to clear out the toxin deposited in the layer. When this is finished, there still may be a hollow space, called a cavitation, with a layer of bone on top. This space could fill with toxins. Serious illnesses may arise if this cavitation exists, especially in the wisdom tooth area. Of course, in proceeding with a root canal, this area should be cleaned out, but it can be and is often, missed.

Although more systematic study has to be made of the possible hazards of this technique, clearly it should not be engaged in as thoughtlessly as it has been.

Fluorides

Dentists have been using root canals and mercury in fillings blithely, ignoring the hazards and accepting traditional methods as necessarily reliable. Before the evidence began to accumulate, especially on the dangers posed by mercury, there was no reason for them to doubt the efficacy of what they were doing, since the fillings had proved themselves.

This is not the case for the last topic we wish to take up. As we look into the shady history of fluoridation, we learn that this procedure was tainted from the beginning, pressed on the gullible common people, not by medicine but by public relations men and their industrial paymasters.

Dr. David Kennedy, from the International Academy of Oral Medicine and Toxicology, puts it quite well when he states fluoride is a poison. It kills rats and insects; so, certainly, it will kill bacteria if it is scrubbed on the teeth.

Fifty percent of the people in the United States drink fluoridated water, and 42 of 50 major cities in the United States have fluoridated water. When water is fluoridated there is 1 part to a million in the water. In toothpaste, there is 1,000 parts to a million and in the dental rinses used by dentists, there is 10,000 parts per million.

All this, when the largest study ever conducted in this country on the effects of fluoridation, which looked at 39,000 school children, saw no significant differences in incidence of tooth decay between cities that had fluoridated water and cities that did not. It was found in this study that Butler, Kansas, which had the lowest evidence of dental caries, did not use fluoridation in its water supply.

It has no positive effects, but what about its down side? Fluoride is carcinogenic, and an immune suppressant that causes dental fluorosis (white or brown spots on the teeth). It increases the tendency to hip fracture by poisoning the bones.

HISTORICAL PERSPECTIVE Why did this dangerous substance, with no real protective qualities, become so widely adopted? In the 1940s there was a crisis in the aluminum industry, with big companies such as Alcoa being sued for polluting and killing cattle and other livestock. Edward Bernays, one of the fathers of public relations, and a nephew of Sigmund Freud, came up with the idea of selling the public on the beneficial uses of fluoride, one of the dangerous byproducts of aluminum production. It was said it could prevent dental caries and the publicity campaign would help the public forget the recent aluminum scandals.

The economic motivation behind this sales effort, which was triumphantly successful, was not the millions of dollars that could be made by marketing fluoride products, but the billions that would be saved by industry if it did not have to clean up the fluoride it was putting into the environment.

In a nutshell, companies have fluoride to dispose of so they are using people's bodies as hazardous waste dumps.

The health hazards of the substance have been discussed in a number of places. In 1977, an executive of the National Cancer Society documented that there is a 5 percent increase in cancer in communities that began fluoridating their water.

An even more notorious study and an attempt to suppress it involved Dr. William Marcus, a senior science advisor at the Environmental Protection Agency's Office of Drinking Water. He read a study that was done to test the dangers of fluoridation concluding there was an increase of bone cancers in animals that took fluorides. In April 1990, he went to a meeting at Research Triangle Park where the National Toxicology Program was to review the study and found that the program's staff had downgraded every cancer reported in the study.

Dr. Marcus stated that in 25 years in the field, he had never seen such a downgrading. Occasionally one or two cancers would be downgraded, usually for terminological reasons, but nothing like this. He returned to his office and asked an investigator to look into it and the investigator found that scientists at the program had been coerced into making these downgrades.

He wrote what is now called the May Day memo, calling the public's attention to this chicanery and was subsequently dismissed from his job. He won a whistle blower's lawsuit brought because of his unlawful firing and was reinstated.

Fluoride is a poisonous substance brazenly passed off as health enhancing.

A FINAL THOUGHT Thus we see proper care of teeth depends on eating sensibly and on being aware of the lurking dangers of accepted practices in dentistry. You should think carefully and consider alternative medical strategies before filling your mouth with silver fillings and having root canals. And you almost should be careful before you turn on the tap; your water may be poisoned with fluoride.

64

Hair Care

Before World War II, Karl Popper came out with a book revolutionizing ways of thinking about science. Where previous philosophers thought there was a way to prove a theory correct, he said this was impossible; the best one could hope for was that it would not be proven wrong. In fact the strongest theory, in his definition, was the one for which it could be said: There were many failed attempts to prove it erroneous.

Nowadays in science you start with a theory and then see whether you can substantiate the theory or see if it has no merit. In good science, you try to disprove more than prove yourself. If you cannot disprove yourself, then pretty much you have made your point.

Is it possible that the reason we lose our hair, and that our skin gets droopy, our nails brittle and fungusy, and our gums bleed more easily as we age is because we have done so little to feed the immune system and our overall body chemistry?

Throughout history, men and women have been concerned about their hair, for religious reasons, social reasons, interpersonal reasons, and for grooming. Sometimes the hair is long, sometimes a person is nearly bald. One thing is for sure, no one looks forward to getting bald. No one is happy about it. People don't like looking down at their feet in the shower and seeing a clump of hair. So I simply kept asking a basic question. Is it possible, using major changes in our diet, lifestyle, amount of exercise, and stress management, to reverse, slow down, or in some way limit the process?

Traditional science says no; if it is in the genes, then it is inevitable. Yes, there has been some small change for those taking the medications, but that is incidental. You might get a little peach fuzz on the site of some former hair, but you pay a price since there are side effects to the medication.

A person had tried the drugs and told me, "My hair was falling out at a pretty fast rate. I was in the Rogaine treatment for five years, and the reason I had to stop it was my blood pressure went up excessively. I was very frustrated. This seemed to be the last stop."

Another man told me, "I wanted to look into this problem of falling or shedding hair, a scaly scalp, and some irritations at the temple and crown. The first thing I did was I went to a dermatologist just to get some consultation. She said I had eczema, dermatitis of a sort. She gave me one direction. She said there was a hot product on the market, monoxodil, that I should try and there should be some results. I tried it for several months and there were no results. Not that it was a waste of money. It was an attempt."

I wanted to see if you could do it without medication, by rebuilding the body chemistry without a magic bullet, salve, potions, or shampoo.

Reasons for Hair Loss

I asked a beautician who has treated hundreds of people's hair whether she saw any connection between the things a person ate and their lifestyle, on the one side, and hair health, on the other.

She told me, "Definitely, I see that when people eat well the hair is healthy looking. It's a reflection of what they eat and the habits they have. Everything is shown in the hair."

Dr. Danise Lehrer, a licensed acupuncturist and a doctor of homeopathy, noted that in traditional Chinese medicine, hair is viewed as a sign of the health of the kidneys, liver, and blood. So if you have healthy hair, then you have healthy blood and healthy energy.

Dr. Martin Feldman, a physician who practices complementary medicine, believes that an overabundance of junk food, processed food, sugar, caffeine, dairy, caffeine, wheat, chicken, additives, salt, yeast, chocolate, alcohol, meat, refined food, preservatives, antacids, and smoking as well as the use of aluminum cookware contribute to hair loss. "Eliminate these and not only will you grow more hair but you will be totally better and will gain longevity and a healthier life span."

Colette Heimowitz, a clinical nutritionist, notes that as alternative physicians and clinicians we have to look at the whole picture and not just at the single symptom of hair loss. We have to constantly replenish our bodies and let the biochemistry and cells function optimally at all times. She adds that the need for replenishment can be seen in light of the danger of free radical molecules in the body.

As mentioned elsewhere in this book, in a free radical pathology, a molecule loses a hydrogen electron and attacks other healthy cells, trying to regain its lost balance. An antioxidant lends a free radical a hydrogen molecule without destroying itself, stopping free radical pathology in its tracks. However, once pathology begins, the radicals duplicate themselves by the billions within a minute, so the antioxidants have to be constantly replenished throughout the day.

A hairstylist put it like this, "Your hair is fed by the bloodstream so if there are any difficulties in that area it will be carried through into the hair and the skin. You could be losing your hair, it could be brittle or dull. Nutrition does have an effect on everything in your body and so your hair is an appendage of what is going on. It is a reflection of who you are."

Hair and skin are last on the list of priorities. Your heart, your liver, your kidneys, your brain are all more important to the body's functioning. Your body has innate knowledge of itself, about what infections or what cancer cells or what viruses are present. It says to itself "I will selectively have to take care of what I can and fight those more important battles first. Whatever is left over I will give to the hair." Well, the average American never has anything left over. They're always drawing more out of the body. There's always a greater assault against the body going on than benefits flowing in.

Nutritional Approaches to Better Hair Health

One clinical nutritionist tells us that for hair and overall body health, we should consume six freshly-prepared green juices a day with organically grown vegetables because, they are free of pesticides, fertilizer and other artificial residues. Also, the soil used in organic farming is very vital and alive and mineral and nutrient rich, far more vital and health-promoting then commercially grown vegetables.

Increased circulation to the scalp is important so exercise should be part of any program, along with juicing, to support the body nutritionally.

I recommend the following four stage program to provide increased vitality to your hair and scalp.

STAGE 1
DAILY PROTOCOL FOR THE FIRST THREE MONTHS
B complex (50 mg)
B_{12} (100 mcg)
garlic (500 mg twice)
aloe (1 oz three times)
protein (9/10th g per kg of body weight) [1 kg = 2.2 pounds]
6 glasses of dark green vegetable juice or 6 scoops of chlorophyll rich powder

STAGE 2
DAILY PROTOCOL FOR THE SECOND THREE MONTHS
sea vegetables (one serving)
flaxseed oil (1 tablespoon)
evening primrose oil (500 mg)

choline and inositol (500 mg twice)
PABA (100 mg)
folic acid (400 mcg)
biotin (500 mcg)

STAGE 3
DAILY PROTOCOL FOR THE THIRD THREE MONTHS
sea vegetables (1 serving)
zinc (50 mg)
I cysteine (500 mg twice)
evening primrose oil (300 mg twice)
pantothenic acid (100 mg twice)
vitamin E (400 IU)
coenzyme Q10 (100 mg twice)
biotin (500 mcg)
choline and inositol (500 mcg)
B complex (50 mg of each)
B_{12} (100 mcg)
silica (150 mg)
PABA (250 mg)
folic acid (800 mcg)
6 glasses of dark green vegetable juice or 3 glasses dark green vegetable
juice and three of green plant extract of 6 scoops of chlorophyll rich powder

STAGE 4
DAILY PROTOCOL FOR THE FOURTH THREE MONTHS
PABA (500 mg)
pantothenic acid (500 mg)
garlic (1,000 mg)
onion (1,000 mg)
sea vegetables (6 oz.)
biotin (500 mcg)
choline (1,000 mg)
inositol (1,000 mg)
niacin (250 mg)
borage oil (500 mg)
omega-3 oil (1,000 mg)
cayenne (5 mg)
protein (9/10th g per kg of body weight [1 kg = 2.2 pounds])
6 glasses of dark green vegetable juice or 3 glasses dark green vegetable
juice and three of green plant extract of 6 scoops of chlorophyll rich powder

Phytochemicals

Dr. Martin Feldman informs us that drugs have potential in genetic-overcoming, like Rogaine, which has been somewhat effective. There are better ways to deal with the problem, however, like extracting phytochemicals in fruits and vegetables via a very low temperature process.

"In a study I did I gave participants as many as 15 to 20 separate fruits and vegetables that were extracted via the low temperature method, giving a total of approximately 300 different phytochemicals per day.

"My study in reversing hair loss did not rely on phytochemicals alone, but was holistic in scope. The program overcomes the genetic threshold through a multiple assault on the problem, by removing stress and doing exercise, becoming vegetarian, and detoxing by removing bad food.

"I should stress that though this approach is multifactorial, phytochemicals are still crucial. We can do it without medication, with phytochemicals, which are probably the medicine of the future."

Excursus on Phytochemicals

Phytochemicals are substances found in edible plants that exhibit potential benefits in the prevention and treatment of disease. There are thousands of phytochemicals in the foods we eat and scientists are just beginning to discover their healing properties. According to the *Journal of the American Dietetic Association* (April 1995): "It is the position of the American Dietetic Association (ADA) that specific substances in foods (e.g., phytochemicals as naturally occurring components and functional food components) may have a beneficial role in health as part of a varied diet. The Association supports research regarding the health benefits and risks of these substances. Dietetics professionals will continue to work with the food industry and government to ensure that the public has accurate scientific information in this emerging field."

The report goes on to say phytochemicals are present in many frequently consumed foods, especially fruits, vegetables, grains, legumes, and seeds, as well as in such less common foods as licorice, soy, and green tea. In addition to naturally occurring phytochemicals, scientists are developing what they call functional foods, which consist of any food or food ingredient providing health benefits beyond the traditional nutrients it contains.

Phytochemicals and functional food components have been associated with the prevention and/or treatment of at least four of the leading causes of death in the country—cancer, diabetes, cardiovascular disease, and hypertension—and with the prevention and/or treatment of other medical ailments including neural tube defects, osteoporosis, abnormal bowel function, and arthritis. Limonene in citrus fruits, for example, is known to increase the production of enzymes that help the body dispose of potentially carcinogenic substances.

Even the National Cancer Institute estimates that one in three cancer deaths are diet related and that eight of ten cancers have a nutrition/diet component.

Phytochemicals have been used by pharmaceutical companies in making many of their products. According to a report in *Business Week* (February 15, 1993), 25 percent of modern pharmaceuticals are derived in some way from plants. The heart medicine digitalis and the cancer drugs vincristine and taxol are just some examples. Pharmaceutical companies may soon be motivated to isolate components in foods into pills or supplement form to market the individual elements for their health benefits. However, due to regulatory problems, such companies will have to market naturally occurring components as drugs.

What makes phytochemicals new in the public ranks is their potential health benefits before people get sick, and the saving of both lives and health-care dollars. Unfortunately, according to Dr. Stephen L. DeFelic, the field is still in its infancy because of too few large-scale clinical trials focusing on the health benefits of foods. Since phytochemicals are not patentable, companies are reluctant to finance long-term studies that could cost as much as $200 million.

Nevertheless, epidemiological evidence and small human trials point to benefits which may well be sleeping giants in the nutrition arena. Such is the case with licorice root. In one USDA study, licorice root, an extract, proved to be 50 times sweeter than sugar without promoting tooth decay. It contains prostaglandin inhibitors that may guard against cancer and ulcers, and it is being pursued by many companies as a food additive.

In another study, Dr. Michael Gould found that d-limonene, the major component of orange peel oil, protects rats against breast cancer. In addition to findings such as these, the ADA report notes that well-designed clinical trials indicate the beneficial effects associated with high fruit and vegetable diets cannot be duplicated by nutritional supplementation alone. Clearly, there are more benefits in the healthy foods we eat than are obtained from the most common nutrients often associated with them such as vitamins C, E, A, beta carotene, and so on.

PART THIRTEEN

Selecting An Alternative Health Practitioner

Ultimately, you are responsible for your own well-being, but having access to proper health care practitioners is an important element in health maintenance. Their educated guidance and treatment can be invaluable, both in times of uncertainty and crisis and for prevention and awareness building during times of complete well-being.

Selecting the right health care professional can be an important decision that will benefit you for the rest of your life. In the first chapter of this final section of the book, we provide an overview on how to go about finding and evaluating such a person. In the following chapter, you will find a comprehensive Resource Guide listing the names, addresses and/or telephone numbers and specialties of hundreds of alternative practitioners. Many of those listed are the very same experts who provided much of the information for this book.

65

General Guidelines

Alternative health practitioners can help define the weak links in your body's structure and function and then direct you toward optimal personal care. There are many different approaches, but some general guidelines are worth mentioning here.

Your Rights as a Patient

A good holistic medical practitioner will perform at least these three basic types of analysis before prescribing any treatment plan:

(1) take a detailed medical history;

(2) perform a physical examination that goes beyond conventional methodologies; and

(3) study carefully the results of appropriate laboratory tests taken at the time of the history taking and the physical examination.

In addition, you have the right to expect that the practitioner includes in his or her repertory, some or all of the following:

♥ as many noninvasive diagnostic techniques as possible;

♥ an awareness of the potential diagnostic value of even very minor signs and symptoms in the prevention of major dysfunction;

♥ a preference for noninvasive over invasive techniques (for example, substances will be administered orally rather than intravenously, except when a condition calls for the more direct route);

♥ a recognition of the importance of strengthening the body's resistive capacities and an interest, wherever possible, in attempting to repair any malfunctioning organ or gland rather than to replace its function through the administering of its secretions;

💙 a tendency, whenever possible, to treat the primary weak link first if more than one has been discovered (for example, if the stomach is producing insufficient hydrochloric acid, resulting in the malabsorption of calcium, among other substances, the resulting calcium deficiency could lead to osteoarthritis, periodontal disease, or skin problems; by treating the hydrochloric acid insufficiency, the physician would be treating the primary weak link);

💙 an approach that treats the person as a whole person, not just a collection of ailing parts;

💙 the demonstrated ability to listen carefully and to skillfully classify any relevant symptoms in order to arrive at the best possible diagnosis;

💙 an orientation toward optimal health and sensitivity to dysfunctions that signal an imbalance in the individual;

💙 familiarity with a combination of approaches to help the person regain balance (for example, in addition to orthodox treatments, the physician's recommendations may include advice about stress reduction and lifestyle changes to reduce or eliminate causative factors in the environment);

💙 a willingness to refer the individual, when the condition warrants, to other medical practitioners whose specialized knowledge in a given area may be necessary to provide the most valuable restorative program; and

💙 a demonstrated awareness of the importance of the individual's own attitudes toward health and disease, and a willingness to communicate openly with the individual.

Your Role as a Patient

The alternative health practitioner should expect you to be an active, committed participant in the process, not a passive, disinterested patient who accepts everything the doctor recommends.

One form of this active participation may be the questions you ask with a view to getting the important information you need to help you in your contributions to the healing process. Some examples are:

What, specifically, is being treated?
How do you know that that's the problem?
What are some realistic goals in my situation?
What is the time frame?
Does every individual with this condition get exactly the same tests,
the same treatments?

What are my weak links?
Are these tests and this treatment relevant to my body and my condition?

The Importance of Commonplace Symptoms

Many people are living with symptoms that, because they are mild and do not constitute a full-blown disease state, are accepted, needlessly, as being an inevitable consequence of getting older. In fact, such people are often told by their conventional physicians: "Nothing is wrong with you. Everything is normal." And yet, the symptoms may be early warnings that something is out of balance.

Gas in the lower bowel (flatulence), belching, heaviness in the stomach, heartburn, and bloating, for example, may all be indicators of a malfunctioning digestive system, depending on their frequency and severity. These conditions are not normal in a healthy state, and they are often correctable.

Similarly, many of the symptoms that accompany delayed allergic reactions (the masked, cyclical allergies) are widely accepted as normal, and therefore to be tolerated for no better reason than "that's the way it is." The failure to recognize a connection between these symptoms and allergies may be due to the fact that they do not appear for upwards of 30 hours after the ingestion of the offending food or chemical substance. Typical symptoms are headache, irritability, anxiety, sudden changes of mood, and excessive fatigue, as well as unexplained body aches and pains. These symptoms may not be severe enough to be labeled as disease states, so the underlying cause is repeatedly overlooked or denied by traditional practitioners. Even when the disorders are recognized, their true significance may still be missed by those who try to reverse the symptoms without addressing the underlying causes for their appearance.

Thus frequent colds, recurring infections, and fatigue are all part of the warning mechanisms used by the body to signal an underfunctioning immune system. But they are rarely recognized as such. The phenomenal sales of cold remedies, for example, reflect how little attention is paid to strengthening the immune system—an approach that would far more effectively reduce the incidence of these disorders.

Types of Practitioners

It has never been my policy to make specific recommendations, to suggest to a person that a specific practitioner is the best doctor for them to see. The quality of a doctor's health care may depend on both the physician and the patient, as well as on their mutual compatibility. This is not something I, or anyone else, could predict in advance. But I still feel that people should be given some direction. So, what I have done here is supplied a directional guide. It is not meant to be a recommendation. Rather, I have offered some general guidelines. I have concentrated on modalities discussed throughout this book that the reader may not have easy access to, including homeopathy, chelation therapy, orthomolecular medicine, acupuncture, clinical ecology, and naturopathy. Chiropractors and osteopaths are not discussed here. Nor are nutritionists, although the experienced holistic nutritionist may be enormously helpful in helping you get the most from your diet.

HOMEOPATHY Homeopathy is based on the principle that what causes illness may follow a law of similars, meaning that by giving a healthy person a dilute amount of that which is a causative agent can in fact help the body rebalance itself. If a person has a head cold, you would give the person a substance that would cause cold symptoms in a healthy person, but in a sick person it helps to cure them. Homeopathy is limited in scope at this time in the United States, although 100 years ago it was the prevailing form of medicine—until allopathic medicine and the American Medical Association in particular launched an intensive drive against it, which culminated in its being virtually banned in this country. Very recently, there has been a renewed interest in homeopathy, and growing numbers of physicians are using its principles.

The homeopath must be a medical doctor in addition to his or her homeopathic specialization. Homeopathy is particularly useful in the treatment of fevers, bacterial infections, toxicity, and the cumulative effects of alcohol, drugs, tobacco, caffeine, or sugar. It is not recommended for cancer, AIDS, or heart disease.

CHELATION THERAPY Chelation therapy is a relatively new medical science, having started only about a quarter of a century ago. There are at this time nearly 1,000 doctors, including many board-certified cardiologists, who are using chelation therapy. The modality involves an intravenous drip of a substance known as EDTA, a chelating agent. The agent helps stimulate the destruction of free radicals, which seem to be a primary causative agent of the aging process itself. By slowing down the destructive potential of these free radicals, it allows the cells to heal themselves. As the cells heal, they are more able to fight off whatever infection or disease affects us. Claims have been made that chelation therapy can open up the arteries. Moreover, objective data has substantiated this. Improvement of vascular circulation in people who had obstructed arteries, especially those to the brain and to the extremities, has been demonstrated following treatment with this modality.

Chelation therapy runs about $100 per visit and patients generally have from 20 to 40 visits, depending on the severity of the condition. People have also begun receiving chelation therapy as a preventative treatment to slow down the aging process, based on the view that free radicals are a primary factor of the aging process. The treatment may be problematic, however, for patients with kidney disease, and renal monitoring is crucial. A physician must be certified as a practicing chelating therapist to perform the therapy.

ORTHOMOLECULAR MEDICINE Orthomolecular physicians and orthomolecular psychiatrists are conventionally trained medical doctors with an additional specialization. The purpose of orthomolecular medicine is the establishment of the right balance of the chemicals naturally occurring in the body. These physicians try to rebalance the chemicals within the body without using synthetic drugs that might interfere with natural processes. Their goal is homeostasis, or balance.

Frequently, orthomolecular physicians use a high-dosage vitamin regimen, far higher than what the average physician would ever presume would be needed. But it is their experience that only with these very high amounts, these megadoses, do they see the best results. For example, orthomolecular psychiatrists have had striking success in the treatment of schizophrenics, putting the condition into remission by using massive doses of niacin (B_3), B_6, and vitamin C—amounts that you would never give a healthy person. Orthomolecular psychiatrists are also better able to treat depression, by examining possible chemical imbalances in the brain. Moreover, orthomolecular physicians have the benefit of being able to use psychoanalysis or psychotherapy if deemed necessary, but that would be as a last resort. The cost of treatment is comparable to that for conventional physicians.

ACUPUNCTURE Acupuncturists work by opening up blocked energy pathways, or meridians, so that healing energy can go directly to a point in the body where it is needed, therefore stimulating the innate natural healing capacity of the body. The acupuncturist, in this country, must also be a medical doctor. Acupuncturists are particularly good for nerve problems, pain, musculoskeletal problems, but not for cancer or heart disease. The cost of treatment may range from $75 to $100 per visit.

CLINICAL ECOLOGY (ENVIRONMENTAL MEDICINE) Clinical ecologists are unique in that they are able to closely examine the relationship between the elements of a person's diet and any symptoms they may be experiencing. For example, a person's irritable bowel may be due to consumption of milk. The clinical ecologist will be able to identify this causative factor. He or she examines all the different foods, inhalants, and liquids that a person consumes to see which one of these, or which combinations, may be causing a physical or mental reaction. This modality has been particularly successful, for example, in the treatment of symptoms of arthritis. Clinical ecologists tend to use a far broader arsenal of treatments than the traditional allergist. Outside of the initial visit, the cost of seeing a clinical ecologist is no more than for a conventional physician, ranging from $40 to $75, depending on the state. The initial visit may vary from $125 to $500, depending on which tests are performed and the time required.

NATUROPATHY Naturopathic physicians can treat most conditions. They are not, however, allowed to perform major surgery (although they can perform minor surgery). Their very extensive background is centered in the botanical sciences, including the use of herbs and tinctures, with a wide variety of natural immune-stimulating properties. The naturopath practices a natural form of health care the traditions of which precede the advent of modern medicine, not unlike the traditional Tibetan physician who must be able to identify nearly 1,000 different healing herbs, mineral sources, and animal sources. The naturopath has years of extensive study in the healing potential of such substances. He or she is also able to understand muscular and skeletal bodily adjustment. Naturopaths use a much broader basis for diagnosis than do conventional allopathic physicians. Finally, the naturopath is usually a very good teacher as well. Not only do you get a therapy, you also generally get an education about the nature of your condition and the rationale behind the therapy. Naturopaths tend to be relatively inexpensive, generally in the neighborhood of $40 to $100 per visit.

66

Resource Guide

Acupressure and Oriental Body Medicine

Acupuncture & Chinese Medicine
The Healing Center
Dr. Yuan Yang, Licensed
Acupuncturist
175 West 72nd Street
New York, NY 10023
212-501-7521

American Oriental Bodywork
Association
Glendale Executive Campus
1000 White Horse Road, Suite 510
Voorhees, NJ 08043
609-782-1616

National Commission for the
Certification of Acupuncturists
1424 16th Street, N.W., Suite 501
Washington, DC 20036
202-232-1404

The American College of
Addictionology and Compulsive
Disorders
5990 Bird Road
Miami, FL 33155
305-661-3474

National Acupuncture Detoxification
Association
Lincoln Hospital
349 E. 140th Street
Bronx, NY 10454
718-993-3100

American Association of Acupuncture
and Oriental Medicine
433 Front Street
Catasququa, PA 18032
610-266-1433

Council of Colleges of Acupuncture
and Oriental Medicine
8403 Colesville Road, Suite 730
Silver Spring, MD 20910
301-608-9175

Alexander Technique

ARIZONA

James E. Coates, Ph.D.
803 West 1st Street, #B
Tempe, AZ
602-829-8738

Georgianne Y. Farness, M. Ed.
812 West Coconino
Flagstaff, AZ
602-774-8056

Harriet Harris
The Hawthorne Apartments
3848 North Third Avenue, #1085
Phoenix, AZ
602-287-9116
hharrisaz@aol.com

Charles Sabghir
HCR-2, Box 757
Tucson, AZ
520-822-1117
chazghir@juno.com

CALIFORNIA

Lona Alexander
4645 Morse Avenue
Sherman Oaks, CA
818-995-7267
MAlexa7582@aol.com

Cheri Alley
1962 15th Street
San Francisco, CA
415-255-6723

Linda Avak
714 Nash Avenue
Menlo Park, CA
650-328-4736

John Baron
1417 A Bridgeway, Suite 6
Sausalito, CA
415-453-1217
jab@wenet.net

Carolyn Behar
1730 Georgina Avenue
Santa Monica, CA
310-393-6970
carolynbehar@webtv.net

Elaine Belle
415 Wellesley Avenue
Mill Valley, CA
415-383-5640

Suzanne Berger
1178½ Wellesley Avenue
Los Angeles, CA
310-826-3912

Simone Biase
734 Wellesley Avenue
Kensington, CA
510-524-4025

Pamela Blanc
3211 Midvale Avenue
Los Angeles, CA
310-470-2993
PBlancAT@aol.com

Anne Bluethenthal
1962 15th Street
San Francisco, CA
415-864-6683

Heidi Brende
1111 Bella Vista Avenue
Pasadena, CA
818-798-1584

Robert Britton
70 Santa Paula Avenue
San Francisco, CA
415-664-5066
britton@infoasis.com

Glenn D. Canin
3674 19th Street
San Francisco, CA
415-487-1361

Maria Carrera
3712 Granada Avenue
San Diego, CA
619-293-3109
Atstudio1@aol.com

Lyn Charlsen
7455 Vista Del Monte
Van Nuys, CA
818-786-3944
LynTeaches@aol.com

Ronit Corry
6189 Stow Canyon Road
Santa Barbara, CA
805-964-9264
escor@west.net

Steve Corry
6189 Stow Canyon Road
Santa Barbara, CA
805-964-9264
escor@west.net

Barbara Coulson
726 Bounty Drive
Foster City, CA
650-572-8151

Galen Cranz, Ph.D.
5862 Birch Court
Oakland, CA
510-658-9330
gcranz@uclink.berkeley.edu

Claire Creese
Claremont Chiropractic Center
2914 Domingo Avenue
Berkeley, CA
510-845-3245
ccreese@earthlink.net

Amy Crocetti
2540 Sutter Street
San Francisco, CA
415-673-7046

Clarissa C. Daniel
70 Santa Paula Avenue
San Francisco, CA
415-664-3286
clarissa@nbn.com

Naomi Davis
851 Pomona, #10
Chico, CA
530-898-9523

Rosemary (Rome) Earle
609 Baywood Road
Alameda, CA
510-522-3888
romeshome@aol.com

Gretchen Elliott
11 Borica Street
San Francisco, CA
415-333-1416
cellopower@aol.com

Darcy Elman
1012 Goldridge Road
Sebastopol, CA
707-824-0931
glenn-darcy@msn.com

Kri Engle
1480 Warrington Road
Santa Rosa, CA
707-584-7318
shanti2u@juno.com

Michal Rabinovich Erez
608 South Burnside Avenue, #1
Los Angeles, CA
213-938-1350
michal8@pacbell.net

Leslie Felbain
1463 30th Avenue
San Francisco, CA
415-731-4132

Michael D. Frederick
P.O. Box 408
Ojai, CA
805-646-8902

Rose Mary Gardner
1134 Crespi Drive
Sunnyvale, CA
408-737-9974
RMGardner1@aol.com

Janet Gee
74 Brady Street, #8
San Francisco, CA
415-252-7070

Ari Gil
3510 Georgia Street
San Diego, CA
619-692-1892

Phyllis M. Gilmore
12 Dickens Court
Irvine, CA
949-856-0809
c/o bhgilmor@uci.edu

Alexander J. P. Gloth
4434 Los Feliz Boulevard, Suite 212
Los Angeles, CA
213-664-6965
medoth@aol.com

Gloria Gotti
3020 Bridgeway, Suite 106
Sausalito, CA
415-332-5686

Josephine Gray
305 Green Street
San Francisco, CA
415-487-7698
jo.gray@usa.net

Doris Green
1811 Pampas Avenue
Santa Barbara, CA
805-569-0235

Elise Guidoux
235 Carmelita Drive
Mountain View, CA
650-961-5674
karenkosh@aol.com

Sydney Laurel Harris
5350 Woodbury
Ventura, CA
805-644-7845
sharris@dynatest.com

Pamela Hartman
14627 Hartsook Street
Sherman Oaks, CA
818-784-0167

Sachiko Hashimoto
951-2 Old County Rd, #275
Belmont, CA
650-533-8335
tmcksh@aol.com

Kay Hogan
101 Gregory Lane, #36
Pleasant Hill, CA
925-676-3696
yakten@slip.net

Charlotte Holtzermann
7128 Flight Avenue
Los Angeles, CA
310-348-9118

Debby Jay
3747 Mound View Avenue
Studio City, CA
818-769-9171
DHJay@aol.com

Sherry Johannes
1038 14th Street, No. 5
Santa Monica, CA
310-284-4878
johannes@lamg.com

Sonja Johnson, R.N.
13548 Centerville Road
Chico, CA
916-893-4355

Rose Adams Kelly
491 Crescent Street, #308
Oakland, CA
510-763-2623

Laura Klein
1519 Virginia Street
Berkeley, CA
510-845-6619
lauraklein@juno.com

Bruce I. Kodish, P.T.
1021 S. Orange Grove Boulevard #101
Pasadena, CA
626-441-4627
bikodish@aol.com

Don Krim
612 North Las Palmas Avenue
Los Angeles, CA
323-466-9746
DonKrim@aol.com

Carolynne Dale Levine
444 Piedmont #221
Glendale, CA
818-243-9608

George Lister
1458 30th Avenue
San Francisco, CA
415-681-1172
ALEXVOCE@aol.com

Carol Longshore
1850 Parkside Drive
Concord, CA
510-685-6710
clongshr@ccnet.com

Eleanor Lyman
Box 291
Bolinas, CA
415-868-1378

Dan Marcus
2501 Pico Boulevard, #604
Santa Monica, CA
310-828-0320

Babette Markus
1913 Thayer Avenue
Los Angeles, CA
310-470-1180
BabetteM@BEAT.cc

Frances Marsden
11317 Otsego Street, #5
N. Hollywood, CA
818-760-6454

Kirsten Marshall
San Francisco, CA
415-831-8116

Stella Moon
471 Corbett Avenue
San Francisco, CA
415-626-4030

Susan Nance
114 Palm Avenue
San Francisco, CA
415-751-5643

Nora Nausbaum
1053 Talbot Avenue
Albany, CA
510-525-6021
listen2@well.com

Sandra Niman
275 Mesa Road
Bolinas, CA
415-868-1208

Bob Odell
200 Lowell Avenue
Palo Alto, CA
415-322-8787

Bruce Oliver
930 Alhambra Boulevard, #270
Sacramento, CA
916-448-7424
piat@sunset.net

Sherry Berjeron Oliver
930 Alhambra Boulevard, #270
Sacramento, CA
916-448-7424
piat@sunset.net

Frank Ottiwell c/o A.C.T.
30 Grant Avenue
San Francisco, CA
415-550-7340
Ottiwell@aol.com

David Page
1930 10th Avenue
San Francisco, CA
415-664-5245

Linda Parker
112 Little Court
Folsom, CA
916-988-0843

Anke Perkert
4130 Manila Avenue
Oakland, CA
510-652-5054

Gary Pettinger
University of California-
San Francisco
500 Parnassus
P.O. Box 0234A
San Francisco, CA
415-476-0350

Heidemarie Pfankuch
16-1 San Gabriel Drive
Chico, CA
530-899-8866
heidi@embo.net

Beth Pierik
115 North Washington Street
Cloverdale,CA
707-894-4521

Giora Pinkas
90 Island Court
Walnut Creek, CA
925-933-0602
alexander_center@hotmail.com

Kari Prindl
362 Lexington Street
San Francisco, CA
415-641-8374

Lisette Rabinow-Palley, MA, OTR
4173 Mentone Avenue
Culver City, CA
310-559-0695
lisetterp@postoffice.worldnet.att.net

Rochelle Reea
P.O. Box 605
Mill Valley, CA
415-789-0816

Rita Rivera
P.O. Box 1373
Felton, CA
831-336-0104
ritariv@aol.com

Shirley Robbins
615 West 9th Street
Claremont,CA
909-626-4322

Jean-Louis Rodrigue
1536 South Rexford Drive
Los Angeles, CA
310-277-0009
JeanLouisR@aol.com

Eleanor Rosenthal
530 Presidio Avenue
San Francisco, CA
415-921-0921
EleanorR@wenet.net

Julie Russell
907 Key Route Boulevard, Suite 4
Albany, CA
510-526-6442

Daryl Schilling
11 Borica Street
San Francisco, CA
415-587-5999
DAndraS@aol.com

Joan Schirle
P.O. Box 305
Blue Lake, CA
707-668-5253
Jschirle@aol.com

Susan Schreier, M.A.
300-A Casitas Avenue
San Francisco, CA
415-566-3726

Laura R. Schreiner
1208 Firmona Avenue
Redondo Beach, CA
310-370-5354
pks@aol.com

Vittoria Segalla
233 Orient
Chico, CA
530-345-7027
vitasan@c-zone.net

Shulamit Sendowski
19108 Lull Street
Reseda, CA
818-886-4153

Robert Shallenberg
2009 Estero Street
Oceanside,CA
760-967-2118
bobshall@subtone.wanet.com

Sally Shallenberg
2009 Estero Street
Oceanside, CA
760-967-2118
bobshall@subtone.wanet.com

Ron Sheredy
381 Bush Street
San Francisco, CA
415-487-6313

Joanne Somerville, DC
3019 Adeline Street
Berkeley, CA
510-548-6229

Jerry Sontag
381 Bush Street, Suite 500
San Francisco, CA
415-434-2542
jerry@mtpress.com

Lana G. Spraker, M.A.
1834 Stoner Avenue #10
Los Angeles, CA
310-479-3646

Judith Stransky
933 20th Street, #A
Santa Monica, CA
310-828-5528

Sandra Sutton
158 Beaumont Avenue
San Francisco, CA
415-221-0977

Carol Swann
1609 Virginia Street
Berkeley, CA
510-848-4435
carolswann@aol.com

Gary Thomas
3021 17th Street
Santa Monica, CA
800-509-5803

Eileen Troberman
1133-E Second Street
San Diego & Encinitas,CA
760-943-9521
ETatAT@aol.com

Bobbi Tryon
1641 Broadway
Chico, CA
916-891-4335

Shel Wagner
911 Palm View Drive
Los Angeles, CA
213-254-4735
ShelWagner@aol.com

Sigrid Wagner
2115 Belmont Lane
Redondo Beach, CA
310-798-5083
sgwagner@ix.netcom.com

Megan Ward
P.O. Box 481
Forest Ranch, CA
916-345-5371

Marcia Werner
56 Hanover Lane, #C1
Chico, CA
530-343-2900

Walton L. White
912 11th Street, Apt H
Santa Monica, CA
310-394-3177

Joanne Wills
4201 Via Marina, #240
Marina Del Rey, CA
310-827-8867
WillsJM@aol.com

Randall Wilson
7234 Sixth Avenue
Tahoma, CA
530-525-5859
avanti@sierranet.com

Kathryn A. Zimmerman
The Studio
771-775 Ocean Avenue
Point Richmond, CA
510-236-9366

Trude Zmoelnig
134 West Alvin Drive, # B
Salinas, CA
831-444-0647
OmegaZ@msn.com

COLORADO

Maedée Duprès
A Living Arts Center
53 East Asbury Avenue
Denver, CO
303-722-1315

Colin Egan
Alexander Technique Institute—
Colorado
880 Hawthorne Place
Boulder, CO
303-449-4143

Gene GeBauer
600 West 123rd Avenue, #4014
Westminster, CO
303-457-4745
meanfeet97@aol.com

Kathy Goodhew, R.N.
2810 7th Street
Boulder, CO
303-449-5834
kathygoodhew@usa.net

Posie Green
8301 West 38th Avenue
Wheat Ridge, CO
303-431-7338
agreenp@ecentral.coom

Trina Jacobson
P.O. Box 3736
Vail, CO
970-949-4019

Joanie Mercer
404 Fairfax Street
Denver, CO
303-333-1218
joanietom@envisionet.net

Mary Lois Misken
5360 Sunset Drive
Littleton, CO
303-797-6013

Vicki Rodgers
171 Sunrise Lane, JSR
Boulder, CO
303-442-3192

Anne Schwerdt
7800 Frying Pan Road
Basalt, CO
970-927-9807

Carol Toensing
2155 Topaz
Boulder, CO
303-449-1838

Victoria Valencia
2245 Floral Drive
Boulder, CO
303-449-7022
valencia@bvsd.k12.co.us

CONNECTICUT

Marta Curbelo
260 West Cedar
Norwalk, CT
212-873-7098

Linda DeLeon
152 East Avenue
Norwalk, CT
203-221-7706

Ilse R. Giebisch
5 Carriage Drive
Woodbridge, CT
203-393-1663

Elizabeth Huebner
46 Obara Drive
Windham, CT
860-456-1529
freake@uconnvm.uconn.edu

Idelle Packer
27A Fairfield Road
Greenwich,CT
203-661-8027
bfarson@aol.com

DISTRICT OF COLUMBIA

Riki Alexander
2943 Tilden Street, N.W.
Washington, DC
202-363-6568
rikidolph@aol.com

Susan Martin Cohen
125 Tennessee Avenue, N.E.
Washington, DC
202-544-2448
smceagle@aol.com

Kathleen Lucatorto
2911 Stephenson Place, N.W.
Washington, DC
202-363-2879

Anne McDonald, MFA, OTR/L
2939 Van Ness Street, N.W., #834
Washington, DC
202-244-3624

Lynn Brice Rosen
3000 Connecticut Avenue, N.W.
Washington, DC
202-333-7702
lnbrosen@aol.com

Nancy Sussman McCarren
4816 Nebraska Avenue, N.W.
Washington, DC
202-244-9337

DELAWARE

Cynthia Morgan
2808 Bexley Court
Wilmington, DE
302-737-7321
cynthiam@brahms.udel.edu

Stanley Tucker
309 Capitol Trail
Newark, DE
302-368-8125

FLORIDA

Tully Hall
8305 Stonebrook Drive
Sanford, FL
407-323-0596
DBBsTbn@aol.com

Corinne Johnston
3203-A 40th Way South
St. Petersburg, FL
727-864-6848

Irene Kaye
1846 Mallory Street, #10
Jacksonville, FL
904-389-8010
irenekaye@mindspring.com

Roberto Mainetti
8125 Crespi Boulevard, #1
Miami Beach, FL
305-861-0424

Marja Scheeres
2811 8th Avenue West
Bradenton, FL
941-748-5754

Don Taber
6440 Ellis Lane
Loxahatchee, FL
561-795-2868
dontaber@freewwweb.com

GEORGIA

Ron Dennis
4246 Peachtree Road, #6
Atlanta, GA
770-454-1177

Wallace Moody, III
Marietta, GA
770-956-9296

HAWAII

Helen Higa
1339 Koko Head Avenue
Honolulu, HI
808-732-1180

Jill Togawa
118 Kaneohe Bay Drive
Kailua, HI
808-254-6483
pmdpjet@aol.com

ILLINOIS

Adeline Anderson
474 Lakewood Boulevard
Park Forest, IL
708-481-8505

Edward Bouchard
2216 W. Palmer Street, Suite 2R
Chicago, IL
773-862 3320
bouchard@flash.net

Rose Bronec
608 E. Burkwood Court
Urbana, IL
217-344-5274
rcarbaug@prairienet.org

Courtney Stephen Brown
3723 North Southport
Chicago, IL
773-878-3865
csbrown@ibm.net

Sherry Cmiel
511 West Clark
Champaign, IL
217-352-1078
blossom@prairienet.org

Connie de Veer
210 Parkview
Bloomington, IL
309-662-8761
chdevee@oratmail.cfa.ilstu.edu

Mary Derbyshire
9231 Springfield
Evanston & Skokie, IL
847-675-0002
maryderby@aol.com

Ruth Don
P.O. Box 258
Kenilworth, IL
312-471-0646

Marilyn Dunsing
2208 South Staley Road
Champaign, IL
217-398-1435
JeanneH175@aol.com

Westley Feaster
604 S. Race, #2N
Urbana, IL
217-344-2080

Kathryn Gault
West Suburban Chicago
Alexander Technique
P.O. Box 4011
Wheaton, IL
800-665-6079

John Henes
1830 Sherman Avenue, Suite 302
Evanston, IL
847-475-3087
j-henes@nwu.edu

Christine Inserra
1923 West Greenleaf Avenue
Chicago, IL
773-338-5016

Robin Kearton
203 South Birch
Urbana, IL
217-384-2946
robstv@soltec.net

Alexander Murray
508 West Washington
Urbana, IL
217-367-3172
admurray@uiuc.edu

Rebecca Nettl-Fiol
6 Genevieve Court
Champaign,IL
217-398-1459
rnettl@uiuc.edu

Melanie Rae Nickolaus
1931 North Howe Street, Apt #3E
Chicago, IL
312-440-7077
melanierae@worldnet.att.net

Robert Resnick
309 South Dixon
Carbondale, IL
618-457-7233

Philip Schalow
2407 Carrelton Drive
Champaign,IL
217-398-8466

Evelyn Shapiro
607 West High Street
Urbana, IL
217-337-6575
esha@prairienet.org

Beth Stein
4538 North Ashland Boulevard
Chicago, IL
773-271-8538
bstein@suba.com

Jeff Tessler
1105 S. New Street
Champaign,IL
217-359-9162

Helene Weisbach
1651 West Olive
Chicago, IL
773-275-6236
weisbac@ibm.net

IOWA

Mary Stuyvesant Eagle
203 Oberlin Street
Iowa City, IA
319-466-4251
mareagl@yahoo.com

LOUISIANA

Nancy R. Gootrad
1015 North Rendon Street
New Orleans, LA
504-482-4094

MASSACHUSETTS

Pamela Bartlett
19 Center Court
Northampton, MA
413-586-2031

Gaye Bennes
11½ Hilliard Street
Cambridge,MA
617-491-0172

Sheldon Berkowitz
85 College Street
South Hadley, MA
413-532-7680
sberkowi@mhc.mtholyoke.edu

Rivka Cohen
10 Bradford Terrace, Apt. 1
Brookline, MA
617-556-4227

Susan Grant Corash
409 Prospect Street
Northampton, MA
413-584-2136
freetomove@msn.com

Ted Dimon
13 Park Avenue
Sommerville, MA
617-876-3434
tdimon@world.std.com

Cathy Hazeltine Fallon
2-3 Warren Road
Stow, MA
978-897-1102
fallons@tiac.net

Laurie Fiscella
227 Montague Road
Leverett, MA
413-548-8132

Stephen L. Forman
P.O. Box 464
Williamsburg, MA
413-582-9000

Jill Geiger
22 Claflin Place
Newton, MA
617-527-7373
geiger@connact.com

Judith Gerratt
201 North Avenue
Weston, MA
781-560-7270

Hannah Ulrike Goertz
345 Harvard Street , #4E
Cambridge, MA
617-441-2975
movewease@aol.com

Lisa Harvey
549 North Farms Road
Northampton, MA
413-585-0405

Millicent Harvey
84 Edgemoor Avenue
Wellesley, MA
781-235-3889

Laura Harwood
993 Memorial Drive, #201
Cambridge, MA
617-876-4907
laurah@channel1.com

Ruth Kilroy
Alexander Technique Training Center
803 Boylston Street
Chestnut Hill, MA
617-734-6898

Kathleen Lawrence
9 Penniman Road
Brookline, MA
617-739-2167

Christine Olson
12 Forbes Avenue
Northampton, MA
413-586-4012
chrolson@hotmail.com

Cheryl Pleskow
126 Williams Street
Northampton, MA
413-584-8793

Betsy Polatin
54 Harvard Avenue
Brookline, MA
617-277-2220
Bpolatin1@aol.com

Julia Priest
22 Roslyn Road
Newton, MA
617-928-0630
priestsinger@att.net

Cecile Raynor
Alexander Technique Associates
124 Harvard Street
Brookline, MA
617-731-8151
617-731-0609

Eckart Schopf
1 Holden Street
Brookline, MA
617-739-2000

Stephanie Segers
94 Pleasant Street
Arlington, MA
781-646-8824
Stephanie@Jacobspatent.com

Abbie Steiner
44 Coles Meadow Road
Northampton, MA
413-585-0567
abjohn@javanet.com

Christine Stevens
59 Grantwood Drive
Amherst, MA
413-549-4881
cmstevens@aol.com

Marie Stroud
5 Walden Street, #6
Cambridge, MA
617-876-7071
mstroud@harvard.edu

Corinne Trabucco
28 Fairfax Street
Burlington, MA
781-272-2939
corinne@connactivity.com

Missy Vineyard
94 Lessey Street
Amherst, MA
413-253-2595
mvine@javanet.com

MARYLAND

Meade Andrews
506 Mississippi Avenue
Silver Spring, MD
301-587-8736

Carol Boggs
6900 Wisconsin Avenue, #700
Bethesda, MD
301-951-4418
cboggs@aol.com

Diana Bradley
40 Columbia Avenue
Takoma Park, MD
301-270-2559
DMBradley@aol.com

Christopher Cherry
2-D Westway
Greenbelt, MD
301-474-2325
kesterford@aol.com

Linda Gunter
1801 Glenallan Avenue
Silver Spring, MD
301-933-3497
rhiscock@marasconewton.com

Nancy Wanich Romita
4412 Wickford Road
Baltimore, MD
410-235-2678
nromita@ibm.net

MAINE

Judith Cornell
30 Munjoy Street
Portland, ME
207-772-1984

Maria Jackson Parker
272 Maine Street
Brunswick, ME
207-729-0839

MICHIGAN

Reinaldo Couto
1075 Barton Drive, #116
Ann Arbor, MI
313-913-4039

Jane R. Heirich
2229 Hilldale
Ann Arbor, MI
734-761-2135
jheirich@umich.edu

Joan Heneghan
120 West 11 Mile Road, Suite 210
Royal Oak, MI
248-547-9373

Clifford Hicks
495 Glen Oaks Drive, Apt. 2D
Muskegon, MI
616-777-2722
hicks@novagate.com

Michelle LaPlace Obrecht
1403 Maywood Avenue
Ann Arbor, MI
734-662-0048
michlap@earthlink.net

Elinore Morin
531 West Oakwood Drive
East Lansing, MI
517-337-2390
morine@pilot.msu.edu

MINNESOTA

Stephanie Chapman
8000 36th Avenue North, #12
Minneapolis/New Hope, MN
612-595-7453

Lisa First
3225 Dupont Avenue, South
Minneapolis, MN
612-822-3504
FIRSTSPOCK@aol.com

Babette Lightner
Downtown Minneapolis
& University of Minnesota
Dept. of Theatre Arts and Dance
Minneapolis, MN
612-729-7127
light002@tc.umn.edu

Brian McCullough
3301 Colfax Avenue South
Minneapolis, MN
612-824-4251
poised@ix.netcom.com

Carol McCullough
3301 Colfax Avenue South
Minneapolis, MN
612-824-4251
poised@ix.netcom.com

James M. Wellman
3621 Blaisdell Avenue South
Minneapolis, MN
612-825-9652

MISSOURI

John Appleton
3354 West Lombard
Springfield, MO
417-831-7131

Kate Frank
4355 Maryland Avenue, #432
St. Louis, MO
314-652-0824

Katherine Mitchell
2011 Blendon Place
St. Louis, MO
314-647-0483
73261.3112@compuserve.com

Patricia A. Wilson
1000 W. 68th Terrace
Kansas City, MO
816-822-2865
duarte8642@aol.com

NORTH CAROLINA

Saura Bartner
6916 Union Grove Church Road
Hillsborough & Chapel Hill, NC
919-967-2528
saura@mindspring.com

Suzanne Faulkner
1711 Lakewood Avenue
Durham, NC
919-403-6848
suzfau@gte.net

Victoria Hyatt
University Drive, #28K
Durham, NC
919-401-0505
vhyatt@worldnet.att.net

Charles Stein, M.M.
200 Harmon Court
Winston-Salem, NC
336-723-8626

NEBRASKA

Robert Rickover
2434 Ryons Street
Lincoln, NE
402-475-4433
robert@alexandertechnique.com

NEW HAMPSHIRE

Deborah Babson
116 Old County Road
Jaffrey, NH
603-532-7582

Lawrence Carter
54 Old Temple Road
Lyndeborough, NH
603-654-5120

Martha Engeman
The Center for Kripalu Yoga &
Creative Dance
Harris Pond, Unit 3
Merrimack,NH
603-886-7308

NEW JERSEY

Pamela Anderson
106 Culberson Road
Basking Ridge, NJ
908-766-6837

Elizabeth Anne Buonomo
49 Morrison Street
Closter, NJ
201-750-2979
EABuonomo@aol.com

Jed Diamond
322 Grand Street, #3L
Hoboken, NJ
201-963-3431
mvg206@is6.nyu.edu

Colleen Higgins
6051 Boulevard East, Apt. 3C
West New York, NJ
201-295-0802

Lauren Jones
20 Nassau Street, Suite 308
Princeton, NJ
609-466-1981

Susan Kramer Loeb
56 Benson Street
Glen Ridge, NJ
201-748-6104

Jean McClelland
101 74th Street, #4
North Bergen, NJ
201-854-7483

Esther Seligmann
59 Gordon Way
Princeton, NJ
609-921-1780

Diann Sichel
7-B Hibben
Faculty Road
Princeton, NJ
609-430-9599

Valerie Van Hoven
21 Broadway
Denville, NJ
201-627-8112
Vhooven@aol.com

NEW MEXICO

Melissa Matson
546 Harkel Road
Santa Fe, NM
505-992-8986

Susan Emmet Reid
29B Old Arroyo Chamiso
Santa Fe, NM
505-820-6615
susanereid@aol.com

Inez Zeller
1E Montoya Circle
Santa Fe, NM
505-989-3326
inez@dsat.com

NEVADA

Vanessa Jones
10 Watkins Way
Yerington, NV
702-463-5549
TAKEOFF@nanosecond.com

NEW YORK

Nina Aledort
14 Prince Street, #2C
New York, NY
212-274-9297
nina@inch.com

Wade Alexander
May through October)
Greystone/430 Caswell Road
Freeville, NY
607-844-9300
wadealxat@earthlink.net

Beret Arcaya
810 Broadway, 2nd Floor
New York, NY
212-677-0022

Joan Arnold
412 11th Street, #2R
Brooklyn, NY
718-768-2746
joanarn@aol.com

Michele Arsenault, M.A.
123 West 77th Street, #5A
New York, NY
212-874-2530
mbsm@interport.net

Pearl Ausubel
262 Central Park West, #12D
New York, NY
212-787-0173

Christine M. Batten
74 MacDougal Street
New York, NY
212-473-3247

Caren Bayer
245 West 14th Street, #3B
New York, NY
212-620-0925

Jacque Lynn Bell
900 West 190th Street, Apt. 10A
New York, NY
212-795-9495

Evangeline Benedetti
90 Riverside Drive, 10F
New York, NY
212-799-5226

Martha Bernard
460 West 22 Street
New York, NY
212-924-1761

Sandra Bernard
113 Park Place
Brooklyn, NY
718-857-4670

Teva Bjerken
360 Fourth Street, #3
Brooklyn, NY
718-788-0062
tevaseth@sprynet.com

Deborah Caplan
365 West End Avenue, #13C
New York, NY
212-724-1372

Robert Lee Cohen
408 West 36th Street, #3-F
New York, NY
212-643-9322

Susan Collinson
Posture in Motion
320 King Street
Chappaqua,NY
914-238-1450
Posturepal@aol.com

Bill Connington
148 East 84th Street, Suite1C
New York, NY
212-517-0020

Alison Courtney
317 West 107th Street, #1B
New York, NY
212-316-1891

Claire C. Cunneen
Tarrytown, NY
914-358-3609
taolife@concentric.net

Karla Diamond
36 Orchard Street
Pleasantville, NY
914-741-5313

Marjorie Dorfman
P.O. Pox 1804
Huntington Station, NY
516-385-4001

Jane Dorlester, CSW
293 Sixth Avenue
Park Slope/Brooklyn, NY
718-788-4991
jdorlester@aol.com

June Ekman
47 West 28th Street, #3
New York, NY
212-686-4316

Gwen Ellison
161 West 54th Street, #504
New York, NY
212-581-8829

Paul W. Farin
The Alexander Studio
419 Lafayette Street, #7
New York, NY
718-783-0460
pfarin@pratt.edu

Allison Foley
110 North 8th Street, #7
Brooklyn, NY
718-218-7146

Neil Friedland
162 9th Avenue
New York, NY
212-691-3502

Billie Daniel Frierson
112 East 19th Street, #5F
New York, NY
212-533-5830

Joan Frost
71 Stephens Road
Tappan, NY
914-365-3497

Sarah Gamble
NY
212-645-0040

Hope Gillerman
32 Union Square East, Room 612N
New York, NY
212-387-0721
hopeg@bway.net

Susan Greene Goodale
39 East 19th Street, #5
New York, NY
212-533-6595

Judith Grodowitz
337 West 21st Street, #5A
New York, NY
212-675-1094
metisnow@aol.com

Alina Holder
30-30 69 Street
Woodside, NY
718-424-4963

Joanne Howell
201 East 17th Street, #12J
New York, NY
212-533-5574

Mary Beth Hraniotis
32 West Searsville Road
Montgomery, NY
914-457-5512

Joy Jacobson
155 East 55th Street, Suite 6C
New York, NY
212-427-4684
Rvelleu@aol.com

Sheilah James
175 Prospect Park SW, Apt. 2A
Brooklyn, NY
718-853-6228

Kim Jessor
114 Fulton Street
New York, NY
718-398-9421
kjessor@spacelab.net

Barbara Kent
444 Central Park West, #11C
New York, NY
212-865-2947
Barakent@aol.com

Laurie Kline
853 Broadway, Suite 1020
New York, NY
212-529-3211

Brian Kloppenberg
155 West 20th Street, #3K
New York, NY
212-924-6875

Cynthia Knapp
306 West 93rd Street, #47
New York, NY
212-222-7663
CynKnapp@aol.com

Jane Kosminsky
41 West 70th Street, #3F
New York, NY
212-724-9755
JBSosmos@aol.com

Thomas Lemens
15 The Parkway
Katonah, NY
914-232-8950

N. Brooke Lieb
317 West 107th Street, #2B
New York, NY
212-866-0679
brookelieb@mindspring.com

Leslie Manes
31 Purchase Street
Rye, NY
914-697-8106
914-669-6717

Gwynne Marshall
623 West End Avenue #1A
New York, NY
212-874-6216
gwynnjef@nyct.net

Hope Martin
15 East 17th Street, 6th Floor
New York, NY
212-243-3867

Ann Sickels Mathews
260 Sickeltown Road
Orangeburg, NY
914-358-4236

Troup Mathews
IRDEAT/74 MacDougal Street
New York, NY
212-473-3247

Hillary Mayers
425 Riverside Drive, #6A
New York, NY
212-663-2586
hillamay@aol.com

Diane McCollough-Young
20 Henry Street, #4A
Brooklyn, NY
718-222-9592
dianeyoung@mindspring.com

Barbara McCrane
304 West 89th Street, #7B
New York, NY
212-875-7134

Patricia McGinnis
344 West 89th Street
New York, NY
212-362-3374

June McIntosh
RR 5, Box 110
Canastota, NY
315-687-5029

Ellen Norman Melamed
484 First Street
Brooklyn, NY
718-788-0780

Jaye Miller
256 West 88th Street
New York, NY
212-877-0428

Kathryn M. Miranda
Mannes College of Music
150 West 85th
New York, NY
201-861-7179
kmmiranda@juno.com

Diana Mullman
New York Center for the Alexander
Technique
853 Broadway at 14th Street
New York, NY
212-734-7875

Steve Neeren
350 West 50th Street, #5G
New York, NY
212-586-3849

Sarnell Ogus
49 Sandra Road
East Hampton, NY
516-324-6218
soil6@juno.com

Charlotte Okie
26 Orchard Street
Pleasantville, NY
914-747-1959

Carlos Osorio
166 Bank Street PHA
New York, NY
212-243-2641

Michael Ostrow
853 Broadway, Suite 1020
New York, NY
212-529-3211

Claudia Peyton
42 Sixth Avenue
Nyack, NY
914-353-4463

Roxolana Podpirka
166-24 15th Drive
Whitestone, NY
718-352-6412

Stefanie Proessl
438 4th Street, Apt 2A
Brooklyn, NY
718-832-2027
prostef@aol.com

Michael Protzel
33 West 16th Street
New York, NY
212-242-4178
protz@superlink.net

Roland Racko
25-AC East 10th Street, #3A
New York, NY
212-254-2393

Jean Rashkind
Soho Center for the Alexander
Technique
225 Lafayette Street, Room 713
New York, NY
212-941-5490
jrashkind@aol.com

Elizabeth Reese
6 Orchard Street
Warwick, NY
914-987-9826
equiart@frontiercomm.net

Samuel S. Reiser, D.D.S.
28 South Washington Avenue
Dobbs Ferry, NY
914-693-2094
drsreiser@aol.com

Cynthia Reynolds
239 Bleecker Street, #3
New York, NY
212-242-8053
cr16@is.nyu.edu

Katherine Reynolds-Cohen
505 East 79th Street, #17 B
New York, NY
212-327-1647

Frances Robertson
Lourdes Wellness Center
1020 Vestal Parkway East
Vestal, NY
607-754-6043
nepalext@nep.net

Janice Stieber Rous
194 Riverside Drive
New York, NY
212-877-9717

Urs Sauer
New York, NY
212-741-3467
Usauer@aol.com

Lauren Schiff
252 West 102 Street, #1
New York, NY
212-971-1925
schiffel@aol.com

Robin Schiff
305 Eighth Avenue, #B2
Brooklyn, NY
718-788-8502

Mollie Schnoll
200 West 16th Street, #6I
New York, NY
212-645-0973

Greg Seel
250 5th Avenue at 28th Street
New York, NY
212-447-5649
JGregS@aol.com

Constance Serchuk
568 Grand Street, #1806J
New York, NY
212-677-1663
alanxm@pipeline.com

Carolyn M. Serota
150 East 37th Street, #4-D
New York, NY
212-683-9078

Daniel Singer
732 Amsterdam Avenue
New York, NY
212-932-1624

Laura Smith
28 8th Avenue
Brooklyn, NY
718-638-1602
rmdinc@earthlink.net

Judith C. Stern
31 Purchase Street
Rye, NY
914-921-2400
neuron123.aol.com

Anne M. Stewart-Frost
267 Oxford Street, #405
Rochester, NY
716-473-8949

Mona Stiles
822 Greenwich Street, #3G
New York, NY
212-741-5036
shelbar@aol.com

Sally Taylor Sullivan
54 Cedar Street
Tappan, NY
914-398-2627

Mona Sulzman
428 Elm Street
Ithaca, NY
607-277-7553

Deborah Tacon
347 Route 340
Sparkill, NY
914-365-1062

Arthur Tobias
127 West 79th Street, Suite 6
New York, NY
212-875-7543

Jane Tomkiewicz
104 East 4th Street, #C2
New York, NY
212-529-2087
JNTMKWCZ@aol.com

Leland Vall
61-19 184th Street
Fresh Meadows, NY
718-321-7316
lelandv@datatone.com

Thomas Vasiliades
403 West 48th Street 3C
New York, NY
212-726-1569

Tony Visconti
1619 3rd Avenue, Apt. # 9KE
New York, NY
212-996-0380
antonyv@aol.com

Nanette Walsh
605 West 112th Street, Apt. 5G
New York, NY
212-663-6338
nanet@ix.netcom.com

Anne Holmes Waxman
124 West 74th Street, #2R
New York, NY
212-787-8198
Annewaxman@aol.com

Nancy Wechter
41 Union Square
New York, NY
212-255-0111

Susan Arthur Whitson
120 Bennett, #5H
New York, NY
212-927-0203

Jessica Wolf
117 West 13th Street
New York, NY
212-691-3941
gess@bestweb.net

Regina Wray
114 Fulton Street, #3W
New York, NY
212-285-1645

Lydia Yohay, C.S.W.
340 West 87th Street, #PH
New York, NY
212/724-5828

Judith Youett
314A North Smith Road
LaGrangeville, NY
914-677-5871
jyouett@aol.com

OHIO

Nancy Crego
3276 Alexandria Drive
Toledo, OH
419-474-0497
ncrego@aol.com

Helen Hobbs
P.O. Box 21032
South Euclid, OH
216-291-4190

Tina Holsapple
1118 Priscilla Lane
Cincinnati, OH
513-321-7551
holsapple@fuse.net

Alan F. Mistler
6584 Wooster Pike
Cincinnati, OH
513-271-7862

Neil Schapera
7445 Fourwinds Drive
Cincinnati, OH
513-891-0415
schapend@email.uc.edu

Vivien Schapera
7445 Fourwinds Drive
Cincinnati, OH
513-891-0415
schapend@email.uc.edu

Jennifer Tinapple
2681 Bahns Drive
Beavercreek, OH
937-429-3845

Lucy Venable
554 South 6th Street
Columbus, OH
614-469-9984
venable.1@osu.edu

OKLAHOMA

Stuart Bell
1421 South Carson Avenue
Tulsa, OK
918-599-8242
SJBELL.aol.com

OREGON

Barbara Conable
Andover Educators
4427 North Willis Boulevard
Portland, OR
503-286-8184

Karen DeWig
654 S.W. Grant Street, #304
Portland, OR
503-464-9428
kdewig@juno.com

Carolene Miller
Mountain Laurel Center for the
Healing Arts
2195 Professional Court
Bend, OR
541-330-9008
doodle@bendnet.com

Dorothy Ormes
1045 Terra Avenue
Ashland, OR
541-482-6234

Sara Padilla
921 S.W. Morrison Street, Suite 538
Portland, OR
503-977-9756

Jocelyn Parrish-Nichols
652 8th Street
Lake Oswego, OR
503-514-2378
enichols@pacifier.com

PENNSYLVANIA

Lelia Calder
31 Dartmouth Circle
Swarthmore, PA
610-543-7789
lelia@craftech.com

Patricia R. Dressler, M.Ed.
2324 Pine Street
Philadelphia, PA
215-732-5799

Diane Gaary
256 West Montgomery Avenue
Haverford, PA
610-642-8267

Jeff Goldman
1807 South 9th Street
Philadelphia, PA
215-327-7783
cjjeff@icdc.com

Celeste Kelly
1720 Delancy Street
Philadelphia, PA
215-552-8558

Pamela Lewis
5812 Northumberland
Pittsburgh, PA
412-421-8409
pl06+@andrew.cmu.edu

Chris Mincer
123 West Linn Street
Bellfonte, PA
814-355-4994

Mary Sickels Seelye
5 Mullen Road
Ambler, PA
215-646-4947

RHODE ISLAND

Heide R. Gerritsen
51 East Manning Street
ProvidenceRI
401-831-4779

Carol Gill
Malik11 Halsey Street
Providence, RI
401-831-0542
amer_malik@postofifice.brown.edu

Mara Sokolsky
377 Cole Avenue
Providence, RI
401-751-9271

TEXAS

Sumi Komo, M.A.
The Alexander Technique Moving
Arts Center (ATMA)
P.O. Box 33176
Austin, TX
512-448-4009

Alice R. Pryor
4703 Hilwin Circle
Austin, TX
512-451-5945
alipryor@onr.com

Phyllis Richmond
700 Tanglewood Lane
Arlington, TX
817-275-1697
pgrichmond@anet-dfw.com

UTAH

Marjean McKenna
1408 Federal Way
Salt Lake City, UT
801-363-3506
marjeana@m1.sprynet.com

Cathy Pollock
893 South McClelland Street
Salt Lake City, UT
801-322-0909
alexander@utah-inter.net

VIRGINIA

Patricia Charmoy Buxton
20006 Bremo Road
Richmond, VA
804-288-1881

Rajal Cohen
Optimal Health Associates
Blacksburg, VA
540-522-2177
rajcohen@usa.net

Hild Creed
110 Monte Vista Avenue
Charlottesville, VA
804-296-3287
hild@rlc.net

Sandra Bain Cushman
100 2nd Street, N.W.
Charlottesville, VA
804-978-7767
sbc@cstone.net

Robin Eastham
Port-a-ferry Farm
Batesville, VA
540-456-8324

Chris Friedman
100 2nd Street, N.W.
Charlottesville, VA
804-296-6250
cfriedman@mindspring.com

Katharine Scott Gilliam
1718 Dairy Road
Charlottesville, VA
804-977-6459
kspiano@aol.com

Marian Goldberg
P.O. Box 449
McLean, VA
703-821-4277
atcwdc@aol.com

Joseph Robert Lee
5433 Shadowwood Drive
Virginia Beach, VA
757-460-4477
jrjlee@earthlink.net

Karen Loving
15706 Fox Chase Lane
Culpeper, VA
540-547-2596
lloving@summit.net

Daria Teresa Okugawa
1021 Sheridan Avenue
Charlottesville, VA
804-977-7186
dokugawa@redlt.com

Joy K. Paoletto
10813 Millington Lane
Richmond, VA
804-741-3476

Suzanne Rice
Arlington, VA
703-527-7329
suzannerice@erols.com

Sally Rogers
4926 Appleberry Lane
Schuyler, VA
804-831-2522

VERMONT

Rupa Cousins
372 Canoe Brook Rd
East Dummerston, VT
802-387-5276
rupa@together.net

Kate Judd
824 Bonnyvale Road
Brattleboro, VT
802-257-1358

Sami Pincus
20 West Canal Street, #230
Winooski, VT
802-655-6610

Maggie Schiele Sullivan
134 Spruce Street
Brattleboro, VT
802-257-2257
navillus@sover.net

WASHINGTON

Jeanne M. Barrett
4110 Stone Way, North
Seattle, WA
206-517-6148

Jane Carr
2614 North 30th Street
Tacoma, WA
253-759-0696

Steve Hurley
10212 5th Avenue, N.E., Suite 200
Seattle, WA
206-524-3455
sph@sph.seanet.com

Marjorie Nelson
2622 Franklin Avenue East
Seattle, WA
206-329-3097

Barbara Nichols
11580 Madison Avenue NE
Bainbridge Island, WA
206-780-0983
barbaranic@aol.com

Sara O'Hare
312 Marietta Ct.
Steilacoom, WA
253-589-2439
saraohare@aol.com

Frank Sheldon
6242 3rd Avenue, N.W., #2
Seattle, WA
206-789-3742
fsheldon@uswest.net

Andrew Zavada
11538 20th Avenue, NE
Seattle, WA
206-440-0084
azavada@msn.com

WISCONSIN

Michael Johnson-Chase
University of Wisconsin-Milwauke
P.O. Box 413
Milwaukee, WI
414-229-3913
mjc@csd.uwm.edu

Jane Peckham
2148 Allen Boulevard, #1
Middleton, WI
608-238-2466
jmpeckham@aol.com

Aromatherapy

ARIZONA

Addesso, Anthony
602-843-9249

Damian, Kate
602-861-3696

Fritsche, Anna Marie
602-494-7332

Kane, Lou Ann
602-934-7929

Magyar, Teri
602-963-7644

May, Kathleen
602-493-3872

Morris, Connie
602-635-2331

Morris, Lance
602-323-7133

New Jenkins, Pat
602-526-8515

Strong, Maria
602-493-3513

CALIFORNIA

Buhler, Ann Marie
818-300-8096

Gardner, Nancy
415-383-7224

Grossman, Michael
714-770-7301

Kahn, Linda Anne
619-457-0191

Luthra, Yugal
916-442-4945

Northrop, Margaret
510-522-0189

Steele, John
818-986-0594

Thomas, Helen DC
707-527-7313

Welke, Lynn
619-225-2197

Zdral, Claudia
510-522-0998

FLORIDA

Carr, Arlene
407-649-8162

D'Costa, Harriet M
813-584-7246

Kratz, Cynthia
407-835-6821

IDAHO

Davis, Annette
208-232-5250

ILLINOIS

Steenvoorden, Marianne
312-296-6700

MASSACHUSETTS

Beaty, Janet
508-772-0222

Lentz, John
413-548-9763

NEW JERSEY

Lindberg, Elisabeth
201-934-1751

PENNSYLVANIA

Cassel, Bonita
215-398-9642

WASHINGTON

Alexander School
206-473-1142

Contento, Elise
206-283-2819

Ayurvedic Medicine

American School of Ayurvedic
Sciences
10025 NE 4th Street
Bellevue, WA 98004
206-453-8022

Ayurvedic Institute
11311 Menaul NE, Suite A
Albuquerque, NM 87112
505-291-2698

Maharishi Ayur-Ved Medical Center
P.O. Box 49667
Colorado Springs, CO 80949-9667
800-843-8332

Biofeedback Training

Association for Applied
Psychophysiology and Biofeedback
10200 West 44th Ave, Suite 304
Wheat Ridge, CO 80033
303-422-8436

Chelation Therapy

ALABAMA

Prosch, Gus Jr. MD
205-823-6180

ALASKA

Denton, Sandra MD
907-563-6200

Manuel, F Russell MD
907-562-7070

Martin, Robert MD
907-376-5284

ARKANSAS

Becquet, Norbert MD
501-375-4419

Gustavus, John
501-758-9350

Wright, William MD
501-624-3312

CALIFORNIA

Belenyessy, Laszlo MD
213-822-4614

Edward, Davids MD
209-783-5068

Gordon, Ross MD
510-526-3232

Jahangirl, M MD
213-587-3218

COLORADO

Denton, Sandra MD
719-548-1600

Fish, James MD
719-471-2273.

Juetersonke, George DO
719-528-1960

CONNECTICUT

Cohen, Alan
203-877-1936

Finnie, Jerrold MD
203-489-8977

Sica, Robban MD
203-799-7733

DISTRICT OF COLUMBIA

Beals, Paul MD
202-332-0370

DELAWARE

Yossif, George MD
302-856-5151

FLORIDA

Dayton, Martin DO
305-931-8484

Haimes, Leonard MD
407-994-3868

Pardell, Herbert DO
305-922-0470

Pynckel, Gary DO
813-278-3377

GEORGIA

Edelson, Stephen MD
404-841-0088

Epstein, David DO
404-525-7333

Gunter, Olover MD
912-336-7343

HAWAII

Arrington, Clifton MD
808-322-9400

IDAHO

McCallum, K Peter MD
208-263-5456

McGee, Charles MD
208-664-1478

Thornburg, Stephen DO
208-466-3517

ILLINOIS

Jenkins, Hugh MD
312-445-6800

Stone, Thomas MD
708-934-1100

Tambone, John R MD
815-338-2345

INDIANA

Darbro, David MD
317-787-7221

Whitney, Norman DO
317-831-3352

Wolverton, George MD
812-282-4309

IOWA

Blume, Horst MD
712-252-4386

KANSAS

Acker, Stevens MD
316-733-4494

Hunsberger, Terry DO
316-275-7128

Neil, Roy MD
913-628-8341

KENTUCKY

Morgan, Kirk MD
502-228-0156

Tapp, John MD
502-781-1483

LOUISIANA

Prakasam, Felix MD
318-226-1304

Whitaker, Joseph MD
318-467-5131

MAINE

Cyr, Joseph
207-868-5273

MARYLAND

Beals, Paul MD
301-490-9911

Brown Christopher, Cheryl MD
410-268-5005

Health Mgmt. Inst.
301-816-3000

MASSACHUSETTS

Cohen, Richard MD
617-829-9281

Janson, Michael MD
508-362-4343

Ruben, Oganesov
617-254-2500

MICHIGAN

Bernard, William DO
313-733-3140

Farris, Lovell DDS
313-861-2100

Modzinski, Leo MD
517-785-4254

MINNESOTA

Carlson, Keith MD
507-247-5921

Dole, Michael MD
612-593-9458

Eckerly, Jean MD
612-593-9458

MISSISSIPPI

Hollingsworth, Robert MD
601-398-5106

Sams, James MD
601-327-8701

Waddell, James MD
601-875-5505

MISSOURI

Dorman, Lawrence DO
816-358-2712

McDonagh, Edward DO
816-453-5940

Sunderwirth, William DO
417-837-4158

MONTANA

Binder, Timothy DC ND
406-363-4041

NEBRASKA

Ilarina Corazon, Ibarra HMD
702-827-1444

Pfau, Terry DO
702-258-7860

Vance, Robert DO
702-385-7771

NEW JERSEY

Harris, Charles MD
908-506-9200

Locurcio, Gennaro MD
908-351-1333

Magaziner, Allan DO
609-424-8222

NEW MEXICO

Krohn, Jacqueline MD
505-662-9620

Shrader, W MD
505-983-8890

Stoesser, Annetter MD
505-623-2444

NEW YORK

Calapai, Christopher MD
516-794-0404

Hoffman, Ronald MD
212-779-1744

Schachter, Michael MD
914-368-4700

Yutsis, Pavel MD
718-259-2122

NORTH CAROLINA

Keith, E Johnson MD
910-458-0606

Laird, John MD
704-252-9833

Wilson, John Jr. MD
704-252-9833

NORTH DAKOTA

Briggs, Brian MD
701-838-6011

Leigh, Richard MD
701-775-5527

OHIO

Aronica, Josephine MD
216-867-7361

Baron, John DO
216-642-0082

Cole, Ted DO
513-779-0300

OKLAHOMA

Anderson, Leon DO
918-299-5039

Farr, Charles MD PhD
405-691-1112

Snitker, Gaylord
918-749-8349

OREGON

Peters, Ronald MD
503-482-7007

Skovsky, Robert ND
503-654-3938

Tyler, Jeffery MD
503-255-4256

PENNSYLVANIA

Burton, Frederick MD
215-844-4660

El-Atteache, Mumduh F
412-547-3576

Schmidt, Robert DO
215-437-1959

SOUTH CAROLINA

Rozema, Theodore MD
803-796-1702

SOUTH DAKOTA

Matheny, Theodore MD
605-734-6958

TENNESSEE

Carlson, James DO
615-691-2961

Reisman, Stephen MD
615-356-4244

VIRGINIA

Collin, Jonathan MD
206-820-0547

Hart, Burton DO
509-927-9922

Huffman, Harold MD
703-867-5242
Washington

Levin, Norman
703-802-8900

Rosenblat, Aldo MD
703-241-8989

Wright, Jonathan MD
206-631-8920

WEST VIRGINIA

Corro, Prudencio MD
304-252-0775

Jellan, Albert MD
304-242-5151

Zekan, Steve MD
304-343-7559

WISCONSIN

Alwa, Rathna MD
414-248-1430

Galvez, Timoteo MD
608-238-3831

Leutner, Thomas DC
414-465-1431

Spaeth, Alan W DDS
414-463-1956

Chiropractic

ALABAMA

Burroughs, George DC
205-476-9000

ALASKA

Connel, Charles DC
907-562-7909

Vaisvil, Sandra DC
907-561-3690

Webb, Gary DC
907-562-6181

ARIZONA

Addesso, Anthony DC
602-843-9249

Boag, Charles DC
602-269-5717

Brimhall, John DC
602-964-5107

Deal, Sheldon DC
602-323-7133

Reade, James DC
602-732-0911

CALIFORNIA

Berry, Linda DC
510-526-6657

Campanelli, Eve Ph.D.
310-548-0906

Chau, Mabel DC
818-956-5165

Cohn, Howard DC
714-668-1112

Dernay, Dan DC
510-682-1234

Eller, H. Lee DC
916-895-1151

Feurstein, Gaie DC
209-431-4571

Friedman, Warren DC
415-459-2550

Geronimo, Rubio
800-388-1083

Kotsonis, Dino DC
805-252-7881

Prins, Charles DC
510-526-6243

Savarese, Vincent DC
818-769-1811

Smith, Steven DC
408-866-8319

Walker, Scott DC
619-753-0107

COLORADO

Birkett, Jerry DC
303-447-9180

Casey, Patrick DC
719-634-2477

Klepper, Gary DC
303-449-7388

Strempel, William DC
303-777-6466

CONNECTICUT

Barone, Alice DC
203-268-7004

Koch, Douglas DC
203-335-8293

Sanna, Julius DC
203-744-7440

FLORIDA

Baker, Thomas DC
407-996-6565

Bloukos, Theodore DC
407-368-2461

Bringas, Barbara DC
305-385-1000

Green, Pamela DC
813-644-8451

Hancock, George DC
813-933-9540

Johnson, Jim DC
305-434-1800

Steven, Corcoran DC
813-592-7767

GEORGIA

Feder, Kenneth DC
404-252-0050

Gordon, Ruth DC
404-916-9800

Haberski, Larry
404-294-5050

Hammer, Jay DC
404-872-8779

Khalsa, Gurusahay DC
404-843-3400

Lee, Linda DC
404-705-9594

Mundale, Mia DC
404-248-1180

Robideau, Robert DC
404-740-8244

HAWAII

Carson, Jacqueline DC
808-934-3233

Felcher, Gerald DC
808-828-6844

Hynes, Karl Sr. DC
808-329-6888

Klein, Robert DC
808-959-4588

ILLINOIS

Berk, Karen DC
312-761-5401

Boudro, Stephen DC
708-544-2700

Case, Amelia DC
312-266-9090

DeStefano, Carl DC
708-858-9780

Distasio, Louis DC
217-544-8118

Donch Elliot, Elizabeth DC
815-433-4112

Maes, Luc Michael DC
708-668-9626

Morantz, Gerald DC
708-331-3329

Orme, Davis DC
309-799-7935

Terry, Mark DC
618-532-5929

INDIANA

Evans, Edward DC
317-541-1114

Hamilton, Thomas DC
812-477-5003

Jackson, Bruce DC
317-827-0393

Mangas, Steven DC
317-247-1717

IOWA

Heise, Forrest DC
319-754-5751

Knutson, Mark DC
319-266-1838

Miller, Don DC
319-393-6530

KANSAS

Dowty, Milton DC
316-684-0550

Miadenoff, Evan DC
913-491-1071

KENTUCKY

Brady, Sean DC
502-458-6165

Hughes, John DC
606-329-9311

LOUISIANA

Beaumont, Sylvia DC
504-861-8000

Guidry, Richard Jr. DC
318-981-2937

MARYLAND

Dale, Constance DC
410-687-4270

Lawrence, Robert DC
410-838-5131

Ozello, Robert DC
301-279-0950

MASSACHUSETTS

Bronstein, Lawrence DC
413-528-2948

DeFilippo, John DC
617-648-4000

Kerner, James DC
617-380-0990

Levesque, Norman DC
413-737-1636

Maykel, William DC
508-832-3248

Orfield, Antonia DC
617-868-8742

MICHIGAN

Boven, Louis DC
616-392-2166

Cordes, John DC
810-647-9005

Deboe, Bruce DC
517-684-3993

Donner, Louis DC
810-682-6513

Goodheart, George DC
313-881-0662

Green, Larry DC
616-754-4617

Heacock, Nancy DC
616-345-3660

Hearon, Colyn DC
517-356-2441

Kalis, Thomas DC
313-382-5222

Koffeman, George DC
517-787-2021

Kraynek, Ronald DC
313-451-1225

Lietz, Charles DC
616-530-3333

Lirot-White, Kathie DC
517-278-5567

Mayo, Joseph Jr. DC
517-764-5305

Morlock, Emil DC
616-532-5291

Ryckman, William DC
810-653-0602

Sayer, Linda DC
313-677-1900

MINNESOTA

Harvey Shapiro, Virginia DC
218-722-4845

Nelson, C Robert DC
612-922-0616

Riabokin, Tatiana DC
612-935-9360

MISSOURI

Anderson, Gary DC
816-425-6311

Conable, Katharine DC
314-991-5655

Duwe, Margaret DC
314-821-6654

Mathis, Shauna DC
501-855-4739

MONTANA

Hager, Robert DC
406-755-1722

NEBRASKA

Engen, Steven DC
308-237-2891

NEVADA

Anderson, Dale DC
702-458-1181

Ediss, John DC
702-882-7085

Francis, Timothy DC
702-221-8870

Robirds, Randall DC
702-646-1150

NEW HAMPSHIRE

Loch, Paul DC
603-772-7888

Nicoletti, A Douglas DC
603-898-5500

Procita, Vincent DC
603-924-3777

NEW JERSEY

Campbell, James DC
201-267-2243

Gibbons, Barbra DC
201-887-0860

Goldstein, Paul DC
908-271-0400

Hildebrandt, Kenneth DC
908-367-0106

Horning, Jeffrey DC
609-778-8688

Kane, John DC
201-744-4904

Kitay, Annalee DC
201-235-0065

Kutschamn, David DC
908-741-4777

Lauria, Paul DC
609-266-1557

Lefkowitz, Harry DC
201-836-7141

Pine, Alan DC
201-567-0700

Pollack, Steven DC
908-244-0222

Schultz, Linda DC
201-489-4325

Serra, Jody DC
908-236-6353

Seugling, Raymond DC
201-696-0500

Smith, Michael DC
908-591-0070

Spreiser, Paul DC
201-334-6053

Teitelbaum, Marianne DC
609-786-3330

Ungaro, Nicholas DC
908-281-7515

Weissman, Robert DC
201-265-3434

Zodkoy, Steven DC
908-308-0099

Zosche, Darren DC
201-543-4001

NEW MEXICO

McClure, Jimmie DC
505-989-9561

McRostie, GP DC
505-988-4210

Ninos, Frank DC
505-334-3633

NEW YORK

Anteby, Samuel DC
718-963-3103

Baker, Donald DC
516-785-8300

Bassman, Larry DC
718-622-3535

Bland, Robert DC
212-246-2330

Bloom, Richard DC
914-425-9575

Borzone, Robert DC
516-496-7766

Briks, Harold DC
914-948-4488

Carlin, Eric DC
212-645-1961

Cohl, Robert DC
315-737-9457

Conway, Lisa DC
516-354-2355

Copperstein, Bruce DC
914-232-9497

Cordaro, Salvatore DC
718-325-8162

Craft, Richard DC
914-647-5430

Davy, John DC
516-867-7997

Esposito, Vincent DC
718-627-1127

Ferentz, Avery DC
212-245-3170

Ferreri, Carl DC
718-253-9702

Freer, Kenneth DC
716-372-6274

French, Loretta DC
212-722-5271

Gizoni, Christine DC
516-589-7814

Golan, Ora DC
718-846-0886

Goldstein, Carol DC
212-489-9396

Gregory, Robert DC
914-623-3939

Gregory, Robert DC
914-638-3399

Hendrickson, Hanna DC
516-669-4673

Herbold, Richard DC
518-371-6431

Heus, Edythe DC
212-505-8680

Hirsch, Richard DC
914-356-0201

Hogan, Wayne DC
518-664-5281

Kearing, Rose Marie DC
516-427-9391

Klein, David DC
212-486-3886

Lang, Harvey DC
718-773-1121

Leroy, Anthony DC
914-354-0005

LiClaire, M DC
516-671-6763

Lynch, Mark DC
516-585-7777

Mafetone, Philip DC
914-628-5000

Manning, Mark DC
718-627-1127

Miller, Columbia DC
718-359-2221

Mindel, Frederick DC
212-752-6770

Moselle, Bruce DC
518-747-5506

Olsen, Mary DC
516-421-1248

Oswald, Steven DC
212-924-2121

Perlman, Eric DC
212-645-0006

Reppert, Diane DC
607-272-4290

Rogowskey, Thomas DC
212-645-1961

Rose, Glenda DC
716-754-9039

Rosen, Marc DC
716-893-8616

Rubenstein, Craig DC
212-213-9494

Shaffner, Michael DC
518-672-4019

Sinett, Sheldon DC
212-752-6770

Tinari, Frederick DC
516-467-8224

Warren, Jaime DC
516-599-0010

Weber, Jeffrey DC
718-376-2300

Weiner, Frederick DC
607-273-9200

Wieczorek, Stanley DC
716-637-2133

Wright, Thomas DC
716-394-2030

NORTH CAROLINA

Dauphine, David DC
704-295-9896

Diener, Mark DC
704-554-1141

Flaherty, Edward DC
919-776-4304

Monnin, Mark DC
704-843-5045

Schmidt, John DC
919-847-3555

Shmit, Walter Jr. DC
919-942-8516

Sisson, William Jr. DC
910-392-3770

Skala, Richard DC
704-364-2243

NORTH DAKOTA

Hestdalen, Darrel DC
701-227-1104

Moon, Derryl DC
701-227-1140

Swanson, William DC
701-748-2136

Thomsen, Robert DC
701-845-2481

OHIO

Carter, Richard DC
614-369-3060

DiPaolo, David DC/ND
419-882-7148

Duckwall, Mark DC
513-767-7251

Duffy, Cecelia DC
216-466-1186

Engel, David DC
419-472-0977

Fedorko, Jeffrey DC
216-494-0422

Hartle, Bruce DC
513-748-0940

Hauserman, Leslie DC
216-251-5444

Kreger, James DC
419-841-4207

Powell, James DC
216-494-5533

West, Lance DC
419-475-4323

OKLAHOMA

Demackiewicz, John DC
405-364-1244

Gdanski, Victor
405-335-5112

Plowman, Paul DC
405-840-5600

OREGON

Cooper, Carol DC
503-393-6071

Dougherty, JJ DC
503-640-2411

Friedman, Nick DC
503-668-3604

Jolley, Barbara DC
503-661-2137

McClure, Steven DC
503-254-1522

Palmer, John DC
503-378-0068

Savard, Carl James DC
503-221-1441

Vrandenburg, Donald DC
503-754-0325

PENNSYLVANIA

Bloom, Glen DC
412-731-9441

Calhoon, Janet DC
717-566-3245

Charron, Richard DC
717-859-3445

Corneal, John DC
814-237-5111

Ferro, Anthony D Jr. C
610-388-2212

Fisher, Li David DC
717-538-5245

Froberg, Warren DC
215-295-4393

Jiga, James DC
717-898-6220

Karpowicz, Alex DC
717-342-0797

Kelley, Justin DC
215-435-8880

Later, William DC
215-293-1660

McCain, William DC
215-345-6888

Rabenau, Robert DC
717-464-2719

Rehrig, Dennis DC
215-566-9040

Reiff, Dennis DC
215-368-5528

Stangl, Alan DC
215-434-7562

Stewart, Roger DC
412-322-1945

Weeks, Skyler DC
717-523-1221

RHODE ISLAND

Bridgham, Clive W DC
401-245-7010

Post, Gary DC
401-789-5008

Redleaf, Roger DC
401-944-6582

SOUTH CAROLINA

Hinson, Lewis DC
803-599-9255

TENNESSEE

Adams, Lawrence DC
615-373-4744

Brennion, William DC
615-356-0876

Markham, Ben DC
615-622-6007

Obersteadt, Louis DC
615-352-4455

Sunshine, Barry DC
615-984-6850

Windham, Sara DC
615-584-0479

TEXAS

Bandy, John DC
512-328-4041

Colwell, Alfred DC
713-351-7343

Connolly, Ken DC
214-618-8227

English, Jolyn DC
210-340-9500

Huneycutt, Arvel DC
817-645-3996

Jackowski, James DC
214-368-8977

Martin, John DC
512-892-3585

Mauldin, Alvin DC
512-447-3332

McCullogh, Tim DC
713-451-6722

Mullins, Roy DC
512-328-4041

Rakowski, Robert DC
713-333-2537

Ram, Lakheeshswar DC
903-581-4393

Rice, Richard DC
214-438-6800

Sanvall, Dale DC
817-861-9400

Schulz, Mark DC
713-541-4402

Scroeter, Tina DC
512-263-5626

Souza, Kipp DC
817-244-1924

Thaxton, Stephen DC
304-788-1922

Tucker, James DC
817-461-9811

UTAH

Brabnham, Korin DC
801-268-8090

Hawkins, Karl DC
801-268-0100

Morgan, Kevin DC
801-583-0900

VERMONT

O'Boyle, Kimberly DC
802-877-3567

Schenck, William DC
802-878-8330

Vreeland, Kurt DC
802-649-3122

VIRGINIA

Carson, Catherine DC
703-273-6106

Erbe, William DC
703-931-2255

Julian, Rose DC
703-689-2300

Kenley, Jack DC
804-473-9900

MacDonald, William DC
703-459-4727

Mowles, Richard DC
703-989-4584

Roselle, Thomas DC
703-698-7117

Schusterman, Dale DC
703-827-0222

Shapiro, Bonnie DC
703-642-8527

Skinner, Joseph DC
703-356-8887

Taylor, James DC
804-520-7246

Thompson, Paul DC
804-422-5866

Weinstein, Alan DC
703-379-2225

WASHINGTON

Green, A Gordon DC
206-483-2320

Stoutenburg, John DC
206-483-5041

Taggart, Michael DC
206-821-1101

WEST VIRGINIA

Jones, E Morgan DC
304-636-3570

WISCONSIN

Bircher, Steven DC
715-723-2696

Borrman, William DC
414-725-4918

Jensen, Jan DC
414-645-1616

Jordan, Craig DC
414-327-6767

Kuehnemann, Herbert DC
414-447-6062

Laden, David DC
608-257-7212

Nelson, Melissa DC
414-743-7255

Vrandenburg, Gene DC
715-723-2696

Wagner, Ronald DC
608-244-0211

WYOMING

White, Paul DC
307-358-5066

Dentistry, Alternative

ALASKA

Connell, Charles DDS
907-562-7909

Miller, Burton DDS
907-277-2600

ARKANSAS

Sinclair, John DDS
501-741-2254

ARIZONA

Ayers, AJ DDS
602-881-8585

Barton, Cecil DDS
602-990-9544

Farnum, Stan DDS
602-721-7874

CALIFORNIA

Alpan, Jack DDS
213-383-3833

Arana, Edward M DDS
408-659-5385

Bleicher, Howard H DDS
818-981-3130

Howe, Frederick DDS
916-334-1730

Kersten, Timothy DDS
916-335-5491

Prescott, Marvin DDS
310-476-8302

COLORADO

Sunshine, Morris DMD
203-374-5777

DISTRICT OF COLUMBIA

National Integrated Health Institute
202-237-7000

FLORIDA

Brody, Marin DDS
305-822-9035

Green, Stevens DDS
305-271-8321

Harrison, James DDS
407-965-9300

Mcllaiwn, Milton DDS
407-293-3185

Parsons, Phillip DDS
904-473-4595

GEORGIA

Dressler, Ronald DDS
404-349-2088

King, Wayne DDS
404-426-0288

IDAHO

Pfost, James DDS
208-375-7786

ILLINOIS

Dieska, Daniel DDS
708-429-4700

Gottlieb, Seymour DDS
708-272-7874

Rothchild, John DDS
708-884-1220

Sukel, Phillip DDS
708-253-0240

IOWA

Allender, Terrance DDS
305-359-3719

KANSAS

Payne, William DDS
316-241-0266

KENTUCKY

Lavely, Robert DMD
502-426-4110

MARYLAND

Somatoro, Eugene DDS
410-964-3118

MICHIGAN

Farris, Lovell DDS
313-861-2100

Lielais, John DDS
810-642-5460

Regiani, David DDS
810-627-4934

Rousseau, Robert DDS
313-642-5460

MINNESOTA

King, Ronald DDS
612-824-0777

Olin, Gary DDS
612-770-8982

MONTANA

Christian, Duane DDS
702-882-4122

Strong, A Gary DDS
406-252-1221

NEW JERSEY

Gilbert, Paul DDS
908-254-7946

Steiner, Alan DDS
201-627-3617

Tortora, John DDS
908-721-0210

NEW MEXICO

Norton, Chris DDS
505-988-1616

Wolfe, Bill DDS
505-292-8533

NEW YORK

Barber, Donald DDS
716-632-7310

Bressack, Norman DDS
516-221-7447

Cantor, Mitchell DMD
516-283-6362

Friedman, Dresla DDS
718-353-3303

Lerner, David DDS
914-265-9643

Sorrin, Bruce DDS
914-338-7200

Winick, Reid DDS
212-867-4223

Wolski, Krystyna DMD
516-484-5871

OHIO

Chanin, Richard DMD
513-729-2800

Westendorf, William DDS
513-923-3839

OKLAHOMA

Plowman, Paul DDS
405-840-5600

OREGON

Thom, Dick
503-526-0397

Willamson, Jeffrey DDS
503-684-4174

PENNSYLVANIA

Gupta, Som DDS
412-828-1920

Krausz, Alan DMD
215-668-2330

Niklaus, Ronald DMD
717-737-3353

Pawk, Michael DDS
412-285-3305

Roeder, Anthony DDS
215-647-7272

Smith, Gerald DDS
215-968-4781

Smith, Steven DMD
215-545-2104

SOUTH DAKOTA

Lytle, Larry
605-342-0989

TENNESSEE

Cobbel, Steven DDS
615-691-2910

TEXAS

McCann, Michael DDS
409-798-9103

Snowden, Jack
817-275-2633

UTAH

Hansen, Joseph DDS
801-753-2322

VIRGINIA

Fischer, Richard DDS
703-256-4441

Whitley, Wayne DDS
703-371-9090

WASHINGTON

Borneman, Ruos
206-293-8451

De Felice, Armand DDS
509-327-7719

Grobins, George DDS
206-564-2722

Kitmoto, Frank
206-842-4772

Mardar, Mitchell
206-367-6453

WISCONSIN

Owen, Allen DDS
414-421-1700

Cook, Douglas DDS
414-842-2083

Energy Medicine

ARIZONA

Ber, Abram MD
602-279-3795

Flagler, Lila NMD
602-721-8821

CALIFORNIA

Alpan, Wendy
213-383-3833

Broadwell, Robert DMD
714-965-9266

COLORADO

Goddard, Sally
303-963-9165

Krakovitz, Rob
303-927-4394

Lange, Andrew ND
303-443-8678

FLORIDA

Zhao, RJ OMD PhD
813-365-8008

HAWAII

Carson, Jacqueline ND
808-934-3233

Kenyon, Paul ND
808-591-2872

ILLINOIS

Pelovska, Eugenia BD
312-296-6700

INDIANA

Sparks, Harold DO
812-479-8228

MARYLAND

Teiterbaum, Jacob
410-224-2222

MASSACHUSETTS

Fagan, Trudy BC
617-964-2551

MISSOURI

Kanion, Dorothy
816-779-4844

NEVADA

Edwards, David MD
702-827-1444

NEW MEXICO

Dean, Willard MD
505-983-1120

Stoesser, Annette MD
505-623-2444

NORTH DAKOTA

Leigh, Richards MD
701-775-5527

OREGON

Bettenburg, Rita ND
503-252-8125

Craddick, Joy MD
503-488-0478

PENNSYLVANIA

Jayalashmi, P MD
215-473-4226

Maulfair, Conrad Jr. DO
215-682-2104

VIRGINIA

Van Landingham, Ruth
703-281-9140

WASHINGTON

Jongaard, Robert ND
206-331-6470

Page, Sarah ACSW
206-361-7306

WISCONSIN

Meyer, Emily
608-249-1206

Environmental Medicine

ALABAMA

Brown, Andrew MD
205-547-4971

Bryan, Don MD
205-663-5840

Goldfarb, Martin MD
205-252-9236

Miller, Joseph MD
205-342-8540

Osmaond, Humphrey MD
205-759-0416

ALASKA

Denton, Sandra MD
907-563-6200

Manuel, Russell MD
907-562-7070

ARIZONA

Cousins, Gabriel DO
602-394-2520

Halcomb, William MD
602-832-3014

Schmutzer, Gene DO
602-795-0292

ARKANSAS

Hedges, Sr., Harold MD
501-664-4810

Kimball, G Howard MD
501-269-4301

Koehn, Laura MD
501-521-3363

Worrell, Aubrey Jr. MD
501-535-8200

Wright, William MD
501-624-3312

CALIFORNIA

Belenyessy, Laszlo MD
213-822-4614

Calabrese, Dorothy MD
714-240-7178

Cathcart, III, Robert MD
415-949-2822

Charles, Alan MD
510-937-3331

Forrest, Steven DC
408-358-2273

Freeman, David MD
818-985-1103

Gard, Zane MD
619-571-0300

Good, Erika MD
415-750-6510

Gunther, Ellen MD
510-841-1677

Kwiker, Michael DO
916-489-4400

Lippman, Cathie MD
310-289-8430

Magin, Sandra OMD
510-525-3016

Mann, Laura OMD
818-702-0717

Marinkovich, Vincent MD
415-327-8380

Plant, Richard DC
619-942-8610

Shamlin, Carol MD
408-378-7970

COLORADO

Denton, Sandra MD
719-548-1600

Duhon, Crawford MD
303-499-9386

Gerdes, Kendall MD
303-377-8837

Van Hardenbroek, Mechteld MD
303-241-8554

Whitcomb, Harold Jr. MD
303-925-5440

CONNECTICUT

Cohen, Alan MD
203-877-1936

D'Adamo, Peter MD
203-661-7375

Germaine, Jacqueline
203-347-8600

Mandell, Marshall MD
203-838-4760

DELAWARE

Groll, Jerome MD
302-645-2833

FLORIDA

Alten, Steve
407-852-9940

Cannon, Stanley MD
305-279-3020

Dooley, Bruce MD
305-527-9355

Haimes, Leonard MD
407-994-3868

Hoover, Kenneth MD
407-679-0662

Melvikov, Eteri MD
813-748-7943

Schoen, Joya MD
305-898-2951

Segler, Marjo MD
407-278-6008

GEORGIA

Boyette, D Morton MD
912-435-7161

Edelson, Stephan MD
404-841-0888

Johnson, G Hugh MD
912-272-8494

HAWAII

Calrk, Wismer VG
808-941-0522

Weing, George MD
808-523-2311

IDAHO

Newbombe, Jr.
208-267-7575

Seeley, Jack MD
208-375-1264

ILLINOIS

Aven, Allen MD
708-253-1070

Hesselink, Thomas MD
708-844-0011

INDIANA

Armer, Robert M MD
317-846-7341

O'Brian, John MD
219-422-9471

Thomas, Robert MD
219-872-5521

IOWA

Kaufmann, Nyle MD
319-338-7862

Riley, V Thomas MD
319-234-5582

Soll, Robert MD
515-247-8750

KANSAS

Emery, Dorothy MS DC
913-682-4848

Hinshaw, Charles MD
316-262-0951

KENTUCKY

Henderson, Nanine DO
502-893-5422

Morgan, Kirk MD
502-228-0156

Parks, John MD
606-254-9001

LOUISIANA

Callendar, Thomas MD
318-233-6022

Cave, Stephanie MD
504-767-7433

MAINE

Hothem, Maurice DO
207-797-4148

Kenney, Bruce DO
207-774-9668

Northrup, Christianne MD
207-846-6163

MARYLAND

Brenner, Arnold MD
410-922-1133

Cook, Paul MD
410-337-2707

Gaby, Alan MD
410-486-5656

MASSACHUSETTS

Janson, Michael MD
617-661-6225

Kaufman, Svetlana MD
508-453-5181

Malladi, R Gopal MD
413-536-2978

MICHIGAN

Bernard, William DO
313-733-3140

Davey, Paula MD
313-662-3384

Petruca, Louis MD
313-864-7400

Walker, Jerry DO
313-292-5620

MINNESOTA

Brauer, William MD
612-871-2611

Sweere, Edward DC
507-345-3323

MISSISSIPPI

Glasgon, Thomas MD
610-234-1791

MISSOURI

Bart, Gerald MD
314-842-5082

Rowland, James DO
816-361-4077

Schwent, John DO
314-937-8688

MONTANA

Kurtz, Curt MD
406-587-5561

Seymour, Sylvia ND
406-222-0300

Steele, Charles MD
406-727-4757

NEBRASKA

Donovan, Roy DC
308-327-4703

Miller, Otis MD
308-728-3251

NEVADA

Baker, Richard MD
702-382-2099

Gerber, Michael MD
702-826-1900

Milne, Robert MD
702-458-5113

NEW HAMPSHIRE

Moore, Michael MD
603-357-2180

NEW JERSEY

Ali, Majid MD
201-586-4111

Braverman, Eric MD
609-921-1842

Harris, Charles MD
908-506-9200

Magaziner, Alan DO
609-424-8222

NEW MEXICO

Cohen, Harold MD
505-898-7115

Collins, Joseph DO
505-434-4699

Klinghard, D MD
505-988-3086

NEW YORK

Ash, Richard MD
212-628-3113

Beasley, Joseph MD
516-789-7031

Chao, I-Tsu MD
718-998-3331

Cooper, Jack MD
914-279-9300

Cutler, Paul MD
716-284-5140

Feldman, Martin MD
212-744-4413

Schachter, Michael MD
914-358-6800

NORTH CAROLINA

Power, Bhaskar MD
919-535-1411

Roberson, Logan MD
704-235-8312

Wilson, John Jr. MD
704-252-9833

NORTH DAKOTA

Byron, Eugene MD
701-780-6000

Each, Galen MD
701-234-3610

Leigh, Richards MD
701-775-5527

OHIO

Bahr, Richard MD
513-299-8788

Baron, John DO
216-642-0082

Cole, Ted DO
513-779-0300

Datt, Stuart MD
216-261-3040

Nelson, Donald MD
216-836-3016

OKLAHOMA

Davis, John MD
405-843-6619

Dushay, Donald DO
918-744-0228

Gilbert, Gerald MD
405-789-9500

OREGON

Green, III, John MD
503-678-2233

Kalb, John DC
503-482-0625

Peabody, Judy ND
503-324-1616

PENNSYLVANIA

Ellis, Leander MD
215-477-6444

Ferro, Anthony Jr. DC
215-388-2212

Krause, Helen MD
412-366-1661

Wenger, Normen MD
717-222-9595

RHODE ISLAND

Puerini, Albert MD
401-943-6910

Radio, Mary MD
401-353-5888

SOUTH CAROLINA

Cassone, Rocco MD
803-536-5511

Harris, Anthony MD
803-648-7897

Hutton, Martine MD
803-795-8135

TENNESSEE

Bryan, Calvin MD
615-821-1177

Furr, Fred MD
615-693-1502

Neely, William
615-929-WELL

Wanderman, Richard MD
901-683-2777

TEXAS

Archer, Jim DO
210-697-8445

Hazelwood, Robert MD
512-479-0101

Jaekle, Richard MD
214-696-0964

Parker, Gerald DO
806-355-8263

Rush, Charles Jr. MD
817-280-0505

UTAH

Harbrecht, David MD
801-292-8303

Harper, Dennis DO
801-288-8881

Payne, Robert MD
801-269-8817

VERMONT

Anderson, Charles MD
802-879-6544

Lee, Alan MD
802-524-1062

VIRGINIA

Kneer, Robert MD
703-938-2244

Neal, Roger MD
703-628-9547

Wetcher, Stewart MD
804-874-8696

WASHINGTON

Buscher, David MD
206-453-0288

Golan, Ralph MD
206-324-0593

Huntoon, Jennifer DC
206-632-8804

WEST VIRGINIA

Corro, Prudencio MD
304-252-0775

Jellen, Albert MD
304-242-5151

Kostenko, Michael DO
304-253-0591

WISCONSIN

Galvez, T MD
608-238-3831

Kadile, Eleazar MD
414-468-9442

Kroker, George MD
608-782-2027

WYOMING

Smith, Gerald MD
307-632-5589

Enzyme Therapy

Dr. Lita Lee
2852 Williamette Street, Suite 397
Eugene, OR 97405
503-746-7621

Exercise and Fitness Consultants

CALIFORNIA

Levy, Michael
818-783-0097

MARYLAND

Ratzin, Rosemary PA
301-689-1794

NEW YORK

Andre, Turan MT
212-874-6738

OHIO

Draper, Tom
216-238-7411

OREGON

Germain, Kathleen
503-635-6643

WISCONSIN

Faber, William DO
414-464-7680

WASHINGTON

Kennedy, David
206-454-6688

Feldenkrais Method

Feldenkrais Guild
P.O. Box 489
Albany, OR 97321
503-926-0981

Flower Remedies Practitioners

CALIFORNIA

Davis, Deborah
805-969-1992

Moore, Tim
209-229-8202

CONNECTICUT

Cunningham, Paul
203-454-4485

HAWAII

Carson, Jacqueline
808-934-3233

ILLINOIS

Kramer Golden, Anda
312-296-6700

KENTUCKY

Broeingmeyer, Mary DC
800-626-3389

MINNESOTA

Gallagher, Robert
612-824-3157

NEW JERSEY

Osten, Irene
908-382-1245

OHIO

Westendorf, Wm DDS
513-923-3839

OREGON

Dev, Perm ND
503-266-3888

PENNSYLVANIA

Stewart, Roger
412-322-1945

TEXAS

Stoup, Glenda ND
214-480-9355

WASHINGTON

Hammer, Lynda ND
509-548-7090

Jongaard, Robert ND
206-321-6470

Kitamoto, Frank DDS
206-842-4772

Guided Imagery

The Academy for Guided Imagery
P.O. Box 2070
Mill Valley, California 94942
800-726-2070

Hellerwork

The Body of Knowledge /
Hellerwork
406 Berry Street
Mt. Shasta, CA 96067
800-392-3900

Herbalists

ALABAMA

The Healthy Way
205-967-4372

ARIZONA

Ber, Abram MD
602-279-3795

Deloe, Oaul NMD
602-886-9988

Heron, Silena ND
520-282-6909

ARKANSAS

Taliaferro, Melissa
501-447-2599

CALIFORNIA

Broadwell, Robert
714-965-9266

Gentile, Teresa PhD
818-707-3126

Hirsh, Roger OMD
310-319-9478

Zhao, William MD
707-445-2290

COLORADO

Adele, Ruth
719-636-0098

Goodrich, Mary
303-927-9617

Lange, Andrew ND
303-443-8678

CONNECTICUT

Kallenborn, Gabrielle
203-454-5989

Klass, Jeffrey
203-481-5219

Schweitzer, Marvin
203-853-6285

FLORIDA

D'Costa, Harriet MD
813-584-7246

Lam, Nghiem
904-357-8351

Willix, Robert Jr. MD
407-362-0724

ILLINOIS

Bhavnani, Lata Herbal Est
312-296-6700

Mauer, William DO
708-255-8988

INDIANA

Jacques, Frank
317-856-5211

Marton, Joy
812-425-5811

LOUISIANA

Dupois, Sidney PhD
318-394-3350

Fingerman, Eileen MD
317-856-5211

MARYLAND

Beech, Douglas DC
301-469-6700

Porks, Ronald MD
410-486-5656

MASSACHUSETTS

Barton, Shivanatha
617-277-4150

Silbert, Barbara
508-465-0929

Umphress, Cartherine
508-371-1228

MICHIGAN

Bayha, Carl DS
616-668-4730

MINNESOTA

Gallagher, Robert
612-824-3157

Lucking, Andrew ND
612-924-8112

Stowell, Thomas ND
612-644-4436

MISSOURI

Kanion, Dorothy
816-779-4844

MONTANA

Lane, Sarah ND
406-726-3000

NEVADA

Schwartzman, Lynn ND
702-435-7501

NEW JERSEY

Kadar, Peter OMD
201-984-2800

Mintz, Charles MD
609-825-7372

NEW YORK

Alyn, Barbara ND
516-421-4807

Chin, Richard OMD
212-686-9227

NORTH DAKOTA

Briggs, Brian MD
701-838-6011

OKLAHOMA

Frye, Bruce DC
918-250-1072

OREGON

Collins, John G
503-667-1961

Dev, Prem ND
503-266-3888

Stargrove, Mitchell
503-526-0397

PENNSYLVANIA

Frank, Cara
215-438-2977

Mantell, Donald MD
412-776-5610

Stewart, Roger DC
412-322-1945

TEXAS

Manso, Gilbert MD
713-840-9355

Stoup, Glenda ND
214-480-9355

UTAH

Jamison, K Brent
801-467-3007

Nunn, William ND
801-265-0077

School of Natural Healing
800-372-8255

WASHINGTON

Brown, Donald
206-623-2520

Clapp, Debra
206-299-9038

Hole, Linda Chiu MD
509-747-2902

WEST VIRGINIA

Jellen, Albert MD
304-581-5151

Holistic Practitioners and Holistic Nurses

American Holistic Medical Association
and American Holistic Nurses Association
4101 Lake Boone Trail, Suite 201
Raleigh, NC 27607
800-878-3373

Luanne Pennesi, RN, MS
516-921-8475

Homeopathy

ALABAMA

Joan Scott Lowe, RN CCH MPH
2038 22nd Court South
Birmingham, AL 35223
205-871-1288

ARIZONA

Pat Bradley, DVM
65 Sunny Gap Road
Conway, AR 72032
501-329-7727

Joy R Dunn, DVM
1123 Ash
Conway, AR 72032
501-327-4729

Eugenie V Anderson, MD MD(H) FACOG
3411 North Fifth Avenue, Suite 207
Phoenix, AZ 85013
602-264-7630 Fax: 602-264-5803

Stephen S Baer, DDS FAGD FICC-MO
105 Roadrunner Drive, Building 2
Sedona, AZ 86336
520-282-2482 Fax: 520-282-9756

Abram Ber, MD MD(H)
5011 North Granite Reef
Scottsdale, AZ 85250
602-941-2141 Fax: 602-941-4114

Jeffrey H Feingold, NMD
5743 East Thomas Road, Suite 1
Scottsdale, AZ 85251
602-945-8773

Lila Flagler, NMD DHANP CCH
6737 East Camino Principal, Suite C
Tucson, AZ 85715
520-721-8821

Samuel Flagler, NMD DHANP CCH
6737 East Camino Principal, Suite C
Tucson, AZ 85715
520-721-8821

Ed Gogek, MD MD(H)
1118 East Missouri Avenue, Suite A1
Phoenix, AZ 85014
602-404-9057

Louise D Gutowski, NMD
13430 North Scottsdale Road
Suite 102
Scottsdale, AZ 85254
602-443-1600 Fax: 602-483-1203

Cheryl A Harter, MD MD(H)
80 Raintree Road
Sedona, AZ 86351
520-284-9777

Deborah M Heath, DO
5055 North 32nd Street, Suite 200
Phoenix, AZ 85018
602-508-6850 Fax: 602-508-6808

John R Keifer, DC DNBHE FIACA
4431 North Swan
Tucson, AZ 85718
520-577-1717 Fax: 520-577-7766

Paul A Mittman, ND DHANP
Southwest Naturopathic Medical
Center
8010 East McDowell Road
Scottsdale, AZ 85257
602-858-9100 Fax: 602-858-9116

Todd A Rowe, MD(H) DHt CCH
Practitioner's Home Page
5501 North 19th Avenue, Suite 425
Phoenix, AZ 85015
602-864-1776 Fax: 602-864-2949

Bruce H Shelton, MD MD(H)
2525 West Greenway Road
Phoenix, AZ 85023
602-993-1200 Fax: 602-942-3787

Ilene M Spector, DO MD(H)
2802 North Alvernon Way, Suite 200
Tucson, AZ 85712
520-322-6331 Fax: 520-326-2737

Marnie Vail, MD MD(H)
210 North Park Street, Suite 2
Flagstaff, AZ 86001
520-774-6590 Fax: 520-774-6629

Robert J Zieve, MD MD(H)
536 South Marina Street
Prescott, AZ 86303
520-771-2979 Fax: 520-771-1919

CALIFORNIA

David J Anderson, MD DHt
339 Spruce Street, Suite A
San Francisco, CA 94118
415-831-1862 Fax: 415-472-4334

Eliott S Blackman, DO
1956 Union Street
San Francisco, CA 94123
415-921-1446 Fax: 415-929-1299

Howardine Woodall Boehm, RN
Box 1886
Loma Linda, CA 92354
909-799-9647

Sue Boyle, RN
2342 Almond Avenue
Concord, CA 94520
510-602-0582

Stephanie A Chalmers, DVM
DACVD
4918A Sonoma Highway
Santa Rosa, CA 95409
707-538-4643

Peggy S Chipkin, RN FNP CCH
158 East Blithdale Avenue, Suite F
Mill Valley, CA 94941
510-389-8589

Christine C Ciavarella, PA-C
Hahnemann Medical Clinic
828 San Pablo Avenue
Albany, CA 94706
510-524-3117 Fax: 510-524-2447

Karen B Cohen, DC CCH
1709 Seabright Avenue
Santa Cruz, CA 95060
408-425-1422 Fax: 408-425-1444

Marsha Cummings, PA-C CCH
Hahnemann Medical Clinic
828 San Pablo Avenue
Albany, CA 94706
510-524-3117 Fax: 510-524-2447

Keith R DeOrio, MD
1821 Wilshire Boulevard, Suite 100
Santa Monica, CA 90403
310-828-3096 Fax: 310-453-1918

Timothy R Dooley, MD
4095 Jackdaw Street
San Diego, CA 92103
619-297-8641

Tisha Douthwaite, LAc
206 North Pine Street
Ukiah, CA 95482
707-467-0335

Miriam Edelweiss, RN NP
45 San Clemente, B-230
Corte Madera, CA 94925
415-927-9660 Fax: 415-331-7170

Salar Farahmand, CA
16661 Ventura Boulevard, Suite 403
Encino, CA 91436
818-501-2000 Fax: 818-501-3021

Lauren S Feder, MD
415 North Crescent Drive, Suite 100
Beverly Hills, CA 90210
310-247-1531

Oscar Fernandez, FNP
1640 West Mineral King Avenue
Suite 100
Visalia, CA 93291
209-733-5710

Katy Festinger, RN FNP
P.O. Box 93
Caspar, CA 95420
707-964-8114

David R Field, ND LAc
46 Doctors Park
Santa Rosa, CA 95405
707-576-7388 Fax: 707-545-6947

Edwin Carlyle Floyd, DC DNBHE
DACBN
6955 La Tijera Boulevard, Suite C
Los Angeles, CA 90045
310-417-3824 Fax: 310-645-1814

Christopher J Gibney, LAc
185 North Redwood Drive, Suite 220
San Rafael, CA 94903
415-499-3319 Fax: 415-499-8629
Email: atmagroup@aol.com

Bill Gray, MD
413 F Street
Davis, CA 95616
916-756-0567

Asa Hershoff, DC ND
2444 Wilshire Boulevard, Suite 305
Santa Monica, CA 90403
310-829-7122

Richard E Hiltner, MD DHt
169 East El Roblar
Ojai, CA 93023
805-646-1495 Fax: 805-646-8159

Ron Hood, MD
101 Westcoast Road
Redway, CA 95560
707-923-2783 Fax: 707-923-2543

Betty J Idarius, LM
206 North Pine Street
Ukiah, CA 95482
707-463-3739 Fax: 707-468-0205
Email: bidarius@zapcom.net

Ifeoma Ikenze, MD
1030 Sir Francis Drake
Kentfield, CA 94904
415-258-9600 Fax: 415-258-9691

Jessica L Jackson, LAc
810 Healdsburg Avenue
Healdsburg, CA 95448
707-433-7714 Fax: 707-433-4427

Richard Jenkins, MD
1956 Union Street
San Francisco, CA 94123
415-921-1446 Fax: 415-921-0215

Linda C Johnston, MD DHt
7549 Louise Avenue
Van Nuys, CA 91406
818-776-8040 Fax: 818-776-0082

Dianne Jurgensen, DC
16575 Los Gatos-Almaden Road
Los Gatos, CA 95032
408-358-2434 Fax: 408-358-1365

Frances E Kalfus, LAc
1911 Vine Street
Berkeley, CA 94709
510-558-1911

Sandra N Kamiak, MD
(see Saratoga, CA)
San Jose, CA
408-741-1332 Fax: 408-741-5791

Hollis H King, DO PhD
5445 Oberlin Drive, Suite 100
LaJolla, CA 92121
619-587-1822 Fax: 619-587-8967

Mark H LaBeau, DO
3232 Duke Street
San Diego, CA 92110
619-224-3515 Fax: 619-224-6253

Eliza Ladyzhensky, MD
760 South Washburn Street, Suite 21
Corona, CA 91720
909-736-8185 Fax: 909-736-8187

Leslie A Lauterbach, DC DNBHE
7917 Emerson Avenue
Westchester, CA 90045
310-215-9061

Jeff D Lester, DO
135 Monte Vista
Watsonville, CA 95076
408-724-1164 Fax: 408-724-1252

Carol Lourie, LAc
724 Gilman Street
Berkeley, CA 94710
510-526-2028

Don E Lundholm, DVM CVA
10130 Adams Avenue
Huntington Beach, CA 92646
714-964-1605 Fax: 714-965-0765

Dianne G Malik, LAc CCH
12145 Alta Carmel Court, Suite 220
San Diego, CA 92128
619-673-0318

William G Mann, LAc
3202 3rd Avenue
San Diego, CA 92103
619-260-1256

Gregory R Manteuffel, MD
2645 Ocean Avenue, Suite 209
San Francisco, CA 94132
415-841-1040

Randy W Martin, LAc PhD
17000 Ventura Boulevard
Encino, CA 91316
818-905-6171

Roger N Morrison, MD
80 Nicholl Avenue
Port Richmond, CA 94801
510-412-9040

Pamela S Nathan, LAc
P.O. Box 927747
San Diego, CA 92192
619-452-2280 Fax: 619-452-1113

Allen C Neiswander, MD DHt
1508 South Garfield Avenue
Alhambra, CA 91801
818-284-6565

Marcia L Neiswander, RN MNNP
Whitting Professional Center
554 East Foothill, Suite 120
San Dimas, CA 91773
818-801-4972

Maud H Nerman, DO CSPOMM
204 Clement Street
San Francisco, CA 94118
415-460-6310 Fax: 415-455-0937

Randall Neustaedter, OMD LAc
CCH
1779 Woodside Road, Suite 201C
Redwood City, CA 94061
415-299-9170 Fax: 415-299-9173

Laura L Paris, OMD LAc
1502 Montana Avenue, Suite 202
Santa Monica, CA 90403
310-453-0286

Richard P Plant, DC DNBHE CCH
1571 San Elijo Avenue
San Diego, CA 92007
619-942-8610 Fax: 619-634-2750

A J Rice, MD PhD
41651 Sierra Drive
Three Rivers, CA 93271
209-561-4683

Donald S Rich, MD
706 Western Drive
Santa Cruz, CA 95060
408-423-2078

David R Riley, OMD LAc CCH
4711 Fourth Street
San Diego/La Mesa, CA 91941
619-462-7890 Fax: 619-697-9389
Email: rdavid@igc.apc.org

Robert C Rosett, MD
739 Bellarmine Drive
Salinas, CA 93901
408-751-3505

Richard M Schiller, DPM
620 East Washington, Suite 201
Petaluma, CA 94952
707-766-8785

Joseph Sciabbarrasi, MD
1502 Wilshire Blvd., Suite 306
Santa Monica, CA 90403
310-395-2453 Fax: 310-899-0356

Jonathan D Shore, MD DHt
322½ Miller Avenue
Mill Valley, CA 94941
415-389-1837 Fax: 415-383-3464

Sidney Elizabeth Skinner, MSN RN-C FNP
Practitioner's Home Page
284 Noe Street
San Francisco, CA 94117
510-915-9855

David L Stephenson, DDS LAc
Practitioner's Home Page
216 West Cypress Street
Anaheim, CA 92805
714-776-7020 Fax: 714-776-0466

Steven I Subotnick, DPM DC CCH
Family Health Center
15051 Hesperian Boulevard
San Leandro, CA 94578
510-278-9990 Fax: 510-278-6600

Harry F Swope, ND DHANP CCH
P.O. Box 12180
La Crescenta, CA 91224
818-541-9172

Tomes Theodorelos, LicAc
2018 Dale Street
San Diego, CA 92104
619-231-9363

Matthew J Vuksinich, MD
Hahnemann Medical Clinic
828 San Pablo Avenue
Albany, CA 94706
510-524-3117 Fax: 510-524-2447

Meris S Walton, DC
621 Water Street
Santa Cruz, CA 95060
408-469-9500 Fax: 408-469-3044

Corey W Weinstein, MD
1199 Sanchez Street
San Francisco, CA 94114
415-824-4124
Email: coreman@igc.apc.org

Patricia E Wolff, DC MFCC
6 Delfino Place P.O. Box 938
Carmel Valley, CA 93924
408-659-5180

COLORADO

Bonnie Alexandra, DOM LAc
1800 30th Street, Suite 201
Boulder, CO 80301
303-939-8322 Fax: 303-415-0590

Robert D Fitts, DC
145 East 13th Street
Durango, CO 81301
970-259-6854 Fax: 970-247-4535

Mary Frazel, ND
104 East Saint Vrain, Suite 10
Colorado Springs, CO 80903
719-635-2050 Fax: 719-635-2625

Dennis H Kay, MD ABO
6053 South Quebec, Suite 202
Englewood, CO 80111
303-290-9401

Arlene M Kellman, DO
2150 Pearl Street
Boulder, CO 80302
303-444-8337 Fax: 303-444-8393

Kenneth H Koenig, DC DNBHE
FIACA
380 East Lionshead Circle
Vail, CO 81657
970-476-1831 Fax: 970-476-1902

Andrew Lange, ND DHANP
3011 Broadway, Suite 14
Boulder, CO 80304
303-443-8678

John S O'Hearne, MD
728 A Front Street
Louisville, CO 80027
303-666-0733 Fax: 303-666-0735

Teresa J Salvadore, DC DNBHE
730 East Cooper
Aspen, CO 81611
970-920-1247

Jody K Shevins, ND DHANP CCH
5353 Manhattan Circle, Suite 102
Boulder, CO 80303
303-494-3713

CONNECTICUT

Ahmed N Currim, MD PhD
148 East Avenue
Norwalk, CT 06851
203-853-1339

Marcie R Fallek, DVM
248 Alden Street
Fairfield, CT 06430
203-254-8642

Howard G Fine, ND DHANP CCH
4 Cross Highway
Westport, CT 06880
203-221-0216

Pearlyn Goodman-Herrick, ND
DHANP
21 Trails End Road
Weston, CT 06883
203-227-5534 Fax: 203-227-2565

Ronald A Grant, MD
Psychotherapy Only
P.O. Box 1174
Weston/Greenwich, CT 06883
203-227-2402

Paul Herscu, ND DHANP
115 Elm Street, Suite 210
Enfield, CT 06082
860-763-1225 Fax: 860-253-5041

Nancy A Mazur, ND
P.O. Box 1644
Avon, CT 06001
860-675-1011

Harold M Ofgang, ND
57 North Street, Suite 323
Danbury, CT 06810
203-730-CURE Fax: 203-746-3310

Amy B Rothenberg, ND DHANP
115 Elm Street, Suite 210
Enfield, CT 06082
860-763-1225 Fax: 860-253-5041

Charles N Shapiro, RN FNP
48 Knollwood Ave
Stamford, CT 06905
203-461-9102

William E Shevin, MD DHt
370 Riverside Drive
North Grosvenordale, CT 06255
860-928-4040 Fax: 860-923-3055

DISTRICT OF COLUMBIA

S Nathan Berger, DDS
800 Fourth Street SW
Washington, DC 20024
202-554-7811 Fax: 202-554-1666

Margaret E Easter, RN/NP RN-C
MSN
4000 Albemarle Street NW
Suite 202
Washington, DC 20016
202-537-5911

Peter A Martin, ND
2025 "Eye" Street NW, Suite 725
Washington, DC 20006
202-861-0822

Ioana A Razi, MD
3537 R Street NW
Washington, DC 20007
202-333-1774

Andrea D Sullivan, ND DHANP
PhD
4601 Connecticut Avenue NW
Suite 6
Washington, DC 20008
202-244-4545

DELAWARE

David C Ehrenfeld, DDS
710 Greenbank Road
Wilmington, DE 19808
302-994-2582 Fax: 302-994-5151

Shelley R Epstein, VMD
Wilmington Animal Hospital
828 Philadelphia Pike
Wilmington, DE 19809
302-762-2694 Fax: 302-762-1620

Robert H Hall, MD
1509 Gilpin Avenue
Wilmington, DE 19806
302-656-5123

Karen S Phillips, VMD
Wilmington Animal Hospital 828
Philadelphia Pike
Wilmington, DE 19809
302-762-2694 Fax: 302-762-1620

Mitchel E Shapiro, PA-C
1008 Milltown Road
Wilmington, DE 19808
302-994-0565 Fax: 610-566-7691

FLORIDA

Kimberly S Alters, RN DC DNBHE
33 Barkley Circle
Fort Myers, FL 33907
941-939-7645 Fax: 941-939-2644

Teresa M Bernard, MD FACOG
441 Stowe Avenue, Suite 1
Orange Park, FL 32073
904-269-6400

Larry A Bernstein, VMD CVA
751 NE 168th Street
Miami, FL 33162
305-652-5372 Fax: 305-653-7244

William C Blecha, DC DNBHE
692 SE Port Saint Lucie Boulevard
Port Saint Lucie, FL 34984
407-878-1790

Thomas M Bozzuto, DO
1529 Margaret Street
Jacksonville, FL 32204
904-354-0410 Fax: 904-358-6559

Elizabeth V Brinkley, MD
1307 Miccosukee Road, Building A
Tallahassee, FL 32308
904-656-1217 Fax: 904-877-3185

Richard Browne, OMD AP DNBHE
10506 North Kendall Drive
Miami, FL 33176
305-595-9500 Fax: 305-595-2622

Robin L Cannizzaro, DVM CVA
326 49th Avenue North
Saint Petersburg, FL 33703
813-528-0298 Fax: 813-525-7005

Michael A Carrigan, AP DNBHE
20975 Rustlewood Avenue
Boca Raton, FL 33428
561-482-4926

Delores A D'Aprile, LicAc DNBHE
NCCA
T.A.O. Medical Institute
3380 Tamiami Trail, Suite B-1
Port Charlotte, FL 33952
941-764-7500 Fax: 941-743-7577

Martin Dayton, DO MD(H)
18600 Collins Avenue
North Miami Beach, FL 33160
305-931-8484 Fax: 305-936-1849

Joe R Demers, DVM CVA
496 North US 1
Melbourne, FL 32935
407-752-0140 Fax: 407-752-0150

Julia A Eastman, AP
830 Anchor Rode Drive
Naples, FL 34103
941-643-9200 Fax: 941-643-3460

S Cornelia Franz, MD DNBHE
2875 South Orange Avenue
Suite 540
Orlando, FL 32806
407-422-2273 Fax: 407-422-2199

John A Frey, DC DNBHE
2774 First Street
Fort Myers, FL 33916
888-467-2232 toll

Harvey J Grossbard, OMD AP
19022 NE 29th Avenue
Aventura, FL 33180
305-937-2281 Fax: 305-937-2387

Ludwika Harrison, MD OMD
DNBHE
1325 Lenox Avenue
Miami Beach, FL 33139
305-672-6339

Rennie J Harrison, OMD CA
DNBHE
1325 Lenox Avenue
Miami Beach, FL 33139
305-672-6339

Gregory H Heigh, AP DNBHE PhD
11012 North Dale Mabry Highway
Suite 304
Tampa, FL 33618
813-960-0026 Fax: 813-968-6885

Travis L Herring, MD MD(H)
106 West Fern Drive
Orange City, FL 32763
904-775-0525 Fax: 904-775-3911

Jan Elkjaer Jensen, DC
1211 Miccosukee Road
Tallahassee, FL 32308
904-222-2952 Fax: 904-877-0845

Roger L Johansen, DC
800 East Bay Drive, Suite P
Largo, FL 33770
813-581-2774 Fax: 813-581-3199

Rebecca Ann Jones, DC LNC
DNBHE
2921 West Michigan Avenue
Pensacola, FL 32506
850-944-7665

Robert R Karman, OMD AP LAc
16991 NE 20th Avenue
North Miami Beach, FL 33162
800-753-9792

Martin P Keane, AP CCH
1432 9th Street North
Saint Petersburg, FL 33704
813-821-7771 Fax: 813-821-6914

Celestino Lopez, OMD AP DNBHE
1490 West 49th Place, Suite 298
Hialeah, FL 33012
305-558-2744 Fax: 305-558-1499

Luisa N Mosquera, AP DNBHE
940 Lincoln Road, Suite 313
Miami Beach, FL 33139
305-535-6178 Fax: 305-604-8596

Philip K Parsons, DDS
445 South Lawrence Boulevard
P.O. Box 266
Keystone Heights, FL 32656
352-473-4595

Danny Quaranto, CA AP DNBHE
2706 20th Street
Vero Beach, FL 32960
561-778-8877 Fax: 561-778-9509

Marcia C Sasso, DC DNBHE
5663 Coral Gate Boulevard
Coral Springs, FL 33063
954-974-3456 Fax: 954-420-0669

Simone R Speyer, DAc(RI) PT
DNBHE
4835 Hollywood Boulevard, Suite 4
Hollywood, FL 33021
954-986-8500 Fax: 954-986-8900

Russell Swift, DVM
7154 North University Drive
Suite 720
Tamarac, FL 33321
954-720-0794 Fax: 954-720-0978

Mary Lee Tupling, AP
Broward Natural Medicine
1012 East Broward Boulevard
Fort Lauderdale, FL 33301
954-760-4449 Fax: 954-463-0551

Arthur Young, DVM
3003 South Federal Highway
Stuart, FL 34994
561-286-6569 Fax: 561-287-0098

GEORGIA

Milton Fried, MD
4426 Tilly Mill Road
Atlanta, GA 30360
770-451-4857 Fax: 770-451-8492

Edward S Garbacz, MD
3082 Shadowlane Avenue
Atlanta, GA 30305
404-848-0033 Fax: 404-848-0438

Tere Haas, LAc
3730 Dumbarton Road NW
Atlanta, GA 30327
404-364-0640 Fax: 404-231-1968

Alice Christine Merritt, RPh
DNBHE
1730 Dixie Highway
Madison, GA 30650
706-342-0943

HAWAII

Michael L Traub, ND DHANP
75-5759 Kuakini Highway, Suite 202
Kailua Kona, HI 96740
808-329-2114

IDAHO

Brent B Mathieu, ND DHANP
1412 West Washington
Boise, ID 83702
208-338-5590

Todd A Schlapfer, ND
1000 West Hubbard, Suite 120
Coeur D'Alene, ID 83814
208-664-1644 Fax: 208-667-5568

ILLINOIS

Toni L Bark, MD
650 Vernon Avenue
Glencoe, IL 60022
847-835-6207

Francine P Burke, DC
202 West Willow, Suite 101
Wheaton, IL 60148
630-510-1102 Fax: 630-691-8651

Daniel R Dieska, DDS
17726-A Oak Park Avenue
Tinley Park, IL 60477
708-429-4700 Fax: 708-532-5090

Timothy W Fior, MD DHt ABFP
400 East 22nd Street, Suite F
Lombard, IL 60148
630-792-9311

Jerry P Gore, MD
Center for Holistic Medicine
240 Saunders Road
Riverwoods, IL 60015
847-236-1701 Fax: 847-236-1705

Lester H Holze, Jr., DC
2000 Larkin Avenue, Suite 200
Elgin, IL 60123
847-888-4770

Clifford L Kearns, DC DNBHE
2223 West Schaumburg Road
Schaumburg, IL 60194
847-301-8585 Fax: 847-301-8582

Ming-Te Lin, MD AAP ABAI
3235 Vollmer Road, Suite 142
Flossmoor, IL 60422
708-957-7937 Fax: 708-957-7975

Anita B Pride, DC
2003 Round Barn Road
Champaign, IL 61821
217-352-9108 Fax: 217-352-9105

John A Rothchild, DDS
1585 North Barrington Road
Suite 106
Hoffman Estates, IL 60194
847-884-1220 Fax: 847-884-1638

Dane J Shepherd, DO
55 East Washington, Suite 1630
Chicago, IL 60602
312-782-9153 Fax: 312-782-9306

Joel R Shepperd, MD
Center for Integral Health
400 East 22nd Street, Suite F
Lombard, IL 60148
630-792-9311

Phillip P Sukel, DDS
1640 North Arlington Heights Road,
Suite 201
Arlington Heights, IL 60004
847-253-0240 Fax: 847-253-0305

Prabha V Vaidya, MD MPH
Center for Holistic Medicine
240 Saunders Road
Riverwoods, IL 60015
847-236-1701 Fax: 847-236-1705

Claudia M Weddaburne-Bossie, MD
Center for Integral Health 400 East
22nd Street, Suite F
Lombard, IL 60148
630-792-9311

Raul A Zavaleta, DC
A Center for Whole Care 202 West
Willow Street, Suite 101-C
Wheaton, IL 60187
630-510-1153 Eng

INDIANA

Carolyn S Blakey, DVM
1831 West Main Street
Richmond, IN 47374
765-966-0015 Fax: 765-935-9043

Robert R Canida, DDS
904 East First Street
Madison, IN 47250
812-265-2083 Fax: 812-265-2177

Mark N Goren, MD
822 West First Street
Bloomington, IN 47403
812-332-5040 Fax: 812-332-1219

Lee A Harris, MD FACOG
3217 Lake Avenue
Fort Wayne, IN 46805
219-424-6919 Fax: 219-424-0747

KANSAS

Sara J Jernigan, DC
The Next Generation Wellness
Center 545 North Woodlawn
Witchita, KS 67208
316-686-5900 Fax: 316-686-0417

KENTUCKY

Victoria R Snelling, DC
6002 Brownsboro Park Boulevard
Louisville, KY 40207
502-899-9950

LOUISIANA

Adriana B Sagrera, DVM
802 Octavia Street
New Orleans, LA 70115
504-899-9510

MASSACHUSETTS

Elisa Adams, DC
10 Muzzey Street
Lexington, MA 02173
617-674-2500

Nancy A Bronstein, DC DNBHE
15 Mahaiwe Street
Great Barrington, MA 01230
413-528-2948 Fax: 413-528-5404

Edward H Chapman, MD DHt
FAAFP
91 Cornell Street
Newton Lower Falls MA 02162
617-244-8780 Fax: 617-244-6850

Savitri Clarke, LicAc CCH
97 Lowell Road
Concord, MA 01742
508-369-3604 Fax: 508-287-4536

Stephen M Driscoll, DC
2956 Falmouth Road
Osterville, MA 02655
508-420-1160 Fax: 508-420-3245

Lauren B Fox, RN/NP
426 Boxberry Hill Road
East Falmouth, MA 02536
508-563-1115

Samuel Gladstone, MD
12 Dickinson Street
Amherst, MA 01002
413-253-2300 Fax: 413-256-0464

Steven P Goldsmith, MD
153 Prichard Street
Fitchburg, MA 01420
508-342-1796

Kathleen L Grandison, MD DHt
West County Physicians
25 Heath Stage Road
Shelburne Falls, MA 01370
413-625-9717

Lisa A Harvey, MD
11 Swift River Road
Cummington, MA 01026
413-634-5626

Leonard M Horowitz, MD
7 Federal Street
Danvers, MA 01923
508-777-8553

Stephen H Howard, LicAc
150 Harvard Road
Stow, MA 01775
508-897-5979

Kacenka L Hruby, MD
23 Nutting Avenue
Northampton, MA 01060
413-586-2137

Cynthia McMahon King, LicAc RPh
25 Stow Road
Boxboro, MA 01719
978-263-4026

Dorsie R Kovacs, DVM
Monson Small Animal Clinic
125 Palmer Road
Monson, MA 01057
413-267-5141

Janet L Levatin, MD
1101 Beacon Street, Suite 5E
Brookline, MA 02146
617-738-4600

Jeffrey Levy, DVM
71 Ashfield Road
Williamsburg, MA 01096
413-268-3000 Fax: 413-268-0333

Christine F Luthra, MD CCH
54 Rockview Street
Jamaica Plain, MA 02130
617-524-3892

Jeffrey A Migdow, MD
P.O. Box 2372
Lenox, MA 01240
413-448-3446 Fax: 413-448-3384

Richard Moskowitz, MD DHt CCH
173 Mount Auburn Street
Watertown, MA 02172
617-923-4604

Patricia E Murphy, RNCS MSN
221 Washington Street
Gloucester, MA 01930
508-281-5225

Keith W L Rafal, MD
326 Union Street, Suite 2
Franklin, MA 02038
508-553-9922

Larry L Raffel, RN
219 Massachusetts Avenue, Suite O
Arlington, MA 02174
617-484-2544

Barbara S Silbert, DC ND
172 State Street, Suite 1
Newburyport, MA 01950
978-465-0929

Richard J Weintraub, MD
1400 Centre Street, Suite 105
Newton, MA 02159
617-630-8100

Sarah French Williams, DC
97 Lowell Road
Concord, MA 01742
978-369-3604 Fax: 978-287-4536

Betty Wood, MD
24 Minot Avenue
Acton, MA 01720
508-635-0605

MARYLAND

Anthony M Aurigemma, MD
4401 East-West Highway, Suite 202
Bethesda, MD 20814
301-654-7537

Premala E Brewster-Wilson, PhD
LN CCH
7606 23rd Avenue
Hyattsville, MD 20783
301-422-1188

Ronald K Buttery, RN PhD
Bleach & Associates 2255 Crain
Highway
Waldorf, MD 20602
301-843-4923

Grace L Calabrese, DVM
P.O. Box 245
Phoenix, MD 21131
410-557-6040

Christina B Chambreau, DVM
908 Cold Bottom Road
Sparks, MD 21152
410-771-4968

Harold D Goodman, DO
8609 Second Avenue, Suite 405B
Silver Spring, MD 20910
301-565-2494

Peter Hinderberger, MD
4801 Yellowwood Avenue
Baltimore, MD 21209
410-367-6263 Fax: 410-367-1961

Monique Maniet, DVM
4820 Moorland Lane
Bethesda, MD 20814
301-656-2882 Fax: 301-656-5033

Willow T M Moore, DC ND
10806 Reisterstown Road, Suite 1E
Owingmills, MD 21117
410-356-4600

Francine K Rattner, VMD
85 West Central Avenue
Edgewater, MD 21037
410-956-2932 Fax: 410-956-3755

Nader E Soliman, MD DAAPM
9707 Medical Center Drive
Suite 200
Rockville, MD 20850
301-251-2335 Fax: 301-972-4671

Carvel G Tiekert, DVM
2214 Old Emmorton Road
Bel Air, MD 21015
410-569-7777 Fax: 410-569-2346

David G Wember, MD DHt
26 Guy Court
Rockville, MD 20850
301-424-4048

MAINE

Mary H File, RN CCH
110 Auburn Street
Portland, ME 04103
207-878-8333 Fax: 207-878-0152

Dayton F Haigney, MD
21 Liberty Street
South Berwick, ME 03908
207-384-2828

Judith K Herman, DVM
95 Northern Avenue
Augusta, ME 04330
207-623-1177 Fax: 207-623-5227

Devra M Krassner, ND
On Balance 4 Milk Street
Portland, ME 04101
207-773-2517

Jerr Roberts, DDS
686 Brighton Avenue
Portland, ME 04102
207-773-2882

Dirk B Vandersloot, MD
17 Masonic Street
Rockland, ME 04841
207-596-0991

MICHIGAN

Kathleen Anzicek, DO
12337 East Michigan Avenue
Grass Lake, MI 49240
517-522-8403 Fax: 517-522-4275

Dennis G Charnesky, DDS
4101 John R Road, Suite 100
Troy, MI 48098
248-680-0775 Fax: 248-680-1108

Dennis K Chernin, MD MPH
2345 South Huron Parkway
Ann Arbor, MI 48104
313-973-3030

Nancy Eos, MD
P.O. Box 417
Lakeland, MI 48143
517-522-8403 Fax: 517-522-4275

Robert N Israel, MD
2282 Springport Road, Suite B
Jackson, MI 49202
517-782-5700

Patricia E Kelly, MD
311 South Fifth Avenue
Ann Arbor, MI 48104
734-995-5982

Gregory Kruszewski, RN CCH
410 South Main Street, Suite 104
Romeo, MI 48065
810-752-7241

E Paul Lockwood, DC DNBHE
PhD
4509 Downing Street, Box 36
Cass City, MI 48726
517-872-2765

James R Neuenschwander, MD
412 Longshore
Ann Arbor, MI 48105
734-995-3200 Fax: 734-995-4254

Margaret Ann Paris, RN FNP
7269 West Grand River Avenue
Brighton, MI 48116
810-229-2312

Ann H Petrou, DC
2330 East Stadium
Ann Arbor, MI 48103
313-971-5683

John M Simon, DVM CVA
410 North Woodward Avenue
Royal Oak, MI 48067
810-545-6630 Fax: 810-545-7979

MINNESOTA

Sharon D Goosmann, DC
200 4th Street SW, Suite 22
Willmar, MN 56201
612-235-9194

Richard J Hruby, DO
3601 Park Center Boulevard
Saint Louis Park, MN 55416
612-920-0844

G William Jones, MD
19644 Cleary Road NW
Anoka, MN 55303
612-753-1377 Fax: 612-753-4746

Jacob I Mirman, MD DHt
5117 France Avenue South
Minneapolis, MN 55410
612-931-9281 Fax: 612-935-5494

MISSOURI

Mary E Hart, RN RN-C
23 North Gore
Webster Groves, MO 63119
314-961-6631 Fax: 314-961-4796

James L Rowland, DO HMD
P.O. Box 1258
3919 SW Linden Lane
Lee's Summit, MO 64082-4544
816-361-4077

Christian Wessling, MD DHt
23 North Gore, Suite 209
Webster Groves, MO 63119
314-961-6631 Fax: 314-961-4796

Rajiv L Yadava, DO
2345 Dougherty Ferry Road
St. Louis, MO 63122
314-984-2712 Fax: 314-966-9202

MONTANA

Donald R Beans, RN LAc PhD
The Medicine Tree
56 Old Highway 93
Saint Ignatius, MT 59865
406-745-3600

John K Harshman, DVM
1201 Pennsylvania Street
Chinook, MT 59523
406-357-2936 Fax: 406-357-3367

Michael H Lang, ND
P.O. Box 1473
Ennis, MT 59729
406-682-5000

Edward J Mullins, OMD CA
3115 Second Avenue North
Billings, MT 59101-2002
406-259-5555

NORTH CAROLINA

Alice A Coblentz, MD
4 Farrwood Avenue
Asheville, NC 28804
704-258-9089

Susan R Delaney, ND
301 West Weaver Street
Carrboro, NC 27510
919-932-6262 Fax: 919-932-7947

Mark J Eisen, MD
900 Airport Road, Suite A
Chapel Hill, NC 27514
919-967-9452 Fax: 919-932-5200

Shara E Eisen-Hecht, DC
910 Constitution Drive, Suite 109
Durham, NC 27705
919-382-2997

Charles E Loops, DVM
38 Waddell Hollow Road
Pittsboro, NC 27312
919-542-0442 Fax: 919-542-0535

James E Schacht, DVM CVA
6400 East Independence Boulevard
Charlotte, NC 28212
704-535-6688 Fax: 704-535-6669

Todd A Smith, DC
3410 Healy Drive
Winston-Salem, NC 27103
910-760-9355

NEBRASKA

Randall S Bradley, ND DHANP
7447 Farnam Street
Omaha, NE 68114
402-391-6714

NEW HAMPSHIRE

Kristy L Fassler, ND DHANP
500 Market Street, Suite 1F
Portsmouth, NH 03801
603-427-6800 Fax: 603-427-2801

Pamela J Herring, ND DHANP
CCH
46 South Main Street
Concord, NH 03301
603-228-0407 Fax: 603-228-3058

George W Tarkleson, DVM
123 Main Street
Colebrook, NH 03576
603-237-8871

NEW JERSEY

Kishan C Agarwal, MD
450 Plainfield Road
Edison, NJ 08820
908-494-9500

Paul Bahder, MD DHt CCH
8 Governors Lane
Princeton, NJ 08540
609-924-3132

Bonnie L Camo, MD
35 Emerald Road
Kendall Park, NJ 08824
732-422-1585 Fax: 732-422-8576

Irene Catania, ND
119 First Street
Hohokus, NJ 07423
201-444-4900

James F Claire, DO
1600 South Burnt Mill Road
Voorhees, NJ 08043
609-627-5600 Fax: 609-627-9007

Kathleen G Daggett, RN FNP MSN
TLC Healthcare
230 North Maple Avenue
Marlton, NJ 08053
609-985-0590

Paul Gilbert, DDS FAGD
123 Dunhams Corner Road
East Brunswick, NJ 08816
732-254-7946 Fax: 732-254-0287

Lynn Krokenberger, RN CCH
952 Route 518
Skillman, NJ 08558
609-924-7337 Fax: 609-924-7828

Gennaro E Locurcio, MD ABFP
DHt
610 Third Avenue
Elizabeth, NJ 07202
908-351-1333 Fax: 908-351-3740

Cathy Ostroff, DC
248 Columbia Turnpike
Florham Park, NJ 07932
201-822-2529 Fax: 201-822-2760

Sidney B Shane, MD
746 Valley Road
Wayne, NJ 07470
201-694-7711

David J Shuch, DDS
11 Route 206, Suite 201
Augusta, NJ 07822
201-579-7400

Pratap C Singhal, MD DHt CCH
431 Washington Avenue
Belleville, NJ 07109
201-759-2241

Howard C Weiss, MD MPH
28 Walnut Street
Madison, NJ 07940
201-301-1770

NEW MEXICO

Lia Bello, RN FNP CCH
HC81 Box 6023
Questa, NM 87556
505-586-1166
Email: liabello@laplaza.org

B Dee Blanco, DVM
P.O. Box 5865
Santa Fe, NM 87502
505-986-3434

Mary Alice Cooper, MD
204 Carlisle NE
Albuquerque, NM 87106
505-266-6522

Lucinda J Dykes, MD FAAP
422 Medico Lane, Suite C
Santa Fe, NM 87505
505-820-6234 Fax: 505-982-1473

Janet Greene, MD
422 Medico Lane, Suite C
Santa Fe, NM 87505
505-982-1910 Fax: 505-982-1473

Raul Griego, MD
P.O. Box 9177
Albuquerque, NM 87119
505-890-5020

Rowan O Jackson, DOM CCH
2311 Calle Brocha
Santa Fe, NM 87505
505-474-5547

Kathryn S Keith, MD
Las Clinicas del Norte, Box 307
Oho Caliente, NM 87530
505-581-4728 Fax: 505-581-4789

Ralph J Luciani, DO MD(H) PhD
2301 San Pedro NE, Suite G
Albuquerque, NM 87110
505-888-5995

David S Riley, MD MD(H)
539 Harkle Road, Suite A
Santa Fe, NM 87505
505-989-9018 Fax: 505-989-3236

Stephen P Weiss, MD DABFP
1472½ South Saint Francis Drive
Santa Fe, NM 87501
505-989-1602 Fax: 505-982-8611

NEVADA

Carol L Barlow, MD HMD MD(H)
2225 East Flamingo Road, Suite 301
Las Vegas, NV 89119
702-731-3117

David A Edwards, MD HMD
MD(H)
6490 South McCarran Boulevard,
Suite C-24
Reno, NV 89509
702-827-1444 Fax: 702-827-2424

Corazon I Ibarra, MD HMD
6490 South McCarran Boulevard,
Suite C-24
Reno, NV 89509
702-827-1444 Fax: 702-827-2424

Terry G Pfau, DO HMD
2810 West Charleston, Suite 55
Las Vegas, NV 89129
702-258-7860

Daniel F Royal, DO HMD
2501 North Green Valley Parkway
Suite D-132
Henderson, NV 89014
702-433-8800 Fax: 702-433-8823

Flemming F Royal, MD HMD
3663 Pecos McLeod
Las Vegas, NV 89121
702-732-1400 Fax: 702-732-9661

NEW YORK

Anthony M Aurigemma, MD
200 Central Park South
New York, NY 10019
212-246-5610

William L Bergman, MD
500 Broadhollow Road
Melville, NY 11747
516-249-0011

Anthony D Capobianco, DO AOB-
SPOMM AOBFP
20 Landing Road
Glen Cove, NY 11542
516-671-5017 Fax: 516-671-5076

John D Capobianco, DO CSPOMM
20 Landing Road
Glen Cove, NY 11542
516-848-7155 Fax: 516-671-5076

Paul J Capobianco, DO
20 Landing Road
Glen Cove, NY 11542
516-671-5017 Fax: 516-671-5076

Ronald W Dushkin, MD
115 West 86th Street
New York, NY 10024
212-873-1616

Rebecca Elmaleh, MD ABFP
103 Fifth Avenue, 4th Floor
New York, NY 10003
212-229-9718

Marcie R Fallek, DVM
451 East 83rd Street, Suite 5B
New York, NY 10028
212-330-7061

Josephine L Favini, MD PhD
2909 Buffalo Road
Rochester, NY 14624
716-426-4434

Michele Bruno Galante, MD
31 Cragmere Road
Suffern, NY 10901
914-369-6900 Fax: 914-369-6911

Martin P Goldman, MD
838 Pelhamdale Avenue, Suite P
New Rochelle, NY 10801
914-632-3333

Lauri J Grossman, DC
58 Marion Drive
New Rochelle, NY 10804
914-235-3838

Kamau B Kokayi, MD NCCA
53 8th Avenue
Brooklyn, NY 11217
718-399-6194 Fax: 718-399-2295

Joel Kreisberg, DC DNBHE
3 Main Street
Chatham, NY 12037
518-392-7975 Fax: 518-392-6456

Levi H Lehv, MD
1 Hilltop Place
Monsey, NY 10952
914-426-5179

Gennaro E Locurcio, MD ABFP
DHt
112 Lexington Avenue
New York, NY 10016
212-696-2680 Fax: 212-696-2694

Larry Malerba, DO
122 Maple Avenue P.O. Box 588A
Altamont, NY 12009
518-861-5856 Fax: 518-861-5901

Mitchel H Mernick, MD
15 Park Avenue
New York, NY 10010
212-686-0901 Fax: 212-686-0950

Patricia A Muehsam, MD
2 East 75th Street
New York, NY 10021
212-946-5700 Fax: 212-861-1155

Roseanne Nenninger, ND
Dogwood Professional Center
Route 25A
Wading River, NY 11792
516-929-7320 Fax: 516-929-3998

Steve Nenninger, ND
109 Randall Avenue
Port Jefferson, NY 11777
516-331-0161

Stephen A Nezezon, MD
Center for Health & Holistic
Medicine 78 Fifth Avenue
New York, NY 10011
212-633-0390

Harold M Ofgang, ND
50 Park Avenue
New York, NY 10016
212-684-2290

Margaret B Ohlinger, DVM
3800 County Route 6
Alpine, NY 14805
607-387-5104

Julie A Plezbert, DC DNBHE
2360 State Route 89
Seneca Falls, NY 13148
315-568-3195 Fax: 315-568-3015

Stefanie Pukit, DC CCH
20 West 20th Street, Suite 1002
New York, NY 10011
212-206-8100 Fax: 212-675-4562

Lloyd C Reiter, DC DNBHE
98 Maple Avenue, Suite 306

OHIO

Suzanne T Croteau, DO
1099 West 2nd Street
Xenia, OH 45385
937-376-5644 Fax: 937-376-8409

James Cuckovich, DC CCSP
1600 Salt Springs Road
Warren, OH 44481
330-824-2662

David C Fabrey, MD
800 Compton Road, Suite 24
Cincinnati, OH 45231
513-521-5333 Fax: 513-521-5334

Douglas J Falkner, MD
2475 Lee Boulevard, Suite 1C
Cleveland Heights, OH 44118
216-321-4400

Michael C Garn, MD DHt DABFP
650 Graham Road, Suite 101
Cuyahoga Falls, OH 44221
330-923-3060 Fax: 330-923-8675

Donn W Griffith, DVM
3859 West Dublin-Granville Road
Dublin, OH 43017
614-889-2556 Fax: 614-761-3623

Carolen L Koleszar, RN BSN
6600 North High, Suite B
Worthington, OH 43085
614-848-9710 Fax: 614-848-9720

Philip C Robbins, DO CCH
131 Portsmouth Street
Jackson, OH 45640-1623
614-286-1889
Email: robbins@zoomnet.net

Michael Somerson, DO CSPOMM
423 West Main Street
Tipp City, OH 45371
513-667-2222 Fax: 513-667-5321

Jeffrey J Starre, MD
P.O. Box 157
Winesburg, OH 44690
330-359-7878

Mark Thomas, MD DABFP
Family First Care Center 2580 Shiloh
Springs Road, Suite B
Trotwood, OH 45426
937-837-5171 Fax: 937-854-0400

OREGON

Adrienne M Borg, ND
74 East 18th Avenue, Suite 12
Eugene, OR 97401
541-686-3330

John G Collins, ND DHANP
800 SE 181st Avenue
Portland, OR 97233
503-667-1961 Fax: 503-669-4263

Katherine M Dahlke, MD MPH
1312 East Burnside
Portland, OR 97232
503-234-7299 Fax: 503-234-9639

Bruce A Dickson, ND DHANP
CCH
1900 North Highway 99 West
Suite A
McMinnville, OR 97128
503-434-6515 Fax: 503-472-5723

Andrew W Elliott, ND
260 East 15th Avenue, Suite B
Eugene, OR 97401
541-343-0571 Fax: 541-465-9332

Durr Elmore, ND CCH
14653 South Graves Road
Mulino, OR 97042
503-829-7326

Deborah L Gordon, MD
987 Siskiyou Boulevard
Ashland, OR 97520
541-482-0342 Fax: 541-482-6986

Mark Immel, ND DHANP
1525 12th Street, Suite 4B
Florence, OR 97439
541-997-6255

Keith W Kale, DO
800 SE 181st Avenue
Portland, OR 97233
503-667-1961

Thomas A Kruzel, ND
800 SE 181st Avenue
Portland, OR 97233
503-667-1961

Meredith L Lowry, DO
1730 NE 42nd Avenue
Portland, OR 97213
503-460-9081 Fax: 503-287-5691

William P Mehan, ND
27636 SE Haley Road
Boring, OR 97009
503-663-0596 Fax: 503-663-4069

Stephen A Messer, ND DHANP
400 East 2nd Avenue, Suite 105
Eugene, OR 97401
541-343-2384 Fax: 541-485-3602

Joseph T Morgan, MD FAAP
FAAEM
1750 Thompson Road
Coos Bay, OR 97420
541-269-0333 Fax: 541-269-7389

Rodney Schaffer, MD DHt
400 East 2nd Avenue, Suite 105
Eugene, OR 97401
541-484-9229 Fax: 541-485-3602

Duncan Soule, MD
1312 East Burnside Street
Portland, OR 97214
503-234-7299 Fax: 503-234-9639

Mitchell Bebel Stargrove, ND LAc
4720 SW Watson Avenue
Beaverton, OR 97005
503-526-0397 Fax: 503-643-4633

PENNSYLVANIA

Bonnie C Bennett, DO MPH
3900 City Line Avenue, Suite 109
Philadelphia, PA 19131
215-477-4066

Franne R Berez, MD AK
1926 Murray Avenue
Pitttsburgh, PA 15217
412-422-5433

Philip L Bonnet, MD
1086 Taylorsville Road
Washington Crossing, PA 18977
215-321-8321

Harris B Brody, CA
605 Louis Drive, Suite 509
Warminster, PA 18974
215-443-9990 Fax: 215-443-9957

Ira S Cantor, MD
Pikeland Village Square, Route 113
Phoenixville, PA 19460
610-933-1688 Fax: 610-983-0698

Michael W DiPalma, ND
The Village at Newtown Medical
Center
2700 South Eagle Road
Newtown, PA 18940
215-579-1300

Athena K Farrell, DC
422 Upper Stump Road
Chalfont, PA 18914
215-997-5055

Sarah M Fisher, MD
Lotus Medical Arts Center
530 South 2nd Street, Suite 108
Philadelphia, PA 19147
215-627-3001 Fax: 215-627-0362

Charles H Grande, DO
218 West Moody Avenue
New Castle, PA 16101
412-658-5654 Fax: 412-652-1109

Nand Kishore Gupta, MD AK
1442 Street Road
Bensalem, PA 19020
215-639-7363

Todd A Hoover, MD
915 Montgomery Avenue, Suite 200
Narbeth, PA 19072
610-667-2138

Marcia S Kesten, DC DNBHE
4530 Baltimore Avenue
Philadelphia, PA 19143
215-386-6998

Deva Kaur Khalsa, VMD CVA
1724 Yardley-Langhorne Road
Yardley, PA 19067
215-493-0621 Fax: 215-493-1944

Edward C Kondrot, MD
239 Fourth Avenue
2020 Investment Building
Pittsburgh, PA 15222
412-281-0447 Fax: 412-281-3660

Stephen A Nezezon, MD
Integrative Therapies
955 Main Street
Honesdale, PA 18431
717-253-8020 Fax: 717-251-3652

Lucy (Lea) Nitskansky, MD
9369 Hoff Street
Philadelphia, PA 19115
215-698-1042

Peter J Prociuk, MD DABIM
Route 82, P.O. Box 444
Unionville, PA 19375
610-347-1311 Fax: 610-347-1412

Lynne A Robinson, RN CRNP MSN
21 Cynwyd Road
Bala Cynwyd, PA 19004
610-667-8290

Brian T Schneider, ND LAc
617 North Bethlehem Pike
P.O. Box 53
Spring House, PA 19477
215-654-9520

Mitchel E Shapiro, PA-C
3740 West Chester Pike
Newtown Square, PA 19073
610-359-7575

C Edgar Sheaffer, VMD
47 North Railroad Street
P.O. Box 353
Palmyra, PA 17078
717-838-9563 Fax: 717-838-0377

James L Vanemon, DC
327 Allegheny Street
Jersey Shore, PA 17740
717-398-0670

Karene P Villaronte, RN CAAPM
BSN
2417 Welsh Road, Suite 205
Philadelphia, PA 19114
215-676-4080 Fax: 215-676-4408

Patricia A Whittaker, VMD CAC
370 Tree Lane
Aspers, PA 17304
717-677-9543 Fax: 717-677-6562

RHODE ISLAND

Steven P Goldsmith, MD
297 Wickenden Street
Providence, RI 02903
401-272-1170

Victoria E Malchar, DC
33 College Hill Road Building 30C
Warwick, RI 02886
401-826-7600 Fax: 401-822-1226

SOUTH CAROLINA

Jacqueline Fabien-Boutrouille, MD
208 Scott Street
Mount Pleasant, SC 29464
803-886-5608 Fax: 803-856-2381

Jeanne R Fowler, DVM CVA
409 Old Buncombe Road
Travelers Rest, SC 29690
864-834-7334

Roger S Jaynes, DC DNBHE
1521 Augusta Street
Greenville, SC 29605
864-232-0082 Fax: 864-232-1884

TENNESSEE

Corinne S Rovetti, RN-C FNP
6925 Sevierville Pike
Knoxville, TN 37920
423-573-0945

Victoria R Snelling, DC
(See Louisville, KY)
Nashville, TN

TEXAS

Lawrence M Cohen, MD
2515 McCullough Avenue, Suite 103
San Antonio, TX 78212
210-733-0990 Fax: 210-733-9603

Patricia A Cooper, DVM
1951 Lexington Street
Houston, TX 77098
713-520-5588 Fax: 713-523-8345

Robert C Ehle, DC
5408 Bell, Suite 150
Amarillo, TX 79109
806-355-5800 Fax: 806-355-1400

Walter T Eidson, DC DNBHE
1833 West Pioneer Parkway
Arlington, TX 76013
817-784-1177 Fax: 817-472-7520

Louis H Esquivel, MD DABFP
2515 McCullough, Suite 103
San Antonio, TX 78212
210-733-6300

William F Falconer, DVM
8509 Zyle Road
Austin, TX 78737
512-288-5400 Fax: 512-288-5402

Jason W Kwee, MD
M&S Tower, Suite 624
730 North Main Street
San Antonio, TX 78205
210-226-3000

Judith J Pruzzo-Hawkins, RPh CCH
8345 Walnut Hill Lane, Suite 220
Dallas, TX 75231-4262
214-373-5154 Fax: 214-691-8432

Karl Robinson, MD
4200 Westheimer, Suite 100
Houston, TX 77027
800-637-5275 Fax: 713-877-8035

James R Snow, DC DNBHE
11615 Forest Central, Suite 105
Dallas, TX 75243
214-341-0400

Ricardo B Tan, MD
3220 North Freeway
Fort Worth, TX 76111
817-626-1993

UTAH

William A Nunn, ND
345 East 4500 South, Suite H
Murray, UT 84107
801-265-0077

VIRGINIA

Lia Bello, RN FNP CCH
Alternative Health Care
6048 Chicory Place
Alexandria, VA 22310
703-921-0378
Email: liabello@laplaza.org

Richard M Evans, RN CRRN BSN
5923 Augusta Drive
Springfield, VA 22150
703-866-1234 Fax: 703-569-2963

Richard D Fischer, DDS FAGD
FIAOMT
4222 Evergreen Lane
Annandale, VA 22003
703-256-4441 Fax: 703-354-1631

Mitchell A Fleisher, MD FAAFP
Rockfish Center, Suite 1
P.O. Box 303
Nellysford, VA 22958
804-361-1896 Fax: 804-361-1928

Elizabeth J Greve, RN
108 Applegate Drive
Sterling, VA 20164
703-435-1059

Frank W Gruber, MD
2200 Colonial Avenue, Suite 6
Norfolk, VA 23517
804-640-1107 Fax: 804-640-8061

George A Guess, MD DHt
10411 Courthouse Road, Suite B
Spotsylvania/Fredericksburg,
VA 22553
804-295-0362 Fax: 804-295-0798

Joyce C Harman, DVM
311-E Gay Street
P.O. Box 488
Washington, VA 22747
540-675-1855 Fax: 540-675-1447

Jordan A Kocen, DVM
6136 Brandon Avenue
Springfield, VA 22150
703-569-0300 Fax: 703-866-4962

Alan M Smith, MD LAc FAAFP
5718 Courthouse Road
Prince George, VA 23875
804-862-4414 Fax: 804-862-3203

Vincent J Speckhart, MD MD(H)
902 Graydon Avenue, Suite 2
Norfolk, VA 23507
757-622-0014 Fax: 757-622-9808

Sidney H Storozum, DVM
1400 Main Street
Lynchburg, VA 24521
804-845-1242

Barry L Swedlow, DPM FACFO
3623 Old Forest Road
Lynchburg, VA 24501-2906
804)385-9393

David G Wember, MD DHt
4910A South 31st Street
Arlington, VA 22206
703-578-3825

Craig A Zunka, DDS
107 West 4th Street
Front Royal, VA 22630
540-635-3610 Fax: 540-635-3510

VERMONT

Lydia W Faesy, ND RN
73 Main Street, Suite 41
Montpelier, VT 05602
802-229-2038

George Glanzberg, VMD
White Creek Road RR 1 Box 373
North Bennington, VT 05257
802-442-8714

Julian J Jonas, CA CCH
Saxtons River Natural Healthcare
Main Street, P.O. Box 515
Saxtons River, VT 05154
802-869-2883

Dhyano C Pierson, MD
168 Battery
Burlington, VT 05401
802-862-0836

John R Roos, MD MPH
2 Church Street, Suite 2B, Box 17
Burlington, VT 05401
802-864-7967

WASHINGTON

Brenda Beeley, LAc
P.O. Box 1339
Suquamish, WA 98392-1339

Jane A Bernstein Pearson, ND
18820 Front Street, Suite 414
P.O. Box 1664
Poulsbo, WA 98370
360-697-7070

Arlin E Brown, MD ABPN
7600 NE 41st Street, Suite 310
Vancouver, WA 97232
360-253-6425 Fax: 360-253-3196

Anthony Calpeno, ND DHANP
CCH
4111A Bridgeport Way West
Tacoma, WA 98466
253-565-2444 Fax: 253-565-0684

Linda I Chiu-Hole, MD DHt
2814 South Grand Boulevard
Spokane, WA 99223
509-747-2902

Sally A Goodwin, MD ABFP
3677 Woodland Hall Lane
Clinton, WA 98236
360-579-1586

Jennifer Jacobs, MD MPH
23200 Edmonds Way, Suite A
Edmonds, WA 98026
206-542-5595 Fax: 206-368-0843

Christopher Jayne, ND
Integrated Natural Health Center
618 Cherry Street
Port Townsend, WA 98368
360-385-1929 Fax: 360-385-1926
Email: cjayne@chiron-h.com

Barbara Kreemer, ND
311 Blaine Street
Seattle, WA 98109
206-281-4282

Judyth L Reichenberg-Ullman, ND
DHANP MSW
The Northwest Center for
Homeopathic Medicine
131 3rd Avenue North
Edmonds, WA 98020
425-774-5599 Fax: 425-670-0319

Robert M Schore, MD DHt
7715 Meridian Avenue North
Seattle, WA 98103
206-525-8722

Robert W Ullman, ND DHANP
The Northwest Center for
Homeopathic Medicine
131 3rd Avenue North
Edmonds, WA 98020
425-774-5599 Fax: 425-670-0319

Lucy Vaughters, PA-C CCH
The Evergreen Clinic
23200 Edmonds Way
Edmonds, WA 98020
206-542-5595

H Jonathan Wright, DVM
7327 South Cedar Road
Spokane, WA 99224
509-443-0803

Jane Laura Doyle, DVM
3774 Valley Road
Berkeley Springs, WV 25411
304-258-5819 Fax: 304-258-5955

C P Negri, OMD DAc(WV) CCH
364 High Street
Morgantown, WV 26505
304-291-5053

Hydrotherapy

**(INTERNATIONAL ASSOCIATION
OF COLON HYDROTHERAPY)**

Thomas Alba
109B Stratford Drive
Williamsburg, VA 23185
757-220-1392

Clarie Alden
1403 NW 85th Street
Seattle, WA 98117
253-572-5100

Patricia Allen
972-252-5779

Connie J. Allred
ALLRED TECHNIQUE
11739 Washington Blvd.
Los Angeles, CA 90066
310-390-5424

Kristina Amelong
ROSE CHIROPRACTIC COMPLETE
HEALTH CARE
2148 Atwood Avenue
Madison, WI 53704
608-249-2188

Gregory Bacon
NEW CHOICE PLUS
1978 S. Garrison
Lakewood, CO 80227
303-989-6889

Mark Baker, D.C.
BAKER CHIROPRACTIC &
ACUPUNCTURE CENTER
11588 St. Charles Rock Road
Bridgeton, MO 63044
314-291-4401

Judy Barber
HEALTH—HYDROTHERAPY
CENTER
915 E. Ocean Blvd.
Stuart, FL 34994
561-286-3650

Rochelle Barbour
ROSELLE CHIROPACTIC GROUP
8316 Arlington, Suite 400
Fairfax, VA 22031
703-698-7117

Jeanelle M. Barry, RH
BARRY HEALTH THERAPY
8316 Blondo Street, #210
Omaha, NE 68134-6339
402-391-0117

Margaret Battles
757 Titus Avenue
Rochester, NY 14617
716-342-6823

Carylann Bautz
P.O. Box 277
Sommerdale, NJ 08083
609-374-1931

JoAnn Baxter
CORPORATE WELLNESS CENTER
The Executive Mews, Suite I-48
Cherry Hill, NJ 08003
609-489-0505

Delois Bennett
URBAN OASIS
11420 Engleside
Detroit, MI 48205
313-521-7918

France Bergeron
ALLRED TECHNIQUE, INC.
11739 Washington Blvd.
Los Angeles, CA 90066
310-390-5424

Myroslava Bertalan
1326 E. Evelyn
Hazel Park, MI 48030
248-584-3214

Pamela Best
THE BEST BODY COMPANY
700 19th Street, Suite 105
Virginia Beach, VA 23451
757-422-6113

Chris Birchall
COLON HYDROTHERAPY
ASSOCIATES
1150 Old US Hwy 1 South, Suite 3
Southern Pines, NC 28387
910-692-9229

Jae Bird
JAE BIRD BOTANICALS
& BODYWORK
P.O. Box 22088
Sante Fe, NM 87502-2088
505-986-0775

Walter Blake
P.O. Box11664
Berklely, CA 94712
510-465-9545

Grace Bonnell
BODY, MIND & SPIRIT CENTER
25211 Via Sistine
Valencia, CA 91355
805-253-3074

Dawn Bork
RENEE BORK, RMT
P.O. Box 3293
Bryan, TX 77805-3293
409-778-0493

Gayle Bradshaw
HOLISTIC ENCHILADA
4861 Campbell Avenue, #2
San Jose, CA 95130
408-866-7380

Karen Brady
BRADY CHIROPRACTIC OFFICE
7886 Lincoln Way West
Saint Thomas, PA 17252
717-369-3996

Florence Branch
HEALING WATER COLON
HYGIENE
2530 Nevels Road
College Park, GA 30349
770-996-0784

Sheila Branch
HEALING WATER COLON
HYGIENE
2530 Nevels Road
College Park, GA 30349
770-996-0784

Annette R. Bray, R.N.
A & B NEUROMUSCULAR
THERAPIES
183 Badman Road
Green Lane, PA 18054-2404
215-257-7629

Kristina Breidenbach
SEE SPIRIT THERAPY
601 Don Canuto
Santa Fe, NM 87501
505-982-6187

Terry Briceño
2774 Bryant Drive
Broomfield, CO 80020
303-439-9041

Julie A. Briggs
195 W. Columbia River Hwy
Clatskanie, OR 97016
503-728-4732

Geri Brown
524 St. Ann's Drive
Laguna Beach, CA 92651
949-494-6516

Irina Bukshteyn
4470 Debracy Pl
Tucker, GA 30084
770-908-2305

Annette Buxton-Bacon
NEW CHOICES +
1978 S. Garrison Street, #7
Lakewood, CO 80227
303-989-6889

Donna Carmony
P.O. Box 963
San Andreas, CA 95249
209-754-0727

Dolores Casarella
FLORIDA MEDICAL MASSAGE
2300 SE 4th Avenue
Ft. Lauderdale, FL 33316
954-898-5712

Dorothy Cato
NEW HORIZONS IN HEALTH
726 Stephen Terrace
Neptune, NJ 07753
732-922-6299

Laura Centorrino
3180 NW 12th Street
Gainsville, FL 32609
904-373-6028

Dr. Milton Chandler, DN
CHANDLER HEALTH EMPORIUM
8 South Michigan Avenue, #820
Chicago, IL 60643
312-782-2285

Henry Chang
4213 N. Rosemead Blvd.
Rosemead, CA 91770
626-451-0588

Phil Chapman
HEALTH BY NATURE
940 Exley Lane
Willits, CA 95490
707-459-6998

Suzanne Childre
SUZANNE CHILDRE'S ASSOC.
l535 6th Street, #105
Santa Monica, CA 90401
310-576-6360

Barbara Chivvis
LONG ISLAND SCHOOL OF
COLON HYDROTHERAPY
21 West Nicholai Street
Hicksville, NY 11801
516-822-6722

Shirley Cho, R.N.
SHAM SHANG HEALTH CENTER
837 S. Kingsley Drive
Los Angeles, CA 90005
213-487-6009

Debra Christian-Foster
C.C.C. CENTRE
1413 Crescent Drive
Tyler, TX 75702, USA
903-592-3900

Liu Chu
TRA-HEALTH INC.
4213 N. Rosemead Blvd.
Rosemead, CA 91770
626-451-0588

Diana Clark
MONTGOMERY COLON
HYDROTHERAPY
2735 Highland Avenue
Montgomery, AL 36107
334-264-6116

Alan D. Clemence
HEALTH THERAPIES
3379 Churchview Avenue
Pittsburgh, PA 15227-4305
412-882-4139

Brenda Cohen
LIVING WATERS SPA THERAPIES
2 Lynxholm Ct.
Hyannis, MA 02601
508-778-8444

Michelle Corrao
414-278-8922

Meredith Craft
109B Stratford Dr
Williamsburg, VA 23185
757-220-1392

Marlene Cupit
BACK TO BASICS
100 W. Southlake Blvd., Suite 144
Southlake, TX 76092,
817-421-1004

Lori Curtis
BEAUTIFUL ACCENTS
5329 Diplomat Circle
Orlando, FL 32810
407-628-5881

Christine Davis
2719 Arcaro Ct
Decatur, GA 30034

Norma Davis
HARMONY THERAPY CENTER
750 S. Orange Ave
Sarasota, FL 34203
941-957-1376

Sarah Decker
COLON CARE CENTER
The Wellness Center
120 S. Main Street
West Lebanon, NH 03784
603-298-8588

Linda DeKam
HEALTH MANAGEMENT
1301 Airport Drive, Suite B
Bakersfield, CA 93308
805-391-0187

Connie Deter
FOR BETTER HEALTH
4221 N. 800 W.
Frankton, IN 46044
765-734-1226

Deborah DiCarlo
9952 E. DelMonte
Gold Canyon, AZ 85219-6899
602-671-5793

Alice DiMaggio
1043 Stuart Street, Suite, #1
Lafayette, CA 94549
925-284-1564

Linda Dolese
167 Main Street
Metuchen, NJ 08840
732-525-0911

Joel Doti
WEST PACIFIC-BODYCENTRE
434 N. Lakeview Avenue
Anaheim, CA 92807
714-998-8079

Rhonda Doud
THE MASTERS NATURAL
ALTERNATIVES II
2904 Moody Lane
Burlington, IA 52601
319-754-6235

Sandra Duggan
TO YOUR HEALTH
2000 General Booth Blvd., Suite 202
Virginia Beach, VA 23454
757-563-9333

Carolyn Dye
MASSAGE THERAPY
BY CAROL & ASSOC
1241-D West Main Street
Tupelo, MS 38801
601-842-6599

Janae Dykstra
TACOMA NATURAL HEALTH
919 S. 10th Street
Tacoma, WA 98405
253-572-5100

Pamela J. Elwell
CAPE COD COLON
HYDROTHERAPY
766 Falmouth Road
Unit A-1, Suite A
Mashpee, MA 02649
508-539-3777

Monica Escalante
11939 Swearingen Drive
Austin, TX 78758
512-836-4212

Jeri Evans
COLON HYDROTHERAPY
924 Buena Vista Street
Duarte, CA 91010
818-359-4662

Donna Evenson, R.N.
DONNA FAYE, INC.
311 S. Naperville Road
Wheaton, IL 60187
630-510-2110

Harry Farris
5212 Madison Ave, Suite B
Indianapolis, IN 46227
317-786-0718

Judith K. Fenley
HARMONIZING HEALTH CENTER
299 N. Edison Street
Graton, CA 95444
707-829-0984

Martha Flannery
11 Calle Medico, Suite 6
Santa Fe, NM 87505
505-983-8722

Dorothy D. Fleisher
FLEISHER THERAPY CENTER
861 N Venetian Drive
Miami, FL 33139-1012
305-374-8240

Donna Florimonte
P.O. Box 255
Waverly, PA 18471
717-563-2565

Kathleen G. Flynn
PANACEA
22706 Aspan, Suite #302
Lake Forest, CA 92630
714-951-7631

AnneMarie Furfaro
336-454-6204

Joyce Gadberry
P.O. Box 397
Winchester, CA 92956
800-799-7127

Marjorie Gatlin
10108 Leona Avenue
Leona Valley, CA 93551
805-270-1766

Alice Gauthier, RN
ALTERNATIVE HEALTH CARE
4720 South 25th Street
Ft. Pierce, FL 34981
561-468-0844

Maxine Giles-Norman
BACK TO BASICS
1631 Carolina Avenue
Orangeburg, SC 29115
803-536-2100

Millie Girouard
THE CENTER
6301 25th Street
Groves, TX 77619
409-963-3338

Maria Goldenberg
NATURAL HEALTH & NUTRITION
CENTER
2221 Ocean Avenue
Brooklyn, NY 11229
718-336-2818

Evelyn L. Gordon
THE HEALING SOURCE & SELF
HELP CENTER
1459 Ogden Street
Denver, CO 80218
303-863-9670

Patricia E. Gosling
3031 Poplar Creek Drive, S.E. , #103
Kentwood, MI 49512
616-949-9573

Phyllis N. Gottshall, RN
VIBRANT BODIES
41516 Kalhia St
Murrieta, CA 92562
909-696-0854

Jean Grandoit
GRANDOIT CENTER
2176 Nostrand Ave
Brooklyn, NY 11210
718 -859-3222

Suzanne Gray
RENEW LIFE CLINIC
1007 N. MacDill Avenue
Tampa, FL 33607
813-871-3200

Jerry Green
HEALTH REFLEXTIONS
1550 W. Rosedale, Suite 206
Ft. Worth, TX 76103
817-870-2042

Nancy Guess
EXQUISITE FACIALS & MORE
1207 N. Sixth Street
Longview, TX 75601
903-234-9033

Willow Gurtler
4745 N. First Avenue
Tucson, AZ 85718
520-293-5399

Scheryle Gusby
8445 Rising Sun Drive
Corryton, TN 37721
423-933-3080

Linda L. Hadley
NATURAL HEALTH CENTER
11155 W. Edna Street
Boise, ID 83713
208-322-9376

Teena Hakeem
222-4 Swing Road
Greensboro, NC 27409
336-851-5250

Lori Hallquist, M.Sc, D. N., Ph.D.
CENTER FOR ENZYME THERAPY
543 3rd Street, Suite C-2
Lake Oswego, OR 97034
503-635-4413

Katherine Hamming
44990 27th Street
Mattawan, MI 49071
616-668-5321

Patricia Hartman
NEW AGE HEALTH SPA
Rt 55
Neversink, NY 12765
914-985-7601

Daisy R. Hawkins
TOTAL HEALTH MINISTRIES
917 Kranzel Drive
Camp Hilll, PA 17011
717-975-9115

Tiffany Hawkins
NATURAL REJUVENATION, INC.
3185 N. High School Road
Indianapolis, IN 46224
317-290-1544

Terri Hawkins, N.D., Ph.D.
NATURAL REJUVENATION, INC.
3185 N. High School Road
Indianapolis, IN 46224
317-290-1544

Vanessa J. Haycock
1509 S. Robert Street
Boise, ID 83705
208-383-4833

Lois Heckman
VIBRANT LIFE
740 North Cleveland Avenue
Loveland, CO 80538
970-669-2332

Alicia Hoffer
ALTERNATIVE THERAPY CENTER
12042 Blanco Road, #10
San Antonio, TX 78216
210-349-3630

Gloria Holder
ACCESS HEALTH
4036-A Plank Road
Fredericksburg, VA 22407
540-786-0525

Darlene J. Holloway
ALTERNATIVE HEALTH CENTER
OF CARY
919 Kildair Farm Road
Cary, NC 27511
919-380-0023

Kathleen S. Hosner
4925 E. Aire Libre Avenue
Scottsdale, AZ 85254
602-787-8838

Norma Howard
12 Spruce Road
Amityville, NY 11701
516-789-5097

Nancy Huberth
NORTHSHORE LOTUS HEALTH
CENTER
23 Railroad Avenue
Swampscott, MA 01907
781-592-8175

Jenifer Jackson
5401 9th Avenue South
Birmingham, AL 35212
205-222-7600

Constance Jones
CONSTANCE JONES
& ASSOCIATES
214 Market Street
Brighton, MA 02135
617-787-5040

Tess Jones
209 Harvard Street, #306
Brookline, MA 02146
617-964-5406

Loree Jordan
LTJ & ASSOCIATES
321 Los Gatos Road
Saratoga, CA 95008
408-379-9488

Linda Kalbach
LOWER CAPE COLON
HYDROTHERAPY, INC.
129 Route 28
West Harwich, MA 02671
508-430-9921

Jeffrey Karls
THE WELLHOUSE CENTER
6562 Lake Road
Windsor, WI 53598
608-846-4862

Andre Kastin
KASTIN HEALING ARTS CENTER,
LLC
12732 Washington Blvd., Suite B
Los Angeles, CA 90066
310-574-6622

May Kastin
KASTIN HEALING ARTS CENTER
12732 Washington Blvd., #B
Los Angeles, CA 90066
310-574-6622

Stephanie Kato
ALLRED TECHNIQUE
11739 Washington Blvd.
Los Angeles, CA 90066,
310-390-5424

Haya Khoury
HEALTH CONNECTIONS CENTER,
INC.
530 S. 2nd Street
Philadelphia, PA 19147
215-627-6000

Joyce Kiger
Road1, Box 137
Spraggs, PA 15362
724-435-7146

Uzi Kira
THE HEALING MASSAGE, INC.
8254 SR 84
Ft. Lauderdale, FL 33324
954-476-7770

Helen Kirby, R.N.
HAYLA INNER VENDICH RAVS
151 Mifflin Road
Millersburg, PA 17061
717-362-2067

Valerie Knowles
VALERIE KNOWLES
750 So. Orange Avenue
Sarasota, FL 34236
941-957-9376

Bradley L. Kolbo
TACOMA NATURAL HEALTH
CLINIC
919 S. 10th Street
Tacoma, WA 98405
253-572-5100

Cherie Kolbo
NATURAL HEALTH CLINIC
3164 Mapu Pl.
Kihei, HI 96753
808-874-1490

Russell Kolbo, DC, ND
919 S. 10th Street
Tacoma, WA 98405
253-572-5100

Lillette J. Koleno
TO-HEAL COLON
HYDROTHERAPY OFFICES
209 Oakdale Drive
So. Amherst, OH 44001
216-322-9096

Yakov Koyfman
4470 Debracy Pl
Tucker, GA 30084
770-908-2305

Anke Meta Krosch
IDYLLWILD CHIROPRACTIC
CLINIC
54185 Pine Crest
Idyllwild, CA 92549
909-659-4663

Vanisa Krula
OMEGA PREVENTATIVE
HEALTH CARE
420 N. Nimitz Hwy., Suite 200
Honolulu, HI 96817
808-531-2013

Rose Mary Laskow
EARTH SPRING WELLNESS
CENTER
354 Dover Milton Road
Oak Ridge, NJ 07438
201-697-3530

Lynda Law
P.O. Box 224
Clementon, NJ 08021
609-489-0505

Paddy Lazar
ALLS WELL THAT ENDS WELL
316 NE 28th Avenue
Portland, OR 97232
503-230-0812

Susan Lenczyk
AB CENTER FOR
NEUROMUSCULAR THERAPIES
183 Badman Road
Green Lane, PA 18962
215-257-6868

Lena Leon
15349 Los Gatos Blvd.
Los Gatos, CA 95032
408-358-2537

Sharron Louie
LUMA SUN—NATURAL HEALTH
CENTER
6360-2 E Thomas Road, Suite 222
Scottsdale, AZ 85251
602-947-5771

Laura Mahan
6711 SE Reedway
Portland, OR 97206
503-771-0998

Jamie Marlow
PASSAGE TO WELLNESS
8724 N. Dixie Drive, Suite 2
Dayton, OH 45414
937-890-6990

Lisa Maroni
RHODE ISLAND COLON
HYDROTHERAPY
234 Main Street
East Greenwich, RI 02818
401-886-7171

Jill Marty
TACOMA NATURAL HEALTH
CLINIC
919 S. 10th Street
Tacoma, WA 98405
253-572-5100

Judith Marty
TACOMA NATURAL HEALTH
CLINIC
919 S. 10th Street
Tacoma, WA 98405
253-572-5100

Marie Mauger
BETTER LIVING INFO SERVICE
P.O. Box 899
Arcata, CA 95518
707-822-6144

Alouette Mayer
204 Westridge Drive
Columbia, MO 65203
573-449-0842

Caitlyn Mayfair
314 26th Street
Virginia Beach, VA 23451-3115
757-422-6113

Paul Mazur
INSTITUTE FOR STRUCTURAL
INTEGRATIVE STUDIES
364 Boylston Street
Boston, MA 02116
617-266-0112

Karen McGinnis
PERSHING OAKS BODY CARE
7859 N. Pershing Avenue
Stockton, CA 95215
209-952-1098

Karen McKenzie
NATURAL HEALTH CENTER
403 S. Water
Silverton, OR 97381
503-873-6051

Patricia McLaughlin
HEALING ARTS & RESOURCE
CENTER
3434 Davenport Avenue
Saginaw, MI 48602
517-792-9411

Rebecca McMahon
933 W.3rd Avenue, #106
Spokane, WA 99204
509-747-1447

Tana Meadows
COLON HYDROTHERAPY OF THE
CAPITAL REGION
188 Spring Street, Suite 1
Albany, NY 12203-1317
518-462-1628

Eleanor Rebecca Medsker
106 North Creek Drive
Quinbt (Florence), SC 29506
803-669-5794

Tsai Mei-Yu
4213 N. Rosemead Blvd., #D
Rosemead, CA 91770
626-285-9190

Grace H. Melby
HEALTH ESSENTIALS
10413 Alden Road
Harvard, IL 60033
815-648-4544

Talya Meldy
ALLRED TECHNIQUE
11739 Washington Blvd.
Los Angeles, CA 90066
310-390-5424

Mireya Mendez
2603 Longwood
Pearland, TX 77581
281-482-2105

Wendy Middleton
FOR THE HEALTH OF IT
183 Sargent Ct.
Monterey, CA 93940
408-373-5979

Michele Miglino, L.M.T. ,C.C.T.
A COLON CARE CENTER
817 SE 9th St
Deerfield Beach, FL 33441-5633
954-421-0703

Anne Miller
BODY HARMONY
2000 Van Ness Avenue, Suite 504
San Francisco, CA 94109
415-563-6630

Jane Miller
2474 North George St
York, PA 17402
717-852-0266

Lucy Miller
COMM. NATURAL FOODS/
LANCASTER HEALTH ASSOC.
1065 W. Main St
New Holland, PA 17557
717-656-7222

Amanda Milosavljevic
TOTAL HEALTH SERVICES
455 Broadway
Hot Springs, AR 71901
501-624-1248

Carolyn Lee Minx
GO WITH THE FLOW
807 Stockbridge
Kalamazoo, MI 49001
616-349-8431

Kaye Moberg
TOTAL WELLNESS
MEDICAL CENTER
9887 W. Bell Road
Sun City, AZ 85351
602-977-0077

Tanya Molinelli
HOLISTIC LIFE CENTER
7396 Harbor Glenn
Stone Mountain, GA 30087
770-413-7734
Email: hlc@bellsouth.net

Martha Montero
A CHOICE FOR HEALTH
1101 W. Moana Lane, Suite 12
Reno, NV 89509
702-829-8122

Margie Morgan
714 East Franklin
Hillsboro, TX 76634
254-582-0484

Betty J. Morosko
MOROSKO'S
2305 Oak Lane
Suite 119, Building 4A
Grand Prairie, TX 75051
972-263-3133

Dianne M. Muldowney
COLONICS FOR HEALTH
1 S. 055 Summit Ave
Oakbrook Terrace, IL 60181
630-495-8782

Magdolna Muller, ND
LIVING WATERS
WELLNESS CENTER
7777 Sunrise Blvd, Suite 1100
Citrus Heights, CA 95610
916-723-2300

Zahra Nafez
CLINIC FOR ALTERNATIVE
HEALTH
106 Russell Street, Unit, #3
Hadley, MA 01035
413-586-9951

Lila E. Nau
CONSTANCE JONES
& ASSOCIATES
214 Market Street
Brighton, MA 02135
617-787-5040

Shona L. Nelson
BARRY HEALTH THERAPY
8316 Blondo Street, #210
Omaha, NE 68134-6339
402-391-0117

Alla Netchitailo
HOLISTIC MED. OF MSMD., INC
8264 Santa Monica Blvd
Los Angeles, CA 90046
213-650-1789

Christine Newberry
INTEGRATED HEALTH
THERAPIES
40 N. 29th Street, #113
Oakland, CA 94609
510-287-5439

Juliana Njinimbam
309 Poplar Lane
Mauldin, SC 29662
864-234-0058

Troy Norman
NATURAL WELLNESS THERAPY
CENTER
10110 Sahara Drive
San Antonio, TX 78216
210-308-8193

Joyce Ochoa
FEEL BETTER COMPANY
507 Benine Road
Westbury, NY 11590
718-783-5344

Teresa Orozco
"ANUHEA" B&B
3164 Mapu Pl
Kikei, HI 96753
808-874-1490

Sandra L. Outerbridge
RENEW LIFE CLINIC
447 S. Nove Road
Ormond Beach, FL 32174
904-615-9491

Paramdevi
CENTER FOR EFFECTIVE LIVING
665 Fox Run Heights
Waynesville, NC 28721
704-926-6014

Jacqueline Anne Parker
ASPEN HEALTH WORKS
305 Unit H AABC
Aspen, CO 81611
970-920-4666

Char Parrott
THE MASTERS NATURAL
ALTERNATIVES
201 Abbott Lane
Branson, MO 65616
417-336-0807

Nancy J. Peck
HEALING TOUCH COLON
HYDROTHERAPY
1463 Oakfield Drive, Suite 110
Brandon, FL 33511
813-651-3507

Marie L. Pence
INNERGY
345 Knechtel Way, NE, Suite 202
(Garden Plaza Bld.)
Bainbridge Island, WA 98110
206-824-4505

Paula Pence
THE HERB SHOP
614 E. Market
Rockport, TX 78358
512-729-0746

Sheena Pope, ND
8520 Price Road
Holland Patent, NY 13354
315-339-1916

Joanne Priaulx
COLON HEALTH SERVICES
874 B. W. Eau Gallie Blvd
Melbourne, FL 32935
407-242-1713

Susan Putt
TODAY'S WAY WELLNESS
MINISTRIES
R.D. 3 Box 359
Huntingdon, PA 16652
814-643-1559

Charil Quiñones
THERAPY ALTERNATIVES
3501 N. MacArther
Irving, TX 75062
972-256-2577

Vonda Rankin
1226 Fern Ave
Imperial Beach, CA 91932
619-546-8804

Suzanne Rasmussen
HEALTHY WAY OUT
701 W. Coral Road
Stanton, MI 48888-9493
517-762-5245

Janice Reed
ADVANCED HEALTH CENTER
1611 N.State Street
Bellingham, WA 98226
360-715-9010

Naima Reynolds
NAIMA'S TOTAL BODY THERAPY
195 Southwest 15 Road, Suite 501
Miami, FL 33129
305-854-9010

Mary Rice
915-366-3347

Amy Riesing
NATURAL HEALTH SERVICES, INC.
1428 N. Farwell
Milwaukee, WI 53202
414-278-8922

Brian Rizzieri
BREAKTHROUGH IN HEALING
CENTER
2639 Parkmont Lane S.W., Suite A
Olympia, WA 98502
360-943-6512

Armando Rodriguez
WE CARE HEALTH RETREAT
18000 Long Canyon Road
Desert Hot Springs, CA 92240
760-251-2261

Trisha Rossi, N.D.
THE NATURAL ALTERNATIVE
CENTER, INC.
310 West 72nd Street
Dr. Office Entrance
New York, NY 10023
212-580-3333

Dee Rowe
CENTER FOR HOLISTIC
MEDICINE
810 53rd Avenue W.
Bradenton, FL 34207
941-727-7711

Annalia Russell
Practitioner's Home Page
FOUNDATION FOR WHOLENESS
924 Encinitas Blvd.
Encinatas, CA 92024-5394
760-632-9990

Muhanad Saada
MT. OF OLIVES HEALTH CENTER
734 W. 23rd Street
Panama City, FL 32405
850-784-9001

Sam Saba
INTEGRATED MEDICAL CENTER
7023 Little River Tpke., #207
Annandale, VA 22003
703-941-3606

Shirley Saylors-Clarkson
AGAPE FELLOWSHIP CENTER
3501 Severn Avenue, Suite 19
Metairie, LA 70002
504-887-9092

Cindy Secrest
TOTAL HEALTH MINISTRIES
917 Kranzel Drive
Camp Hill, PA 17011
717-795-9950

Juanita Selman
TEXAS HEALTH ENHANCEMENT,
INC.
P.O. Box 61150
Midland, TX 79711
915-520-5993

Elisa Ramirez Sharps
EAST BAY COLON HYGIENIST
INSTITUTE
401 29th Street, Suite 113
Oakland, CA 94609
510-287-5439

Cathy Shea, LMT, LCT
SHEA EDUCATIONAL GROUP, INC.
13878 Oleander Avenue
Juno Beach, FL 33408
561-627-3560

Sheila Shea
INTESTINAL HEALTH INSTITUTE
4427 E. 5th Street
Tucson, AZ 85711
520-325-9686

Sandy Shirley, L.V.N
ALLRED TECHNIQUE
11739 Washington Blvd.
Los Angeles, CA 90066
310-390-5424

Chen Shuchao
TRA-SOL HEALTH, INC.
4213 N. Rosemead Blvd., #E
Rosemead, CA 91770
626-331-4133

Rosemarie Siciliano
4 YOUR HEALTH
609 N. Scottsdale Road, Suite A
Scottsdale, AZ 85257
602-994-4378

Jill Simons
ALLS WELL THAT ENDS WELL
316 NE 28th Avenue
Portland, OR 97232
503-230-0812

Effie Skinner
17110 Cottonwood Canyon Road
Yakima, WA 98908
509-966-7306

Linda T. Skinner, R.N.
HEALTH SPRINGS
101 Manning Drive
Charlotte, NC 28209
704-553-1422

Kay L. Slick, RN, LMT
KAY SLICK BODYWORKS
5015 SE Hawthorne, Suite B
Portland, OR 97215
503-234-5675

Jalene Smith
BREAKTHROUGHS IN HEALING
CENTER
2639 Parkmont Lane SW
Olympia, WA 98502
360-943-6512

Judy Smith
BODY HEALTH
20351 Irvine Avenue, Suite C-4
Santa Ana Heights, CA 92707
714-662-7613

Sandra Smith
GARLAND COLONIC CENTER
401 W. Centerville Road, Suite 3
Garland, TX 75041
972-278-3984

Trisha Smith
HEALQUEST 2000
HEALING CENTER
11263 Reading Road
Cincinnati, OH 45241
513-936-8141

Jeffery Snyder
A CHOICE FOR HEALTH
1101 W. Moana Lane, Suite 12
Reno, NV 89509
702-829-8122

Michelle Sobel
THE CENTER FOR NATURAL
HEALING
1103 S. Washington
Royal Oak, MI 48067
248-543-2020

Steve Solomon
1100 Warburton Avenue, Apt 5G
Yonkers, NY 10701
914-969-2371

Denise Souza
COLON HYDROTHERAPY CENTER
972 State Road
Westport, MA 02790
508-675-4153

Linda Stowe
ANNOINTED MASSAGE THERAPY
111 S. Glenstone, Suite 2-203
Springfield, MO 65804
417-832-1962

Patricia A. Stranahan
NATURAL HEALING CENTER, INC
243 Church Street, Suite 100-D
Vienna, VA 22180
703-938-4868

Joan Sughrue, RN, MEd
AWARENESS CENTER
1240 Johnson Ferry Place, Suite 70-B
Marietta, GA 30068
770-977-9959

Lexa Allin Sutherland
AMERICAN INSTITUTE
OF MASSAGE THERAPY
2101 N. Federal Highway
Ft. Lauderdale, FL 33305
954-568-6200

Mike Sutherland
AMERICAN INSTITUTE
OF MASSAGE THERAPY
2101 N. Federal Highway
Ft. Lauderdale, FL 33305
305-568-6200

Margaret Szalata
ADVANCED THERAPIES
1777 Fordham Blvd.
Chapel Hill, NC 27516
919-967-2323

Maya Tai
3441 Cahaunga Blvd. West, Suite 7
Los Angeles, CA 90068
323-512-5493

Bonnie Tetro
SERENITY WELLNESS CENTER
35 Lebanon Ave
Colchester, CT 06415
860-537-6357

Connie Thrush
THE DOO DROP
2386-B E. Buchanan Road
Ithaca, MI 48847
517-875-8634

Jeri C. Tiller
MIND BODY NATUROPATHIC
INSTITUTE
10911 West Ave
San Antonio, TX 78213
210-342-7444

Misty Tiller
MIND BODY NATUROPATHIC
INSTITUTE
10911 West Ave
San Antonio, TX 78213
210-342-7444

William Tiller, N.D.
MIND BODY NATUROPATHIC
INSTITUTE
10911 West Ave
San Antonio, TX 78213
210-342-7444

Tom Tiller III
MIND BODY NATUROPATHIC
INSTITUTE
10911 West Ave
San Antonio, TX 78213
210-342-7444

Marilee Tolen, RN
CORPORATE WELLNESS
CONSULTANTS, INC.
1930 E. Marlton Pike, Suite I-48
Cherry Hill, NJ 08011
609-489-0505

Virginia Tracey
NATURAL THERAPY ASSOCIATES
380 Smith Road
Sedona, AZ 86336
520-204-2874

Cassilda Tucker
HARMONY OF BODY & SELF
5232 Forest Ln., Suite 131
Dallas, TX 75240
214-826-2449

Karen Utter
NATURAL SOLUTION
5205-I Davis Blvd
FortWorth, TX 76180
817-485-9717

Gail Van Treeck
NATURAL HEALTH SERVICES, INC.
1428 N. Farwell
Milwaukee, WI 53202
414-278-8922

Cindy Van-Valen
CINDY JACKSON VAN-VALEN
2563 Western Ave, Park Place Plaza
Guilderland, NY 12084
518-456-8805

Clarisa Vargas
RADIANCE DAY SPA
46-05 Cass Street
San Diego, CA 92109
619-272-6337

Carol Ann Vice, R.N.
INTERNAL HEALTH
1815 W. Charleston Blvd., Suite 5
Las Vegas, NV 89102
702-471-0088

Marilynn Volkoff
HEALTH ESSENTIALS
1563 63rd Avenue, NE
Salem, OR 97301
503-581-6171

Andraa VonBoeselager
COLONICS WITH CARE
2885 E Aurora Avenue, #3
Boulder, CO 80303
303-541-9909

Gwen Wade
WEHINGER CHIROPRACTIC
WELLNESS CENTER
3151 Olin Ave
San Jose, CA 95117-1635
408-246-5242

Peggy Walla
WALLA WELLNESS CENTER
3627 Farquhar
Los Alamitos, CA 90720
562-493-2324

Leigh Warlick
EVERGREEN HOLISTIC HEALTH
1014 East Main Street
Franklin, NC 28734
704-349-3178

Jenne Watkins
MCMAHON & WATKINS—
COLON HYDROTHERAPY
933 W. 3rd
Spokane, WA 99204
509-747-1447

Brenda F. Watson
RENEW LIFE, INC.
401 E. Spruce Street
Tarpon Springs, FL 34689
813-937-6625

Roxanne Watson
CENTER FOR ADVANCED
MEDICINE
4403 Manchester Avenue, Suite 107
Encinitis, CA 92024
619-632-9042

Challen W. Waychoff, N.D.
HEAVENLY WATER
46060 National Road W., Suite 9
St. Clairsville, OH 43950
740-695-9188

Brenda White
COMPREHENSIVE HEALTH CARE
76 West 125th Street
New York, NY 10026
212-410-7822

Linda S. Whitney
INTEGRATIVE HEALTH SERVICES
36 Lincoln Street
Greenfield, MA 01301
413-772-1963

Susan Wiersema
SHEPHERD OF HOPE CLINIC
5085 Anna Drive
Traverse City, MI 49686
616-946-7360

Cynthia Wilkins
FROM THE HEART COLON
HYDROTHERAPY CLINIC
3134 Nahehahe Place
Kihei, HI 96753
808-875-1375

Jean A. Woodilla
900 Eighth Avenue South
Naples, FL 34102
941-435-0899

Beata-Maria Worsham
BEATE'S HOLISTIC
BALANCE STUDIO
100 W. Main Street, Suite #2
Tustin, CA 92680
714-703-3945

Chien Kuo Yao
TRA-SOL HEALTH, INC.
4213 N. Rosemead Blvd., #E
Rosemead, CA 91970
626-285-9961

Susan Yarnovich
8920 Mathew NE
Albuquerque, NM 87112

Jessica Zaccaro
TRANSFORMATIONAL
HEALTH SERVICES
Venice, CA 90405
310-821-4480

Natalya Znamenok
WELLNESS CENTER
1761 E. 12th Street
Brooklyn, NY 11229
718-376-8331

Hypnotherapy

Michael Ellner, D.D., Ph.D.
212-580-3471

Internation Medical and Dental
Hypnotherapy Association
4110 Edgeland, Suite 800
Royal Oak, MI 48073
810-549-5594
800-257-5467 (outside Michigan)

The American Society of Clinical
Hypnosis
2200 East Devon Avenue, Suite 291
Des Plaines, Illinois 60018
708-297-3317

Light Therapy

Environmental Health & Light
Research Institute
16057 Tampa Palms Blvd., Suite 227
Tampa, FL 33647
800-544-4878

Society for Light Treatment and
Biological Rhythms
10200 W 44th Avenue, Suite 304
Wheat Ridge, CO 80033
303-424-3697

Massage Therapy Associations

American Massage Therapy
Association
820 Davis Street, Suite 100
Evanston, IL 60201
708-864-0123

Associated Bodywork & Massage
Professionals
28677 Buffalo Park Road
Evergreen, CO 80439-7347
303-674-8478 or 800-458-2267
303-674-0859 (fax)

Music and Sound Therapy Associations

The American Association
for Music Therapy
P.O. Box 80012
Valley Forge, PA 19484
610-265-4006

The National Association
of Music Therapy
8455 Colesville Road, Suite 930
Silver Spring, MD 20910
301-589-3300

Myotherapy

Bonnie Prudden Pain Erasure
7800 E Speedway
Tuscon AZ 85710
800-221-4634

Naturopathy

(FOLLOWING ARE MEMBERS OF THE AMERICAN ASSOCIATION OF NATUROPATHIC PHYSICIANS (AANP))

ALASKA

Cary Jasper, ND
1407 W. 31st Avenue, 4th Floor
Anchorage, AK 99503
907-276-4611

Torrey Smith, ND
1407 W. 31st Avenue, 4th Floor
Anchorage, AK 99503
907-276-4611

Mary Minor, ND
3201 C. Street
Anchorage, AK 99503
907-567-2330

L. Hope Wing, ND
520 E. 34th Avenue, Suite 305
Anchorage, AK 99503-4116
907-561-2330

Tim Hagney, ND
3201 C. Street, Suite 602
Anchorage, AK 99504
907-563-6200

Daniel Young, ND, LAc
10928 Eagle River Road, Suite 254
Eagle River, AK 99577
907-694-5522

Madeleine Morrison-Young, ND
10928 Eagle River Road, Suite 254
Eagle River, AK 99577
907-694-5522

Toby Wheeler, ND
P.O. Box 2289
Homer, AK 99603-2289
907-235-5954

Patton Pettijohn, ND
P.O. Box 878894
Wasilla, AK 99687
907-276-5077

Ruth Bar-Shalom, ND, LAc
222 Front Street
Fairbanks, AK 99701
907-451-7100

John Soileau, ND
222 Front Street
Fairbanks, AK 99701-3145
907-451-7100

Emily Kane, ND, LAc
418 Harris Street, #329
Juneau, AK 99801
907-586-3655

ALABAMA

Deborah Carter, ND
503 State Street, Suite #3
Muscle Shoals, AL 35661
256-386-9804

ARIZONA

Michael Cronin, ND
2524 N. 53rd Street
Phoenix, AZ 85008
602-990-7424

Ann Manby, NMD
3543 N. Seventh Street
Phoenix, AZ 85014
602-222-3578

Dana Keaton, ND
5333 N. 7th Street, Suite C-221
Phoenix, AZ 85014
602-266-4670

Renee Waldman, BA, ND
4710 N. 31st Way
Phoenix, AZ 85016

Tilli Williams, ND
5333 N. 7th Street, Suite C221
Phoenix, AZ 85016
602-266-4955

John Oxley, ND
6130 N. 16th Street
Phoenix, AZ 85016
602-970-0000

Teresa Vesco, ND
4710 N. 31st Way
Phoenix, AZ 85016

Marianna Fisher, ND
5743 E. Indian School Road
Phoenix, AZ 85018
602-994-8474

Larry Abel, ND
36633 N. 21st Street
Phoenix, AZ 85027
602-595-9358

Karsten Alexandria, ND
13832 N. 32nd Street, Suite C2-4
Phoenix, AZ 85032
602-493-2273

Konrad Kail, ND, PA-C
13832 N. 32nd Street, Suite C2-4
Phoenix, AZ 85032
602-493-2273

Ian Bier, ND, LAc
2150 W. Devonshire Street
Mesa, AZ 85201

Jennifer Trask, ND
540 N. May, #2100
Mesa, AZ 85201

Bruce Davis, ND
1004 E. Jensen
Mesa, AZ 85203
602-962-7893

Scott Luper, NMD
845 S. 21st Street
Mesa, AZ 85204
602-920-0000

Pat Hallman, ND
2112 E. Lehi Road
Mesa, AZ 85213
602-668-0307

Rick Chester, ND, RPh
590 N. Alma School Road, Suite 11
Chandler, AZ 85224
602-963-4410

Gilberto Leon, Jr., ND, BA
1257 W. Warner, Suite A-1
Chandler, AZ 85224
602-857-3484

Karen Van Der Veer, NMD
7950 E. Camelback Road, #206
Scottsdale, AZ 85251
602-945-8407

Theresa Ramsey, ND
7375 E. Stetson, #100
Scottsdale, AZ 85251
602-945-7770

Hope Farmer, ND
6219 East Rose Circle
Scottsdale, AZ 85251

Laryn Callaway, ND
3414 N. 62nd Pl.
Scottsdale, AZ 85251

Serene Wai-Mei Loh, NMD
6505 E. Osborn Road, #243
Scottsdale, AZ 85251
602-990-9635

Mary Ellen O'Brien, ND
P.O. Box 8073
Scottsdale, AZ 85252-8073

Chris Beltran, ND
10301 N. 70th Street, #103
Scottsdale, AZ 85253
602-596-0915

Louise Gutowski, ND
13430 N. Scottsdale Road, Suite 102
Scottsdale, AZ 85254
602-443-1600

Debi Smolinski, ND
7502 E. Kimsey Lane
Scottsdale, AZ 85257

Daniel Rubin, ND
7502 E. Kimsey Lane
Scottsdale, AZ 85257
602-481-7683

Clark Hansen, ND
8040 East Morgan Trail, Suite 23
Scottsdale, AZ 85258
602-991-5092

Christine Madsen, NMD
8300 N. Hayden Road, Suite 207
Scottsdale, AZ 85258
602-596-0671

Jeffrey Feingold, ND
7227 E. Shea Blvd.
Scottsdale, AZ 85260
602-998-8736

Allyn Krieger-Fiedler, ND
16650 E. Hawk Drive
Fountain Hills, AZ 85268
602-816-1600

Kelly Hannigan, RN, ND
14650 Love Court
Fountain Hills, AZ 85268

Kevon Arthurs, ND
P.O. Box 3881
Scottsdale, AZ 85271-3881
619-490-9860

David Macallan, ND
P.O. Box 3881
Scottsdale, AZ 85271-3881
619-490-9860

Kareen O'Brien, ND
2140 E. Broadway Road
Tempe, AZ 85282
602-858-9100

Paul Mittman, ND
2140 E. Broadway Road
Tempe, AZ 85282
602-858-9100

Farra Swan, ND, LM
2435 E. Southern, Suite 8
Tempe, AZ 85282
602-820-0911

Nick Buratovich, NMD
2435 E. Southern Avenue, #9
Tempe, AZ 85282
602-831-0717

Alan Christianson, ND
1402 N. Miller Road, Ste F-6
Scottsdale, AZ 85297
602-425-9224

John Brewer, BA, DC, ND
5002 W. Glendale Avenue, Suite 101
Glendale, AZ 85301-2791
602-937-4756

Debbie Jacques, ND
1858 Paseo San Louis, Suite H
Sierra Vista, AZ 85635
520-459-5210

Nancy Aton, NMD
5813 N. Oracle
Tucson, AZ 85704
520-293-3751

Judy Hutt, ND
268 E. River Road, Suite 130
Tucson, AZ 85704
520-887-4287

Bruce Sadilek, ND
6336 N. Oracle Road, Suite 163
Tucson, AZ 85704-2944

Stacey Kargman, NMD
540 West Prince, Suite A
Tucson, AZ 85705
520-293-5400

J. Lyn Patrick, ND
540 W. Prince Road, Suite A
Tucson, AZ 85705
520-293-5400

Lance Morris, ND, BA
1601 N. Tucson Blvd., Suite 37
Tucson, AZ 85716
520-322-8122

Jorge Badillo-Cochran, ND
1601 N. Tucson Blvd.
Tucson, AZ 85716
520-322-8122

Teri Davis, ND
11505 E. Camino Del Desierto
Tucson, AZ 85747
520-886-7721

Shana Turrell, ND
800 W. Forest Meadows, #249
Flagstaff, AZ 86001

Mark James, ND
809 N. Humphreys
Flagstaff, AZ 86001
520-774-1770

Mary Poore, ND
809 N. Humphreys
Flagstaff, AZ 86001
520-774-1770

Judith Petersen, ND, BS
P.O. Box 126
Joseph City, AZ 86032
520-288-3920

Marley Robertson, ND
315 W. Goodwin
Prescott, AZ 86303
520-778-6169

Debora Chelson, ND
315 W. Goodwin Street
Prescott, AZ 86303
520-445-4995

Michael Vesely, NMD
15 Cindy Lane
Sedona, AZ 86336
520-203-0807

Eric Yarnell, ND
2081 W. Highway 89A, #1C
Sedona, AZ 86336
520-282-6909

Brenna Hatami, ND
15 Cindy Lane
Sedona, AZ 86336
520-203-0807

Silena Heron, ND
2081 W. Hwy. 89A
Sedona, AZ 86336
520-282-6909

Frank Sweet, ND
1731 Mesquite, #5
Lake Havasu City, AZ 86403
520-453-9525

CALIFORNIA

Bridget O'Bryan, ND
1411 5th Street, Suite 405
Santa Monica, CA 90401
310-458-0400

Pamela Durgin, ND, DC
612 Santa Monica Blvd.
Santa Monica, CA 90401
310-576-6176

Holly Castle, ND
1821 Wilshire Blvd., Suite 300
Santa Monica, CA 90403
310-453-9591

Marcus Laux, ND
P.O. Box 1577
Santa Monica, CA 90406-1577
310-306-2220

Bonnie Marsh, ND, CNM
937 S. Coast Hwy. 101, Suite 205
Encinitas, CA 92024
760-436-3455

Mark Stengler, ND
3142 Vista Way, Suite 205
Oceanside, CA 92057
760-966-6385

Angela Stengler, ND
3142 Vista Way, Suite 205
Oceanside, CA 92057
760-966-6385

Jacqueline Carson, ND
2496 E. Street, Suite 300
San Diego, CA 92102-2024
619-236-8285

Subhash Gharmalkar, ND, LAc
1530 Baker Street, Suite G
Costa Mesa, CA 92626-3752
949-437-7710

Robert Abell, ND, LAc
24953 Paseo De Valencia, Suite 16C
Laguna Hills, CA 92653
949-206-9090

Prudence Broadwell, ND, LAc
18837 Brookhurst Street, #210
Fntn Valley, CA 92708
714-965-9266

Robert Broadwell, ND, LAc
18837 Brookhurst Street, #210
Fntn Valley, CA 92708
714-965-9266

Luc Maes, DC, ND
19 E Mission Street, Suite A
Santa Barbara, CA 93101
805-563-8660

Zoe Wells, ND
891 Pismo Street
San Luis Obispo, CA 93401
805-541-2614

Robert Reynolds, ND, PhD
P.O. Box 754
Santa Ynez, CA 93460

Audra Foster, ND
1010 Cass Street, Suite D-7
Monterey, CA 93940
831-373-0141

Carl Hangee-Bauer, ND, LAC
1615 20th Street
San Francisco, CA 94107
415-643-6600

Dean Botz, ND
1536 Grove Street
San Francisco, CA 94117

Marcel Hernandez, ND
4153 B El Camino Way
Palo Alto, CA 94306
650-857-0226

Connie Hernandez, ND
4153 B El Camino Way
Palo Alto, CA 94306
650-857-0226

Christopher Henderson, ND
290 Chestnut Avenue
Palo Alto, CA 94306

Ilene Dahl, ND, LAc
2342 Almond Avenue
Concord, CA 94520
510-602-0582

Ellen Potthoff, DC, ND
200 Gregory Lane, #B1
Pleasant Hill, CA 94523
510-603-7300

Sally LaMont, ND, LAc
500 Tamal Plaza, Suite 507
Corte Madera, CA 94925
415-927-7015

Judy Lee, ND
455 Los Gatos Blvd., Suite 107
Los Gatos, CA 95032
408-358-3544

Michele Goodwin, ND, CMP
555 Soquel Avenue, Suite 260-H
Santa Cruz, CA 95062
408-459-9206

J. Claire Green, ND
4778 Holly Street
Santa Rosa, CA 95404
707-544-5546

David Field, ND, LAc
46 Doctors Park Drive
Santa Rosa, CA 95405
707-576-7388

Mary Wheeler, ND
P.O. Box 6901
Eureka, CA 95502

Heidi Hook, ND
6615 Bear River Lane
Auburn, CA 95602

James Mally, ND
112 Douglas Blvd.
Roseville, CA 95678
916-782-1275

Priscilla Monroe, RN, ND
2600 Capital Avenue, Suite 213
Sacramento, CA 95816
916-448-9927

Jon Kvenvolden, ND
4220 H Street
Sacramento, CA 95819
916-491-5170

Jeanette Abel, ND
P.O. Box 1042
Corning, CA 96021
808-969-7848

CANADA

Theresa Maclean, ND
139 Union Street
Berwick, NS, Canada B0P 1E0
902-538-8733

Dan Smith, ND
3 Hillborne Ct. RR, #4
Uxbridge, ON, Canada L9P 1R4
905-852-7961

Chris Turner, ND
459 William Avenue
Winnepeg, MB, Canada R3A0J5
204-956-1555

Paul Conyette, ND
2637 Victoria Avenue
Brandon, MB, Canada R7B 0M9
204-727-3524

Stefan Kuprowsky, ND, BSc, MA
RR1 Box 50 Pacific Shores
Nanoose Bay, BC, Canada V0R 2R0
250-468-7133

Gudrun Tonskamper, ND
#304 1493 Johnston Road
White Rock, BC, Canada V4B3Z4
604-536-1400

S. Craig Wagstaff, ND
11270 Hwy. 97N
Winfield, BC, Canada V4V 1H8
250-766-3633

Jim Chan, ND
#101 3380 Maquinna Drive
Vancouver, BC, Canada V5S4C6
604-435-3786

Dorothy Fairley, BSW, ND
2021 W. 4th Avenue, Suite 250
Vancouver, BC, Canada V6J IN3
604-738-2205

Valerie Farina, ND
1960 W. 7th Avenue, #310
Vancouver, BC, Canada V6S 1T1
604-738-6219

Ina Wong,
#8-310 Goldstream Avenue
Victoria, BC, Canada V8X 4N4
250-478-4057

COLORADO

Lori Olaf, ND
6558 S. Yosemite Circle
Greenwood Village, CO 80111
303-694-5757

Debra Rouse, ND
255 Detroit Street
Denver, CO 80206
303-322-9294

Steve Rissman, ND
210 University Blvd., Suite 440
Denver, CO 80206
303-321-0222

Jenny Demeaux, RNC, ND, LM
1673 Fillmore Street
Denver, CO 80206
303-331-6919

Carrie Louise Daenell, ND
2222 E. 18th Avenue
Denver, CO 80206
303-333-3733

Rena Bloom, ND
1181 S. Parker Road, Suite 101
Denver, CO 80231
303-337-4884

Jacob Schor, ND
1181 S. Parker Road, Suite 101
Denver, CO 80231
303-337-4884

James Rouse, ND
3285 30th
Boulder, CO 80301
303-449-1330

Nancy Rao, ND, LAc
3005 47th Street, Suite F-2
Boulder, CO 80301
303-545-2021

Tara Skye Goldin, ND
4770 Baseline, Suite220
Boulder, CO 80302
303-494-4433

Jody Shevins, ND, DHANP
5353 Manhattan Circle, Suite 102
Boulder, CO 80303
303-494-3713

Erik Flatland, ND Dipl.Ac
2885 Aurora Avenue, Suite 27
Boulder, CO 80303
303-447-1339

Johannah Reilly, ND
2660 13th Street
Boulder, CO 80304
303-541-9600

Michele Loewe, ND
607 10 Street, Suite 105
Golden, CO 80401
303-215-1669

Virginia Osborne, ND
P.O. Box 774135
Steamboat Springs, CO 80477
970-879-8569

Clare Wykert, ND
504 S. College Avenue
Fort Collins, CO 80524
970-495-9067

Clinton Pomroy, ND
2160 W. Drake Road, Suite A-1
Fort Collins, CO 80526
970-484-6390

Glen Nagel, ND
104 E. St. Vrain, Suite 10
Colorado Springs, CO 80903
719-635-2050

Edith Sucher, ND
712 S. Tejon Street
Colorado Springs, CO 80903
719-634-0292

Mary Frazel, ND
104 E. St. Vrain, Suite 10
Colorado Springs, CO 80903
719-635-2050

William Nelson, ND
1422 N. Hancock Avenue
Suite 5 South
Colorado Springs, CO 80903
719-635-4776

Ruth Adele, ND
1625 W. Uintah Street, Suite I
Colorado Springs, CO 80904
719-636-0098

Louise Edwards, ND, LAc
929 E. 3rd Avenue
Durango, CO 81301
970-247-2043

James Massey, BS, ND
755 E 2nd Avenue, Suite C
Durango, CO 81301-5210
970-259-7979

Rick Jensen, ND
835 Colorado Avenue
Grand Junction, CO 81501
970-248-9520

CONNECTICUT

Nancy Mazur, ND
P.O. Box 1644
Avon, CT 06001
860-675-1011

Paul Herscu, ND, DHANP
115 Elm Street, Suite 210
Enfield, CT 06082
203-763-1225

Amy Rothenberg, ND, DHANP
115 Elm Street
Enfield, CT 06082
203-763-1225

Lucia Coletta, ND, BA
139 Hazard Avenue, #3
Enfield, CT 06082
860-749-1941

Whitney Miller, ND
126 Boston Post Road
East Lyme, CT 06333-1039
860-691-1166

Deirdre O'Connor, ND
12 Roosevelt Avenue
Mystic, CT 06355
860-572-9566

Bert Schwarz, ND
12 Rossevelt Avenue
Mystic, CT 06355

Christine Girard-Couture, ND
130 Division Street
Derby, CT 06418
203-732-1138

Tammy Alex, ND
35 Boston Street, #4
Guilford, CT 06437
203-453-0122

Kathleen Riley, ND
P.O. Box 65, 31 Hawleyville Road
Hawleyville, CT 06440
203-426-2306

Michael Kane, ND
87 Bernie O'Rourke Drive
Middletown, CT 06457
860-347-8600

Enrico Liva, ND
87 Bernie O'Rourke Drive
Middletown, CT 06457
860-347-8600

Mary Markow, ND
87 Bernie O'Rourke Drive
Middletown, CT 06457
860-347-8600

Keli Samuelson, ND
87 Bernie O'Rourke Drive
Middletown, CT 06457
860-347-8600

Jacqueline Germain, ND
87 Bernie O'Rourke Drive
Middletown, CT 06457
860-347-8600

Eric Secor, ND,MSA
87 Bernie O'Rourke Drive
Middletown, CT 06457
860-347-8600

Cathryn Flanagan, ND
12 Spencer Plains Road
Old Saybrook, CT 06475
860-399-1212

Andrew Rubman, ND
900 Main Street South
Southbury, CT 06488-2217
203-262-6755

Michael Petreycik, ND
P.O. Box 747
Stratford, CT 06497
203-333-8916

James Sensenig, ND
2558 Whitney Avenue
Hamden, CT 06518
203-230-2200

Robin Ritterman, ND
2558 Whitney Avenue
Hamden, CT 06518
203-230-2200

Ron Hobbs, ND
221 University Avenue
Bridgeport, CT 06601
203-576-4110

Jennifer Brett, ND, DiplAc
998 Nichols Avenue
Stratford, CT 06614
203-377-1525

Robert Murphy, ND
118 Migeon Avenue
Torrington, CT 06790
860-482-4730

Michelle Pouliot, ND
118 Mijun Avenue
Torrington, CT 06790
860-482-4730

Debra Gibson, ND
51 Sherman Hill Road, Suite A 104-B
Woodbury, CT 06798
203-266-4007

Sherry Stemper, ND
18 Old Route 7
Brookfield, CT 06804
203-740-7745

Harold Ofgang, ND
57 North Street, Suite 323
Danbury, CT 06810
203-798-0533

Sandoval Melim, PhD, CNS, PCS, ND
1500 Boston Post Road, 2nd Floor
Darien, CT 06820
203-656-6635

Susanna Reid, PhD, ND
1500 Boston Post Road, 2nd Floor
Darien, CT 06820
203-656-6635

Victoria Zupa, ND
762 Post Road
Darien, CT 06820
203-275-6599

John Farrell, NMD
239 Glenville Road
Greenwich, CT 06831
203-531-8230

Daniel Heller, ND
112 Main Street
Norwalk, CT 06851
203-845-0734

Marvin Schweitzer, ND
1 Westport Avenue
Norwalk, CT 06851
203-847-2788

Christopher Fabricius, ND
21 Ann Suite AC-1
Norwalk, CT 06854
203-299-0143

Kathryn Foulser, ND
158 Danbury Road, #1
Ridgefield, CT 06877

Howard Fine, ND DHANP CCH
4 Cross Highway
Westport, CT 06880
203-221-0216

Lawrence Caprio, ND
830 Post Road E.
Westport, CT 06880
203-226-4167

Gabriele Kallenborn, ND
61 Edgewater Common Lane
Westport, CT 06880
203-454-5989

Pearlyn Goodman-Herrick, ND, DHANP
21 Trails End Road
Weston, CT 06883
203-227-5534

Peter D'Adamo, ND
2009 Summer Street
Stamford, CT 06905
203-348-4800

DISTRICT OF COLUMBIA

Andrea Sullivan, PhD, ND
4601 Connecticut Avenue N.W., #6
Washington, DC 20008
202-244-4545

Michelle Cochran, ND, MW
4820 Reno Road, N.W.
Washington, DC 20008
202-237-0717

Monique Lai, ND
4801 Wisconsin Avenue N.W.
Washington, DC 20016
202-244-1310

FLORIDA

Ember Carianna, ND
1900 S. Olive Avenue
W. Palm Beach, FL 33401-7726
561-835-6821

GEORGIA

John Davis, ND
1241 Virginia Avenue NE, #C-4
Atlanta, GA 30306
404-325-7734

HAWAII

John Turetzky, ND
99-128 Aiea Heights Drive, #501
Aiea, HI 96701
808-487-8833

Mary Lynn Garner, ND, DHANP
P.O. Box 1152
Captain Cook, HI 96704-1152
808-334-6294

Kevin Davison, ND, LAc
444 Hana Hwy., Suite, #211
Kahului, HI 96732
808-871-4722

Michael Traub, ND, DHANP
75-5759 Kuakini Hwy., #202
Kailua-Kona, HI 96740
808-329-2114

James Niehaus, PA, SA, ND
P.O. Box 1858
Kapaa, HI 96746
808-822-2707

Miles Greenberg, ND
1420 Kanepoonui Road
Kapaa, HI 96746-9046
808-245-2277

Anne-Marie Lambert, ND
P.O. Box 688
Kealakekua, HI 96750-0688
808-323-3370

Steven Dubey, ND
3093 Akahi Street
Lihue, HI 96766
808-245-2277

Laura O'Neal, ND
P.O. Box 98
Lahaina, HI 96767
808-661-5432

David Kern, ND
P.O. Box 567
Makawao, HI 96768
808-572-6091

Nathan Ehrlich, ND
P.O. Box 756
Makawao, HI 96768
808-572-1388

Nima Rosepiper-Meeker, ND
3543-B Baldwin Avenue
Makawao, HI 96768

Julie Holmes, ND
651 Omaopio Road
Kula, HI 96790
808-878-3267

James Howard, ND
1188 Bishop Street, Suite 1408
Honolulu, HI 96813
808-536-8891

Jason Uchida, ND
181 South Kukui, Suite 207
Honolulu, HI 96813
808-545-2093

Karen Tan, ND, LAc
615 Piikoi Street, Penthouse #2
Honolulu, HI 96814
808-593-9445

Jack Burke, ND, DHANP
615 Piikoi Street, Penthouse #2
Honolulu, HI 96814
808-593-9445

Hazel Ogawa-Lerman, ND
1150 S. King Street, Suite 404
Honolulu, HI 96814
808-597-8109

Laurie Steelsmith, ND, LAc
4211 Waialae Avenue, Suite 401
Honolulu, HI 96816
808-737-0414

Lori Kimata, ND
2569 Ipulei Way
Honolulu, HI 96816
808-735-5433

IDAHO

Brent Mathieu, ND, BS, DHANP
1412 W. Washington
Boise, ID 83702
208-338-5590

Joan Haynes, ND
1612 W. Jefferson Street
Boise, ID 83702
208-338-0405

Karen Erickson, ND, LM
1509 South Roberts, Suite 101
Boise, ID 83705
208-383-4833

Todd Schlapfer, ND
1000 W. Hubbard, Suite 120
Coeur D'alene, ID 83814
208-664-1644

Curt Eastin, DDS, ND
1000 W. Hubbard, Suite 120
Coeur D'Alene, ID 83814
208-664-1644

Alan Miller, ND
501 S. Lincoln
Sandpoint, ID 83864
208-265-1342

Kathleen Head, ND
2013 Janelle Way
Sandpoint, ID 83864
208-263-1337

Gabrielle Duebendorfer, ND
2023 Sandpoint West Drive
Sandpoint, ID 83864
208-265-2213

ILLINOIS

Julie Martin, ND
273 Market Square, #14
Lake Forest, IL 60045
847-735-9142

Timothy Birdsall, ND
2520 Elisha Avenue
Zion, IL 60099
847-872-6067

Hugh Jenkins, ND, DC
2148 W 95th Street
Chicago, IL 60643-1120
773-445-6800

Laurence Grey, ND, MD
5528 N. Chester Avenue, #1N
Chicago, IL 60656
905-725-7000

Pamela Taylor, ND
Suite 706, Fifth Avenue Building
Moline, IL 61265-7910
309-797-3271

KANSAS

Stanley Beyrle, ND
1101 N. West Street
Wichita, KS 67203
316-942-2220

LOUISIANA

Joanie Goss, ND
P.O. Box 144
Lacassine, LA 70650-0144
318-588-4249

Andrea Neri, ND
P.O. Box 12533
Alexandria, LA 71315
318-443-3322

MASSACHUSETTS

Margaret Wakefield, ND
P.O. Box 351
Tyringham, MA 01264
413-237-0972

Jodie Tonelli-Chapin, ND
232 Chandler
Worcester, MA 01609
508-754-2707

Janet Beaty, ND
56 Winthrop Street
Concord, MA 01742
978-369-2266

Paul Rajcok, MA, ND
6 Courthouse Ln., Suite 16
Chelmsford, MA 01824
978-452-3776

Barbara Silbert, DC, ND
172 State Street, #1
Newburyport, MA 01950
978-465-0929

Shiva Barton, ND, LAc
186 Alewife Brook Parkway
Cambridge, MA 02138
617-876-2660

Lynn Hsu, BS, ND, MS
824 Boylston Street, Suite 101
Chestnut Hill, MA 02167
617-739-1001

Geffin Falken, ND
1073 Hancock Street, Suite 103
Quincy, MA 02169
617-448-0095

Joan-Ellen Macredis, ND
63 Moraine Street, #18
Belmont, MA 02178
617-489-9835

Barry Taylor, ND
270 Winter Street
Weston, MA 02193
781-237-8505

Anne McClenon, ND, LM
116 Court Street
Plymouth, MA 02360
508-830-1644

Elizabeth Wotton, ND, LM
116 Court Street
Plymouth, MA 02360
508-830-1644

Peter Glidden, ND
P.O. Box 1300
Barnstable, MA 02630
508-362-7089

Maria Perillo, ND
62 A Cranberry Hwy.
Orleans, MA 02653
508-255-8686

Paul Giordano, DC, ND
101 President Avenue
Fall River, MA 02720
508-324-9999

MARYLAND

Angela Duncan, ND
907 Hudson Avenue, #3
Takoma Park, MD 20912

Willow Moore, ND, DC
10806 Reisters Town Road, #1E
P.O. Box 684
Owingsmills, MD 21117
410-356-4600

Steven Sinclair, ND
1305 Pennsylvania Avenue
Hagerstown, MD 21742
301-714-0500

Giselle Lai, ND
1305 Pennsylvania Avenue
Hagerstown, MD 21742
301-714-0500

MAINE

Sarah Ackerly, ND
171 Park Row
Brunswick, ME 04011
207-798-3993

Julie Taylor, ND, LAc
171 Park Row
Brunswick, ME 04011
207-798-3993

Richard Maurer, ND
34 Cumberland Street
Brunswick, ME 04011
207-721-8400

Priscilla Skerry, ND, RT
66 Pearl Street
Portland, ME 04101
207-772-5227

Devra Krassner, ND
4 Milk Street
Portland, ME 04101
207-773-2517

Janet Ballard, ND
220 Water Street, Suite 3
Hallowell, ME 04347
207-621-4100

Laura Bridgman, ND
142 Hammond Street, Suite 5
Bangor, ME 04401
207-941-0981

Laralee Jasper-Litov, ND
35 Harden Avenue
Camden, ME 04843
207-236-0036

MICHIGAN

Suzie Zick, ND
111 N. First Suite1
Ann Arbor, MI 48104
734-994-6315

MINNESOTA

Helen Healy, ND
905 Jefferson Avenue, #202
St. Paul, MN 55102
612-222-4111

Amrit Devgun, BSc, ND
658 Selby Avenue, 2nd Floor
St. Paul, MN 55104
612-227-1803

John Hauser, ND
3016 Portland Avenue
Minneapolis, MN 55407-1527
612-824-7585

Andrew Lucking, ND
5032 Xerxes Avenue S.
Minneapolis, MN 55410
612-926-1549

Karla Lilleberg, ND
1521 Northway Drive, Suite 112
St. Cloud, MN 56303
320-654-0871

Kristi Hawkes, ND
1413 Broadway
Alexandria, MN 56308
320-762-4295

MONTANA

Roberta Bourgon, ND
328 Grand Avenue
Billings, MT 59101
406-259-5096

Margaret Beeson, ND
328 Grand Avenue
Billings, MT 59101-5923
406-259-5096

Mona Morstein, ND, DHANP
518 9th Street South
Great Falls, MT 59405-2114
406-727-6680

Michael Bergkamp, ND, LAc
516 Fuller Avenue
Helena, MT 59601
406-442-2091

Nancy Aagenes, ND, LAc
330 Eleventh Avenue
Helena, MT 59601
406-442-8508

Elisabeth Kirchhof, ND, BA, BS
203 Haggerty Lane
Bozeman, MT 59715
406-586-8244

Michael Lang, ND
P.O. Box 1473
Ennis, MT 59729
406-682-5000

Nancy Dunne-Boggs, ND
715 Kensington Suite 24a
Missoula, MT 59801
406-728-8544

Amy Haynes, ND
521 S. 2nd W.
Missoula, MT 59801
406-721-2147

Sarah Lane, ND
210 N. Higgins, Suite 222
Missoula, MT 59802
406-549-0005

Jamison Starbuck, JD, ND
210 N. Higgins, Suite 222
Missoula, MT 59802
406-549-0005

Timothy Binder, ND, DC, LAc
173 Blodgett Camp Road
Hamilton, MT 59840
406-363-4044

Hillery Daily, ND
413 State Street
Hamilton, MT 59840
406-375-0167

Ann Waltz, ND, CA
322 2nd Avenue W, Suite B
Kalispell, MT 59901
406-756-0308

Steven Gordon, ND
333 Baker Avenue
Whitefish, MT 59937
406-863-9300

NORTH CAROLINA

Susan Delaney, ND
301 Weaver Street
Carrboro, NC 27510
919-932-6262

Priscilla Evans, ND
P.O. Box 69
Cary, NC 27512
919-604-2235

Preeta Kuhlman, ND
Blue Ridge Plaza, Suite 203
Raleigh, NC 27607
919-781-3978

Tim Kuhlman, ND
Blue Ridge Plaza, Suite 203
Raleigh, NC 27607
919-781-3978

Jay Wrigley, ND, BA
1201 East Boulevard
Charlotte, NC 28203
704-332-1201

Leang Eap, ND
6548 Carmel Road, #124
Charlotte, NC 28226
704-544-8681

Stephen Barrie, ND
63 Zillicoa Street
Asheville, NC 28801-1074
828-253-0621

Mary James, ND
27 Spring Hollow Circle
Asheville, NC 28805
828-253-0621

NORTH DAKOTA

Conradine Zarndt, ND
C/O Margaret Zarndt
New Salem, ND 58563

NEBRASKA

Ranall Bradley, ND, DHANP
7447 Farnam Street
Omaha, NE 68114
402-391-6714

NEW HAMPSHIRE

Shirley Snow, ND
755 Straw Hill
Manchester, NH 03104-1681
603-644-4525

Liam McClintock, ND,MAcOM
401 Gilford Avenue, Suite 250
Gilford, NH 03246
603-524-9261

Pamela Herring, ND, DHANP,
CCH
46 S. Main Street
Concord, NH 03301
603-228-0407

Christine Kuhlman, ND, CNM,
MPH
35 West Street
Concord, NH 03301
603-224-0000

Nina Iselin, ND
Main Street
Dublin, NH 03444
603-563-7066

Maureen Williams, ND
P.O. Box 70
Lyme, NH 03768-0070
603-643-4818

Leon Hecht, III, ND, BS
500 Market Street, Suite 1F
Portsmouth, NH 03801-3456
603-427-6800

Kristy Fassler, ND, DHANP
500 Market Street, #1F
Portsmouth, NH 03801-3456
603-427-6800

James D'Adamo, ND, DC
44-46 Bridge Street
Portsmouth, NH 03801-3902
416-968-0496

Carole Robinson, ND
P.O. Box 887
Exeter, NH 03833
603-772-1800

NEW JERSEY

Donald Brown, ND
180 Wyoming Avenue
Maplewood, NJ 07040
973-762-0840

Irene Catania, ND
119 First Street
Ho-Ho-Kus, NJ 07423
201-444-4900

Jack Larmer, ND
34 Bussell Court
Dumont, NJ 07628
201-385-7106

NEW MEXICO

Catherine Stauber, DC,
ND,DHANP
1904 N. Gonzales
Las Vegas, NM 87701
505-454-9525

NEVADA

J. Leandra Even, ND
2810 W. Charleston Blvd., #F-55
Las Vegas, NV 89102
702-258-7860

NEW YORK

Kelly Cohen, ND
1431 Vian Avenue
Hewlett, NY 11557
212-995-5379

Roseanne Nenninger, ND
109 Randall Avenue
Port Jefferson, NY 11777
516-331-0161

Steve Nenninger, ND
109 Randall Avenue
Port Jefferson, NY 11777
516-331-0161

Ashley Lewin, ND
27 Locust Street
Wading River, NY 11792
516-929-3950

Kristin Stiles, ND
200 Front Street
Vestal, NY 13850
607-754-6877

Robert Johnson, BS, ND
120 Allens Creek Road
Rochester, NY 14618-3306

OHIO

Donn Griffith, NMD
3859 W Dublin-Granville Road
Dublin, OH 43017
614-889-2556

OKLAHOMA

Michael Leu, ND, RPh
3100 S. Elm Place Suite B
Broken Arrow, OK 74012
405-327-5064

OREGON

Dickson Thom, DDS, ND
4770 SW Watson Avenue
Beaverton, OR 97005
503-520-8859

Mitchell Stargrove, ND, LAc
4720 SW Watson Avenue
Beaverton, OR 97005
503-526-0397

Jack Daugherty, ND, DC, BS
12195 SW Allen Blvd.
Beaverton, OR 97005
503-646-0697

Ravinder Sahni, ND, DC, BMS
9570 SW Beaverton Hillsdale Hwy.
Beaverton, OR 97005-3309
503-641-8503

David Shefrin, ND
Beaver Creek Business Park
Beaverton, OR 97006
503-644-7800

Chris Meletis, ND
2708 SW 199th Pl.
Aloha, OR 97006-2262
503-231-1825

Linda Meloche, ND, LAc
8070 SW Hall
Beaverton, OR 97008
503-643-0156

William Mehan, ND
27636 SE Haley Road
Boring, OR 97009
503-663-0596

Kimberley Horner, MS, ND
13233 SE Shannon View Drive
Clackamas, OR 97015

Maureen Barnhart, ND
8800 SE Sunnyside Road, Suite 111
Clackamas, OR 97015
503-654-3225

Jennifer Reid, ND
657 NE Hood Avenue
Gresham, OR 97030
503-519-4680

Corey Resnick, ND
2204-8 NW Birdsdale
Gresham, OR 97030
503-661-5401

Amber Ackerson, ND, LMT
2204-8 NW Birdsdale
Gresham, OR 97030
503-661-5401

Pamela Jeanne, ND, RN
22400 SE Stark Street
Gresham, OR 97030
503-669-2997

Kenneth Rifkin, ND, LAc
338 SW 2nd Street
Lake Oswego, OR 97034
503-636-2975

Jacob Farin, ND
560 First Street, Suite 204
Lake Oswego, OR 97034
503-636-2734

Kathleen Germain, ND, MS, LAc
545 1st Street
Lake Oswego, OR 97034
503-635-6643

Noel Peterson, ND
560 1st Street, Suite 204
Lake Oswego, OR 97034
503-636-2734

Anna MacIntosh, PhD, ND
545 1st Street
Lake Oswego, OR 97034
503-631-8621

Durr Elmore, ND, DHANP
P.O. Box 990
Mulino, OR 97042
503-829-7326

Bozena Celnik, ND
19633 SW 67th Avenue
Tualatin, OR 97062

Richard Brinkman, ND
4320 Calaroga Drive
West Linn, OR 97068-1008
800-640-0848

Victoria Larson, ND
10000 SE 222nd Avenue
Gresham, OR 97080-8717
503-658-7130

Kevin Wilson, ND
150 NE 3rd Avenue
Hillsboro, OR 97124-3150
503-648-0484

Bruce Dickson, ND, DHANP
1900 N. Hwy. 99 W. Suite A
McMinnville, OR 97128
503-434-6515

Larry Herdener, ND
415 E. 3rd Street
Mcminnville, OR 97128-4612
503-434-6170

Kathleen Flewelling, ND
2647 Hwy 101 N.
Seaside, OR 97138
503-717-1770

Erin Lommen, ND
4444 SW Corbett Avenue
Portland, OR 97201
503-224-4003

Gary Weiner, ND
4444 SW Corbett Avenue
Portland, OR 97201
503-224-4003

Dohn Kruschwitz, MDND
4444 SW Corbett Avenue
Portland, OR 97201
503-224-8476

Jared Zeff, ND
1099 SW Columbia, Suite 300
Portland, OR 97201
503-221-9974

Guru Sandesh Khalsa, ND
049 SW Porter Street
Portland, OR 97201
503-499-4343

Catherine Downey, ND
049 SW Porter Street
Portland, OR 97201
503-499-4343 ext. 256

Richard Barrett, ND
049 SW Porter Street
Portland, OR 97201
503-255-4860

Susan Roberts, ND
4444 SW Corbett Avenue
Portland, OR 97201-4207
503-224-4003

Samantha Brody, ND
2307 SE Tibbets
Portland, OR 97202
503-231-8322

Steven Sandberg-Lewis, ND
6315 SE 15th Avenue
Portland, OR 97202
503-255-7355

Peggy Rollo, ND, LAc
833 SW 11th Suite612
Portland, OR 97205
503-223-7067

Katharina Torri, ND
P.O. Box 3706
Portland, OR 97208-3706

Michelle Suber, ND
1915 NW Northrup
Portland, OR 97209
503-224-4876

Tori Hudson, ND
2067 NW Lovejoy
Portland, OR 97209
503-222-2322

Steven Bailey, ND
2606 NW Vaughn
Portland, OR 97210
503-224-8083

Bradley Bongiovanni, ND
2515 NW Overton
Portland, OR 97210
503-255-7355

Arianna Staruch, ND
1715 NW 23rd Avenue
Portland, OR 97210
503-227-3828

Keyena Nishawa, ND
5827 NE 31st Avenue
Portland, OR 97211

Sara Hazel, ND
P.O. Box 11272
Portland, OR 97211

Sonja Petterson, ND
3412 NE Fremont Street
Portland, OR 97212
503-255-7355

Mary Caselli, ND
1823 NE 13th
Portland, OR 97212
503-335-8983

Bernie Bayard, ND
1722 NE Schuyler
Portland, OR 97212
503-288-9793

Jonna Alexander, ND
635 NE 78th
Portland, OR 97213
503-256-0931

Audrey Bergsma, ND
912 NE 71st Avenue
Portland, OR 97213

Lori Von Der Heydt, ND
4445 NE Fremont
Portland, OR 97213
503-249-7752

Rene Minz, MD, ND
4110 SE Hawthorne Blvd., #139
Portland, OR 97214
503-234-1531

David Naimon, ND
1825 SE 12th Street, #3
Portland, OR 97214

Martin Milner, ND
1330 SE 39th Avenue
Portland, OR 97214
503-232-1100

Stephen Austin, ND
1330 SE 39th Avenue
Portland, OR 97214
503-232-1100

Karen Frangos, ND
1919 SE 35th Pl.
Portland, OR 97214-5801

Jeffrey Baker, ND
8037 SE Main Street
Portland, OR 97215

Deah Baird, ND
415 SE 68th Avenue
Portland, OR 97215

Mary Scott, ND
1835 SE 50th Avenue
Portland, OR 97215
503-232-4047

Lowell Chodosh, ND, LAc
1922 SE 42nd
Portland, OR 97215
503-231-6476

Barbara MacDonald, ND
7735 SE Morrison Street
Portland, OR 97215
503-255-7355 ext237

Russell Marz, ND
2002 SE 50th Avenue
Portland, OR 97215
503-233-0585

Patricia Timberlake, ND, MSW,
LCSW
1835 SE 50th Avenue
Portland, OR 97215
503-236-1366

Nancy Scarlett, ND
11231 SE Market Street
Portland, OR 97216
503-255-7355 x106

Alexandra Gayek, ND
8316 SE Yamhill
Portland, OR 97216
503-261-9010

Joseph Coletto, ND, LAc
10525 SE Cherry Blsm. Drive
Portland, OR 97216
503-254-3566

Susan Allen, ND
8602 SE Taylor Street
Portland, OR 97216
503-257-9754

Rosetta Koach, ND
11000 SE Stephens Street
Portland, OR 97216-3234

Sierra Levy, ND
5247 N. Haight
Portland, OR 97217
503-335-0292

Rita Bettenburg, ND
10360 NE Wasco Street
Portland, OR 97220
503-252-8125

Elizabeth Collins, ND
10360 NE Wasco
Portland, OR 97220
503-252-8125

Thomas Abshier, ND
1414 NE 109th
Portland, OR 97220
503-255-9500

Nora Tallman, ND
10360 NE Wasco Street
Portland, OR 97220
503-252-8125

Suzanne Lawton, BA, ND
4041 NE 99th Avenue
Portland, OR 97220
503-252-2612

Katherine Zieman, ND, LM
10360 NE Wasco
Portland, OR 97220
503-252-8125

Barbara Betcone Jolley, ND, DC
4610 SW Beaverton Hillsdale Hwy.
Portland, OR 97221-2910
503-245-3444

Louise Tolzmann, ND
3436 SE Johnson Creek Blvd.
Portland, OR 97222
503-255-7355 x169

Joyce Ho, ND
6501 SE King Road
Milwaukie, OR 97222
503-777-9839

Stacey Raffety, RN, LAc, ND
9830 SW McKenzie
Tigard, OR 97223
503-639-1712

David Greenspan, ND
11509 SW Pacific Hwy.
Tigard, OR 97223
503-293-1151

Lori Horan, ND
8625 SW Inez Street
Tigard, OR 97224

Jacqueline Jacques, ND
1600 SW Cedar Hills Blvd., Suite
102
Portland, OR 97225
503-644-4446

Rick Marinelli, ND, MAcOM
1600 SW Cedar Hills Blvd.
Portland, OR 97225
503-644-4446

Beverly Yates, ND
2161 NE Broadway
Portland, OR 97232
503-280-1950

Suzanne Scopes, ND
316 NE 28th
Portland, OR 97232
503-230-0812

Holly Zapf, ND
1444 NE Broadway
Portland, OR 97232
503-460-0630

Patricia Meyer, ND
800 SE 181st Avenue
Portland, OR 97233
503-667-1961

Thomas Kruzel, ND
800 SE 181st Avenue
Portland, OR 97233
503-667-1961

Brian Maccoy, ND
19125 SW Stark
Portland, OR 97233
503-491-1067

John Collins, ND DHANP
800 SE 181st Avenue
Portland, OR 97233
503-667-1961

Jan Selliken Bernard, ND
9350 SE Dundee Ct.
Portland, OR 97266
360-906-1180

Robert Sklovsky, Pharm D, ND
6910 SE Lake Road
Milwaukie, OR 97267
503-654-3938

Dan Carter, ND
P.O. Box 33961
Portland, OR 97292
503-255-7355

Andrew Perry, ND, BA, LMT
410 Lancaster Drive N.E., Suite B
Salem, OR 97301
503-364-1441

Alex Serkalow, ND
859 Medical Center Drive NE
Salem, OR 97301
503-588-2333

Paul Anderson, ND
1115 Liberty Street SE
Salem, OR 97302
503-365-0377

Linda Taylor, ND
1447 Liberty Street SE
Salem, OR 97302
503-910-7771

Michael Jacobs, ND, MS, PT
804 SW 4th Street
Corvallis, OR 97333
541-757-7660

K.E. Edmisten, ND, LAc
344 SW 7th Street, Suite B
Newport, OR 97365
541-265-6378

Elizabeth Dickey, MSW, ND
132 E. Broadway, Suite 420
Eugene, OR 97401
541-465-1155

Stephanie Wilson, ND
1755 Coburg Road, Building 2
Eugene, OR 97401
541-683-9357

Adrienne Borg, ND
74 E 18th Avenue, Suite 12
Eugene, OR 97401
503-686-3330

Stephen Messer, ND, DHANP
400 East 2nd Street, #105
Eugene, OR 97401
503-343-2384

Daniel Hardt, ND
280 W. 11th Avenue
Eugene, OR 97401-3031
503-683-4404

Karen Kunkler, ND
1965½ Monroe Street
Eugene, OR 97405

Julie Parke, ND
15 S. 6th Street
Cottage Grove, OR 97424
541-942-8399

Sharol Marie Tilgner, ND
P.O. Box 279
Creswell, OR 97426
541-895-5152

Mark Immel, ND, DHANP
1525 12th Street, Suite 4b
Florence, OR 97439
541-997-6255

Joseph Kassel, ND LAc
25632 Jeans Road
Veneta, OR 97487
541-935-3453

Linda Herrick, ND, LAc
586 Glenwood Drive
Ashland, OR 97520
541-482-0409

Deborah Frances, ND, RN
316 SE 8th Street
Grants Pass, OR 97526
541-474-0503

John Hahn, ND, DPM
334 NE Irving Avenue, Suite 104
Bend, OR 97701
541-385-0775

Sheila Myers, ND, LAc
711 NE Irving
Bend, OR 97701
541-385-6249

Howard Reingold, ND
365 NE Greenwood Suite 3
Bend, OR 97701
541-389-6935

Mark Cooper, ND, LAc
61555 Parrell Road
Bend, OR 97702
541-389-4600

John Winters, ND
1606 6th Street
La Grande, OR 97850
541-963-7289

PENNSYLVANIA

Steve Kutlesa, ND
495 North Hermitage Road
Hermitage, PA 16148
724-981-4144

Brian Freeman, ND
3913 Market Street
Camp Hill, PA 17011
717-730-9066

Michael Reece, ND
4233 Oregon Pike
Ephrata, PA 17522
717-859-4222

Gregory Pais, ND, DHANP
837 Washington Blvd.
Williamsport, PA 17701
717-320-0747

Steven Nemeroff, ND
3 Abington-Executive Park
Clarks Summit, PA 18411
717-585-4040

Michael DiPalma, ND
2700 South Eagle Road
Newtown, PA 18940
215-579-1300

PUERTO RICO

Milva Vega Garcia, ND
Avenue Fagot, #81
Ponce, PR 00731
787-840-3793

Madhavi Torres-Cabret, PT, ND
1603 Ponce De Leon Suite123
San Juan, PR 00909
787-722-4365

Efrain Rodriguez, ND
Calle Lodi 571, Urb. Luarca
Rio Piedres, PR 00924
787-751-4682

RHODE ISLAND

Jill Sanders Stanard, ND
469 Angell Street
Providence, RI 02906
401-455-0546

SOUTH DAKOTA

Lauri Aesoph, ND
717 S. Duluth Avenue
Sioux Falls, SD 57104
605-339-9080

TENNESSEE

Scott Olson, ND
1110 17th Avenue S., Suite #2
Nashville, TN 37212
615-321-7221

TEXAS

Stephen Sporn, ND
13740 Midway Road, Suite 506
Dallas, TX 75244
972-490-3703

Rajesh Vyas, ND
3725 Durwood Drive
Beaumont, TX 77706-3708
409-896-5466

Candice Jackson, ND
335 Roundabout
Kerrville, TX 78028
830-895-1727

Terry Rudd, ND
2414 Lakeview, Suite 6
Amarillo, TX 79109
806-359-1003

U.S. VIRGIN ISLANDS

Lynda Clark, ND
Box 25479
Christiansted, USVI 00824
340-773-4594

UTAH

Todd Cameron, ND
975 N. Main Street, Suite 1
Layton, UT 84041
801-593-6653

Ulrich Knorr, ND
502 S. State Street
Orem, UT 84058
801-224-5780

Leslie Peterson, ND
502 S. State Street
Orem, UT 84058
801-224-5780

Cordell Logan, PhD, ND
9265 S 1700 W., #A
West Jordan, UT 84088
801-562-2211

William Allen Nunn, ND, BA, BS
345 E. 4500 S. Suite H
Murray, UT 84107
801-265-0077

Katherine Ruggeri, ND, BA
201 East 500 South
River Heights, UT 84321
801-753-5987

VIRGINIA

Stephanie Story, ND
P.O. Box 1087
Virginia Beach, VA 23451
757-428-7979

VERMONT

Susan Kowalsky, ND
P.O. Box 851
Norwich, VT 05055
802-649-1064

Kathleen Audette, ND
185 North Street
Bennington, VT 05201
802-442-7000

Jody Noe, MS, ND
1063 Marlboro Road
Brattleboro, VT 05301
802-254-9332

Donna Powell, ND, LAc
41 Main St
Burlington, VT 05401
802-863-7099

Molly Fleming, ND
41 Main St
Burlington, VT 05401
802-863-7099

William Warnock, ND
2 Harbor Road
Shelburne, VT 05482
802-985-8250

Lorilee Schoenbeck, ND
2 Harbor Road
Shelburne, VT 05482
802-985-8250

Bernie Noe, ND
73 Main Street, Suite 41
Montpelier, VT 05602
802-229-2038

Lydia Faesy, ND
73 Main Street, Suite 41
Montpelier, VT 05602
802-229-2038

Donna Caplan, ND
28 East State Street
Montpellier, VT 05602
802-229-2635

WASHINGTON

Joanna Forwell, ND
1200 112th NE, #A-100
Bellevue, WA 98004
425-688-8818

Elizabeth Freeman, RN, ND, BS
10603 NE 14th Street
Bellevue, WA 98004
425-454-0908

Paula Baruffi, ND
9236 SE Shorland Drive
Bellevue, WA 98004
425-644-6048

Sheila Dunn-Merritt, ND
2025 112th Avenue NE
Building 2, Suite 300
Bellevue, WA 98004
425-452-9366

Michael Murray, ND
1540 140th Avenue
Bellevue, WA 98005-4516
425-644-6048

Sigrid Penrod, ND
14777 NE 40th Street, Suite 206
Bellevue, WA 98007
425-882-2089

Carlo Calabrese, ND, MPH
14500 Juanita Drive NE
Bothell, WA 98011
425-602-3160

Eric Jones, ND
14500 Juanita Drive NE
Bothell, WA 98011
206-823-1300

Leanna Standish, PhD, ND
14500 Juanita Drive NE
Bothell, WA 98011
425-602-3166

Joseph Pizzorno, Jr., ND
14500 Juanita Drive NE
Bothell, WA 98011
425-602-3003

Sarah Ringdahl, ND
14500 Juanita Drive
Bothell, WA 98011
425-602-3386

Pamela Snider, ND
14500 Juanita Drive NE
Bothell, WA 98011
206-523-9585

Robert Ullman, ND, DHANP
131 Third Avenue N.
Edmonds, WA 98020
425-774-5599

Judyth Reichenberg-Ullman, ND,
MSW
131 3rd Avenue N
Edmonds, WA 98020
425-774-5599

Kasra Pournadeali, ND
21701 76th Avenue W., Suite 302
Edmonds, WA 98026
425-744-1780

Dean Neary, ND
21200 72nd Avenue W
Edmonds, WA 98026
425-775-3717

Craig Baldwin, ND
23700 Edmonds Way
Edmonds, WA 98026
425-775-6001

Richard Kitaeff, ND, CA, DiplAc
23700 Edmonds Way
Edmonds, WA 98026
425-783-2873

Cheryl Wood, ND
7614 195th Street SW
Edmonds, WA 98026-6260
425-778-5673

David Wood, ND, BS
7614 195th Street SW
Edmonds, WA 98026-6260
425-778-5673

Steve MacPherson, ND
85 NW Alder Pl Suite C
Issaquah, WA 98027
425-391-1080

Davis Lamson, ND
515 West Harrison
Kent, WA 98032
253-854-4900

Robert Martinez, ND, DC, BS
11417 124th Avenue NE, Suite 103
Kirkland, WA 98033
425-828-6232

Mark Groven, ND
10203 116th Avenue NE
Kirkland, WA 98033
206-834-4112

Michael Woo, ND
11811 NE 128th Street, Suite 202
Kirkland, WA 98034
425-821-8118

Walter Crinnion, ND
11811 N.E. 128th, #202
Kirkland, WA 98034
425-821-8118

Jonathan Prousky, ND
12520 101st Way NE, #5
Kirkland, WA 98034
360-651-9355

Joni Olehausen, ND
P.O. Box 1627
Kent, WA 98035
253-854-4900 x161

Carol Vincent- Hall, ND
5031 212th Street SW
Lynnwood, WA 98036-7732

Leah Stebbens, ND
16260 NE 85th Street
Redmond, WA 98052
425-883-6565

Lisa Ann Azzopardi, ND
11025 SW 238th Street
Vashon Island, WA 98070
206-938-9890

Fran Brooks, ND
P.O. Box 1921
Vashon Island, WA 98070
206-463-5611

Sherry Jo-Kerchner, ND
2366 Eastlake Avenue E, #317
Seattle, WA 98102
206-323-7864

Melissa Mcclintock, ND
123 Boylston Avenue E., Suite B
Seattle, WA 98102
206-323-2378

James Wallace, ND
1307 N 45th Street, Suite 200
Seattle, WA 98103
206-632-0354

Jenefer Huntoon, ND
1329 N. 45th Street
Seattle, WA 98103
206-632-8804

Pamela Houghton, ND
6303 Phinney Avenue N.
Seattle, WA 98103
206-789-4066

Bonnie Reay, LMP, ND
1603 N. 46th, #103
Seattle, WA 98103

Trina Doerfler, ND, DC
4649 Sunnyside North, #350
Seattle, WA 98103
206-632-8670

Cathy Rogers, ND
4649 Sunnyside North, #300e
Seattle, WA 98103
206-527-5522

Marie Adams, ND
3931 Bridge Wy N.
Seattle, WA 98103
206-545-1310

William Wulsin, ND, MA, LAc
753 N 35th Street, Suite 302
Seattle, WA 98103
206-632-0411

Stephen Bucklew, ND
P.O. Box 31063
Seattle, WA 98103-1133

Stephen King, ND, DHANP
5502 34th Avenue NE
Seattle, WA 98105
206-522-0488

Bruce Milliman, ND
5312 Roosevelt Way NE
Seattle, WA 98105
206-525-8015

Sheryl Kipnis, ND, DHANP
5502 34th Avenue NE
Seattle, WA 98105
206-522-0488

Judy Christianson, ND
1102 NW 64th
Seattle, WA 98107
206-782-6521

Marleen Haverty, ND
1120 NW 63rd Street
Seattle, WA 98107
206-632-0354

Irvin Miller, ND
1153 NW 51st
Seattle, WA 98107-5126
206-781-4677

William Mitchell, ND
518 1st Avenue N., Suite 28
Seattle, WA 98109
206-284-6040

Barbara Kreemer, ND
311 Blaine
Seattle, WA 98109
206-281-4282

Styliani Kondilis, ND
2225 Queen Anne Avenue N.
Seattle, WA 98109
206-378-1712

Bill Caradonna, ND, RPh
311 Blaine Street
Seattle, WA 98109
206-524-2421

Rebecca Wynsome, ND
150 Nickerson Suite 211
Seattle, WA 98109
206-283-1383

Laura Flanagan, ND
605 29th Avenue East
Seattle, WA 98112
206-860-7896

Richard Posmantur, Jr., ND, LM,
LAc
2705 E. Madison
Seattle, WA 98112
206-328-7929

Felice Barnow, ND, LM, RN
2705 E. Madison
Seattle, WA 98112
206-328-7929

Douglas Lewis, ND
9111 Roosevelt Way NE
Seattle, WA 98115
206-525-8078

Agnes Yabuki, ND
3716 NE 75th, #303
Seattle, WA 98115

Keri Brown, ND
6308½ 18th Avenue NE
Seattle, WA 98115

Karen Coshow, BA, ND
8043 Ravenna Avenue N.
Seattle, WA 98115
206-729-0907

Nancy Mercer, ND
7114 Roosevelt Way NE
Seattle, WA 98115
206-526-0203

Linda Warren, ND
7746 18th Avenue NE
Seattle, WA 98115
206-525-5257

David Bove, ND, CA
6520 17th Avenue NE
Seattle, WA 98115
206-526-8384

Mylinh Vo, ND
1815 NE 82nd Street
Seattle, WA 98115
206-283-1383

Bobbi Lutack, ND
2008 NE 65th Street
Seattle, WA 98115
206-729-0907

Jill Fresonke, ND
8521 15th Avenue NE
Seattle, WA 98115
206-525-3735

Lisa Meserole, ND
420 NE Ravenna Blvd.
Seattle, WA 98115
206-527-6355

Robert May, ND
8029 Brooklyn Avenue NE
Seattle, WA 98115
206-632-0354

Jeana Kimball, ND
4141 California Avenue SW
Seattle, WA 98116
206-938-1393

Ralph Wilson, ND
3419 61st Avenue SW
Seattle, WA 98116
206-634-3679

Molly Linton, ND
1409 NW 85th Street
Seattle, WA 98117
206-781-2206

Christy Lee-Engel, ND, LAc
600 W. Mcgraw, #1
Seattle, WA 98119
206-285-4625

Brad Lichtenstein, ND
600 W. Mcgraw, #1
Seattle, WA 98119
206-285-4625

Que Areste, ND
1122 E. Pike, #806
Seattle, WA 98122
206-328-2926

Marian Small, ND, LAc, RN
1523 E. Madison
Seattle, WA 98122
206-322-4416

Eileen Stretch, ND
726 Broadway Suite 301
Seattle, WA 98122
206-726-0034

Cynthia Phillips, ND
726 Broadway, Suite 301
Seattle, WA 98122
206-726-0034

Cindy Breed, ND
211 Euclid Avenue
Seattle, WA 98122

Lise Alschuler, ND
726 Broadway, Suite 301
Seattle, WA 98122
206-726-0034

John Hibbs, ND
1523 E. Madison Street
Seattle, WA 98122-4013
206-322-4416

Jane Guiltinan, ND
211 Euclid Avenue
Seattle, WA 98122-6527
206-632-0354 x105

Morgaine Donna Hager, ND
14330 12th Avenue NE, #318
Seattle, WA 98125

Linnea Thompson, ND
14300 32nd Avenue NE, #203
Seattle, WA 98125

Nancy Roberts, ND
14546 Greenwood Avenue N.
Seattle, WA 98133
206-362-3250

Judy Atwell, ND
16324 Fremont Avenue N.
Seattle, WA 98133

Eva Urbaniak, ND
5236 California Avenue SW, Suite D
Seattle, WA 98136
206-938-9505

Tom Ballard, ND
2006 19th Avenue S.
Seattle, WA 98144
206-726-0034

Kenneth Harmon, ND
1835 SW 152nd Street
Seattle, WA 98166
206-243-5252

Herbert Schuck, ND
12610 Des Moines Memorial Drive
#202
Seattle, WA 98168
206-248-0061

Laura Martin, ND
2520 Colby Avenue
Everett, WA 98201
425-257-9713

Dean Howell, ND
1827 37th Street
Everett, WA 98201
425-252-6066

Corina Going, ND
1809 100th Pl. S.E. Suite B
Everett, WA 98208
425-337-5004

Melanie Whittaker, RN, ND
713 SE Everett Mall Way, #D
Everett, WA 98208
425-290-5309

Miechelle Poulos, ND
1809 100th Pl. S.E. Suite B
Everett, WA 98208
425-337-5004

Barbara Davies, ND
1809 100th Place SE Suite B
Everett, WA 98208
425-337-5004

W. Hunter Greenwood, ND, DC
1116 17th Street
Anacortes, WA 98221
360-293-6277

Laura Shelton, ND
1707 F Street
Bellingham, WA 98225
360-734-1560

Rachelle Herdman, MD, ND
1919 Broadway, Suite 204
Bellingham, WA 98225
360-734-0045

Mark Steinberg, ND
1919 Broadway, #206
Bellingham, WA 98225-3239
360-738-3230

Robert Jangaard, ND
P.O. Box 130
Freeland, WA 98249
360-331-6470

Rhonda Summerland, ND
P.O. Box 115
Index, WA 98256-0115
360-793-1033

Gary Bachman, ND, RN, LMP
1910 Riverside Drive, #5
Mt Vernon, WA 98273
360-424-3460

Magda Mische, ND, RPh
P.O. Box 22 /Olga Road
Olga, WA 98279
360-376-5454

Mary Griffith, RN, ND
5122 Olympic Drive NW, #B104
Gig Harbor, WA 98335
253-851-7550

Steven Davis, ND
5603 38th Avenue NW
Gig Harbor, WA 98335-8218
253-857-5544

Jane Bernstein Pearson, ND
P.O. Box 1664
Poulsbo, WA 98370
360-697-7070

Mark Swanson, ND
720 E. Washington Street
Sequim, WA 98382
360-683-1110

Linda Dyson, ND, RN, LM
17610 49th Street E.
Sumner, WA 98390
253-926-2229

Owen Miller, ND
1530 South Union, Suite 4
Tacoma, WA 98405
253-752-2558

Paul Reilly, ND
3620 Sixth Avenue
Tacoma, WA 98406
253-752-4544

Joseph Cates-Carney, ND
4325 Tacoma Avenue S.
Tacoma, WA 98408

Anthony Calpeno, DC, ND, CAc,
DHANP
4111-A Bridgeport Way W.
University Place, WA 98466
253-565-2444

Thomas Young, ND
8909 Gravelly Lake Drive SW
Tacoma, WA 98499-3109
253-584-1144

Dennis Sklar, ND
3726 Pacific Avenue SE, Suite A
Olympia, WA 98501-2170
206-754-8576

Jon Dunn, ND
2617-B 12th Ct. SW, #6
Olympia, WA 98502-9702
360-352-7880

Robin Moore, ND
3627 Ensign Road, Suite B
Olympia, WA 98506
360-459-9082

Suzanne Adams, ND
3627 Ensign Road, Suite B
Olympia, WA 98506
360-459-9082

Patricia Hastings, ND
4324 Martin Way, Suite B
Olympia, WA 98516
360-438-2882

Jennifer Booker, ND
6326 Martin Way, E. Suite 205
Olympia, WA 98516
360-491-2111

Pierre Wise, ND
301 Ocean Avenue
Raymond, WA 98577
360-942-3956

Jill Stansbury, ND
408 E. Main Street
Battle Ground, WA 98604
360-687-2799

Anne Scott, ND
316 E. Fourth Plain Blvd., Suite B
Vancouver, WA 98661
360-750-4642

Cheryl Deroin, ND
3606 Main Street, Suite 202
Vancouver, WA 98663
360-695-7699

Kevin Murray, ND, LAc
316 East 4th Plain Blvd., #B
Vancouver, WA 98663
360-750-4642

Meed West, ND
1612 NE 78th Street
Vancouver, WA 98665
360-573-3223

Elyssa Harte, ND
40 Major Creek Road
White Salmon, WA 98672
509-493-3835

Jacqueline Thomas, ND
1214 5th Street
Wenatchee, WA 98801
509-665-0867

Andrea Black, ND
138 Buzzard Lake Road
Okanagan, WA 98841
509-826-1164

Sierra Breitbeil, ND
P.O. Box 993
Winthrop, WA 98862
509-996-3970

Randy Sandaine, ND
143 Garden Homes Drive
Colville, WA 99114
509-685-2300

Letitia Watrous, ND, BS
W. 1137 Garland Avenue
Spokane, WA 99205
509-327-5143

Neural Therapy

The American Academy of Neural
Therapy
1468 South St. Francis Drive
Santa Fe, NM 87501
505-988-3086

Nutrition

**FOLLOWING ARE THE CHAPTER HEADS
OF THE INTERNATIONAL AND AMERICAN
ASSOCIATIONS OF CLINICAL
NUTRITIONISTS IAACN))**

CALIFORNIA

Robert J. Marshall, Ph.D., CCN
Pacific Research Systems
1010 Crenshaw Blvd., Suite 170
Torrance, CA 90501
Phone: 310-320-1132
Fax: 310-320-7557

FLORIDA

Martin Dayton, MD, DO, CCN
Medical Center, Sunny Isles
18600 Collins Avenue
North Miami Beach, FL 33160
Phone: 305-931-8484
Fax: 305-936-1849

ILLINOIS

Jack O. Taylor, MS, DC, CCN
Dr. Taylor's Wellness Center, Inc.
3601 Algonquin Road, Suite 801
Rolling Meadows, ILL 60008
Phone: 847-222-1192
Fax: 847-423-3541

NEW YORK

Joan A. Friedrick, Ph.D., CCN—
Acting President
Life-Line Nutritional Services, Inc.
P.O. Box 482
Bronxville, NY 10708
Phone: 914-423-3531
Fax: 914-423-3531

OREGON

I.F. Kelly, DC, CCN—
Acting President
P.O. Box 2150
Newport, OR 97365
Phone: 541-265-5132
Fax: 541-265-8680

RHODE ISLAND

Joyce Martin, DC, RN, CCN—
Acting President
708 Reservoir
Smithfield, RI 02917
Phone: 401-942-0600
Fax: 401-943-0604

TEXAS

Gay Langham-McNally, CCN
Clinical Profiles, Inc.
3102 Oak Lawn, Suite 620
Dallas, TX 75219
Phone: 214-522-6885
Fax: 214-522-6883

Orthomolecular Medicine

The Huxley Inst. for Biosocial
Research
American Academy of
Orthomolecular Medicine
900 North Federal Highway
Boca Raton, FL 33432
800-847-3802

Osteopathy

American Academy of Osteopathy
3500 DePauw Boulevard, Suite 1080
Indianapolis, IN 46268
317-879-1881
Fax: 317-879-0563

Rolfing Practitioners

ALABAMA

Dean R. Bowden, M.S.
Certified Rolfer
Rolf Movement Practitioner
Huntsville, AL 35801
Office: 256-882-9777
Fax: 256-882-9188
Residence: 256-883-5092
DRBowden@aol.com

J. Thomas West, Ph.D.
Certified Advanced Rolfer
Huntsville, AL 35801
205-534-2560
Fax: 205-536-5508
westjt@eckerd.edu

Charles Whetsell, Ph.D.
Certified Rolfer
Birmingham, AL 35242
205-408-9479

ALASKA

Duffy Allen Begich
Certified Rolfer
Rolf Movement Practitioner
Anchorage, AK 99501
907-278-3982

David Brickell, M.S.
Certified Advanced Rolfer
Juneau, AK
907-586-3834 and
Fairbanks, AK 99708
907-479-3709

Mark I. Hutton
Certified Rolfer
Soldotna, AK 99669
907-260-1914
huttonm@aol.com

Linda C. Jordan, M.Sc.
Certified Advanced Rolfer
Anchorage, AK 99524
907-272-6147
lcj@alaska.net

Barbara Maier
Certified Advanced Rolfer
Anchorage, AK 99503
Office: 907-562-0926
bmaier@alaska.net

Gabriele Mehnert
Certified Rolfer
Sterling, AK 99672
907-262-1915
gabriele@alaska.net
and
Soldotna, AK 99669
Office: 907-262-4544

Gwin A. Moerlein
Certified Advanced Rolfer
Anchorage, AK 99507
907-345-3317

Paul C. Van Alstine
Certified Rolfer
Anchorage, AK 99501
907-272-7027

Gail L. Boerwinkle
Certified Rolfer
Anchorage, AK 99508
907-562-2158

Barbara Kavanagh M.A.
Certified Advanced Rolfer
Anchorage, AK 99503
Office: 907-566-0865

Judith Stohl
Certified Advanced Rolfer
Anchorage, AK 99508
907-278-6227
907-566-4641

ARIZONA

Jim D. Asher
Certified Advanced Rolfer
Rolf Movement Practitioner
Tucson, AZ
520-299-3802
funnybone5@aol.com

Ulrike Boecker
Certified Rolfer
Phoenix, AZ 85208
Residence: 602-404-7224
and Scottsdale, AZ 85257
Office: 602-994-0343

Joe Breck
Certified Rolfer
Rolf Movement Practitioner
Tucson, AZ 85704
520-297-3777
ljbreck@gci-net.com

Bob Brill
Certified Advanced Rolfer
Sedona, AZ 86336
520-282-2856
800-677-1519
bobbrill@sedona.net

Casey J. Clark
Certified Rolfer
Prescott, AZ 86303
Office: 520-541-7591

Clay Cox, Ph.D.
Certified Advanced Rolfer
Tucson, AZ 85712-3646
Residence: 520-323-0188
Fax: 520-323-0188
tucsonrolfer@juno.com

Susan Holland
Certified Rolfer
Rolf Movement Practitioner
Flagstaff, AZ 86002
Residence: 520-556-3056
Office: 520-774-5865

William J. Kamer
Certified Advanced Rolfer
Phoenix, AZ 85019
602-808-1448
darlenekamer@hotmail.com

Suzanne Lucas
Certified Rolfer
Phoenix, AZ 85032
Office: 602-404-8483
Residence: 602-246-2533

Helen Luce
Certified Advanced Rolfer
Tucson, AZ 85716
520-326-7543
Fax: 520-326-9775
LUZ1311@azstarnet.com

Jeffrey Maitland, Ph.D.
Certified Advanced Rolfer
Scottsdale, AZ 85258
Messages: 602-945-4032
Fax: 602-922-8783
Office: 602-922-1376
JMaitland@aol.com

Owen Marcus, M.A., Lic.
Certified Advanced Rolfer
Scottsdale, AZ 85251
602-949-1185
owenmarcus@juno.com

Terry Scott Martin, M.A.
Certified Advanced Rolfer
Phoenix, AZ 85020
Residence: 602-331-1388
and Phoenix, AZ
Phoenix: 602-331-1388

Deanna Melnychuk
Certified Rolfer
Rolf Movement Practitioner
Phoenix, AZ 85032
602-404-1338
Rolfer@abilnet.com
and Phoenix, AZ 85028
Office: 602-494-3037

Stephen Mettner
Certified Advanced Rolfer
Tempe, AZ 85281
Office: 602-966-1776
Residence: 602-667-0249

Linda K. Mills
Certified Rolfer
Tucson, AZ 85749
602-745-1570

Matthew Oren
Certified Rolfer
Phoenix, AZ 85018
602-954-7171
poren98892@aol.com

David E. Robinson
Certified Rolfer
Paradise Valley, AZ 85253
602-998-7477
and Scottsdale, AZ 85258
602-922-1376

Patti A. Selleck
Certified Rolfer
Glendale, AZ 85301
Office: 602-915-3533
CaringHands@juno.com

Lee Stanley
Certified Rolfer
Tucson, AZ 85703
520-882-9899
Fax: 520-620-9332
rolfer@azstarnet.com
http://www.azstarnet.com/~rolfer/ind
ex.html

Kirsten Tinning
Certified Rolfer
Flagstaff, AZ 86001
520-525-3541
Limited Practice

Dr. Nancy O'Toole Gokmen
Certified Rolfer
Tucson, AZ 85718
520-299-7969
Fax: 520-299-7958
ngokmen@aol.com

Lee Horwin, Ph.D.
Certified Rolfer
Phoenix, AZ
800-971-8978

Linda Lindy-Navasaitis
Certified Rolfer
Tucson, AZ 85745
520-743-2010
irolf@theriver.com
Arkansas, AR
Limited Practice

Marie Dunkel
Certified Rolfer
Hot Springs, AR 71913
501-617-9591
mdunkel@hsnp.com

Richard Rossiter
Certified Advanced Rolfer
Little Rock, AR 72207
501-663-8100
rhr@rossiter.com

CALIFORNIA

David Adams
Certified Rolfer
Santa Monica, CA 90405
310-664-9503
rolfworks@aol.com

Carol Agneessens, M.S.
Certified Advanced Rolfer
Rolf Movement Practitioner
Capitola, CA 95010-3454
408-479-8221
Fax: 408-479-8233

Bob Alonzi
Certified Advanced Rolfer
Santa Monica, CA 90401
Office: 310-451-3250
BobRolfer@aol.com
and Encino, CA 91316
Office: 818-906-2770

Christopher Amodeo
Certified Advanced Rolfer
Costa Mesa, CA 92627
714-646-ROLF
IROLFU@aol.com
and Laguna Beach, CA 92651
714-497-5446

Kathleen Atkinson, R.N.
Certified Rolfer
Rolf Movement Practitioner
Carmel, CA 93922
408-484-9480
kiatkinson@earthlink.net

Michael Baker
Certified Advanced Rolfer
Solana Beach, CA 92075
619-755-7405
mbaker@ucsd.edu

Bridget Beck
Certified Advanced Rolfer
Santa Rosa, CA 95405
Office: 707-575-6852
bridgetbec@aol.com

Jeff Belanger
Certified Advanced Rolfer
Sausalito, CA 94965-1710
415-331-5443
Jeffbel@aol.com

Joe Bennington
Certified Rolfer
Venice, CA 90291
310-392-5013

Mary Bond
Certified Advanced Rolfer
Rolf Movement Practitioner
Los Angeles, CA 90041
213-254-0963
merrybe@flash.net

Nuria L. Bowart
Certified Rolfer
San Francisco, CA 94110-4727
415-821-6659
sweetea@earthlink.net

Renee Branch-Wagner
Certified Advanced Rolfer
Pacific Palisades, CA 90272
310-454-2644

Mark Caffall, Ph.D.
Certified Advanced Rolfer
Leucadia, CA 92023

Cheryl L. Campbell
Certified Rolfer
Laguna Beach, CA 92651
714-644-4840
714-499-6624
and Newport Beach, CA 92660
Office: 714-644-4840

Kathleen Cheek
Certified Rolfer
San Rafael, CA 94901
Office: 415-789-8263
kcheek6055@aol.com

Lynda Connelly-Richardson, RPT
Certified Advanced Rolfer
Monterey, CA 93940
408-373-5045

Bob Craven
Certified Advanced Rolfer
San Diego, CA 92109
Office: 619-483-7106
Residence: 619-280-0062
and Palm Springs, CA

Giovanna D'Angelo
Certified Advanced Rolfer
St. Helena, CA 94574
rickbrennan@yahoo.com
and Corte Madera, CA
Res/Office: 707-963-5774

William Deane
Certified Rolfer
Fountain Valley, CA 92708
714-964-5911
and San Luis Obispo, CA 93401
805-544-3009

Georgette Maria Delvaux-Salveson, D.C.
Certified Advanced Rolfer
Berkeley, CA 94708
Office: 510-548-8270
Fax: 510-548-9257
Emergency: 510-548-9326
delvaux@aol.com

Mark P. Donahue
Certified Rolfer
Cotati, CA 94931-4477
707-792-2380
Drowa@svn.net

Beverly Ensing
Certified Rolfer
San Luis Obispo, CA 93405
805-544-6670

Raym Ensing
Certified Advanced Rolfer
San Luis Obispo, CA 93401
805-545-0370

Margaret Eyles
Certified Rolfer
Rolf Movement Practitioner
San Luis Obispo County, CA
and Los Osos, CA 93402
Office: 805-528-2547
and Cayucos, CA 93430
Office: 805-528-2547
Residence: 805-995-2140

Daniel Frank
Certified Rolfer
Santa Barbara, CA 93101-3351
805-965-3707

Sherwood Fulmor
Certified Rolfer
Leucadia, CA 92024
Office: 619-623-9058
Residence: 760-942-1177

Howie Gaynor
Certified Rolfer
Rolf Movement Practitioner
Santa Barbara, CA 93101
805-568-0999

Victor Geberin
Certified Advanced Rolfer
Solana Beach, CA 92075-1802
619-481-8113
Fax: 619-481-8118
Geberin@io-online.com

Richard Goodstein
Certified Advanced Rolfer
Santa Barbara, CA 93105
805-569-3081
jrpri@erols.com

Marie Jo Graziadei
Certified Rolfer
Mill Valley, CA 94941
Office: 415-388-9617
Grazia@infoasis.com

Timothy A. Greenstreet
Certified Advanced Rolfer
Soquel, CA 95073
831-462-2105
agreenstreet@earthlink.net

Per Haaland
Certified Advanced Rolfer
Soquel, CA 95073
Office: 831-462-2600
and Los Gatos, CA
Office: 831-395-1105

Jai Haissman
Certified Rolfer
San Francisco, CA 94115
Office: 415-828-8725
Fax: 415-383-4731
jairolf@concentric.net
and Mill Valley, CA 94941
Office: 415-828-8725
Fax: 415-383-4731

Kathryn Kuper Harris
Certified Rolfer
Rolf Movement Practitioner
Santa Barbara, CA 93111
805-967-8920

Don Hazen, D.C.
Certified Advanced Rolfer
Berkeley, CA 94707
510-528-1514
hazen@best.com

Allan Herranen
Certified Rolfer
San Francisco, CA 94123
415-563-3972

Kathy Holler
Advanced Rolfer
Rolf Movement Practitioner
West Covina, CA 91792
626-810-6058
Fax: 626-912-9149
kathyholler@juno.com

James Hrisikos
Certified Rolfer
San Rafael, CA 94903
415-507-0259
hrisikos@well.com

Julia Ireland
Certified Advanced Rolfer
Sausalito, CA 94965
415-331-6816
INYOI@aol.com

Ms. Shawnee Isaac-Smith
Certified Rolfer
Venice, CA 90291-2870
Office: 310-581-2500
Fax: 310-452-6272

Helen G. James, M.A., P.T.
Certified Advanced Rolfer
Clovis, CA 93612-2234
Office: 209-299-7784
Home & Fax: 209-299-0723
helenj@csufresno.edu

Steve James
Certified Rolfer
San Diego, CA 92107-3642
619-454-9357

Robert Janda D.C.
Certified Rolfer
Costa Mesa, CA 92627
Office: 714-515-9900
sierra1@pe.net

Vivian Jaye
Honorary Rolfer
Rolf Movement Practitioner
Monterey, CA 93940
408-655-1714
VJAYE@aol.com

Michael Kilgroe
Certified Advanced Rolfer
Palo Alto, CA 94306
650-326-0360

Clinton Kramer
Certified Rolfer
San Francisco, CA
74653.2163@compuserve.com

David John Krizman
Certified Rolfer
Rolf Movement Practitioner
Santa Cruz, CA 95061
408-602-6013
and Santa Cruz, CA 95060
Office: 408-460-0860

Ms. Hadidjah Lamas
Certified Rolfer
Los Angeles, CA 90064
310-473-6229

Bill Peter LeGrave
Certified Rolfer
Palm Springs, CA 92264-1364
760-322-5373
blegrave@aol.com
and Desert Hot Springs, CA
760-251-2261 and
Lake Forrest & Laguna Beach, CA
714-830-7840

Jennifer C. Mark
Certified Rolfer
Rolf Movement Practitioner
San Fransisco, CA 94115
415-289-2068
bodywork@pacbell.net

Pilar Martin Espin
Certified Advanced Rolfer
Soquel, CA 95073
Residence: 408-462-2600

Kevin McCoy
Certified Advanced Rolfer
San Francisco, CA 94118
415-567-2384
Office: 415-668-5332
goodhealer@aol.com

Jason Mixter, MFCC
Certified Advanced Rolfer
Rolf Movement Practitioner
San Francisco, CA 94115
Office: 415-567-0620
Residence: 510-204-9767
mixter@aol.com

Lindsey Morin, D.C.
Certified Rolfer
Mendocino, CA 95460
Residence: 707-937-1425
Office: 707-937-2225
lmorindc@mcn.org

Michael Wm. Murphy
Certified Advanced Rolfer
Rolf Movement Practitioner
Palo Alto, CA 94301
Office: 650-328-4072
MurphyRolf@aol.com

Gael Ohlgren
Certified Advanced Rolfer
Rolf Movement Practitioner
Delmar, CA 92014
619-481-1488
Fax: 619-481-6630
gaelo@aol.com

Ben Ohs
Certified Advanced Rolfer
Sacramento, CA 95816
916-444-7862
and Davis, CA 95616
Residence: 916-756-9399

Julie Paul
Advanced Rolfer
Tarzana, CA 91335
818-705-8194
maleuse@earthlink.net

Jerry Perkins
Certified Advanced Rolfer
Petaluma, CA 94952
707-769-7424
www.satsong.com

Trevor Plaugher
Certified Rolfer
Santa Barbara, CA 93108
TJCall@aol.com

R. Grant Powers
Certified Advanced Rolfer
Costa Mesa, CA 92627
Office: 949-642-7618
RGP@aol.com
and Laguna Beach, CA 92651
949-494-4146
Fax: 949-494-4904

Karen S. Price
Certified Advanced Rolfer
Palo Alto, CA 94306
650-324-8863

Arthur Riggs
Certified Advanced Rolfer
Oakland, CA 94619
510-482-9427
Fax: 510-482-6489
artriggs@aol.com

Barbara Robinson
Certified Advanced Rolfer
Huntington Beach, CA 92648
714-962-5951
brabraa@flash.net

Robert Robinson
Certified Advanced Rolfer
Sacramento, CA 95816
Office: 916-447-4329
71064.3413@compuserve.com

Harvey Ruderian
Certified Rolfer
Topanga, CA 90290-4265
310-455-0774

Gene R. Sage
Certified Advanced Rolfer
San Anselmo, CA 94960
415-457-6843
and Mill Valley, CA

Karen Sallovitz
Certified Advanced Rolfer
Aptos, CA 95003
408-685-8609
karen@cruzio.com

Michael Salveson
Certified Advanced Rolfer
Berkeley, CA 94708
Office: 510-548-8270
Fax: 510-548-9257
SalvesonM@aol.com

Bruce Schonfeld
Certified Advanced Rolfer
Rolf Movement Practitioner
Santa Monica, CA 90401
310-395-3555

James Schwartz
Certified Advanced Rolfer
Rolf Movement Practitioner
Mill Valley, CA 94941
415-381-2204
JamesJS@aol.com
and Novato, CA 94945-1722
415-898-5148
and San Rafael, CA 94901
Office: 415-902-8462

Donald Setty
Certified Advanced Rolfer
Los Angeles, CA 90069
213-656-0479

Benjamin Shield, Ph.D.
Certified Rolfer
Los Angeles, CA 90034
310-446-1800
BenShield@aol.com

Lillian Jane Shoupe
Certified Rolfer
Sacramento, CA 95821
Office: 916-489-7805
lillian@2xtreme.net
www.2xtreme.net/amrita

Charles G. Siemers, B.S.
Certified Advanced Rolfer
Santa Monica, CA 90401
310-395-8088
ZenBones@aol.com
and Manhattan Beach, CA 90266
310-545-0288

Lin Silver
Certified Rolfer
Paradise, CA 95969
916-877-1936
and Chico, CA 95928
916-896-0701

Douw Smith
Certified Rolfer
Fairfax, CA 94978
514-451-1884
desmondD@aol.com

COLORADO

Steven Altschuler, M.S.W.
Certified Advanced Rolfer
Boulder, CO 80303
303-447-9939
303-322-9294
eurobe@aol.com
and Denver, CO 80206
303-322-9294
303-447-9939

Jim D. Asher
Certified Advanced Rolfer
Rolf Movement Practitioner
Boulder, CO 80302
303-443-6415
funnybone5@aol.com
and Denver, CO 80206
303-377-6464

Jeff Bailey
Certified Rolfer
Rolf Movement Practitioner
Boulder, CO 80303
303-499-9402
Yogarolf@aol.com

Laura J. Barnes
Certified Rolfer
Longmont, CO 80501
Office: 303-682-3161
villagerolfer@seqnet.net
www.seqnet.net/~villagerolfer

Joe Bennington
Certified Rolfer
Boulder, CO 80304
Appts: 310-392-5013

Mirella "Mimi" Berger
Certified Advanced Rolfer
Rolf Movement Practitioner
Boulder, CO 80302
303-447-0476
Fax: 303-440-3971

Sue D. Boatwright
Certified Rolfer
Rolf Movement Practitioner
Golden, CO 80401
Voice Mail: 303-271-3438
Fax: 303-279-3993
Residence: 303-279-3994
and Denver, CO 80203
Voice Mail: 303-271-3438

Don Bruce
Certified Rolfer
Rolf Movement Practitioner
Boulder, CO 80304
303-546-6556
DonBruce@idcomm.com
and Boulder, CO 80302
303-449-1831

Francoise Lajoie Brunette
Certified Rolfer
Boulder, CO 80302-4540
303-448-0640

Edward "Eagle" Butler, M.A.
Certified Advanced Rolfer
Aspen, CO 81612
970-920-9738
970-925-9102
and Denver, CO 80224
303-753-9598

Victoria Cashman
Certified Advanced Rolfer
Longmont, CO 80503-8739
303-530-1325

Wells Christie
Certified Rolfer
Boulder, CO 80303
303-554-1913
wells@indra.com

Mary P. Dalles, Ph.D.
Certified Rolfer
Niwot, CO 80544-0428
Residence: 303-652-3898
Office: 303-652-9097
mdalles@bouldernews.infi.net

Carol Anne Doehner, R.N., BSN
Certified Rolfer
Rolf Movement Practitioner
Longmont, CO 80501
303-651-6196
rncwhite@juno.com

Jack Donisvitch
Certified Rolfer
Denver, CO 80220-4438
303-399-5133
and Denver, CO 80206
Office: 303-388-8523
and Boulder, CO 80302

Delbert M. Dorn
Certified Rolfer
Denver, CO 80218
Phone/Fax: 303-861-8411
deldorn@earthlink.net
and Greenwood Village, CO 80111
Phone/Fax: 303-861-8411

Nanette Litten Earley
Certified Rolfer
Arvada, CO 80003
303-425-7298

Patrick Ellinwood
Certified Advanced Rolfer
Rolf Movement Practitioner
Boulder, CO 80304
Office: 303-545-5792
Residence: 303-443-7952
PEllinwood@aol.com

Sara Forbes
Certified Rolfer
Boulder, CO 80304
303-247-1886
and Denver, CO 80203
303-247-1886

Liz Gaggini, M.A.
Certified Advanced Rolfer
Rolf Movement Practitioner
Boulder, CO 80301
303-786-9794
Fax: 303-415-1072
LGRolfer@aol.com

Ric Galanits
Certified Rolfer
Denver, CO 80203
303-860-1569
RGalanits@aol.com

Jane Harrington, M.A.
Certified Advanced Rolfer
Rolf Movement Practitioner
Boulder, CO 80301
303-447-2760
janech@worldnet.att.net

Robert Heller
Certified Rolfer
Denver, CO 80226
Residence: 303-988-6667

Kim Hourston
Certified Rolfer
Lafayette, CO 80026
303-664-9515

Ken Jamititus
Certified Rolfer
Boulder/Loveland/Longmont, CO
303-931-KENJ

Roger T. Jordan, M.S.
Certified Advanced Rolfer
Longmont, CO 80503
303-449-2788
Fax: 303-473-0554
jorda84@ibm.ne

Teresa Y. Kappers-Wright
Certified Rolfer
Rolf Movement Practitioner
Arvada, CO 80004
Office: 303-420-7223
Voicemail: 303-382-3810
and Denver, CO 80203
Office: 303-420-7223
Voicemail: 303-382-3810
and Westminster, CO 80003
Office: 303-650-9710
Office: 303-420-7223
Voicemail: 303-382-3810

Marianne G. Korosy
Certified Rolfer
Ft. Collins, CO 80526
Office: 970-481-7531
Residence: 970-204-9050
MKoros@aol.com

Vickie Kovar
Certified Rolfer
Rolf Movement Practitioner
Lakewood, CO 80228
303-989-6895
sci@ecentral.com

Robin Kratschmer
Certified Rolfer
Boulder, CO 80303
303-554-0574
rakrolfs@bouldernews.infi.net

Debra Kuresman
Certified Advanced Rolfer
Rolf Movement Practitioner
Boulder, CO 80304
303-440-7357
DebKures@aol.com

Melanie Lee Lancaster
Rolfer
Boulder, CO 80304
303-546-6068

Barbara Dee Leach, R.N.
Certified Advanced Rolfer
Rolf Movement Practitioner
Grand Junction, CO 81501
970-243-4472

Jeffery M. Linn
Certified Rolfer
Denver, CO 80218
303-863-0391
JLinn24538@aol.com
http://members.aol.com/JLinn24538/
index.html

Til Luchau
Certified Advanced Rolfer
Rolf Movement Practitioner
Lafayette, CO 80026
Phone: 303-499-8811
Fax Svc: 303-494-2778
TilLuchau@aol.com
and Lafayette, Boulder, Denver, CO
Phone: 303-499-8811
Fax: 303-494-2778

Melissa Luzung
Certified Rolfer
Rolf Movement Practitioner
Denver, CO 80202
303-454-8013
Voice Mail: 303-839-2194

Shari MacCallum
Certified Advanced Rolfer
Boulder, CO 80302
Residence: 303-473-0732
ShariMac@hotmail.com
and Denver, CO 80203
Office: 303-830-2994

Douglas Martin, M.B.S.
Certified Advanced Rolfer
Colorado Springs, CO 80903-3422
Office: 719-635-8877

Jonathan S. Martine
Certified Advanced Rolfer
Rolf Movement Practitioner
Boulder, CO 80302
303-443-2681
Mobile: 303-641-3416
JSMartine@aol.com
and Denver, CO 80210
303-443-2681
Mobile: 303-641-3416

Michael Mathieu
Certified Rolfer
Ft. Collins, CO 80526
970-221-2728
tstone@peakpeak.com

Ray McCall
Certified Advanced Rolfer
Rolf Movement Practitioner
Boulder, CO 80304
303-449-9477
rkmc@aol.com
and Denver, CO 80203
303-449-9477

Dameron Midgette
Certified Rolfer
Rolf Movement Practitioner
Boulder, CO 80302
Office: 303-473-0484
dameronm@rolfingsi.com
http://www.rolfingsi.com

Bret Nye, M.D.
Certified Advanced Rolfer
Bellvue, CO 80512
Residence: 970-484-8842
KYGR73A@Prodigy.com
and Loveland, CO 80537
970-669-2849

Ruth Oaks
Certified Rolfer
Niwot, CO 80503
303-652-3037
Pager: 303-448-3296
colorado@bouldernews.infi.net
and Boulder, CO 80302
Office: 303-652-3037
Pager: 303-448-3296
Fax: 303-652-8308

Joy Om
Certified Advanced Rolfer
Nederland, CO 80466
303-449-8664
303-258-0717
joy@indra.com
and Boulder, CO
303-449-8664

Jim Pascucci
Certified Advanced Rolfer
Boulder, CO 80301
Office: 303-581-0530
JPascu@aol.com
and Loveland, CO
Office: 970-495-3407
and Denver, CO
Office: 303-581-0530

Suzanne Picard
Certified Rolfer
Rolf Movement Practitioner
Boulder, CO 80303
Office: 303-494-3281

Joy Ptasnik, B.S.,R.N.
Certified Advanced Rolfer
Englewood, CO 80110
Residence: 303-789-0494
Fax: 303-781-2843

Pamela H. Rankin
Certified Rolfer
Rolf Movement Practitioner
Boulder, CO 80302
Office: 303-938-9189
Residence: 303-440-3435

Darrell Sanchez, M.A.
Certified Advanced Rolfer
Denver, CO 80210
303-447-1539
darsan@ibm.net
and Boulder, CO 80302
303-447-1539

Tim Shafer
Certified Rolfer
Rolf Movement Practitioner
Ft. Collins, CO 80525-6614
Office: 970-229-1925
Fax: 970-493-1903
rolfer@frii.com

Eric F. Shapiro
Certified Rolfer
Boulder, CO 80306-7524
303-447-0051
yties1@hotmail.com

Don Sisolak
Certified Rolfer
Rolf Movement Practitioner
Colorado Springs, CO 80903
Office: 719-578-0504
Rolfspace@aol.com

Lance C. Slaughter
Certified Advanced Rolfer
Boulder, CO 80304
303-443-8223

Donna Splane
Certified Rolfer
Denver, CO 80206
Office: 303-449-0643
and Boulder, CO 80302
303-449-0643

Heather Starsong
Certified Advanced Rolfer
Rolf Movement Practitioner
Boulder, CO 80304
303-449-6208
hstarsong@compuserve.com

Patricia Stepan
Certified Rolfer
Boulder, CO 80303
303-444-8227

Patricia Stevens, M.S.
Certified Advanced Rolfer
Colorado Springs, CO 80903-3422
Office: 719-635-8877

Marekah Stewart
Certified Advanced Rolfer
Denver, CO
303-321-1795

Pam Stoffer
Certified Rolfer
Boulder, CO 80302-7602
303-449-1831
pstoffer@bouldernews.infi.net

Charles Swenson
Certified Advanced Rolfer
Ft. Collins, CO 80524
Office: 970-493-6939

Elizabeth H. Swenson
Certified Advanced Rolfer
Ft. Collins, CO 80524
Office: 970-493-6939
and Ft. Collins, CO 80524
Office: 970-472-5000

Douglas Tapp
Certified Advanced Rolfer
Colorado Springs, CO 80904
719-444-8814

Jim Terrien
Certified Advanced Rolfer
Denver, CO 80209
303-320-ROLF

Cathy McAnsh Ulrich, P.T.
Certified Rolfer
Rolf Movement Practitioner
Ft. Collins, CO 80525
Office: 970-223-8808
Residence: 970-225-1364
cathpt@ix.netcom.com

William Vidal
Certified Advanced Rolfer
Wheatridge, CO 80033
303-420-6170
303-786-9203

Betty Jean Wall, Ph.D.
Certified Advanced Rolfer
Rolf Movement Practitioner
Boulder, CO 80302
303-449-6407

Michael Washburn
Certified Rolfer
Boulder, CO 80301
303-516-0671

Janice K. Wedmore
Certified Rolfer
Rolf Movement Practitioner
Crested Butte, CO 81224
Phone & Fax: 970-641-4802
wedpula@rmi.net

Gary C. Weidner
Certified Advanced Rolfer
Rolf Movement Practitioner
Grand Junction, CO 81501
970-241-7256
and Glenwood Springs, CO 81601
970-945-0280
and Vail, CO 81657
970-476-0444

Kate Zorensky
Certified Rolfer
Durango, CO 81301
970-247-4554
kstarz@ix.netcom.com
Limited Practice

Kim Anderson
Certified Rolfer
Rolf Movement Practitioner
Boulder, CO 80302-6646
303-938-1686
kimnconi@idcomm.com

Mary "Marijah" Baldwin
Certified Rolfer
Rolf Movement Practitioner
Littleton, CO
303-798-7860
and Denver, CO 80236
303-798-7860
and Boulder, CO
303-798-7860

Gary Burns
Certified Rolfer
Longmont, CO 80503
303-682-9352
jukilo@csd.net

Kit E. Cohan
Certified Rolfer
Lakewood, CO 80228
303-988-0502
shabel@ecentral.com

Bryan Devine
Certified Rolfer
Boulder, CO 80302
Office: 303-449-0659
bdevine99@hotmail.com

Sandra Ebling
Certified Advanced Rolfer
Boulder, CO 80301
303-444-4102
Sandebling@aol.com
and Littleton, CO
303-694-2247

Michelle Hagen
Certified Rolfer
Rolf Movement Practitioner
Boulder, CO 80301
Office: 303-402-9088 x3
Residence: 303-698-2690

Hal Paris
Certified Advanced Rolfer
Boulder, CO 80304
303-449-0773

Anngwyn St. Just, R.N., Ph.D.,
L.P.C.
Certified Rolfer
Lyons, CO 80540
Office & Fax: 303-823-9733
Residence: 303-823-9732
Anngwyn@aol.com

Elizabeth M. Vann, B.A.
Certified Rolfer
Loveland, CO 80538
Office: 970-663-5478

Ramone Yaciuk
Certified Advanced Rolfer
Boulder, CO 80303-6526
303-499-7644

CONNECTICUT

Irwin August, D.O., ED.D.
Certified Advanced Rolfer
Madison, CT 06443-0547
860-823-6321 Ext. 2396

Francoise Lajoie Brunette
Certified Rolfer
Litchfield, CT
Appts: 303-448-0640

Anne Dahlberg Kowalczyk, M.A.
Certified Advanced Rolfer
Ivoryton, CT 06442
860-767-0070
annedk@snet.net

William Kaye
Certified Advanced Rolfer
Norwalk, CT 06854
Residence: 203-838-9792
Office: 203-855-8734
wkaye@concentric.net

Sharon Sklar
Certified Advanced Rolfer
West Hartford, CT 06110-1757
860-561-4337
and Avon, CT 06001
860-675-1011

Mary C. Staggs, M.S.
Certified Advanced Rolfer
Mystic, CT 06355-0127
860-536-0750
staggsrolf@aol.com

Craig Swan
Certified Rolfer
Cos Cob, CT 06807
203-629-2620
cswan01@set.net

DELAWARE

Ellen Freed
Certified Advanced Rolfer
Rolf Movement Practitioner
Wilmington, DE 19806-4003
Office: 302-425-4344
Residence: 302-421-8228
freedmi@msn.com

Chris D. Key, Ph.D.
Certified Advanced Rolfer
Newark, DE 19715
302-368-3638
jgkey@udel.edu

DISTRICT OF COLUMBIA

Joy Belluzzi
Certified Advanced Rolfer
Chevy Chase, MD 20815
Office: 301-654-5025

Rebecca Carli-Mills, M.F.A.
Certified Advanced Rolfer
Rolf Movement Practitioner
Silver Spring, MD 20910
Office: 301-585-3328
Residence: 301-585-6690
CarliMills@aol.com

David Delaney
Certified Advanced Rolfer
Washington, DC
Appts: 202-627-6421
DGDelaney@aol.com

Steve Hancoff, L.C.S.W.
Certified Advanced Rolfer
Silver Spring, MD 20904-3029
301-622-2058
Fax: 301-622-2382
SHX2@aol.com

Hubert Ritter
Certified Rolfer
Washington, DC 20009
202-986-2050
703-497-4437
301-236-4614
hritter@mindspring.com
http://www.mindspring.com/~hritter

G. Cosper Scafidi
Advanced Rolfer
Alexandria, VA 22314
Office: 703-998-0474
Fax: 703-836-2667
xascia@aol.com

William Short, M.S.
Certified Advanced Rolfer
Rolf Movement Practitioner
Washington, DC 20009
202-328-3441

Diane Tredway Stroud, P.T.
Certified Advanced Rolfer
Arlington, VA 22201
Office: 703-527-8446
mdstroud@erols.com

David C. Swetz
Certified Rolfer
Alexandria, VA 22302
Appts: 703-845-5493
and Prince Frederick, MD 20678
Appts: 410-286-3030

Sharon Wheeler-Hancoff
Certified Advanced Rolfer
Rolf Movement Practitioner
Silver Spring, MD 20904-3029
301-622-2058
Fax: 301-622-2382
SHX2@aol.com
and Fairfax, VA
540-989-1617
and Fairfax, VA
703-989-1617

FLORIDA

Michelle Arsenault
Certified Rolfer
Seminole, FL 34646
Office: 813-560-3335

Thomas J. Burke
Certified Rolfer
Wellington, FL 33414
561-790-6956

David Clark
Certified Advanced Rolfer
Brandon, FL 33510-4109
Office: 813-661-3662
813-677-5067
helixinc@tampa.mindspring.com

Thom Coker
Certified Rolfer
Stuart, FL 34995
Office: 561-286-2639

Candace Cressor
Certified Rolfer
Rolf Movement Practitioner
Tampa, FL 33606
Office: 813-251-1367
ccressor@juno.com

Donna Jo Cross-Sutherland
Certified Advanced Rolfer
Naples, FL 34103
941-435-4900
Fax: 941-262-6754

Janis G. Davis, M.D.
Certified Advanced Rolfer
St. Petersburg, FL 33705
813-896-8807

Carolyn Dombroski, R.N.
Certified Rolfer
Sarasota, FL 34236
Phone/Fax: 941-953-6875
rdombroski@home.com

Emily Flowers
Certified Rolfer
Clearwater, FL 34620
Office: 813-538-4188
emily.rolfs@juno.com

Ms. Sydney Ellen Frasca
Certified Advanced Rolfer
Tampa, FL 33614-2869
Office: 813-933-6229

Suzanne Kelsall
Certified Advanced Rolfer
Winter Haven, FL 33880
941-297-5539
and Naples & Marco Isl., FL 33940
941-642-9326

Eileen Kepper
Certified Advanced Rolfer
Altamonte Springs, FL 32701
Office: 407-339-2309
and Longwood, FL 32750

Michael Kilmartin, Ph.D.
Certified Advanced Rolfer
Sarasota, FL 34236
Office: 941-955-1020
941-951-7765

Caryn T. King
Certified Rolfer
Cocoa, FL 32922
Office: 407-636-4548
and Tavernier, FL 33070
305-852-1614

Judi Macy, RN
Certified Rolfer
St. Petersburg, FL 33734
813-521-1476
jmacy30056@aol.com

Robyn Martin
Certified Rolfer
Winter Park, FL 32792
407-647-0445
ROBYNROLF@aol.com

Miraa Joanne Neill, LMT
Certified Advanced Rolfer
Hawthorne, FL 32640-8014
Office: 352-373-5505

Patricia Nelson
Certified Rolfer
Ft. Lauderdale, FL 33301
954-522-8807
and Stuart, FL
954-522-8807

Lynne Odekirk
Certified Advanced Rolfer
Vero Beach, FL 32968-3270
561-562-4062

M. Breck Parker, J.D.
Certified Rolfer
Clearwater, FL 34619
Residence: 813-797-4124
and S. Naples, FL 33940
813-261-0236

Keith Parmenter
Certified Rolfer
Pompano Beach, FL 33062
561-368-6753
and Boca Raton, FL 33433
Office: 561-368-6753

Jeff Reisman
Certified Rolfer
Miami, FL 33130
305-285-6991
Pager: 305-352-1626

Ronald A. Thompson
Certified Advanced Rolfer
Tampa, FL 33604
Office&Fax: 813-933-6868
IRolf@aol.com

J. Thomas West, Ph.D.
Certified Advanced Rolfer
St. Petersburg, FL 33705
Phone/Fax: 813-867-8875
westjt@eckerd.edu
Limited Practice

Eileen Allman
Certified Rolfer
Rolf Movement Practitioner
Port Charlotte, FL 33952-2307
941-629-9567

Donald Curry
Certified Advanced Rolfer
Lake Worth, FL 33461
and Ft. Lauderdale, FL 33301
Appts: 305-463-5430

Dr. Gladys Man, Ph.D.
Certified Advanced Rolfer
Hollywood, FL 33019-3711
954-920-6569

Margaret F. Scott
Certified Rolfer
Melbourne Beach, FL 32951
Office: 407-952-4387
pegscott@iu.net
and Melbourne, FL 32901
Residence: 407-984-1270

Michael Shea, Ph.D.
Certified Advanced Rolfer
Juno Beach, FL 33408
407-627-7327
sheagroup@aol.com

Georgia, GA

Raymond J. Bishop, Jr., Ph.D.
Certified Rolfer
Rolf Movement Practitioner
Woodstock, GA 30188
Residence: 770-591-8115
Office: 404-257-1257

Julie Salazar
Certified Rolfer
Rolf Movement Practitioner
Atlanta, GA 30329
Office: 770-401-3108
Cyclecraz@aol.com

Libby Eason Sener
Certified Advanced Rolfer
Rolf Movement Practitioner
Atlanta, GA 30345
Office: 404-315-0099
libbyeason@aol.com

Caroline Widmer, Ph.D.
Certified Advanced Rolfer
Atlanta, GA 30324-2563
404-266-1992
Fax: 404-266-8536
caroline_i._widmer@atlmug.org
Limited Practice

Linda Crocker, N.D.
Certified Rolfer
Roswell, GA 30076
770-641-6557

HAWAII

Richard Diehl, M.Ed., L. Ac.
Certified Advanced Rolfer
Honolulu, HI 96815
808-923-4041

Leland Everett
Certified Rolfer
Rolf Movement Practitioner
Kamuela, HI 96743
808-885-5866

Anne F. Hoff
Certified Rolfer
Makawao, Maui, HI 96768
808-572-6699
Fax: 808-572-1371

Sally J. Klemm M.Ed.
Certified Advanced Rolfer
Rolf Movement Practitioner
Honolulu, HI 96815
808-732-4828
SJKlemm@aol.com

Mars Celeste Lang
Certified Rolfer
Honomu, HI 96728
808-963-5451

James Lawson
Certified Rolfer
Kailua, HI 96734
808-262-9017

Angela Ledington-Fischer, P.T.
Certified Rolfer
Kapaa, Kauai, HI 96746
Office: 808-822-0551
Cell Phone: 808-635-1657

Michael Misha-E. Noonan
Certified Rolfer
Rolf Movement Practitioner
Honolulu, HI 96816-0925
808-732-4828
migraine@lava.net
and Honolulu, HI 96816
Cell: 808-388-6600
808-739-3884

Doris Xenia Resch
Certified Rolfer
Honolulu, HI 96821
808-377-9752
lanhnl@worldnet.att.net

Kim Schaefer, R.N.
Certified Rolfer
Rolf Movement Practitioner
Kapaa, Kauai, HI 96746
808-822-1151
schaefr@aloha.net

Marianne Broz Wassel, M.Ed.
Certified Advanced Rolfer
Honolulu, HI 96813
Office: 808-545-7653

Charles Winchell
Certified Rolfer
Kapaa, Kauai, HI 96746
808-822-7663
Limited Practice

Rebecca Lux
Certified Rolfer
Rolf Movement Practitioner
Kapaau, HI 96755
Office: 808-935-8720
808-889-5236
rjdlux@ilhawaii.net

Rosemary Shoong
Certified Advanced Rolfer
Lahaina, Maui, HI 96761
808-667-7609
808-667-7296

IDAHO

Owen Marcus, M.A., Lic.
Certified Advanced Rolfer
Sandpoint, ID 83864
208-265-8440
owenmarcus@juno.com

Ron Murray
Certified Advanced Rolfer
Sand Point, ID

Glennette O'Rourke, M.A.
Certified Advanced Rolfer
Boise, ID
Appts: 208-336-3362
gio1r@aol.com

Lissa Poynter
Certified Rolfer
Ketchum, ID 83340
Office: 208-725-0303
Fax: 208-726-9648
Residence: 208-726-2350
pnutpop@aol.com

Martha Vandivort, M.A.
Certified Rolfer
Boise, ID 83712
208-338-0284
mbvandiv@micron.net

ILLINOIS

Robert G. Ahrens, M.S.W.
Certified Advanced Rolfer
Evanston, IL 60202
847-328-7174
Robahrens@aol.com

John Cottingham, P.T.
Certified Advanced Rolfer
Champaign, IL 61821
217-355-5721
jcottingha@aol.com

Allan Davidson, M.A.
Certified Advanced Rolfer
Chicago, IL 60622
773-486-6857
nosdivad@ais.net

Barbara Drummond, PT
Certified Rolfer
Rolf Movement Practitioner
Waukegan, IL 60085
Office: 847-336-3066
Residence: 847-244-7659
Redrolf1@aol.com
and Brookfield, IL 60513
Office: 847-336-3066

Thomas Earnest, Jr.
Certified Advanced Rolfer
Chicago & Suburbs, IL
x6740: 800-927-2527

David C. Englund
Certified Rolfer
Rolf Movement Practitioner
Niles, IL 60714
847-965-3448
mrerolfu@aol.com

Karen Giles
Certified Rolfer
Downer's Grove, IL 60516
Office: 630-434-9960

Heidi Massa
Certified Rolfer
Rolf Movement Practitioner
Chicago, IL 60614
Residence: 773-975-5946
hmassa@enteract.com
and Chicago, IL 60610
Office: 312-943-5808

Brian Moore
Certified Advanced Rolfer
Evanston, IL 60202
Office: 800-282-1222
BMoore2967@aol.com

Grace A. Powers
Certified Rolfer
Carbondale, IL 62901
618-529-5465
gpowerbit@aol.com
and Makanda, IL 62958
618-529-5465

Donald Soule, M.A.
Certified Advanced Rolfer
Chicago, IL
Office: 312-645-1880
dcsoul@inland.com
Limited Practice

Ms. Bjorg Holte
Certified Rolfer
Urbana, IL 61801
217-344-9245

Sol Warkov, M.F.A.
Certified Rolfer
Glen Ellyn, IL
Office: 630-515-5597
and Chicago, IL
630-515-5597
Indiana, IN

Dan Dyer
Certified Rolfer
Indianapolis, IN 46220-3136
317-925-9572

John Maurer
Certified Rolfer
Bloomington, IN 47401
812-339-2784

Jane Hale McSpadden
Certified Advanced Rolfer
New Paris, IN 46553-9610
219-831-4037

Dan Somers
Certified Advanced Rolfer
Indianapolis, IN 46220
317-259-4205

IOWA

Ralph Bianco
Certified Advanced Rolfer
Fairfield, IA 52556
515-472-9048
Rolfer@lisco.com

Judith Clinton
Certified Advanced Rolfer
Iowa City, IA 52240
910-793-1930

Ron Petit, M.A.
Certified Rolfer
Marshalltown, IA 50158
Office: 515-752-6255

Glenn Watt
Certified Rolfer
Fairfield, IA 52556
515-472-9299
wattsup@kdsi.net
and Iowa City, IA
x33: 319-338-1129

KANSAS

Elaine Brewer
Certified Rolfer
Lawrence, KS 66044
Office: 785-749-2740
Residence: 785-841-2216

Karla Darnstaedt, M.A.
Certified Rolfer
Fairway, KS 66205
Office: 913-432-2600

Kent Dickinson
Certified Rolfer
Rolf Movement Practitioner
Lenexa, KS 66215
Office: 913-438-2239
Residence: 913-268-0965
KCRolfer@worldnet.att.net

Carol Rasor
Certified Rolfer
Rolf Movement Practitioner
Lawrence, KS 66044
Office: 785-843-5854

Larry Redding, M.S.
Certified Advanced Rolfer
Lawrence, KS 66047-2955
Office: 785-841-8481
Residence: 785-841-1838
Limited Practice

Jack Windhorst
Certified Rolfer
Manhattan, KS 66502
913-776-9804
Kentucky, KY

Mary Agneessens
Certified Rolfer
Versailles, KY 40383
606-873-6348

John Maurer
Certified Rolfer
Louisville, KY 40207
502-895-2230

Wanda Sucher
Certified Advanced Rolfer
Rolf Movement Practitioner
Crescent Springs, KY 41017
606-341-8907

LOUISIANA

John R. DeMahy, R.N.
Certified Advanced Rolfer
New Orleans, LA 70119
504-488-7555
jdemahy@bellsouth.net

Allen Frost
Certified Rolfer
Rolf Movement Practitioner
Thibodaux, LA 70301
504-447-4118
agfrost@juno.com

Kathy Rooney
Certified Advanced Rolfer
Rolf Movement Practitioner
New Orleans, LA 70124
504-486-8936
DeltaKar@aol.com

John H. Schewe, M.S.
Certified Advanced Rolfer
New Orleans, LA 70119
504-488-6174
JHSchewe@sprintmail.com

MAINE

Becky Dacus
Certified Rolfer
Auburn, ME 04210
Office: 207-784-6582
bdacus@cybertours.com
and Auburn, ME 04210
207-784-2188

Paul Gordon, M.A.
Certified Advanced Rolfer
Eliot, ME 03903
Office: 207-439-8522
GordonRolf@aol.com
www.openfaucet.com/gordon.html

Lily Hill
Certified Advanced Rolfer
Rolf Movement Practitioner
Camden, ME 04843
207-763-3811

Marilyn B. Huss
Certified Rolfer
Rolf Movement Practitioner
Brunswick, ME 04011
207-725-7801

Michael C. Morrison, M.S.
Certified Rolfer
Portland, ME 04102
207-871-8002
mcmorrison@compuserve.com

Thomas Myers
Certified Advanced Rolfer
Scarborough, ME 04074
Office/Fax: 207-883-2756
888-546-3747
kinesis@ime.net

Carol Wu
Certified Rolfer
Yarmouth, ME 04096
207-847-9205

Annie Wyman
Certified Rolfer
Rolf Movement Practitioner
Portland, ME 04102
Off&Res: 207-772-0965
tribe@javanet.com

MARYLAND

Michael R. Alwood
Certified Rolfer
Rolf Movement Practitioner
Baltimore, MD 21209
Office: 410-367-7300
ironhand@trail.com

Joy Belluzzi
Certified Advanced Rolfer
Chevy Chase, MD 20815
Office: 301-654-5025

Tessy Brungardt
Certified Advanced Rolfer
Rolf Movement Practitioner
Baltimore, MD
Office: 410-367-7300
TESSYB@aol.com
and
Hampstead, MD 21074
410-239-1514

Rebecca Carli-Mills, M.F.A.
Certified Advanced Rolfer
Rolf Movement Practitioner
Silver Spring, MD 20910
Office: 301-585-3328
Residence: 301-585-6690
CarliMills@aol.com

Steve Hancoff, L.C.S.W.
Certified Advanced Rolfer
Silver Spring, MD 20904-3029
301-622-2058
Fax: 301-622-2382
SHX2@aol.com

Holly Howard
Certified Advanced Rolfer
Baltimore, MD 21209
Office: 410-367-7300
HollyHow@aol.com

Larry Kofsky
Certified Rolfer
Owings Mills, MD 21117
410-356-5937
and Baltimore, MD

Hubert Ritter
Certified Rolfer
Washington, DC 20009
202-986-2050
703-497-4437
301-236-4614
hritter@mindspring.com

G. Cosper Scafidi
Certified Advanced Rolfer
Alexandria, VA 22314
Office: 703-998-0474
Fax: 703-836-2667
xascia@aol.com

William Short, M.S.
Certified Advanced Rolfer
Rolf Movement Practitioner
Washington, DC 20009
202-328-3441

David C. Swetz
Certified Rolfer
Alexandria, VA 22302
Appts: 703-845-5493
and Prince Frederick, MD 20678
Appts: 410-286-3030

Francis Wenger, M.D.
Certified Advanced Rolfer
West River, MD 20778
410-867-2742
301-261-5748

Sharon Wheeler-Hancoff
Certified Advanced Rolfer
Rolf Movement Practitioner
Silver Spring, MD 20904-3029
301-622-2058
Fax: 301-622-2382
SHX2@aol.com
and Fairfax, VA
540-989-1617
Limited Practice

Bren Jacobson
Certified Advanced Rolfer
Annapolis, MD 21401
410-224-4877
BrenJaco@bigfoot.com
www.cybermall2000/stores/multipure

Debra Savage
Certified Rolfer
Valley Lee, MD 20692
301-994-9819
evocycles@olg.com
and onardtown, MD 20650
x3: 301-475-0312

MASSACHUSETTS

Dennis S. Bailey
Certified Rolfer
Marshfield, MA 02050-4113
781-834-0748

Paul Gordon, M.A.
Certified Advanced Rolfer
Cambridge, MA 02139
617-864-2727
GordonRolf@aol.com
www.openfaucet.com/gordon.html

Ross W. Hackerson, M.A.
Certified Advanced Rolfer
Northampton, MA 01060
413-587-0403
800-409-9344
ross@northeasthealth.com
www.northeasthealth.com

Eric Jacobson
Certified Rolfer
Arlington, MA 02174
781-643-6874
ejcbsn@aol.com

Chris D. Key, Ph.D.
Certified Advanced Rolfer
Nantucket, MA 02554
508-228-2491
jgkey@udel.edu

Ellen Landauer
Certified Advanced Rolfer
Northampton, MA 01060
413-586-0869

Dick Larson, Ph.D., L.Ac.
Certified Advanced Rolfer
Rolf Movement Practitioner
Northampton, MA 01062
Office: 413-582-0123
larsons@javanet.com

Charles Maier
Certified Advanced Rolfer
Northampton, MA 01060
413-586-0869

Thomas Myers
Certified Advanced Rolfer
Boston, MA
888-546-3747
kinesis@ime.net

Aline Newton, M.A.
Certified Advanced Rolfer
Rolf Movement Practitioner
Cambridge, MA 02139
Phone&Fax: 617-661-6409
aline@world.std.com

William M. Redpath, M.F.A., M.Ed.
Certified Advanced Rolfer
Lexington, MA 02173-8025
Phone&Fax: 781-861-0184
redpathw@tiac.net
www.tiac.net/users/redpathw

Richard Shaw
Certified Advanced Rolfer
Northampton, MA 01060
413-586-8252
rcshaw@hotmail.com

Lenaye Siegel-Hudock
Certified Advanced Rolfer
Marblehead, MA 01945
Office: 617-631-2420
lenaye@shore.net

Betty Jean Wall, Ph.D.
Certified Advanced Rolfer
Rolf Movement Practitioner
Woods Hole, MA 02543
508-540-1079

Garret Whitney
Certified Advanced Rolfer
Concord, MA 01742
978-371-2188
gw@world.std.com
and Brighton, MA 02135
978-371-2188
Limited Practice

Joseph M. Laur
Certified Advanced Rolfer
Wendell, MA 01379
Residence: 978-544-0001
seedjoe@aol.com
www.seedsys.com
New Hampshire, NH

Ticia Agri
Certified Advanced Rolfer
Exeter, NH 03833
603-778-6247
Fax: 603-778-3962
ticia@nh.destek.net

Bruce Dow
Certified Rolfer
Rolf Movement Practitioner
Concord, NH 03301
603-225-3595
BruceDow@aol.com
and Keene, NH
603-225-3595

Jane Halle Esselstyn
Certified Rolfer
Hanover, NH 03750
603-643-4948

Kevin K. Frank
Certified Advanced Rolfer
Ashland, NH 03217-9505
603-968-9585
kkfrank@cris.com
and Concord, NH
603-968-9585

Paul Gordon, M.A.
Certified Advanced Rolfer
Portsmouth, NH
207-439-8522
617-864-2727
GordonRolf@aol.com
www.openfaucet.com/gordon.html

Suzy Reed
Certified Rolfer
Sanbornton, NH 03269
603-286-4331
rsreed@lr.net

MICHIGAN

Leland Austin, M.A.
Certified Advanced Rolfer
Ann Arbor, MI 48103
734-741-0038
LelandSF@aol.com

Kim Tillen Hicks, P.T.
Certified Rolfer
Milford, MI 48381-4042
248-685-0405

Neil G. King, P.T.
Certified Advanced Rolfer
Rochester, MI 48307
248-651-8085

Allan J. Kupczak
Certified Rolfer
Milford, MI 48381
248-685-1035

Karen Parker, M.A., C.S.W.
Certified Rolfer
Birmingham, MI 48009-6600
Office: 248-647-5877

Kathleen L. Strauch, J.D.
Certified Advanced Rolfer
Rolf Movement Practitioner
Southfield, MI 48034
248-354-3484
and
East Lansing, MI 48823
517-351-9240

Jim Z. Tavrazich, P.T.
Certified Rolfer
Bloomfield Hills, MI 48304
248-332-8122

Anthony Zimkowski, Ph.D.
Certified Advanced Rolfer
Lambertville, MI 48144
(and Detroit Area), MI
Office: 313-856-6806
Residence: 313-856-1698
Limited Practice

Cori Terry
Certified Rolfer
Kalamazoo, MI 49007-3205
616-388-5310
Lambertville, MI 48144
and Detroit, MI
Office: 313-856-6806
Residence: 313-856-1698

MINNESOTA

Olixn Adams
Certified Rolfer
Minneapolis, MN 55414
612-331-3530

Briah Anson, M.A.
Certified Advanced Rolfer
Rolf Movement Practitioner
St. Paul, MN 55102
612-228-9569

Teresa Dalseth
Rolf Movement Practitioner
Saint Paul, MN 55105-3329
612-222-4247

Siana Goodwin
Certified Advanced Rolfer
Rolf Movement Practitioner
Minneapolis, MN 55414
Office: 612-379-3895
SianaB@aol.com

Roger Hartley
Certified Advanced Rolfer
Rolf Movement Practitioner
Duluth, MN 55803
218-724-6812
RHartwise@aol.com
http://nnic.com/roger.html

Lance Hauge
Certified Rolfer
Hopkins, MN 55343
612-930-0916

Sandy Henningsgaard, R.N.
Certified Advanced Rolfer
Stillwater, MN 55082
612-430-3716
SandyHenn@aol.com
http://www.continuumrolfing.com
and Minneapolis, MN 55414
612-331-3530

Wayne M. Henningsgaard, M.A.
Certified Advanced Rolfer
Stillwater, MN 55082
612-430-3716
SandyHenn@aol.com
http://www.continuumrolfing.com
and Minneapolis, MN 55414
612-331-3530

Cindy Jamieson
Certified Rolfer
Excelsior, MN 55331
612-474-1576
Fax: 612-474-1048
jamduff@aol.com

Ron Petit, M.A.
Certified Rolfer
Richfield, MN 55423-2309
612-436-3845
612-861-6129

Mark Powell
Certified Rolfer
Minneapolis, MN 55405
Office: 612-872-6055
and Minneapolis, MN 55408
Residence: 612-381-1391

Ursula Weltman
Certified Rolfer
Minneapolis, MN 55414
Office: 612-331-3530
http://www.continuumrolfing.com

MISSOURI

B.J. Clark
Certified Rolfer
Independence, MO 64052-1935
Residence: 816-461-5350
and Independence, MO 64055
Office: 816-254-0606

Karla Darnstaedt, M.A.
Certified Rolfer
Fairway, KS 66205
Office: 913-432-2600

Deborah A. Nuckolls
Certified Rolfer
Kansas City, MO 64111
816-753-4888
debbie@thirdwave.net

Grace A. Powers
Certified Rolfer
St. Louis, MO
Appts: 618-529-5465
gpowerbit@aol.com

Judith Mayanja
Certified Advanced Rolfer
Kansas City, MO 64114

MONTANA

Marilyn Faye Beech
Certified Rolfer
Missoula, MT 59801
Office: 406-728-7777
mbeech@montana.com

Noel Clark
Certified Advanced Rolfer
Bozeman, MT 59715
406-585-5995
thumper@mcn.net

R. Kerrick Murray
Certified Advanced Rolfer
Helena, MT 59601
Office: 406-431-4246
TollfreeMT: 888-570-8550
Residence: 406-723-6779
and Butte, MT 59701
Office: 406-782-8550
TollfreeMT: 888-570-8550

Rob Stevens, D.P.M.
Certified Rolfer
Whitefish, MT 59937
406-862-9028
Office: 406-862-8768
Fax: 406-862-8391
stevensr@cyberport.net
Limited Practice

Michael C. Stabile
Certified Rolfer
Bozeman, MT 59715
Phone/Fax: 406-586-7295
Limited Practice
816-333-8931
New Hampshire, NH

Ticia Agri
Certified Advanced Rolfer
Exeter, NH 03833
603-778-6247
Fax: 603-778-3962
ticia@nh.destek.net

Bruce Dow
Certified Rolfer
Movement Teacher
Concord, NH 03301
603-225-3595
BruceDow@aol.com
and
Keene, NH

Jane Halle Esselstyn
Certified Rolfer
Hanover, NH 03750
603-643-4948

Kevin K. Frank
Certified Advanced Rolfer
Ashland, NH 03217-9505
603-968-9585
kkfrank@cris.com
and
Concord, NH
603-968-9585

Paul Gordon, M.A.
Certified Advanced Rolfer
Portsmouth, NH
207-439-8522
617-864-2727
GordonRolf@aol.com

NEW JERSEY

Richard D. Bruder
Certified Rolfer
Westfield, NJ 07090-3621
908-233-6321

Chuck Carpenter
Certified Advanced Rolfer
Milltown, NJ 08850
908-422-8029
Fax: 908-821-6516
and New York, NY 10001
212-307-5367

David Frome P.T.
Certified Advanced Rolfer
Montclair, NJ 07042
Office: 201-509-8464
and
New York, NY 10025
Office: 212-529-1901

Ms. Joey Joann-George
Certified Rolfer
Belle Mead, NJ 08502
Office: 908-874-0596

Steven Glassman
Certified Advanced Rolfer
Englewood Cliffs, NJ 07632
201-816-8333
and
Nyack, NY 10960
914-353-3160

Diane Kuschel
Certified Rolfer
High Bridge, NJ 08829
Residence: 908-638-5409
dan.devenio@worldnet.att.net
and Clinton, NJ 08809
Office: 908-735-7403
Fax: 980-735-4949

Caroline May
Certified Rolfer
Stockton, NJ 08559
609-397-2500

George J. Smyth
Certified Advanced Rolfer
Ocean City, NJ
717-426-3085

Ruth Solomon M.A.
Certified Advanced Rolfer
N. Brunswick, NJ 08902
908-821-6868

Ron Spechler
Certified Rolfer
Closter, NJ 07624
201-767-9251
and Mountain Lakes, NJ
201-402-8510

Edward Toal
Certified Rolfer
Gibbstown, NJ 08027
609-423-5662
ETOAL4@aol.com

Sheila Toal
Certified Rolfer
Gibbstown, NJ 08027
609-423-3087
sheialtoal@aol.com
Limited Practice

Karen Hedley M.F.A.
Certified Rolfer
Westwood, NJ 07675
201-722-0989
76744.3274@compuserve.com

Gil Hedley Jr., Ph.D.
Certified Rolfer
Westwood, NJ 07675
201-722-0989
76744.3274@compuserve.com

Julia Ireland
Certified Advanced Rolfer
Moorestown, NJ 08057-2200
609-235-1684
INYOI@aol.com

NEW MEXICO

Michael R. Alwood
Certified Rolfer
Rolf Movement Practitioner
Santa Fe, NM 87504
505-984-3177
ironhand@trail.com

Carter Beckett
Certified Advanced Rolfer
Santa Fe, NM 87505
505-983-5457

Valerie Berg
Certified Rolfer
Albuquerque, NM 87109
Office: 505-881-6509
vberg@flash.net

James G. Blackburn II
Certified Rolfer
Rolf Movement Practitioner
Ruidoso, NM 88345
Residence: 505-257-9425
Office: 505-257-7555
Office: 505-627-7109
villagerolfer@seqnet.net

Constance A. Buck
Certified Rolfer
Santa Fe, NM 87501
505-982-4718

John Deckebach
Certified Advanced Rolfer
Silver City, NM 88061
505-538-0050
and Gila, NM 88038
505-535-2400

Juli Ditto
Certified Rolfer
Rolf Movement Practitioner
Placitas, NM 87043
505-867-2775
jmditto@aol.com

Thomas Earnest, Jr.
Certified Advanced Rolfer
Albuquerque, NM 87108
Office: 505-268-2772
x6740: 800-927-2527
and Albuquerque, NM 87120-4620
Residence: 505-899-2949

Brian Fahey, Ph.D.
Certified Advanced Rolfer
Albuquerque, NM 87106
505-243-7458

Giselle Genilla
Certified Rolfer
Santa Fe, NM 87501
Phone/Fax: 505-989-4662
gisgenillard@webtv.net
and Santa Fe, NM 87505
Residence: 505-989-9100

Jill Gerber
Certified Rolfer
Santa Fe, NM 87501
505-984-8830
twoboos@roadrunner.com

Marilyn Grimes
Certified Advanced Rolfer
Rolf Movement Practitioner
Ranchos de Taos, NM 87557
505-758-4439
and Taos area, NM
505-758-4439

Hallie Hardenstine
Rolf Movement Practitioner
Albuquerque, NM 87111
505-294-2334

Linda Holley, Ph.D.
Certified Rolfer
Albuquerque, NM 87114-1937
Office: 505-897-9524

Kristen Kuester, M.F.A.
Certified Advanced Rolfer
Santa Fe, NM 87501
505-989-7529

Scott Mackenzie
Certified Rolfer
Monticello, NM 87939-0038
505-894-5082

Andree Neumeister
Certified Advanced Rolfer
Santa Fe, NM 87501
505-982-1368
acnooo@earthlink.net

David Receconi
Certified Rolfer
Santa Fe, NM 87504-2708
505-982-7724

Elisabeth K. Rimann
Certified Rolfer
Santa Fe, NM 87505
Office: 505-982-5868
Fax: 505-995-0500
Residence: 505-983-2250
erimann@ix.netcom.com

Robert Schrei
Certified Advanced Rolfer
Glorieta, NM 87535-9602
505-983-7213
rjschrei@roadrunner.com

William Smythe
Certified Advanced Rolfe
Santa Fe, NM 87501
505-982-2295
Fax: 505-982-1130
WDSmythe@aol.com

Jan Henry Sultan
Certified Advanced Rolfer
Santa Fe, NM 87501
505-983-8847
Fax: 505-988-5200
JHSultan@aol.com

Michael J. Wick
Certified Rolfer
Truth or Consequences, NM 87901-1091
505-894-9582

Christopher B. Wilson
Certified Rolfer
Algodones, NM 87001
505-891-1462
Cell: 505-450-6414
NPRN58A@Prodigy.com

Don Wolvington
Certified Advanced Rolfer
Santa Fe, NM 87505-1706
505-438-6008
dwolvton@rt66.com

Robert B. Younger, M.A.
Certified Rolfer
Albuquerque, NM 87110
Office: 505-889-3333
Residence: 505-268-7778
RBYounger@aol.com
Limited Practice

Allen Heaton
Certified Advanced Rolfer
Mountainair, NM 87036
505-423-3262

Sabina Schulze
Certified Rolfer
Santa Fe, NM 87501-2211
505-982-4183
ralphsab@concentric.net

Bill Zimmer, Ph.D.
Certified Advanced Rolfer
Albuquerque, NM 87106
505-266-6699

NEW YORK

Sam Adams
Certified Rolfer
New York, NY 10014
212-807-6827

Helga Birth
Certified Rolfer
Movement Teacher
Rochester, NY 14607
Office: 716-271-2920

John Botsford
Certified Rolfer
Rochester, NY 14607
Office: 716-461-9519
Residence: 716-288-1556

Chuck Carpenter
Certified Advanced Rolfer
Milltown, NJ 08850
908-422-8029
Fax: 908-821-6516
and New York, NY 10001
212-307-5367

Bonnie Clark
Certified Rolfer
Movement Teacher
West Harrison, NY 10604
Office: 914-285-9298
bonclark@worldnet.att.net

David Delaney
Certified Advanced Rolfer
New York, NY 10003
Office: 212-627-6421
Voice Mail: 212-969-0552
DGDelaney@aol.com
and Hudson, NY 12534
518-822-1210
Fax: 518-822-0336

David Frome P.T.
Certified Advanced Rolfer
Montclair, NJ 07042
Office: 201-509-8464
and New York, NY 10025
Office: 212-529-1901

Steven Glassman
Certified Advanced Rolfer
Englewood Cliffs, NJ 07632
201-816-8333
and Nyack, NY 10960
914-353-3160

Tom Gustin
Certified Advanced Rolfer
Southampton, NY 11968-5033
516-287-6564

Dorothy Hunter
Certified Advanced Rolfer
Movement Teacher
New York, NY 10024
Office: 212-724-6963

William Kaye
Certified Advanced Rolfer
New York, NY 10001
Office: 212-268-8705
wkaye@concentric.net

David Keffer
Certified Rolfer
New York, NY 10023
212-957-1978

Laurie Latner
Certified Rolfer
Pittsford, NY 14534
716-248-9110

Nancy Leone
Certified Advanced Rolfer
Orchard Park, NY 14127
716-662-1955

Margaret Ann Markert
Certified Rolfer
New York, NY 10023
212-580-0135

H. Simon Msadoques
Certified Rolfer
Cheektowaga, NY 14225
716-631-3413

John Murphy
Certified Rolfer
Movement Teacher
New York, NY 10021
212-744-3552
Voice Mail: 212-465-3104

Glennette O'Rourke M.A.
Certified Advanced Rolfer
Baldwinsville, NY 13027
315-638-2429

Darcey Ortolf Ph.D.
Certified Rolfer
New York, NY 10011
212-727-8561

Barbara A. Pelc
Certified Rolfer
S. Wales, NY 14139
716-457-1312

Kayte Ringer M.A.
Certified Advanced Rolfer
New York, NY 10014
212-929-1602

Gary J. Robb
Certified Rolfer
Movement Teacher
Buffalo, NY 14213
716-885-3329

Judith Roberts
Certified Rolfer
Movement Teacher
New York, NY 10024
212-580-7644

Kali Rosenblum
Certified Rolfer
Bearsville, NY 12409
914-679-2335

R. Louis Schultz Ph.D.
Certified Advanced Rolfer
Movement Teacher
New York, NY 10014
212-924-2610
RLou1@aol.com

Kristin S. Sloth
Certified Rolfer
Oneonta, NY 13820
607-433-2536
607-432-7817

Kevin Smith
Certified Advanced Rolfer
Bearsville, NY 12409
914-679-2335

Beth Ullmann-Franzese
Certified Advanced Rolfer
New York, NY 10007
212-346-9621
and Bronx, NY 10465

Don Van Vleet
Certified Advanced Rolfer
New York, NY 10128
212-369-8038

Carol Wu
Certified Rolfer
Pleasantville, NY 10570-2702
914-741-2623
ratel@bestweb.net

Paul Zimmerman
Certified Advanced Rolfer
Waterport, NY 14571
716-682-9720
Limited Practice

Howard Finkelson
Certified Rolfer
New York, NY 10023
212-877-1123

Lisa Tackley
Certified Advanced Rolfer
Albany, NY 12220-0320
518-475-7560

NORTH CAROLINA

Jennifer E. Albrecht
Certified Rolfer
Raleigh, NC 27615
919-847-7201
JEAlbrecht@aol.com

Nathan Boniske
Certified Advanced Rolfer
Asheville, NC 28801
828-252-7451
Naugual@aol.com

Rodney Buchner, M.A. Psych.
Certified Advanced Rolfer
Rolf Movement Practitioner
Mill Spring, NC 28756
704-894-3146
and Hendersonville, NC

Judith Clinton
Certified Advanced Rolfer
Wilmington, NC 28403
Office: 910-763-6878
Voicemail: 910-452-6779
Residence: 910-793-1930

Candace Frye
Certified Rolfer
Greenville, NC 27858
Office: 919-353-1121
and Greenville, NC 27836
919-830-2934

Brian D. Hopkins
Certified Advanced Rolfer
Durham, NC 27705
Office: 919-286-5877
Residence: 919-479-2130
Fax: 919-286-9627

Bill Morrow
Certified Rolfer
Summerfield, NC 27358
336-643-6779

Cameron Nims
Certified Advanced Rolfer
Chapel Hill, NC 27516
919-929-4111
cnfs@earthlink.net

Ellen Presnell, R.N.
Certified Rolfer
Rolf Movement Practitioner
Asheville, NC 28801-3609
828-258-2833

Marsha Presnell-Jennette
Certified Advanced Rolfer
Rolf Movement Practitioner
Raleigh, NC 27605
Office: 919-821-3760

Kathy Rooney
Certified Advanced Rolfer
Rolf Movement Practitioner
Greensboro, NC 27410
Office: 336-852-7315
Fax: 336-852-4413
DeltaKar@aol.com
and Summerfield, NC 27358-9213
Residence: 336-643-7878

Shannon Warwick
Certified Advanced Rolfer
Asheville, NC 28801
Office: 828-285-0564
shannonw@buncombe.main.nc.us
and Hendersonville, NC 28792
704-749-1460 and
Saluda, NC 28773
Limited Practice

Judith Bradt
Certified Rolfer
Chapel Hill, NC 27514
Residence: 919-929-1211
Office: 919-929-8222
rolfer@intrex.net

Polly Lucas
Advanced Rolfer
Rolf Movement Practitioner
Asheville, NC 28804

OHIO

Kim Hourston
Certified Rolfer
Athens, OH
614-593-8155

Austin McElroy
Certified Rolfer
Granville, OH 43023-9675
Office: 614-587-2902
Residence: 614-587-1629
acmcelroy@nextek.net
and Cleveland, OH
Office: 614-587-2902
and Columbus, OH
Office: 614-587-2902

Ruth Mendelsohn
Certified Rolfer
Cleveland, OH 44124
216-464-5826
ruthmend@apk.net

Brian Moore
Certified Advanced Rolfer
Cleveland and Dayton, OH
800-282-1222
BMoore2967@aol.com

Jason Perry
Certified Rolfer
Toledo, OH 43605
419-693-2007

Larry Stone
Certified Advanced Rolfer
Worthington, OH 43085
614-268-1557

Wanda Sucher
Certified Advanced Rolfer
Rolf Movement Practitioner
Cincinnati, OH 45236
513-984-8636

OKLAHOMA

Kay Blanchard
Certified Rolfer
Tulsa, OK 74135-2206
918-749-4559

Erik Dalton, Ph.D.
Certified Advanced Rolfer
Oklahoma City, OK 73122
405-728-7711
Fax: 405-721-7666

Dan Gentry
Certified Rolfer
Oklahoma City, OK
405-749-1363
and Oklahoma City, OK 73162-7443
Residence: 405-721-4345

Annie Heartfield Hartzog
Certified Rolfer
Tulsa, OK 74104
Home & Fax: 918-748-8173
aheart@tulsa.oklahoma.net
and Tulsa, OK 74114
Office: 918-630-7533

Jo Evelyn "Jody" Seay
Certified Advanced Rolfer
Tulsa, OK
918-835-5927

OREGON

Jeffrey Burch, M.S.
Certified Advanced Rolfer
Eugene, OR 97404
541-689-1515
darkwood@rio.com

Kerry Khalsa Haladae
Certified Rolfer
Portland, OR 97214-3057
nrh0prs@pioneer.net
and Portland, OR
503-642-4527

Karl D. Jackson
Certified Rolfer
Bend, OR 97702
541-317-1521
karldjack@aol.com

Karen Lackritz
Certified Advanced Rolfer
Eugene, OR 97401
Office: 541-345-2926
Residence: 541-343-4157
KLackritz@aol.com

Ellyn V. Lindquist
Certified Rolfer
Portland, OR 97215
503-777-6054
Office: 503-636-2734
elliecr@teleport.com

Ron McComb
Certified Advanced Rolfer
Portland, OR
503-226-7653
ronraven@aol.com
and Salem, OR
503-581-0658

Martha Pfleeger
Certified Rolfer
Portland, OR 97204
503-228-1715

Jan Rizzo
Certified Advanced Rolfer
Portland, OR 97214
Office: 503-234-8331
jrizzo@linkport.com

Jo Evelyn "Jody" Seay
Certified Advanced Rolfer
Portland, OR 97282-0213
Office: 503-231-1156

Diane L. Sullivan
Certified Rolfer
Bend, OR 97701
541-388-4167
Limited Practice

Karl Humiston, M.D.
Certified Rolfer
Albany, OR 97321
541-926-9594
humiston@peak.org

Jeff W. Ryder, D.C.
Certified Rolfer
Portland, OR 97201
503-464-0226

PENNSYLVANIA

Linda L. Grace, M.A.
Certified Advanced Rolfer
Movement Teacher
Philadelphia, PA 19146-1506
Phone: 215-985-1263
Fax: 215-985-0167
LLG3@aol.com

Bill Harvey
Certified Advanced Rolfer
Philadelphia, PA 19144
Office: 215-438-3773
Fax: 215-848-8588
wjh4@aol.com

Dorothy Hunter
Certified Advanced Rolfer
Movement Teacher
Point Pleasant, PA 18950
215-297-8816

Judy Madjecki
Certified Rolfer
Philadelphia, PA 19119
215-849-3121

Warren Miles
Certified Rolfer
Movement Teacher
Allentown, PA 18102
610-770-9476

John Murphy
Certified Rolfer
Movement Teacher
Scotrun, PA 18332
717-629-6246

George J. Smyth
Certified Advanced Rolfer
Marietta, PA 17547
717-426-3085

Susan Stone
Certified Rolfer
Huntingdon Valley, PA 19006
215-782-1664
215-947-3611
Limited Practice

Thomas A. Kriczky, D.C.
Certified Rolfer
Blue Bell, PA 19422
Office/Fax: 215-628-8874

RHODE ISLAND

Steve Cavanagh
Certified Advanced Rolfer
Saunderstown, RI 02874
Res/Fax: 401-294-9660

Gregory Knight
Certified Rolfer
Rolf Movement Practitioner
Pawtucket, RI 02860-5733
401-724-8426

Joe Wheatley
Certified Rolfer
West Greenwich, RI 02817
401-397-4428

SOUTH CAROLINA

Rodney Buchner, M.A. Psych.
Certified Advanced Rolfer
Rolf Movement Practitioner
Spartanburg, SC
Appts: 704-894-3146

Betsy Culpepper, R.N.
Certified Rolfer
Clemson, SC 29631
864-653-3314
betsycu@aol.com

Brian D. Hopkins
Certified Advanced Rolfer
Columbia, SC 29204
803-256-6456

Tabitha R. Mountjoy
Certified Rolfer
Charleston, SC
Office: 843-556-5533

Ellen Presnell, R.N.
Certified Rolfer
Rolf Movement Practitioner
Greenville, SC 29615
864-322-7641
South Dakota, SD

Charlie Evander, P.T.
Certified Advanced Rolfer
Yankton, SD 57078
605-665-7434

TENNESSEE

Les Kertay, Ph.D.
Certified Advanced Rolfer
Chattanooga, TN 37403
Office: 423-265-2455
Fax: 423-265-8336
Residence: 423-847-9018
shrink@atlcom.net

Deborah Starrett
Certified Advanced Rolfer
Nashville, TN
Office: 615-356-5888
dstarrett@aol.com

Thomas E. Walton
Certified Rolfer
Movement Teacher
Germantown, TN 38183-1164
Memphis: 901-759-9696
Residence: 901-377-3915

Neil Williams
Certified Rolfer
Cookeville, TN 38506
931-432-4292
and Cookeville, TN 38506
Office: 931-526-5852
and Nashville, TN 37212
Office: 615-385-1312

Nina McIntosh, MSW
Certified Rolfer
Memphis, TN 38107
Office: 901-680-1177
Residence: 901-272-2555
ninamac@aol.com

TEXAS

Brian Beard
Certified Rolfer
Rolf Movement Practitioner
Austin, TX 78746
Office: 512-306-1992

Norma Bell, R.N.
Certified Advanced Rolfer
Rolf Movement Practitioner
Austin, TX 78746
Office: 512-328-4424
Fax: 512-328-5114
rolfer@texas.net
and Austin, TX 78733
512-263-9661

Randall D. Bonifay
Certified Rolfer
Dallas, TX 75208-3953
Residence: 214-942-3441

Sandy Collins, R.N.
Certified Rolfer
Austin, TX 78746
Office: 512-327-9824
Messages: 512-479-9341
SCDancer@aol.com

Steven A. Collins
Certified Advanced Rolfer
Austin, TX 78746
Office: 512-327-9824
Residence: 512-892-5010
Wherever@aol.com
and Victoria, TX 77901
Office: 512-578-0566
Residence: 512-892-5010

Doris T. Fausett, D.C.
Certified Rolfer
Monahans, TX 79756
Office: 915-943-4892

Nicholas French, M.A.
Certified Advanced Rolfer
Dallas, TX 75229
Office: 214-357-7571
Fax: 214-351-1233

Linda Gaddy
Certified Rolfer
Fort Worth, TX 76116
Home: 817-613-0507
Office: 817-377-4750
Fax: 817-377-0720

Allison Hubbard
Certified Rolfer
Austin, TX 78705
512-482-0821

Sam Johnson
Certified Rolfer
Dallas, TX 75231
214-360-0624
scj@why.net

Adrian Kellar
Certified Rolfer
Victoria, TX 77901
Office: 512-576-1518

Mary Elizabeth Kimberlin
Certified Rolfer
Plano, TX 75023
Office: 972-392-7653
mkmbrln@cyberramp.net
and Dallas, TX 75214
Residence: 214-874-0393

Jan Liebsch
Certified Rolfer
Kingwood, TX 77345-1824
Office: 281-360-0473
Residence: 281-360-9617
AMBRA652@msn.com

Chuck Lustfield, Ph.D.
Certified Advanced Rolfer
Dallas, TX 75229
214-902-8900
cdl2@airmail.net

Andrew Robert MacKenzie, R.N.
Certified Rolfer
Humble, TX 77346-1838
Residence: 281-812-4132

Randy Mack
Certified Advanced Rolfer
Austin, TX 78731
Office: 512-371-3940
Fax: 512-371-0939
rmack2@earthlink.net

Kathleen McBride Lallier
Certified Rolfer
Rolf Movement Practitioner
Bandera, TX 78003
Office: 830-510-4366
klallier@texas.net

Michael Laird McIver
Certified Advanced Rolfer
Houston, TX 77027
Office: 713-621-6619
Fax: 713-840-8959
McRolf@aol.com

David McQueen, M.A.
Certified Advanced Rolfer
Rolf Movement Practitioner
El Paso, TX 79902
Office: 915-544-5710
Residence: 915-533-5048

Richard Merbler
Certified Rolfer
Garland, TX 75042
972-216-4618
and Dallas, TX 75240
Office: 972-392-7653
Fax: 972-789-1589

Rita Millett Mikel
Certified Advanced Rolfer
Boerne, TX 78006
830-336-2322

Richard A. Mintz
Certified Advanced Rolfer
Austin, TX 78746
Office: 512-327-9107
rmintz@swbell.net

Wiley Patterson, M.D.
Certified Rolfer
San Antonio, TX 78240
Office: 210-558-9593

Kathy Purvis
Certified Rolfer
Rolf Movement Practitioner
Bario, TX 79504
254-725-7259

Dena Roberts, M.Ed.
Certified Rolfer
Austin, TX 78746
512-327-2928
denadoug@aol.com

Jo Evelyn "Jody" Seay
Certified Advanced Rolfer
Dallas, TX 75244
972-392-7188

Ken Solberg
Certified Advanced Rolfer
Dallas, TX 75252
972-599-0308

Deborah Starrett
Certified Advanced Rolfer
Houston, TX 77005
713-523-7447
dstarrett@aol.com

Limited Practice
Patty Sanders
Certified Rolfer
Austin, TX 78723-1326
Residence: 512-459 4402

TENNESSEE

Les Kertay, Ph.D.
Certified Advanced Rolfer
Chattanooga, TN 37403
Office: 423-265-2455
Fax: 423-265-8336
Residence: 423-847-9018
shrink@atlcom.net

Deborah Starrett
Certified Advanced Rolfer
Nashville, TN
Office: 615-356-5888
dstarrett@aol.com

Thomas E. Walton
Certified Rolfer
Movement Teacher
Germantown, TN 38183-1164
Memphis: 901-759-9696
Residence: 901-377-3915

Neil Williams
Certified Rolfer
Cookeville, TN 38506
931-432-4292
and Cookeville, TN 38506
Office: 931-526-5852
and Nashville, TN 37212
Office: 615-385-1312

Nina McIntosh, MSW
Certified Rolfer
Memphis, TN 38107
Office: 901-680-1177
Residence: 901-272-2555
ninamac@aol.com

UTAH

Iginia Valehtina Boccalandro
Certified Rolfer
Salt Lake City, UT 84106
801-461-0448
SFIVBEGI@aol.com

Sibel Iren
Certified Rolfer
Moab, UT 84532
435-259-1907

Ken Jamititus
Certified Rolfer
Salt Lake City/Park City, UT
801-856-ROLF

Judah Robb Lyons
Certified Rolfer
Salt Lake City, UT 84111-2903
Office: 801-355-6363
Residence: 801-654-3023
bluestar@xmission.com

Nancy Ellen Stotz, M.F.A.
Certified Rolfer
Salt Lake City, UT 84102
Office: 801-532-2634
Residence: 801-521-3244

VERMONT

Kevin K. Frank
Certified Advanced Rolfer
Norwich, VT
603-968-9585
kkfrank@cris.com

Jeffry H. Galper, Ph.D.
Certified Advanced Rolfer
Hinesburg, VT 05461
Office: 802-865-4770
Residence: 802-482-2031
www.to-be.com/rolfgalp

Casey Kiernan
Certified Rolfer
Rolf Movement Practitioner
VT
802-863-5073
Casewave@aol.com

Gale Loveitt
Certified Rolfer
South Burlington, VT 05403-6145
802-864-0444
werolf@together.net

Rebecca Riley
Certified Rolfer
Montpelier, VT 05601
802-229-4645

Diane Rodgers
Certified Rolfer
Montpelier, VT 05601
802-223-1425

Betsy Sise, M.S., M.Ed.
Certified Advanced Rolfer
Norwich, VT 05055
802-649-3027
betsise@sover.net

Thom Walker
Certified Advanced Rolfer
South Burlington, VT 05403-6145
802-864-0444
werolf@together.net

VIRGINIA

Svaha Baylin-Woodward
Certified Rolfer
Charlottesville, VA 22902
804-296-7023

Joy Belluzzi
Certified Advanced Rolfer
Chevy Chase, MD 20815
Office: 301-654-5025

Susan Bergman
Certified Rolfer
Rolf Movement Practitioner
Falls Church, VA 22044
703-671-2387

Carol Y. Blanding
Certified Rolfer
Roanoke, VA 24018
540-774-5333

Rebecca Carli-Mills, M.F.A.
Certified Advanced Rolfer
Rolf Movement Practitioner
Silver Spring, MD 20910
Office: 301-585-3328
Residence: 301-585-6690
CarliMills@aol.com

Dale F. Clark
Certified Rolfer
Virginia Beach, VA 23452
Office: 757-422-0774
Residence: 757-422-6062
Pager: 757-939-9104
and Richmond, VA
757-422-0774
and Newport News, VA 23606
757-422-0774

Rose Crawmer
Certified Advanced Rolfer
Rolf Movement Practitioner
Fredericksburg, VA 22401
Office: 540-371-6291
Residence: 540-372-4426
crawmer@erols.com

C. Keith Economidis
Certified Rolfer
Virginia Beach, VA 23451
Office: 757-437-0383
Residence: 757-437-8517
pegecono@pilot.infi.net

Vicki L. Egge
Certified Rolfer
Blacksburg, VA 24062
540-953-0283
rolfer@bnt.com

Steve Hancoff, L.C.S.W.
Certified Advanced Rolfer
Silver Spring, MD 20904-3029
301-622-2058
Fax: 301-622-2382
SHX2@aol.com

Casey Kiernan
Certified Rolfer
Rolf Movement Practitioner
Arlington, VA 22205
703-532-6038
Casewave@aol.com

Hubert Ritter
Certified Rolfer
Washington, DC 20009
202-986-2050
703-497-4437
301-236-4614
hritter@mindspring.com

Elizabeth Salzman
Certified Rolfer
Virginia Beach, VA 23452
757-486-8040
bodyworkrs@aol.com

G. Cosper Scafidi
Certified Advanced Rolfer
Alexandria, VA 22314
Office: 703-998-0474
Fax: 703-836-2667
xascia@aol.com

William Short, M.S.
Certified Advanced Rolfer
Rolf Movement Practitioner
Washington, DC 20009
202-328-3441

Diane Tredway Stroud, P.T.
Certified Advanced Rolfer
Rolf Movement Practitioner
Arlington, VA 22201
Office: 703-527-8446
mdstroud@erols.com

David C. Swetz
Certified Rolfer
Alexandria, VA 22302
Appts: 703-845-5493

Viki Van Wey
Certified Advanced Rolfer
Virginia Beach, VA 23452
Office: 757-422-0774
Residence: 757-422-6062
and Richmond, VA
757-422-0774
and Newport News, VA 23606
757-422-0774

Sharon Wheeler-Hancoff
Certified Advanced Rolfer
Rolf Movement Practitioner
Silver Spring, MD 20904-3029
301-622-2058
Fax: 301-622-2382
SHX2@aol.com

Eva Jo Wu
Certified Advanced Rolfer
Rolf Movement Practitioner
Roanoke, VA 24018
540-989-1617
Fax: 540-989-1618
rolfers@roanoke.infi.net
and Charlettesville, VA
540-989-1617
and Fairfax, VA
540-989-1617

Frank Wu
Certified Advanced Rolfer
Rolf Movement Practitioner
Roanoke, VA 24018
540-989-1617
Fax: 540-989-1618
rolfers@roanoke.infi.net
and Charlottesville, VA
540-989-1617
and Fairfax, VA
703-989-1617

WASHINGTON

Jill Allison Ableson
Certified Rolfer
Seattle, WA 98125
Office: 206-361-7554
Aajillity@aol.com

Gio Aguilera
Certified Rolfer
Bothell, WA 98012
425-486-4135
gioaguil@aol.com

Gerard Allard
Certified Rolfer
Rolf Movement Practitioner
Issaquah, WA 98027
Office&Fax: 425-391-9846
gallard.@cse-net.com
and Bellevue, WA 98005
Office: 425-391-9846

Louise S. Almgren
Certified Rolfer
Seattle, WA 98118
Office: 206-722-5997
LouiseA417@aol.com

Jeanie Birchall, R.N., B.S.N.
Certified Rolfer
Bellingham, WA 98226
360-595-2203
jeabir@aol.com

Lucy Bissell
Certified Advanced Rolfer
Seattle, WA 98115
206-729-9617

Marita Rose Bott
Certified Advanced Rolfer
Olympia, WA 98516
Office: 360-923-0612
Residence: 360-458-2057

Shonnie Carson, R.N., B.S.N.,
A.N.P.
Certified Advanced Rolfer
Port Orchard, WA 98366
360-769-8467

Sherri Cassuto
Certified Advanced Rolfer
Seattle, WA 98103
Office: 206-633-2612
scassuto@nwlink.com

Jamie D. Compton
Certified Rolfer
Bellevue, WA 98004
425-637-8755
jcompton@rolfnet.com
http://www.rolfnet.com
and Wenatchee, WA 98801
509-665-8712

Carola de Keizer
Certified Rolfer
Yelm, WA 98597-2184
360-446-ROLF
Cristal13@webtv.net

Elaine T. Dolan
Certified Rolfer
Bothell, WA 98011
206-485-9181
rolfing1@gte.net

Sarah Emory
Certified Advanced Rolfer
Seattle, WA 98117
206-781-9656

Elizabeth "Lisa" Failor-Howe
Certified Advanced Rolfer
Rolf Movement Practitioner
Olympia, WA 98506
360-923-5747

James Fiorino
Certified Rolfer
Tacoma, WA 98409
253-472-9168

Sarah J. Gengler
Certified Rolfer
Seattle, WA 98107
206-783-8498
tazland@compuserve.com

Diane L. Gilkeson
Certified Rolfer
Pasco, WA 99301
Office: 509-547-8794
Residence: 509-588-1905
DLGhands@aol.com

Kirsten Michelle Grohe
Certified Rolfer
Olympia, WA 98516
360-413-5647

Gregory Hampel
Certified Rolfer
Rolf Movement Practitioner
Seattle, WA 98104
206-587-4567
xtram@aa.net
and Vashon Island, WA 98070
206-463-6609

Rex A. Holt
Certified Advanced Rolfer
Bellevue, WA 98004
425-637-8755
Fax: 425-688-1993

Martha Hope
Certified Rolfer
Bellingham, WA 98225-2535
360-733-7653

Barbara L. Jacobsen
Certified Advanced Rolfer
Bainbridge Island, WA 98110
206-780-9502
and Seattle, WA 98115
206-522-2595

Tina Kaplan-Tesch
Certified Rolfer
Rolf Movement Practitioner
Seattle, WA 98103
206-548-9165
TKTesch@aol.com

Allan M. Kaplan
Certified Advanced Rolfer
Seattle, WA 98103
206-548-9165
AMKaplan@aol.com

Gonya W. Klein, P.T.
Certified Rolfer
Rolf Movement Practitioner
Seattle, WA 98119
206-285-6471
gwk@igc.apc.org

Elizabeth Krull
Certified Rolfer
Rolf Movement Practitioner
Monroe, WA 98272
360-794-4314
lizkrull@worldnet.att.net
and Kirkland, WA 98034
425-821-3394

Carole Gisele LaRochelle
Certified Rolfer
Kent, WA 98032
Office: 425-413-1998
CLCRolfer@compuserve.com
www.aa.net/~mkelly/
and Maple Valley, WA 98038
Residence: 425-413-8070

John Lodge, M.A.
Certified Advanced Rolfer
Redmond, WA 98052
425-883-4692

Ellen D. Madsen
Certified Advanced Rolfer
Olympia, WA 98502
Office: 360-753-8095
Residence: 360-866-1327
EMadsen@aol.com

Michael Maskornick
Certified Advanced Rolfer
Bellingham, WA 98225
360-671-9716

Ron McComb
Advanced Rolfer
Seattle, WA 98104
206-340-1549
ronraven@aol.com
and Richland, WA
509-943-3934
and Spokane, WA
509-943-3934

Shane P. Mettilie
Certified Rolfer
Shoreline, WA 98133-5551

Louise M. Mitchell
Certified Rolfer
Seattle, WA 98125
Office: 206-361-7554

Ron Murray
Advanced Rolfer
Spokane, WA
509-534-2075

Michael Reams
Certified Rolfer
Seattle, WA 98125
206-363-1244

Tom Robinson
Certified Advanced Rolfer
Seattle, WA 98115
206-522-5236
ourzone@msn.com

Todd Romer
Certified Rolfer
Rolf Movement Practitioner
Steillacoom, WA 98388
253-588-1637

Sandy Schneider, MS, MSW
Certified Rolfer
Rolf Movement Practitioner
Seattle, WA 98148
206-244-0665

Leslie Selle
Certified Rolfer
Seattle, WA 98118
Office: 206-725-7039
Residence: 206-723-3720
LRSelle@aol.com

Tom Wing
Certified Advanced Rolfer
Rolf Movement Practitioner
Olympia, WA 98513
360-455-8157
and Seattle, WA
206-343-9709

Jean Keenan Wynia
Certified Rolfer
Spokane, WA 99203
Office: 509-838-2903
Wyoming, WY

Limited Practice
Anne McDermit
Certified Rolfer
Movement Teacher
Jackson, WY 83002
Voice Mail: 307-734-4119

Trager Technique

Mary Able
1020 Urban Street
Golden, CO 80401

Glennda Adair
21851 Herencia
Mission Viejo, CA 92692

Linda Adams
29 Lincoln Place
Rancho Mirage, CA 92270

Shirley Adams
1650 Woodmancy Road
Tully, NY 13159

Henrietta Agney
565 59th Street
Lisle, IL 60532

Michele Agney
307 West Willow
Carbondale, IL 62901

Joe Aguirre
370 Greenway Road
Memphis, TN 38117

Linda Alanen,
1632 D Monroe Street
Madison, WI 53711

Janet Alba
5540 Fernwood Circle
El Paso, TX 79932

Susan Alban
P.O. Box 267
Fredricksburg, TX 78624

Zoe Alexi
429 Waverly Road
North Andoyer, MA 01845

Diane Allen
150 Westford Road , #37
Tyngsboro, MA 01879

Mucie Allred
221 Elmer Avenue
Weirton, WV 26062

Ruth Alpert
303 East Buena Vista, #3
Santa Fe, NM 87501

Donna Anders
1378 Pine Street
Pittsburg, CA 94565

Gail Anderson
P.O. Box 793
Asheville, NC 28802

Gayle Anderson
4670 Aroale Street
Sarasota, FL 34232

Lisa Anderson
P.O. Box 367
Paauilo, HI 96776

Martin Anderson
74 Egmont, #6
Brookline, MA 02446

Antje Andrea
3924 South Angeline Street
Seattle, WA 98118

Marie Arendt
1556 West Harriet Lane
Anaheim, CA 92802

Marilyn Arnett
22025 Butler Market Road
Bend, OR 97701

Heather Arnold
4113 Idlewild, #2
Austin, TX 78731

Maria Arrington
1400 Echo Lake Road
Bigfork, MT 59911

Stephanie Artz
344 East 6th Street, #2D
New York, NY 10003

Joy Assad
RD. #1, Box 600
New Salem, PA 15468

Carole Austin
805 East Lee Street
Pensacola, FL 32503

Debby Bailey
89 Navratil Road
Willington, CT 06279

Lucy Baker
18532 Firlands Way
Shoreline, WA 98133

Lucie Barbeau
2367 Woolsey Street
Berkeley, CA 94705

Conne Bard
1049 Stratton Place
Elberon, NJ 07740

Nancy Barnes
8315 Willow Run
Fogelsville, PA 18051

Dee Gee Bateman
1762 Broadmoor
Evansville, IN 47714

Gayle Bates
P.O. Box 221
Saxtons River, VT 05154

Mark Bauman
6833 Del Monte Avenue
Richmond, CA 94805

Steve Bear
Ione Beauchamp
6 Carroll Street
Brooklyn, NY 11231

Dodie Becker
2505 Highland Circle
Bethel Park, PA 15102

Guy Bedau
53 Twin Hill Road
Hubbardston, MA 01452

Bud Bedell
5629 SE 44th Avenue
Portland, OR 97206

Jane Begley
14356 Hubbard
Livonia, MI 48154

Charles Behm
312 Monmouth Road
Elizabeth, NJ 07208

David Belch
4562 East Sunrise Drive
Tucson, AZ 85718

Joyce Belmonte
70 Harrison Road
West Chester, PA 19380

Lhesli Benedict
1441 Lincoln Avenue, #D
San Rafael, CA 94901

Patricia Bennett
5614 Parade Ridge
Austin, TX 78731

Bonnie Bergara
P.O. Box 213
Falls City, TX 78113

Elizabeth Berks
222 Saint John Street, #320
Portland, ME 04102

Adrienne Bernardina
1132 Mellan Street, #1
Pittsburgh, PA 15206

Catherine Bertrand
Kripalu Center, Box 793
Lennox, MA 01240

Inger Besman
328 Pleasant Street
Ithaca, NY 14850

Donna Bielby
240 North Main Street
Glen Ellyn, IL 60137

Susan Bissell
212 Overlook Road
Ithaca, NY 14850

Jack Blackburn
5762 27th NE,
Seattle, WA 98105

Laura Blackwood
3700 Shore Drive
Richmond, VA 23225

Lorraine Blake
51 Orchard Street
East Hartford, CT 06108

Linda Boehmer
82 Congress Street
Greenfield, MA 01301

Nanna Bolling
18½ Wolfe Avenue
Colorado Springs, CO 80906

Ana Marie Booth
2012 Stain Glass Drive
Plano, TX 75075

Kenneth Booth
2012 Stain Glass Drive
Plano, TX 75075

Andrea Borak
49 Bay State Road
Pittsfield, MA 01201

Renee Bork
P.O. Box 3293
Bryan, TX 77805

Henry Bornstein
P.O. Box 11214
Berkeley, CA 94712

Christina Bour
4890 Battery Lane, #320
Bethesda, MD 20814

Gerald Bowers
10 South Broad Street
Mechanicsburg, PA 17055

Marcia Bowers
10 S. Broad Street
Mechanicsburg, PA 17055

Ann Bowles
12 Barrington Place
Great Barrington, MA 01230

Yvonne Bowman-Burton
18643 East Cavendish Drive
Castro Valley, CA 94552

Sefla Robin Boyd
P.O. Box 446
Soquel, CA 95073

Helga Brandt-Duval
257 Santa Margarita Avenue
Menlo Park, CA 94025

Lynette Brannon
1825-A Waterston
Austin, TX 78703

Lisa Bregman
4201 Cathedral Avenue NW, #603W
Washington, DC 20016

Theresa Bremer
1164 South Clarion Street
Philadelphia, PA 19147

Lucy Brinew
7 Walter Drive
Jackson, NJ 08527

Charlene Brown
2651 South Bala Drive
Tempe, AZ 85282

Linda Brown
60 Lanes End
Concord, MA 01742

Gary Brownlee
1334 18th Street
Manhattan Beach, CA 90266

Spencer Bryant
11511-17th Avenue NE
Seattle, WA 98125

Thomas Bryant
P.O. Box 172
Silver Lake, NH 03875

Ruth Bucher
3515 Coker, #232
Irving, TX 75062

Carolea Burgess
77 Wildwood Road
Storrs, CT 06268

Bonnie Burgund
504 West John Street
Champaign, IL 61820

Jane Burns
3664 Chestnut Street
Lafayette, CA 94549

Penny Butts
3262 Slate Stone Road
Cable, OH 43009

Beth Cachat
11416 Slater Avenue NE, #203
Kirkland, WA 98033

Catherine Callies
13576 Camino Del Sol, #23
Sun City West, AZ 85375

Carol Campbell
512 Old San Jose Road
Soquel, CA 95073

Dave Campbell
781 Lois Avenue
Sunnyvale, CA 94087

Sandra Canby
2010 Bonhill Drive
Reisterstown, MD 21136

John Canfield
195 Clinton Street
Saratoga Springs, NY 12866

Maxine Carnahan
16 Orchard Drive,
Acton, MA 01720

Mary Caroline
4627 10th Street NW
Albuquerque, NM 87107

Brenda Carpenter
2705-A West Central
Missoula, MT 59804

Alice Cason
2120 Swift Creek Lane
Olympia, WA 98512

Bonita Cassel-Beckwith
5677 Greens Drive
Allentown, PA 18106

Al Cedarholm
1903 Variations Drive NE
Atlanta, GA 30329

Lynn Chadsey
1721 Rucker Avenue
Everett, WA 98201

Holly Chaplin
26 Love Lane
Weston, MA 02193

Mary Chariker
3648 Boywood Road
Graham, NC 27253

Sheryl Charity
8 Rider Avenue
Yonkers, NY 10710

Carol Charles
RR1 Box 170,Warren
VT 05674

Earl Charles
3912 East Weldon Avenue
Phoenix, AZ 85018

Michelle Charles
3912 East Weldon Aveue
Phoenix, AZ 85018

Leanne Chattey
10059 SW Northilla Road
Vashon Island, WA 98070

Mary Chicoine
84 Torrey Street
Easthampton, MA 01027

Fawn Christianson
21721 Granada Avenue
Cupertino, CA 95014

Jerry Chroman
438 NE 72nd Street
Seattle, WA 98115

Claudius Claiborne
440 Mountain View Drive
Staunton, VA 24401

Peggy Clancy
20 Kildare Court
Deerfield, IL 60015

Robert Clark
5405 Purlington Way
Baltimore, MD 21212

Deirdre Clarke
835 Jay Street
Albany, NY 12203

Patsy Cloer
641 Statesville Boulevard, #302
Salisbury, NC 28144

Kathleen Clouse
Route 1, Box 76A
San Mateo, FL 32187

Laurie Coe
2038 West Dixon
Mesa, AZ 85201

Sharmila Cohen-Gold
25 Rosewood Drive
Sag Harbor, NY 11963

Shar Colburn
1387 Turquoise Avenue
Mentone, CA 92359

Susan Coleman
2503 Park Street
Houston, TX 77019

Dana Collins
153 Joshua Road
Divide, CO 80814

Katherine Colman
120 11th Street NE
Washington, DC 20002

Ross Connors-Keith
1770 Felix Avenue
Arcata, CA 95521

Rachel Conrad
1903 Bryan Street
Melbourne, FL 32901

Tricia Conti
9500 Roosevelt Way NE, #203
Seattle, WA 98115

deRon Coppage
106 East Lawson Street
Hahira, GA 31632

Earl Corbitt
4102 Sequoia Trail West
Georgetown, TX 78628

Joan Cordle,
723 Sturgis Drive
Richmond, VA 23236

Shirley Cornell
4534 Onyx Lane
Madison, WI 53714

Nancy Ramani-Costerisan
17 Cone Hill Road
West Stockbridge, MA 01266

Michel Cote
8 SE 2nd Avenue, #402
Miami, FL 33131

Maureen Coughlin
41 Jones Hill Road, #113
West Haven, CT 06516

John Cowlishaw
25860 West 14 Mile Road
Bloomfield, MI 48301

Beverly Cox
5010 Winthrop
Indianapolis, IN 46205

Chris Crary
1112 North 87th Street
Scottsdale, AZ 85257

Michael Crear
292 West 92nd Street, #5C
New York, NY 10025

Celeste Crine
608 B Legion Road
Aston, PA 19014

Robert Croft
1281 Wewdell Avenue
North Fort Myers, FL 33903

Mari-Jean Crossman
P.O. Box 669
Pine, AZ 85544

Patsy Crowell
1662 Barnstead Drive
Reston, VA 20194

Teresa Crowell
1802 Holbrook Street
Oakhurst, NJ 07755

Peggy Cruise
P.O. Box 2283
Paducah, KY 42002

Maxine Cubel
3791 North 700W Street
Anderson, IN 46011

Amy Culver
4407 Stone Mill Drive
Indianapolis, IN 46237

Carol Currens
9611 Copper Creek
Austin, TX 78729

Cheri Curry
823 Riverview Drive
Brielle, NJ 08730

Reeve Curry
108 Beech Pond Road
Wolfeboro, NH 03894

Ursula D'Angelo
P.O. Box 792
Honaunau, HI 96726

Jane Danielson
4501 Louisiana Avenue North
Crystal, MN 55428

Mary Dariano
9395 Kern Avenue
Gilroy, CA 95020

Irene Darpino
254 Lebanon Road
Bridgeton, NJ 08302

Mary Davenport
119 S. Silverlake Street
Oconomowoc, WI 53066

Elizabeth Davies
13 Kushaqua Trail North
Hewitt, NJ 07421

Joan Davis
7118 Sycamore Avenue
Takoma Park, MD 20912

Patricia Dawn
2827 West Avenue L
Lancaster, CA 93536

Marty Dawson
916 SW King, #202
Portland, OR 97205

James Day
21 Whittier Avenue
Trenton, NJ 08618

Peter de Zordo
300 Ewing Terrace
San Francisco, CA 94118

Cheryl Dean
37 Pleasant View Street
Methuen, MA 01844

Renee Dean
P.O. Box 603
Middlebury, VT 05753

Nancy Deckard
297 East Selby Boulevard
Worthington, OH 43085

Sharon Decker
2701 Middle River Drive, #11
Fort Lauderdale, FL 33306

Shiranda Deerwoman
9325 Shoshone Road NE
Albuquerque, NM 87111

Andrea DeSharone
53 Hill Street
Concord, MA 01742

Joseph Dewane
1128 East Fern Drive
Phoenix, AZ 85014

Mary Dewane
1128 East Fern Drive
Phoenix, AZ 85014

Leisha Diane
5054 7th Avenue NE
Seattle, WA 98105

Eileen Dickinson
532 Fourth Street
Ann Arbor, MI 48103

David Dimmack
29 Cavendish Drive
Ambler, PA 19002

James Doherty
10061 Riverside Drive, Box 205
Toluca Lake, CA 91602

Joanna Donovan
1342 Jenifer Street, #1
Madison, WI 53703

Lisa Dorfi
7602 Sycamore Drive
Citrus Heights, CA 95610

Lori Dorman
330 Kempton Road
Glendale, CA 91202

Craig Douglass
2307 Toulouse Drive
Austin, TX 78748

Steven Drapeau
P.O. Box 80387
Fairbanks, AK 99708

Sara Driscoll
73 Montebello Road
Jamaica Plain, MA 02130

Janice Drout
210 North Higgins, #214
Missoula, MT 59802

Anna Duguay-Corsa
483 Spring Street
Harbor Springs, MI 49740

Sylvia Duty
1405 Sunset Avenue Ext.
Asheboro, NC 27203

Leslie Dworkin
132 West Mt. Pleasant Avenue
Philadelphia, PA 19119

Eula Marie Dyson
108 Milton Street
Brooklyn, NY 11222

Julian R. Eagleheart
10905 West 39th Avenue
Wheat Ridge, CO 80033

Patricia Earle
11542 Gold Nugget
College Station, TX 77845

Maryann Eastman
HCR Box 242,Ctr
Chatham, NH 03813

Gail Easton
P.O. Box 703
Rockland, ME 04841

Nancy Ekimoto
45153 Lorimer Street
Lancaster, CA 93534

Dawn Elaine
P.O. Box 217
Glenside, PA 19038

Kathleen Eldridge
52 Fresh Pond Place
Cambridge, MD 02138

Carol Ellen
482 Aster Street
Laguna Beach, CA 92651

Michael Elliff
7717 Westchester Drive
Belleville, IL 62223

Gordon Ellis
2541 C La'I Road,
Honolulu, HI 96816

Rebecca Ellis
2541 C La'I Road
Honolulu, HI 96816

Deanna English-Burdick
Route 2, Box 755
Grangeville, ID 83530

Tracey Eno
11030 Hemlock Drive
Lusby, MD 20657

Marga Enyart
1809 Marble NW
Albuquerque, NM 87104

Lorinda Erb
3030 South Rural Road, Suite 107
Tempe, AZ 85282

Barbara Erbland
203 Elmdorf Avenue
Rochester, NY 14619

Mary Jeanne Ernst
742 Coyote Road
Santa Barbara, CA 93108

Linda Erwin
1896 SW Brooklane Drive
Corvallis, OR 97333

Betty Eshnaur
2005 McArthur Avenue
Colorado Springs, CO 80909

Mark Eucher
P.O. Box 221092
Carmel, CA 93922

Sharon Ewton
601 Stallion Way
El Paso, TX 79922

Janet Fairhurst
Rt. 1, Box 32, 590 East Frontage
San Acacia, NM 87831

Jodi Falk
11 Arnold Avenue 3A
Northampton, MA 01060

Pam Falkowski
312 Cenacle Road
Ronkonkoma, NY 11779

Idominia Falorca
One William Street
Summit, NJ 07901

Elisabeth Farley
P.O. Box 1307
El Prado, NM 87529

Rob Farrar-Koch
810 Anchor Rode Drive
Naples, FL 34103

Judy Fasone
308 South Franklin Street, #1
Richwood, OH 43344

Margee Johnson Faunce
P.O. Box 1255
Koloa Kauai, HI 96756

Sara Feld
64 Rollingwood Lane
Concord, MA 01742

Lisa Feldman
P.O. Box 6535
Kamuela, HI 96743

Charles Ferguson
3718 Ole Mississippi Drive
Kenner, LA 70065

Mary K. Ferreter
1424 37th Street
Sacramento, CA 95816

Katherine Fieber Sodeinde
1133 William Street
State College, PA 16801

Lindsley Field-Kirkland
RR 5, Box 5350
Belfast, ME 04915

Ronald Fine
130 East 5th Street
Media, PA 19063

Hal Fischbeck
924 Douglas Drive
Endwell, NY 13760

John Flanagan
11 Stuyvesant Oval, MG
New York, NY 10009

Heidi Fleischbauer
10313 S.D. Mission Road, #305A
San Diego, CA 92108

Anne Fleming
8 Lackawanna Avenue
Dallas, PA 18612

Jan Fleming
431 Epping Way
Annapolis, MD 21401

Pamela Fleming
719 Field Street
Baltimore, MD 21211

Carol Flint
38533 Madrone Road
Carmel Valley, CA 93924

Shelley Warren Font
62111 Falcon Road
Montrose, CO 81401

Becky Forest
P.O. Box 1405
Paonia, CO 81428

Janet Fortess
225 Columbia Street
Ithaca, NY 14850

Marsha Fortner
P.O. Box 5126
Destin, FL 32540

JoAnn Foulds
825 West Main Street, #19
Hyannis, MA 02601

Ja Link Ka Fountain
25 SE South Street
Pullman, WA 99163

Shelby Frago
1317 Oak Avenue
Davis, CA 95616

Timothy Franc
60 Burnside Avenue
Sommerville, MA 02144

Karen Fraser
P.O. Box 109
Keene, NY 12942

Lowell Freedlund
11801 Old River Road
Rockton, IL 61072

Sherry Frichtl
P.O. Box 523292,
Springfield, VA 22152

William Frick
400 West 43rd Street, #14N
New York, NY 10036

Carla Friedman
704 Belmont Place East, #2
Seattle, WA 98102

Patricia Joy Frisbee
2000 South A1A, #N-502
Jupiter, FL 33477

Betty Fuller
423 Belvedere Avenue
Belvedere, CA 94920

Lorraine Gage
6717 Rubio Avenue
Van Nuys, CA 91406

Russ Gaines
17 Doral Drive
Shalimar, FL 32579

Anne Galbraith
1436 Henry Place
Waukegan, IL 60085

Gilbert Gallego
6015 Independence Way
Alexandria, VA 22312

Charles Ganzon
P.O. Box 58
Pacific Grove, CA 93950

Nancy Rose Gardner
2310 Forest Park Drive, #3
Anchorage, AK 99517

Teresa Garzelloni
336 Indianwood Boulevard
Park Forest, IL 60466

Cleide Gaspar
3700 NE 22nd Avenue, #4
Lighthouse Point, FL 33064

Alicia Gates
8031 Caminito Mallorca
La Jolla, CA 92037

Sandra Gekler
P.O. Box 679
Fairhope, AL 36533

Jeanne Gelineau
2034 Northampton Street
Holyoke, MA 01040

Patricia Geller
601 Huronview
Ann Arbor, MI 48103

Caroline Gelsman
915 Western Avenue
Petaluma, CA 94952

Edith Genteman
38238 North 20th Street
Phoenix, AZ 85027

Frank Gentzke
6439 Hoover Road
Indianapolis, IN 46260

Steffony George
129 South Oxford Street
Brooklyn, NY 11217

Jo Gerhard
P.O. Box 232
Freeland, WA 98249

Veba Gerkins
12741 Amethyst Street
Garden Grove, CA 92845

Barbara Gerry
5000 Royal Marco Way, #336
Marco Island, FL 34145

Jean Gerth
7905 Selle Road
Sandpoint, ID 83864

Cindy Getchonis
P.O. Box 6775
Ithaca, NY 14851

Deborah Getting
3534 SW Skyline Parkway
Topeka, KS 66614

Greta Gibble
Box 396
Solon, ME 04979

Joyce Gibson
10 Powder Horn Court
Holmdel, NJ 07733

Claudia Gilman
Lost River Caverns, P.O. Box M
Hellertown, PA 18055

Tinsley Ginn
250 B Howard Street
Atlanta, GA 30317

John Ginnity
128 East County Road 32
Fort Collins, CO 80525

Gioia Pharo Gioia
7753 Patriot Drive, #27
Annandale, VA 22003

Tony Giordano
15 Colonial Lane
Bellport, NY 11713

Geralyn Giuffrida
1774 Roth Hill Drive
Maryland Heights, MO 63043

Katrina Gleason
P.O. Box 481
Kimberton, PA 19442

Bev Godec
5270 Whip Trail
Colorado Springs, CO 80917

Jane Goerss
405 North Ashland Avenue
Park Ridge, IL 60068

Mercedes Gonzalez
2027 NE Multnomah Street
Portland, OR 97232

James Goodman
131 Corson Avenue
Staten Island, NY 10301

Deb Gordon
4130 Clairmont Road
Atlanta, GA 30341

Judith Gordon
545 North Clarendon Street
Kalamazoo, MI 49006

Kathleen Gordon
4602 Deerfield Circle
Peabody, MA 01960

Regina Gordon
34 Rupert
Monte Vista, CO 81144

Sheila Gradison
P.O. Box 432
Murphys, CA 95247

Deborah Gray
P.O. Box 9514
North Amherst, MA 01059

Lourdes Gray
15 Dolly Lane
Rindge, NH 03461

Jolie Green
5624 Olde Wadsworth Boulevard
Arvada, CO 80002

Karina Green
P.O. Box 1272
Blue Lake, CA 95525

Julie Greene
151 Santa Rosa Avenue
Oakland, CA 94610

Marina Gresham
220 Church Street
Phoenixville, PA 19460

Joe Griffin
912 Goebel Avenue
Savannah, GA 31404

Constance Griffith
1650 East Barbarita Avenue
Gilbert, AZ 85234

Barbara Gross
6218 Woodard Bay Road NE
Olympia, WA 98506

Mary Gudmundson
985 Vernon Road
Columbus, OH 43209

Maxine Forster Guenther
30 Denise Drive
Red Bank, NJ 07701

Deborah Haber
1575 Bedivere Circle
Lafayette, CO 80026

Elizabeth Haehl
1025 Wellington Road
Lawrence, KS 66049

Stanley Haehl
1025 Wellington
Lawrence, KS 66049

David Haines
511 Laurel Street
Lancaster, PA 17603

Elizabeth Haltom
614 South First, #318
Austin, TX 78704

Lynne Hamilton
24544 Camino Del Monte
Carmel, CA 93923

Margaret Hamlet
10581 Manitou Park NE
Bainbridge Island, WA 98110

Cathy Hammond
P.O. Box 2896
La Jolla, CA 92038

Marsha Handel
45 Riverside Drive, #3B
New York, NY 10024

JoAnn Hangst
1422 Woolsey Street
Schenectady, NY 12303

Heather A. Hankin
6141 Gossard Avenue
East Lansing, MI 48823

Carol Hanlon
9985 Tropical Parkway
Las Vegas, NV 89129

Sigrid Hansen
4789 Heaton Road
Petoskey, MI 49770

Kathryn Hansman-Spice
9857 Waters Meet Drive
Tallahassee, FL 32312

Cynthia Harada
P.O. Box 25423
West Los Angeles, CA 90025

Nancy Harold
1731 Ford Parkway
Saint Paul, MN 55116

Fran Hart
24 LaVonne Drive
Campbell, CA 95008

Sondra Hartmann
207 Center, #2
Ithaca, NY 14850

Roger Hartsell
124 East Fisher Avenue
Greensboro, NC 27401

Marianna Hartsong
1630 Horseshoe Bend
Camp Verde, AZ 86322

Karen Hastings
1706 Silverwood Drive
Tallahassee, FL 32301

Royce Ann Heard
1002 Redbud Lane
Crockett, TX 75835

Beverly Hedegor
239 Main Street, #B-11
Reading, MA 01867

Natasha Heifetz
1678 Shattuck Avenue, #282
Berkeley, CA 94709

Pamela Heleen
24151 Black Bear Lane
Conifer, CO 80433

Penny Helms
5 Chelsea Road
Little Rock, AR 72212

Andrea Hendron
1324 Marengo Court
Naperville, IL 60564

Gae Henry
P.O. Box 11214
Berkeley, CA 94712

Vicki Heppe
RR #2, Box 2256
Saylorsburg, PA 18353

Kathleen Hernandez
597 Gross Dam Road
Golden, CO 80403

Richard Hernandez
5645 Upper Valley
El Paso, TX 79932

Diana Heying
3330 Third Avenue, Suite 304
San Diego, CA 92103

Catherine Hillard
404 Tennessee Avenue
Alexandria, VA 22305

Michael Hillenbrand
213 North 16th, #3
Allentown, PA 18102

Janet Hogan
8315 Hermosa Avenue
Ben Lomond, CA 95018

Rachel Hogancamp
205 Center Street
Ithaca, NY 14850

Catrinka Holland
327 Clay Street
Nevada City, CA 95959

Kathleen Hoover
10076 Bristol Court
Wexford, PA 15090

Sharon Hour
9292 Franz Valley School Road
Calistoga, CA 94515

Alayne Howard
5729 Cantaloupe Avenue
Van Nuys, CA 91401

Theresa Huber
1501 Arizona, 5E
El Paso, TX 79902

Robert Hudgens
907 Akin Avenue
Fort Collins, CO 80521

Sara Huether
14304 Woodcrest Drive
Rockville, MD 20853

Peggy Humphreys
460 West Cedar Drive
Chandler, AZ 85248

Alan Hundley
12 Burton Woods Lane
Cincinnati, OH 45229

Diane Hunt
5096 Easy Street
Tallahassee, FL 32303

Saundra Huntley Bardak
387 Hall Avenue
Saint Paul, MN 55107

Sarah Huntting
1101 18th Avenue
Seattle, WA 98122

Leslie Hutchins
301 South Bedford Street, Suite 217
Madison, WI 53703

Jean Iams
1479 Hopkins Street
Berkeley, CA 94702

Stephen Imbrogno
2201 Leeds Court
West Chester, PA 19382

Softline Information
AltHealthWatch
20 Summer Street
Stamford, CT 06901

Lynn Inouye
P.O. Box 581
Bridgeport, CA 93517

Benjamin Iobst
467 East Main Street
Kutztown, PA 19530

Mary Jean Jaeger
525 Ridgeway Drive
Metairie, LA 70001

Christie James
One Colonial Drive
Kennebunk, ME 04043

Kim James
107 Park Hill Avenue
Columbia, MO 65203

Erica James Razafimbahiny
c/o Lynx Air, P.O. Box 407139
Fort Lauderdale, FL 33340

Nancy Jaqua Dein
1710 Halama Street
Kihei Maui, HI 96753

Kathy Jennings
21 Oakview Circle
Westport, CT 06880

Jeffrey Joel
P.O. Box 70
Kelly, WY 83011

Brian Johnson
243 Ortega Street
San Francisco, CA 94122

Carol Johnson
732 Pierson Drive
Charlotte, NC 28205

Helen (Sandy) Johnson
506 Pine Street
Amhurst, MA 01002

Joy Johnson
398 Millstone Road
Brewster, MA 02631

Leslie Johnson
16040 Old Seward Highway
Anchorage, AK 99516

Melvyn Johnson
501 West Holly
Phoenix, AZ 85003

Reed Svadesh Johnson
15832-34th Avenue NE
Seattle, WA 98155

Sally Johnson
4290 Rosewood Place
Riverside, CA 92506

Sharon Johnson
501-W Holly
Phoenix, AZ 85003

Sheila Merle Johnson
112 Janes
Mill Valley, CA 94941

Clyde Rae Jolie
2708 South Lakeridge Trail
Boulder, CO 80302

Catherine Jolly
1932 6th Avenue, #11
Oakland, CA 94606

Cherie Jones
1632 30th Street NW, #11
Washington, DC 20007

Jill Jones
9397 Crest Drive
Spring Valley, CA 91977

Larry Jones
P.O. Box 179
Jemez Springs, NM 87025

Lenore Jones
26621 Carmel Center Place, #201
Carmel, CA 93923

Phil Jones
4521 North 39th Street
Arlington, VA 22207

Jo-Ann Joseph
15 Rhode Island Avenue
Newport, RI 02840

Marie Judy
P.O. Box 817
Hazelwood, NC 28738

Deane Juhan
105 East Strawberry Drive
Mill Valley, CA 94941

Kate Juliano
130 East 5th Street
Media, PA 19063

Christine Kakehashi
1130 Maycliffe Place
Cincinnati, OH 45230

Sally Cunningham Kane
6928 Steven Miller Drive
Newaygo, MI 49337

Sharon Kantor
8745 SW 155 Terrace
Miami, FL 33157

Stephanie Karpinski
1914 Dundee Road
Rockville, MD 20850

Laurie Kautz
N2218 Pustaver Road
Lodi, WI 53555

Conni Kay
451 Los Gatos Boulevard, #103
Los Gatos, CA 95032

Betty Keathley
533 Bruton Bends, #J
Richardson, TX 75081

Mary Kedl
123 Indian Lane
Oak Ridge, TN 37830

Annette Keenan
5917 State Route 287
West Liberty, OH 43357

Deborah Keil
221 Sandbank Road
Ithaca, NY 14850

Ginny Keith
7800 East Lincoln Drive, #2100
Scottsdale, AZ 85250

Sharad Kelkar
1834 Tewa Road
Sante Fe, NM 87505

Mary Kelly
208-B Villa Garden Drive
Mill Valley, CA 94941

Julie Kennicott
11705 Durrette
Houston, TX 77024

Ellen Kessler
280 West 86th Street, #2R
New York, NY 10024

Dianne Khebreh
5359 West 123rd Street
Hawthorne, CA 90250

Jefferson Kincaid
2926 NE Flanders
Portland, OR 97232

Sharon King Green
305 Laura Springs Drive
Salisbury, NC 28146

Christine Kirk
RD. 1, Box 251
Red Hook, NY 12571

Susanna K. Kirsch
6629 North Majorca Lane East
Phoenix, AZ 85016

Ronan Kisch
3858 Kenwick Drive
Kettering, OH 45429

Susan Kissinger
60 Lake Forest Drive
Saint Louis, MO 63117

Danna Kistner
Box 486, Cairnwood Farm
Bryn Athyn, PA 19009

Steven Kloman
825 Sir Francis Drake
San Anselmo, CA 94960

Margo Knis
204 Victoria Way
Friendswood, TX 77546

Dhori Knud-Hansen
3215 Heidelberg Drive
Boulder, CO 80303

Benna Kolinsky
P.O. Box 381,
Boonville, CA 95415

Susan Komatsu
1111 Spanish Tr.
P.O. Box 1922
Eagar, AZ 85925

Catherine Kord
25 Main Street, #340
Northampton, MA 01060

Annette Krakovitz
4 McKay Circle
Cabin John, MD 20818

Brigitte Kranabitl
P.O. Box 578
Detroit, OR 97342

Davida Krantz
1610 Zining Trail
Smyrna, GA 30080

Charlotte Rose Kreitzer
533 East Lantana Avenue, #412
Camarillo, CA 93010

Dian Krumlauf
1011 W. Cottage Grove
Bloomington, IN 47404

Sabine Kuehner
935A 14th Street
San Francisco, CA 94114

Regina Kujawski
9523 Boca River Circle
Boca Raton, FL 33434

Ruth Kuo
5139 Wetheredsville Road
Baltimore, MD 21207

Mia Kusumadilaga
P.O. Box 795
Hingham, MA 02043

Gabrielle Laden
1244 Rutledge Street
Madison, WI 53703

Laurel Ladwig
3303 Sunset Boulevard
Houston, TX 77005

Mary Laffey Adams
222 Plant Avenue
Webster Groves, MO 63119

David Lamon
22 Huckleberry Lane
Mt. Desert, ME 04660

Jane Langone
819-North 8th Avenue
Maywood, IL 60153

Susan LaRose
15 West Palmer Street
Danielson, CT 06239

Jo Ellen Larsen
25135 Terrace Lantern
Dana Point, CA 92629

Ernest Larson
Box 5165
Bozeman, MT 59717

Jeanne Laskin
122 Daley Road
East Chatham, NY 12060

Michelle Laudadio
10053 Cotton Mill Lane
Columbia, MD 21046

Sarah Lawrence
P.O. Box 145
Montebello, VA 24464

Margaret Ann Lawson
420 Harvard Street
Rochester, NY 14607

Lluvia Lawyer
O Box 488
Dixon, NM 87527

Lucinda Lea
5916 Greene Street
Philadelphia, PA 19144

Michael Lear
827 Wilbur Street
Easton, PA 18042

Michele LeBrett
4055 Redwood Avenue, #M112
Los Angeles, CA 90066

Annie LeBus
P.O. Box 2453
44460 Little Lake Road
Mendocino, CA 95460

Robin Lee
18714 Cleveland Avenue
Salinas, CA 93906

Catherine LeFevre
100 Lincoln Village Circle, #114
Larkspur, CA 94939

Val Leoffler
320 Liberty Street
Santa Cruz, CA 95060

Cindy Leonard
1946 Elizabethtown Road, #3
Elizabethtown, PA 17022

Leslie Leonelli
155 West 71st Street, #1B
New York, NY 10023

Dena Phyllis Lerner
15323 Weddington Street, #107
Van Nuys, CA 91411

Anne Leslie
2326 North Spaulding, #2A
Chicago, IL 60647

Sonja Leszinski
3557 Lookout Court, Apt. 446,
Oceanside, CA 92056

Elaine Levenson
2004 Brickell Court
Virginia Beach, VA 23454

Jonathan Levy
8714 Garfield Street
Bethesda, MD 20817

Lorraine Lewis
107 Morningside Drive
Carrboro, NC 27510

Julie Lienert
1861 Striplin Road
Nicolaus, CA 95659

Aaron Liskin
1401 Saint Edwards Drive, #218
Austin, TX 78704

Jack Liskin
1333 South Genesee Avenue
Los Angeles, CA 90019

Elizabeth Lockley
P.O. Box 2483
Providence, RI 02906

Debra Lolmaugh
702 Montana
San Antonio, TX 78203

Janet K. Long
12901 Brookpark Road
Oakland, CA 94619

Stacey Longanecker
11405 Daisy Lane,
Glenn Dale, MD 20769

Erika Lorinez-Taveras
132 East 45th Street, #6H
New York, NY 10017

Cindy Lovell
6890 Royal Palm Boulevard, #H-105
Margate, FL 33063

Betsy Wright Loving
12014 246 Street NE
Arlington, WA 98223

Becky Lundin
P.O. Box 7603
Olympia, WA 98507

Rita Lustgarten
332 Richardson Drive
Mill Valley, CA 94941

Eugenia Luvizaro
8301 A Pershing Drive
Playa Del Rey, CA 90293

Kari Lygren
P.O. Box 344, Carlton Way
Milton MIlls, NH 03852

Volina Lyons
420 Sunrise Avenue
Lake Bluff, IL 60044

Maria Rose MacDonald
30 8th Avenue
Dayton, KY 41074

Sage Madrone Self
385 Harmony Way
Oviedo, FL 32765

Ronald Maier
206 West Kelsey Street
Bloomington, IL 61701

Wendy Maiorana
4318 Fessenden Street NW
Washington, DC 20016

Louis Major
P.O. Box 254611
Patrick AFB, FL 32925

Barbara Majoros
DPO 301, P.O. Box 2005
New Brunswick, NJ 08903

Celia Maluf
4000 Towerside Terrace, #1711
Miami, FL 33138

Rachel Mann
626 Cobblestone Drive
Wilmington, NC 28405

Laura Marks
2565 Guilford Road
Cleveland Heights, OH 44118

Graeme Marsh
5806 Lokelani Road
Kapaa, HI 96746

Becca Martin
505 Montclaire Drive NE
Albuquerque, NM 87108

Joy Martin
P.O. Box 805
Evansville, IN 47705

Ann Martin-Janus
4969 Barnett Shoals Road
Athens, GA 30605

Deborah Martyn
P.O. Box 1424
Eastsound, WA 98245

Carolyn Mason
1506 Queens Court
Claremont, CA 91711

Judith Masur
5 Gavilan Place
Santa Fe, NM 87505

Cynthia Matcha
2930 North 46th Street, #406
Phoenix, AZ 85018

Valarie Matinjussi
11220 South East 204th
Kent, WA 98031

Marilyn Mattson
1630 South Cook Street
Denver, CO 80210

Joan Maute
P.O. Box 1987
Kamuela, HI 96743

Mary Mayhew
14415 Woodcrest Drive
Rockville, MD 20853

Ann McAlhaney
11421 SW 61st Street
Miami, FL 33173

Joy McCombe
476 Malaga Way
Pleasant Hill, CA 94523

Bill McCormick
4515 Marcy Lane, #235
Indianapolis, IN 46205

Elleva Joy McDonald
18111 Covington Path
Minnetonka, MN 55345

Linda McDonald
P.O. Box 6935
Chandler, AZ 85246

Benny McGehee
1024 Quinault Drive,
El Paso, TX 79912

Daniel McGovern
215 West 90th Street, #12D 8
New York, NY 10024

Terri McIntyre
4788 Clothier Way
Sacramento, CA 95841

Gail McKinley
4500 9th Avenue NE, Suite 340
Seattle, WA 98105

Vincent McKone
495 Central Drive
Southern Pines, NC 28387

Jane McLaughlin
P.O. Box 101
Valley Farm Road
Millbrook, NY 12545

John-Paul McMullen
423 South Orange Street, #3
Media, PA 19063

David McNeely
P.O. Box 14343
Evansville, IN 47728

Chris Meacham
315 Peakview
Manitou Springs, CO 80829

Carol Mecko
712-11th Street SW
Little Falls, MN 56345

Mindy Melemed
80 Adelphi Street,
Brooklyn, NY 11205

Patricia Menoche
15 Lakeside Drive,
Plainville, MA 02762

Abbie Mercurio
5 Aiden Court,
Palm Beach Gardens, FL 33418

Franklin Merillat
7921 NW 202 Avenue
Alachua, FL 32615

Mary Metcalf
P.O. Box 505, 8840 East Road
Redwood Valley, CA 95470

Bonnie Meyer
7008 Anaqua Drive
Autin, TX 78750

Emily Meyer
2152 Linden Avenue
Madison, WI 53704

Susanne Michaud
1206 North 43rd Street
Seattle, WA 98103

Beth Michelson
2204 NW 8th Court
Gainesville, FL 32609

Ann Mick
54 Washington Avenue
Northampton, MA 01060

Betsy Milberg
101 Sunny Hills Drive
San Anselmo, CA 94960

Irene Miller
2115 Peach Street
Morgantown, WV 26505

Judyth Miller
5155 East 10th Avenue
Apache Junction, AZ 85219

Michele Mills
832 Sante Fe Avenue
Albany, CA 94706

Linda Mizer
3303 Orleans Drive
Columbus, OH 43224

Marlis Moldenhauer
1707 North Prospect Avenue, #4B
Milwaukee, WI 53202

Michael Moody
411½ Orange Road
Montclair, NJ 07042

Barbara Moore
3654 Lois Drive
Hood River, OR 97031

Dianne Moore
P.O. Box 147
Van Wyck, SC 29744

Edie Moore
994 Avondale Avenue
Cincinnati, OH 45229

Vivis Moore
P.O. Box 692,
Brookhaven, MS 39602

Sarah Moran
225 Evergreen Street, Box 1373
Duxbury, MA 02331

Elizabeth Moreland
5508 Guilford Avenue
Indianapolis, IN 46220

Judith Morgan
484 Fall Creek Terrace
Felton, CA 95018

Cynthia Moseley
557 West Bear Springs
Pipe Creek, TX 78063

Sonja Mountain
514 Ocean Avenue
Melbourne Beach, FL 32951

Brenda Mountjoy
2915 Providence Road, #450
Charlotte, NC 28211

Marylou Mowrer
P.O. Box 3746
Pagosa Springs, CO 81147

Marilynne Moyers
368 Rose Street
Danville, CA 94526

Maria Moyles
87 Manhattan Boulevard
Islip Terrace, NY 11752

Becky Mulkern
P.O. Box 99, East Side Road
Conway, NH 03818

K. Tyler Mullins
400 North Mill Road
Addison, IL 60101

Stephani Murdoch
402 Woodland Road
Easton, PA 18042

Margo Murray
2394 Camino Pintores
Sante Fe, NM 87505

Terry Nathanson
P.O. Box 591
Port Jefferson, NY 11777

Dianne Navarro-Springborn
5030 Snider Road
Brutus, MI 49716

Pearl Neff
739 North Columbus Street
Lancaster, OH 43130

Barbara Nehman
416 Brook Glen Drive
Richardson, TX 75080

Carol Nelson
238 Hoyt Street
Hudson, WI 54016

Gloria Luz Nelson
1402 East Skyline Drive
Madison, WI 53705

Sam Nettles
P.O. Box 40407
Tuscaloosa, AL 35404

Susan Garner New
1805 38th Avenue
Seattle, WA 98122

Donald Nichols
9901 North Oracle Road, #8204
Tuscon, AZ 85737

Mary Ann Nickerson
20 Captain Jones Way
Eastham, MA 02642

Deborah Niebuhr
571 East Howard Street
Winona, MN 55987

Anna Nisson
4086 Acreage Lane
Sebastopol, CA 95472

Mary Kent Norton
398 Ridgely Avenue
Annapolis, MD 21401

Joyce Nuttall
227 West Main Street
Lock Haven, PA 17745

Lisa Nymark
113 East Falls Street
Ithaca, NY 14850

Itara O'Connell
5335 College Oak Drive, #112
Sacramento, CA 95841

Marlena O'Hagan Buzzell
14 Portland Street
Fryeburg, ME 04037

Siste O'Malia
1921 Bloomfield Highway
Farmington, NM 87401

Peg O'Rourke
1825 NE 56th Avenue
Portland, OR 97213

Maryann O'Sullivan
3635 Majestic Avenue
Oakland, CA 94605

Kathryn Ochs
9117 Fordham
Indianapolis, IN 46268

Martha Ohrenberger
RR 1, Box 66 A
Penobscot, ME 04476

Betsy Oldenburg
106 Lucas Park Drive
Greensboro, NC 27455

Paula Ondov
6101 Running Springs Road
Ukiah, CA 95482

Mary Openlander
430 W. Jefferson
Kirkwood, MO 63122

Robert Orzel
P.O. Box 888
Blue Hill, ME 04614

Barbara Osborne
10931 East Desert Senna Drive
Tucson, AZ 85748

Eileen Osborne
1198 Worlidge Court
Marietta, GA 30068

Mabel Padilla
1835 Broadway SE
Albuquerque, NM 87102

Shaun Pankoski
800 1st Avenue North, #36
Seattle, WA 98109

Martha Partridge
512-17th Street, First Floor
Brooklyn, NY 11215

Susan Patashny
360 West Hudson Street
Long Beach, NY 11516

Marjorie Patrick
4922 Palo Alto SE
Albuquerque, NM 87108

Luisa Cristina Pestana
11977 Kiowa Avenue, #307
Los Angeles, CA 90049

John Peterson
12823 Sage Terrace
Germantown, MD 20874

Patricia Peterson
2131 Hillcrest Road
Redwood City, CA 94062

Caroline Petree
174 Radcliffe Road
Island Park, NY 11558

Malissa Petrock
1716 Fair Street
Ann Arbor, MI 48103

Teresa Phipps
8586 Grandbury Place Cove
Cordova, TN 38018

Nathalie Pickering
10085 County Road 24
Watertown, MN 55388

Karen Piehutkoski
1296 Newport Road
Ann Arbor, MI 48103

Freddie Pipkin
9307 Rolling Oak Trail
Austin, TX 78750

Tathagata Pitaka
16140 Matilija Drive
Los Gatos, CA 95030

Tammy Podgis
520 Route 103 E
Warner, NH 03278

Paula Pohlmann
1418-A Fifth Street
Berkeley, CA 94710

Richard Polishuk
3914 Burke Avenue North
Seattle, WA 98103

James Pond
1264 A Page Street
San Francisco, CA 94117

Barbara Porro
4982 West 60th Terrace
Mission, KS 66205

Randy Porter
914 North 5000 West
Westpoint, UT 84015

Betty Post
34 Lorrie Lane
Lawrenceville, NJ 08648

Connie Pounders
P.O. Box 1774
Kitty Hawk, NC 27949

Sharon Priven
725 Kains Avenue
Albany, CA 94706

Diana Proctor
Old Temple Road
RR1 Box 46
Lyndedoro, NH 03082

Daniel Quat
36 Barstow Road, #1M
Great Neck, NY 11021

Alvina Quatrano
48 Main Avenue, #2
Ocean Grove, NJ 07756

Phyllis Quinn
674 Main Street
Branford, CT 06405

Jim Quist
23150 McDougal Lane
Richland Center, WI 53581

Elfriede Rabbat
2740 SW 22nd Avenue, #1608
Delray Beach, FL 33445

Jonathan Ramljak
9A Farrar Street
Cambridge, MA 02138

Hannah Rappaport
8461 Valley Circle Boulevard
West Hills, CA 91304

Mary Redmond
139 South 600 East
Salt Lake City, UT 84102

Charles Reedy
14802 Newport Avenue, #11D
Tustin, CA 92780

Jane Reichert
4129 Wyoming Street
Saint Louis, MO 63116

Samuel Reiser
28 South Washington Avenue
Dobbs Ferry, NY 10522

Sandra Remus
585 Moorland Road, #302
Madison, WI 53713

Claudette Renner
1620 Whitefield Road, #4
Pasadena, CA 91104

Karen Rezny
1715 Cromwell Hill
Austin, TX 78703

E'Layne Rhiannon
9601-57 Miccosukee Road
Tallahassee, FL 32308

Roxanne Rhodes
Box 181, 555 Waverly Lane
Bryn Athyn, PA 19009

Julia Rice
20400 Frederick Road B-1
Germantown, MD 20876

Alice Richards
2507 Gaywood Drive
Pittsburgh, PA 15235

Peggy Richards
4227 North Jokane Road
Scottsdale, AZ 85251

Carmen Richardson
9639 W. Chatfield Avenue, Unit B
Littleton, CO 80128

Donna Richardson
8 Low Hill Lane
Lexington, SC 29072

Cheryl Rigas
18 Beechnut Terrace
Ithaca, NY 14850

Patricia Riley
6555 NE Bell Street
Suquamish, WA 98392

Ann Ritter
100 Wedgedale Avenue
Greensboro, NC 27403

Karen Roberts
5903-2 Montgomery Street
Baltimore, MD 21207

Lynn Roberts
35522 Orangelawn
Livonia, MI 48150

Paula Roberts
94 Wynmere Drive
Horsham, PA 19044

June Robinson
304 East Lullwood
San Antonio, TX 78212

Martha Robrahn
40298 Goldside Drive
Oakhurst, CA 93644

Debora Robson
2117 Brookwood Street
Harrisburg, PA 17104

Laureen Rodriguez
20-68 26th Street, #1A
Astoria, NY 11105

Celeste Rogers
2801 E. Sweetwater Avenue
Phoenix, AZ 85032

Elizabeth Rohack
8191 White Rock Circle
Boynton Beach, FL 33436

Rosalba Rojas-Currier
297 Euclid Avenue
Hackensack, NJ 07601

Jill Winter Rose
20100 NE 23rd Court
North Miami Beach, FL 33180

Kate Rose
740 Hillpine Drive NE
Atlanta, GA 30306

Colleen Ross
30 Excelsior Lane, #3
Sausallito, CA 94965

Virginia Roth
26 Sutton Drive
Boynton Beach, FL 33436

Gail Rothman
6503 North Miltary Trail, #1102
Boca Raton, FL 33496

Robbin Rubano
119 North Oakland Street
Lakewood, NJ 08701

Connie Ruble
244A Old Fort Road
Fairview, NC 28730

Joan Rudholm
5581 South Newmark
Parlier, CA 93648

Shirley Ruppert
734 Linden Street
Bethlehem, PA 18018

Ella Russell
P.O. Box 84
Elk, CA 95432

Fumiko Ryan
3881 Sirius Drive
Huntington Beach, CA 92649

Raymond Ryan
320 Cedar Street, #319
Seattle, WA 98121

Sheila Ryan
2016 Travis Circle
Tallahassee, FL 32303

Daniel Rybold
200 Sunset Way
Muir Beach, CA 94965

Gary Sachs
P.O. Box 73
Sharon, VT 05065

Susan Sacks
11 Borden Place
Livingston, NJ 07039

Karen Salinas
1613 Drake Avenue
Austin, TX 78704

Alfred Salomon
12 Thrumont Road
West Caldwell, NJ 07006

Jan Sandman
18 Pearl Street
Montpelier, VT 05602

Peggy Sankot
P.O. Box 496
Hawi, HI 96719

Linda Savage
Route 1, Box 109B
Sandia, TX 78383

Mary Kate Sawert
50 Chof Trail
Flagstaff, AZ 86001

Pepper Sbarbaro
2108 Eunice Street
Berkeley, CA 94709

Mary Lou Schaeffer
362 Hannon Avenue
Monterey, CA 93940

Suzanne Schevene
P.O. Box 956
Goldendale, WA 98620

Susan Schiedel
327 Jefferson Avenue, #2
Miami Beach, FL 33139

Janet Schmidt
10 Wolf Ridge Lake
Toxaway, NC 28747

Bill Scholl
1308 Alta Vista,
Austin, TX 78704

Patricia Schuckert
3518 Garfield Avenue South
Minneapolis, MN 55408

Don Schwartz
21 Locust Avenue
Mill Valley, CA 94941

John Samuel Scott
1731 "S" Street NW, #7
Washington, DC 20009

Leigh Sebera
12720 Burson Drive
Manchaca, TX 78652

Debra Seglund
1776 Ygnacio Valley Road, #104
Walnut Creek, CA 94598

Judy Rose Seibert
2317 Peggy Lane
Silver Spring, MD 20910

Sally Sestokas
14 Hill Road
Belmont, MA 02178

Catherine Seufert
1005 Chestnut Hill Road
Cambridge, NY 12816

Janice Shaheen
30 Dickinson Avenue
Nyack, NY 10960

Dominique Shelton
P.O. Box 218
Kihei, HI 96753

Kitty Sherrill
335 North Bost Street, #4
Statesville, NC 28677

Letitia Short
4361 Coffman Court
Casper, WY 82604

Skip Short
152 Montowese Street
Branford, CT 06405

Clifford Shulman
41 West 70th Street, #3F
New York, NY 10023

Deborah Simon Block
115 Camino Del Mar
P.O. Box 494
Inverness, CA 94937

Carole Sinclair-Thompson
P.O. Box 932
Chadds Ford, PA 19317

Nancy Sine
83 Terrace Avenue
Point Richmond, CA 94801

Peggy Singleton
7409 Grovewood Court
Orlando, FL 32818

Forresta Skinner
4827 Walnut Street
Oakland, CA 94619

Marva Sletten
660 Peck Avenue
Fort Myers, FL 33919

Steven Sloan, c/o AWI
P.O. Box 429
Rincon, PR 00677

Emily Slonina
19961 North Denaro Drive
Glendale, AZ 85308

Jan Smeigh
380 Granville Square
Worthington, OH 43085

Kelle Smith
c/o Finger Lakes School, 1251
Trumans
Ithaca, NY 14850

Pat Smith
709 Mississippi Avenue
El Paso, TX 79902

Richard Smith
629½ Park Avenue
South Pasadena, CA 91030

Pat Snider
1010 University Avenue, #714
San Diego, CA 92103

Judith Spater
4389 Philipps Road NE
Granville, OH 43023

Valerie Spencer
2711 7th Avenue
Pueblo, CO 81003

Beth Sperry
100 Lincoln Village Circle, #203
Larkspur, CA 94939

Barbara Ebright Spiller
1024 North Swope Avenue
Colorado Springs, CO 80909

Francine Spindel
1324 Acequia Borrada
Santa Fe, NM 87505

Carolyn Spinelli
305 Shetlands Lane
Glen Burnie, MD 21061

Agnes Spisak
14108 Arlis Avenue
Cleveland, OH 44111

Joe Springer
2149 Champions Drive
La Place, LA 70068

Jill Stallard Sames
8725 Alaska Avenue SE
Caledonia, MI 49316

Deirdre Steel
7138 Calder Avenue
Sebastopol, CA 95472

Janet Steele
240 West 98th Street, #14B
New York, NY 10025

Janine Stein
2410 19th Avenue
Port Huron, MI 48060

Jeannette Stelzenmuller
3537 Victoria Road
Birmingham, AL 35223

Jill Stephens
943 East River Spur
Priest River, ID 83856

Kathleen Sterner
1106 West Wyoming Street
Allentown, PA 18103

Bonnie Stetson
32 West 86th Street, #1-C
New York, NY 10024

Andrea Stevens
300 West Washington Avenue
Fairfield, IA 52556

Katherine Stewart
6510 Union Deposit Road
Harrisburg, PA 17111

Renee Stewart
841 NE 86th Street
Seattle, WA 98115

Deborah Stockton
1875 Commonwealth Avenue
Auburndale, MA 02166

Adrienne Stone
629½ Park Avenue
South Pasadena, CA 91030

Sara Strasburger
1611 North State Street
Bellingham, WA 98225

Susan Straus-Kroll
3102 Eisenhauer Road, #B-14
San Antonio, TX 78209

Charlene Strawn
1005 Ashburn Street
College Station, TX 77840

Petro Strelakos
6325 23rd Avenue N.E., #3
Seattle, WA 98115

Lynn Stull
2497 Sierra Drive
Upland, CA 91784

Wendy Stupka
5702 Buffalo Avenue
Valley Glen, CA 91401

Julia Sullivan
P.O. Box 2790
Santa Fe, NM 87504

Sharon Sullivan
44 Lunn Avenue
Bergenfield, NJ 07621

Barbara Surface
2617 Ramsey Road
Raleigh, NC 27604

Sylvia Surrette
26 Northern Avenue
Lynn, MA 01904

Jennifer Swan
29 Elm Street, #1
Brookline, MA 02146

Marilyn Swanson
22207 Del Valle
Woodland Hills, CA 91364

Andy Swenson
1567 Murray Circle
Los Angeles, CA 90026

Beverly Swope
4315 Valerie
Bellaire (Houston), TX 77401

Allen Symonds
P.O. Box 396
Fairlee, VT 05045

Michelle Synnestvedt
73 North Delaware Avenue
Yardley, PA 19067

Nancy Talian-Portela
602 Holly Ridge Road
Severna Park, MD 21146

Shannon Tate
317 Kingsbury Drive
Waynesboro, VA 22980

Russ Taylor
2017 Bluebonnet Lane, #206
Austin, TX 78704

Madeleine Terry
112 North Cottonwood Drive
Richardson, TX 75080

Nancy Thomas
2242 Mulberry Hill Road 1
Annapolis, MD 21401

Wanita Thompson
P.O. Box 1227
Mesilla, NM 88046

Heidi Timms
3090 Norvell Road
Grass Lake, MI 49240

Bunni Tobias
24842 Oak Creek
Lake Forest, CA 92630

Roger Tolle
292 West 92nd Street, #5C
New York, NY 10025

Regina Touhey,
2077 Center Avenue, #9E
Fort Lee, NJ 07024

Paul Tousignant
427 Snakehill Road
Poestenkill, NY 12140

Ted Towne
1835 Vallejo Street, #201
San Francisco, CA 94123

Lisa Tracy
5515 Ridgewood Cove
Mound, MN 55364

Tomaj Trenda
P.O. Box 32
Puunene, HI 96784

Wendy Tryon
Main Road, 369
Monterey, MA 01245

Kathryn Tufano
68 West 10th Street, #37
New York, NY 10011

Jessica Turken
105 East Strawberry Drive
Mill Valley, CA 94941

Kathleen Ullmann
455 East 51st Street, #3D/E
New York, NY 10022

Sue Unger
P.O. Box 804
Calistoga, CA 94515

Thomas Valenzano
2770 SW 15th Street
Deer Field Beach, FL 33442

Suzanna Valerie
P.O. Box 635
Volcano Hawaii, HI 96785

Barbara Vamvalis
296 Housatonic Street
Lenox, MA 01240

Ethel Van Dam
704 South Casey Key Road
Nokomis, FL 34275

Wilhelmina Van de Poll
9218 Laurel Oak Drive
Bethesda, MD 20817

Jan Van Erp
9910-213 Shelbourne
Gaithersburg, MD 20878

Ted Van Noord
4315 Inverness
Dexter, MI 48130

Claire Van Valkenburg
4526 Illinois Street, #9C
San Diego, CA 92116

Marlaina Vance
32 Lakes Edge Drive
Smyrna, GA 30080

Melanie Vestal
4025 Acreage Lane
Sebastopol, CA 95472

Allison Victor
9520 SW 8th Avenue
Portland, OR 97219

Susan Vinton
4640 NW 28th Avenue
Boca Raton, FL 33434

Carolyn Amala Viola
203 Mountain Road
Ringoes, NJ 08551

Nancy-Noel Voll
7100 Sunset Way, #201 West
Saint Petersberg Beach, FL 33706

Leo Wagner
402 East Main Street
Montfort, WI 53569

Flay Wahl
416 4th Street
Langley, WA 98260

Susan Waide
2209 Lawnmont, #105
Austin, TX 78756

Ruth Waite
504 Valley Road
Terre Haute, IN 47803

Phyllis Waldhutter
607 Dunwich Way
Baltimore, MD 21221

Scott Waldron
361 East 10th Street, #53
New York, NY 10009

JennTara Ward
7074 Mardel Apt. Rear
Saint Louis, MO 63109

Robert Breck Warwick
20433 Londelius Street
Canoga Park, CA 91306

Patricia Waters
207 South Butler Avenue
Indianapolis, IN 46219

Ilene Watrous
131 Cranbury Road
Princeton Junction, NJ 08550

Ric Watson
1911 Pierce Street NE
Minneapolis, MN 55418

Cathie Wegrzyn
5402 Moonlight Lane
La Jolla, CA 92037

Elizabeth Weick
8003 Mandan Road, #101
Greenbelt, MD 20770

Lauren Weisman
P.O. Box 282
North Cambridge, MA 02140

Kathy Weliever
6408 South Emerson
Indianapolis, IN 46237

Peggy Weller
3841 Flory Avenue
Dayton, OH 45405

Cheryl Wells
6130 Highway 16
Forestville, CA 95436

Harriet Wayne Wells
184 Middle Road
Newbury, MA 01922

Joy Wells
P.O. Box 586
Annandale, NJ 08801

Gina Weston
251 Route 1
Carmel, CA 93923

Lynne Weynand
705 Tamarack Drive
Canyon Lake, TX 78133

Barbara Whan
21 Fox Hollow Road
Rhinebeck, NY 12572

Nancy Wharton
5944 South Kipling, Suite 301
Littleton, CO 80127

Catherine Wheeler
4409 North Hamblin
Flagstaff, AZ 86004

James Wherry
12 Sarafian Road
New Paltz, NY 12561

Anne White
P.O. Box 638
Davidson, NC 28036

Marian Whitney
7650 Teller Street
Arvada, CO 80003

Susan Whittaker
39 Howard Street, Apt. 2
Portland, ME 04101

William Whittaker
230 Clayton Street, #2
San Francisco, CA 94117

Lee Whittier
P.O. Box 161
Woodstock, VT 05091

June Wieder
330 West 85th, #4D
New York, NY 10024

Suzy Wienckowski
5558 Hellner Road
Ann Arbor, MI 48105

Bonnie Wiesel
P.O. Box 1309
Salida, CO 81201

Elizabeth Wieshofer
509 East 83rd Street, #3W
New York, NY 10028

Cherie Wilcox
5886 Stow Road
Fowlerville, MI 48836

Arlene Wilder
1031 Poplar Drive
Falls Church, VA 22046

Blanche Williams
P.O. Box 398674
Miami Beach, FL 33239

Neil Williams
1201 Ashlawn Court
Fort Collins, CO 80525

Elaine Williams-Smith
838 West 880 North
Orem, UT 84057

Suzanne Wilner-Mariner
750 Jasmine Street
Denver, CO 80220

Ann Windau
651 B Turney Road, #139
Bedford, OH 44146

Linda Wise
5555 Morningside, #214A
Houston, TX 77005

Sandra Wolf
3444 NW 5th Court
Plantation, FL 33325

Wallie Wolfgruber
433 6th Street, #2
Brooklyn, NY 11215

Heidi Lyn Wood
P.O. Box 175
Boulder, CO 80306

Dorothy Workman
8114 NE 9th Street
Vancouver, WA 98664

Karen Wright
14512 Hollyhock Way
Burtonsville, MD 20866

Nancy Wright-Gray
Box 582
Sterling, MA 01564

Susan Wrzalinski
8191 N. State Road 135
Morgantown, IN 46160

Amy Wuest
202 Yorkshire Lane
Victoria, TX 77904

Margaret Wyche
7440 Watercrest Road
Charlotte, NC 28210

Kevin Wynkoop
319 Harbor Place
P.O. Box 846
Frankfort, MI 49635

Sherry Wynne
435 North Adoline
Fresno, CA 93728

Beth Yancy
803-C Divisidero Street,
San Francisco, CA 94115

Andrew Yavelow
General Delivery
Kamuela, HI 96743461

Lori Yelensky
114 Crescent Place
Ithaca, NY 14850

John and Rene Zahourek
2198 West 15th Street
Loveland, CO 80538

Anne Zanes
290 Riverside Drive, #15A
New York, NY 10025

Maryann Zimmermann
5130 La Jolla Bouleva Road, #3M
San Diego, CA 92109

Gertrude Zukowski
334 San Mateo Boulevard
Titusville, FL

Veterinary Medicine

American Holistic Veterinary
Medicine Association
2214 Old Emmorton Road
Bel Air, MD 21015
410-569-0795

Yoga

International Association of Yoga
Therapists
109 Hillside Avenue
Mill Valley, CA 94941
415-383-4587

Index